AF669008

Postgraduate
MEDICINE

Postgraduate MEDICINE

Volume 3

Editor-in-Chief

Gurpreet S Wander MD DM FACC FAMS
Professor and Head of Cardiology
Hero DMC Heart Institute
Dayanand Medical College and Hospital
Ludhiana, Punjab, India

Section Editors

PK Deb	Cardiology
SK Sharma	Clinical Medicine
Surinder K Jindal	Pulmonary Medicine
Ajay Kumar	Gastroenterology
Vivekanand Jha	Nephrology
Rohini Handa	Rheumatology
Jyotirmoy Pal	General Medicine
Gagandeep Singh	Neurology
Dhruva Chaudhry	Critical Care
Sanjay K Bhadada	Endocrinology
Bibhuti Saha	Infectious Diseases

Associate Editors

Rajesh Mahajan
NK Singh

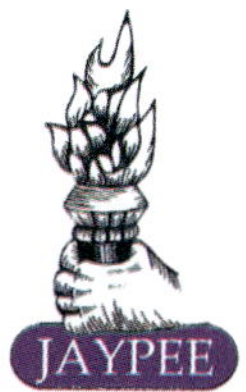

JAYPEE BROTHERS MEDICAL PUBLISHERS
The Health Sciences Publisher
New Delhi | London

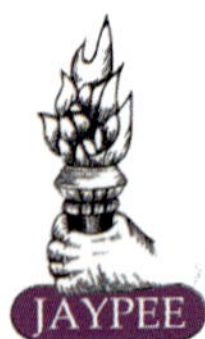

Jaypee Brothers Medical Publishers (P) Ltd

Headquarters
EMCA House
23/23-B, Ansari Road, Daryaganj
New Delhi 110 002, India
Landline: +91-11-23272143, +91-11-23272703
+91-11-23282021, +91-11-23245672
E-mail: jaypee@jaypeebrothers.com

Corporate Office
Jaypee Brothers Medical Publishers (P) Ltd.
4838/24, Ansari Road, Daryaganj
New Delhi 110 002, India
Phone: +91-11-43574357
Fax: +91-11-43574314
E-mail: jaypee@jaypeebrothers.com

Overseas Office
JP Medical Ltd.
83, Victoria Street, London
SW1H 0HW (UK)
Phone: +44-20 3170 8910
Fax: +44(0)20 3008 6180
E-mail: info@jpmedpub.com

Website: www.jaypeebrothers.com
Website: www.jaypeedigital.com

Inquiries for bulk sales may be solicited at: jaypee@jaypeebrothers.com

Postgraduate Medicine / *Gurpreet S Wander*

First Edition: **2022**

ISBN: 978-93-90595-46-4

Printed at: Sanat Printers

DEDICATED TO

Dr Harjit Singh

(1926–2018)

Professor and HOD Medicine
Government Medical College
Patiala, Punjab, India

"My father who taught me the value of hard work and integrity"

Dr BK Sharma

(1937–2021)

Professor and HOD Medicine
Postgraduate Institute of Medical Education and Research
Chandigarh, India

"My teacher in MD medicine from whom I learned bedside manners"

Dr SB Khurana

(1938–2011)

Professor and HOD Medicine
Dayanand Medical College Hospital
Ludhiana, Punjab, India

"Who taught me that practice of clinical medicine needs common sense and simple thinking"

Dr Siddharth N Shah

(1946–2021)

Past President API
Mumbai, Maharashtra, India

"From whom I learned how to work with others in a team with mutual respect"

Smt Raman Vij

(1957–2021)

W/o Sh Jitender Pal Vij and M/o Mr Ankit Vij
New Delhi, India

"Who was the driving force and inspiration for the Jaypee Brothers Medical Publishers (P) Ltd"

Editor-in-Chief

Section Editors

Associate Editors

CONTRIBUTORS

VOLUME 3 (SECTION 9–12)

Section 9: Nephrology (Section Editor: Vivekanand Jha)

Ajay Kher MD DM
Consultant Nephrologist
Vishwasth Clinic
Noida, Uttar Pradesh, India

Anantharam Jairam MD DM
Professor of Nephrology
St John's Medical College Hospital
Bengaluru, Karnataka, India

Arpana Iyengar MD DM
Professor of Pediatric Nephrology
St John's Medical College Hospital
Bengaluru, Karnataka, India

Arpita Ray Chaudhury MD DM
Professor of Nephrology
Institute of Postgraduate of Medical
Education and Research
Kolkata, West Bengal, India

Arunkumar S MD DM
Assistant Professor
Department of Nephrology
All India Institute of Medical Sciences
New Delhi, India

Ashwani Kumar PhD
Postdoctoral Research Associate
Department of Histopathology
Postgraduate Institute of Medical
Education and Research
Chandigarh, India

Ashwini Balasaheb Gadde MD DNB
Associate Consultant
Department of Nephrology and
Transplant Medicine
Medanta – The Medicity
Gurugram, Haryana, India

Dinesh Khullar DM FACP FRCP
Chairman, Nephrology and Renal
Transplant Medicine
Max Super Speciality Hospital
Saket, New Delhi, India

Divya Bajpai MD DM
Associate Professor
Department of Nephrology
Seth GSMC and KEM Hospital
Parel, Mumbai, Maharashtra, India

Gopesh K Modi MD DM
Consultant Physician and Nephrologist
Director, Samarpan Kidney Center
Bhopal, Madhya Pradesh, India

Indu Ramachandra Rao MD DM
Associate Professor
Department of Nephrology
Kasturba Medical College, Manipal
Manipal Academy of Higher Education
Manipal, Karnataka, India

Kristin George MD DM
Senior Resident
Department of Nephrology
All India Institute of Medical Sciences
New Delhi, India

Manisha Sahay MD DM
Professor and Head
Department of Nephrology
Osmania Medical College
Hyderabad, Telangana, India

Manish Rathi MD DM MAMS FRCP
Professor, Department of Nephrology
Postgraduate Institute of Medical
Education and Research
Chandigarh, India

Mayuri Trivedi MD DM
Assistant Professor
Department of Nephrology
Lokmanya Tilak Municipal Medical
College, Mumbai, Maharashtra, India

M Sreelatha MD DM
Professor and Head
Government Medical College
Kozhikode, Kerala, India

Narayan Prasad MD DM
Professor and Head
Department of Nephrology
Sanjay Gandhi Postgraduate Institute
of Medical Sciences
Lucknow, Uttar Pradesh, India

Natarajan Gopalakrishnan MD DM
Professor and Head
Madras Medical College
Chennai, Tamil Nadu, India

Pallavi Prasad MBBS MD DNB
Associate Consultant
Department of Nephrology
Sri Ramachandra Institute of Higher
Education and Research
Chennai, Tamil Nadu, India

Pranaw Kumar Jha MD DNB FASN
Director
Department of Nephrology and
Transplant Medicine
Medanta – The Medicity
Gurugram, Haryana, India

Raja Ramachandran MD DM
Associate Professor
Department of Nephrology
Postgraduate Institute of Medical
Education and Research
Chandigarh, India

Ravindra Prabhu Attur MD DM
Professor and Head of Unit
Department of Nephrology
Kasturba Medical College
Manipal Academy of Higher Education
Manipal, Karnataka, India

Ritambhra Nada MD MNAMS
Professor
Department of Histopathology
Postgraduate Institute of Medical
Education and Research
Chandigarh, India

R Jayasurya MD DM
Consultant Nephrologist
Apollo Gleneagles Hospital
Kolkata, West Bengal, India

Ruju Gala DM
Assistant Professor
Department of Nephrology
GMC and JJ Hospital
Mumbai, Maharashtra, India

Sandeep Mahajan MD DM
Professor
Department of Nephrology
All India Institute of Medical Sciences
New Delhi, India

Santosh Varughese MD DM
Professor and Head
Department of Nephrology
Christian Medical College
Vellore, Tamil Nadu, India

Shankar Prasad Nagaraju MD DM
Professor and Head of Nephrology
Kasturba Medical College, Manipal
Manipal Academy of Higher Education
Manipal, Karnataka, India

Snehal Gaikwad MD DM
Consultant Nephrologist
King Edward memorial Hospital
Pune, Maharashtra, India

Sreejith Parameswaran MD DNB DM
Professor of Nephrology
JIPMER, Puducherry, India

S Shiri MD DM
Senior Resident
Department of Pediatric Nephrology
St John's Medical College Hospital
Bengaluru, Karnataka, India

Suceena Alexander MD DM
Professor and Head
Department of Nephrology
Christian Medical College
Vellore, Tamil Nadu, India

UK Sharma MD DM
Physician and Nephrologist, Paras Hospital, Gurugram, Haryana, India

Valentine Lobo MD DM
Consultant Nephrologist
King Edward memorial Hospital
Pune, Maharashtra, India

Vijay Kher MD DM FAMS
Chairman
Department of Nephrology and Transplant Medicine
Medanta – The Medicity
Gurugram, Haryana, India

Vijoy Kumar Jha MD DNB DM
Physician and Nephrologist
Command Hospital Airforce
Bengaluru, Karnataka, India

Vinay Sakhuja MD DM
Director, MSSH, Mohali
Emeritus Professor
Department of Nephrology
Postgraduate Institute of Medical Education and Research
Chandigarh, India

Vivek Kumar MD DM
Associate Professor
Department of Nephrology
Postgraduate Institute of Medical Education and Research
Chandigarh, India

Section 10: Neurology (Section Editor: Gagandeep Singh)

Abhilash Somasundaram MD DM
Resident, Institute of Neurology
Madras Medical College
Chennai, Tamil Nadu, India

Achal K Srivastava MD DM FRCP
Professor of Neurology
All India Institute of Medical Sciences
New Delhi, India

Ajay Garg MD DM
Professor of Neuroradiology
All India Institute of Medical Sciences
New Delhi, India

Amol Nanak Singh MBBS Intern
Department of Internal Medicine
Dayanand Medical College and Hospital
Ludhiana, Punjab, India

Birinder Singh Paul MD DM
Professor of Neurology
Dayanand Medical College and Hospital
Ludhiana, Punjab, India

Deepa Avadhani MD
Resident, Institute of Neurology
Madras Medical College
Chennai, Tamil Nadu, India

Devangi Desai MD
Professor of Medicine
Shree Krishna Hospital and Pramukhswami Medical College
Karamsad, Anand, Gujarat, India

Dhananjay Duberkar MD DM
Consultant Neurologist
Sahyadri Hospital
Nashik, Maharashtra, India

Dimple Dawar BOT MOT (Neurology)
Senior Occupational Therapist
Department of Neurology
Christian Medical College and Hospital
Ludhiana, Punjab, India

Divyani Garg MD DM
Department of Neurology
Lady Hardinge Medical College
New Delhi, India

Gagandeep Singh MD DM
Professor and Head
Department of Neurology
Dayanand Medical College and Hospital
Ludhiana, Punjab, India

Guhan Ramamurthy MD DM
Assistant Professor of Neurology
Madras Medical College
Chennai, Tamil Nadu, India

Gunchan Paul MBBS MD
Associate Professor
Department of Critical Care Medicine
Dayanand Medical College and Hospital
Ludhiana, Punjab, India

Ivy Anne Sebastian MD DM
Consultant, Department of Neurology
St Stephen's Hospital
New Delhi, India

Jagarlapudi MK Murthy MD DM
Clinical Director and Chief of Neurology
CARE Institute of Neurosciences
CARE Hospitals, Banjara Hills
Hyderabad, Telangana, India

Jayantee Kalita DM FIAN FAMS
Professor of Neurology
Sanjay Gandhi Postgraduate Institute of Medical Sciences
Lucknow, Uttar Pradesh, India

Jeyaraj Durai Pandian MD DM
Principal and Professor of Neurology
Christian Medical College
Ludhiana, Punjab, India
Honorary Professor, The George Institute for Global Health, Sydney

Karthika Ajit MD
Resident, Institute of Neurology
Madras Medical College
Chennai, Tamil Nadu, India

K Ravi Kumar MD
Resident, Institute of Neurology
Madras Medical College
Chennai, Tamil Nadu, India

Lakshmi Narasimhan Ranganathan
MD DNB DM PhD FRCP
Director and Professor of Neurology
Institute of Neurology
Madras Medical College
Chennai, Tamil Nadu, India

Manish Modi MD DM
Professor
Department of Neurolgy
Postgraduate Institute of Medical Education and Research
Chandigarh, India

Manjit Matharu PhD FRCP
Associate Professor and Honorary Consultant Neurologist
Headache and Facial Pain Group
University College London (UCL) and The National Hospital for Neurology and Neurosurgery
London, United Kingdom

Michlene R Passeri MD
PGY IV Neurology Resident
Barrow Neurological Institute
Phoenix, Arizona, United States

Mohammed Faruq MBBS PhD
Principal Scientist
Genomics and Molecular Medicine
CSIR-Institute of Genomics and Integrative Biology
New Delhi, India

MV Padma Srivastava MD DM FRCP
Professor, Head of Neurology
Chief, Neurosciences Center
All India Institute of Medical Sciences
New Delhi, India

Neeraj Balani MD DM
Assistant Professor
Department of Neurology
Postgraduate Institute of Medical Education and Research
Chandigarh, India

Rahul Yadav DNB
Consultant Neurologist
Shree Krishna Hospital and Pramukhswami Medical College
Karamsad, Anand, Gujarat, India

Rajinder K Bansal MD DM
Professor of Neurology
Dayanand Medical College and Hospital
Ludhiana, Punjab, India

Rakesh K Singh DM DNB
Honorary Assistant Professor
Department of Neurology
Sir JJ Hospital, Grant Medical College
Consultant Neurologist
Jupiter Hospital
Mumbai, Maharashtra, India

Ram N Narayan MD CRND
Assistant Professor, Neurology
Barrow Neuroimmunology Division
Assistant Professor of Neurology
University of Arizona School of Medicine, Phoenix, Arizona
United States

Raviteja Kakarla MBBS MD DM
Senior Resident
Department of Neurology
Christian Medical College and Hospital
Ludhiana, Punjab, India

Salwa Kamourieh MBBS MRCP
Headache and Facial Pain Group
University College London (UCL)
Queen Square Institute of Neurology and The National Hospital for Neurology and Neurosurgery
Queen Square, London, UK

Sanjay Cheema MBBS MRCP
Consultant Neurologist
Headache and Facial Pain Group
University College London and The National Hospital for Neurology and Neurosurgery
London, United Kingdom

Satish V Khadilkar MD DM
Dean, Senior Consultant Neurologist
Bombay Hospital Institute of Medical Sciences
Emeritus Professor of Neurology
Sir JJ Hospital, Grant Medical College
Mumbai, Maharashtra, India

Shrivarthan R MD
Resident
Institute of Neurology
Madras Medical College
Chennai, Tamil Nadu, India

S Mahesh Kumar DNB
Consultant, Aravind Eye Hospitals and Postgraduate Institute of Ophthalmology
Madurai, Tamil Nadu, India

S Meenakshi-Sundaram MD DM
Associate Professor of Neurology
Department of Neurosciences
Apollo Speciality Hospitals
Madurai, Tamil Nadu, India

Soaham Desai DM
Sr Consultant Neurologist and Professor and Head (Neurology)
Shree Krishna Hospital and Pramukhswami Medical College
Karamsad, Anand, Gujarat, India

Sundaram Challa MD
Basavatarakam Indo American Cancer Hospital and Research Institute
Banjara Hills
Hyderabad, Telangana, India

Usha K Misra MD DM
Director of Neuroscience
Apollomedics Super Speciality Hospitals
Lucknow, Uttar Pradesh, India

Vedantam Rajshekhar MCh
Professor of Neurosurgery
Department of Neurological Sciences
Christian Medical College Hospital
Vellore, Tamil Nadu, India

Vibhor Pardasani MD DM
Assistant Professor
Department of Neurology
Bombay Hospital Institute of Medical Sciences, Mumbai, Maharashtra, India

Vikram Aglave DM
Lecturer
Department of Neurology
Sir JJ Hospital, Grant Medical College
Mumbai, Maharashtra, India

Vineeth Jaison MBBS MD DM
Associate Professor
Department of Neurology
Christian Medical College and Hospital
Ludhiana, Punjab, India

Vishnu VY MD DM
Assistant Professor
Department of Neurology
All India Institute of Medical Sciences
New Delhi, India

Yogeesh PM MD DM
Senior Resident
Department of Neurology
All India Institute of Medical Sciences
New Delhi, India

Section 11: Pulmonary Medicine (Section Editor: Surinder K Jindal)

Abhishek Goyal MD DM
Associate Professor
Department of Pulmonary Medicine
All India Institute of Medical Sciences
Bhopal, Madhya Pradesh, India

Aditya Jindal DNB FCCP DM
Senior Consultant and Intervention Pulmonologist, Jindal Clinics
Chandigarh, India

Anant Mohan MD PhD FAMS FRCP
Professor and Head
Department of Pulmonary, Critical Care and Sleep Medicine
All India Institute of Medical Sciences
New Delhi, India

Avishek Kar MD
Fellow Sleep Medicine
Department of Pulmonary Medicine
All India Institute of Medical Sciences
Bhopal, Madhya Pradesh, India

Balamugesh T MD DM
Professor of Pulmonary Medicine
Christian Medical College
Vellore, Tamil Nadu, India

Barney J Isaac MBBS Dip NB
Professor of Pulmonary Medicine
Christian Medical College
Vellore, Tamil Nadu, India

Chitra Veluthat DNB
Assistant Professor
Department of Pulmonary Medicine
St John's Medical College
Bengaluru, Karnataka, India

D Behera MD FCCP FAMS FNCCP FICP FICA FAPSR FICS MNAMS
Padma Awardee
Professor and Ex-HOD, Department of Pulmonary Medicine, Postgraduate Institute of Medical Education and Research, Chandigarh, India

Deepak Aggarwal MD
Professor of Pulmonary Medicine
Govt Medical College and Hospital
Chandigarh, India

Deepak Talwar MD DM
Director and Chair
Metro Centre for Respiratory Diseases
Noida, Uttar Pradesh, India

DJ Christopher DTCD DNB FICS FRCP FCCP
Professor of Pulmonary Medicine
Christian Medical College
Vellore, Tamil Nadu, India

Irfan Shekh MD
Senior Resident
Pulmonary, Critical Care and Sleep Medicine
All India Institute of Medical Sciences
New Delhi, India

Irshad Ahmad Banday MD
Fellow
Interventional Pulmonary-Radiology
All India Institute of Medical Sciences,
New Delhi, India

Javid Ahmad Malik MD DM
Professor and Head
Department of Pulmonary Medicine
SKIMS- Medical College
Srinagar, Jammu and Kashmir, India

Karan Madan MD DM
Associate Professor
Department of Pulmonary, Critical
Care and Sleep Medicine
All India Institute of Medical Sciences
New Delhi, India

Kavitha Venkatnarayan MD DM
Assistant Professor
Department of Pulmonary Medicine
St John's Medical College
Bengaluru, Karnataka, India

Ketaki Barve Utpat MD DM
Assistant Professor
Department of Pulmonary Medicine
Topiwala National Medical College and
BYL Nair Hospital
Mumbai, Maharashtra, India

Khushboo Saxena DNB
Fellow-Sleep Medicine
Department of Pulmonary Medicine
All India Institute of Medical Sciences
Bhopal, Madhya Pradesh, India

Mansi Gupta MD DNB DM
Associate Professor
Department of Pulmonary Medicine
Sanjay Gandhi Postgraduate Institute
of Medical Sciences
Lucknow, Uttar Pradesh, India

Mohammad Azizur Rahman MD
Professor of Respiratory Medicine
Under Faculty of Medicine, Dhaka
University, Dhaka, Bangladesh

Navneet Singh MD DM FRCP
Additional Professor
Department of Pulmonary Medicine
Postgraduate Institute of Medical
Education and Research
Chandigarh, India

Pajanivel Ranganadin MD DM
Professor and Head
Department of Pulmonary Medicine
Mahatma Gandhi Medical College and
Research Institute (MGMCRI)
Puducherry, India

Pawan Tiwari MD DM
Assistant Professor
Department of Pulmonary
Critical Care and Sleep Medicine
All India Institute of Medical Sciences
New Delhi, India

Priya N MBBS MD
Assistant Professor
Department of Pulmonary Medicine
Christian Medical College
Vellore, Tamil Nadu, India

Priya Ramachandran MD DNB
Professor of Pulmonary Medicine
St John's Medical College
and Hospital
Bengaluru, Karnataka, India

Raja Dhar MD DM
Director and Head of Department
Department of Pulmonology
CK Birla Hospitals
Kolkata, West Bengal, India

Randeep Guleria MD DM
Director
All India Institute of Medical Sciences
New Delhi, India

Ranjan Kumar Behera MS
Senior Resident
Department of Ophthalmology
Postgraduate Institute of Medical
Education and Research
Chandigarh, India

Saurav Verma MD
Senior Resident
Department of Medical Oncology
Dr B R Ambedkar Institute Rotary
Cancer Hospital
All India Institute of Medical Science
New Delhi, India

Shyam Krishnan MD DM
Consultant Pulmonologist
CK Birla Hospitals
Kolkata, West Bengal, India

SK Chhabra MD DM
Ex-Director Professor
Vallabhbhai Patel Chest Institute
Senior Consultant and Head
Department of Pulmonary, Sleep and
Critical Care Medicine
Primus Superspeciality Hospital
New Delhi, India

Surinder K Jindal MD
Medical Director, Jindal Clinics
Emeritus-Professor
Postgraduate Institute of Medical
Education and Research
Chandigarh, India

Srinivas Rajagopala MD DM
Professor of Pulmonology
PSG Institute of Medical Sciences and
Research, Coimbatore, Tamil Nadu, India

Surendra K Sharma MD PhD FNASc
Adjunct Professor
Department of Molecular Medicine
Jamia Hamdard Institute of Molecular
Medicine, Jamia Hamdard (Deemed-
to-be-University)
Hamdard Nagar, New Delhi, India

Tarang Kulkarni MD DM
Consultant Pulmonologist
Jupiter Hospital
Kolkata, West Bengal, India

Tejas M Suri MD DM
Senior Resident, Department of
Pulmonary, Critical Care and Sleep
Medicine, All India Institute of Medical
Sciences, New Delhi, India

Trinath Dash DNB MNAMS FCCP
Joint Director
Jawahar Lal Nehru Hospital
Bhilai Steel Plant, Steel Authority of
India, Bhilai, Chhattisgarh, India

Uma Devaraj DNB (Inter Med, Resp Dis)
Professor of Pulmonary Medicine
St John's Medical College and Hospital
Bengaluru, Karnataka, India

Uma Mohan Krishnaswamy MD DM
Professor and Head
Department of Pulmonary Medicine
St John's Medical College
Bengaluru, Karnataka, India

Vartika Mathur MSc MPhil PhD
Assistant Professor
Sri Venkateswara College
New Delhi, India

Vijay Hadda MD FCCP FISCCM
Associate Professor
Pulmonary, Critical Care and Sleep Medicine, All India Institute of Medical Sciences, New Delhi, India

Vishwanath Upadhyay PhD Scholar
Department of Molecular Medicine
Jamia Hamdard-Institute of Jamia Hamdard (Deemed-to-be-University)
Hamdard Nagar, New Delhi, India

Section 12: Rheumatology (Section Editor: Rohini Handa)

Amita Aggarwal MD DM FNASc FAMS
Professor and Head
Department of Clinical Immunology and Rheumatology
Sanjay Gandhi Postgraduate Institute of Medical Sciences
Lucknow, Uttar Pradesh, India

Amit Kansal MD DM
Consultant Rheumatologist
KARE Clinic
Ludhiana, Punjab, India

Ashok Kumar MD FRCP (London)
Director and Head
Department of Rheumatology
Fortis Flt Lt Rajan Dhall Hospital
Vasant Kunj, New Delhi, India

Binoy J Paul MD PhD DNB FRCP (Edin)
Professor of Medicine and Chief of Rheumatology, KMCT Medical College
Kozhikode, Kerala, India

Debashish Mishra MD DM
Consultant Rheumatologist
IMS and SUM Hospital
Bhubaneswar, Odisha, India

Kushagra Gupta MD
Fellow in Rheumatology
Fortis Flt Lt Rajan Dhall Hospital
Vasant Kunj, New Delhi, India

Latika Gupta MD DM
Assistant Professor
Department of Clinical Immunology and Rheumatology
Sanjay Gandhi Postgraduate Institute of Medical Sciences
Lucknow, Uttar Pradesh, India

Liza Rajasekhar MD DM
Professor
Nizam's Institute of Medical Sciences
Hyderabad, Telangana, India

Molly Mary Thabah MD
Additional Professor of Medicine
Jawaharlal Institute of Postgraduate Medical Education and Research
Puducherry, India

Prithvi Sanjeevkumar Gaur MBBS
Student, Smt Kashibai Navale Medical College and General Hospital
Pune, Maharashtra, India

Ramakrishna Rao Uppuluri MD
Consultant Rheumatologist
Sri Deepti Rheumatology Centre
Hyderabad, Telangana, India

Ramya Aithala MD DM
Associate Professor
Department of Clinical Immunology and Rheumatology
St John's Medical College Hospital
Bengaluru, Karnataka, India

Reeta James MD
Associate Professor of Medicine
KMCT Medical College
Kozhikode, Kerala, India

Renu Saigal MD FICP FRCP FACP
Professor, Department of Medicine
JNU IMSRC, Jaipur, Rajasthan, India

Rohini Handa MD DNB FAMS FRCP
Professor and Senior Consultant
Department of Rheumatology
Apollo Indraprastha Hospitals
New Delhi, India

Rudrarpan Chatterjee MD DM
Senior Resident of Clinical Immunology and Rheumatology
Sanjay Gandhi Postgraduate Institute of Medical Sciences
Lucknow, Uttar Pradesh, India

Sakir Ahmed MD DM
Associate Professor, Clinical Immunology and Rheumatology
Kalinga Institute of Medical Sciences
Consultant Rheumatologist
Pradyumna Bal Memorial Hospital
Bhubaneswar, Odisha, India

Sarit Sekhar Pattanaik MD DM
Assistant Professor
Department of Rheumatology
SCB Medical College
Cuttack, Odisha, India

Shefali K Sharma MD
Additional Professor
Clinical Immunology and Rheumatology Wing
Department of Internal Medicine
Postgraduate Institute of Medical Education and Research
Chandigarh, India

SJ Gupta FRCP FICP
Senior Consultant Rheumatologist
Apollo Indraprastha and Sant Parmanand Hospitals
New Delhi, India

Sreejitha KS DM
Senior Resident
Nizam's Institute of Medical Sciences
Hyderabad, Telangana, India

Sripurna Deepti Challa MD MMed Rheumatology
Speciality Doctor, Rheumatology
Wrightington, Wigan and Leigh NHS Foundation Trust England

Subramanian Shankar MD DNB MNAMS FICP FRCP
Consultant Medicine and Clinical Immunology
Department of Rheumatology and Clinical Immunology
O/o DGAFMS and Army Hospital (R and R), New Delhi, India

Ved Chaturvedi MD DM
Professor
Rheumatology and Clinical Immunology, GRIPMER, Delhi
Senior Consultant Rheumatology
Sir Ganga Ram Hospital
New Delhi, India

Vikramraj Jain MD DM
Consultant and Head
Clinical Immunology and Rheumatology
Bhagwan Mahaveer Jain Hospital
Bengaluru, Karnataka, India

Vineeta Shobha MD DM
Professor and Head
Department of Clinical Immunology and Rheumatology
St John's Medical College Hospital
Bengaluru, Karnataka, India

Vivek Vasdev MD DNB
Professor, HOD and Consultant
Department of Geriatrics
Armed Forces Medical College
Pune, Maharashtra, India

CONTENTS

VOLUME 1

SECTION 1: CLINICAL MEDICINE

SECTION 2: GENERAL MEDICINE

GENERAL TOPICS

GERIATRICS

SECTION 3: INFECTIOUS DISEASES

BASIC CONSIDERATIONS

BACTERIAL INFECTIONS

VIRAL INFECTIONS

CORONAVIRUS INFECTION

OTHER INFECTIONS

SECTION 4: CRITICAL CARE

VOLUME 2

SECTION 5: CARDIOLOGY

SECTION 6: ENDOCRINOLOGY AND METABOLIC DISORDERS

SECTION 7: GASTROENTEROLOGY

SECTION 8: HEMATOLOGY AND ONCOLOGY

HEMATOLOGY

ONCOLOGY

VOLUME 3

SECTION 9: NEPHROLOGY

SECTION 10: NEUROLOGY

SECTION 11: PULMONARY MEDICINE AND TUBERCULOSIS

Free Online Resources

1. **E-version of the book chapters:** Kindly refer to the back side of the front cover to redeem the scratch code on http://www.emedicine360.com **and access the E-version.** All the chapters in the printed version can be accessed online.

2. **MCQs:** Each chapter in the printed book is followed by 5–10 MCQ's. These MCQ's have 4–5 options and one correct answer. They are from the contents of the chapter. You are advised to solve these after reading the whole chapter.

   In order to access MCQs in the E-version, kindly click the link given at the end of each chapter on www.emedicine360.com.

3. **E-Chapters:** Free elaborated E-version of the following 6 chapters is available on http://www.emedicine360.com
   - e-15 (CH-15): Chest X-ray Evaluation and Some Spotters
   - e-23 (CH-23): Electronic Health Records, Artificial Intelligence, and Big Data—Role in Medicine
   - e-38 (CH-38): Prevention and Management of Infection in Transplant Recipients
   - e-48 (CH-48): Other Virus Infections—Chikungunya, Hantavirus, Nipah Virus, and Zika Virus
   - e-88 (CH-88): Noninvasive Cardiac Imaging
   - e-118 (CH-118): Endocrine Tumors and Malignancies

4. **Videos:** Some of the chapters have videos. These videos can be accessed online in respective chapters.
   - ch-28: Falls in Elderly
   - ch-89: Cardiac Catheterization and Coronary Angiography
   - ch-185: Seizures and Epilepsy
   - ch-193: Movement Disorders: The Clinical Vignette

CHAPTER 163

Signs, Symptoms and Laboratory Tests of Kidney Disease

Raja Ramachandran, Vinay Sakhuja

ABSTRACT

In patients with kidney disease, the signs and symptoms are often vague, nonspecific, or absent till a substantial compromise in renal functions occurs. The findings may be local, the systemic effect of kidney disease, or may reflect as abnormal urinary findings. Considering the latency in clinical presentation, the physician must be aware of early symptoms of kidney disease and order structured investigations. Urine examination is the cornerstone for evaluating kidney disease, followed by serum creatinine, electrolytes, and ultrasound examination of the kidneys and urinary tract. A kidney biopsy is critical for knowing the exact status of the kidneys, followed by structured serological investigation for accurate classification.

"Cure the symptoms, cure the disease"

—Michael Crichton

INTRODUCTION

Kidney disease encompasses a spectrum of acute, subacute, and chronic diseases. For an early and precise diagnosis of the kidney disease, the physician needs to be aware of the various ways in which kidney disease presents. A detailed history and clinical examination, including urine analysis, paves the way for structured investigations from routine screening to specific tests. The standard tests include serum creatinine, blood urea, serum electrolytes, and ultrasound examination of the kidneys. An accurate classification of kidney disease mandates a renal biopsy (light microscopy, immunofluorescence, and *case-by-case-based* electron microscopy) with appropriate serological and radiological investigations.

CLINICAL PRESENTATION

Patients with kidney disease seek medical attention for:

- Sign(s) and/or symptom(s) suggestive of kidney disease
- A systemic disease known to affect the kidneys/urinary tract
- Urinary, biochemical, or radiological abnormalities suggestive of kidney disease despite being asymptomatic.

FEATURES SUGGESTIVE OF KIDNEY DISEASE

The following are the features to suggest disorders of kidney or urinary tract:

- Abnormalities in urine composition
- Disorders of urine volume
- Edema and hypertension
- Disorders of micturition
- Renal mass
- Pain originating from the renal tract
- Uremia

ABNORMALITIES IN THE URINE COMPOSITION

Proteinuria: An average adult excretes about 150 mg of protein in his urine daily and the *Tamm-Horsfall* protein accounts for 70% of this. Various clinical conditions like fever, exercise, pregnancy, dehydration, acute illness, and heat injury result in a transient increase in the proteinuria. Proteinuria is often the first and most typical manifestation of kidney disease in both children and adults. The basis for various classification of proteinuria includes quantity (nephrotic or non-nephrotic), pathophysiological (glomerular, tubular, and overflow), posture (constant or orthostatic), type (selective or nonselective), and association with other urinary abnormalities (isolated proteinuria or with hematuria).

The basis for the pathophysiological aspect of proteinuria is the compartment of the kidney primarily affected by the disease process. Patients with proteinuria of the glomerular etiology, have a protein excretion rate (PER) of over 2 g/day and the most dominant fraction is the albumin. On the contrary, patients with tubular disease have a PER of <2 g/day composed of a variety of low-molecular-weight proteins. Overflow proteinuria is a result of protein produced in excessive amount filtered by the glomeruli, overwhelming the resorptive capabilities of the renal tubules and consequently appearing in the urine. The example of overflow proteinuria includes multiple myeloma, hemolysis, rhabdomyolysis, and leukemia. Orthostatic proteinuria (proteinuria in an upright position, with normal PER while recumbent) is the most common cause of proteinuria in children and is a benign condition.

Albumin fraction of the proteinuria is detected by dipstick examination; in patients with no albuminuria on dipstick examination, but significant proteinuria on the sulfosalicylic acid test is suggestive of overflow proteinuria, most commonly light chains. Currently, most laboratories use dye-binding (calorimetric) technique to assess the PER.

Hematuria: It may be visible to the naked eye or only on microscopic examination. Hematuria can arise from any part of the urinary tract. Description of hematuria is according to the following parameters:

- *Gross*: Presence of red or brown (depending on the pH) urine due to presence of erythrocytes is gross hematuria. Bright red urine with the passage of clots is usually suggestive of active bleeding from the lower urinary tract, however, can be rarely seen with renal cell carcinoma.
- *Microscopic hematuria*: Urine that is normal to the naked eye, but has abnormal quantities of erythrocytes on microscopic examination. Microscopic hematuria: ≥3 erythrocytes per high-power field in a spun urinary sediment (or any erythrocyte on unspun urine). Further classification of hematuria includes persistent or intermittent, symptomatic or asymptomatic and initial, terminal, or uniform.

One needs to distinguish true hematuria from other causes of red/brown urine. The close mimicker to hematuria is hemoglobinuria or myoglobinuria. Upon allowing to settle, patients with hematuria have a clear supernatant with sediments settling to the bottom, however, in hemoglobinuria and myoglobinuria, the supernatant is red/brown and the tests positive for heme (dipstick testing).

It is vital to localize the *origin of hematuria*, glomerular vs. nonglomerular. Patients with glomerular origin need to be evaluated and managed differently as compared to those with urological causes of hematuria. Identification of dysmorphic (fragmented and distorted erythrocytes, as observed on phase-contrast microscopy) erythrocytes, cellular casts, proteinuria with or without compromised renal function point to renal (most common glomerular) etiology. Dysmorphic erythrocytes (≥40% of all erythrocytes) on phase-contrast microscopy are specific for the glomerular origin of hematuria. Acanthocytes [≥5% of excreted red blood cells (RBCs)], a particular form of dysmorphic erythrocyte (ring-shaped RBCs with vesicle-shaped protrusions), are most predictive of glomerular etiology. Patients with dysmorphic erythrocytes on urine examination with PER of >500 mg/day, will need to undergo renal biopsy for an etiological diagnosis. In patients with bleeding arising from the urinary tract need to undergo ultrasonography of the urinary tract followed by computed tomography (CT) scan and cystoscopy.

DISORDERS OF URINARY VOLUME

Oliguria: Considering an average solute intake and maximal urine concentrating ability of 600 and 1,200 mOsm/kg, respectively, a urine output of 500 mL is required to achieve the excretory goal. Urine output less than that required to excrete the average daily solute intake with maximal concentration defines oliguria. Numerically, oliguria is urine output <400 mL/day. In patients admitted under supervision, Kidney Disease Improving Global Outcome (KDIGO) defines oliguria as urine output of <0.5 mL/kg/h (for at least 6 h), despite adequate hydration.

Before the KDIGO guidelines, prerenal oliguria is *defined as* reduced urine output consequential to decreased renal perfusion despite normal kidneys and urinary tract, secondary to a reduction (blood or body fluid loss), normal (sepsis), or increased (cardiac tamponade, congestive heart failure, cor pulmonale, or severe hypoalbuminemia) extracellular fluid. In the absence of obvious signs of fluid overload (elevated jugular venous pulse, edema or crackles in lower lung fields), a saline challenge followed by 100–200 mg of furosemide may help in distinguishing prerenal from the intrinsic cause of renal failure.

A broad spectrum of kidney disease (*intrinsic causes*) results in oliguria. The most common cause is acute tubular necrosis secondary to toxic or ischemic insult. Acute glomerulonephritis, acute kidney disease (AKD), and acute pyelonephritis can cause acute onset oliguria. The approach to acute kidney injury (AKI) is mentioned elsewhere. Oliguria is also a manifestation of advanced chronic kidney disease (CKD). Obstruction to urine flow (*postrenal*) can also result in oliguria. The common causes include calculi and benign prostatic hyperplasia (BPH). Other rare causes include retroperitoneal fibrosis, sloughed renal papillae in papillary necrosis, bladder/prostatic carcinoma. Intrarenal obstruction can be due to crystals (uric acid or cystine or drugs) or casts (light chain casts in multiple myeloma).

Anuria: Failure of the kidneys to produce any urine. In routine practice, a urine output of <100 mL/day defines anuria. Most of the causes of oliguria can also result in transient anuria. However, the obstruction of the urinary tract and vascular system, renal cortical necrosis (secondary to vascular insult), and antiglomerular basement membrane disease are the traditional causes of anuria. Duplex ultrasonography is critical in the evaluation of acute onset anuria.

Polyuria: A urine output exceeding 3 L/day in adults and 2 L/m^2 in children, defines polyuria. One needs to distinguish polyuria from nocturia and an increase in the frequency of micturition. Polyuria may be divided into three groups: (1) Solute diuresis (urine osmolality >300 mOsm/kg); (2) Water diuresis (urine osmolality <150 mOsm/kg); (3) Mixed (urine osmolality 150–300 mOsm/kg). Water deprivation tests help to distinguish diuresis which is due to decreased antidiuretic hormone (ADH) secretion by the posterior pituitary or resistance of the distal nephron to ADH.

Nocturia: The definition of nocturia is variable, from waking at night to void urine to waking up at night, two or more times to pass urine. Two or more voids at night are associated with poor health-related quality of life. The former definitions are pertinent to common urological conditions like BPH. However, in the context of CKD, the passage of large volume of urine between 6 pm and 6 am, with ratio approaching 1:1 in <60 years of age and below 0.6:1 in elderly indicates nocturia. Pathogenesis in CKD includes solute natriuresis secondary to loss of nocturnal dipping in blood pressure.

EDEMA AND HYPERTENSION

- Hippocratic medicine reports edema as a sign of disease. Starling duly explained the pathophysiology of edema. Edema is initially noticed in the feet and ankles at the end of the day and periorbital region upon awakening in patients with kidney disease (change after recumbency). The extent of edema graded as 1+- edema in feet and ankles, 2+- up to knees, 3+- thighs, and 4+- anasarca or the whole body. The edema is pitting in nature and resolves quickly compared to other fluid overload states like congestive heart failure and is often associated with pleural effusion and ascites.
- Edema formation will depend on the imbalance between the opposing forces determining the transcapillary exchange of fluids. An increase in the capillary hydrostatic pressure, reduction of intracapillary oncotic pressure, or a reduction in the absorption of lymphatic fluids leads to edema. Edema in advanced CKD is due to an increase in salt and water resorption. Other cause of edema in CKD, includes drug-induced like dihydropyridine calcium channel blockers (nifedipine and amlodipine) and nonsteroidal anti-inflammatory drugs. Also, edema of kidney disease needs differentiation from other systemic causes, mainly cardiac- and liver-related. History of paroxysmal nocturnal dyspnea, elevated jugular venous pressure, gallop rhythm, and hepatojugular reflux suggests cardiac cause and gastrointestinal bleed, spider naevi, palmer erythema, gynecomastia, and testicular atrophy point to chronic liver disease.
- Patients with glomerulonephritis, ischemic renal disease, autosomal dominant polycystic kidney disease, and advanced CKD have resistant or refractory hypertension. The hypertension may precede advanced renal failure by many years. In patients with type 1 diabetes mellitus (T1DM), hypertension is a consequence of onset of diabetic nephropathy, however, hypertension may precede onset of albuminuria in type 2 diabetes mellitus (T2DM). Patients with CKD have the lack of nocturnal dipping of their blood pressure.

DISORDERS OF MICTURITION

- *Dysuria*: It is defined as discomfort while voiding urine. Dysuria is a common complaint in elderly male and is a presenting symptom for multiple conditions. The most frequent cause of dysuria is BPH and urinary tract infections (UTIs) viz. prostatitis, urethritis, cystitis, or epididymitis.
- Frequency in micturition often accompanies dysuria. Isolated dysuria is a feature of reduced bladder capacity, which may be secondary to chronic infection resulting in fibrosis, pelvic mass, or gravid uterus.
- The *frequency-dysuria* complex is commoner in females. The pain felt from inside is suggestive of urethritis/cystitis, whereas pain in labia indicates vaginal infection. In men, perineal or rectal pain suggests prostatitis, also terminal dysuria and pyuria are strong pointers to prostatitis.
- Elderly males with BPH have poor stream and prolonged voiding time.
- Women, with symptoms consistent with uncomplicated cystourethritis, may be treated without obtaining urine culture. However, in all others, a urinary sediment examination, followed by culture is the first step in the evaluation of *frequency-dysuria* complex. A sterile pyuria is indicative of *Mycobacterium* tuberculosis infection, chlamydia, or protozoal infection.

Hematuria is suggestive of renal stone disease or bladder neoplasms. A cystourethroscopy may be further required to evaluate bladder pathology. A diagnosis of vesicoureteric reflex or urethral pathology may be confirmed on voiding cystourethrogram. A four-specimen culture (first 10 mL of voided urine, midstream specimen, prostatic secretions, and first 10 ml of voided postmassage) confirms prostatic infection is underused by both nephrologists/urologists and primary care physicians. Some centers do two-step procedure (pre- and postmassage) for the diagnosis of prostatic infections.

UREMIC SYMPTOMS

- Physiological adaptive mechanism accounts for the vast anatomical and physiological reserve in patients with CKD. The above-mentioned allow the patient to remain asymptomatic despite the loss of as much as 80% of the renal parenchyma. Uremia indicates symptomatic renal failure and can involve virtually any organ system, and the clinical presentation is variable.
- Failure of the endocrine functions of the kidney manifests as anemia and bone disease. Renal tubular acidosis, both proximal and distal, can be a manifestation of CKD. Clinical manifestations of secondary hyperparathyroidism include pruritus, spontaneous tendon rupture, bone pain (common in patients with osteomalacia and osteitis fibrosa) and fracture, bone deformities (rickets in children, adults with severe osteomalacia and in those with slipped epiphysis due to secondary hyperparathyroidism), growth retardation, and skin ulceration and tissue necrosis. Soft tissue and vascular calcification is also a feature of chronic uremia, more commoner in older patients with long-standing diabetes mellitus and those on chronic ambulant peritoneal dialysis.

PAIN FROM URINARY TRACT

- The capsule of the kidneys and the pelvicalyceal system is sensitive to pain. Pain produced by sudden obstruction and the resultant dilatation of the urinary tract results in renal colic.

Typical renal colic (due to calculi, clot, sloughed papillae, or foreign body) originates from the flank and extends downward. Nausea, vomiting, and even paralytic ileus may accompany renal colic. As compared to intestinal colic, renal colic pain is constant with a *crescendo-decrescendo* pattern. The pain suddenly disappears with the resolution of the obstruction. Pain originating from the pelvicalyceal system or pelvic ureteric junction is felt in the loin, radiating to the upper abdomen. Pain originating in the midureter is felt in the flank, radiating downward and obstruction in the lower ureter can cause a referred pain to the anterior abdomen, groin including, ipsilateral testicle or vulva. Obstruction to the ureterovesical junction mimics trigone irritation and presents with *frequency-dysuria* complex.

RENAL MASS

- The incidence of renal mass is highest in children and over 50 years of age. Etiologically renal mass is classified as congenital/hereditary, inflammatory, traumatic, and neoplastic disease.

A strong family history or presence of cysts in liver/other organ are suggestive of hereditary cause. Presence of fever, flank pain, and pyuria indicates an inflammatory pathology. Hematuria, fever, weight loss point to neoplastic etiology. Renal mass is detected on ultrasonography, occasionally is large enough to be palpable. Contrast CT scan/magnetic resonance imaging (MRI) helps in characterization of the mass. Contrast ultrasound may be useful to differentiate clear cell carcinomas from nonclear cell carcinomas. Heterogeneous echotexture, delayed washout, and quantitative lesion peak intensity on contrast ultrasound are useful to predict clear cell carcinoma.

SYNDROMES IN NEPHROLOGY

Conventionally, patients with kidney diseases are diagnosed with one of the ten clinical syndromes, which serve as a focal point for further evaluation. The syndromes are constellation of symptoms, and many of them may be a part of multiple syndromes. The syndromic approach aids in appropriate planning for various diagnostic strategies. The clinical syndromes are:

Acute nephritic syndrome: The syndrome is characterized by short history of hematuria (with erythrocyte casts and dysmorphic erythrocytes), hypertension, oliguria, edema, and renal dysfunction. The most common cause of acute nephritic syndrome is postinfectious glomerulonephritis. Most of the children recover spontaneously; however, up to 20% may have residual kidney damage and progress to CKD. Patients with persisting urinary abnormalities, renal dysfunction, and/or persisting hypocomplementemia beyond 4–6 weeks should undergo kidney biopsy.

Nephrotic syndrome: PER of >3.5 g/1.73 m^2/day in adults and >40 mg/m^2/h in children, with hypoalbuminemia, edema, hyperlipidemia defines nephrotic syndrome. A wide variety of primary and secondary glomerular disease causes nephrotic syndrome. Minimal change disease and focal segmental glomerulosclerosis/primary membranous nephropathy are the most common cause of nephrotic syndrome in children and adult, respectively.

Asymptomatic urinary abnormalities: Detection of abnormal urine sediments (hematuria, pyuria, or subnephrotic proteinuria) on testing for unrelated reasons viz. health insurance, occupational screening, pregnancy and while evaluating nonrenal diseases.

Acute kidney injury: An abrupt decline in the glomerular filtration rate (GFR) over few hours to 7 days. The KDIGO guidelines define AKI as any increase in serum creatinine by ≥0.3 mg/dL within 48 hours or increase in serum creatinine to ≥1.5 times baseline, which is known or presumed to have occurred within the prior 7 days, or urine volume <0.5 mL/kg/h for 6 hours. An attempt to identify the cause of AKI is critical, as the time line and the trajectory of renal recovery depend on the reversal of the pathophysiological process. AKI increases the risk of CKD by many folds. AKI, which persists beyond 7 days to 3 months is called *Acute Kidney Disease*. AKD was also known as rapidly progressive renal failure.

Chronic kidney disease: Persistence of kidney damage (inferred on urinary sediment examination, kidney biopsy, or radiological imaging) or a reduction in the renal function for 3 months or more defines CKD. In the absence of data suggesting reduced GFR for 3 months, presence of anemia, resistant hypertension, renal osteodystrophy, left ventricular hypertrophy on echocardiography, and bilateral shrunken kidneys suggest CKD.

Urinary tract infection: Presence of any fever, dysuria, frequency, urgency, lower abdominal or loin pain, with a demonstration of significant bacteriuria (10^5 colonies/mL). A colony count of 10^3 or fewer colony-forming unit (CFU)/mL from untreated patients is uncommon with urinary tract infection. Presence of 200 CFU/mL from a suprapubic aspirate ensures the purity of growth and would need antimicrobial susceptibility testing. Acute pyelonephritis is a clinical condition characterized by fever, flank pain, and other signs and symptoms of systemic illness like chills, rigors, malaise, nausea, and vomiting.

Obstructive uropathy: Urinary blockage can occur at the renal pelvis, ureter, bladder, or urethra. Obstruction of the bladder or urethra presents with a poor urinary stream with prolonged voiding time, and hesitancy or dysuria and ultrasonography reveal postvoid residual urine (practical definition >50% of the prevoid urine). The common cause of lower urinary tract obstruction is BPH in elderly or urethral stricture and posterior urethral valve in children.

Hypertension: Renoparenchymal hypertension is the most common cause of secondary hypertension. American College of Cardiology (ACC) and Joint National

Committee-8 (JNC 8) define hypertension as blood pressure over 130/80 and 140/90 mm Hg, respectively. Renoparenchymal hypertension is also the most common cause of resistant and refractory hypertension. Also, there are emerging evidence to suggest the pathogenic role of the kidney in primary or essential hypertension. Renal artery stenosis is common in patients with coronary artery disease and peripheral artery disease and contributes to preexisting hypertension in these cases and adversely affects the long-term outcome.

Nephrolithiasis: Renal or ureteral stone is a common clinical problem. The presentation is variable ranging from renal colic, hematuria, and acute onset anuria to asymptomatic or vague abdominal pain. Up to 80% of the stones are calcium-related, and stone analysis is critical for determining the composition. Patients with recurrent stone formation mandate metabolic evaluation.

Renal tubular defects: Often, tubular dysfunction is a manifestation of either glomerular or tubulointerstitial disease. However, isolated renal tubular defects may manifest due to inherited or acquired renal disease. The abnormalities may result from proximal or distal tubular dysfunction or sometimes, both. Patients with proximal tubular dysfunction present with Fanconi syndrome. Those with distal tubular dysfunction present with hypokalemia-related muscle weakness, nephrocalcinosis or renal osteodystrophy.

CONCLUSION

Urine examination, serum creatinine, sodium, potassium, and ultrasonography are the cornerstones for the assessment of the structural and functional status of the kidney. Urine examination is considered as an extension of clinical examination. Serum creatinine, though not an ideal biomarker of renal function, is the most pragmatic marker available to date. Creatinine clearance estimates the GFR. Complete blood count, urine examination, blood urea, serum creatinine, and ultrasonography constitute the basic investigations. Specialized tests in patients with kidney disease include kidney biopsy, serological testing for autoimmune disease (anti-nuclear factor and antineutrophil cytoplasmic antibody), serum and urine protein electrophoresis, free light chain assay, and color Doppler to assess renal vessels.

RECOMMENDED READINGS

1. Becker GJ, Garigali G, Fogazzi GB. Advances in Urine Microscopy. Am J Kidney Dis. 2016;67(6):954-64.
2. Bolenz C, Schröppel B, Eisenhardt A, Schmitz-Dräger BJ, Grimm MO. The Investigation of Hematuria. Dtsch Arztebl Int. 2018;115(48):801-7.
3. Carroll MF, Temte JL. Proteinuria in adults: a diagnostic approach. Am Fam Physician. 2000;62(6):1333-40.
4. Cavanaugh C, Perazella MA. Urine Sediment Examination in the Diagnosis and Management of Kidney Disease: Core Curriculum 2019. Am J Kidney Dis. 2019;73(2):258-72.
5. O'Neill WC. Renal relevant radiology: use of ultrasound in kidney disease and nephrology procedures. Clin J Am Soc Nephrol. 2014;9(2):373-81.
6. Sharp VJ, Barnes KT, Erickson BA. Assessment of asymptomatic microscopic hematuria in adults. Am Fam Physician. 2013;88(11):747-54.

CHAPTER 164

Acute Kidney Injury and Rapidly Progressive Renal Failure

Manisha Sahay

ABSTRACT

Acute kidney injury (AKI) and rapidly progressive renal failure (RPRF) are important causes of sudden onset of renal dysfunction. Kidney size is normal. AKI is acute (hours to days) and cause of renal failure is apparent while onset of RPRF is subacute (days to weeks) and many times the cause is unclear. Renal biopsy helps in diagnosis of RPRF. Management of AKI is based on fluid management and dialysis. RPRF may need specific treatment in the form of immunosuppression. Identification of cause and rapid treatment is essential for good outcome.

"The easiest thing is to react, the second easiest is to respond but the hardest thing is to initiate"

—Seth Godin

DEFINITIONS

ACUTE KIDNEY INJURY

- Acute kidney injury is an abrupt decline in renal function (occurs in hours to days). Mostly etiology is known and AKI improves over 2–3 weeks. Kidney size is normal.
- Acute kidney injury is most commonly defined by rise in creatinine. Standardized definitions for AKI include the risk, injury, failure, loss, end-stage renal disease criteria (RIFLE), Acute Kidney Injury Network (AKIN) criteria, and Kidney Disease Improving Global Outcomes (KDIGO) classification (not graded). Presently AKI is defined as per KDIGO criteria mentioned in **Table 1**. Baseline creatinine is defined as the lowest serum creatinine value in the last 3 months.

Some limitations of AKI criteria include:

- These criteria include: (1) changes in creatinine and creatinine clearance or (2) changes in urine output. These two changes do not correspond to the same degree of AKI severity. Oliguric AKI patients have threefold increased risk of undergoing renal replacement therapy (RRT) as compared to non-oliguric AKI patients. If both criteria are fulfilled, there is 20-fold higher risk of RRT.
- Acute kidney injury criteria depend on changes in serum creatinine. However, creatinine does not accurately reflect renal function.
- Estimation of changes in creatinine clearance is difficult in patients who do not have a "baseline" serum creatinine (before disease onset). Here baseline glomerular filtration rate (GFR) can be taken as 120 mL/min/1.73 m^2. Another option is to use published minimum and maximum normative serum creatinine for age and gender.

RAPIDLY PROGRESSIVE RENAL FAILURE

Rapidly progressive renal failure is a syndrome of progressive renal impairment of seemingly unknown etiology occurring over few days to weeks. These patients present slower than AKI, but duration is shorter than that of chronic kidney disease (CKD), i.e., <3 months. Patients with RPRF, like those of AKI, have normal-sized kidneys, while the presence of small contracted echogenic kidneys establishes the diagnosis of CKD.

ETIOLOGY

ACUTE KIDNEY INJURY

Acute kidney injury may be community acquired (CA-AKI) as is seen in low-resource countries (LRCs) or may be hospital acquired (HA-AKI) mostly as a part of multiorgan failure and sepsis or due to nephrotoxic drugs. HA-AKI is seen >48 hours after admission in noncritically ill patients and is most frequently due to exposure to nephrotoxins. Underlying comorbidities may be seen. CA-AKI is defined as AKI developing within 48 hours of hospital admission and may be due to tropical infections, e.g., malaria, dengue etc., and is generally reversible. AKI may also be classified as either prerenal, renal or postrenal (**Table 2**). In developed countries AKI is seen in intensive care unit (ICU) setting with multiorgan failure, postcardiac surgery, malignancy, or transplantations. The causes of tropical AKI are shown in the **Table 3**.

RAPIDLY PROGRESSIVE RENAL FAILURE

Rapidly progressive renal failure encompasses a heterogeneous group of clinical syndromes. The renal histopathology shows lesions affecting any or a combination of the three traditional renal compartments: glomerular (RPGN), tubulointerstitial, or vascular. World Health Organization defines rapidly progressive glomerulonephritis (RPGN)/rapidly progressive nephritic syndrome as an abrupt or insidious onset of macroscopic hematuria, proteinuria, anemia, and rapidly progressing renal failure. The diseases causing RPRF are listed in **Table 4**. Same disease can present with AKI or as RPRF depending on the rapidity of presentation. It is essential to properly work up cases of RPRF so that the exact diagnosis is established. Time is a valuable factor since if the appropriate treatment is not initiated, then the patient may progress

TABLE 1 RIFLE, AKIN, and KDIGO criteria for AKI.

AKI stage	Serum creatinine criteria: KDIGO	RIFLE	AKIN	Urine output
1 (R)	Increase ≥0.3 mg/dL within 48 hours or ≥1.5- to 2-fold from baseline	Increase × 1.5 baseline or GFR decrease >25%	Increase 1.5–1.9 times from baseline or ≥0.3 mg/dL increase within 48 hours	<0.5 mL/kg/h for 6–12 hours
2 (I)	2.0–2.9 times from baseline	Increase × 2 from baseline or GFR decreased >50%	Increase >2- to 3-fold from baseline	<0.5 mL/kg/h for 12 hours
3 (F)	3.0 times from baseline or increase in serum creatinine to ≥4.0 mg/dL or initiation of renal replacement therapy or, in patients <18 years, decrease in eGFR to <35 mL/min/1.73 m^2	Increase × 3 from baseline, or serum creatinine >4 mg/dL with an acute rise >0.5 mg/dL or GFR decreased >75%	Increased >300% (>3-fold) from baseline, or ≥4.0 mg/dL with an acute increase of ≥0.5 mg/dL or on renal replacement therapy	<0.3 mL/kg/h for 24 hours or anuria for 12 hours

(AKIN: acute kidney injury network; KDIGO: kidney disease improving global outcomes; RIFLE: risk, injury, failure, loss, end-stage renal disease criteria)

TABLE 2 Causes of AKI.

Mechanism	Etiology
Prerenal causes:	
Decreased intravascular volume	• True volume depletion—dehydration, hemorrhage, diuretics, burns, DKA • Low effective intravascular volume—shock, nephrotic syndrome, cirrhosis
Decreased cardiac function	Heart failure, arrhythmias
Peripheral vasodilation	Sepsis, anaphylaxis, antihypertensive medication
Renal vasoconstriction	Sepsis, nonsteroidal anti-inflammatory drugs, ACE inhibitor
Hyperviscosity	Polycythemia
Intrinsic causes:	
Tubular injury (acute tubular necrosis)	Prolonged ischemia, nephrotoxins, hypotension, sepsis, myoglobinuria, hemoglobinuria
Renal vascular diseases	Hemolytic uremic syndrome, vasculitis, thrombosis
Interstitial diseases	Interstitial nephritis, infections, malignant infiltrations
Glomerulonephritis	Post-infectious glomerulonephritis, rapidly progressive glomerulonephritis, Henoch Schönlein purpura
Postrenal	Posterior urethral valves, neurogenic bladder

to irreversible end-stage renal disease (ESRD) needing life-long RRT. RPRF may in fact be considered as "renal emergency". Hence the role of the physician, who sees the patients in the initial stages, is vital to ensure optimal management of RPRF. The traditional approach to a patient namely history, physical examination, and appropriate investigations, all play a vital role in the diagnostic work-up. Ultimately kidney biopsy is required in most patients.

EPIDEMIOLOGY

Acute kidney injury can affect patients of all ages including newborns as well as children and elderly. Estimates suggest that 13.3 million people worldwide are affected by AKI annually, 85% of whom live in developing

TABLE 3 AKI in tropics.

Infections	Malaria, dengue, scrub typhus, leptospirosis, hepatitis, gastroenteritis, HIV, IRGN
Indigenous medicines	Heavy metals and herbal medicines
Heat stress	
Poisoning	Mushrooms, marking nut
Pregnancy AKI	Preeclampsia, puerperal sepsis, obstetric hemorrhage
Bites and stings	Sea snakes, cobra, viper and krait, wasps, bee
Chemicals	Copper sulfate, hair dye (paraphenylenediamine)

(IRGN: infection-related glomerulonephritis)

TABLE 4 Causes of rapidly progressive renal failure (RPRF).

Glomerular (RPGN)	ANCA-positive vasculitis	• Granulomatosis with polyangiitis (Wegener granulomatosis) • Microscopic polyangiitis (MPA) • Renal-limited necrotizing crescentic glomerulonephritis (NCGN) • Eosinophilic granulomatosis with polyangiitis (EGPA; Churg–Strauss syndrome)
	Immune complex RPGN	• Postinfectious (staphylococci/streptococci) • Collagen vascular disease • Lupus nephritis • Henoch-Schönlein purpura (immunoglobulin A and systemic vasculitis) • Immunoglobulin A nephropathy (no vasculitis) • Mixed cryoglobulinemia • Membranoproliferative glomerulonephritis • Fibrillary glomerulonephritis • C3 GN • Idiopathic
	Anti-GBM	• Goodpasture syndrome (lung and kidney involvement) • Anti-GBM disease (only kidney involvement)
Vascular	HUS	
Interstitium	• Acute tubulointerstitial nephritis • Atheroembolic disease • Multiple myeloma • Obstruction	

(ANCA: antineutrophil cytoplasmic antibody; GBM: glomerular basement membrane; HUS: hemolytic uremic syndrome; RPGN: rapidly progressive glomerulonephritis)

countries. AKI occurs in 5% of noncritically ill hospitalized patients. A multinational epidemiological study using KDIGO criteria showed that the incidence of AKI in the ICU was 57.3%, AKI may be seen in 80% of patients on ventilator.

Rapidly progressive renal failure has varying etiologies. The annual prevalence of patients with antineutrophil cytoplasmic antibody (ANCA)-associated vasculitis is 17.1 per million. Anti-glomerular basement membrane (GBM) antibody disease is rare, estimated to occur in fewer than one case per million population. The annual incidence of hemolytic uremic syndrome (HUS) is approximately 2.2 cases per 100,000 population. In unselected autopsy series, the frequency of atheroembolic disease is generally low, ranging from 0.8% to 4.4%. A retrospective study from the Spanish Registry of patients with RPRF, in whom kidney biopsy was done, has shown that crescentic glomerulonephritis accounted for 33% cases, acute interstitial nephritis (AIN) 11%, immunoglobulin A (IgA) 9%, acute tubular necrosis (ATN) 5%, and lupus nephritis, postinfectious glomerulonephritis (PIGN), myeloma kidney, and thrombotic microangiopathy (TMA) approximately 3% each.

In a North Indian study analyzing biopsies in AKI, ATN was seen in 30%, AIN 30%, crescentic GN 15%, and TMA 5%.

RISK FACTORS

Elderly, Age, comorbidities, sepsis, hypotension, and nephrotoxic drug use are important risk factors for AKI and RPRF. Some may have genetic predisposition, e.g., Anti-GBM, ANCA, and atypical HUS.

CLINICAL PRESENTATION

Symptoms:

- Patients may present with oliguria, swelling, breathlessness, encephalopathy, and seizures. Some patients may have anuria. Oliguria in children and adults means urine output <0.5 mL/kg/h for >6 hours. Polyuria, i.e., urine output >3 mL/kg/h may be seen in those with ATN and those with nephrotoxic AKI. Hematuria may be seen in glomerulonephritis.
- Sometimes the symptoms are nonspecific and may include vomiting, oliguria, poor appetite, and swelling.
- History of gastroenteritis may suggest prerenal AKI while nephrotoxic drug intake may suggest drug-induced AKI. Bloody diarrhea may be seen in childhood HUS while adult HUS may be atypical with complement abnormalities. Pharyngitis or skin infections may suggest infection-related glomerulonephritis (IRGN), common in children. In adults, IRGN may be seen with MRSA infections with dominant IgA deposits. Rash and joint pains may point towards autoimmune diseases. ANCA vasculitis and lupus nephritis may present with multisystem symptoms including respiratory (breathlessness, hemoptysis, nasal or oral ulcers, and chest infiltrates), musculoskeletal (joint pains), neurological, skin manifestations, (rash) etc. ANCA vasculitis occurs in older age group while anti-GBM has a bimodal presentation. Anti-GBM disease due to antibodies to glomerular basement membrane may have pulmonary renal syndrome with hemoptysis and renal failure (Goodpasture syndrome). American Rheumatology Association (ARA) and Systemic Lupus International Collaborating Clinics (SLICC) criteria may be used for diagnosis of lupus nephritis.

On examination, edema may be seen especially periorbital edema. Signs of volume depletion (loss of skin turgor, cold extremities, and dry mucosa) may be seen in prerenal AKI. Rash, digital ischemia may be seen in autoimmune diseases and vasculitis, palpable kidneys in renal vein thrombosis or hydronephrosis. Hypertension is a feature of glomerulonephritis. Livedo reticularis and Hollenhorst's plaques may be seen in cholesterol embolism. Cause of AKI should be determined whenever possible (KDIGO—not graded).

LABORATORY INVESTIGATIONS

Complete urine examination: Urine examination is very essential and is called a liquid renal biopsy.

Urine examination is normal in prerenal or postrenal AKI. In intrarenal causes of AKI/RPRF urine examination provides a wealth of information. Protein may be positive in glomerular disease. Hematuria with dysmorphic RBC (>40%) and RBC casts indicate glomerulonephritis. Acanthocytes are dysmorphic RBC with blebs on them. More than 5% acanthocytes indicate glomerular hematuria. Telescoped urine showing a mixture of RBC casts or granular casts and broad casts is characteristic of SLE nephritis. Muddy brown casts and epithelial cell casts are a feature of ATN. Pyuria (urine WBC >5/HPF) indicates infection or ATIN. Urine eosinophils indicate ATIN. Uric acid crystals may be seen in acute urate nephropathy which may be seen in tumor lysis syndrome.

- *Urine indices* can help to differentiate prerenal or postrenal and intrarenal diseases:
  - *Urine specific gravity* <1.010 is seen in ATN due to loss of concentrating ability. Urine specific gravity >1.020 suggests prerenal disease.
  - *Urine osmolality*: Patients with ATN have urine osmolality < 350 mOsmol/kg, whereas patients with prerenal disease have values >500 mOsmol/kg. The maximum urine concentration increases from 400 mOsmol/kg in the first few days after birth to 1,200 mOsmol/kg at 1 year of age.
  - *Fractional excretion of Na–*

    $$\text{Fe Na \%} = \frac{\text{UNa} \times \text{SCr}}{\text{SNa} \times \text{UCr}} \times 100$$

    Fe Na < 1% is seen in prerenal AKI while >2% is seen in ATN. In preterms the corresponding values are <2% and >2.5%. Fe urea may also be used (<35% prerenal while >50% is renal). These parameters are not useful in those on diuretics.
  - *Blood urea—serum creatinine*: In prerenal AKI urea: creatinine ratio is high (Urea:Creatinine 40:1) due to reabsorption of urea.

- *Fluid challenge* 10–20 mL/kg of normal saline (NS) may be diagnostic as well as therapeutic.

Blood biochemistry:

- *Serum creatinine and urea* are elevated beyond normal.
- *Electrolytes*: There may be hyperkalemia, hypocalcemia, hyperphosphatemia, and high anion gap metabolic acidosis. Hypocalcemia, hyperphosphatemia, hyperuricemia, and hyperkalemia may occur in tumor lysis syndrome. Hypocalcemia and hyperphosphatemia may be seen in rhabdomyolysis. Hyponatremia (dilutional) or hypernatremia due to dehydration or excess sodium administration may be seen.

Complete blood picture: Presence of anemia generally indicates CKD. However, anemia may be seen in AKI due to HUS or blood loss. Eosinophilia may be seen in drug-induced AKI. Leukocytosis may reflect infection.

Peripheral smear may reveal schistocytes and thrombocytopenia in case of HUS.

Liver function test (LFT): Indirect hyperbilirubinemia may be seen in hemolytic anemias while hepatitis may be seen in viral infections.

Erythrocyte sedimentation rate: Although a nonspecific finding, the rate is usually elevated with active disease.

C-reactive protein: Levels are elevated and correspond with disease activity.

Electrocardiogram (ECG) may show tall peaked T-waves, prolonged PR interval, flattened P waves, widened QRS complex, ventricular tachycardia, and fibrillation in hyperkalemia.

Ultrasound shows a normal kidney size. The renal echotexture may be altered. There may be pelvicalyceal dilatation in case of obstruction. Small kidney size indicates CKD.

Other tests are done if AKI is not resolving; etiology of AKI is not clear or if RPRF is suspected:

- Lactate dehydrogenase (LDH) may be elevated in case of hemolysis.
- *Complement studies including C3, C4, CH50, and AH50*: Hypocomplementemia is seen in patients with poststreptococcal glomerulonephritis (PSGN).
- Lactate dehydrogenase and creatine phosphokinase (CPK) may be high if muscle injury. High LDH may occur in HUS.

Serological tests are indicated in RPRF. These include ANA, double-stranded DNA, and complement levels in SLE nephritis. ANCA titers both C (cytoplasmic) and P (perinuclear) titers in granulomatous polyangiitis and microscopic polyangiitis, respectively. ANA should be done by indirect immunofluorescence (IIF) and enzyme immunoassay (EIA). The labeling characteristics (cytoplasmic or perinuclear) are obtained by IIF, and identification of the specific target antigen with EIAs: enzyme-linked immunosorbent assay (ELISA), fluorescence enzyme immunoassay (FEIA), and chemiluminescent enzyme immunoassay (CLEIA). Direct antigen testing for proteinase 3 (PR3) and myeloperoxidase (MPO) can be performed.

- *ANCA with ELISA subtyping*: More than 80% of patients with microscopic polyangiitis are ANCA-positive. Of patients with granulomatosis with polyangiitis, 90% are ANCA-positive and most have cANCA with PR3 specificity, especially in pulmonary involvement. However, ANCA type and specificity is not pathognomonic for each of these clinical syndromes because some patients with granulomatosis with polyangiitis are pANCA-positive and some patients with microscopic polyangiitis are cANCA-positive. Some cases of ANCA-positive disease are induced by drugs (e.g., propylthiouracil, hydralazine, allopurinol, penicillamine, minocycline, rifampicin, and levamisole). Anti-PTX3 aAbs were present in nearly 40% of patients studied including in patients without detectable MPO and PR3 ANCA.
- Anti-GBM antibodies are elevated in Anti-GBM disease.
- *Cryoglobulins*: Cryoglobulin titer result should be negative.
- Antiphospholipid antibody (APLA)
- *Hepatitis profile*: Hepatitis B is associated with polyarteritis nodosa and hepatitis C is associated with mixed cryoglobulinemia.
- *Urine and serum protein electrophoresis*: Perform this in any middle aged or elderly person presenting with rapidly progressive glomerulonephritis to exclude the presence of light chain disease or overt multiple myeloma as a cause of the clinical findings.

Renal biopsy is done if there is nonrecovery of renal functions within 2 weeks or if the renal failure is unexplained or rapidly progressive. Renal biopsy is helpful in diagnosis and is done after stabilization. Dialysis may be required before biopsy if the renal function is impaired. Because the sensitivity and the specificity of ANCA testing for pauci-immune glomerulonephritis is only 80–90%, a renal biopsy is recommended in RPGN to establish a definite diagnosis and to determine the severity of the disease. The initiation of therapy should not be delayed for biopsy results to be obtained.

- Biopsy may show diffuse, proliferative, necrotizing glomerulonephritis with crescents on light microscopy in cases of RPGN. Crescent is the hallmark of RPGN (**Figs. 1** and **2**). Immune fluorescence helps differentiate between the causes for RPGN. Linear basement membrane staining is seen in anti-GBM disease. Immune deposits may be seen in immune complex glomerulonephritis (ICGN), lupus nephritis, Henoch-Schönlein purpura (HSP) nephritis, and cryoglobulinemia (**Fig. 3 A** and **B**). Linear deposits are seen in anti-GBM (**Figs. 4 A** and **B**). ANCA-related GN is characterized by pauci-immune glomerulonephritis (**Figs. 5 A** and **B**). Mesangiolysis with thrombi can be seen in TMA (**Fig. 6**) and interstitial inflammation in AIN.

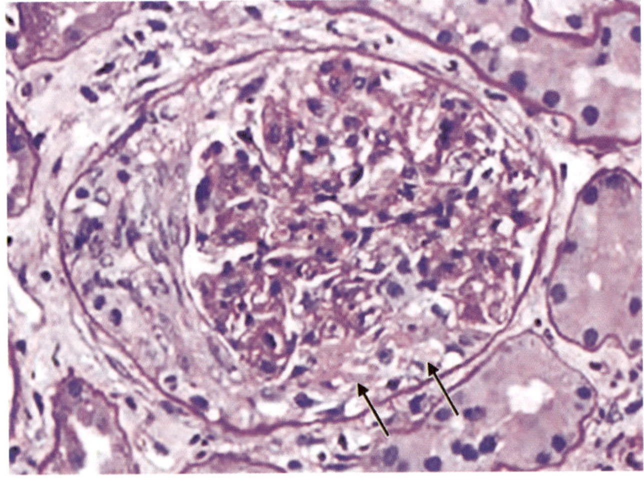

(LM: light microscopy; PAS: periodic acid–Schiff)

FIGURE 1: Crescentic glomerulonephritis (LM, PAS stain).

FIGURE 2: Immune complex deposits.

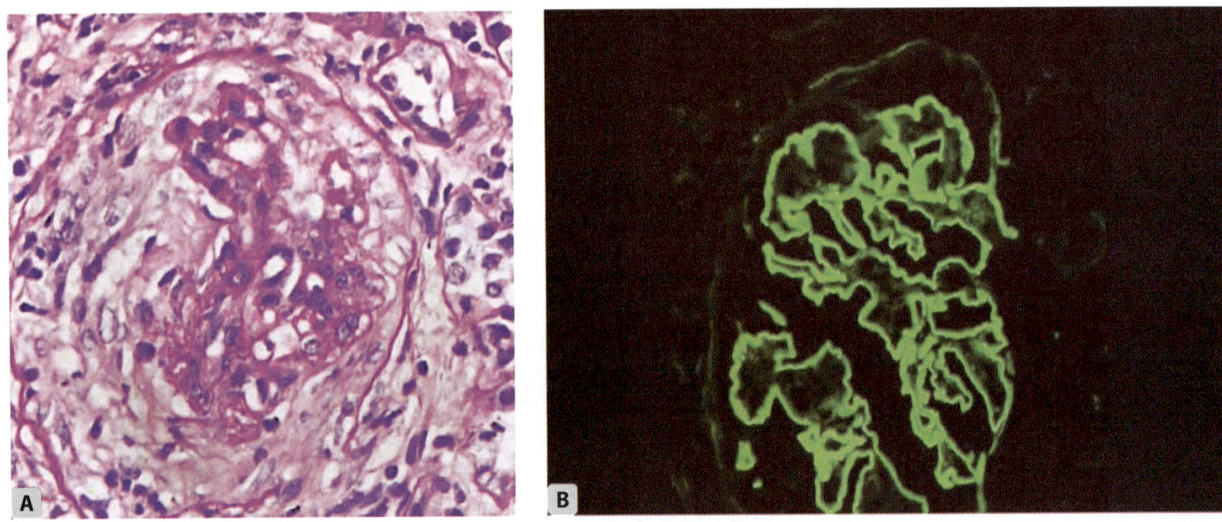

FIGURES 3 A & B: Anti GBM disease. (A) Light microscopy; **(B)** Linear deposits on immunofluorescence.

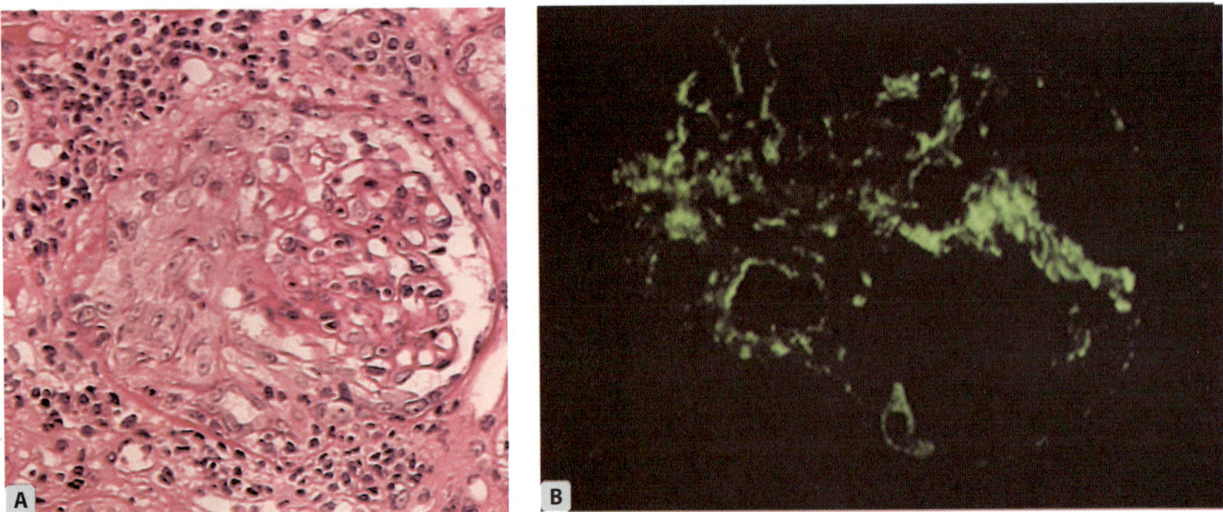

FIGURES 4 A & B: (A) Light microscopy showing crescents (B) pauci immune deposits on immunofluorescence.

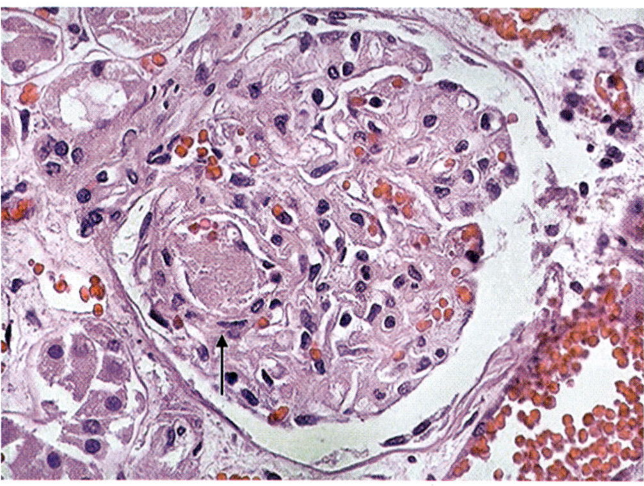
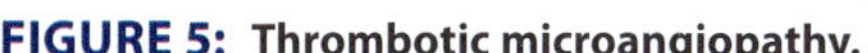

FIGURE 5: Thrombotic microangiopathy.

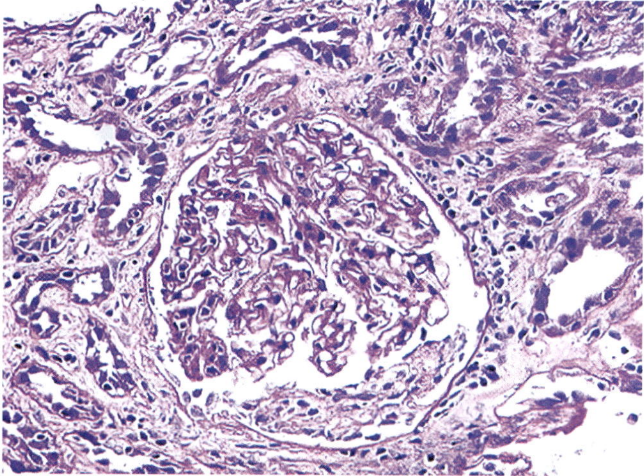

FIGURE 6: Acute interstitial nephritis.

TABLE 5 Differential diagnosis.

Suspected diagnosis	Clinical clues	Diagnostic testing
Prerenal AKI	History of volume loss, hypotension, dehydration, shock	Urine indices—Fe Na, urine osmolality
Renal AKI: • Glomerulonephritis	Hypertension, hematuria	Urine protein, urine sediment—RBC, casts, serology-ASO, ANA, C3
• *Tubulointerstitial nephritis*	History of drug intake, rash	Eosinophils in urine, granular casts
• Vasculitis	• Vasculitis • Hemolytic uremic syndrome	• ANCA • Schistocytes on smear, low platelets, anemia, high LDH, high bilirubin
Postrenal	History of lithuria, renal colic, hematuria, urine retention	Hydronephrosis on USG

(AKI: acute kidney injury; ANA: antinuclear antibody; ANCA: antineutrophil cytoplasmic antibody; ASO: antistreptolysin O; LDH: lactate dehydrogenase; RBC: red blood cell; USG: ultrasonography)

DIFFERENTIAL DIAGNOSIS

The differential diagnoses of AKI/RPRF are described in **Table 5**.

TREATMENT

Correction of hypovolemia: This initial fluid management depends on the status of intravascular volume. Volume can be assessed clinically by body weight, fluid intake, volume of urine and stool, vital signs, and lower extremity edema. Serum chemistries, chest X-ray, and lung ultrasound are also useful.

For the hypovolemic patient, a fluid bolus of 0.9% saline at 10 mL/kg of body weight is given over 30 minutes after which the patient is assessed for urine output and bolus is repeated if necessary. If the urine output increases (5–10 mL/kg of urine, over 1–3 hours) and renal function improves, then prerenal azotemia is likely. Crystalloids are preferred [KDIGO (2B)] and balanced saline solutions are better. NS causes hyperchloremic metabolic acidosis. However, overzealous administration of fluid causes fluid overload and can increase the mortality. Vasopressors along with fluids are used for AKI with shock. (1C) Protocol-based management is suggested in septic shock (2C):

- For the euvolemic patient, fluid management includes giving ongoing fluid losses plus insensible fluid (400 mL/m^2/day) plus fluid volume that equals the previous urine output volume and then assess for urine production and improvement in renal function.
- For the hypervolemic patient, IV fluid is restricted, and the patient is given intravenous (IV) frusemide (2–4 mg/kg IV; maximum 5 mg/kg/day). Fluid overload exceeding 10–20% fluid overload is a critical threshold for poor outcome. Diuretics are only indicated for treatment of fluid overload. (2C).
- For hypotension, fluid resuscitation is done if hypotension is due to hypovolemia. Norepinephrine is recommended if hypotension persists after volume replacement.

Correction of dyselectrolytemia: Specific management is provided for hyponatremia, hyperkalemia, hypocalcemia, and metabolic acidosis. Hyperkalemia is corrected by calcium gluconate, insulin dextrose drip, IV sodium bicarbonate, nebulization with beta 2 agonists, and administration of K-binding resins.

Diet: Nutrition should not be overlooked in AKI. Energy intake of 30–35 kcal/kg body weight/day is recommended in combination with a daily protein intake of 0.7–1 g/kg. Protein intake should be increased on dialysis. Dietary sodium, potassium, and phosphate are usually restricted. The enteral route is preferred over parenteral route. (2C) Insulin is recommended in critically ill patients to keep sugars between 110 and 149 mg/dL. (1C)

Hypertension due to fluid overload is treated with IV frusemide. Patients with severe hypertension and encephalopathy are treated with IV hydralazine (0.2 mg/kg loading dose, 5–20 mg every 4 h) or IV labetalol 0.2–1 mg/kg, maintenance 0.4–3 mg/kg. Less severe hypertension can be treated with nifedipine 0.25–0.5 mg/kg up to 10 mg per dose.

Stop nephrotoxins: Medications that may adversely affect renal function, e.g., nonsteroidal anti-inflammatory drugs (NSAIDs), angiotensin-converting enzyme inhibitor (ACEI), angiotensin receptor blocker (ARB), aminoglycosides, heavy metals, and calcineurin inhibitors should be stopped. Dose modification can be done for renally excreted drugs. Routine use of diuretics is not indicated except in case of fluid overload. Diuretics convert oliguric to nonoliguric renal failure and may help in overloaded patients. However, they do not hasten recovery; also these may cause AIN and AKI.

Pulmonary edema: Prior to dialysis of patients with pulmonary edema all IV fluids should be stopped. They should be nursed propped up on bed, 100% oxygen at 3–4 L/min should be given to keep oxygenation > 92% along with IV frusemide at 5 mg/kg and IV morphine at 0.1 mg/kg.

Uremic bleeding can be treated by desmopressin and estrogen and RBC and platelet transfusions.

Dialysis: Indications of dialysis are mentioned in **Box 1**. Early initiation of RRT does not reduce mortality when compared with standard or late initiation in adults. The following modalities are available for the provision of RRT:

- Peritoneal dialysis (PD)
- Intermittent HD
- Continuous renal replacement therapies (CRRT):
    - Continuous venovenous hemodialysis (CVVHD)
    - Continuous venovenous hemofiltration (CVVH)
    - Continuous venovenous hemodiafiltration (CVVHDF)
- Prolonged intermittent renal replacement therapy (PIRRT) is defined as intermittent RRT performed over a prolonged period of time (>6 hours) using conventional HD machines.
- Several trials in adults have demonstrated no difference in survival between CRRT and HD.

Peritoneal dialysis: In patients <10 kg usually peritoneal dialysis (PD) is preferred though HD machines are available even for dialysis for newborns and infants. PD can be done with minimal equipment and can be done at bedside. It is a useful modality in very small children and those with hemodynamic instability. However, PD is absolutely contraindicated if there are diaphragmatic defects.

BOX 1 Indications of dialysis.

Dialysis is indicated if:

- BUN > 100 mg/dL
- >15% fluid overload
- Oliguria not responding to diuretics
- Need for adequate nutrition, if nutrition is compromised by fluid restriction or electrolyte abnormalities
- Need for giving large volumes of medications or blood products if >10% fluid overload
- Life-threatening metabolic derangements that are refractory to medical management, i.e.,:
    - Hyperkalemia >6.5 mmol/L
    - Severe intractable acidosis (plasma bicarbonate <10 mmol/L)

Dialysis may also be done for:

- Severe hyponatremia (Na < 118 mmol/L with oliguria)
- Severe hypernatremia (Na > 160 mmol/L with oliguria)
- Severe hypocalcemia [total Ca (corrected) <1.75 mmol/L, ionized Ca < 0.8 mmol/L] not responding to therapy
- Severe hyperphosphatemia (PO_4 >1.7 mmol/L)
- Hyperuricemia (serum uric acid >15 mg/dL) if medical measures fail

Hemodialysis: Hemodialysis for AKI is done in the hospital and needs dialysis machines and water processing plant. Anticoagulation is required for HD and hemodynamic stability is mandatory. Consumables include the dialyzer, blood tubing, and catheters.

Continuous renal replacement therapies or PD are more suitable for hemodynamically unstable patients as opposed to intermittent HD. Bioimpedance spectroscopy, echocardiographic measurements of inferior vena cava, and lung ultrasound to assess B lines are another tool to detect hypervolemia. Blood volume monitoring can be conducted during dialysis and ultrafiltration rate can be adjusted.

Specific treatment for rapidly progressive renal failure: Since the causes of RPRF are very heterogeneous, the treatment is varied. The specific treatment modalities for the various causes of RPRF are shown in the **Table 6**. For those patients whose biopsy shows severe tubular atrophy or interstitial fibrosis or glomerulosclerosis, those >70 years, and those patients of anti-GBM disease with dialysis-dependent renal failure aggressive immunosuppression may not be indicated.

PROGNOSTIC FACTORS

Sepsis AKI and AKI with multiorgan dysfunction is associated with poor outcomes. Patients with severe AKI (stages 2 and 3) and fluid overload have worse outcomes.

Among various causes of RPRF, anti-GBM with hemoptysis and dialysis-dependent renal failure has a poor prognosis. Also late presentation with changes of chronicity on biopsy carries a poor prognosis. IRGN and AIN have a good prognosis.

TABLE 6 Treatment of rapidly progressive renal failure (RPRF).

ANCA vasculitis	Induction: • Methyl prednisolone • Cyclophosphamide or rituximab • Mycophenolate if no organ threatening disease • Plasmapheresis if organ threatening disease, alveolar hemorrhage or associated with anti-GBM Maintenance: • Rituximab • AZA • Mycophenolate • Methotrexate	• Induction for 3 months • Maintenance 18 months
Anti-GBM	• Methyl prednisolone and steroids 6 months • Cyclophosphamide 2–3 months • Plasmapheresis till anti-GBM titers persist	No maintenance
Multiple myeloma	• Chemotherapy • Melphalan, bortezomib, carfilzomib, lenalidomide, thalidomide	

SLE nephritis	Induction:
	• NIH protocol:
	  ◦ Cyclophosphamide and steroids
	  ◦ Monthly cyclophosphamide pulses
	• ELNT protocol:
	  ◦ Fortnightly 500 mg cyclophosphamide for 6 doses
	• Mycophenolate and steroids
	• Rituximab
	• IVIG
	Maintenance:
	• Mycophenolate
	• AZA
	• Cyclosporin/tacrolimus
		Total induction and maintenance 36 months

IgA nephritis/Henoch-Schönlein purpura nephritis	ACEI/ARB/steroids	
Infection-related glomerulonephritis	Control of BP	
Acute interstitial nephritis	Withdrawal of offending drug ± steroids	
Thrombotic microangiopathy (TMA)	Plasmapheresis for thrombotic thrombocytopenic purpura (TTP) and eculizumab for HUS	
Obstruction	Relief of obstruction	

(AZA: azathioprine; ELNT: Euro-Lupus Nephritis Trial; GBM: glomerular basement membrane; HUS: hemolytic uremic syndrome; IVIG: intravenous immunoglobulin; NIH: National Institute of Health)

OUTCOMES

Acute kidney injury is an independent risk factor for mortality with 15% mortality in hospitalized patients, 30% mortality in ICU, and 1–5% in nonhospitalized AKI. Severe AKI was associated with an increased risk of death by day 28 after adjustment of confounding variables (e.g., primary diagnosis, coexisting conditions at baseline, mechanical ventilation, and vasoactive therapy). AKI can progress to CKD (20%), recurrent AKI, and hypertension. KDIGO guidelines suggest evaluation of AKI survivors within 3 months after the onset of AKI to assess for resolution and/or CKD (Not graded).

Untreated RPRF progresses to CKD and ESRD.

PREVENTION OF ACUTE KIDNEY INJURY

Prevention in community: Identifying the causes of AKI, understanding what resources are available to treat patients at risk for AKI, developing education programs to increase the awareness of the importance of early diagnosis and treatment of AKI, and developing appropriate treatment strategies. The International Society of Nephrology has set a goal of eliminating preventable deaths from AKI by 2025—the "0X25" initiative, especially in LRCs by implementing above strategies.

Prevention in hospital setting: Avoid nephrotoxic drugs. If the drug is mandatory, then the dose and interval should be titrated as per the GFR. Volume expansion with NS is also helpful in preventing AKI due to hemoglobinuria, myoglobinuria, tumor lysis, radiocontrast agents, and other nephrotoxic drugs.

Contrast agents should be used only if mandatory in the lowest possible dose. Low osmolal contrast is preferred. Hydration is the key to prevention of contrast nephropathy. Saline 1 mL/kg/h can be given for 12 hours before procedure. In case of emergency, sodium bicarbonate 3 mL/kg/h 1 hour before and 6 mL/kg/h for 6 hours after can be used. (1A) The KDIGO guidelines recommend N-acetyl cysteine (NAC) to prevent contrast-induced AKI in high-risk patients, i.e., those with underlying CKD (1B).

RECENT ADVANCES

Novel biomarkers, such as cystatin C, neutrophil gelatinase-associated lipocalin (NGAL), kidney injury molecule-1 (KIM-1), interleukin-18 (IL-18), and fibroblast growth factor 23 (FGF23) may help in early diagnosis of AKI and may allow for early intervention before rise of serum creatinine; however, their clinical use is limited.

RECOMMENDED READINGS

1. Kidney disease: Improving Global Outcomes (KDIGO) Acute Kidney Injury Work group. KDIGO clinical practice guideline for acute kidney injury. Kidney Int Suppl. 2012;2:1-138.
2. KDIGO Glomerulonephritis guidelines. Kidney Int Suppl. 2012;2:209.
3. KDIGO. Glomerulonephritis guidelines. 2020.
4. Bhowmik D, Sinha S, Gupta A, Tiwari SC, Agarwal SK. Clinical approach to rapidly progressive renal failure. J Assoc Physicians India. 2011;59:38-41.
5. Lopez-Gomez JM, Rivera F, Spanish Registry of Glomerulonephritis. Renal biopsy findings in acute renal failure in the cohort of patients in the Spanish registry of glomerulonephritis. Clin J Am Soc Nephrol. 2008;3:674-81.
6. Birdman E, Jha V, Sitprija V. AKI in tropics. In: Feehally J, Floege J, Tonelli M, Johnson RJ (Eds). Comprehensive Clinical Nephrology, 6th edition. Philadelphia: Mosby An Imprint of Elsevier; 2019. pp. 802-10.
7. Jennette JC, Falk RJ. Renal and systemic vasculitis. In: Feehally J, Floege J, Tonelli M, Johnson RJ (Eds). Comprehensive Clinical Nephrology, 6th edition. Philadelphia: Mosby An Imprint of Elsevier; 2019. pp. 290-306.
8. Brady HR, O'Meara YM, Brenner BM. Glomerular diseases. In: Kasper DL, Braunwald E, Fauci AS, Hauser SL, Longo DL, Jameson JL (Eds). Harrison's Principles of Internal Medicine, 16th edition. New York: McGraw-Hill Medical Publishing Division; 2005. pp. 1674-93.
9. Nachman PH, Jennette CJ, Falk RJ. Primary glomerular disease. In: Brenner BM (Ed). Brenner & Rector's The Kidney, 8th edition. Philadelphia: Saunders An imprint of Elsevier; 2008. pp. 987-1066.
10. Noris M, Ruggenenti P, Remuzzi G. Thrombotic microangiopathies including hemolytic uremic syndrome (HUS). In: Feehally J, Floege J, Tonelli M, Johnson RJ (Eds). Comprehensive Clinical Nephrology, 6th edition. Philadelphia: Mosby An Imprint of Elsevier; 2019. pp. 343-56.
11. Rossert JA, Fischer EA. Acute interstitial nephritis. In: Feehally J, Floege J, Tonelli M, Johnson RJ (Eds). Comprehensive Clinical Nephrology, 6th edition. Philadelphia: Mosby An Imprint of Elsevier; 2019. pp. 729-37.
12. DhamejaN, DASbMA, NarrendranAP, ArvindGupta. A clinicopathological study of acute kidney injury from a tertiary care centre. Indian J Sci Res. 2017;15(1): 13-9.

CHAPTER 165

Acid-base and Electrolytes

Ashwini Balasaheb Gadde, Ajay Kher

ABSTRACT

Acid-base and electrolyte disorders are common disorders that are seen every day. Management of these disorders requires evaluation of the severity of the disorder, evaluation for cause, and treatment to correct the disorder. In most situations, all of these are happening at the same time. It is important to understand some of the basic physiologic principles to understand how disease states overwhelm them to lead to these disorders.

Most of the times, multiple acid-base and electrolyte abnormalities coexist. A simultaneous and systematic evaluation may point toward a broader systemic disease, making definitive management feasible.

This chapter tries to summarize these for each of these disorders and provides references for more exhaustive review at the end.

"The most complicated skill is to be simple"

—Dejan Stojanovic

ACID-BASE DISORDERS

Evaluation of acid-base disorders starts with evaluation of the ABG (arterial blood gas). A stepwise/systematic approach to evaluation of ABG is shown in **Table 1**, with renal and respiratory compensation in **Table 2**, anion gap and delta/delta in **Figure 1**, and some examples in **Table 3**. Once the evaluation is done, the diagnosis of simple or mixed acid-base disorders is made. Each of these disorders has a small differential and the cause is usually apparent on history or examination and if not readily apparent requires some additional workup. Management is mostly focused on treatment of the underlying cause and occasionally requires additional interventions.

TABLE 1 Arterial blood gas evaluation.

Steps	
pH	Acidemia/alkalemia
pCO_2/HCO_3	Metabolic or respiratory
Compensation	**Table 2**: Compensated or second disorder
Anion gap and delta/delta	Increased anion gap or normal anion gap. If increased anion gap, then delta/delta to assess for additional nongap acidosis or metabolic alkalosis (**Fig. 1**)
Why	Write the final simple or mixed disorders. Evaluate for cause of disorder(s)

METABOLIC ACIDOSIS

Metabolic acidosis is a disorder with a low pH and reduced bicarbonate. It is important to note that a low bicarbonate by itself is not enough to diagnose metabolic

TABLE 2 Renal and respiratory compensation.

Disorder	Primary change	Compensatory change
Metabolic acidosis	Decreased HCO_3	5/4 (1.2) mm Hg decrease in pCO_2 for every 1 mEq/L decrease in HCO_3
Metabolic alkalosis	Increased HCO_3	3/4 (0.7) mm Hg increase in pCO_2 for every 1 mEq/L increase in HCO_3
Acute respiratory acidosis	Increased pCO_2	1 mEq/L increase in HCO_3 for every 10 mm Hg increase in pCO_2
Chronic respiratory acidosis	Increased pCO_2	4 mEq/L increase in HCO_3 for every 10 mm Hg increase in pCO_2
Acute respiratory alkalosis	Decreased pCO_2	2 mEq/L decrease in HCO_3 for every 10 mm Hg decrease in pCO_2
Chronic respiratory alkalosis	Decreased pCO_2	4 mEq/L decrease in HCO_3 for every 10 mm Hg decrease in pCO_2
Memory tool		*5/4, 3/4, 1, 4, 2, 4*

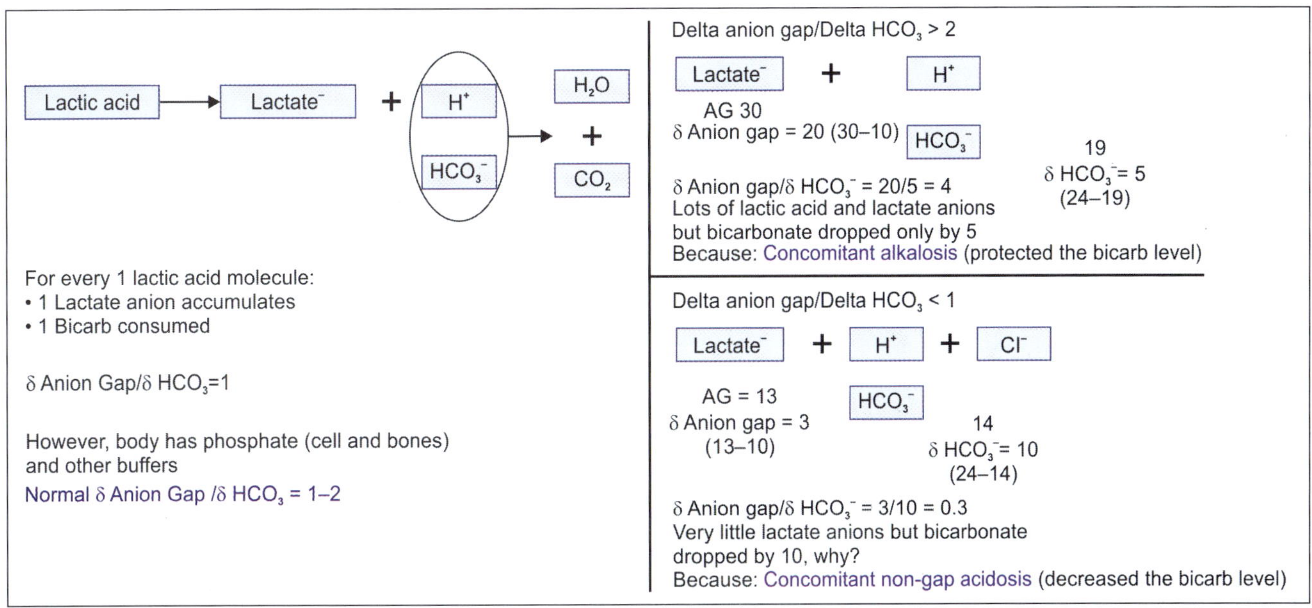

FIGURE 1: **Anion gap and delta/delta.**

TABLE 3 Examples of ABG analysis.

Steps	Example 1	Example 2	Example 3	Example 4	Example 5	Example 6
pH/pCO_2 pO_2/HCO_3 $Na:Cl:HCO_3$	7.22/20 100/8 140:102:8	7.22/20 100/8 140:122:8	7.47/46 80/32 140:100:32	7.17/80 60/28 140:102:28	7.45/30 80/20 140:110:20	7.37/34 100/19 140:91:19
pH	Acidemic	Acidemic	Alkalemic	Acidemic	Alkalemic	Normal
pCO_2/HCO_3	Metabolic	Metabolic	Metabolic	Respiratory	Respiratory	Metabolic
Compensation	$5/4 \times 16 = 20$ pCO_2 should be = 40–20 Appropriate	$5/4 \times 16 = 20$ pCO_2 should be = 40–20 Appropriate	$3/4 \times 8 = 6$ pCO_2 should be = 40 + 6 Appropriate	For acute: 1 for every 10, so for 40 increase, HCO_3 should increase by 4 s(24 + 4 = 28) Appropriate	For chronic: 4 for every 10, so for 10 decrease, HCO_3 should decrease by 4 (24 – 4 = 20) Appropriate	$5/4 \times 5 = 6.25$. pCO_2 should be 40–6 = 34 Appropriate
Anion gap and delta/delta	AG = 140 – (102 + 8) = 30 Delta AG/delta HCO_3 = 1.25 (30–10 = 20)/ (24–8 = 16) Delta/delta within 1–2 so no additional disorder	AG = 140 – (122 + 8) = 10 No anion gap and hence no need for delta/ delta	AG = 140 – (100 + 32) = 8 No anion gap and hence no need for delta/ delta	AG = 140 – (102 + 28) = 10 No anion gap and hence no need for delta/delta	AG = 140 –(110 + 20) = 10 No anion gap and hence no need for delta/delta	AG = 140 – (91 + 19) = 30 Delta AG/delta HCO_3 = 4 (30 – 10 = 20)/ (24 – 19 =5) Delta/delta > 2 and hence metabolic alkalosis also present
Why	Anion gap acidosis	Nongap acidosis	Metabolic alkalosis	Acute respiratory acidosis	Chronic respiratory alkalosis	Mixed disorder (anion gap acidosis + metabolic alkalosis)

acidosis as it can be appropriate renal compensation for chronic respiratory alkalosis and hence pH should be assessed prior to making this diagnosis.

The response to an acid load to the body involves:

- Chemical buffering (bicarbonate buffering), the large concentration of bicarbonate compared to other buffers, makes it a vital buffer.
- Rapid removal of produced CO_2 and this capacity is critical to making bicarbonate a good buffering system.
- Renal excretion of acid load.

Renal excretion of acid load consists of the following steps:

- Reabsorption of HCO_3
- Excretion of titratable acid (buffered with phosphate)
- Ammonia (NH_4^+) generation and excretion
- Main regulator is extracellular pH (through intracellular pH).
- Other regulators are renin-angiotensin-aldosterone system (RAAS), potassium, and volume status.

An important step in evaluation of metabolic acidosis is *anion gap* [$Na^+ - (Cl^- + HCO_3^-)$], which indirectly measures anion other than Cl^- and HCO_3. The normal anion gap is approximately 10 and predominantly due to albumin (4 mg/dL) and so in setting of hypoalbuminemia, the normal anion gap decreases by 2.5 for every 1 mg/dL decrease in albumin. Whenever acidosis is secondary to hydrochloric acid, a decrease in bicarbonate is associated with proportionate increase in chloride keeping anion gap normal, also known as hyperchloremic acidosis. When acidosis is secondary to addition of acid other than HCl, a decrease in bicarbonate occurs, which is compensated by increase in another (nonchloride) anion which is measured indirectly by increase in anion gap (**Fig. 1**).

Calculating anion gap helps us narrow the causes; **Table 4** and **Box 1** mention the causes of anion gap and nongap acidosis, respectively. The etiology is self-evident in most patients but may require additional testing for some. In simple anion gap acidosis, decrease in bicarbonate is proportionate to increase in anion gap. Sometimes, this change in bicarbonate and anion gap is disproportionate. Identifying this change with delta/delta helps us to identify coexisting other acid-base disorders (**Fig. 1**) (Refer to examples in **Table 3** for further clarification).

Treatment: It is predominantly focused on correcting the underlying condition. Replacement of bicarbonate will be required for all conditions with nongap acidosis as the bicarbonate has been lost. However, in gap acidosis, conditions in which the accumulated anion is a "potential bicarbonate" (lactic acidosis and ketoacidosis) usually do not require bicarbonate as correction of the underlying condition will allow the liver to metabolize the anion (lactate or ketoacids) and produce bicarbonate, resolving the acidosis.

TABLE 4 Causes of anion gap acidosis with mnemonic.

Mnemonic CAT MUDPILES	Causes	Mnemonic GOLDMARK	Causes
C	• Carbon monoxide • Cyanide • Congenital heart failure	G	Glycols (ethylene and propylene)
A	Aminoglycosides	O	Oxoproline (paracetamol)
T	• Toluene (glue sniffing) • Theophylline	L	L—lactic acidosis
		D	D—lactic acidosis
M	Methanol	M	Methanol
U	Uremia (renal failure)	A	Aspirin
D	• Diabetic ketoacidosis • Alcoholic ketoacidosis • Starvation ketoacidosis	R	Renal failure
P	• Paracetamol/acetaminophen (oxoproline) • Paraldehyde • Phenformin	K	• Diabetic ketoacidosis • Alcoholic ketoacidosis • Starvation ketoacidosis
I	• Iron • Isoniazid • Inborn errors of metabolism		
L	Lactic acidosis (D and L)		
E	Ethylene glycol and ethanol		
S	Salicylates (aspirin)		

BOX 1 Causes of nongap (hyperchloremic) acidosis.

- **GI loss of bicarbonate:**
  - Diarrhea
  - Enteric fistula
  - Pancreatic fistula
- **Renal loss of bicarbonate:**
  - Type 2 (proximal) renal tubular acidosis
- **Renal dysfunction:**
  - Renal failure
  - Type 1 (distal) renal tubular acidosis
  - Type 4 renal tubular acidosis

Ureteral diversions

- **Ingestions:**
  - Ammonium chloride
  - Hyperalimentation fluids

Lactic acidosis is one of the most common causes of anion gap acidosis and can be of two types (**Table 5**). Role of bicarbonate in lactic acidosis is listed in **Table 6**. Treatment of other causes of metabolic acidosis is listed in **Table 7**.

METABOLIC ALKALOSIS

Metabolic alkalosis is defined by high bicarbonate and high pH. As the kidney has a very high capacity for bicarbonate excretion, persistence of metabolic alkalosis requires that there is a limitation in the kidneys capacity to excrete bicarbonate, either due to volume depletion or hypokalemia or both.

Causes of development of metabolic alkalosis and maintenance of metabolic alkalosis are shown in **Table 8**. The etiology of metabolic alkalosis is usually evident on history, if not evident, then usually is either surreptitious vomiting, surreptitious diuretic use, or mineralocorticoid excess. Volume status, urine chloride, urine pH, and urine Na can be useful tests to guide in evaluation of those patients (**Table 9**). Treatment of metabolic alkalosis is based on etiology and can be normal saline for saline responsive (low urine chloride), correction of hypokalemia, aldosterone antagonists, and acetazolamide or dialysis (**Table 9**).

POTASSIUM DISORDERS

Majority of potassium (K) is intracellular and initial buffering (intracellular shifts) of potassium absorbed from diet is critical to ensure that extracellular potassium does not have large shifts post meals (**Figs. 2 A** to **C**).

Renal elimination of potassium is critical for maintaining potassium homeostasis. It is determined by:

- Distal delivery
- Serum potassium
- Aldosterone

Disturbances in these factors can lead to hypokalemia or hyperkalemia (**Table 10**).

TABLE 5	Types of lactic acidosis.
Type A lactic acidosis	• *Tissue hypoperfusion/hypoxia from*: ◦ Hypovolemia ◦ Cardiac failure ◦ Septic shock ◦ Respiratory failure ◦ Cardiopulmonary arrest
Type B lactic acidosis	• Inborn errors of metabolism • Seizures • Alcoholism • Cancer (leukemia, lymphoma and solid organ malignancy) • Congenital mitochondrial defects • Severe liver dysfunction • Thiamine deficiency • Diabetic ketoacidosis • Burns and smoke inhalation • Excessive muscle activity (exercise/ rhabdomyolysis) • Drugs: ◦ Metformin ◦ Paracetamol ◦ Nucleoside reverse transcriptase inhibitors ◦ Propofol ◦ Linezolid ◦ Theophylline ◦ Beta 2-agonists ◦ Cyanide ◦ Cocaine

TABLE 6	Role of bicarbonate in lactic acidosis.
Benefits of bicarbonate	*May prevent*: • Reduced LV contractility • Arrhythmias • Arterial vasodilation + venoconstriction • Impaired responsiveness to catecholamine vasopressors
Risks of bicarbonate	• Raise systemic pCO_2, unless adequately ventilated • May raise local tissue level pCO_2 • Increase lactate production • Hypocalcemia (decreases ionized calcium) • Hypernatremia • Increase extracellular volume
When to give	• pH < 7.1 (with low bicarbonate, usually < 6 mEq/L) • pH 7.1–7.2 with severe acute kidney injury
How to give and monitor	*Goal*: Correct underlying process: • Improve pH > 7.1 • Improve pH > 7.3 if also severe acute kidney injury *Give*: 1–2 mEq/kg sodium bicarbonate as bolus and repeat in 30–60 minutes if pH still below goal as above. If need longer therapy, then can make isotonic bicarbonate (D5W—1 liter with 150 mEq bicarbonate) and infuse it continuously and dialysis if still refractory. *Monitor*: pH • pCO_2 (should be adequately ventilated, if not the pCO_2 should < 15 mm Hg) • Ionized calcium

TABLE 7 Treatment of metabolic acidosis.

Cause of metabolic acidosis	Treatment	Comments
L—lactic acidosis—type A	• Reversal of shock • Bicarbonate therapy as above	
L—lactic acidosis—type B	• Removal of offending agent • Supplementation in case of deficiency	
D—lactic acidosis	• Sodium bicarbonate to correct acidosis • Antimicrobials • Low carbohydrate diet	
Diabetic ketoacidosis	• Normal saline and insulin • Potassium replacement when needed	
Chronic kidney disease	• Oral sodium bicarbonate to keep HCO_3 > 22	
Methanol and ethylene glycol	• Sodium bicarbonate • Fomepizole or ethanol • Hemodialysis (for elevated levels, severe acid-base disturbance or end organ toxicity)	• Calculating osmolar gap helps in diagnosis. • Osmolar gap = measured – calculated osmolarity • Measured osmolarity = (2 × Na) + (BUN/2.8) + (Glucose/18)
Salicylates	• Alkalinization with sodium bicarbonate • Hemodialysis for severe poisoning or for those with AKI or CKD	

Continued...

Continued...

Cause of metabolic acidosis	Treatment	Comments
Type 1 RTA (distal)	• Sodium or potassium salt of bicarbonate or citrate or combination sodium and potassium salt to keep bicarbonate > 22	
Type 2 RTA (proximal)	• Remove offending agent, if possible • Combination of alkali, hydrochlorothiazide, and potassium-sparing diuretic	
Ureteric diversions	• Sodium bicarbonate or sodium/potassium citrate	

(AKI: acute kidney injury; BUN: blood urea nitrogen; CKD: chronic kidney disease; RTA: renal tubular acidosis)

TABLE 8 Causes of development and maintenance of metabolic alkalosis.

Causes of development of metabolic alkalosis	Causes of maintenance of metabolic alkalosis
Hydrogen loss	Effective volume depletion
Gastrointestinal loss: • Vomiting • Nasogastric suction • Antacid therapy • Chloride losing diarrhea	Hypokalemia
Renal loss: • Loop or thiazide diuretics • Bartter or Gitelman disorders • Mineralocorticoid excess • Postchronic hypercapnia	Renal failure (acute or chronic)
Transcellular shift of hydrogen: *Hypokalemia*	Decreased distal tubule delivery of chloride
Retention of bicarbonate: • Exogenous bicarbonate administration or • Its equivalent (acetate/citrate) • Milk-alkali syndrome • Large blood transfusions	
Contraction alkalosis	

Due to the huge adaptability of the renal excretion of potassium (20–400 mEq), diet alone is seldom a cause for hypokalemia or hyperkalemia.

Management: In the management, as is true for other acid-base and electrolyte issues, evaluation and management usually happen simultaneously. Potassium disorders are usually also associated with acid-base disorders and evaluation of acid-base status is essential to evaluate and manage potassium disorders. The key principles are the same for most of them:

- Assess for signs and symptoms of severity
- Assess for etiology
- Treat based on severity and etiology

HYPOKALEMIA

Signs and symptoms of hypokalemia are listed in **Table 11**.

The three most common causes of hypokalemia are vomiting, diarrhea, and diuretics and these are usually self-evident on history and examination. However, if etiology is not clear, a systematic evaluation requires combination of acid-base status with renal potassium excretion to provide the answer (**Flowchart 1**).

Treatment (Table 12): The goals of treatment in hypokalemia are to prevent or treat life-threatening complications (arrhythmias, paralysis, and rhabdomyolysis), replace

TABLE 9 Evaluation and management of metabolic alkalosis.

Evaluation	Differential	Further tests	Management	Comments
Low urine chloride (<20 mEq/L)	• GI loss (vomiting, NG suction, and chloride diarrhea) • Diuretic use (post effect)	Diuretic screen	Normal saline: Normal saline and stop diuretics	Surreptitious diuretic use may have wide swing of urine chloride and may be clue
High urine chloride (>20 mEq/L) with low or normal blood pressure	• Bartter or Gitelman syndrome • Diuretic use (effect on)		• Sodium, potassium, and magnesium supplementation • Potassium-sparing diuretics (spironolactone/eplerenone/amiloride) • Normal saline and stop diuretics	Edematous states: Continue diuretics and add acetazolamide and potassium-sparing diuretics (spironolactone/eplerenone/amiloride)

Continued...

Continued...

Evaluation	Differential	Further tests	Management	Comments
High urine chloride (>20 mEq/L) and hypertension	• Primary hyperaldosteronism • Renovascular hypertension • Exogenous mineralocorticoid • Apparent mineralocorticoid excess • Liddle syndrome • Cushing syndrome (ectopic ACTH)	Renin/ aldosterone	• Variable based on etiology and condition • May need additional testing: CT scans or adrenal vein sampling, Doppler or CT angiography or MR angiography • Potassium-sparing diuretics (spironolactone/eplerenone/ amiloride)	

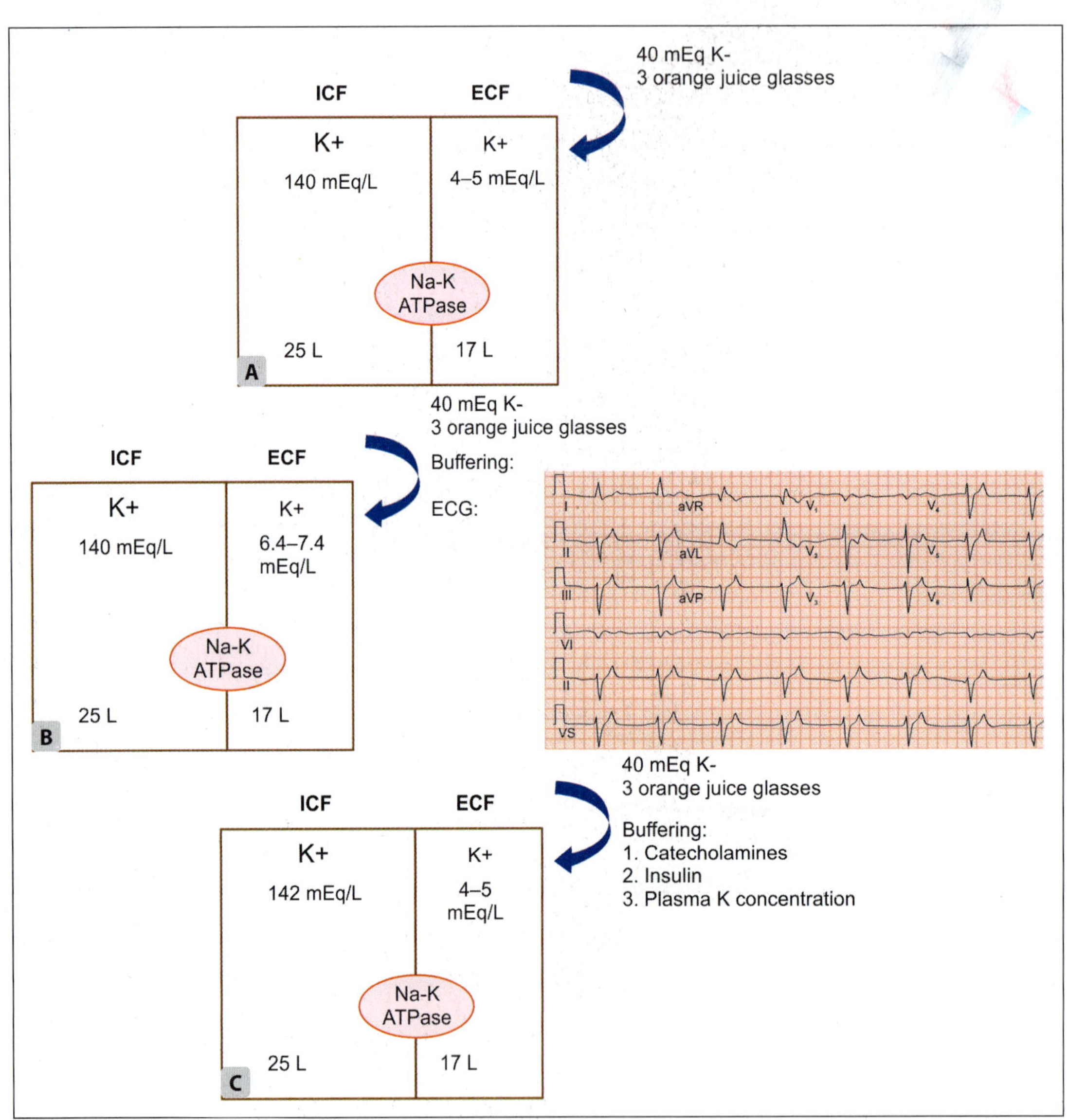

(ECF: extracellular fluid; ICF: intracellular fluid)

FIGURES 2 A to C: Potassium buffering: It is important to recognize the important role played by buffering in daily potassium management of the body. **(A)** Represents the potassium distribution of the body and the person is about to drink three glasses of orange juice (net K load 40 mEq). **(B)** What would happen if there was no buffering of the potassium to the intracellular compartment, significant increase in potassium and lead to bradycardia as shown in the ECG. **(C)** Buffering due to the serum potassium level, insulin, and catecholamines leads to limited increase in serum potassium.

TABLE 10 Causes of hypokalemia and hyperkalemia.

Cause of hypokalemia (serum potassium < 3.5 mEq/L)	Mechanism	Cause of hyperkalemia (serum potassium > 5.5 mEq/L)
	Dietary intake (not usually sole cause)	
Low potassium dietary intake		High potassium dietary intake
	Transcellular shift of K	
Metabolic alkalosis		Metabolic acidosis
Increased insulin		Insulin deficiency
Increased beta-adrenergic activity (stress or medications)		Beta-adrenergic blockade
Periodic paralysis		Periodic paralysis
Cell turnover (treatment of megaloblastic anemia/GM-CSF)		Cell lysis/tissue catabolism Severe exercise
Pseudohypokalemia (e.g., acute leukemia and postblood collection)		Pseudohyperkalemia (during collection—repeated clenching with tourniquet, hemolysis, or postcollection—cell lysis)
Others: • Barium intoxication • Chloroquine intoxication		*Others*: • Succinylcholine • Digitalis overdose
	Renal elimination of potassium	
Loop and thiazide diuretics		Renal failure (acute or chronic)
Gitelman and Bartter syndrome		
	Mineralocorticoid	
Primary mineralocorticoid excess: • Primary hyperaldosteronism (adenoma, hyperplasia, and carcinoma) • Cushing disease (some cases) • Exogenous mineralocorticoid (fludrocortisone) • Hyperreninism (renal artery stenosis and renin-producing tumor) • Glucocorticoid remediable hyperaldosteronism • Hypersecretion of deoxycorticosterone or other mineralocorticoid • Licorice or other mineralocorticoids		*Decreased RAAS*: • Hyporeninemic hypoaldosteronism • NSAIDS • ACE inhibitors/ARBs • Calcineurin inhibitors *Decreased adrenal synthesis*: • Low cortisol (primary adrenal insufficiency, congenital adrenal hyperplasia) • Normal cortisol (heparin, isolated hypoaldosteronism, postadrenal adenoma removal) *Aldosterone resistance*: • Potassium-sparing diuretics • Pseudohypoaldosteronism
Liddle syndrome		Selective potassium secretion defects
• Ampho B • Hypomagnesemia		Type 1 RTA
• Polyuria • Salt-wasting nephropathies	Distal delivery/flow	Volume depletion (true or effective)
	Nonrenal causes	
Vomiting (urinary K loss contributes)	Increased GI loss	
Diarrhea		
	Dialysis	

TABLE 11	Signs and symptoms of hypokalemia.
Muscle weakness	• Starts with lower extremity and can progress to trunk and upper extremity • Respiratory failure—respiratory muscle weakness • Intestinal ileus (Pseudo-obstruction) • Rhabdomyolysis
Cardiac arrhythmias	• *ECG changes*: Delayed ventricular repolarization, depression of ST-segment, decrease in amplitude of T waves and increase in amplitude of U waves (especially V_4–V_6) • Premature atrial or ventricular beats, sinus bradycardia, atrioventricular blocks, ventricular tachycardia, or ventricular fibrillation.

potassium loss (if actual deficit and not due to transcellular shifts), and diagnose and treat underlying cause. It is important to recognize whether the hypokalemia is due to transient potassium loss (renal or gastrointestinal) for which potassium replenishment and resolution of underlying cause is appropriate or whether this a steady state (Bartter, Gitelman, hyperaldosteronism, and stable diuretic doses with need for continued use) where supplementation is unlikely to correct the hypokalemia and hence potassium-sparing diuretics (amiloride/triamterene) or mineralocorticoid antagonists (spironolactone/eplerenone) are more appropriate. Another important aspect is the amount of potassium deficit (if not due to transcellular shift) required to cause a serum potassium of 3 mEq/L is 200–400 mEq and 2 mEq/L is 400–800 mEq.

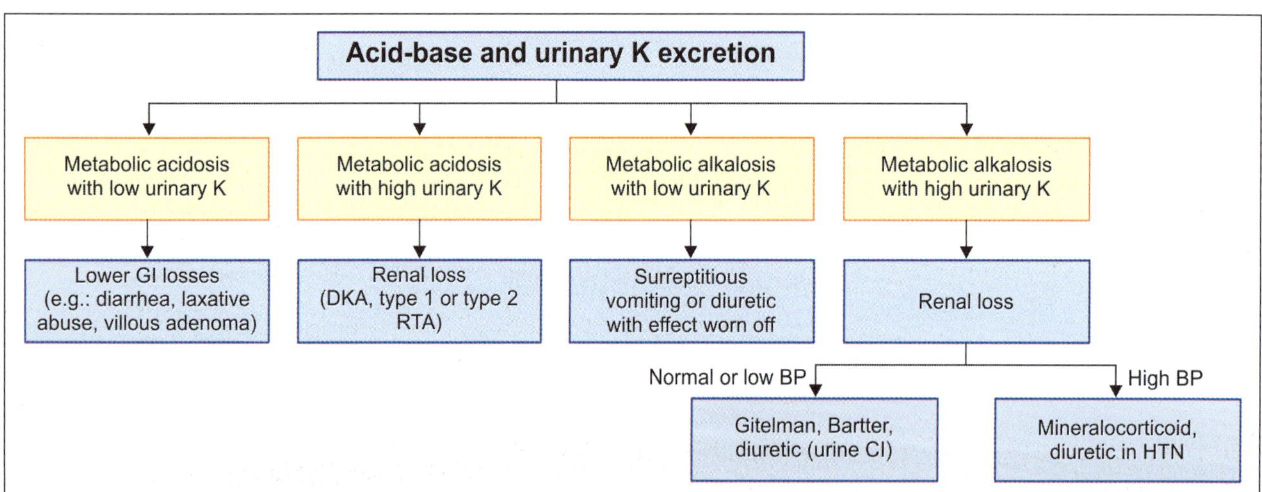

FLOWCHART 1: Diagnostic algorithm for hypokalemia.

TABLE 12	Treatment of hypokalemia.	
Principle	**Degree or cause**	**Treatment**
Prevent or treat life-threatening complications	Severe hypokalemia	• Intravenous potassium chloride (20–40 mEq/L of saline solution or dextrose). Usually at the rate not more than 10 mEq/h (central vein) • Avoid dextrose if possible as will increase endogenous insulin and lead to transcellular shift of potassium and worsen hypokalemia • Additional oral potassium should be provided as larger quantities can be provided through this route • Frequent monitoring is needed as ongoing losses not accounted in deficit estimate
	Mild-moderate hypokalemia (3–3.5 mEq/L)	Oral potassium chloride of 60–80 mEq/day. However, larger amounts may be needed if potassium loss is expected to continue
Diagnose and correct underlying cause	• Low dietary intake	Augment diet
	• Transcellular shift	Correct shift, supplement potassium only if severe symptoms (e.g., paralysis) as likely overshoot later
	• Renal elimination ◦ Diuretics	Stop if possible, if continued need, then add potassium-sparing diuretics (amiloride/triamterene/spironolactone/eplerenone)
	◦ Mineralocorticoid	• Remove mineralocorticoid if possible (e.g., adenoma, licorice) or add mineralocorticoid antagonist or potassium-sparing diuretic (amiloride/triamterene) • Supplementing with oral or IV potassium is unlikely to significantly alter potassium as these patients are at "steady state"

HYPERKALEMIA

The causes of hyperkalemia are listed in **Table 10**.

Signs and symptoms of hyperkalemia are listed in **Table 13**

Treatment of hyperkalemia is focused on three steps (**Table 14**):

1. If membrane instability, then stabilize the membrane (IV calcium gluconate/calcium chloride)
2. Shift potassium intracellularly, if membrane instability and need time to implement/derive benefit from step 3.
3. Remove potassium from body

Currently new exchange resins are available and may be used for treatment or prevention of hyperkalemia, (**Table 15**). There are concerns of intestinal necrosis with sodium polystyrene sulfonate and hence it should be used judiciously and should be avoided in certain conditions (**Box 2**).

TABLE 13	Signs and symptoms of hyperkalemia.
Muscle weakness	• Begins with lower extremity and ascends to trunk and upper extremity • Paralysis
Cardiac arrhythmia	• ECG changes (**Fig. 2 B**) Peaked T waves, wide PR interval, wide QRS duration, Loss of P waves and then sinusoidal wave • Sine-wave or cardiac standstill • Ventricular fibrillation

VOLUME AND WATER PHYSIOLOGY

Plasma osmolality is a tightly regulated parameter, total body water being the primary determinant of it. Disorders of water balance can present as hypo-osmolar state or as hyperosmolar state. As sodium is the major extracellular electrolyte, any change in total body water, leads to changes in serum osmolality present as change in *sodium concentration.* It is critical to recognize that plasma osmolality is regulated by handling of water in the body and hence hyponatremia and hypernatremia are water problems and not sodium problems. In contrast, the total content of sodium in the body dictates the ECF (extracellular fluid volume) and hence is the main determinant of that volume and hence edema/volume overload is a sign of too much sodium content in the body, while volume depletion is due to sodium loss and it is regulated in the body by sodium retention or excretion (**Table 16**).

HYPONATREMIA: SERUM NA < 136 MMOL/L

In setting of hyponatremia, the antidiuretic hormone (ADH) release stops and kidneys excrete hypotonic urine with a urine osmolality (UOsm) 50–100 mOsm/L, thus eliminating free water and returning osmolarity to normal.

When there is hyponatremia, despite UOsm < 100, it means water intake is more than kidneys ability to excrete,

TABLE 14	Treatment of hyperkalemia.	
Step 1: Stabilize the membrane (if no ECG changes and hyperkalemia is not severe, can skip step 1)	• *IV calcium gluconate* or calcium chloride • Usual dose 10 mL of 10% calcium gluconate	• Continue to monitor ECG and continue to repeat calcium every 5 minutes till ECG changes reversed • Calcium chloride has three times the calcium of calcium gluconate but requires central line for administration
Step 2: Shift potassium into the cell • If hyperkalemia is not severe and there is enough time for step 3 to work, then can skip step 2	• *Glucose and insulin* • *Usual dose*: 10 units of regular insulin with 30–50 g of glucose	• Impact starts in minutes, peaks at 30–60 minutes and lasts 4–6 hours with a lowering of 0.5–1.5 mEq/L (if hyperglycemia is present, can give insulin alone)
	• *Sodium bicarbonate* • *Usual dose*: 50 mEq given over 5 minutes	• Impact starts in 1 hour and lasts 4–6 hours, with lowering of 0.5 mEq/L • Impact is low in patients with renal failure and those who don't have metabolic acidosis
	• *Beta2-adrenergic agonists* • *Usual dose*: Antihyperkalemic dose is 10–20 mg of albuterol over 10 minutes	• Impact starts in 60–90 minutes and lasts 4–6 hours with a lowering of 0.5–1.5 mEq/L • Tachycardia and angina can be precipitated and so avoid in active coronary disease
Step 3: Removal from the body	***Diuretics***	• Loop or thiazide diuretics or their combination, if there is enough renal function • If not volume overloaded, then may combine with IVF (normal saline or bicarbonate) to increase distal delivery
	Cation-exchange resins	• Sodium polystyrene, patiromer, and sodium zirconium cyclosilicate • Take time to act and need active gut motility, risk of intestinal necrosis, hence avoid in conditions listed in **Box 2**
	Dialysis	May be needed for those with limited or no renal function

TABLE 15 Exchange resins for hyperkalemia.

Potassium-binding agent	Usual dosing	Exchanges	Concerns
Sodium polystyrene sulfonate	15 g given one to four times a day	• Exchanges potassium for sodium • Also binds magnesium and calcium	• Intestinal necrosis • Electrolyte abnormalities (hypokalemia). Fluid overload if sensitive to sodium • GI symptoms
Patiromer	8.4 g daily and increase dose weekly in 8.4 g increments	• Exchanges potassium for calcium • Also binds magnesium	• Hypomagnesemia and hypokalemia • GI symptoms
Sodium zirconium cyclosilicate	10 g thrice a day for first 48 hours, maintenance doses from 5 g alternate day to 15 g daily (adjust in 5 g increments)	• Exchanges potassium for hydrogen and sodium	• Edema • Hypokalemia

BOX 2 Conditions to avoid exchange resins.

- Postoperative patients
- Bowel obstruction
- Ileus
- Symptomatic hyperkalemia (due to delay in action)

TABLE 16 Osmolarity regulation and volume regulation.

	Osmoregulation (sodium concentration)	Volume regulation (total sodium)
What sensed	Plasma osmolarity	Effective circulating volume
Sensor	Hypothalamic osmo-receptors	Carotid sinus, afferent arteriole, Atria
Effectors	ADH, thirst	RAAS, natriuretic, ADH, sympathetic
Affected	Water excretion, Water intake	Urinary sodium excretion or sodium retention
Disorder	• Hyponatremia (too much water) • Hypernatremia (water depletion)	• Volume overload (too much sodium) • Volume depletion (sodium depletion)

condition known as "primary polydipsia" as person needs to drink >12 L water per day on normal dietary osmolar intake (600 mOsm). An alternate reason is poor solute intake ("tea and toast" hyponatremia or "beer potomania") in which low solute intake combined with normal or high water intake can overwhelm the kidneys capacity to excrete free water.

In the setting of hyponatremia, a urine osmolality >100 implies that ADH is present and leading to defect in renal water excretion. **Table 17** explains an algorithmic approach to hyponatremia, if there is significant renal failure [(acute kidney injury (AKI) or chronic kidney disease (CKD)], then this evaluation is not needed as the impaired free water excretion capacity of the kidney is due to the impaired renal function itself.

As seen in **Table 17**, effective circulatory blood volume (ECBV) assessment is needed in evaluation and management of hyponatremia. In some patients, it may be difficult to assess the effective volume, with only clinical assessment especially in cirrhotic and heart failure patients on diuretics and dynamic evaluation with IVC assessment pre- and postdiuretics or volume may guide management. Fractional uric acid excretion (FE UA > 12%) and plasma copeptin level may also help for diagnosis of syndrome of inappropriate antidiuretic hormone (SIADH).

Clinical presentation:

- Rapidity of onset and degree of hyponatremia determine symptoms
- *Acute* (onset <48 h) severe (<125) hyponatremia causes cerebral edema. Symptoms can vary from nausea, vomiting, lethargy, and dysgeusia to confusion, hallucinations, seizures, and coma.
- *Chronic* hyponatremia is generally asymptomatic due to brain cell adaptation. However, there may be subtle symptoms and can result in falls, especially in elderly.

Management: Acute hyponatremia with cerebral edema is a medical emergency, while in chronic hyponatremia, brain cell adaptation has occurred and acute increase in extracellular tonicity can cause osmotic demyelination syndrome (ODS). As previous laboratory investigations are not always available, differentiation between acute and chronic hyponatremia on the basis of time is not always feasible. Presence and severity of symptoms rather than duration can be used to decide treatment plans. **Table 18** explains the stepwise treatment options for management of hyponatremia.

HYPERNATREMIA: SERUM NA > 145 MMOL/L

Hypernatremia occurs because of net free water loss; it may or may not be associated with sodium loss. However, as thirst is the strong defensive mechanism against hypernatremia and strong stimulus for water intake.

TABLE 17 Algorithmic approach to hyponatremia.

	Approach	Investigation needed	Explanation
Step 1	*Identify true (hypoosmolar) hyponatremia*	Serum osmolality	Serum osmolality < 275 mOsm/L • If normal osmolality—it is known as pseudohyponatremia which is a laboratory artifact and can be due to paraproteinemia or hypertriglyceridemia • High osmolality—evaluate for hyperosmolar states secondary to other osmoles like glucose, mannitol, and sucrose • Serum sodium concentration should be corrected by increasing serum Na+ by 1.6 mmol/L for every 100 mg/dL increase in the serum glucose concentration and by 4 mmol/L for glucose concentration > 400 mg/dL • If osmolality is increased due to elevated urea, as urea is an ineffective osmole, remove the contribution of urea and then reassess osmolality
Step 2	*Assess for presence or absence of ADH*	Urine osmolality UOsm (mOsm/L)	• UOsm < 100 implies that there is no ADH and kidneys are eliminating free water appropriately (cause: primary polydipsia, tea and toast, or beer potomania) • UOsm > 100: ADH is present—proceed to step 3
Step 3	*Is ADH secretion appropriate (due to real or effective volume depletion) or inappropriate?*	ECBV assessment: • History and clinical examination • Urine Na *Optional*: • Serum uric acid • FE UA • Plasma copeptin level	• Urine Na low (<20) with signs of volume depletion—true volume depletion—cause (GI loss—vomiting and diarrhea) • Urine Na low (<20) with signs of edema—effective volume depletion (Cause: cirrhosis, heart failure, and nephrotic syndrome) • Urine Na high (>40) with normal volume assessment—SIADH (syndrome of inappropriate antidiuretic hormone), exclude hypothyroidism and hypocortisolism prior to labeling SIADH as presentation can be same

TABLE 18 The stepwise treatment options for management of hyponatremia.

Treatment of acute hyponatremia	Treatment of chronic hyponatremia
Goal: Rise of Na 4–6 mmol/L in first 4 hours and then rise in Na < 10 mmol/L in 24 hours ***Hypertonic saline (3%):*** Can be given as continuous infusion or as fixed intermittent boluses (usually 100 mL) Volume of hypertonic saline to reach a predefined increase in Na can be estimated using the Adrogué–Madias or Barsoum–Levine formulae For 24 hour correction with 3% saline rate—[0.5 × weight (kg)] mL/h can be used In patients with hypovolemic hyponatremia, correcting volume with normal saline may be sufficient ***Higher risk of ODS*** In hypokalemia, alcoholism, malnutrition, or liver disease ***Risk of autocorrection*** It is more in primary polydipsia patients and hypovolemic patients where ADH is suppressed after volume correction In both these group of patients, desmopressin 1 or 2 μg IV or subcutaneously can be used either proactively or reactively to avoid overcorrection	***Goal***: Slower correction rate of 6–8 mmol/L/day can be used. Treatment is based on cause: ***Primary polydipsia***: Limit fluids ***Tea and toast***: Increase solute intake ***True volume depletion***: Normal saline ***Effective volume depletion (heart failure, cirrhosis etc.)***: Continue diuretics, limit salt, and increase protein intake ***SIADH***: *Treatment should be based on the degree of ADH production (urine osmolality) and can combine the following*: ***Free water restriction:*** *<1 L/day* Two things to consider—urine osmolality and solute intake E.g., if solute intake is 600 mOsm (normal dietary intake) and urine osmolality is 300 mOsm/L, person will produce 2 liter of urine at least to excrete the solute load. If we restrict water intake to 1 L, net water excretion will be a liter and hyponatremia will improve. However, if solute intake is 300 mOsm and urine osmolality is 600 mOsm/L, then there will only 500 mL urine output and 1 L water restriction alone will not correct hyponatremia ***Increase the solute intake***: In the above mentioned patient, if we increase the solute load to 900 mOsm, he will produce 1.5 L of urine rather than 500 mL of urine and in combination of 1 L water restriction, would be enough to correct hyponatremia High salt diet (1 g of salt = 17 mEq Na) High urea diet (1 g urea = 16.7 mOsm)

Continued...

Continued...

Treatment of acute hyponatremia	Treatment of chronic hyponatremia
	Decrease the urine osmolality with loop diuretics: If urine osmolality is high, >600 for example, then use of low dose loop diuretics (10–20 mg of furosemide, multiple times a day, will limit urine osmolarity to ~300 mOsm/L). This will result in more free water excretion and in combination with increased solute intake and water restriction would correct hyponatremia
	Tolvaptan: Block vasopressin type 2 receptors in collecting duct principal cells and therefore induce aquaresis Generally used at dose of 7.5–15 mg/day (can be titrated) Studied in SIADH, heart failure, or liver cirrhosis Studies have not shown any morbidity or mortality benefit from its use, though it is effective at raising serum sodium Risk of overcorrection—important to start in inpatient setting, with close monitoring during the first 24 hours and counsel the patient regarding liberal fluid intake

TABLE 19 Causes for hypernatremia.

Pathophysiology	Causes
Total body water loss > total sodium loss	• *Renal loss*: Osmotic diuresis, postobstructive diuresis, loop diuretics, and diuretic phase of ATN • *Extrarenal loss*: Osmotic diarrhea and excessive sweating
Free water loss (total body sodium remains unchanged)	• Central diabetes insipidus (CDI) • Nephrogenic diabetes insipidus (NDI) • Insensible losses (fever and tachypnea), poor water intake
Increased total body sodium (TBW variable)	Administration of hypertonic saline solutes (recently IV fosfomycin administration has become the important cause) primary aldosteronism, inadvertent use of isotonic solutions in patients with impaired urinary concentrating ability

TABLE 20 Management of hypernatremia.

Step 1: Acute vs. chronic hypernatremia	• Cutoff of 48 hours is used for differentiation • Slower correction is needed to avoid risk of cerebral edema, especially in chronic hypernatremia • A reduction of <8–10 mEq/L/day in serum sodium concentration is appropriate in the majority of cases (though recently complications of overcorrection have been challenged)
Step 2: Calculate free water deficit (FWD) *= TBW × (serum Na/140 – 1)* • TBW is estimated as 60 or 50% of lean body weight in men and women, respectively • Ongoing renal and extrarenal losses need to be added to this, to ensure appropriate rate of correction	• Calculate FWD needed to decrease serum sodium levels by 8–10 mEq/L/day to avoid overcorrection • This FWD should be replaced with proper solution as per patient's clinical status • Normal/half normal (0.45%) saline can be used in severely hypovolemic patients • Free water through oral/RT, 5% dextrose solution can be used in euvolemic/mildly hypovolemic patients • In hypervolemic patients, free water replacement (intravenous glucose solution) plus furosemide can be used
Adrogue-Madias formula can be used to roughly predict change in serum Na after fluid administration, though frequent monitoring of serum Na is necessary for titration of therapy to avoid over- or undercorrection	

Hypernatremia occurs only if there is inability to drink in response to that thirst stimuli. More commonly occurs in elderly, neonates, or in critically ill patients (**Table 19**).

Evaluation:

- *In setting of hypernatremia, a urine osmolality >300 generally rules out complete/partial diabetes insipidus*
- Urine osmolality will also help us identify patients with osmotic diuresis.
- *Total solute excretion = UOsm × 24 hour urine volume (L)*
- Normal diet contains 600-900 mOsm/day. So excretion more than this indicates osmotic diuresis due to glucose, urea, hypertonic saline, mannitol etc.

Clinical presentation: Hypernatremic patients are generally hypovolemic, except the third category mentioned above who can be hypervolemic. Orthostatic hypotension, lethargy is followed by altered mentation, ataxia, stupor, and coma in severe cases (serum Na > 160). Focal neurological deficit has been reported rarely. Diabetes insipidus presents with polyuria and polydipsia.

Management: Management of hypernatremia is given in **Table 20**.

RECOMMENDED READINGS

1. Palmer BF. Approach to fluid and electrolyte disorders and acid-base problems. Prim Care. 2008;35(2):195-213.
2. Hoorn EJ, Zietse R. Diagnosis and treatment of hyponatremia: Compilation of the guidelines. J Am Soc Nephrol. 2017;28(5):1340-9.
3. Sterns RH. Treatment of severe hyponatremia. Clin J Am Soc Nephrol. 2018;13(4):641-9.
4. Liamis G, Filippatos TD, Elisaf MS. Evaluation and treatment of hypernatremia: A practical guide for physicians. Postgrad Med. 2016;128(3):299-306.
5. Palmer, BF, Clegg DJ. Diagnosis and treatment of hyperkalemia. Cleveland Clin J Med. 2017:84(12): 934-42.
6. Jaber S, Paugam C, Futier E, Lefrant JY, Lasocki S, Lescot T, et al. Sodium bicarbonate therapy for patients with severe metabolic acidemia in the ICU (BIACR-ICU) a multicentre, open label, randomized controlled phase 3 trial. Lancet. 2018:392:31-40.
7. Rose B, Post T. Clinical Physiology of Acid Base and Electrolyte Disorders. US: McGraw Hill Education/ Medical; 2001.
8. Berend K, de Vries AP, Gans RO. Physiological approach to assessment of acid-base disturbances. N Engl J Med. 2014:371:1434-45.
9. Kraut J, Madias NE. Lactic acidosis. N Engl J Med. 2014:371:2309-19.

CHAPTER 166

Glomerular Diseases

Natarajan Gopalakrishnan, M Sreelatha

ABSTRACT

Glomerular diseases can be idiopathic or secondary to a host of causes like infections, drugs, toxins, connective tissue diseases, and metabolic diseases like diabetes, malignancies, and inherited diseases. Clinical presentation and prognosis vary depending on etiology and pathology. Glomerulonephritis contributes for 14% of chronic kidney disease in India. This chapter briefly discusses the primary glomerular diseases.

Clinical presentations of glomerular diseases are given in (**Table 1**). Common glomerular diseases are discussed one by one in the order of their occurrence and signficiance otherwise.

"Today is yesterday's effect and tomorrow's cause"

—Phillip Gribble

TABLE 1 Clinical presentations of glomerular diseases.

Acute nephritic syndrome	
Primary	IgA nephropathy, C3 glomerulopathy, Alport's syndrome
Secondary	Infection-related glomerulonephritis and lupus nephritis
Nephrotic syndrome	
Primary	Minimal change disease, focal segmental glomerulosclerosis, membranous nephropathy, and IgA nephropathy
Secondary	Diabetes mellitus, lupus nephritis, amyloidosis, and monoclonal immunoglobulin deposition diseases

Continued...

Continued...

Rapidly progressive glomerulonephritis	
Type I	Anti-GBM disease
Type II	Infection-related glomerulonephritis, lupus nephritis, and IgA nephropathy
Type III	ANCA associated vasculitis

(ANCA: antineutrophil cytoplasmic antibody; GBM: glomerular basement membrane; Ig: immunoglobulin)

MINIMAL CHANGE NEPHROPATHY SYNDROME

Minimal change nephropathy (MCN), described initially by Munk in 1913 as lipoid nephrosis, is the prototype of (NS). The incidence of MCN is more common in Asians than in the Western population.

EPIDEMIOLOGY

It is the most common cause for NS in children, contributing to about 70–90% of NS in <10 years and 50% of NS in adults. It contributes to 10–15% of cases of primary NS in adults with male to female ratio of 2:1 to 3:1.

ETIOPATHOGENESIS

Although the exact pathogenesis of MCN syndrome (MCNS) remains unclear, multiple lines of evidence suggest dysregulation of a T cell subset and the presence of circulating factors. Mutations and polymorphisms of various genes have been implicated in the pathogenesis of MCNS including heterozygous mutation of nephrin, podocin and interleukin-4 (IL-4) and IL-13. Drugs such as gold, lithium, nonsteroidal anti-inflammatory drugs (NSAIDs), viral and parasitic infections, tumors including Hodgkin lymphoma and thymoma, and allergies to certain substances are known to cause MCNS. Recent evidence also suggests a role for IL-13 and angiopoietin-like factor 4 (ANGPTL4) as potential permeability factors. Factors commonly associated with MCNS are given in **Box 1**.

CLINICAL FEATURES

Abrupt onset of nephrotic-range proteinuria, hypoalbuminemia, hypercholesterolemia, and edema is the cardinal clinical features of MCN. Hematuria, hypertension, and renal failure are distinctly unusual. After initial response to steroids, 25% will go into long-term remission, 25–30% will have infrequent relapses (less than two relapses in initial 6 months of initial response or less than four relapses in any 1-year period) and the remaining 50% will have either a frequently relapsing (two or more relapses within 6 months of initial response or four or more relapses in any 1-year period), steroid dependent (two or more consecutive relapses while on tapering dose of steroids or within 2 weeks of stopping steroids) or steroid resistant (no response to adequate dose of steroids after 8 weeks in children and 16 weeks in adults) clinical course.

BOX 1 **Common associations with minimal change nephrotic syndrome.**

- **Primary:**
  - T-cell dysregulation
  - Presence of circulating permeability factors:
    - Active isoform of hemopexin
    - Interleukin-13
    - Angiopoietin-like 4 over-production (ANGPTL4)
- **Secondary**:
  - Infections
    - Viral
    - Parasitic
  - Drugs
    - NSAIDs
    - Gold
    - Lithium
    - Ampicillin
    - Rifampin
  - Tumors
    - Hodgkin disease
    - Lymphomas and leukemia
    - Thymoma
    - Solid tumors
  - Allergies
  - Secondary to systemic diseases
    - SLE
    - Following HSCT

(HSCT: hematopoietic stem cell transplantation)

PATHOLOGY

Light microscopy remains normal (**Fig. 1**), though mild mesangial expansion in the glomerulus and protein and lipid reabsorption droplets in tubular epithelium may be seen in some cases. Immunofluorescence (IF) is usually negative. Focal presence of interstitial fibrosis and tubular atrophy in a young patient and focal, segmental well-defined staining in IF for C3 and immunoglobulin M (IgM) should raise suspicion for unsampled focal segmental glomerulosclerosis (FSGS). Electron microscopy (EM) shows diffuse foot process effacement.

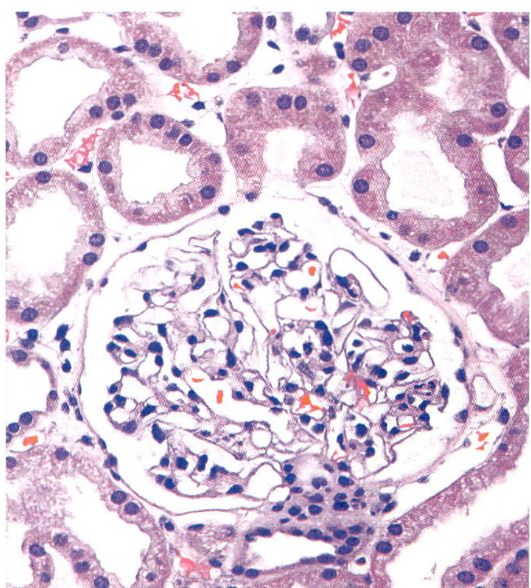

FIGURE 1: Minimal change disease.

MANAGEMENT

The drug of choice for the initial episode is prednisone or prednisolone at a dose of 1 mg/kg/day up to a maximum of 80 mg/day, for a period of 4–16 weeks until remission is achieved, followed by a taper over 6 months. Infrequent relapsers are treated with the same initial dose and duration as that of the first episode for the relapses. Those with relative contraindications to steroids or frequently relapsing/steroid-dependent NS are treated with oral cyclophosphamide or calcineurin inhibitors (CNIs). Oral cyclophosphamide is given at a dose of 2–2.5 mg/kg/day for 8 weeks. Mycophenolate mofetil (MMF) is indicated in frequently relapsing/steroid-dependent NS, if they are intolerant to alkylating agents or CNIs. Those who are steroid-resistant are treated with CNIs such as tacrolimus.

Supportive therapy includes renin–angiotensin–aldosterone system (RAAS) blockade, salt and water restriction, dyslipidemia control, antihypertensives, and anticoagulation, if the serum albumin < 2 g/dL. Lifestyle modification, regular physical activity, and weight reduction are found to be useful.

FOCAL SEGMENTAL GLOMERULOSCLEROSIS

Focal segmental glomerulosclerosis has different underlying etiologies, sharing a common theme of podocyte injury and depletion. FSGS contributes significantly to the end-stage renal disease (ESRD) burden in the younger population. The classification of FSGS is constantly undergoing changes due to explosion of knowledge in recent times.

EPIDEMIOLOGY

Focal segmental glomerulosclerosis is the most common cause of NS in adults aged < 40 years in India with 5-fold increase in frequency over last five decades. Annual incidence rates of FSGS range from 0.2 to 1.8/100,000 population per year with incidence in men 1.5-fold higher than in women.

ETIOPATHOGENESIS

Primary FSGS is mediated by circulating permeability factors like soluble urokinase plasminogen activated receptor (suPAR), cardiotrophin-like cytokine factor 1 (CLCF1), apolipoprotein A1B (Apo A1B), and anti-CD40 antibody which are toxic to the podocytes and cause podocyte dysfunction. Conditions associated with increased single-nephron glomerular filtration rate (GFR) induce podocyte stress resulting from mismatch between the glomerular load and glomerular capacity, and cause an adaptive form of FSGS. The pathology can start with normal or elevated estimated GFR (eGFR) as seen in obesity and cyanotic congenital heart disease or decreased GFR as seen in reflux nephropathy and renal anomalies. Genetic mutations causing FSGS like NPHS1, NPHS2, and APOL-1 polymorphism are increasingly recognized as causative factors. Infections by human immunodeficiency virus (HIV), cytomegalovirus (CMV), and parvovirus and drugs like bisphosphonates, lithium, interferon, and anabolic steroids injure the podocyte and cause FSGS.

CLINICAL FEATURES

Abrupt-onset NS is the most common presentation of primary FSGS, which is seen in 100% of patients with primary FSGS. Other manifestations include micro-hematuria (50%), hypertension (20%), reduced GFR (25–50%), and tubular dysfunction (glycosuria, amino-aciduria, phosphaturia, and concentrating defects). In secondary FSGS, proteinuria (subnephrotic to nephrotic range proteinuria) without edema and normal serum albumin is frequently seen. Exceptions include HIV-associated nephropathy (HIVAN) and bisphosphonate-induced FSGS, which can present with NS. Characteristic clinical features and pathological features of various forms of FSGS are given in **Table 2**.

PATHOLOGY

Focal segmental glomerulosclerosis initially affects the juxtamedullary/inner cortical glomeruli. This is due to the higher blood flow and higher blood pressure of juxtamedullary area. Being a focal pathology, the sensitivity of renal biopsy depends on the number of glomeruli sampled, with >20 glomeruli generally considered adequate. FSGS is classified into five variants by the Columbia classification which is based on light microscopic findings—NOS (**Fig. 2**) (not otherwise specified), perihilar, cellular, tip, and collapsing.

Immunofluorescence may reveal nonspecific trapping of IgM and C3 in areas of segmental sclerosis. EM shows diffuse foot process effacement of >80% in primary FSGS and <80% in secondary FSGS though it does not rule out primary FSGS.

MANAGEMENT

Immunosuppressive therapy should be offered only in idiopathic FSGS associated with clinical features of NS. Immunosuppression should not be used in adults with

FSGS of undetermined cause or in those with secondary FSGS. Corticosteroids are recommended as the first-line immunosuppressive treatment for primary FSGS. CNIs can be considered as first-line therapy for patients with relative contraindications or intolerance to high-dose corticosteroids (e.g., uncontrolled diabetes, psychiatric conditions, and severe osteoporosis). For steroid-resistant FSGS, CNIs are the recommended first-line treatment; if there is a partial or complete remission, CNI treatment is continued for at least 12 months, followed by a slow taper. A combination of CNIs and MMF along with low-dose steroids is used in patients who are resistant to CNIs.

TABLE 2 Differentiating features of primary versus maladaptive focal segmental glomerulosclerosis (FSGS).

	Primary FSGS	Maladaptive FSGS
Clinical features	Abrupt onset edema	No edema
Proteinuria	Nephrotic range	Subnephrotic to nephrotic range
Serum albumin	<3 g/dL	>3 g/dL
Light microscopy	• Glomerulomegaly less common • In early disease often no other damage	• Glomerulomegaly more common • Perihilar variant common • Global glomerulosclerosis and other scarring
Electron microscopy	• Diffuse foot process effacement (>80%)* • Foot process width (>1,500 nm)	• Segmental foot process effacement (<80%) • Shorter foot process width

*Segmental foot process effacement does not rule out primary FSGS.

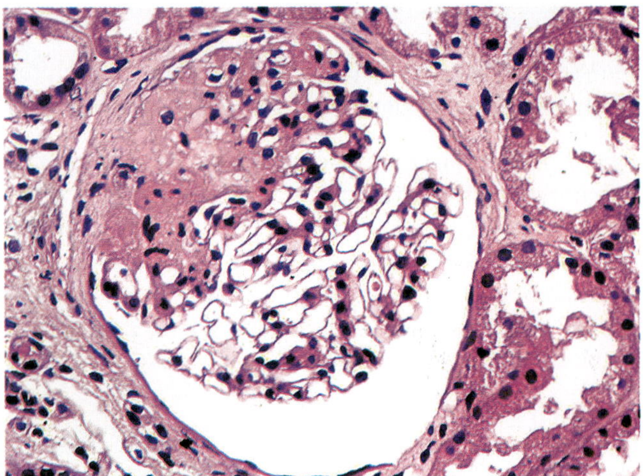

FIGURE 2: Focal, segmental glomerulosclerosis, and H&E stain.

Other therapies being studied for resistant cases include rituximab, abatacept, plasma exchange, and low-density lipoprotein (LDL) apheresis.

Spontaneous remission of proteinuria occurs in >20%. The degree of proteinuria is a strong predictor of long-term outcome. Renal survival at 10 years in patients with non-nephrotic range proteinuria is around 90% (it is important not to initiate immunosuppression in these patients at the outset), whereas it is 41% for nephrotic patients not in remission. Collapsing variant and presence of significant interstitial fibrosis and tubular atrophy indicate poor prognosis.

MEMBRANOUS NEPHROPATHY

Membranous nephropathy (MN) is one of the most common causes of idiopathic NS in adults.

EPIDEMIOLOGY

The peak incidence occurs during fourth and fifth decade, with a male female ratio of 2:1. MN is characterized by diffuse immune complex (IC) deposition in subepithelial location in the glomerular basement membrane (GBM).

ETIOPATHOGENESIS

As with other forms of NS, the causes of MN may be either primary or idiopathic or secondary (**Table 3**).

Primary MN is a "renal-limited" autoimmune disease. In experimental animal models, circulating antibodies against the podocyte antigen "megalin" is formed (this antigen is not found in humans). An endogenous or planted antigen called M-type phospholipase A2 receptor (PLA2R), located on the podocyte is the cause of most cases of idiopathic MN in humans. The ICs deposit in the subepithelial location space, the complement system is activated, and the membrane attack complex C5b-9 inserts onto the podocyte causing injury. GBM expansion occurs by overproduction of GBM components like type IV collagen and laminin resulting in the characteristic basement membrane thickening. Podocyte injury results in proteinuria. Anti

TABLE 3 Secondary causes of membranous nephropathy.

Etiology	Examples of diseases
Infections	HBV, HCV, HIV, filariasis, and malaria
Malignancy (paraneoplastic syndrome)	Carcinoma lung, prostate, and CLL
Autoimmune diseases	SLE, thyroiditis, and rheumatoid arthritis
Drugs	NSAID, D-penicillamine, mercury, and gold
Alloimmune diseases	Graft vs. host disease, transplant glomerulopathy

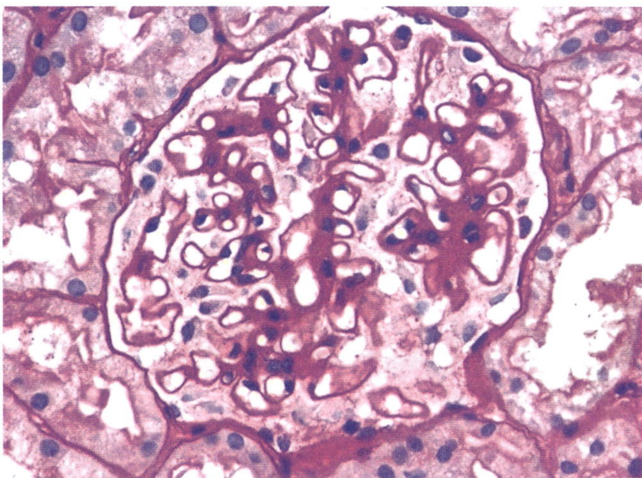

FIGURE 3: Membranous nephropathy (H&E stain).

Courtesy: Dr Anila Abraham Kurien, Renopath, Centre for Renal and Urological Pathology, Chennai.

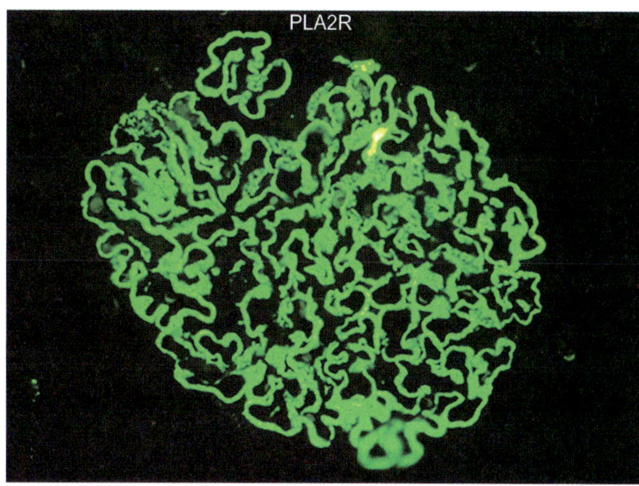

FIGURE 4: Membranous nephropathy—immunofluorescence [phospholipase A2 receptor (PLA2R) staining].

M-PLA2R antibody is not found in secondary MN and other glomerular diseases. Therefore, antibody to PLA2R is a useful biomarker for idiopathic MN which is present in about 75% of patients. In addition, kidney biopsy staining for PLA2R by IF reveals positivity in 60–85% of patients with idiopathic MN.

Thrombospondin type-1 domain-containing 7A (THSD7A) is a transmembrane protein expressed on podocytes and may be the causative antigen in about 10% of patients with idiopathic MN in whom anti-PLA2R antibody is absent. IgG4 antibodies traverse the GBM and form "in-situ" ICs with PLA2R.

Other antigens implicated include neural epidermal growth factor-like 1 (NELL-1), neutral endopeptidase, semaphorin 3B (SEMA3B), and cationic bovine serum albumin (cBSA).

PATHOLOGY

Light microscopy reveals uniformly thickened glomerular capillary wall on hematoxylin and eosin (H&E) stain (**Fig. 3**), along with spikes and "pinhole" lesions on the basement membrane best seen on Jones methenamine silver stain. IF shows diffuse granular deposits of IgG4 along the GBM. IF staining for PLA2R antigen is strongly positive in most patients with idiopathic MN (**Fig. 4**).

CLINICAL FEATURES

Most patients present with NS. Hypertension and microhematuria are present in about 30–40% of patients. Male gender, severe proteinuria, persistence of NS for >6 months, low GFR at presentation, and hypertension are poor prognostic factors. A detailed evaluation to rule out secondary causes has to be carried out. As mentioned above, MN can occur as a paraneoplastic manifestation and at times, it may precede malignancy.

MANAGEMENT

Because of the chronic nature of the disease and tendency for spontaneous remissions in about 30% of cases, treatment should be tailored for the individual patient. The main therapeutic approaches include:

- Conservative treatment with RAAS blockade [using angiotensin-converting enzyme (ACE) inhibitors and angiotensin receptor blockers (ARBs)] for their antiproteinuric action. Decision regarding conservative treatment or need for immunosuppression is based on initial response to conservative therapy.
- Corticosteroids therapy
- Alkylating agents like cyclophosphamide

Indications for immunosuppression [as per Kidney Diseases Improving Global Outcomes (KDIGO) guidelines] are:

- Nephrotic syndrome with persistent proteinuria > 4 g/day despite 6 months of antihypertensive and antiproteinuric therapy
- Presence of severe disabling life-threatening symptoms related to NS
- Rise in serum creatinine > 30% within 6–12 months from diagnosis, but eGFR not <25–30 mL/min/1.73 m^2.

The immunosuppressive regimen used is the modified Ponticelli regime. This consists of a 6-month treatment schedule using steroids and cyclophosphamide alternately at monthly intervals. During months 1, 3, and 5, intravenous methylprednisolone 1 g/day is given for the first 3 days followed by oral prednisolone 0.5 mg/kg/day from day 4 to day 30. During months 2, 4, and 6, oral cyclophosphamide (1.5 mg/kg/day) is given for 30 days each.

In the case of secondary MN, the management is essentially treatment of the underlying disease while continuing general supportive treatment and antiproteinuric measures.

INFECTION-RELATED GLOMERULONEPHRITIS

INTRODUCTION

Infection-related glomerulonephritis (IRGN) is an immune-mediated glomerular disease due to nonrenal infections. There have been significant changes in epidemiology, clinical presentation, and outcome of IRGN during the past two decades. From being a prototype of IC-mediated acute glomerulonephritis affecting exclusively children with invariably good prognosis, it is increasingly becoming a disease of adults with less favorable prognosis. In children, glomerulonephritis usually occurs about a week after pharyngitis or cutaneous infection. Hence, it used to be referred to as "postinfectious" glomerulonephritis. But, in most adults, there is ongoing infection at the time of diagnosis. Hence, the term "infection-related glomerulonephritis" is preferred.

EPIDEMIOLOGY

Adult IRGN has a male preponderance. Diabetes, alcoholism, and severe malnutrition are predisposing factors. Infections of respiratory tract, skin, teeth and periodontal sites, urinary tract, infective endocarditis, and visceral abscess can be associated with IRGN.

ETIOPATHOGENESIS

In children, *Streptococcus* is the most common preceding infection whereas in adults, nonstreptococcal bacteria like *Staphylococcus* and gram-negative bacteria are also increasingly reported. Complement activation consequent to plasmin activation or defect in regulating mechanisms of alternative complement pathway is implicated in the pathogenesis. Circulating antigen–antibody ICs is deposited in subendothelial and/or mesangial regions. In-situ ICs formed by antibodies directed against bacterial or intrinsic glomerular antigens via "molecular mimicry" result in subepithelial deposits and activation of the alternative complement pathway. The resultant complement activation in glomeruli leads to the generation of chemotactins C3a and C5a, recruitment of neutrophils and monocytes, and leukocyte-mediated injury.

CLINICAL FEATURES

The clinical manifestations of adult IRGN are notably similar to childhood IRGN. In both age groups, symptomatic patients most commonly manifest acute nephritic syndrome, with new onset hematuria, proteinuria, edema, hypertension, and reduced renal function. Hypertension is present in 60–84% of adult patients at presentation. The degree of proteinuria varies from 1 to 3 g/day, with a quarter to a third of patients having full NS. Almost all patients have microhematuria with or without red blood cell casts. Hypocomplementemia is present in 35–80% of adults with IRGN. In most patients, C3 is depressed with or without depression of C4. Usually, serum complement levels normalize within 2 months. While most affected children recover completely, the prognosis is less favorable in adults with a fraction of them progressing to chronic kidney disease.

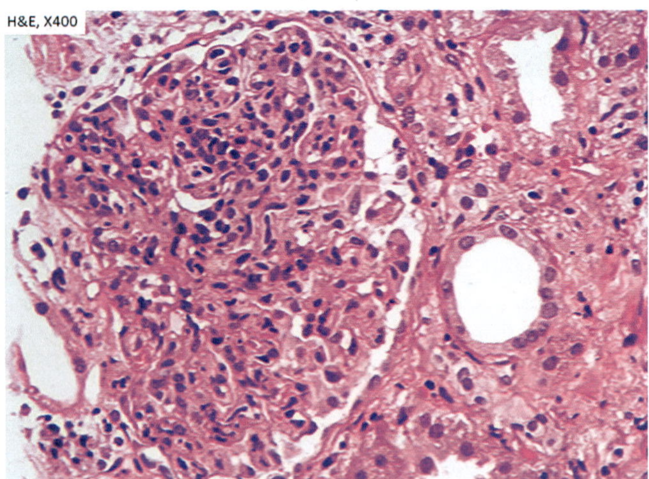

FIGURE 5: Infection-related glomerulonephritis (diffuse proliferative glomerulonephritis).

PATHOLOGY

- *Light microscopy*: The most common histological pattern of injury is diffuse endocapillary proliferative and exudative glomerulonephritis with numerous intracapillary neutrophils (**Fig. 5**). Crescentic and necrotizing glomerulonephritis is rare, occurring in around 5% of cases.
- *Immunofluorescence*: IF typically reveals C3-dominant or codominant glomerular staining. In most cases, there is coarsely granular mesangial and glomerular wall staining, resembling the "starry sky pattern." IgG is usually the most frequent Ig deposited. In individuals with underlying diabetes and staphylococcal infections, dominant presence of IgA is frequently reported, which is referred to as "IgA dominant IRGN."
- *Electron microscopy*: EM study shows scattered large subepithelial electron-dense deposits, which exhibit a characteristic "hump-shaped" appearance in most cases.

MANAGEMENT

The treatment of IRGN should include eradication of infection and management of complications of nephritis. Focus of infection has to be diligently searched. Treatment of acute nephritic syndrome includes antihypertensive drugs, diuretics, and dietary salt restriction. In patients with persistent moderate or heavy proteinuria, renin-angiotensin system (RAS) blockade is recommended to slow disease progression. The role of immunosuppressive therapy in the treatment IRGN is doubtful. Despite the frequent use of steroids for the treatment of adult IRGN for renal insufficiency with or without crescentic disease, none of the studies found a beneficial effect of steroids on outcome.

IMMUNOGLOBULIN A NEPHROPATHY

Immunoglobulin A nephropathy (IgAN) is the most common primary glomerulonephritis worldwide. It was previously known as Berger's disease.

EPIDEMIOLOGY

The highest prevalence of IgAN is seen in developed countries in East Asia, particularly nations like Japan, Korea, and Taiwan, where urinalysis is frequently used as a screening tool. The incidence is higher in children and young adults.

ETIOPATHOGENESIS

The primary abnormality in IgAN is the presence of high serum levels of galactose-deficient IgA1 (Gd-IgA1). This elicits an autoimmune response, resulting in the production of autoantibodies to the Gd-IgA1, culminating in the deposition of ICs in the kidneys. These then cause complement and mesangial cell activation, which eventually result in glomerular inflammation.

CLINICAL FEATURES

Immunoglobulin A nephropathy is often first detected by asymptomatic urinary abnormalities, identified by routine urinalyses. The classic presentation, however, is synpharyngitic macroscopic hematuria which occurs in association with an upper respiratory tract infection. There is no latent period between the upper respiratory tract infection and the onset of macroscopic hematuria (unlike poststreptococcal glomerulonephritis).

Immunoglobulin A nephropathy also often presents as progressive chronic kidney disease, with some patients only presenting at ESRD. Less common presentations include acute kidney injury (AKI) and rapidly progressive glomerulonephritis (RPGN).

PATHOLOGY

The diagnosis of IgAN is only made on renal biopsy, and is defined by the presence of dominant or codominant IgA on IF, with deposits predominantly occurring in the mesangium. The light microscopic findings may range from mesangial expansion (M), endocapillary hypercellularity (E), segmental sclerosis (S), varying degrees of interstitial fibrosis and tubular atrophy (T), and occasionally crescents (C). These findings, together, constitute the "Oxford classification" system of IgAN, also known as the MEST-C score, which has prognostic implications.

MANAGEMENT

Multiple studies have demonstrated the efficacy of RAS blockade (in the form of ACE inhibitors or ARBs) in lowering proteinuria and retarding the rate of progression of renal failure. There is increasing evidence that short courses of steroids can play a significant role in reducing proteinuria and progression to ESRD. Several other therapies have also been suggested, including fish oil, tonsillectomy, azathioprine, and MMF.

CRESCENTIC GLOMERULONEPHRITIS

Rapidly progressive glomerulonephritis is a renal syndrome that is characterized by a deterioration of renal function that occurs over days to weeks. This is in contrast to AKI which occurs over hours to days. The histologic hallmark of RPGN is crescentic glomerulonephritis.

Crescentic glomerulonephritis is an aggressive inflammatory lesion of the glomerulus that is characterized by focal breaks in the GBM, which allows the influx of various inflammatory mediators and leukocytes into the Bowman's space. These then stimulate the proliferation of the parietal epithelial cells, which fill the Bowman's space, producing a "crescent" around the glomerular tuft. Crescent, by definition, is presence of two or more layers of cells in the Bowman's space (**Fig. 6**).

CLASSIFICATION

The diseases that present as a RPGN are classified based on the IF pattern on renal biopsy:

- Linear GBM Ig staining—anti-GBM disease
- Granular staining for Ig and complement—IC diseases such as lupus nephritis, IgAN, and IRGN
- Absence of staining for Ig and complement ("pauci-immune")—anti-neutrophil cytoplasm antibody (ANCA)-associated vasculitides, which include granulomatosis with polyangiitis (GPA), microscopic polyangiitis (MPA), eosinophilic granulomatosis with polyangiitis (EGPA), and renal-limited vasculitis

CLINICAL PRESENTATION

Rapidly progressive glomerulonephritis is a nephrological emergency that sometimes presents in a misleadingly insidious manner, but quite often announces itself by its rapidly-evolving, catastrophic, clinical course. Urine output often falls rapidly and patients may even become anuric. Other organ systems may also often be affected, depending on the underlying disease with pulmonary hemorrhage occurring in the setting of ANCA vasculitis, anti-GBM disease, and occasionally

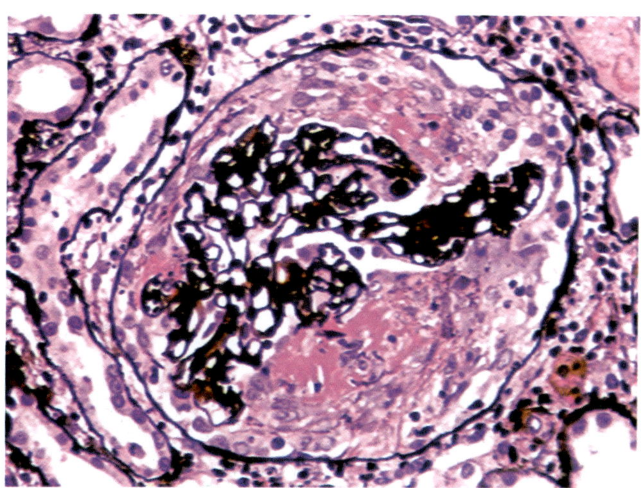

FIGURE 6: Crescentic glomerulonephritis.

SLE. A urinalysis often reveals proteinuria and an active urinary sediment with dysmorphic red blood cells, and occasionally red cell casts.

MANAGEMENT

Immunosuppression with intravenous pulse methylprednisolone, along with a cyclophosphamide pulse, is often instituted as soon as the diagnosis is suspected, without waiting histological confirmation. A tissue diagnosis by renal biopsy is performed as soon as it becomes safe to undertake the procedure, and subsequent therapy is dictated by the underlying cause of the RPGN.

ANTIGLOMERULAR BASEMENT MEMBRANE DISEASE

Anti-GBM disease is characterized by circulating antibodies to the GBM and deposition of IgG (rarely IgA) along the GBM. It can occur as a renal limited disease (anti-GBM glomerulonephritis) or as a pulmonary–renal vasculitic syndrome (Goodpasture syndrome).

EPIDEMIOLOGY

Incidence of anti-GBM disease shows a bimodal distribution, with the first peak in the second or third decade, more commonly associated with pulmonary hemorrhage, and the second peak in sixth or seventh decade, more often presenting with renal-limited disease.

PATHOGENESIS

The antigen against which antibodies are directed is, the noncollagenous domain (NC1) of type IV collagen (90% α3 chain), however, the antigenic epitopes are generally cryptic and are exposed when hexameric NC1 denatures to dimers and monomers. It is presumed that environmental factors such as exposure to hydrocarbons, tobacco smoke, respiratory infections, and endogenous oxidants can expose these cryptic Goodpasture antigens. About one-third of patients with Goodpasture syndrome also have circulating myeloperoxidase (MPO) ANCAs.

CLINICAL FEATURES

The onset of renal anti-GBM disease is typically characterized by an abrupt, acute glomerulonephritis with severe oliguria or anuria. There is a high risk of progression to ESRD, if appropriate therapy is not instituted immediately. Goodpasture syndrome is characterized by life-threatening pulmonary hemorrhage concurrent with glomerulonephritis (far more common among smokers). Kidney involvement typically causes an acute nephritic syndrome with hematuria and proteinuria.

PATHOLOGY

The diagnostic laboratory findings are detection of circulating antibodies to GBM, specifically the α3-chain of type IV collagen (95%). The diagnosis may be aided by increased diffusing capacity of carbon monoxide due to alveolar hemorrhage. Renal biopsy in 97% patients of anti-GBM disease shows some degree of crescent formation, and 85% of patients have crescents in >50% of the glomeruli. These crescents are typically of uniform morphology on light microscopy. The most severely injured glomeruli have glomerular necrosis, circumferential cellular crescents, and extensive disruption of Bowman's capsule, which over time evolves into glomerular sclerosis and fibrous crescents. IF showing linear staining of the GBM for IgG (rarely IgA) is indicative of anti-GBM glomerulonephritis. EM findings usually reflect those seen on light microscopy.

MANAGEMENT

The standard treatment for anti-GBM disease is intensive plasmapheresis combined with corticosteroids and cyclophosphamide. About 40% patients progress to ESRD despite aggressive treatment. The subset of patients associated with vasculitis has a relatively better prognosis. Once remission is achieved, recurrence of the disease is rare. Similarly, recurrence of anti-GBM disease is rare postrenal transplantation, but experience suggests that patients should wait for 6 months and until serum antibodies are undetectable to undergo kidney transplantation.

MEMBRANOPROLIFERATIVE GLOMERULONEPHRITIS

The kidney responds to injurious stimuli in a limited number of histological patterns. Membranoproliferative glomerulonephritis (MPGN) is one such *pattern of injury* that is seen on light microscopy when tissue from a renal biopsy is examined. It is not a diagnosis, but merely represents a common pattern of the renal injury, in response to a variety of disease entities.

PATHOLOGY

Pathologically, it is characterized by lobular accentuation of the glomerular tuft (**Fig. 7 A**), and characteristic double contouring of the GBM (**Fig. 7 B**). This occurs because the podocytes are stimulated to produce a "neomembrane," which results in a duplication of the existing basement membrane. This double contouring is best appreciated by stains that highlight the basement membrane—the Jones methenamine silver stain and the Periodic Acid-Schiff (PAS) stain.

CLASSIFICATION

The classification of MPGN has undergone significant restructuring in the recent past, based on the increasing recognition that MPGN does not represent a disease entity *per se*, but rather just a pattern of injury.

The current classification is based on the findings on IF.

- Immunofluorescence showing Igs with or without complement deposition (immune-complex diseases):
  - Autoimmune diseases such as lupus nephritis
  - Infection-related glomerulonephritis

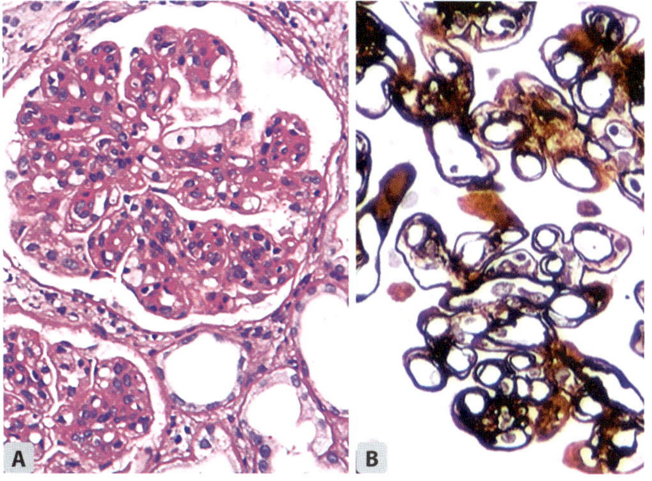

FIGURES 7 A & B: Membranoproliferative glomerulonephritis: **(A)** H&E stain; and **(B)** Silver stain.

- Immunofluorescence showing dominant complement deposition without Ig deposition:
  - Dense deposit disease (DDD)
  - C3 glomerulonephritis (C3GN)
- Immunofluorescence showing no staining for Igs or complements:
  - Chronic thrombotic microangiopathy
  - Antiphospholipid antibody syndrome
  - Nephropathy associated with hematopoietic stem cell transplantation
  - Chronic renal allograft nephropathy
  - Malignant hypertension

MANAGEMENT

The management of MPGN depends on the underlying etiology.

C3 GLOMERULOPATHIES

C3 glomerulopathies are a type of complement-mediated MPGN caused by dysregulation and persistent activation of the alternate complement pathway. There are two main entities: (1) C3GN and (2) DDD.

EPIDEMIOLOGY

Dense deposit disease affects both children and young adults. In older adults, it is associated with monoclonal gammopathy. C3GN, unlike DDD, affects older individuals.

ETIOPATHOGENESIS

Mutations in the genes encoding complement regulatory proteins or antibodies against these proteins are also seen in some patients. C3 nephritic factor that stabilizes the C3 convertase is present in circulation in the majority of patients, leading to persistent activation of the complement pathway.

CLINICAL FEATURES

- *Dense deposit disease*: Almost all patients have proteinuria with or without hematuria. Two-thirds of patients present with nephrotic range proteinuria. Acute nephritic syndrome is another common modality of presentation. Variable degrees of renal insufficiency often occur. Ocular drusen and acquired partial lipodystrophy can be seen in some patients.
- *C3 glomerulonephritis*: Clinical manifestations are less well defined. Two-thirds of the affected individuals have microscopic hematuria and hypertension, and one-third have NS.

PATHOLOGY

- *Light microscopy*: Most cases show a membranoproliferative pattern of injury (MPGN) with increase in mesangial matrix and cells, capillary wall thickening with double contouring, and endocapillary hypercellularity leading to glomerular lobulation. Endocapillary hypercellularity may affect most glomeruli as in a diffuse proliferative glomerulonephritis seen in IRGN. Crescent formation is also not uncommon.
- *Immunofluorescence*: C3 deposits along the glomerular or tubular basement membrane, and in the mesangium, at least two orders of magnitude greater than that of other immune reactants.
- *Electron microscopy*: DDD is characterized by sausage-shaped, wavy, densely osmophilic deposits within the GBM (**Fig. 8**). Such electron dense materials are absent in C3GN.

INVESTIGATIONS

Serum C3 levels are low in approximately 80% of patients with DDD and 50% of patients with C3GN. Serum C3NeF is present in the majority of patients with DDD, but is not a characteristic feature limited to DDD. Genetic study for mutations of complement-regulating factors aids in diagnosis.

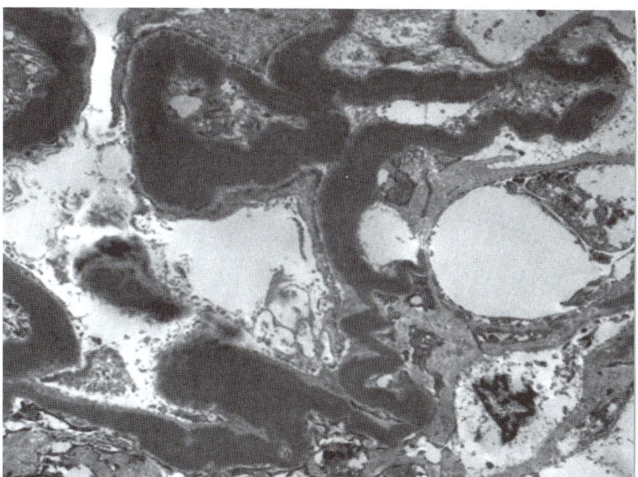

FIGURE 8: Dense deposit disease (electron microscopy).

MANAGEMENT

The treatment modalities for C3 glomerulopathies are not clearly defined as the disease entity is comparatively new and well-conducted trials are lacking. KDIGO Controversies Conference recommends that all patients should receive optimal blood pressure control medications. Those with moderate disease defined as proteinuria >500 mg/day despite supportive therapy may be given MMF or prednisolone, and those with severe disease with proteinuria >2 g/day or progressive renal failure should receive methylprednisolone pulses and other anticellular immunosuppressants. Progression to end-stage renal failure occurs in 50% of patients with either DDD or C3GN within 10 years.

ALPORT SYNDROME

Alport syndrome is an inherited disorder of defective collagen in basement membranes causing hereditary nephritis, which inevitably progresses to ESRD by the second to fourth decade of life. It is frequently associated with hearing loss and ocular abnormalities, and usually manifests in children or young adults.

ETIOPATHOGENESIS

In the mature kidney, collagen type IV is composed of heterotrimers of six possible α-chains, GBM contains collagen type IV α3α4α5. There are three genetic forms of hereditary nephritis: (1) X-linked (COL4A5), (2) autosomal (COL4A3/A4), and (3) digenic (COL4A3/A4/A5). Majority of cases are transmitted via X-linked inheritance. Mutations in COL4A5 on Xq22-24 chromosome (encoding α5-subunit) are responsible for more frequent forms of hereditary nephritis. The identified mutations include deletions, insertions, substitutions, and duplications.

CLINICAL FEATURES

Males are predominantly affected and can present with persistent microscopic hematuria, episodic gross hematuria, and flank pain. Nephrotic-range proteinuria, hypertension, and slow progression to ESRD are the natural course of the disease. Females are usually carriers and may have only microscopic hematuria, but up to 20% have been reported with progression to renal failure. Sensorineural deafness is seen in 30–50% of patients and is almost always associated with renal failure. Anterior lenticonus is virtually pathognomonic of Alport and other ocular abnormalities including keratoconus, spherophakia, cataracts, and retinitis pigmentosa also have been documented.

PATHOLOGY

Light microscopy and IF on renal biopsy are nonspecific, with segmental to diffuse mesangial proliferation and matrix expansion and interstitial foam cells. The cardinal electron microscopic abnormality is variable thinning, thickening, basket-weaving, and lamellation of the GBM giving it a characteristic "split and splintered" appearance.

MANAGEMENT

There is no proven therapy for Alport syndrome. Protein reduction strategies and control of hypertension might slow the progression of the disease and renal replacement therapy may be necessary in patients with hereditary nephritis. Patients who receive renal allografts usually develop anti-GBM antibodies toward collagen epitopes absent in their native kidney, however, overt Goodpasture syndrome is rare and graft survival is better.

RECOMMENDED READINGS

1. Kidney International Supplements. (2012). KDIGO Clinical practice guideline for glomerulonephritis. [online] Available from https://kdigo.org/wp-content/uploads/2017/02/KDIGO-2012-GN-Guideline-English.pdf
2. Rosenberg AZ, Kopp JB. Focal segmental glomerulosclerosis. Clin J Am Soc Nephrol. 2017;12: 502-17.
3. Indian Society of Pediatric Nephrology, Gulati A, Bagga A, Gulati S, Mehta KP, Vijayakumar M. Management of steroid resistant nephrotic syndrome. Indian Pediatr. 2009;46(1):35-47.
4. Bagga A. Revised guidelines for management of steroid-sensitive nephrotic syndrome. Indian J Nephrol. 2008;18(1):31-9.
5. Rodrigues JC, Haas M, Reich HN. IgA Nephropathy. Clin J Am Soc Nephrol. 2017;12(4):677-86.
6. Nasr SH, Radhakrishnan J, D'Agati VD. Bacterial infection-related glomerulonephritis in adults. Kidney Int. 2013;83(5):792-803.

CHAPTER
167

Chronic Tubulointerstitial Disorders and Obstructive Nephropathy

Suceena Alexander, Santosh Varughese

ABSTRACT

Chronic tubulointerstitial disorders of the kidney are caused by immune- or non-immune mediated damage of the tubulointerstitial compartment persisting beyond 3 months. These typically cause a slowly progressive disease with low-grade proteinuria with little or no elevation of the blood pressure, no decrease in urine output or edema. Some common causes are drugs, infections, and genetic and in many cases, the etiology is unknown. Management depends on early diagnosis and focusses on slowing the progression of disease.

Both congenital and acquired causes may lead to obstruction to flow of urine in the kidney and urinary tract causing obstructive nephropathy. The causes may be structural or functional, intrinsic or extrinsic, and lead to acute or chronic obstructive nephropathy. The treatment depends on etiology and chronicity and in general focuses on relieving the obstruction, slowing progression of disease, and on alleviation of lower urinary tract symptoms, if present.

"Research is creating new knowledge"

—Neil Armstrong

CHRONIC TUBULOINTERSTITIAL DISORDERS

Chronic tubulointerstitial disorders are caused by known or unknown entities that cause either immune-mediated or nonimmune-mediated damage of the tubulointerstitial compartment of the kidney and are persistent beyond 3 months duration. Immune-mediated disorders are otherwise called as "chronic interstitial nephritis".

PREVALENCE AND PRESENTATION

It can account up to 30% of chronic kidney disease (CKD) in adults and up to 10% in children. Any age group may be affected and depends on many factors such as specific etiology, geographic region, demographic characteristics, occupational hazards, environmental exposures etc. Since, most people are asymptomatic or have nonspecific symptoms, delay in diagnosis is common. Usual presentation is a slowly progressive disease with low-grade proteinuria and normotension or mild-to-moderate hypertension depending on the stage of CKD. Most people are nonoliguric, do not have edema or volume overload, and may present with salt losing nephropathies. Tubular dysfunction may manifest as Fanconi syndrome.

ETIOLOGY

The etiology is varied but the most common is caused by medication or drug exposure. The various causes are listed in **Table 1**.

Drug or medication induced: Most common medications are beta-lactam antibiotics and nonsteroidal anti-inflammatory drugs (NSAIDs). Rifampicin can cause sudden onset symptoms and severe interstitial nephritis. This is characterized by chronic interstitial nephritis and papillary necrosis due to chronic ingestion of NSAIDs. Phenacetin was particularly associated with this disorder and its withdrawal in the 1990s led to a marked decrease in the incidence of analgesic nephropathy.

Infection related: The various causes are listed in **Table 1**. In renal transplant recipients, interstitial nephritis can be caused by polyomavirus or cytomegalovirus and increases the risk of graft rejection. Bone marrow transplant recipients can have a necrotizing form of interstitial nephritis caused by adenovirus. Epstein–Barr virus infections are associated with tubulointerstitial nephritis and uveitis (TINU) syndrome in children and adults.

Systemic inflammatory disorders: Interstitial nephritis is also associated with inflammatory bowel disease, systemic lupus erythematosus, sarcoidosis, Sjögren's disease, TINU syndrome etc. Immunoglobulin G4 (IgG4)-associated multiorgan autoimmune disease can also cause interstitial nephritis characterized by infiltration of IgG4-positive plasma cells and C3 deposition.

Genetic: Some patients with tubulointerstitial nephritis can have antitubular basement membrane antibodies against tubulointerstitial nephritis antigen (TIN-ag) which is an extracellular matrix basement membrane protein. Deletion of the *TIN-ag* gene *hTIN-ag* localized

TABLE 1	Etiology of tubulointerstitial nephritis.
Drug related	Antimicrobials
	NSAIDs
	Others
Infections	
Viral	Cytomegalovirus, hepatitis, HIV, Epstein–Barr virus, hantavirus, and polyomavirus
Bacterial	*Salmonella, Streptococcus, Yersinia, Brucella,* and leptospirosis
Fungal	Histoplasmosis
Parasitic	Leishmania and toxoplasma
Immune-mediated	Sarcoidosis
	Systemic lupus erythematosus
	Sjögren's disease
	Inflammatory bowel disease
Idiopathic	
TINU	
Granulomatous tubulo-interstitial nephritis	Medications
	Sarcoidosis
	Tuberculosis
	Bacterial/Fungal infections
	TINU
	Granulomatosis with polyangiitis

(TINU: tubulointerstitial nephritis and uveitis)

on chromosome 6 can lead to the disease manifestation. Autosomal dominant tubulointerstitial kidney disease has recently been described and disorders in four genes have been identified till date—*Uromodulin, Renin, Hepatocyte nuclear factor-1B,* and *Mucin-1.*

PATHOPHYSIOLOGY

In acute interstitial nephritis, the interstitial edema, infiltration with lymphocytes and plasma cells, and tubular dysfunction leads to an acute fall in estimated glomerular filtration rate (eGFR). If this damage persists, it can lead to accumulation of extracellular matrix leading to interstitial fibrosis and tubular atrophy leading to irreversible renal function impairment as seen in chronic interstitial nephritis. Nephron loss leads to compensatory hyperfiltration in the remaining nephrons and eventual progressive CKD.

The patho-mechanism in drug-induced interstitial nephritis is immune-mediated and similar to an allergic reaction. This is substantiated by the following observations:

- It is not dose dependent
- It can recure after rechallenging of the drug
- The presence of eosinophils in the interstitium
- There can be systemic manifestations
- It occurs only in a minority of patients exposed to the drug.

In granulomatous tubulointerstitial nephritis, the infiltrating cells form granulomas that are usually non-necrotic and consist of multinucleated giant cells. Tuberculosis can cause caseating granulomas in the interstitium. Over time the granulomas are replaced by fibrotic tissue and their presence does not correlate with poor prognosis compared to nongranulomatous interstitial nephritis.

LABORATORY MANIFESTATIONS

The serum creatinine may be increased and the urine analysis may show hematuria and sterile pyuria. There will be no dysmorphic red blood cells (RBCs) or cellular casts. The proteinuria is tubular in nature and usually <1.5 g/day. Anemia is seen in moderate-to-severe renal dysfunction and is generally disproportionate to the degree of renal impairment. Fanconi syndrome can have electrolyte abnormalities, metabolic acidosis, aminoaciduria, glycosuria, and elevated fractional excretion of sodium along with mild proteinuria.

RADIOGRAPHIC MANIFESTATIONS

The ultrasound of kidney may show the following features in advanced stages depending on the etiology:

- Small echogenic kidneys
- Calcifications in the renal papillae
- Irregular contour of the kidneys, especially in analgesic nephropathy
- Tuberculosis may affect unilateral kidney and may have extrarenal manifestations such as contracted bladder and calcifications of the vas deferens, seminal vesicles, or prostate.
- Medullary sponge kidneys have calcifications restricted to the medulla.

Computed tomography (CT) is more sensitive, but usually not required for diagnosis or management.

HISTOPATHOLOGY

- *Light microscopy*: Lymphoplasmacytic infiltration is predominantly seen in the tubulointerstitial space and is out of proportion to the interstitial fibrosis and tubular atrophy. The infiltrate contains CD4/CD8 T cells, B cells, and plasma cells. The glomerular compartment may show evidence of secondary damage such as periglomerular fibrosis, ischemic wrinkling of glomerular basement membrane, or secondary sclerosis. Vessels can have sclerosis or hyalinosis (**Fig. 1**).
- *Immunofluorescence*: No specific pathology.
- *Electron microscopy*: No specific pathology.

TREATMENT

- *Non-pharmacological interventions*:
  - *Diet*: Restrict salt to 4 g/day if there is hypertension, increase salt if there is salt wasting with normo- or hypotension. Restrict potassium if there is hyperkalemia or in advanced stages of renal impairment.

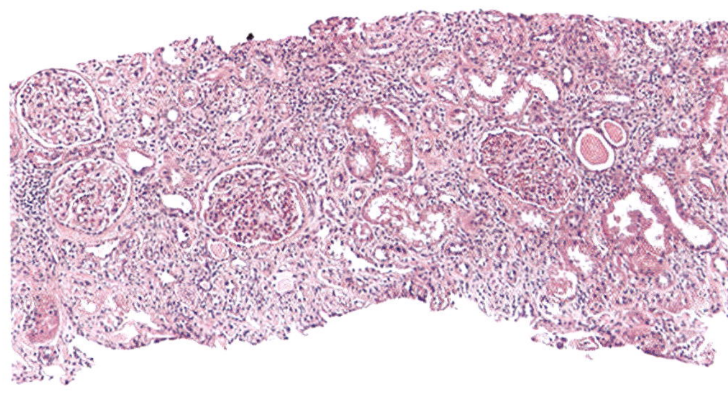

FIGURE 1: Light microscopy—hematoxylin and eosin stain.

Source: Fogo AB, Lusco MA, Najafian B, Alpers CE. AJKD Atlas of Renal Pathology: Chronic Interstitial Nephritis. Am J Kidney Dis. 2017;70:e1-e2.

Restrict fluids if there is edema in advanced stages. Restrict protein intake to 0.8–1 g/kg/day.

- Exercise and maintain body mass index (BMI) within limits.

- Supplementation of potassium/magnesium/phosphorous/citrate if there is accompanying renal losses.
- Avoidance of the agents causally linked to the kidney disease, e.g., analgesic intake, heavy metals, and herbal medications.
- Treatment of the underlying etiology with specific medications, e.g., steroids in sarcoidosis and antituberculous therapy.
- Optimal control of hypertension and proteinuria with maximally tolerated dose of renin–angiotensin system blockers.

PROGNOSIS

The general course of the disease depends on the stage of CKD at presentation and the underlying etiologies. It is generally a chronic and slowly progressive disease. Early identification can improve outcomes. Prolonged low molecular weight proteinuria is associated with poor long-term prognosis.

CHRONIC KIDNEY DISEASE OF UNCERTAIN ETIOLOGY (CKDu)

This entity describes CKD in endemic hot spots worldwide and was first described in South America as "Mesoamerican nephropathy". Other related terms are chronic kidney disease of unknown/uncertain etiology (CKDu) or chronic kidney disease of nontraditional cause (CKDnT). It is seen in young agricultural workers and is thought to be related to poor living conditions, occupational exposure to heat stress, recurrent hypovolemia, and loss of minerals. Initially described in El Salvador and Nicaragua, CKDu hot spots have been reported from Sri Lanka, Tunisia, and India (in the states of Goa, Odisha, and Andhra Pradesh). It is unclear whether the pathogenesis in the different regions is the same as interstitial inflammation and vascular changes are much more severe in CKDu outside the Mesoamerica. Some of the risk factors postulated for CKDu are enlisted below:

- Agriculture or manual labor in hot and humid climate
- Exposure to agrochemicals and pesticides
- Male gender
- Low socioeconomic class
- Use of rehydrating drinks containing sugar
- Family history of CKD
- Exposure to silica
- Rampant use of NSAIDs
- Infections with unknown viruses
- Genetic factors

The pathogenesis is not known with certainty. Repeated episodes of acute kidney injury (AKI) secondary to dehydration or chronic tubulointerstitial nephritis due to infectious or toxic exposures are postulated. Many other contributing factors such as inorganic arsenic, cadmium, hard water, pesticides, and mycotoxins have been suggested. On laboratory analysis, most common abnormalities are elevated serum creatinine and leukocyturia. There is absence of proteinuria and hematuria. Kidney biopsy shows extensive tubular atrophy and fibrosis with extensive chronic glomerular changes such as glomerulosclerosis and glomerular tuft hypertrophy. There is no specific treatment and is directed towards preventing the progression of CKD.

OBSTRUCTIVE NEPHROPATHY

When the flow of urine in the kidney and urinary tract is impeded due to structural or functional changes of the urinary tract, the resultant kidney disease is called *obstructive nephropathy*. The obstruction may be acute or chronic or intrinsic or extrinsic. The etiology varies with age and gender. Fetal urinary tract obstruction usually gets picked up on routine antenatal ultrasonography. Congenital abnormalities of kidney and urinary tract (CAKUT) are more common in boys under 10 years of age and are associated with progressive CKD. Between 10 and 20 years, the incidence in both sexes is similar and above 20 years of age, there is a female preponderance contributed by obstruction from gynecological neoplasms and pregnancy. Calculi occur more commonly in men between 10 and 30 years of age. In men older than 60 years, prostatic hypertrophy and carcinoma cause obstruction. It is estimated that nearly a third of men over the age of 50 years have obstructive symptoms.

ETIOLOGY

It is useful clinically to classify the causes of urinary tract obstruction as being either congenital or acquired. *The congenital causes* are of importance in adults as they may cause CKD and end-stage kidney disease (ESKD). Of these, posterior urethral valves, neurogenic bladder and pelviureteric junction (PUJ) obstruction (especially when bilateral) have consequences that last throughout the child's adult life. In addition, the kidneys may be dysplastic leading to reduction in renal function

Acquired causes of obstructive nephropathy may be intraluminal, intramural, or extrinsic. Among the intraluminal causes, crystals (from drugs such as indinavir, acyclovir, or uric acid after chemotherapy in hematological malignancies) or casts (e.g., light-chain protein casts in patients with myeloma) are the most important ones. Intramural causes of obstruction may be either functional (e.g., vesicoureteric or PUJ obstruction and bladder dysfunction due to neurogenic bladder) or anatomic (e.g., urethral strictures, malignant and benign bladder masses, and transitional cell carcinoma of ureters). A more comprehensive list of causes is given in **Table 2**.

PATHOGENESIS AND PATHOLOGY

The knowledge of the pathogenesis of obstructive nephropathy is derived from mouse models of ureteral obstruction. Chronic obstruction has deleterious effects on both glomerular and tubular function. Obstruction results in increased proximal tubular pressure. This is soon followed by production of vasodilatory prostaglandins that causes afferent arteriolar dilatation. The resultant increase in glomerular capillary pressure is insufficient to overcome the raised tubular pressure, and the lowered pressure gradient in the glomeruli causes the glomerular filtration rate (GFR) to decrease. When the obstruction is chronic, the renal blood flow falls as a result of elevated levels of angiotensin II and thromboxane A2. These have effects on tubular function as do the reduced nitric oxide (NO) and elevated antidiuretic hormone (ADH). This results in reduced aquaporin expression, decreased number of tubular sodium transporters, and medullary concentration gradient is lost. The kidney's handling of fluids and electrolytes is hampered with inability to concentrate urine, impaired distal acid secretion leads to hyperchloremic acidosis and hyporeninemic hypoaldosteronism.

Structural changes accompanying obstruction are tubular dilation that preferentially affects the distal nephron, tubulointerstitial fibrosis, and atrophy with loss of nephron number. Ultrastructurally, there is apoptosis and increase in myofibroblasts in the interstitium and extracellular matrix. These are mediated by angiotensin II, transforming growth factor-β, and galectin-3, the latter two being released from macrophages (**Flowchart 1**).

CLINICAL FEATURES

In untreated disease or if there is delay in treatment, progressive CKD and ESKD is inevitable, especially in patients with bilateral obstruction a single kidney or if obstruction is bilateral. It is estimated that obstruction of less than a fortnight of obstruction is potentially reversible while >12 weeks results in irreversible structural damage and decreased residual GFR despite relief of obstruction. This makes early recognition of disease, prompt diagnosis, and initiation of treatment essential.

It is important to bear in mind that slowly progressive obstruction may occur without any symptoms. A variety of symptoms are possible depending on site of obstruction—upper versus lower urinary tract, degree of obstruction, and its duration. Complete obstruction to the flow of urine causes oliguria and AKI whereas resistance to ADH in partial obstruction may present either with polyuria and polydipsia or the urine output may vary greatly.

TABLE 2 Causes of urinary tract obstruction.

Level of obstruction	Obstruction within the lumen	Obstruction within the wall	Extrinsic compression
Kidney	• Stones • Sloughed papillae	• Cysts • Tumors • Anatomical abnormalities (e.g., PUJ obstruction)	Lower pole renal vessels crossing at PUJ
Ureter	Stones	• Tumors • Stricture (malignant, postsurgery or postradiotherapy) • Tuberculous, and schistosomiasis • Anatomical abnormalities, e.g., vesicoureteric junction obstruction	• Tumors • Retroperitoneal fibrosis • Retrocaval right ureter (congenital) • Pancreatitis and inflammatory bowel disease (rare)
Bladder/bladder neck	• Stones • Clot retention	• Tumors • Functional obstruction (diabetes, neurological damage to bladder, and drugs)	Pelvic tumors
Urethra	• Stones • Blood clots (after catheterization or surgery)	• Stricture (postinfective or postsurgical) • Congenital urethral valves • Tumors	Prostate enlargement

(PUJ: pelviureteric junction)

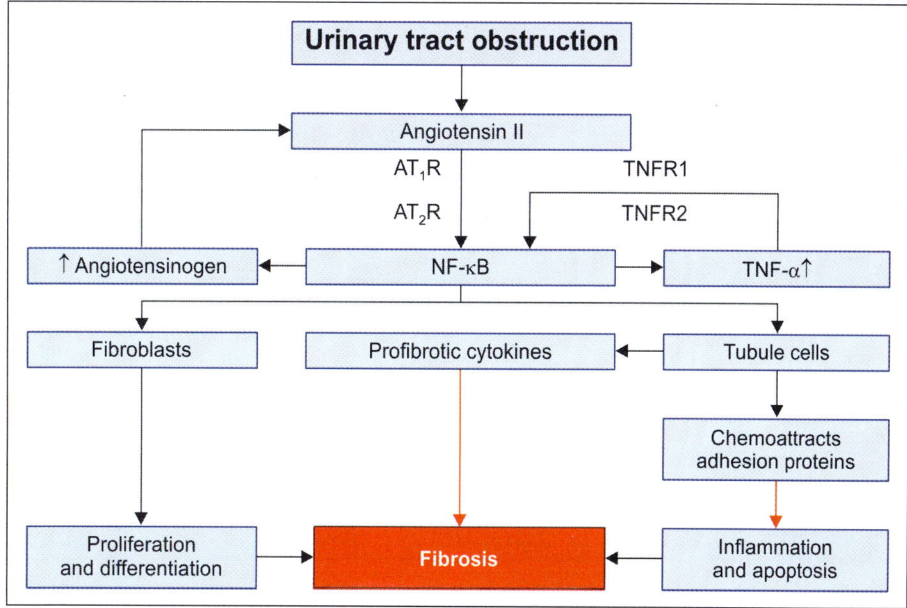

(NF-κB: nuclear factor kappa B; TNF-α: tumor necrosis factor-α)

FLOWCHART 1: Urinary tract obstruction leads to irreversible renal damage.

Obstruction due to ureteric calculi causes pain that results from stretch to the lumen of the collecting system. The site of obstruction determines the site of radiation of pain, i.e., obstruction in the upper ureter or renal pelvis, there may be pain and tenderness in the ipsilateral flank and obstruction in the lower ureter, pain radiates to groin. Classic renal colic is a severe crescendo flank pain of variable duration. The resultant trauma to the mucosa may cause hematuria. Hematuria may also indicate bleeding from an obstructive malignancy and the resultant clot may obstruction and/or colicky abdominal pain.

Although a distended bladder or enlarged, palpable, and hydronephrotic kidneys may be palpable, routine examination is largely noncontributory. Per rectal or per vaginal examinations may reveal pelvic pathology causing lower urinary tract obstruction.

EVALUATION AND DIAGNOSIS

Clinically, obstructive nephropathy needs to be considered as a possible differential diagnosis and to be excluded in all cases of unexplained renal function impairment, while symptoms and signs may occasionally suggest a diagnosis based on carefully taken history and clinical examination. Crystals on urine microscopy may indicate the type of stone causing obstruction. Bacteriuria is invariable in obstruction. Hematuria occurs in obstruction due to calculi, neoplasms, and with mucosal sloughing. Renal function evaluation and abnormalities in electrolyte and acid-base status must also be looked for.

Imaging is the cornerstone for evaluation of obstructive nephropathy. The simplest and commonly available bedside tool of *ultrasonography* may be sufficient in many instances. Its common uses are in measurement of kidney sizes, detection of altered echogenicity (with respect to the liver and spleen on the right and left sides, respectively), and pelvicalyceal system (PCS) dilatation. Antenatal ultrasonography detects neonatal hydronephrosis. Ultrasonography alone is sufficient for neonates with milder degrees of hydronephrosis without calyceal dilatation (grade 1 and 2) whereas grade 3 and 4 (with moderate and severe PCS dilatation, respectively) are evaluated with voiding cystourethrography as well to help in distinguishing between vesicoureteric reflux and obstruction from posterior urethral valve etc.

Ultrasonography alone is often insufficient to pick up the etiology of obstruction and combination with other imaging modalities is often necessary. Of note, small calculi within the kidney and ureteric calculi are picked up better by *plain abdominal radiography (X-ray)* since about 90% of calculi are radio-opaque with uric acid and xanthine calculi being the exception. The clinician must remember certain important clinical situations where the ultrasonography may not be sensitive in diagnosing obstruction. These are: Early and slowly progressive obstruction caused by encasement of ureters by tumor or retroperitoneal fibrosis; acute obstruction (i.e., <24 h) before dilatation sets in; and with severely reduced urine output (accompanying very low GFR and in severe intravascular volume depletion). Staghorn calculus may cause the obstruction to be missed on ultrasonography by its acoustic shadow masking PCS dilatation.

In renal allograft recipients, sometimes the dense fibrotic tissue may prevent ureters from dilating appreciably and obstruction may be missed. When obstruction is suspected, it is advisable ultrasonography after 24 or 48 hours for confirmation. Using *color Doppler to measure resistive index (RI)* may be helpful in evaluation of obstructive nephropathy, though RI may be altered in several other conditions as well.

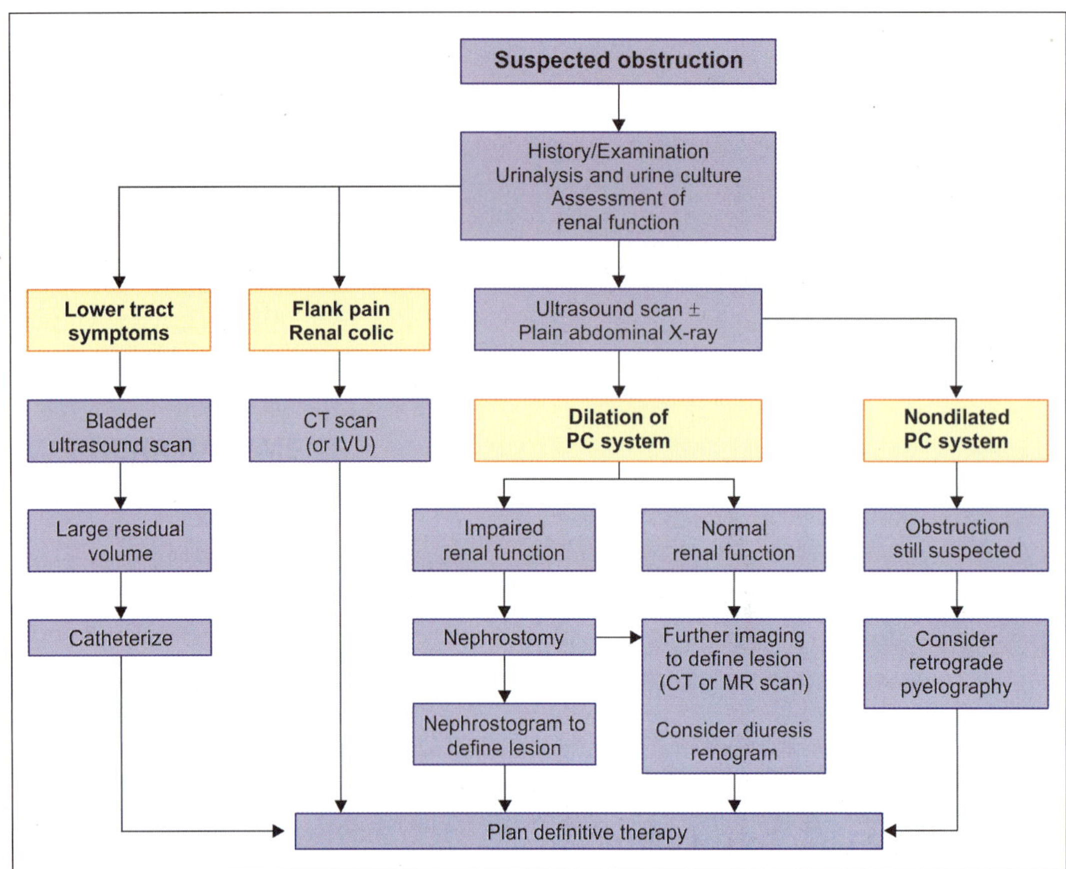

(CT: computed tomography; IVU: intravenous urography; MR: magnetic resonance; PC: pelvicalyceal)

FLOWCHART 2: Investigation and management of suspected urinary tract obstruction.

RI is calculated as the ratio of the difference between the peak systolic velocity and end-diastolic velocity to the peak systolic velocity. RI > 0.7 is seen in obstructive nephropathy due to increased vascular resistance present. The other utility of ultrasonography is in evaluation of bladder emptying in patients with lower urinary tract symptoms. Bladder outflow obstruction is suspected if the postvoid residual volume in the bladder is >50 mL (>100 mL if older than 65 years) and further evaluation by urodynamics is warranted.

Both contrast-enhanced and unenhanced CT and magnetic resonance imaging (MRI) are other imaging tools used for diagnostic evaluation. Intravenous urography (IVU) is less commonly used as the radiation exposure is high and administration of intravenous nephrotoxic contrast agents is required. CT scans are very useful in detection of ureteric calculi, obstructing lesions, and for contributory retroperitoneal or pelvic conditions. MRI improves upon the accuracy provided by the CT. MRI with urography (MRU) provides information on the anatomy and function of the kidneys and if there is hyperfiltration to compensate for the obstruction.

Technetium-99m mercaptoacetyltriglycine (^{99m}Tc-MAG3) with furosemide showing hold-up of isotope is sometimes used in diagnosis and follow-up. Cystoscopy and retrograde pyelography, the latter done under general anesthesia are useful procedures for definitive histopathological diagnosis (from biopsy of the lesion) and for interventions such as dilatation and stent placement.

TREATMENT

In general, rapid relief of obstruction is the objective of therapy (**Flowchart 2**). Close collaboration is needed between nephrologists and urologists in management of these patients. In addition to relief of obstruction, associated renal dysfunction and acid-base and electrolyte abnormalities need to be addressed. Postobstructive diuresis is another important consideration. Dialysis may be required at least temporarily in patients with hyperkalemia or rarely with fluid overload.

Prior to definite surgical treatment, immediate relief of obstruction frequently requires bladder catheterization or rarely suprapubic cystostomy when obstruction occurs distal to bladder, cystoscopy and ureteral stent placement or more commonly percutaneous nephrostomy is done to relieve upper urinary tract obstruction. Definitive treatment including treatment of underlying condition may require a multidisciplinary approach.

RECOMMENDED READINGS

1. Joyce E, Glasner P, Ranganathan S, Swiatecka-Urban A. Tubulointerstitial nephritis: diagnosis, treatment, and monitoring. Pediatr Nephrol. 2017;32(4):577-87.
2. Obrador GT, Levin A. CKD Hotspots: Challenges and Areas of Opportunity. Semin Nephrol. 2019;39(3):308-14.
3. Almaguer M, Herrera R, Orantes CM. Chronic kidney disease of unknown etiology in agricultural communities. MEDICC Rev. 2014;16(2):9-15.
4. Lissauer D, Morris RK, Kilby MD. Fetal lower urinary tract obstruction. Semin Fetal Neonatal Med. 2007;12(6):464-70.
5. Chevalier RL, Forbes MS, Thornhill BA. Ureteral obstruction as a model of renal interstitial fibrosis and obstructive nephropathy. Kidney Int. 2009;75(11):1145-52.
6. Wang G, Li C, Kim SW, Ring T, Wen J, Djurhuus JC, et al. Ureter obstruction alters expression of renal acid-base transport proteins in rat kidney. Am J Physiol-Ren Physiol. 2008;295(2):F497-506.
7. Henderson NC, Mackinnon AC, Farnworth SL, Kipari T, Haslett C, Iredale JP, et al. Galectin-3 Expression and Secretion Links Macrophages to the Promotion of Renal Fibrosis. Am J Pathol. 2008;172(2):288-98.
8. Ricardo SD, Diamond JR. The role of macrophages and reactive oxygen species in experimental hydronephrosis. Semin Nephrol. 1998;18(6):612-21.
9. Ravanan R, Tomson CR. Natural History of Postobstructive Nephropathy: A Single-Center Retrospective Study. Nephron Clin Pract. 2007;105(4):c165-70.
10. Belarmino JM, Kogan BA. Management of neonatal hydronephrosis. Early Hum Dev. 2006;82(1):9-14.
11. Mostbeck GH, Zontsich T, Turetschek K. Ultrasound of the kidney: obstruction and medical diseases. Eur Radiol. 2001;11(10):1878-89.
12. Granata A, Zanoli L, Clementi S, Fatuzzo P, Di Nicolò P, Fiorini F. Resistive intrarenal index: myth or reality? Br J Radiol. 2014;87(1038):20140004.
13. Grattan-Smith JD, Little SB, Jones RA. MR urography evaluation of obstructive uropathy. Pediatr Radiol. 2008;38(S1):S49-69.
14. Gallagher KM, Hughes J. Urinary tract obstruction. In: Johnson RJ, Feehally J, Floege J (Eds). Comprehensive Clinical Nephrology, 6th edition. Edinburgh: Elsevier; 2019. p. 708.
15. Yaqoob MM, Bennett-Richards K, Junaid I. The patient with urinary tract obstruction. In: Turner NN, Lameire N, Goldsmith DJ, Winearls CG, Himmelfarb J, Remuzzi G (Eds). Oxford Textbook of Clinical Nephrology, 4th edition. Oxford, United Kingdom: Oxford University Press; 2016. pp. 2854-70.

CHAPTER 168 Hypertension, Diabetes, and Kidney Disease

Anantharam Jairam, Vijoy Kumar Jha

ABSTRACT

Diabetes, hypertension (HTN), and kidney diseases are closely interlinked diseases. HTN may be due to multiple factors in the setting of renal dysfunction like sodium retention and fluid overload, increased sympathetic nervous system activity, activation of the renin–angiotensin–aldosterone system (RAAS), and other complications of chronic kidney disease (CKD). The main strategies in the management of HTN in kidney diseases include dietary salt restriction, diuretic therapy, and initiation of RAAS blockers. Poorly controlled HTN will lead to significant cardiovascular (CV) morbidity and mortality. It also accelerates the worsening of renal dysfunction leading to end-stage kidney disease (ESKD). However, no clinical trials have shown that adequately controlled blood pressure (BP) will slow the progression of CKD.

Diabetic nephropathy (DN) is the most common cause of ESKD worldwide. The standard management of patients with DN includes CV risk reduction with lifestyle modification, statins and antiplatelet drug, adequate blood sugar and BP control, and RAAS inhibitors. RAAS inhibitors are considered the single best drug in preventing and slowing the progression of DN. In recently published CV outcome trials, new drugs like sodium-glucose cotransporter-2 (SGLT-2) inhibitors have been found to have reduction in albuminuria and reduction in the occurrence of a composite renal outcome.

"Everything is interlinked"

—H Zendage

INTRODUCTION

Diabetes mellitus (DM) and HTN are the most common causes of ESKD.

Hypertension increases the risk for kidney disease onset and its progression, CV morbidity, and mortality. In this chapter, we will discuss briefly the kidney diseases related to HTN, DM, and their relationship with each other.

HYPERTENSION AND KIDNEY DISEASE

The relationship between HTN and kidney disease particularly, CKD is cyclic.

Uncontrolled HTN is a risk factor for developing CKD, rapid progression of CKD, and is the second leading cause of ESKD after DN.

Progressive renal disease exacerbates poorly controlled HTN due to volume overload and increased peripheral vascular resistance.

HYPERTENSION AS A RISK FACTOR FOR KIDNEY DISEASE

Chronic hypertension leading to chronic kidney disease: Nephrosclerosis seen with normal aging is exacerbated with chronic HTN. Hypertensive nephrosclerosis is a kidney disease associated with long-standing HTN.

Risk factors: Black race, poorly controlled HTN, and underlying renal dysfunction or CKD.

Presentation of hypertensive nephrosclerosis is usually with long history of HTN, slowly progressive elevations in the blood urea nitrogen (BUN) and plasma creatinine concentration and mild proteinuria. Proteinuria or renal dysfunction is preceded by long history of HTN.

Diagnosis of benign hypertensive nephrosclerosis: Characteristic clinical features, evidence of target organ damage by HTN in the form of hypertensive retinopathy, left ventricular hypertrophy, and the exclusion of other renal diseases, are the mainstay of diagnosis.

A kidney biopsy is not performed routinely.

Characteristic histological features in kidney biopsy are intimal thickening and luminal narrowing of the large and small renal arteries and the arterioles in the glomeruli. Presence of both focal global and focal segmental glomerulosclerosis is seen.

Effective treatment of the HTN usually slows renal injury progression. The role of angiotensin-converting enzyme (ACE) inhibitors and angiotensin receptor blockers (ARBs) in patients with benign nephrosclerosis without proteinuria is not clear.

Severe hypertension causing acute kidney injury: Severe HTN may occasionally cause acute kidney injury (AKI) (acute hypertensive nephrosclerosis and malignant nephrosclerosis).

Characterized by a recent history of HTN and elevated serum creatinine. Characteristic histological findings are fibrinoid necrosis of small arterioles and "onion skinning" of small renal arteries.

The glomerular ischemia due to renal vascular disease activates renin-angiotensin system (RAS) exacerbating HTN.

Acute kidney injury may sometimes require dialysis. The improvement in renal function may be seen with long-term BP control.

Acute hypertensive nephrosclerosis has become uncommon with the availability of effective antihypertensives.

Hypertension accelerating progressive renal damage in chronic kidney disease: Patients with CKD, both diabetic and nondiabetic, are more susceptible to BP elevations due to impairment of the renal autoregulatory mechanisms. Vascular pathology often is not prominent in the setting of CKD. Histologically, there is an accelerated segmental or global glomerulosclerosis on the background of underlying renal disease.

The mechanisms by which glomerular HTN and hypertrophy accelerate glomerular injury may be direct endothelial cell damage, detachment of the glomerular epithelial cells from the glomerular capillary wall, and increased strain on the mesangial cells stimulating to produce cytokines and more extracellular matrix.

Aldosterone, whether of local or systemic origin, as a result of excess mineralocorticoid receptor stimulation and nonhemodynamic effects of angiotensin II, may also contribute to progressive renal injury.

HYPERTENSION IN KIDNEY DISEASE

The pathogenesis of HTN varies with the different etiologies of renal dysfunction (e.g., glomerular versus vascular) and with the disease duration (acute vs. chronic).

Hypertension in acute glomerular disease: Patients with acute glomerulonephritis (GN) are found to be edematous due to increased sodium retention and increased sodium reabsorption in the collecting tubules. BP elevation is primarily due to fluid retention. There is a RAAS inhibition and atrial natriuretic peptide (ANP) release in acute GN. Diuretic (particularly loop diuretics) is preferred as initial therapy in patients with reduced glomerular filtration rate (GFR). In case of persistent high BP, ACE inhibitors may be effective, though this is low-renin HTN.

Hypertension in acute vascular disease: In acute vascular diseases, such as vasculitis or scleroderma renal crisis, HTN is very common. The elevation in BP results from ischemia-induced activation of RAS rather than volume expansion. ACE inhibitors are preferred as initial antihypertensive therapy.

Hypertension in chronic kidney disease: The prevalence of HTN in CKD ranges from 60 to 90% depending on the CKD stage and its cause. Uncontrolled HTN is associated with a higher risk for CV morbidity and mortality.

Pathophysiology of hypertension in CKD: Several factors including neural and hormonal changes contribute to elevated BP in patients with CKD (**Flowchart 1**)

*Normal and abnormal BP in CKD (**Table 1**)*:

- An office BP < 120/80 mm Hg is considered to be normal as per the recent American Heart Association/American College of Cardiology (AHA/ACC) guidelines.
- Definitions of normal and abnormal BP based on the 2017 AHA/ACC guideline in patients with CKD are as given in **Table 1**. The apparatus used for BP measurement in some clinical trials and the various methods of BP measurement are summarized in **Table 2**.
- Resistant and refractory HTN in CKD stages 4 to 5 are common, for which multiple classes of antihypertensive agents are frequently needed. Most guidelines [including Kidney Disease: Improving Global Outcomes (KDIGO)] continue to recommend treatment of HTN based on office measured BPs in adults with CKD.

Hypertension workup in CKD:

- Additional workup for other causes of HTN is warranted, if there are reasons to suspect a secondary cause of HTN, if the onset of elevated BPs occurred before the onset of renal dysfunction or CKD, uncontrolled malignant HTN that is out of proportion to the CKD stages, a person with

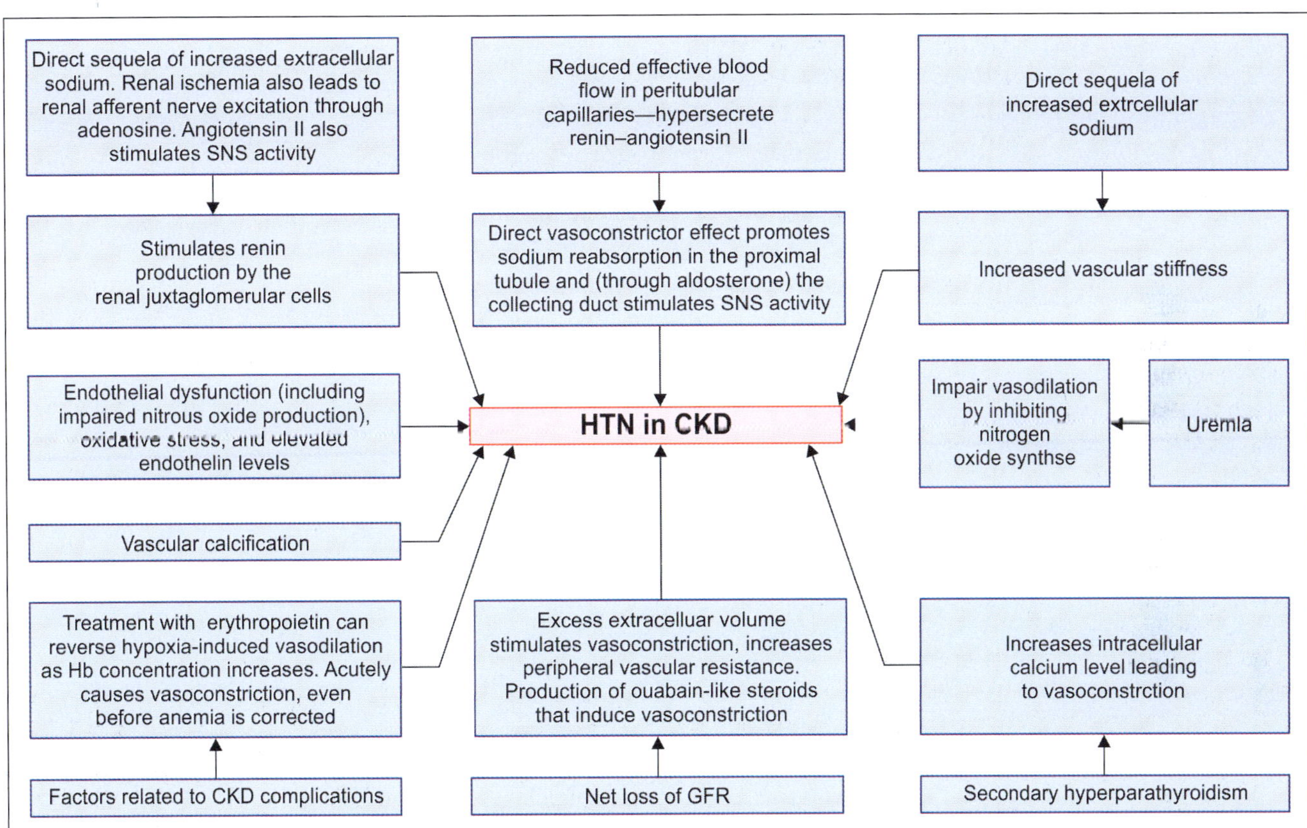

(CKD: chronic kidney disease; GFR: glomerular filtration rate; Hb: hemoglobin; SNS: sympathetic nervous system)

FLOWCHART 1: Pathophysiology of hypertension (HTN) in CKD.

TABLE 1 Definitions of normal and abnormal BP based on the 2017 AHA/ACC guideline in patients with CKD.

BP classification	Office BP	Daytime ABPM or Home BP
Normal or elevated BP	120 to <130/80 mm Hg	120 to <130/80 mm Hg
Sustained hypertension	≥130/80 mm Hg	≥130/80 mm Hg
White coat hypertension	≥130/80 mm Hg	<130/80 mm Hg
Masked hypertension	<130/80 mm Hg	≥130/80 mm Hg
Difficult to control BP	**Definition**	
Resistant hypertension	Receiving >3 antihypertensive agents, one of which is a diuretic, without adequate BP control	
Refractory hypertension	Receiving ≥3 antihypertensive agents, one of which is a thiazide-type diuretic and another of which is spironolactone, without adequate BP control	

(ABPM: ambulatory blood pressure monitoring; ACC: American College of Cardiology; AHA: American Heart Association)

TABLE 2 The apparatus used for BP measurement in some clinical trials and the various methods of BP measurement.

Study	Observer	Device description	Measurements	Time interval between measurements	Resting position	Position	Arm	Cuff
ACCORD (2007, 2010)		Automated blood pressure monitor (Omron 907)	Average of three readings			Seated		
SPRINT (2017)	Unattended	Automated manometer (Omron 907)	Average of three readings	1 minute	After 5 minutes of rest	Seated		Proper cuff size
HOPE-3 (2016)		Automatic blood pressure monitor (Omron HEM-711DLXCAN) or mercury sphygmomanometer	Average of two readings	At least 1 minute	After 5 minutes of rest	Seated	Right arm	Evenly tight

Types of BP measurement	Advantages	Remarks
Home BP measurement	More practical, two readings should be taken at each sitting, twice a day. Useful adjunct for improving BP control, especially if combined with telehealth counseling	Automated devices that have been validated should be used, and individuals should be trained
Ambulatory BP measurement (ABPM)	• Preferred for the confirmation of abnormal BPs • Stronger association between BPs obtained from ABPM with CV and renal outcomes • Allows for assessment of appropriate nocturnal physiologic dipping (BP should decrease by >10% during sleep) and BP variability • Both nocturnal hypertension and nondipping status have also been associated with higher risk for adverse CV outcomes, as well as CKD progression • A substantial proportion of patients with CKD has white coat (10–20%) and masked hypertension (10–30%), which would not be detected in the absence of ABPM	• During 24-hour ABPM, an appropriate-size BP cuff is worn for 24 hours, with measurements taken every 15–20 minutes during the daytime and every 30–60 minutes during sleep • When available, elevated BPs obtained using an appropriate technique in the clinic can be confirmed with 24-hour ABPM • Useful for confirmation of BP control and help detect hypotension that may be occurring outside the office setting in symptomatic patients
Office BP measurement	• Most clinical BP measurements are obtained in the office • Commonly used during treatment decisions • All major adult clinical trials data related to the effect of BP treatment on renal and CV outcomes have used BPs obtained in the clinic setting under standardized protocols with serial measurements	• Standardized fashion after 5 minutes of quiet rest using a validated device that is routinely calibrated • The cuff should be placed on the arm at the level of the atrium with the correct cuff size (the bladder of the cuff should encircle 80% of the arm), and the patient should be sitting with feet flat on the ground and back supported by a chair at least two readings should be obtained

(CV: cardiovascular)

good BP control suddenly worsens with hypertensive emergency or urgency, or resistant/refractory HTN. Asymmetric kidney sizes, diminishing GFR [estimated (eGFR)] with ACE inhibition or ARB, abdominal bruit, or flash pulmonary edema may give a clue for the presence of renovascular HTN.

- The initial screening test for renal artery stenosis is Doppler ultrasonography. To detect ≥ 60% reduction in renal artery diameter, a peak systolic velocity cutoff of 180–200 cm/s has been proposed. Three randomized trials that compared medical therapy and renal angioplasty with stenting in patients with atherosclerotic renal artery stenosis have not demonstrated differences in mortality, CV events, or progression of CKD. Factors that may increase the chances of improving BP control with revascularization are recent onset/progression of HTN, resistant HTN, and flash pulmonary edema. Patients with a solitary kidney and renal artery stenosis or bilateral renal artery stenosis with worsening kidney function may also be benefitted from revascularization.

Management of hypertension in CKD:

Nonpharmacologic therapy:

- DASH (Dietary Approaches to Stop Hypertension) diet: Diets rich in fruits and vegetables and low in saturated or unsaturated fats can lead to moderate declines in BP by ~10 mm Hg. DASH diet is associated with lower risk of ESKD in individuals with stage 3 CKD and HTN. In more advanced CKD, high-potassium intake may be difficult as it will increase the risk of hyperkalemia. Reducing sodium intake also has the added benefit of reducing proteinuria. Weight loss can reduce BP by ~ 5 mm Hg for every 5 kg weight loss and bariatric surgery may be a potential option. BP can be further improved with both aerobic and isometric resistance exercise.

- Renal denervation: The role of renal denervation for the treatment of resistant (or refractory) HTN among patients with CKD is unclear. Few studies showed remarkable reductions in BP (>30 mm Hg), albuminuria and progression of CKD with renal denervation.

Pharmacological therapy:

- Angiotensin-converting enzyme inhibitors and ARBs are the antihypertensive agents of choice especially in the presence of concurrent albuminuria (albumin excretion >300 mg/day). The combination of these two is not effective at slowing the progression of CKD or reducing CV events in patients with CKD (with or without diabetes). The combination may predispose to hyperkalemia and AKI. The use of ACE inhibitors or ARBs with aldosterone antagonists needs to be monitored carefully for hyperkalemia.
- Diuretics are considered an optimal second-line class of antihypertensive agents for most patients with CKD, especially in the setting of volume overload. Loop diuretics are preferred diuretics in reduced GFR. Thiazide and thiazide-like diuretics through indirect vasodilatory mechanisms act as effective antihypertensive agents. Diuretics may not be considered as the antihypertensive agent of choice for polycystic kidney disease as these drugs lead to volume depletion and vasopressin release contributing to cyst enlargement.
- Nondihydropyridine calcium channel blockers (CCBs) (e.g., diltiazem or verapamil) are also considered as good antihypertensives as these drugs have antiproteinuric effects. Other classes of antihypertensive agents, such as β-blockers may be indicated in patients with cardiac disease. Regimens that include a diuretic or spironolactone may be considered in resistant HTN. In these cases, confirmation of the accuracy of BP measurements and adherence to BP medications is important. The optimal first-line agent for patients with CKD in the absence of albuminuria is debated and may be selected based on concurrent indications. SGLT-2 inhibitors also possess antihypertensive effects and reduce the risk of adverse CV and kidney disease outcomes.

Effect on outcomes and treatment targets: There is strong observational evidence that uncontrolled HTN is associated with worse renal and CV outcomes across all age groups. However, it is still less clear whether the intensive lowering of BP slows GFR reduction. Patients with CKD are at elevated CV risk and HTN is one of the leading risk factors for CV events and stroke. Recommended BP target for patients with CKD in absence of significant proteinuria was <140/90 mm Hg for the last many years. As a result of the publication of the SPRINT trial in 2017, the AHA/ACC released new guidelines recommending a <130/80 mm Hg BP target for patients with CKD regardless of the degree of proteinuria present. However, the appropriate BP target for patients with CKD who do not fit the SPRINT inclusion criteria (including those with DM) is still debatable. BP targets should be individualized given the potential risks and benefits of treatment. In the setting of pregnancy in CKD, the optimal BP target is unclear. Agents acceptable for use during pregnancy include nifedipine, labetalol, and methyldopa. RAAS inhibitors are contraindicated during pregnancy.

Recent trials and meta-analysis related to HTN are summarized in **Table 3**.

ESC/ESH 2018 Guidelines: The clinical considerations and strategies for the treatment of HTN in CKD patients and recommendations (derived from 2018 european society of cardiology/european society of HTN (ESC/ESH) guidelines for the management of arterial HTN) are as follows.

Clinical considerations:

- Albuminuria reduction has been considered as a therapeutic target.
- Whether reducing albuminuria prevents CVD, remains unclear.
- Chronic kidney disease patients should follow lifestyle advice, especially sodium restriction.
- Loop diuretics should replace thiazide diuretics when the eGFR is <30 mL/min/1.73 m^2.
- It is expected for eGFR to reduce by 10–20% in patients treated for HTN.
- Careful monitoring of blood electrolytes and eGFR is essential.

Recommendations:

- In patients with diabetic or nondiabetic CKD, it is recommended that an office BP of ≥140/90 mm Hg be treated with lifestyle advice and BP-lowering medication (IA).
- In patients with diabetic or nondiabetic CKD, it is recommended to lower systolic BP (SBP) to a range of 130 to <140 mm Hg (IA).
- Individualized treatment should be considered according to its tolerability and impact on renal function and electrolytes (IIa C).
- Renin–angiotensin–aldosterone system blockers are more effective at reducing albuminuria and are recommended as part of the treatment strategy in hypertensive patients in the presence of microalbuminuria or proteinuria (IA).
- A combination of an RAS blocker with a CCB or a diuretic is recommended as initial therapy (IA).
- A combination of two RAS blockers is not recommended (IIIA).

TABLE 3 Recent trials and meta-analysis related to hypertension.

Trials (Year)	Design	Follow-up and outcome	Conclusion
SPRINT (2015)	Randomized controlled, open-label trial conducted at 102 clinical sites in the United States	9,361 participants with an SBP of 130 mm Hg or higher, presenting with an increased CV risk, but without diabetes, were randomly assigned to an SBP target of <120 mm Hg (intensive treatment) or <140 mm Hg (standard treatment). Patients with diabetes mellitus, polycystic kidney disease, and a history of stroke were excluded along with patients with heavy proteinuria (>1 g/day urine protein excretion). The primary composite outcome was MI, other ACS, stroke, HF, or death from cardiovascular causes	• The study was stopped early after a median follow-up of 3.26 years because of a statistically significant 25% reduction of the primary composite outcome in the intensive-treatment group, compared with the standard-treatment group • All-cause mortality, a secondary outcome, was also significantly lower in the intensive treatment group, with separation in mortality becoming apparent at about 2 years • Higher rates of serious events with the intensive treatment group than the standard treatment group, including hypotension, syncope, electrolyte abnormality, and AKI
CKD—SPRINT (JASN, 2017)	Randomized controlled, open-label trial conducted at 102 clinical sites in the United States	• Of the total SPRINT cohort (n = 9,361), 2,646 participants (28.3%) had CKD at baseline • Randomly assigned to a systolic BP target of <120 mm Hg (intensive group; n = 1,330) or <140 mm Hg (standard group; n = 1,316)	Among patients with CKD and hypertension without diabetes, targeting an SBP < 120 mm Hg compared with <140 mm Hg reduced rates of major cardiovascular events and all-cause death without evidence of effect modifications by CKD or deleterious effect on the main kidney outcome
Meta-analysis (JAMA, 2017)	A systemic review and meta-analysis Association of Intensive Blood Pressure control and Kidney Disease Progression in Nondiabetic Patients with Chronic Kidney Disease	Nine randomized clinical trials with 8,127 patients and a median follow-up of 3.3 years	Targeting BP below the current standard did not provide additional benefit for renal outcomes compared with standard treatment during a follow-up of 3.3 years in patients with CKD without diabetes. However, non-Black patients or those with higher levels of proteinuria might benefit from the intensive BP-lowering treatments
ACCORD BP trial (2010)	Randomized trial conducted at 77 clinical sites. The trial enrolled 10,251 high-risk participants with type 2 diabetes mellitus. 4,733 participants were also randomly assigned (in a 2-by-2 factorial design) to either intensive or standard BP control (the ACCORD blood-pressure trial)	A total of 4,733 participants with type 2 diabetes were randomly assigned to intensive therapy, targeting a systolic pressure of <120 mm Hg, or standard therapy, targeting a systolic pressure of <140 mm Hg. The primary composite outcome was nonfatal myocardial infarction, nonfatal stroke, or death from cardiovascular causes. The mean follow-up was 4.7 years	In patients with type 2 diabetes mellitus at high risk for cardiovascular events, targeting a systolic blood pressure of <120 mm Hg, as compared with <140 mm Hg, did not reduce the rate of a composite outcome of fatal and nonfatal major cardiovascular events

(ACS: acute coronary syndrome; AKI: acute kidney injury; BP: blood pressure; CKD: chronic kidney disease; CV: cardiovascular; HF: heart failure; MI: myocardial infarction; SBP: systolic blood pressure)

DIABETES AND KIDNEY DISEASE

Diabetic kidney disease (DKD) and DN are the leading cause of ESKD. Diabetes accounts for 30–50% of the incident cases of ESKD in India. 30–40% of patients with diabetes develop DN.

Diabetic kidney disease in diabetic patients can be from many diverse causes, including hypertensive nephrosclerosis and unresolved AKI. *DN* refers to specific pathologic structural and functional changes in diabetic patients from the effects of DM on the kidney.

The risk of DN is likely polygenetic and the interplay of several genes may be involved. Its prevalence varies among racial and ethnic groups.

PATHOPHYSIOLOGY OF DIABETIC NEPHROPATHY

The diabetic milieu leads to the generation and circulation of advanced glycation end products, elaboration of growth factors, hemodynamic and hormonal changes, release of reactive oxygen species, and inflammatory mediators. All these changes result in glomerular hyperfiltration and HTN, renal hypertrophy, and glomerular composition alteration manifesting clinically as proteinuria/albuminuria and HTN.

Pathologically, the kidneys undergo several changes, including the mesangial deposition of extracellular matrix, glomerular basement membrane thickening, proliferative changes, and tubular atrophy resulting in interstitial fibrosis and glomerulosclerosis.

With the onset of diabetes, kidney size and weight increase by an average of 15%. This increased size remains even after progressive renal dysfunction.

The classic pathologic lesion of DN is nodular glomerulosclerosis. These typical acellular nodules are positive by periodic acid–Schiff stain. They are reported in 10–50% of biopsy specimens from diabetic patients. A far more common lesion is the diffuse glomerular lesion with diffuse mesangial matrix expansion. There are prominent arteriolar lesions involving both the afferent and efferent vessels. After some time, hyaline material replaces the entire vessel wall structure.

NATURAL HISTORY OF DIABETIC NEPHROPATHY

After the diagnosis of type 1 DM (T1DM), proteinuria appears after 11–23 years, serum creatinine starts to increase after 13–25 years, and ESKD develops after 18–30 years. Microalbuminuria (30–300 mg/g creatinine) is noted to precede the onset of overt proteinuria (macroalbuminuria > 300 mg/g creatinine) in most diabetic patients, occurring 5–10 years after the diagnosis. It is very difficult to assess the timing of DM onset in type 2 DM (T2DM). In T2DM, a patient may present for the first time at the time of diagnosis with proteinuria and may have DN on kidney biopsy.

Proteinuria is considered as the single biggest predictor of eGFR deterioration and DN progression. Based on studies of untreated patients with T1DM and Pima Indians with T2DM, the rate of GFR loss can be to the order of 7–12 mL/min/1.73 m^2 per year. Treatment with RAS inhibitors has reduced this rate of decline to 3–6 mL/min/1.73 m^2 per year. CV death was thought to be more frequent than the progression of kidney disease to ESKD. However, in a more recent analysis of participants in two large multinational renal clinical trials in patients with established advanced DN and proteinuria, the risk for ESKD was significantly more common than CV death. Multiple therapies aimed at reducing the complications of DM have reduced the rate of macrovascular complications.

Recent reports have noted that up to 25% of patients with T2DM and diminished kidney function have little or no proteinuria despite having biopsy-proven DN. This may be due to the impact of long-term RAS inhibitor therapy, underdiagnosed unresolved AKI, or other factors.

DIAGNOSIS OF DIABETIC NEPHROPATHY

There is a decreased likelihood of DN in the case of significant albuminuria before 5 years or after 25 years duration of T1DM. 95% of patients with T1DM and DN also have diabetic retinopathy. Seven-field fundus photos must be obtained to rule out retinopathy. Diabetic retinopathy is concordant with DN in only about 60–65% of T2DM. If a diabetic patient has retinopathy, the onset of proteinuria in the usual timeframe and no evidence to support another proteinuric disease, it is unlikely that an alternative diagnosis will be found.

Difference between DN due to T1DM/T2DM:

- Timing of DN onset in patients with T2DM is difficult to assess.
- The patient may present for the first time with proteinuria and on kidney biopsy has DN and diagnosed to be T2DM thereafter.
- Cardiovascular disease (CVD) and death due to cardiac illness
    - Increased risk from the onset of T2DM and early DN
- Elevated risk for CVD is minimal—
    - Until the renal disease is advanced in T1DM

When do we suspect nondiabetic causes of CKD in DM?

- Absence of retinopathy
- Fast deterioration of GFR
- Rapidly increasing proteinuria
- Active urinary sediments
- Refractory HTN
- Signs or symptoms of other systemic illness

How DN differs from other CKD:

- Anemia and mineral bone disorder develop earlier in DN.
- Predominant tubulointerstitial damage affects the peritubular interstitial cells and reduced erythropoietin production.
- Diabetic nephropathy patients are predisposed to adynamic bone disease.
- Deaths due to CVDs and infections are highly prevalent and compete with progression to ESKD.
- Problems with vascular access
- Hemodynamic instability during hemodialysis

TREATMENT OF DIABETIC NEPHROPATHY

Standard treatment of DN patients can be divided into four major areas: (1) *cardiovascular risk reduction, (2) glycemic control, (3) BP control, and (4) inhibition of RAS.*

Cardiovascular events and renal function deterioration are higher with increasing BP and are reduced progressively with optimal BP control. The current Kidney Disease Outcomes Quality Initiative (KDOQI) guideline recommends a goal BP < 130/80 mm Hg, whereas the Eighth Joint National Committee (JNC 8) guidelines recommend a goal BP < 140/90 mm Hg for most diabetic patients, but with individualization. The current evidence strongly supports the use of RAS-blocking agents in DN. Although RAS blockade with more than 1 agent may be effective in reducing proteinuria, the adverse event profile (hyperkalemia, AKI, and increased CV events) and no benefit in preventing ESKD preclude its use for DN treatment. The third-generation mineralocorticoid receptor antagonist *finerenone* has shown albuminuria reduction in DN without a significant safety concern. Recently, two studies, designed as CV safety studies, EMPAREG outcome (Empagliflozin, Cardiovascular Outcomes, and Mortality in Type 2 Diabetes) and CANVAS (Canagliflozin Cardiovascular Assessment Study) have demonstrated albuminuria reduction and a reduction in the occurrence of a composite renal outcome. Recent outcome trials and one meta-analysis with SGLT-2 inhibitors are summarized as in **Table 4**. Other interventions presently under investigation for the therapy of DN include uric acid-lowering and bicarbonate therapy.

TABLE 4 Recent outcome trials and meta-analysis with SGLT-2 inhibitors.

Trials/Study	Main inclusion criteria	Main cardiovascular outcomes	Main renal outcomes
• **DECLARE-TIMI 58** • DAPA 10 mg or placebo once daily • $n = 7{,}160$, eGFR = 85.2 mL/min/1.73 m^2 • Median follow-up: 4.2 years	• Type 2 diabetes mellitus, HbA1c 6.5–12.0%, established atherosclerotic CVD or multiple risk factors for atherosclerotic CVD • Creatinine clearance ≥60 mL/min	17% reduction of the composite of cardiovascular death or hospitalization for heart failure. No effect on MACEs	47% reduction of renal-specific composite outcome
• **EMPA-REG OUTCOME** • EMPA 10 mg, EMPA 25 mg, or placebo once daily, $n = 7{,}020$, eGFR = 74.1 mL/min/1.73 m^2 • Median follow-up: 3.1 years	• Type 2 diabetes mellitus, HbA1c 7.0–9.0% without glucose-lowering therapy or HbA1c 7.0–10.0% with stable glucose-lowering therapy • BMI ≤ 45 kg/m^2, established CVD, eGFR ≥ 30 mL/min/1.73 m^2	14% reduction of composite of death from CV causes, nonfatal myocardial infarction or nonfatal stroke	39% reduction of renal-specific composite outcome
• **CANVAS** • CANA 300 mg, CANA 100 mg or placebo once daily $n = 10{,}142$, eGFR = 76.5 mL/min/1.73 m^2 • Median follow-up: 2.4 years	• Type 2 diabetes mellitus, HbA1c 7.0–10.5% • Established CVD or two or more risk factors for CVD • eGFR ≥ 30 mL/min/1.73 m^2	14% reduction of composite of death from CV causes, nonfatal myocardial infarction or nonfatal stroke	40% reduction of renal-specific composite outcome
• **CREDENCE** • CANA l00 mg or placebo once • daily, $n = 4401$ • eGFR = 85.2 mL/min/1.73m^2 • Median follow-up: 2.6 years	• Type 2 diabetes mellitus, ≥30 years of age, HbA1c 6.5–12.0% • Established CKD: eGFR 30–90 mL/min/1.73 m^2 and urinary ACR 300–5,000 mg/g	31% reduction of composite of CV death or hospitalization for heart failure	34% reduction of renal-specific composite outcome
• **DAPA-CKD** • Dapagliflozin 10 mg or placebo once daily, $n = 4304$ • Median follow-up: 2.4 years	• Type 2 diabetes mellitus (67.51%) • eGFR = 25–75 mL/min/1.73 m^2 and urinary ACR 200–5,000 mg/g	Hazard ratio for the composite of death from cardiovascular causes or hospitalization for heart failure was 0.71 (95% CI, 0.55–0.92; $p = 0.009$)	The hazard ratio for the composite of a sustained decline in the estimated GFR of at least 50%, ESKD, or death from renal causes was 0.56 (95% CI 0.45–0.68; $p < 0.001$). The effects of dapagliflozin were similar in participants with type 2 diabetes mellitus and in those without type 2 diabetes mellitus
• Association of SGLT-2 Inhibitors With Cardiovascular and Kidney Outcomes in Patients with Type 2 Diabetes (JAMA 2020) • Data from six trials comprised 46,969 unique patients with type 2 diabetes mellitus, including 31,116 (66.2%) with atherosclerotic CV disease	Meta-analysis: A total of six randomized. placebo-controlled CV and kidney outcomes trials of SGLT-2 inhibitors in patients with type 2 diabetes mellitus were identified, with contributory data from nine publications	SGLT-2 inhibitors were associated with a reduced risk of major adverse CV events. HHF/CV death-associated risk reduction for HHF was consistent across the trials, whereas significant heterogeneity of associations with outcome was observed for CV death	Reduced risk of kidney outcomes (HR 0.62; 95% CI 0.56–0.70; Q statistic, $p = 0.09$). with no significant heterogeneity of associations with outcome

(HHF: hospitalization for heart failure; MACE: major adverse cardiovascular event)

TABLE 5 Difference in HTN between type 1 DM and type 2 DM.

Type 1 DM	Type 2 DM
• Incidence of HTN rises from 5% at 10 years, 33% at 22 years, 70% at 40 years • BP increases within few years after onset of microalbuminuria • BP increases progressively with progression of renal disease	• 40% already hypertensive on diagnosis • 50% patients—elevated BP before onset of moderately increased albuminuria • Increased CV morbidity and mortality

TABLE 6 Studies showing benefits of HTN treatment in DM.

Study	Outcome
UKPDS (UK Prospective Diabetes Study)	Reduction in diabetes-related endpoints including microvascular disease, death, and stroke; reduction in significant deterioration in retinopathy and visual acuity
HOT (Hypertension Optimal Treatment)	Relative risk of CV events reduced
ADVANCE (Action in diabetes and vascular disease: Preterax and Diamicron MR controlled Evaluation)	A lower rate of major macrovascular or microvascular events, lower rate of CV mortality and all-cause mortality
Meta-analysis	Reduced mortality, CV disease, MI, and stroke

TABLE 7 Goal BP in diabetic nephropathy.

2017 ACC/AHA guidelines	<130/80 mm Hg	To maintain DBP ≥ 60 mm Hg in older adults
2017 ADA consensus report	Endorse highest level of evidence for <140 mm Hg	Attaining lower BP (125–130 mm Hg) should be attempted, if tolerated to prevent CV events

(ACC: American College of Cardiology; AHA: American Heart Association; ADA: American Diabetes Association)

ADDITIONAL THERAPEUTIC STRATEGIES

Doses of oral hypoglycemic agents and insulin must be reduced with decreased GFR. Metformin is contraindicated in patients with eGFRs < 30 mL/min/1.73 m^2 due to its association with severe lactic acidosis in these patients. Patients with DN irrespective of kidney function are at increased risk for hyperkalemia and metabolic acidosis due to type IV renal tubular acidosis. This can be treated with low-potassium diet, diuretics, and base supplementation. These patients are also at increased risk for developing AKI from iodinated radiocontrast administration, volume depletion, or NSAIDs use.

DIABETES AND HYPERTENSION

Difference between HTN in T1DM and T2DM is given in **Table 5**. Studies showing the benefit of HTN treatment are given in **Table 6**. Goal BP in DM as per recent guidelines is given in **Table 7**.

RECOMMENDED READINGS

1. Umanath K, Lewis JB. Update on diabetic nephropathy: Core curriculum 2018. Am J Kidney Dis. 2018;71:884-95.
2. Ku E, Lee BJ, Wei J, Weir MR. Hypertension in CKD: Core curriculum 2019. Am J Kidney Dis. 2019;74:120-31.
3. Whelton PK, Carey RM, Aronow WS, Casey DE Jr, Collins KJ, Himmelfarb CD, et al. 2017 ACC/AHA/AAPA/ABC/ACPM/AGS/APhA/ASH/ASPC/NMA/PCNA Guideline for the prevention, detection, evaluation, and management of high blood pressure in adults: executive summary: a report of the American College of Cardiology/American Heart Association Task Force on Clinical Practice Guidelines. J Am Soc Hypertens. 2018;12: 579.e1-579.e73.
4. Cheung AK, Rahman M, Reboussin DM, Craven TE, Greene T, Kimmel PL, et al. Effects of intensive BP control in CKD. J Am Soc Nephrol. 2017;28:2812-23.
5. Dwyer JP, Lewis JB. Nonproteinuric diabetic nephropathy: when diabetics don't read the textbook. Med Clin North Am. 2013;97:53-8.
6. Rodriguez-Iturbe B, Romero F, Johnson RJ. Pathophysiological mechanisms of salt-dependent hypertension. Am J Kidney Dis. 2007;50:655-72.
7. KDOQI. KDOQI Clinical Practice Guidelines and Clinical Practice Recommendations for Diabetes and Chronic Kidney Disease. Am J Kidney Dis. 2007;49: S12-154.
8. Campese VM. Pathophysiology of resistant hypertension in chronic kidney disease. Semin Nephrol. 2014;34:571-6.

CHAPTER

169 Infections and Kidney

Arunkumar S, Kristin George, Sandeep Mahajan

ABSTRACT

Infections are common causes of kidney disease worldwide particularly so in tropical countries. All types of infections—bacterial, viral, fungal, parasitic, and protozoal infections can involve the kidney to varying degrees. Renal involvement is a result of hemodynamic perturbations, direct microbial invasion of renal tissue, or a consequence of immune mediated injury and can affect any one or all of the renal compartments.

High burden of infectious diseases in developing countries like India is a major contributor of acute kidney injury (AKI). AKI is commonly seen in severe malaria, leptospirosis, dengue fever (DF), and more recently in emerging infections like scrub typhus. Cross-border transportation and blurring of geographical boundaries increase the risk of newer infections and emergence of hitherto uncommon infections. Potential for complete recovery with early detection and appropriate therapy mandates thorough knowledge about these conditions and concerted effort to improve outcomes. In this chapter, we provide a brief overview about the mechanisms, clinical presentation, and management of common infective conditions associated with kidney involvement.

"We don't grow when things are easy, we grow when we face challenges"

—Anonymous

INTRODUCTION

Infection-associated kidney disease is an important cause of morbidity and mortality worldwide. Tropical and developing countries like India offer suitable environment for subsistence of microorganisms and their vectors increasing the likelihood of contracting infections. This coupled with prevailing socioeconomic factors predisposes a vast majority to infections and their complications. It is important to recognize these complications early, as timely detection and treatment are curative and limit renal injury.

Almost all groups of microorganisms—bacteria, viral, fungal, parasitic, and protozoal organisms can affect the kidney. All the renal compartments namely, glomeruli, tubules, interstitial, and vascular compartment can be affected leading to a variety of clinical manifestations (**Table 1**). Renal abnormalities range from asymptomatic urinary abnormalities to frank glomerular disease, from mild increase in creatinine to severe AKI requiring renal replacement therapy.

APPROACH TO A PATIENT

Patients with infections frequently present with febrile illness with a combination of clinical features which are mostly overlapping and often nonspecific. There is no characteristic feature to differentiate all infections. This is where a watchful scrutiny of the locoregional factors combined with thorough medical history and careful physical examination helps in narrowing the differential diagnosis. History should include the chronology of events, anything suggestive of contact with infectious agent—exposure to livestock and animal habitat during outdoor activities, insect bites, and a complete travel history of

TABLE 1 Various infectious agents associated with renal involvement.

Bacteria	Virus	Parasite	Fungus
• *Streptococcus* • *Staphylococcus* • *Mycobacterium* • *Escherichia coli* • *Salmonella* • *Legionella*	• Dengue • Hantavirus • Hepatitis viruses (A, B, and C) • HIV • Cytomegalovirus • Parvovirus • EBV	• Malaria • Filariasis • Leishmaniasis • Schistosomiasis • Hydatid disease • Toxoplasmosis	• *Candida* • Mucormycosis • Aspergillosis

(EBV: Epstein–Barr virus; HIV: human immunodeficiency virus)

patient and attenders. Physical examination for skin lesions, bite marks, "eschar", and lymphadenopathy and systemic examination to assess fluid status and organ-specific complications have to be performed.

MECHANISM OF RENAL INVOLVEMENT

Infection-associated kidney injury can result due to direct effect of the causative organism or due to indirect systemic effects. Direct invasion and damage to the tubules, acute tubular necrosis, tubulointerstitial nephritis, endothelial damage and thrombotic microangiopathy, immune complex deposition, and complement-mediated glomerular damage are the major modes of direct renal involvement. Indirect effects on kidney are due to hemodynamic effects as a consequence of dehydration and hypovolemia, cytokine release and vasodilatory shock, hemolysis, and rhabdomyolysis. Renal infarction can occur due to thrombotic microangiopathy due to disseminated intravascular coagulation (DIC) or due to angioinvasive infections like mucormycosis. Apart from the infections per se, treatment with antibiotics and other drugs can cause or precipitate renal failure. It is usually a combination of all these factors which cause kidney injury. The various mechanisms of renal involvement in infections are depicted in **Flowchart 1**.

Though the list of infections is vast, we have limited our discussion to the most common infections in the Indian context. Studies from India have shown that infections are a major cause of renal dysfunction accounting for 20–50% of all cases of AKI. The important causes of such AKI are malaria, leptospirosis, dengue, and scrub typhus.

MALARIA

Malaria is the most prevalent endemic parasitic infection in tropical countries of Asia, Latin America, and Africa. It causes considerable morbidity and mortality and AKI is

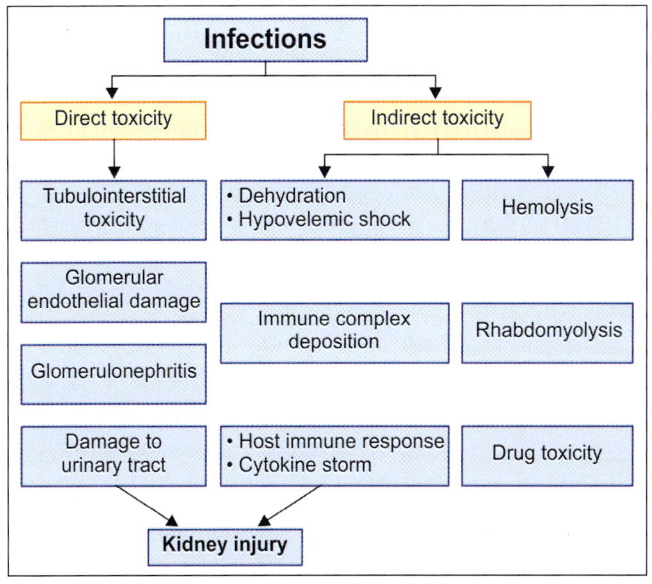

FLOWCHART 1: Mechanism of renal involvement in infectious diseases.

a well-known dreaded complication. Kidneys are affected in infections with *Plasmodium falciparum*, *P. vivax*, and *P. malariae*. Malaria contributes to about 2–39% of total hospital admissions for AKI. In those with severe infection, up to 60% can develop AKI.

Though *P. falciparum* has traditionally been the major cause of complicated malaria and AKI, in recent years, there has been increase in such cases due to *P. vivax*. In a study from North India, almost 60% of hospitalized patients with severe malaria had *P. vivax* infection and 36% of them developed AKI. AKI is more common in nonimmune individuals and hence travelers to endemic regions are more prone to fatal infection.

PATHOPHYSIOLOGY

While *P. vivax, P. ovale*, and *P. knowlesi* infect young red blood cells (RBCs) and *P. malariae* infects older erythrocytes, *P. falciparum* infects RBCs of all ages and hence produces heavy parasitemia. Infected erythrocytes have decreased deformability, exhibit cytoadherence causing sequestration which affects the microcirculation. Exaggerated/dysregulated host immune response and combined Th1 and Th2 activation result in the production of several proinflammatory cytokines like tumor necrosis factor, interleukins [IL-1, IL-6, IL-8 and interferon gamma (IFN-γ)], and vasoactive mediators in severe malaria.

Malarial AKI is a result of ischemia and hypoxia and is seen with heavy parasitemia, intravascular coagulation, hemolysis, and/or rhabdomyolysis. These factors super-added to the hypovolemia due to febrile dehydration and low intake of fluids causes AKI. The infected erythrocytes block the glomerular capillaries and result in acute tubular injury. Malarial antigens have been demonstrated on glomerular endothelium and medullary capillaries. There are recent reports of *P. vivax* presenting with thrombotic microangiopathy manifesting as fibrinoid necrosis and acute cortical necrosis in the kidneys. *P. malariae* is associated with glomerulonephritis with presence of malarial antigen and immune complex deposits in the glomeruli.

CLINICAL FEATURES

Malaria presents with high grade periodic fever, chills, headache, malaise, and occasionally jaundice. Cerebral malaria, jaundice, AKI, and acute respiratory distress syndrome (ARDS) are seen in severe cases. AKI occurs at the end of the 1st week and oliguria is reported in two-thirds of the cases. Malarial AKI can be an isolated complication following infection or can present as a part of multiorgan failure. Favorable outcomes are seen more commonly in isolated cases. Severe acidosis, hypoglycemia, and hypotension are frequently seen and timely management of these complications improves the prognosis of patients. Male gender, hemoglobin (Hb) < 7.5 g/dL, hyperbilirubinemia, and thrombocytopenia (<25,000/mcL) at baseline are associated with development of AKI. Hemoglobinuria is seen in patients with intravascular hemolysis. Fluid and electrolyte disturbances are common with hyponatremia seen in about three-fourths of all patients.

DIAGNOSIS AND MANAGEMENT

Diagnosis of the malaria is made by the demonstration of the parasite in a thick blood smear. Newer antigen-based card tests can also be used for quick diagnosis and in resource-limited settings. In patients who present with AKI after other acute complications subside, peripheral smear examination does not reveal parasites and hence immunochromatographic tests and antibody-based card tests have to be used to establish the diagnosis. The most common histologic feature in renal biopsy is acute tubular necrosis, while acute cortical necrosis is seen in severe cases. Interstitial nephritis, glomerulonephritis (*P. malariae*), and thrombotic microangiopathy (*P. vivax*) can be seen in some cases.

Artemisinin-based combination therapies are the recommended treatment and should be started as soon as a diagnosis is made. Artesunate has high efficacy and does not need dose modification in the presence of renal dysfunction. Aggressive management of complications including timely renal replacement therapy is essential for recovery of renal function and improved survival. Exchange blood transfusion and erythracytapheresis can be attempted in patients with heavy parasitemia. Mortality rate of malarial AKI is 10–50% and is often dependent on locoregional factors and severity of infection. Survivors of severe malarial AKI may have residual renal impairment with slow progression to chronic kidney disease (CKD) and have to be on follow-up. *P. malariae,* which causes chronic quartan malaria in the African regions, may present with nephrotic syndrome which responds poorly to antimalarial treatment and also to immunosuppressive therapy.

LEPTOSPIROSIS

Leptospirosis is a zoonotic disease caused by the spirochete of the genus *Leptospira*. Infection is transmitted to humans through contact with contaminated water or animal urine. Seasonal outbreaks occur after rains and flooding. Occupational exposure is seen in sewer workers, farmers, abattoir workers, veterinarians, garbage collectors, and pet traders. World Health Organization (WHO) has classified leptospirosis as a reemerging infectious disease in both developed and developing nations.

Though most of the infections are mild, recovering completely with appropriate treatment, some develop AKI and multiorgan dysfunction which can be life threatening. Studies from India have shown AKI to be present in 15–60% of leptospirosis affected patients. In a study from Southern India, it was seen that hypotension, acidosis, tachypnea, thrombocytopenia, and infection with serovar Pyrogenes increase the risk of AKI. Present interest in leptospiral kidney involvement has been spurred by the finding of leptospiral seropositivity in CKDu (CKD of unknown origin) hotspots suggesting probable role of leptospiral kidney disease in future development of CKD.

PATHOPHYSIOLOGY

Tissue injury in leptospirosis is due to a combination of the direct effects of *Leptospira* and the host-immune response. The outer membrane of *Leptospira interrogans* contains lipopolysaccharide (LPS), cytotoxic glycolipoprotein (GLP), and lipoproteins. It has tropism for kidney with these endotoxins primarily affecting tubulointerstitial cells. The effect of GLPs on tubular Na^{+}- K^{+} ATPase results in urinary concentrating defects, hypokalemia, and AKI. The spirochete membrane proteins also cause injury to the glycocalyx and endothelium contributing to AKI.

CLINICAL PRESENTATION

Classic clinical presentation is biphasic—initial *leptospiremic phase* lasts 5–7 days and is characterized by nonspecific, transient flu-like symptoms that resolve spontaneously or can be completely asymptomatic. This is followed by the *immune phase,* characterized by increase in cytokines, immunoglobulin M (IgM) antibodies, and multiorgan involvement. Patients develop AKI during the second phase of illness, along with jaundice, upper gastrointestinal bleed, arrhythmia, and pulmonary hemorrhage. This severe presentation of leptospirosis with icterus is referred to as *Weil's disease.* AKI is classically nonoliguric with hypokalemia. The severity of AKI is associated with increasing mortality. Tubulointerstitial nephritis with tubular dysfunction and electrolyte wasting is characteristic of leptospiral kidney involvement.

DIAGNOSIS AND MANAGEMENT

The diagnosis of leptospirosis needs correlation of clinical and epidemiological information and serological tests to confirm the diagnosis. Microscopic agglutination test (MAT) is highly sensitive and specific making it the gold standard for serologic diagnosis. The solid-phase assay to detect IgM antibodies though commonly used cannot be interpreted in endemic areas where IgM can last for longer periods. Polymerase chain reaction (PCR)-based tests to detect leptospiral DNA are a promising diagnostic tool limited by cost and technical support. Urine examination may show varying proteinuria (<1 g/day), hematuria, leukocyturia, and granular casts.

Though role of universal antibiotic therapy is debated, antibiotic therapy with penicillin, cephalosporins or doxycycline is often prescribed. Mild cases may not require antibiotic therapy. Adequate supportive care including management of dyselectrolytemia and adequate fluid replacement is important. For patients with severe disease manifestations, intensive care therapy is needed with respiratory support and optimal renal replacement therapy. AKI is an independent prognostic factor for patients with severe disease.

DENGUE FEVER

Dengue is a common mosquito borne illness predominantly affecting the tropics and subtropics. The dengue virus belongs to the genus *Flavivirus* is an RNA arbovirus, transmitted by the bite of female *Aedes aegypti* mosquito. There are four serotypes of the dengue virus (DEN1 to DEN4) and immunity to one does not provide lifelong immunity to the other serotypes. Reinfection with a different serotype is associated with severe clinical manifestations, likely due to cross-reactive antibodies. Though often a self-limited febrile illness, severe forms of dengue can result in significant mortality. Studies have reported AKI in 1–15% of patients with severe dengue with mortality of 10–50%.

PATHOPHYSIOLOGY

The presence of non-neutralizing antibodies following prior infection (different serotype) results in formation of immune complexes which further results in antibody-dependent enhancement and thereby release of various cytokines and interleukins. The resultant capillary leakage and fluid loss lead to shock, decreased kidney perfusion, and acute tubular necrosis. Dengue viral antigens have been demonstrated in tubular epithelial cells suggesting direct effects. Rhabdomyolysis, myositis, multiorgan failure, and direct viral invasion are the other pathogenic determinants of renal involvement.

CLINICAL PRESENTATION

The dengue virus has an incubation period of 3–14 days and typically presents with fever, arthralgia, and rash. Clinically, dengue is classified into undifferentiated fever, DF, dengue hemorrhagic fever (DHF), and dengue shock syndrome (DSS) by the WHO. Common clinical presentation is high grade fever, myalgia, arthralgia, headache, retroocular pain, and rash. In the severe forms, patient develops plasma leakage (pleural effusion, ascites), hypotension, hemorrhage, shortness of breath, and shock. Kidney involvement in dengue manifests as AKI, proteinuria (can be nephrotic), hemolytic uremic syndrome, electrolyte abnormalities, and glomerulonephritis.

Risk factors for development of AKI include trans-aminitis, hypoalbuminemia, multiorgan dysfunction, rhabdomyolysis, use of inotropic agents, concomitant viral or bacterial infection, and delayed hospitalization.

DIAGNOSIS AND MANAGEMENT

Clinical suspicion in patients with acute febrile illness has to be supported by serological investigations to diagnose dengue. A reverse transcription-PCR (RT-PCR) or the NS1 test is useful in the 1st week of infection while late cases are better diagnosed with antibody tests.

Treatment is mainly supportive with adequate fluid therapy and avoiding nonsteroidal anti-inflammatory drugs. Fluid is returned to intravascular compartment from the third space during recovery phase of dengue and this has to be monitored as overhydration during this phase can precipitate heart failure in susceptible patients. The high rate of mortality among patients with DSS (15%) is significantly reduced with optimal management.

SCRUB TYPHUS

Scrub typhus is a neglected tropical disease endemic in Asia caused by the rickettsia *Orientia tsutsugamushi*. Despite the high prevalence and a case fatality rate of 30% in severe cases, it is underdiagnosed and underreported as a cause of acute febrile illness and hence designated as a reemerging disease by the WHO. Multiple reports from India suggest that kidneys are commonly affected in scrub typhus with AKI reported in 10–60% of all patients. Urinary abnormalities are seen in 40–80% of typhus-infected patients.

CLINICAL FEATURES AND MANAGEMENT

Humans are infected by the larval forms (chiggers) of infected trombiculid mite. The bite site evolves into an eschar, which is pathognomonic of scrub typhus infection and can ulcerate to form a black crust. The clinical picture consists of fever, skin rash, myalgia, and gastrointestinal symptoms. In severe cases, multiorgan involvement with jaundice, AKI, ARDS, myocarditis, meningitis, septic shock, and DIC can develop. Patients with thrombocytopenia, hypoalbuminemia, and requirement of intensive care are more prone to develop AKI. Volume depletion and resulting decrease in renal perfusion are the most important reasons for AKI. Other mechanisms described are direct tubular toxicity, interstitial nephritis, rhabdomyolysis, and thrombotic microangiopathy due to DIC.

Serological assays are commonly used to diagnose scrub typhus. Commonly used tests include Weil–Felix test, enzyme-linked immunosorbent assay (ELISA), immunofluorescence assays, and recently the RAD diagnostic tests. Nucleic acid test (NAT) though the gold standard is not widely available and hence cases may be missed by routine serology. Treatment with doxycycline or azithromycin is highly effective and patients recover with timely antibiotic therapy. Patients with multiorgan involvement and renal failure have high mortality especially when not treated with optimal antibiotics.

HANTAVIRUS

Hantaviruses belong to the Bunyaviridae family of enveloped single-stranded RNA viruses. Their important distinction from other viral hemorrhagic agents is their worldwide distribution. The virus is rodent-borne and transmission is via aerosols of rodent excreta, saliva, and urine. Hantaviruses are classified into two main groups: (1) "Old World" group causing hemorrhagic fever with renal syndrome (HFRS) common in Europe and Asia and (2) the "New World" group causing hantavirus pulmonary syndrome (HPS) commonly seen in the Americas. There has been shown to be considerable overlap between these syndromes and geographical location in recent times. Many new hantaviruses have been discovered in the last decade worldwide but the pathogenic significance is still uncertain. Studies from India suggest hantaviral infection to be prevalent from around the year 2000 and retrospective studies have yielded serological (IgG) positivity in undifferentiated febrile illness.

PATHOPHYSIOLOGY

Hantaviruses are endotheliotropic and cause generalized vascular injury and increased permeability. Viral glycoprotein interaction with integrins on host immune cells elicits a strong host immune response. Kidney involvement is characterized by severe blood stasis and leakage in the outer medulla along with extensive interstitial hemorrhage and occasionally necrosis in the deeper medulla. The virus targets the tight junction protein in the glomeruli and results in damage to podocytes and proteinuria.

CLINICAL FEATURES

After the incubation period ranging from 1 to 5 weeks, HFRS classically presents with a febrile phase characterized by influenza-like symptoms with conjunctival suffusion and petechial rash. This is followed by the hypotensive phase which proceeds to the oliguric phase. The oliguric phase is characterized by worsening thrombocytopenia and shock accounting for 30–50% of all mortality. Diuretic phase follows in survivors wherein renal function improves and patients recover completely during the convalescent phase. Proteinuria starts early in febrile phase but is often self-limited subsiding by the diuretic phase. Respiratory failure as a result of diffuse capillary leak syndrome and noncardiogenic pulmonary edema can be seen in a subset of patients.

DIAGNOSIS AND MANAGEMENT

Diagnosis is made on the basis of serological tests as the viremic phase is limited and direct detection of virus is often not possible. IgM and/or IgG antibodies are detected by ELISA or immunofluorescence assays. Supportive therapy is the primary mode of treatment. Though ribavirin has been tried, the therapeutic efficacy is uncertain and may be useful only in the early phase when the diagnosis per se would be uncertain.

FILARIASIS

Lymphatic filariasis is widespread in tropical and subtropical regions and is common in the Indian subcontinent. Most of the cases are caused by *Wuchereria bancrofti* and *Brugia malayi*. Though asymptomatic in most cases, the acute symptomatic patient presents with lymphadenitis. Persistent obstruction of lymphatic vessels by adult worms and ensuing inflammation results in chronic filariasis characterized by in lymphedema, hydrocoele, and elephantiasis. Obstruction and rupture of lymph vessels result in chyluria seen in chronic cases. Rarely gross hematuria may occur in patients with filarial chyluria. The renal involvement in filariasis includes glomerulonephritis (immune complex mediated) with varying degrees of hematuria and proteinuria.

The diagnosis depends mainly on a combination of history, clinical examination, and detection of microfilariae in peripheral blood or urine in acute cases. Diethylcarbamazine (DEC) and ivermectin are the commonly used antifilarial drugs.

COMPLICATED URINARY TRACT INFECTION

Urinary tract infections (UTIs) are the most common bacterial infection both in the in-patient setting and in the community. Based on the extent of involvement and severity, they are classified into uncomplicated and complicated UTI. Though definitions have evolved over time with multiple definitions over the years, uncomplicated UTI occurs in healthy nonpregnant women and readily responds to antibiotic therapy. Complicated UTI refers to cystitis or pyelonephritis in a patient with underlying functional or structural abnormalities of the genitourinary tract.

Most cases of UTIs are due to the colonization of the urogenital tract with perineal and rectal flora. The most common organisms include *Escherichia coli, Klebsiella, Pseudomonas, Proteus*, enterococci, or *Staphylococcus* species. Certain organisms are more common in a given clinical situation—pseudomonal UTI in in-patients with/without instrumentation and *Staphylococcus saprophyticus* in young healthy women.

CLINICAL FEATURES AND MANAGEMENT

Symptoms of cystitis like dysuria, urinary frequency, and urgency along with systemic features like fever or flank pain, nausea, vomiting, and costo-vertebral angle tenderness suggestive of pyelonephritis. Elderly patients can present with only delirium or a febrile illness with no localization. At times, complicated UTI can present as undifferentiated sepsis or even septic shock. The virulence of infecting organism and the host immunity decides the severity of UTIs.

An appropriately collected urine specimen is vital for diagnosis. Significant bacteriuria is defined by counts of $\geq 10^5$ CFU/mL in a midstream urine sample or $\geq 10^4$ CFU/mL if an "in and out" catheter urine sample is taken. Treatment should not be delayed, if the clinical presentation is strongly suggestive of UTI and broad-spectrum antibiotics based on local sensitivity pattern should be initiated after collecting urine samples for microscopy and culture. Patients with mild symptoms can be managed as outpatients with fluoroquinolones or cephalosporins such as cephalexin or amoxicillin/clavulanic acid. Those with more severe presentation or failed initial therapy should be started on parenteral cephalosporins, piperacillin and tazobactam, fluoroquinolones, or carbapenems. Aminoglycoside can be added with close monitoring of kidney function. Failure to respond to therapy by 48–72 hours is an indication to repeat cultures, add/change antibiotics, and evaluate for a possible obstructive component.

Ultrasonography and CT scans may be needed in cases of suspected perinephric abscess, obstructive causes like stone, or urinary retention and should be undertaken in all patients who fail to respond to the appropriate antibiotic treatment. Treatment should be continued for 7 days in case of mild presentation and 14 days in severe cases or those with persisting symptoms. It may be extended to 3–4 weeks depending on the clinical response. In patients with genitourinary abnormalities and recurrent UTI, long-term suppressive antibiotic therapy may be needed.

CONCLUSION

Renal involvement is common in various infections and is prevalent worldwide. The mechanism of renal involvement is multifactorial consisting of direct renotoxic effect, hemodynamic disturbances, effects of systemic host immune response, and adverse effect of therapeutic agents. Socioeconomic development with better control of infections will reduce the burden of kidney disease. Most of the causes of kidney disease are incurable and cannot be prevented. However, infections are probably the only preventable cause of kidney disease and potentially curable with timely management. Advances in diagnostic testing with widespread availability of point-of-care tests to diagnose infections and detect renal dysfunction early are the need of the hour. The role of residual renal disease following infections in adding to the prevalence of CKD and end-stage renal disease (ESRD) requires further long-term studies and disease-specific registries. All treating physicians should be sensitized to the importance of renal involvement and importance of follow-up to manage those with persisting and progressive kidney disease.

RECOMMENDED READINGS

1. Jha V, Parameswaran S. Community-acquired acute kidney injury in tropical countries. Nat Rev Nephrol. 2013;9(5):278-90.
2. Turner N, Lameire N, Goldsmith DJ, Winearls CG, Himmelfarb J, Remuzzi G. The patient with infections causing renal disease. In: Jha V (Ed). Oxford Textbook of Clinical Nephrology, Volume 2. Oxford: Oxford University Press; 2015. pp.1545-625.
3. Anghan H, Sethi P, Soneja M, Mahajan S, Wig N. Clinical and laboratory features associated with acute kidney injury in severe malaria. Indian J Crit Care Med. 2018;22(10):718-22.
4. Jha V, Prasad N. CKD and infectious diseases in Asia Pacific: Challenges and opportunities. Am J Kidney Dis. 2016;68:148-60.
5. Prasad N, Patel MR. Infection-induced kidney diseases. Front Med. 2018;5:327.
6. Mishra SK, Das BS. Malaria and acute kidney injury. Semin Nephrol. 2008;28:395-408.
7. Mallhi TH, Khan AH, Adnan AS, Sarriff A, Khan YH, Jummaat F. Incidence, Characteristics and Risk Factors of Acute Kidney Injury among Dengue Patients: A Retrospective Analysis. PLoS One. 2015;10(9):e0138465.
8. Patel ML, Himanshu D, Chaudhary SC, Atam V, Sachan R, Misra R, et al. Clinical characteristic and risk factors of acute kidney injury among dengue viral infections in adults: A retrospective analysis. Indian J Nephrol. 2019;29(1):15-21.
9. Oliver J, Macdowell M. The renal lesion in epidemic hemorrhagic fever. J Clin Invest. 1957;36(1 Pt 2):99-133.
10. Ferluga D, Vizjak A. Hantavirus Nephropathy. J Am Soc Nephrol. 2008;19(9):1653-8.
11. Peter JV, Sudarsan TI, Prakash JAJ, Varghese GM. Severe scrub typhus infection: clinical features, diagnostic challenges and management. World J Crit Care Med. 2015;4:244.
12. Wagenlehner FM, Bjerklund Johansen TE, Cai T, Koves B, Kranz J, Pilatz A, et al. Epidemiology, definition and treatment of complicated urinary tract infections. Nat Rev Urol. 2020;17(10):586-600.

CHAPTER 170 Hereditary and Congenital Kidney Diseases

Dinesh Khullar, Pallavi Prasad

ABSTRACT

Hereditary disorders of kidney include glomerular diseases, cystic diseases, and disorders of renal tubule. A hereditary basis of renal disease should be suspected in patients of pediatric age group, in those with family history of kidney disease or families with history of consanguineous marriages. Disorders may be monogenic, polygenic, or associated with chromosomal abnormalities. Congenital abnormalities of kidney or urinary tract (CAKUT), which are also the most common cause of end-stage renal disease (ESRD) in pediatric population have a polygenic basis.

Glomerular disorders include congenital nephrotic syndrome, Alport syndrome, and thin basement membrane disease. Cystic disorders may be autosomal dominant (AD)—autosomal dominant polycystic kidney disease (ADPKD), von Hippel–Lindau (VHL) syndrome, tuberous sclerosis (TS) or autosomal recessive (AR)— nephronophthisis (NPHP) and autosomal recessive polycystic kidney disease (ARPKD). Disorders of renal tubule include Bartter syndrome, Gitelman syndrome, diabetes insipidus, and renal tubular acidosis (RTA).

"Your genetics load the gun. Your lifestyle pulls the trigger"

—Mehmet Oz

INTRODUCTION

Inherited or congenital renal abnormalities are the cause of ESRD in approximately 10% of adults and nearly all children who undergo renal replacement therapy. Accurate diagnosis of genetic disorders is not only important for the appropriate treatment of patients but also to make them aware regarding the risk of transmission of disease to their offspring. Renal disorders with a genetic basis include monogenic disorders, polygenic disorders, and chromosomal disorders.

MONOGENIC DISORDERS

Monogenic renal inherited disorders can be grouped under the following headings:

- Glomerular disorders
- Cystic disorders
- Disorders of renal tubule (acid-base, electrolyte, and water handling)
- Other systemic disorders with renal manifestations.

GLOMERULAR DISORDERS

Inherited nephrotic syndrome:

- Nephrotic syndrome may be idiopathic, secondary, or have a genetic basis.
- Approximately 30% cases of steroid resistant nephrotic syndrome younger than 25 years of age have a genetic basis for their disease, the percentage can go as high as 70% in age group 0–3 months.

Genetics:

- Mutations in more than 50 genes, which encode for various proteins essential for the function of glomerular filtration barrier, have been identified to be the genetic basis of such inherited nephrotic syndrome.
- Most mutations are inherited in autosomal recessive (AR) pattern, some maybe autosomal dominant (AD). Some of the important mutations are enlisted in **Table 1** and illustrated in **Figure 1**.

Clinical features: An inherited cause of nephrotic syndrome should be suspected when:

- Nephrotic syndrome occurs at age < 1 year
- Steroid resistant nephrotic syndrome in children and adolescents
- Family history of nephrotic syndrome
- Family history of consanguineous marriage

Treatment:

- Once a causative mutation is identified, immunosuppressive therapy (steroids, cyclophosphamide etc.) is generally discontinued.
- All patients must receive angiotensin-converting enzyme (ACE) inhibitor/angiotensin receptor blocker (ARB) and supportive therapy.
- Renal transplantation may be offered in case of ESRD.
- Patients with some mutations (*PLCE1*, *INTS1*, and *INTS2*) may respond to steroids or cyclosporine. Some patients respond to specific therapies like COQ 10 supplementation (*COQ* mutation) and vitamin B12 supplementation (*ARGHDIA* mutation).

Alport syndrome:

- Alport syndrome is caused by defects in type IV collagen, which is composed of a heterotrimer of α chains 3, 4, and 5.
- Type IV collagen is an important constituent of basement membrane, the cochlea, cornea, lens capsule, and retina.
- Prevalence is 1 in 50,000 individuals.

Genetics:

- It has multiple modes of inheritance, X-linked being the most common (85%) due to mutation in *COL4A5*.
- It may also be AR and AD (*COL4A3*, *COL4A4*—both on chromosome 2).
- Patients with *MYH9* mutations may have similar clinical presentation.

Clinical features:

- Renal:
  - Hematuria and proteinuria in first two decades of life; may progress to renal failure in second to third decade of life.
  - Females may be affected with increasing age even in X-linked forms (40% have ESRD by age 80 years)

TABLE 1 Genes causing inherited nephrotic syndrome.

Recessive gene (gene product)	Dominant gene
• *NPHS1* (nephrin)—Finnish variety • *NPHS2* (podocin) • *PLCE1* • *LAMB2* • *COQ6*	• *INF2* • *TRPC6* • *ACTN4* • *WT1*

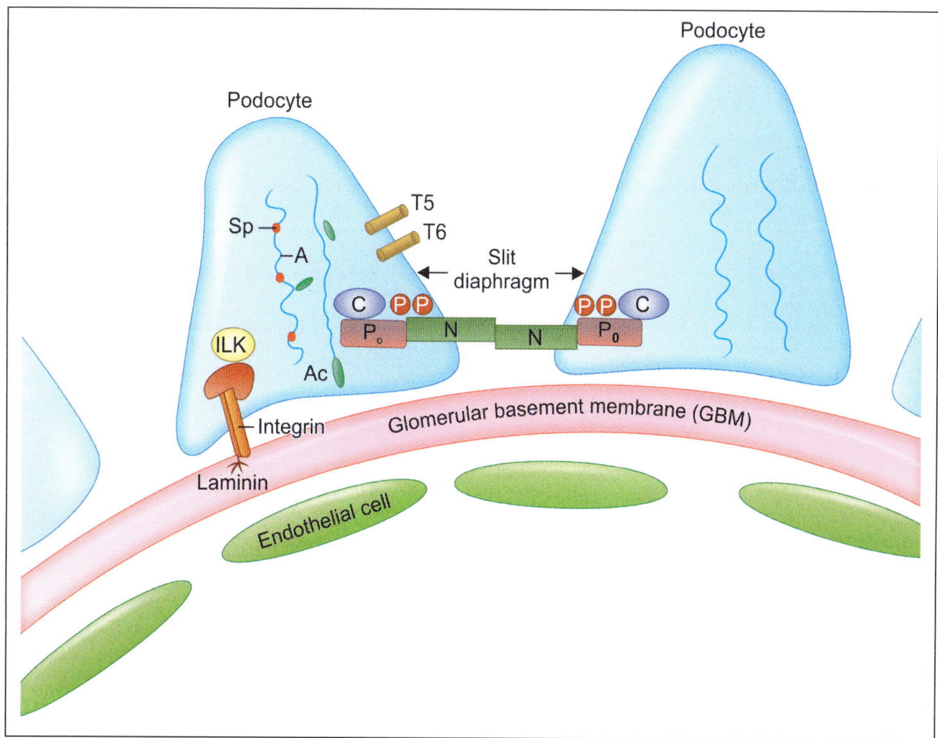

(A: actin; Ac: actinin; C: CD2-associated protein; ILK: integrin linked-kinase; N: nephrin; Po: podocin; P: phosphate; S: synaptopodin; T5: TRPC5; T6: TRPC6)

FIGURE 1: Podocyte structural proteins which may cause inherited nephrotic syndrome. The figure shows some important structural proteins which maintain podocyte structure. Mutation in any one of more than 52 genes encoding podocyte proteins may cause inherited nephrotic syndrome.

- Kidney biopsy—light microscopy shows focal segmental glomerulosclerosis (FSGS) in most patients, foam cells may be present.

  Electron microscopy is diagnostic with glomerular basement membrane (GBM) thinning, splitting, and lamellation with a "basket weave pattern."
- Auditory manifestations: High frequency hearing loss may be detected (by audiometry) in late adolescence or adulthood.
- Ocular lesions:
  - It may have anterior lenticonus and corneal vesicles (both detected by slit-lamp examination).
  - Macular flecks (detected on ophthalmoscopy)
- Hematological manifestations: Macrothrombocytopenia and leukocyte inclusions may occur in patients with *MYH9* mutation. Patients have similar clinical presentation as Alport syndrome with hereditary nephritis and sensorineural deafness in the absence of collagen IV mutations.

Treatment:
- Renin-angiotensin-aldosterone system (RAAS) blockade helps in delaying the progression to ESRD. ACE inhibitors should be started in all patients who are detected to have proteinuria.
- Ophthalmology and ear, nose, and throat (ENT) consultations should be taken.
- Renal transplantation is a viable option for patients. Careful donor selection should be done since females from the family might also be affected.
- Anti-GBM glomerulonephritis occurs rarely after transplantation since COL4A5 is perceived as a new antigen by the immune system.

Thin basement membrane disease: It is the most common cause of isolated persistent microhematuria in children and adults with a prevalence of 1–2%.

Genetics: Inheritance is AD with involvement of *COL4A3* or *COL4A4* (chromosome 2).

Clinical features:
- Generally presents as asymptomatic microscopic hematuria ± proteinuria; episodic macrohematuria may occur with upper respiratory tract infections.
- Overt proteinuria and hypertension (HT) occur in 30%. ESRD is rare.
- Kidney biopsy reveals thinning of GBM (<250 nm in adults) on electron microscopy. Light microscopy is unremarkable.

Treatment:
- Patients should be reassured that it is a benign disease.
- Blood pressure (BP) monitoring and urine analysis should be done every 1–2 years.

C3 glomerulopathy and atypical hemolytic uremic syndrome:

- Mutations in the various genes coding for alternate complement pathway proteins and their regulators may occur, inheritance is generally AR.
- Manifests either as a membranoproliferative glomerulonephritis with C3 deposits or as a thrombotic microangiopathy with hemolytic uremic syndrome (HUS).
- Treatment of C3 glomerulopathy is with RAAS blockers; steroids with mycophenolate may be needed in severe cases. Eculizumab is treatment of choice in atypical HUS.

CYSTIC DISORDERS

Autosomal dominant polycystic kidney disease:

- It is a multisystemic disorder with cyst formation in bilateral kidneys, liver, pancreas, and other organs.
- Prevalence is 1 in 400—1 in 1,000 live births.
- It is responsible for 2.6% cases of chronic kidney disease (CKD) in India (as per Indian CKD registry data).

Genetics:

- The genes implicated in ADPKD are:
  - PKD1 coding for polycystin 1 (16p13.3) in 78% cases
  - PKD2 coding for polycystin 2 (4q21) found in 7% cases
- Mutations in *GANAB* and *DNAJB11* also are responsible for ADPKD—like phenotype in a small percentage of patients.
- Inheritance is in an AD pattern.

Pathogenesis:

- Polycystins 1 and 2 are transmembrane proteins present in primary cilia and endoplasmic reticulum; involved in the detection of extracellular signals to primary cilia and in cell-to-cell contact.
- There is overactivation of cyclic adenosine monophosphate/protein kinase C (c-AMP/PKC) and mammalian target of rapamycin (mTOR) pathways in ADPKD leading to increased fluid secretion and cell proliferation resulting in cyst formation

Clinical features:

- Renal:
  - Bilateral renal enlargement with multiple diffuse bilateral renal cysts is pathognomonic of ADPKD. The number of cysts on each side increases with age and is rarely present in childhood and adolescence.
  - Polyuria due to impaired concentrating capacity
  - Cyst hemorrhage may be localized to cyst causing pain, or may cause gross hematuria.
  - Cyst infection may present with pyelonephritis-like features, urine culture may be negative, if infection is confined to the cyst.
  - Nephrolithiasis: It is present in 20% patients.
  - Pain: It may be due to cyst hemorrhage, infection, stones, or due to increase in cyst size.
  - Renal failure: With gradual replacement of functional renal parenchyma with cysts, there is drop in the glomerular filtration rate (GFR).

    End-stage renal disease develops in early in PKD 1 (Fifth to sixth decade) as compared to PKD 2 (seventh to eighth decade). A higher height-adjusted total kidney volume (htTKV) for age also predicts faster epidermal GFR (eGFR) decline.
- Hypertension:
  - It may be present in patients with normal renal function and in all patients with ESRD.
  - Compression of blood vessels by the enlarging cysts causes local activation of intra-renal RAAS and subsequent HT.
- Liver:
  - About 50–90% patients have multiple hepatic cysts.
  - Generally asymptomatic; may present with pain due to stretching of liver capsule or mass effect of cysts causing compression of nearby structures.
- Cysts in other organs: Pancreas, spleen, seminal vesicles, and meninges may have cysts.
- Vascular:
  - Intracranial aneurysms ("berry" aneurysms) may be present, more common in those with a family history of aneurysms.
  - Generally asymptomatic but may cause compression of adjacent structures causing cranial nerve palsies; may rupture to cause subarachnoid hemorrhage (SAH).
  - Risk factors for SAH include size >1 cm, family history of SAH and posterior circulation aneurysm.
  - Indications for screening for intracranial aneurysm:
    - A family history of aneurysm or SAH
    - Previous aneurysm rupture
    - Preparation for major elective surgery
    - High-risk occupations
- Cardiac: It may have mitral or aortic regurgitation.
- Other possible manifestations:
  - Colonic diverticulosis
  - Bronchiectasis

Diagnosis:

- The diagnosis of ADPKD in an individual with a positive family history primarily relies on imaging.
- The revised unified criteria for diagnosis of ADPKD by renal ultrasound are given in **Table 2**.
- Magnetic resonance imaging (MRI) or computed tomography (CT) scan (<5 cysts) may be used to definitely exclude disease in young patients.
- Genetic testing has a role in patients with equivocal imaging results, atypical cases, those with a negative family history or in cases where diagnosis at an early age is required as for living kidney donors.

TABLE 2 Revised ultrasound criteria for diagnosis of ADPKD.

Age (in years)	Criteria for diagnosis
15–39	≥3 cysts, unilateral or bilateral
40–59	≥2 cysts in each kidney
≥60	≥4 cysts in each kidney

(ADPKD: autosomal dominant polycystic kidney disease)

Treatment: All patients of ADPKD need to be monitored for cyst growth and for complications of the disease. TKV by MRI is a good marker to monitor cyst growth.

All patients should be treated with:

- Antihypertensives for BP control (RAAS blockers)—target BP ≤ 110/75 mm Hg (18–50 years)
- Restriction of sodium and caffeine intake
- Hydration to maintain low urine osmolality

Novel agents for ADPKD:

- Tolvaptan:
  - Recommended in patients with a rapid increase in TKV or rapid decline in eGFR
  - TEMPO 3:4 and REPRISE trials demonstrated the benefit in rate of eGFR decline in patients treated with tolvaptan.
  - Side effects include liver toxicity, hypernatremia, and hyperuricemia.
- Mammalian target of rapamycin inhibitors: Failed to show benefit in clinical trials despite encouraging results in animal models of PKD.
- Somatostatin analogs (lanreotide and octreotide): May decrease the rate of TKV increase but no effect on rate of eGFR decline.

End-stage renal disease:

- Dialysis—patients do better than other patients due to preserved hemoglobin concentration.
- Transplantation—modality of choice. Pretransplant native nephrectomy may occasionally be required. Careful donor selection needed to rule out ADPKD in related donors.

Intracranial aneurysms:

- Asymptomatic, <7 mm—no intervention, yearly monitoring of aneurysm size
- About 7–10 mm—surgical intervention based on location and prior history of SAH
- About >10 mm or symptomatic—coiling or clipping of aneurysm

  Complications like cyst infection, pain, renal stones, and cyst hemorrhage can be managed with medical ± surgical interventions, depending on the severity of involvement.

Other inherited cystic disorders of kidney: Other important inherited cystic disorders are summarized in **Table 3**. An approach to diagnosis of a patient with bilateral renal cysts has been summarized in **Flowchart 1**.

TABLE 3 Inherited cystic diseases of the kidney (excluding ADPKD).

	Autosomal dominant cystic kidney diseases (ADPKD excluded)				Autosomal recessive cystic kidney diseases	
	Von Hippel–Landau syndrome	**Tuberous sclerosis**	**Medullary sponge kidney**	**Autosomal dominant tubulointerstitial kidney disease**	**Autosomal recessive polycystic kidney disease**	**Nephronophthisis**
Age at presentation	Generally adults (30–40 years)	Older children Adults (10–30 years)	Adults (30–40 years)	Adults (30–60 years, variable)	Perinatal/ infancy	Three age groups of presentation: 1. Infantile 2. Juvenile 3. Adolescent
Site and type of cysts	Multiple cystic RCC	Few to multiple cysts, enlarged kidneys, and angiomyolipoma	Medullary	Small multiple cysts at corticomedullary junction	Multiple cortical + medullary, enlarged kidneys	• Biopsy reveals varying degrees of interstitial fibrosis and cysts at cortico-medullary junction • No visible cysts on gross examination
	Generally normal, may be impaired rarely	Normal	Normal	Impaired	Severely impaired	Impaired with chronic interstitial nephritis like presentation

Continued...

Continued...

	Autosomal dominant cystic kidney diseases (ADPKD excluded)				Autosomal recessive cystic kidney diseases	
Other renal manifestations			Multiple renal stones, recurrent UTI, renal tubular acidosis, and nephrocalcinosis	Hyperuricemia may be present		
Other organ manifestations	• Pheochromocytoma • Retinal and CNS hemangioblastoma	Facial angiofibroma, Café-au-lait macules, shagreen patch, retinal nodular hamartomas, and CNS cortical tubers (seizures, low IQ)	CAKUT or structural abnormalities of other organs	Gout (UMOD mutation) Maturity onset diabetes (HNF 1β)	Non-obstructive intrahepatic biliary duct dilatation, congenital hepatic fibrosis	• Retinitis pigmentosa (Senior–Loken syndrome) • Oculomotor apraxia (Cogan syndrome) • Cerebellar vermis aplasia (Joubert syndrome)
Gene and chromosome (*encoded protein*)	VHL—Chr 3p25 (*VHL protein*)	TSC1—Chr 9q34 (*tuberin*) TSC2—Chr 16p13 (*hamartin*)	RET—Chr 10q11 (*RET protein*) GDNF—Chr5p13 (*glial-derived neurotropic factor*) (May also be a sporadic illness)	MUC1—Chr 1q2 (*mucin*) UMOD—Chr16p12 (*uromodulin*) REN—Chr 1q32 (*renin*) HNF1β—Chr 17q12 (*hepatocyte nuclear factor 1β*)	PKHD1—Chr 6p21 (*fibrocystin*)	NPHP1—20—various chromosomes (*nephrocystins*)

(ADPKD: autosomal dominant polycystic kidney disease; CAKUT: congenital abnormalities of kidney or urinary tract; RCC: renal cell carcinoma)

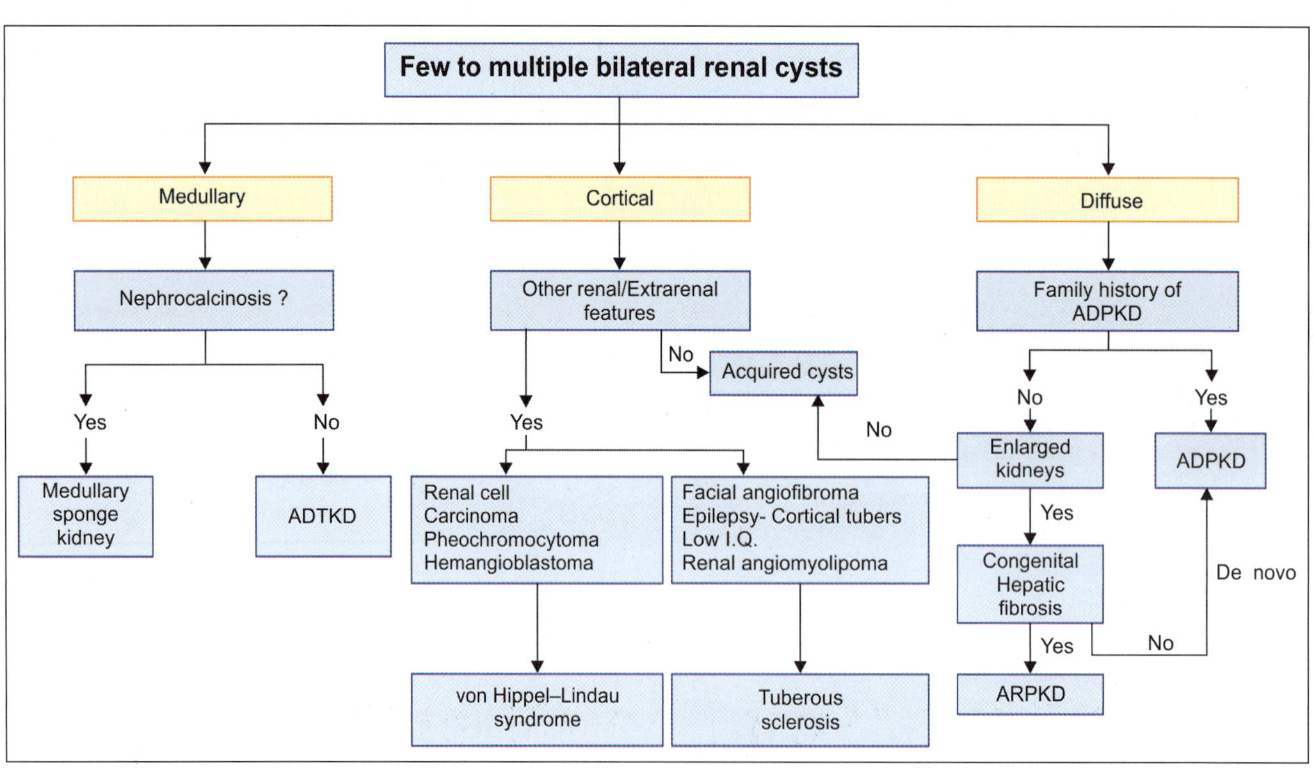

(ADTKD: autosomal dominant tubulointerstitial kidney disease; ADPKD: autosomal dominant polycystic kidney disease; ARPKD: autosomal recessive polycystic kidney disease; IQ: intelligence quotient)

FLOWCHART 1: Differential diagnosis of a patient with bilateral renal cysts.

Source: Adapted from Irazabal MV, Torres VE. Cystic diseases of the kidneys. In: Lerma EV, Sparks MA, Topf JM (Eds). Nephrology Secrets. Philadelphia: Elsevier; 2018.

RENAL TUBULAR FUNCTION ABNORMALITIES

Disorders of acid-base handling:

- Acid-base abnormalities with genetic basis include Fanconi syndrome, proximal RTA, and distal RTA.
- These abnormalities can also occur due to acquired causes including exposure to drugs, autoimmune diseases, and certain environmental exposures. Hence treatable causes should be ruled out before labeling a patient as a genetically inherited disease.

Table 4 lists the abnormalities in acid-base balance with their genetic basis and associations.

Disorder of sodium handling:

- This may include loss of function or gain of function mutation of genes encoding for sodium transport or handling. They may cause either HT or salt wasting/hypotension.

Table 5 showcases important monogenic disorders of sodium handling causing HT and **Table 6** describes important monogenic salt-wasting syndrome.

Figures 2 and **3** explain the pathophysiology of Bartter syndrome and Gitelman syndrome, respectively.

Disorder of phosphate handling—hypophosphatemic rickets:

- This is a disorder of renal phosphate wasting giving rise to vitamin D-resistant rickets.
- Inheritance is most commonly X-linked (*PHEX* gene) but may be AD or recessive.
- Laboratory findings include normal calcium, low phosphate, low-normal vitamin D levels, and high FGF-23 levels.
- Treatment is with phosphate and vitamin D supplements.
- Burosumab is the drug of choice for untreated X-linked hypophosphatemic rickets.

TABLE 4 Inherited acid-base abnormalities.

	Fanconi syndrome	Proximal RTA	Distal RTA
Inheritance	AR or X-linked	AR or AD	AR or AD
Protein defect	Generalized proximal tubular dysfunction	• Na-HCO_3 transporter • Carbonic anhydrase II	• Anion exchanger • H+ ATPase
Possible associations	• AR—cystinosis, tyrosinemia, galactosemia, and Wilson disease • X-linked—Lowe syndrome, Dent disease	• AR—ocular abnormalities (band keratopathy, cataract, and glaucoma), osteopetrosis, and cerebral calcification • AD—short stature, osteomalacia	Sensorineural deafness
Metabolic/ electrolyte defects	• Mild acidosis • Hypokalemia • Hypophosphatemia (rickets, osteomalacia) • Aminoaciduria • Renal glycosuria	• Metabolic acidosis (with urine pH < 5.5) • Hypokalemia • Bicarbonaturia	• Metabolic acidosis (with urine pH > 5.5) • Hypokalemia • Hypercalciuria • Nephrolithiasis
Treatment	• Treatment of primary disease • Alkali replacement • Potassium replacement • Vitamin D therapy	Alkali replacement	• Alkali replacement • ± Potassium replacement

(AD: autosomal dominant; AR: autosomal recessive; RTA: renal tubular acidosis)

TABLE 5 Monogenic forms of hypertension.

	Liddle syndrome	Glucocorticoid remediable aldosteronism	Syndrome of apparent mineralocorticoid excess
Inheritance	AD	AD	AR
Gene defect	ENaC	CYP11B1/CYP11B2	11β-hydroxysteroid dehydrogenase 2
Clinical features	• Hypertension • ↓Serum K, ↑HCO_3 • ↓Renin, ↓ Aldosterone	• Hypertension • ↓Serum K, ↑HCO_3 • ↓Renin, Normal or ↑Aldosterone • Urine 18-oxocortisol+, 18-hydroxycortisol +	• Hypertension • ↓Serum K, ↑HCO_3 • ↓Renin, ↓ Aldosterone • ↑Urinary cortisol/cortisone ratio
Treatment	ENaC inhibitors—amiloride and triamterene	Glucocorticoids	Spironolactone and ENaC inhibitors

(AD: autosomal dominant; AR: autosomal recessive; ENaC: epithelial sodium channel)s

TABLE 6 Monogenic salt-wasting syndromes.

	Bartter syndrome	Gitelman syndrome
Inheritance	AR/AD (type V)	AR
Site of defect	TAL of LOH	Distal convoluted tubule
Age of presentation and symptoms	• Antenatal/neonates • Polyhydramnios • Polyuria, polydipsia, failure to thrive, muscle cramps, and salt craving ± sensorineural deafness	• Adolescents • Often asymptomatic or with mild symptoms like muscle cramps • Incidental detection
BP and electrolyte abnormalities	• Low BP • ↑HCO_3, K↓, Mg normal/↓, urinary Ca↑	• Low BP • ↑HCO_3, K↓, Mg ↓↓, urinary Ca↓
Treatment	• Potassium supplementation • Aldosterone antagonist • NSAIDs	• Potassium supplementation • Magnesium supplementation
Tip to remember	Same effect as loop diuretics	Same effect as thiazide diuretics

(AD: autosomal dominant; AR: autosomal recessive; TAL: thick ascending limb; LOH: loop of Henle)

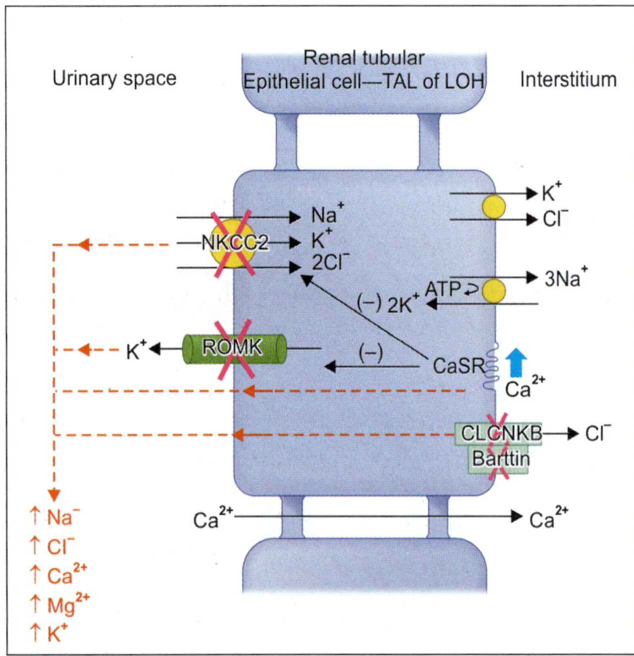

(NKCC2: Na-K-2Cl channel; ROMK: renal outer medullary potassium channel; CLCNKB: chloride channel; Barttin: subunit of CLCNKB, (-): inhibitory signal; X: protein with loss of function, ↑: protein with gain of function)

FIGURE 2: Bartter syndrome. It occurs due to mutations encoding proteins involved in sodium transport in the thick ascending limb of loop of Henle. Loss-of-function of NKCC2 (type I), ROMK (type II), CLCNKB (type III), Barttin (type IV), or a gain-of-function of calcium-sensing receptor (Type V) may cause Bartter syndrome. There is loss of sodium, potassium, chloride, magnesium, and calcium in urine.

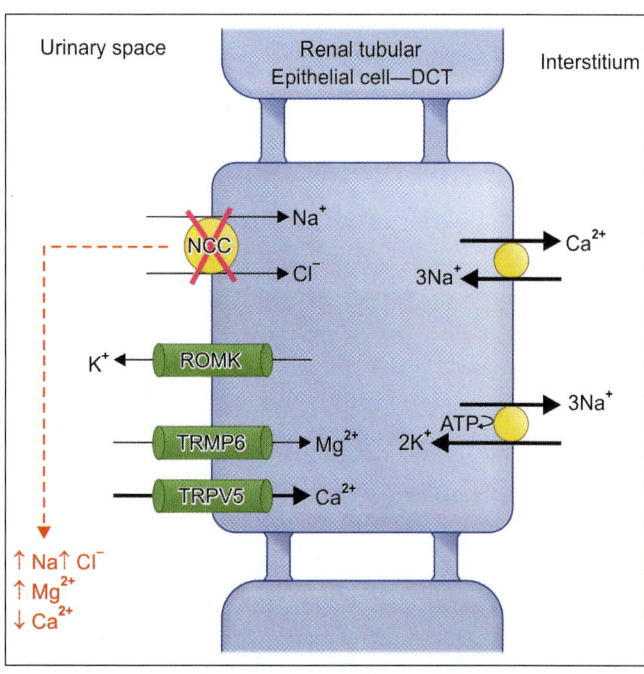

(NCC: sodium chloride cotransporter; ROMK: renal outer medullary K channels; TRMP6: magnesium channel; TRPV5: calcium channel; X: protein with loss of function)

FIGURE 3: Gitelman syndrome. It occurs due to mutation in the gene encoding Na-Cl cotransporter protein in the distal convoluted tubule. This leads to loss of sodium and chloride in urine, along with urinary magnesium wasting due to inhibition of TRMP6. Increased calcium reabsorption via TRPV5 channel and proximal tubular calcium reabsorption lead to hypocalciuria.

Disorder of water handling—nephrogenic diabetes insipidus:

- This is an X-linked/AR illness secondary to loss of function mutation of gene coding for aquaporin V2.
- Clinical features include early dehydration episodes, hypernatremia, and hyperthermia in the first few weeks of life.
- Early recognition with aggressive volume replacement can prevent complications.

OTHER SYSTEMIC MONOGENIC DISORDERS WITH RENAL MANIFESTATIONS

Sickle cell nephropathy:

- Autosomal recessive inheritance with mutation in gene coding for β chain of hemoglobin
- Red blood cell (RBC) sickling causes medullary hypoperfusion and ischemia.
- Renal manifestations may include polyuria, isosthenuria, proteinuria, secondary FSGS, and papillary necrosis.
- Treatment is with ACE inhibitor/ARB in those with proteinuria; hydroxyurea may have a role in prevention of disease.

Fabry disease nephropathy:

- X-linked mutation in GLA gene (encoding α-galactosidase)
- Glycolipid accumulation leads to microvascular involvement causing acroparesthesias, gastrointestinal symptoms, angiokeratomas in "bathing trunk" distribution and corneal dystrophy in adolescents and cardiac disease, kidney failure, and strokes in middle age.
- Renal involvement with proteinuria, tubular dysfunction, and renal biopsy shows "zebra bodies"; ESRD occurs in fourth to fifth decade.
- About 0.2% of males on hemodialysis have unrecognized Fabry disease.
- *Treatment*: Enzyme replacement therapy

Primary hyperoxaluria:

- Autosomal recessive inherited mutation in *AGXT* gene (type 1), *GRHPR* gene (type 2), and *HOGA* gene (Type 3)
- Type 1 is the most common type of hyperoxaluria (in 80% cases).
- Defect in hepatic peroxisomal glyoxylate metabolism due to a deficiency in alanine glyoxylate aminotransferase (type 1).
- Accumulation of oxalate may occur in various organs including kidneys (causing nephrocalcinosis and nephrolithiasis), joints, retina, heart etc.
- Patients may present with ESRD due to recurrent renal stones.
- *Diagnosis*: Typical clinical picture combined with high serum or urinary oxalate levels helps to clinch the diagnosis. Confirmatory diagnosis is made by estimation of enzyme activity on liver biopsy or by gene analysis.
- *Treatment*: Early treatment may be done with high dose pyridoxine which prevents oxalate deposition in kidney and other organs; in case of ESRD, a combined liver + kidney transplantation is warranted.

POLYGENIC DISORDERS

These consist of conditions which have polygenic susceptibilities with or without environmental influences playing a role in their pathogenesis.

It may consist of structural abnormalities like CAKUT or glomerular disorders like *APOL1* nephropathy, immunoglobulin A (IgA) nephropathy etc.

CONGENITAL ABNORMALITIES OF KIDNEY AND URINARY TRACT

- These are a group of structural malformations of the kidney and genitourinary tract present at birth.
- Congenital abnormality of the kidney and urinary tract is the most common cause of ESRD in pediatric population.

Genetics:

- More than 40 genes have been identified with a role in causing CAKUT (including HNF1B, PAX-2, RET, REN etc.).
- There is incomplete penetrance and significant phenotypic variability.
- Environmental factors (like maternal hyperglycemia and use of ACE inhibitors) also contribute to the pathogenesis of CAKUT.

Clinical features: CAKUT may be classified as follows:

- Aplasia (agenesis)
- Simple hypoplasia (decreased renal size and nephron number)
- Dysplasia ± cysts (malformation of tissue elements)
- Isolated dilatation of the renal pelvis ± ureters (collecting system)
- Anomalies of position (ectopic kidney and horseshoe kidney).

  Presentation may be at different age groups depending on severity and type of renal involvement.
- *In utero*: Detected on fetal ultrasonography incidentally or presenting as oligohydramnios
- *Perinatal*: Associated with pulmonary hypoplasia, posterior urethral valves (PUVs), and prune belly syndrome
- *Childhood and adolescence*: Recurrent UTI in cases of vesicoureteric reflux (VUR). Renal impairment may ensue. CAKUT-related ESRD frequently develops in second or third decade of life.
- *Adulthood*: Incidental detection on imaging (unilateral renal agenesis and horseshoe kidney)

Associated abnormalities of other systems include colorectal abnormalities leading to bowel dysfunction and spinal abnormalities (myelomeningocele).

Treatment:

- Treatment depends on the type of CAKUT.
- Corrective surgeries may be needed as in PUV (treated by transurethral resection or fulguration of valves), vesicoureteral reflux (VUR) (intraureteric dextranomer injection or ureteric reimplantation).
- Some like ureteric duplication, horseshoe kidney, and ectopic kidney may not require any treatment until complicated by either obstruction or progressive renal impairment.

APOL1 NEPHROPATHY

- Two variants of the *APOL1* gene (G1 and G2) have high prevalence in people of African descent.

- The presence of *APOL1* gene mutations predisposes carriers to a variety of renal diseases including FSGS, human immunodeficiency virus (HIV)-associated nephropathy, and HT-related ESRD, although the mutated gene in itself is not considered causative.
- Inheritance of two risk alleles further increases the risk of renal disease and hence it is said to be inherited in AR pattern.

CHROMOSOMAL DISORDERS

- Renal structural abnormalities are often found in aneuploidy, which refers to an abnormal gene dosage. This can be either in the form of whole chromosome trisomy/monosomy or partial monosomy/trisomy due to gene deletion/duplication.
- Syndromic features in the form of abnormal facial features, growth problems, birth defects, and developmental disabilities are often present. Such patients should be screened with an ultrasound for renal structural abnormalities.
- Some of the common chromosomal abnormalities with their renal defects are enlisted below:
  - *Trisomy 21 (Down syndrome)*: Hydronephrosis, multicystic kidneys, and renal agenesis
  - *Monosomy X (Turner syndrome)*: Horseshoe kidney and ureteral duplication
  - *Deletion7q11 (Williams syndrome)*: Asymmetric kidneys, solitary kidney, and reflux

GENETIC TESTING IN RENAL DISORDERS

- The role of genetic testing in renal diseases varies depending on the type of the disease.
- In families with a known mutation, genetic analysis may not be needed in each family member and diagnosis can often be made with typical phenotypic presentation. It may, however, be needed in cases with genotype-phenotype mismatch or atypical presentations, in living kidney donors for patients with known or suspected inherited renal disorder and for pregnancy counseling.
- Genetic testing may be done in various ways like single gene testing (e.g., ADPKD), gene panel testing (e.g., inherited nephrotic syndrome), or whole exome sequencing (undiagnosed disorder with broad differential diagnoses).

CONCLUSION

Inherited and congenital renal disorders are an important cause of ESRD in pediatric as well as adult population. A detailed history (including family history) and thorough examination often point towards a genetic basis of disease. Relevant radiologic, biochemical and genetic analyses help in clinching the diagnosis. Accurate diagnosis is important for management since many of these conditions have well-established targeted therapies.

RECOMMENDED READINGS

1. Mehta L, Jim B. Hereditary Renal Diseases. Semin Nephrol. 2017;37(4):354-61.
2. Kumar BH, Krishnamurthy S, Chandrasekaran V, Jindal B, Ananthakrishnan R. Clinical spectrum of congenital anomalies of kidney and urinary tract in children. Indian Pediatr. 2019;56(7):566-70.
3. Lipska-Ziętkiewicz BS, Ozaltin F, Hölttä T, Bockenhauer D, Bérody S, Levtchenko E, et al. Genetic aspects of congenital nephrotic syndrome: a consensus statement from the ERKNet-ESPN inherited glomerulopathy working group. Eur J Hum Genet. 2020;28(10):1368-78.
4. Chebib FT, Perrone RD, Chapman AB, Dahl NK, Harris PC, Mrug M, et al. A Practical guide for treatment of rapidly progressive ADPKD with tolvaptan. J Am Soc Nephrol. 2018;29(10):2458-70.
5. Irazabal MV, Torres VE. Cystic diseases of the kidneys. In: Lerma EV, Sparks MA, Topf JM (Eds). Nephrology Secrets. Philadelphia: Elsevier; 2018, pp. 293-306.
6. Bockenhauer D. Inherited disorders of sodium and water handling. In: Feehally J, Floege J, Tonelli M, Johnson RJ (Eds). Clinical Comprehensive Nephrology, 6th edition. Philadelphia: Elsevier; 2019, pp. 575-85.
7. Schlondorff J, Pollak MR. Inherited Disorders of the Glomerulus. In: Yu AS, Chertow GM, Luyckx VA, Marsden PA, Skorecki K, Taal MW, Wasser WG (Eds). Brenner and Rector's The Kidney, 11th edition. Philadelphia: Elsevier; 2020. pp. 1434-49.

CHAPTER 171

Systemic Diseases and Kidney

Manish Rathi, Arpita Ray Chaudhury

ABSTRACT

Kidney involvement in systemic diseases contributes significantly to the mortality and morbidity and also changes the treatment approach to the disease. This chapter covers three broad groups of diseases which commonly present with renal involvement: (1) Systemic vasculitis; (2) Dysproteinemia and kidney diseases; and (3) Autoimmune diseases. Last two decades of hard work from immunologists, renal pathologists, and clinicians in the field of nephrology, rheumatology, and hematology have added important insights into the pathogenesis and translation of those insights into treatment approach with clinical trials. Kidney Disease: Improving Global Outcomes (KDIGO) had reviewed the clinical trials from time to time and published updated treatment recommendation in 2020, which we have mostly picked up as treatment approach for most of the diseases. Due to space constraint, we have put lots of information in Flowcharts and Tables which are not repeated in the text and those should be considered as an important adjunct to the text.

"When suffering happens, it forces us to confront life in a different way than we normally do"

—Philip Yancey

INTRODUCTION

This chapter on systemic disorders and kidney attempts to update the clinical, laboratory, and histologic aspects of renal manifestations of several systemic disorders and to improve the diagnostic, prognostic, and the management skills of postgraduate trainees. The systemic disorders where renal involvement is important in diagnosing the disease early and in changing and guiding the therapy are discussed particularly highlighting the need to recognize the syndrome and build a clinically relevant differential diagnosis.

RENAL AND SYSTEMIC VASCULITIS

Many of these diseases have important renal manifestations that may present with proteinuria with or without hematuria, rapidly progressive glomerulonephritis (RPGN), and/or with acute kidney injury (AKI). Some of them have recent changes in diagnostic approach and change in management guidelines. We have followed updated KDIGO guidelines for disease management. We hope the summarized approach will make trainees more interested for additional reading.

Vasculitides can be classified as large vessel, medium vessel, and small vessel vasculitis and 2012 Chapel Hill Conference Consensus provided the standard nomenclature to be used unambiguously throughout the world (**Flowchart 1**). Large vessel vasculitis (Takayasu's disease) or medium vessel vasculitis (polyarteritis nodosa) may involve kidney, but most commonly and consistently kidneys are affected by small vessel vasculitis. Small vessel vasculitis encompasses a group of diseases characterized by necrotizing inflammation of small vessels (i.e., arterioles, capillaries, and venules) and little or no deposition of immune complexes in the vessel wall (pauci-immune). Occasionally, medium-sized vessel may be involved. Glomerular capillary involvement with these conditions manifests as pauci-immune focal and segmental necrotizing and crescentic glomerulonephritis (NCGN). Active pauci-immune small vessel vasculitis is typically associated with circulating antineutrophil cytoplasmic antibodies (ANCAs), and granulomatous with polyangiitis (GPA), microscopic polyangiitis (MPA), and eosinophilic granulomatosis with polyangiitis (EGPA) are three diseases included under antineutrophil cytoplasmic antibody (ANCA)-associated vasculitis (AAV).

ANTINEUTROPHIL CYTOPLASMIC ANTIBODY-ASSOCIATED VASCULITIS (TABLE 1)

The pauci-immune vasculitis is often associated with circulating ANCA, either myeloperoxidase (MPO)-ANCA or proteinase 3 (PR3)-ANCA depending on the target antigen. About 90% of patients with small vessel vasculitis or NCGN have ANCA, directed primarily to the neutrophil granule proteins MPO or PR3. 10% NCGN patients may be ANCA negative.

Microscopic polyangiitis, GPA, and renal limited pauci-immune crescentic glomerulonephritis all are associated with ANCA, involving kidney in >80% cases. EGPA is also a small vessel disease with low ANCA positivity and less renal involvement (20%) with eosinophilia in peripheral blood and asthmatic bronchopulmonary manifestations.

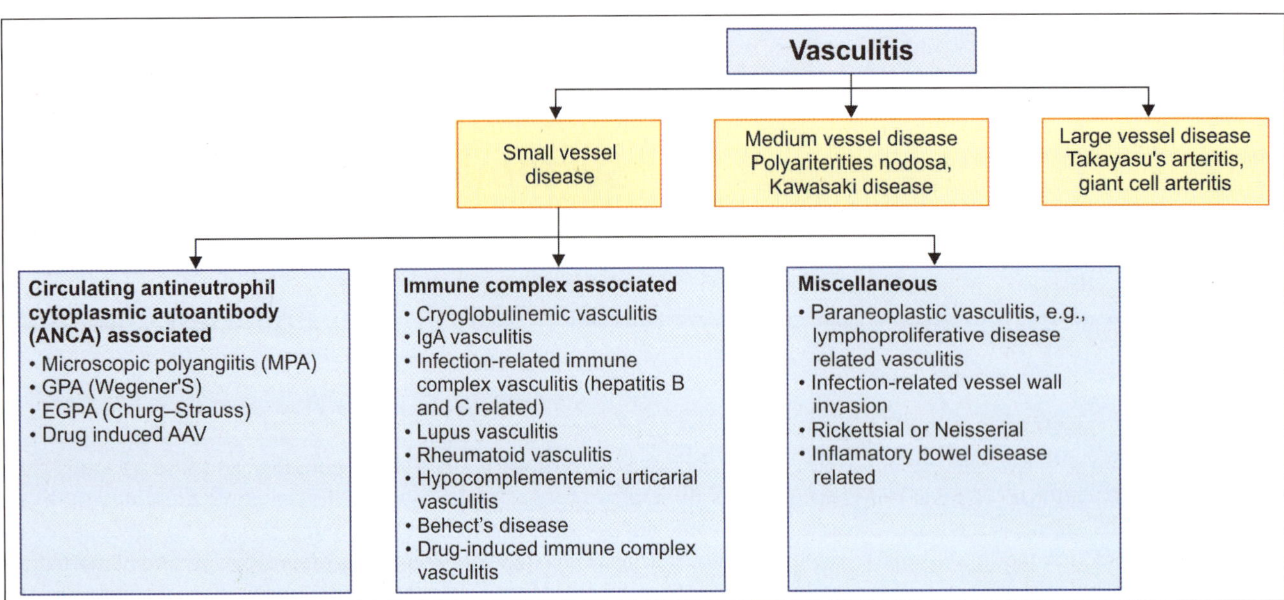

(AAV: antineutrophil cytoplasmic antibody-associated vasculitis; EGPA: eosinophilic granulomatosis with polyangiitis; GPA: granulomatous with polyangiitis)

FLOWCHART 1: Chapel Hill Consensus Conference 2012 classification of vasculitis.

TABLE 1 Definition and subclassification of ANCA vasculitis.

• Small vessel vasculitis • ANCA-associated small vessel vasculitis • Necrotizing vasculitis, with few or no immune deposits, predominantly affecting small vessels, capillaries, venules, arterioles, small arteries associated with MPO-ANCA, PR3-ANCA, and some patients even ANCA negative	
Microscopic polyangiitis (MPA)	Necrotizing inflammation of small vessels without granulomatous inflammation. Necrotizing GN is common and pulmonary capillaritis often occurs
Granulomatosis with polyangiitis (GPA)	Necrotizing inflammation of small vessels with granulomatous inflammation invading upper and lower respiratory tract, along with necrotizing GN
Eosinophilic granulomatosis with polyangiitis (EGPA)	Eosinophil rich necrotizing granulomatous inflammation of upper and lower respiratory tract. ANCA positive small percentage, when necrotizing GN is present. Associated with asthma and eosinophils

(ANCA: antineutrophil cytoplasmic antibody; GN: glomerulonephritis; MPO: myeloperoxidase; PR3: proteinase 3)

Clinical and experimental evidence suggests a pathogenesis driven by ANCA-induced activation of neutrophils and monocytes, followed by activation of alternative complement pathway leading to destructive necrotizing vascular and extravascular inflammation. The pathogenic transformation of naturally occurring autoantibodies might be triggered by commensal or pathogenic microbes, drugs, exogenous or endogenous autoantigen complementary peptides, or dysregulated autoantigen expression.

Diagnosis depends upon recognizing syndromic (RPGN) presentation and demonstration of ANCA in serum and confirmation by renal biopsy [both light microscopy LM) and immunofluorescence (IF)] (**Flowchart 2**).

The updated consensus statement about ANCA detection recommends (1) Antigen specific assay should be Elisa based , not indirect IF based (2) in patients with high clinical suspicion, a negative or weakly positive antigen-specific assay should be repeated and if still negative renal biopsy should be pursued to establish diagnosis.

Histology: Light microscopy usually reveals crescents in various stages; cellular, fibrous and fibrocellular, and varying degrees of tubulointerstitial scarring. IF adds by documenting few or no immune deposits in glomeruli or vessel wall (**Figs. 1 A** and **B**).

Diagnosis of relapses and monitoring: The persistence of ANCA positivity, an increase in ANCA levels, and a change in ANCA from negative to positive are only modestly predictive of future disease relapse and should not be used to guide treatment decisions. Therefore, monitoring includes regular screening for urinalysis, 24-hour urine protein or urine protein to creatinine ratio (UPCR), and renal function.

Outcome prediction and treatment decision cannot be accurately done either from type or titer of ANCA or from histopathologic scoring. There had been several attempts to attribute a renal risk score to guide treatment decision on the basis of focal (>50% normal glomeruli), crescentic (>50% cellular crescents), mixed (<50% normal glomeruli with no predominant lesion), and sclerotic class disease (>50% globally sclerosed glomeruli) which confirmed best and worst renal outcomes in focal and sclerotic class disease, respectively. Another risk scoring that incorporates. Both histopathologic (% of normal glomeruli,

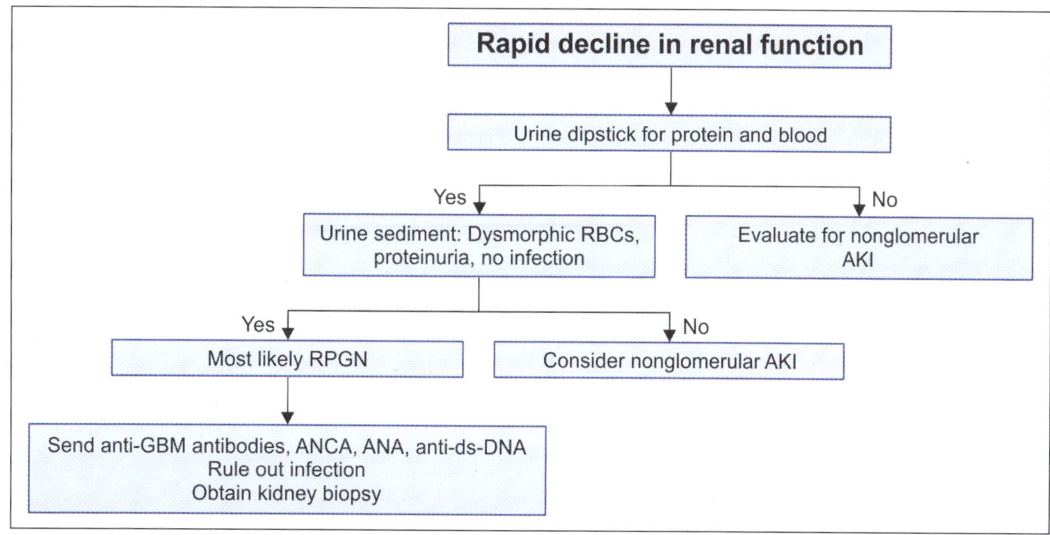

(ANCA: antineutrophil cytoplasmic antibody; ds-DNA: double-stranded deoxyribonucleic acid)

FLOWCHART 2: RPGN diagnostic workup.

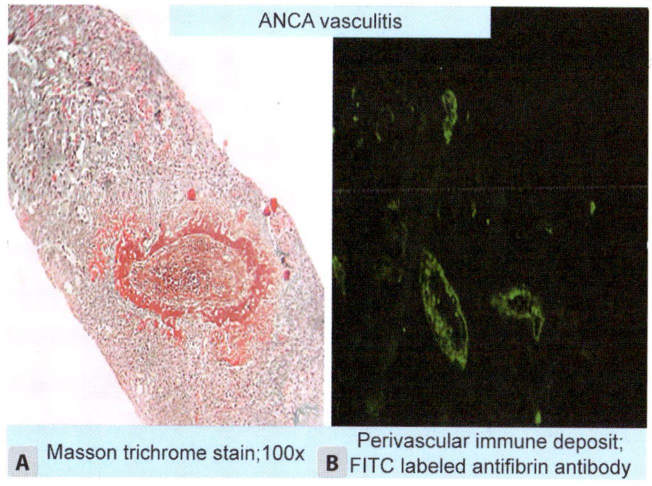

(ANCA: antineutrophil cytoplasmic antibody; FITC: fluorescein isothiocyanate; IF: immunofluorescence)

FIGURES 1 A & B: Crescent in ANCA vasculitis with significant interstitial fibrosis and tubular atrophy (IFTA). IF shows paucity of immune deposit with antifibrin antibody positivity.

% of interstitial fibrosis, and tubular atrophy) with clinical parameters [estimated glomerular filtration rate (eGFR) at diagnosis] has been attempted recently which looked at the end-stage kidney disease (ESKD) rates at the end of 3 years. The common observation of these prediction tools identifies *proportion of normal glomeruli in the kidney biopsy specimen as a strong predictor of long-term outcome.*

Clinical presentation (Table 2): The disease is common in middle aged and elderly. Indian patients manifest the disease at third or fourth decade, a decade earlier than Western cohort, without any male preponderance as reported in West. The renal presentation is usually a RPGN continuous decline in kidney function over weeks, ongoing proteinuria with the presence of dysmorphic red cells in the urine, and red cell casts. Generalized nonspecific symptoms attributable to systemic inflammations such as malaise and fever, myalgia and arthralgia, and anorexia and weight loss are often present. Other organ involvement signs and symptoms also may be present. The frequency of other organ involvement is useful to subclassify AAV and differentiate from other vasculitis (**Table 2**). Upper and lower airway involvement, which is most common in GPA and EGPA but also seen in MPA, manifests as cough and hemoptysis caused by necrotizing granulomatous inflammation of pulmonary tissue, which together with renal presentation becomes an important differential of pulmonary renal syndrome. In MPA and GPA, the patients may have alveolar capillaritis leading to diffuse alveolar hemorrhage (DAH), a severe manifestation of the disease.

Treatment (Tables 3 and 4): Antineutrophil cytoplasmic antibody vasculitis with GN is associated with very poor outcomes without therapy. Treatment with corticosteroids and cyclophosphamide (CYC) has dramatically improved the short- and long-term outcomes of ANCA vasculitis associated with systemic disease. Treatment with immunosuppressive therapy is indicated in all cases of ANCA vasculitis with or without renal involvement. The rare possible exception is the patients with severe kidney-limited disease, in the absence of extrarenal manifestations of small vessel vasculitis.

The treatment may be divided in two phases: (1) Remission induction therapy where high dose immunosuppressants are used to control severe disease activity for short period of initial 6–9 months; and (2) Maintenance therapy where long-term immunosuppression is used in relatively lower dose to decrease relapse risk and drug-related adverse effects. Maintenance therapy is recommended once the patient achieves remission, as the disease is characterized by relapses once immunosuppression is abruptly withdrawn. Remission is defined as normalization or stabilization of creatinine within 25% of the baseline

TABLE 2 Differences of organ system involvement in ANCA vasculitis subclassification.

Organ system involvement in small vessel vasculitis Frequency of involvement (%), frequency of ANCA positivity (%)			
	Microscopic polyangiitis (MPA)	Granulomatosis with polyangiitis (GPA)	Eosinophilic granulomatosis with polyangiitis (EGPA)
Kidney (RPGN and CKD)	90	90	20
Skin/cutaneous (purpura and nodule)	40	40	40
Lungs (hemoptysis and asthma)	50	90	90
Ear nose throat (otitis media, sinusitis, and subglottic stenosis)	35	90	70
Musculoskeletal (myalgia and arthralgia)	60	60	50
Neurologic (peripheral neuropathy)	30	50	40
Gastrointestinal (abdominal pain and bloody diarrhea)	50	50	40
ANCA positivity	• MPO-ANCA 50% • PR3-ANCA 40% • ANCA negative 10%	• PR3-ANCA 70% • MPO-ANCA 25% • ANCA negative 5%	• ANCA negative 55% • MPO-ANCA 40% • PR3-ANCA 5%

(ANCA: antineutrophil cytoplasmic antibody; CKD: chronic kidney disease; MPO: myeloperoxidase; PR3: proteinase 3; RPGN: rapidly progressive glomerulonephritis)

TABLE 3 Immunosuppressive drug dosing for AAV remission—induction.

Oral cyclophosphamide	Intravenous cyclophosphamide	Rituximab	Rituximab cyclophosphamide	MMF

• 2 mg/kg × 3 months
• If required up to 6 months
 	
• Reduction for age and GFR
  ◦ >60 years 1.5 mg/kg
  ◦ >70 years 1 mg/kg
  ◦ GFR < 30 mL/min reduce 0.5 mg/kg/day
	• 15 mg/kg (2, 4, and 6 weeks, then 9, 12, 15, 18, and 21 weeks, if required
	
	• Reduction for age GFR
	  ◦ >60 years 12.5 mg/kg
	  ◦ >70 years 10 mg/kg
	  ◦ GFR < 30 mL/min reduce 2.5 mg/kg/day
		• 375 mg/m^2 weekly × 4 weeks
		Or
		• 1 g/m^2 weekly × 2 weeks
			• 375 mg/m^2 weekly × 4 weeks and cyclophosphamide 15 mg/kg week 0 and 2
			Or
			• Rituximab 1 g/m^2 weekly × 2 weeks and IV cyclophosphamide 500 mg × 6 doses 2 weekly
				• 2,000 mg/day in divided doses may be increased up to 3,000 mg for poor response

(AAV: antineutrophil cytoplasmic antibody-associated vasculitis; GFR: glomerular filtration rate; IV: intravenous; MMF: mycophenolate mofetil g/day)

TABLE 4 Immunosuppressive drug dosing for AAV remission—maintenance.

Rituximab	Azathioprine	MMF
• 500 mg infusion at remission, then every 6 months three doses, 6, 12, and 18 months Or • 1,000 mg infusion at remission, then at 4, 8, 12, and 16 months	• 1.5–2 mg/kg at remission then for 1 year same dose, decrease 25 mg every 3 months up to 2 years Or • 1.5–2 mg/kg/day for 18–24 months, then 1 mg/kg up to 4 years then taper by 25 mg every 3 months	• 2,000 mg/day at remission in divided doses for 2 years

(AAV: antineutrophil cytoplasmic antibody-associated vasculitis; MMF: mycophenolate mofetil)

value and absence of dysmorphic hematuria along with decline of proteinuria.

Early initiation of immunosuppressives is associated with better outcome, particularly with RPGN presentation, so treatment should be initiated in appropriate clinical presentation with MPO/PR3-ANCA positivity without waiting for biopsy.

Remission induction therapy includes use of high-dose glucocorticoids with intravenous (IV) CYC or rituximab. The addition of CYC to corticosteroids in induction therapy improved the remission rate from about 55% to about 85%, and decreased the relapse rate 3-fold.

The optimum dose, route of administration, and duration of CYC treatment were well studied in a long-term study by the European Vasculitis Society (EUVAS) investigators; pulsed IV regimens are equivalent to daily oral treatment for initial disease control and are associated with lower incidence of adverse events such as leukopenia, though at the potential cost of increased relapse risk during long-term follow-up.

Rituximab is preferred in children, adolescents, females, and males with concern about fertility, and in relapsing disease particularly with PR3 positivity, while CYC is a choice in severe GN (serum creatinine > 350 mmol at diagnosis) with or without lung hemorrhage and in patients with cost concern (**Table 4**). Rituximab failed to decrease adverse effects, so induction with mycophenolate mofetil (MMF) was also attempted in patients without severe disease. Mycophenolate, though noninferior to induce remission, failed to decrease adverse events in comparison with CYC and was associated with more relapses. So mycophenolate may be considered as a choice in nonorgan-threatening disease or MPO-ANCA positive disease with low risk for relapse. Addition of plasmapheresis to standard immunosuppressive regimen in AAV with RPGN presentation with or without DAH was being practiced with benefit of reducing ESKD in long term, with low quality. The recently reported PEXIVAS trial concluded a trend towards benefit in patients with severe lung hemorrhage, not in ESKD reduction. It may have a place in refractory disease or patients intolerant to other therapies.

Glucocorticoids are very important adjunct to therapy to improve outcome, but also increases the risk of infection. Early tapering of steroid may reduce the sepsis-related serious adverse events while maintaining efficacy compared to high-dose steroids. Newer treatment includes trials with C5a inhibitor avacopan which may have a steroid-sparing role.

Remission maintenance therapy is used to prevent relapse and ESKD in long term, using reduced dose steroid and an additional immunosuppressive agent for an extended period. After CYC-based induction, azathioprine has been used as standard therapy and proved to be superior to MMF maintenance. Exact duration of maintenance therapy is not defined, but 4 years maintenance is associated with less relapse and lesser ESKD progression compared to 2 years maintenance therapy.

Rituximab (500 mg every 6 months for 3–4 doses) has become a new option for maintenance. When compared to azathioprine 2 mg/kg/day regimen, rituximab is proved to be more effective and superior to azathioprine in maintaining remission. Whether fixed dose rituximab or tailored dose based on CD19 cell count or ANCA monitoring will be better for relapse-free remission and better outcome is not yet decided. Rituximab may be a choice for older frail people, patients intolerant to azathioprine, and in relapsing PR3 positive disease.

Treatment of refractory disease may include plasmapheresis and higher dose of glucocorticoids in addition to IV CYC.

Prophylaxis for treatment complications: Cotrimoxazole is used daily single dose for prevention of *Pneumocystis jiroveci*. Oral antifungal lozenges or rinse and nasal mupirocin to decrease staphylococcal carrier state may reduce relapse risk.

Patients who progress to ESKD may undergo renal transplantation at least 6 months after disease remission. Persistence of ANCA should not delay transplantation. The relapse rate is 0.02–0.03 per patient year and is not influenced by presence of ANCA at the time of transplantation.

ANTI-GLOMERULAR BASEMENT MEMBRANE DISEASE

Anti-glomerular basement membrane (anti-GBM) disease is a rare small vessel vasculitis that affects the capillary beds of the kidneys and lungs. Several terminologies associated with this disease involving lung and kidney remain confusing to students, which have been described in **Table 5**. The disease is well recognized in Asian population, rare in Africans, and in Europe incidence is about 1.6 in 1 million.

TABLE 5 Terminologies important in relation to anti-GBM disease.

Term	Definition	Mechanism and diseases
Pulmonary renal syndrome	Renal and respiratory failure	Causes of Goodpasture syndrome and nonimmune causes such as pulmonary edema, cardiorenal syndrome, infectious causes like hantavirus infection
Goodpasture syndrome	RPGN and alveolar hemorrhage	ANCA vasculitis, lupus nephritis, catastrophic APLA syndrome, IgA vasculitis, HSP, rheumatoid vasculitis, and cryoglobulinemia
Anti-GBM disease	Disease associated with antibodies specific for GBM any component	Example is Alport patients developing antibodies to components of GBM
Goodpasture disease	Disease associated with antibodies specific for GBM alpha 3(IV)/NC1 domain	May cause lung hemorrhage, RPGN, or both, autoimmunity to the specific alpha 3(IV)/NC1
Alport syndrome post-transplant anti-GBM disease	Disease associated with anti-GBM antibodies developed in Alport syndrome patients after transplantation	Immunity to foreign antigen of donor GBM, usually alpha 3/5 collagen IV NC1 domain

(APLA: antiphospholipid antibody; HSP: Henoch–Schönlein purpura; IgA: immunoglobulin A)

It is a model autoimmune disease, being characterized by the presence of directly pathogenic autoantibodies directed against antigens in the NC1 domains of collagen IV in the glomerular and alveolar basement membranes. The recent observation of spatial and temporal clustering of cases suggests that environmental factors, including infection, may trigger disease in genetically susceptible individuals [inheritance of human leukocyte antigen (HLA)-DR15 is consistently associated with disease susceptibility, whereas HLR-DR1, -DR7, and -DR9 are negatively associated with disease risk]. Anti-GBM disease with pulmonary involvement is more frequent in men (about 80%) and typically occurs during the second decade. Anti-GBM GN may present either as an isolated kidney disease or as a pulmonary-renal syndrome (Goodpasture disease). If untreated, anti-GBM disease has very high morbidity with almost all patients progressing to ESKD and can have significant mortality. In patients with Goodpasture syndrome, mortality rate was 96% before the introduction of immunosuppression and 47% despite being treated with immunosuppression. The cornerstone of the treatment is rapid removal of the pathogenic autoantibodies and suppression of their production to prevent further kidney and pulmonary injury.

Clinically the disease presents as rapidly progressive crescentic GN and about 80% of patients have crescents in half or more of their glomeruli. In patients who present with a suspected RPGN and lung hemorrhage, serologic testing for the presence of anti-GBM antibodies should be done urgently using commercially available enzyme-linked immunoassays (**Flowchart 3**). The immunoassays for anti-GBM antibodies may be negative in up to 10% of patients, and in these individuals, diagnosis may be established only by kidney biopsy demonstrating linear immunoglobulin G (IgG) deposition along the GBM. Diagnosis of diffuse alveolar hemorrhage is usually suspected clinically and confirmed by the high-resolution computed tomography (CT) scans. Bronchoscopy may demonstrate hemosiderin filled macrophages and telltale sign of alveolar hemorrhage, but are often unnecessary and may be difficult to perform in critically ill and unstable patients. Diagnosis should be made without delay and kidney biopsy findings (**Figs. 2 A to D**) should be reported to the clinician by the pathologist on the day of the biopsy.

Current treatment guidelines recommend that in patients with alveolar hemorrhage or crescentic GN with <100% crescents on the kidney biopsy specimen, anti-GBM disease should be treated with plasma exchange, cytotoxic immunosuppression, and glucocorticoids. As it is a rare disease, controlled studies are not available. Observational studies show that it is effective when initiated before the onset of anuric and/or dialysis-dependent renal failure. The rationale for therapy is to clear, the existing antibodies by plasmapheresis to prevent tissue injury and to suppress formation of autoantibodies using CYC and using steroid as an effective agent for reducing tissue inflammation. KDIGO guidelines suggest that in the absence of lung hemorrhage, when 100% of glomeruli on the kidney biopsy specimen are affected by crescent formation, recovery from dialysis is so unlikely that treatment is unlikely and there may be withheld. Two large observational French studies have documented beneficial role of plasmapheresis, high-dose steroids, and oral CYC in severe anti-GBM disease with favorable 1-year and 5-year patient survival, age >60 years and number of plasma exchanges (eight sessions was the cutoff number for 95% positive predictive value for survival) correlated with overall survival after multivariate analysis. Serum creatinine > 5.6 mg/dL at diagnosis was predictive of dialysis dependence. Optimum route of CYC IV versus oral showed therapeutic equivalence (**Table 6**).

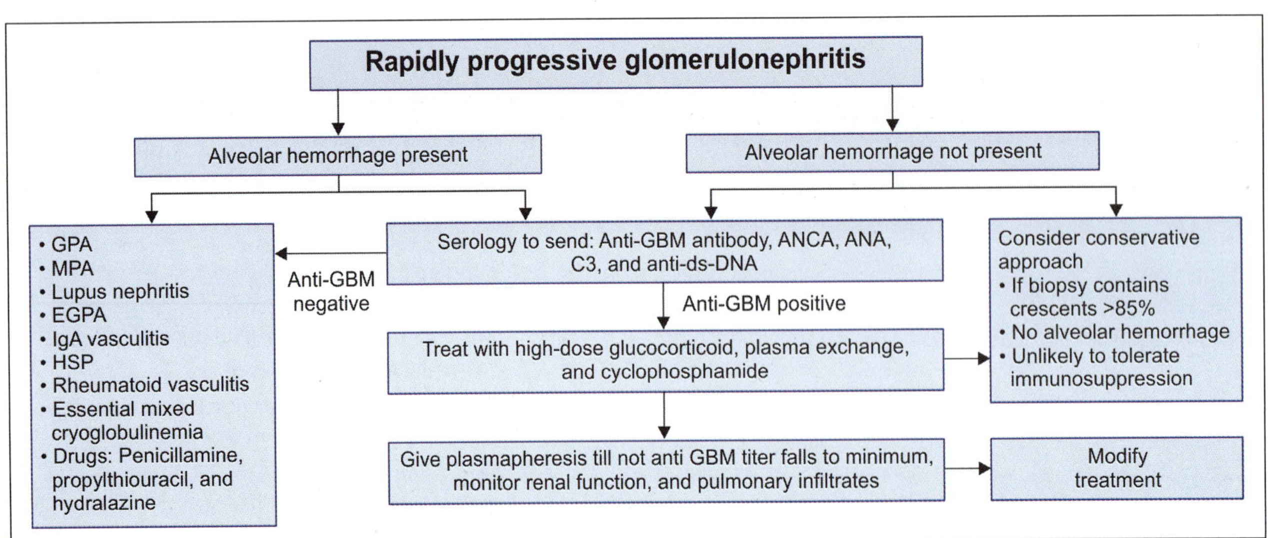

(EGPA: eosinophilic granulomatosis with polyangiitis; GPA: granulomatous with polyangiitis; HSP: Henoch–Schönlein purpura; IgA: immunoglobulin A; MPA: microscopic polyangiitis)

FLOWCHART 3: Pulmonary renal syndrome workup.

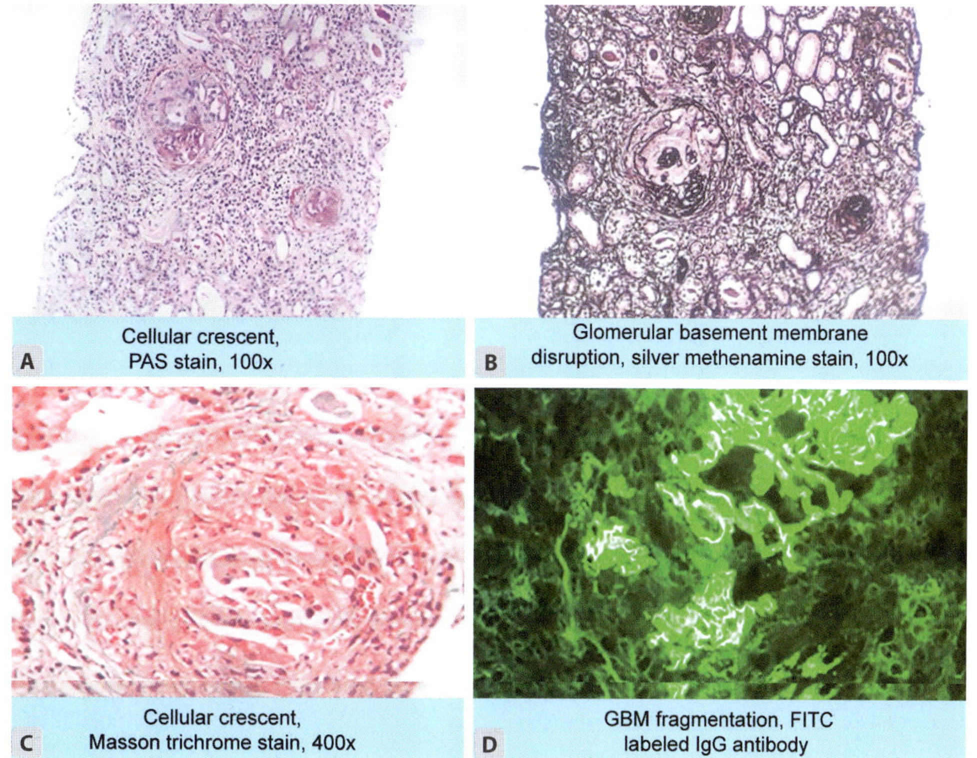

(FITC: fluorescein isothiocyanate; IF: immunofluorescence; IgG: immunoglobulin G; PAS: periodic acid–Schiff)

FIGURES 2 A to D: Anti-glomerular basement membrane (GBM) disease: Upper panel shows cellular crescent in PAS and silver stain with silver stain highlighting disruption of GBM. Masson's trichrome shows the same crescent without any fibrous change. IF shows ruptured basement with IgG deposition.

TABLE 6 Treatment of anti-GBM disease.

Intervention	Dosing	Duration
Plasmapheresis	40–50 mL/kg of ideal body weight to be removed daily against 5% albumin FFP to be added after PP in patients with DAH or after kidney biopsy	Until circulating anti-GBM antibody become negative usually 14 days
Cyclophosphamide	• 2–3 mg/kg orally per day (2 mg/kg in people >55 years of age) • Experience with IV cyclophosphamide limited • Experience with rituximab or MMF in patients not tolerating cyclophosphamide limited	For 3 months
Glucocorticoids	• Pulse methylprednisolone 1,000 mg/day × 3 days • Then 1 mg/kg/day • Reduce to 20 mg/day by 6 weeks	For 6 months

(DAH: diffuse alveolar hemorrhage; FFP: fresh frozen plasma; GBM: glomerular basement membrane; IV: intravenous)

Electively not to treat decision is taken if there is oliguric renal failure with >85% crescents on biopsy, no alveolar hemorrhage, or risk of immunosuppression is high in the individual.

The poor kidney outcome in patients presenting with dialysis-dependent renal failure highlights the need for more rapid and effective treatments in anti-GBM disease. In a murine model of anti-GBM disease, IgG-degrading enzyme of *Streptococcus pyogenes* (IdeS) treatment reduced glomerular inflammatory cell infiltration and albuminuria. It may come up as effective therapy as it is an endopeptidase which cleaves all IgG subclasses and has potential anti-inflammatory action.

DOUBLE POSITIVE DISEASE

It is well recognized that anti-GBM disease may coexist with ANCA, particularly MPO-ANCA. Some studies have suggested better outcome in double positive diseases while others have shown similar outcome. A recently published multicenter European study comparing double positive patients with isolated anti-GBM disease and AAV have documented important observations: (1) Double positive patients mostly presented with severe disease (dialysis dependent and pulmonary hemorrhage) features of anti-GBM disease, but had trend towards recovery of renal function more like AAV; and (2) Long-term follow-up showed that they have relapse like AAV, which no single positive anti-GBM patient did have.

DYSPROTEINEMIA AND KIDNEY INVOLVEMENT DISEASES

These diseases are caused by clonal expansion of plasma cells and B cells with deposition of nephrotoxic monoclonal immunoglobulins or their components secreted by these cells in glomerulus and tubulointerstitium of the kidney. The glomerular capillaries are a favorite site for abnormal misfolded and aggregated protein as happens in amyloidosis. The clonal expansion may meet the criteria of overt hematologic (multiple myeloma plasma cells) or lymphoblastic (systemic lymphoma, lymphoplasmacytic lymphoma, and B cells) malignancy or may not meet the criteria of malignancy-related complications. When renal biopsy reveals kidney lesions but they do not meet tumor definition criteria or tumor complications are absent, they are classified as monoclonal gammopathy of renal significance (MGRS).

The *diagnosis of dysproteinemic kidney disease* is picked up by kidney biopsy (**Figs. 3 A** to **D**) that demonstrates injury caused directly (i.e., *with evidence of monotypic staining on IF microscopy*) or indirectly by the monoclonal immunoglobulin. Hematologic evaluation involves measuring paraprotein levels in the serum [by serum protein electrophoresis, serum immunofixation, and serum k-l free light chain (FLC) assay] and urine (by urine immunofixation and urine protein electrophoresis), and bone marrow biopsy is often required to diagnose the underlying clonal cell process. Additional studies are peripheral blood flow cytometry and radiologic imaging. Both the conditions are associated with significant mortality and morbidity (**Flowchart 4**).

The renal and extrarenal features of various dysproteinemic diseases have been summarized in **Table 7**, along with the diagnostic measures to detect the underlying paraprotein and/or the clone. While light chain cast nephropathy is a myeloma-defining condition and definitely mandates oncotherapy, many other renal limited dysproteinemia with monoclonal gammopathy needs clone-directed therapy because if the patient progresses to renal failure, untreated the disease may recur after transplantation, and even renal deterioration may be stabilized with therapy. The diagnostic approach starting from LM, IF, and electron microscopy along with tests to identify the clone or paraprotein behind has been shown in **Flowchart 4**. Some lesions such as light chain cast nephropathy, amyloidosis associated with monoclonal immune globulin deposition, monoclonal immunoglobulin deposition (MID) disease, and light chain proximal tubulopathy have higher likelihood of (a rate of 90–100%) paraprotein detection as well as clone detection, whereas proliferative GN with monoclonal immunoglobulin deposition (PGN-MID) is associated with 40–60% chances of clone or paraprotein detection.

For cast nephropathy, therapy is directed to rapid lowering of FLC level within 21 days with bortezomib-based regimen and various forms of extracorporeal therapies have

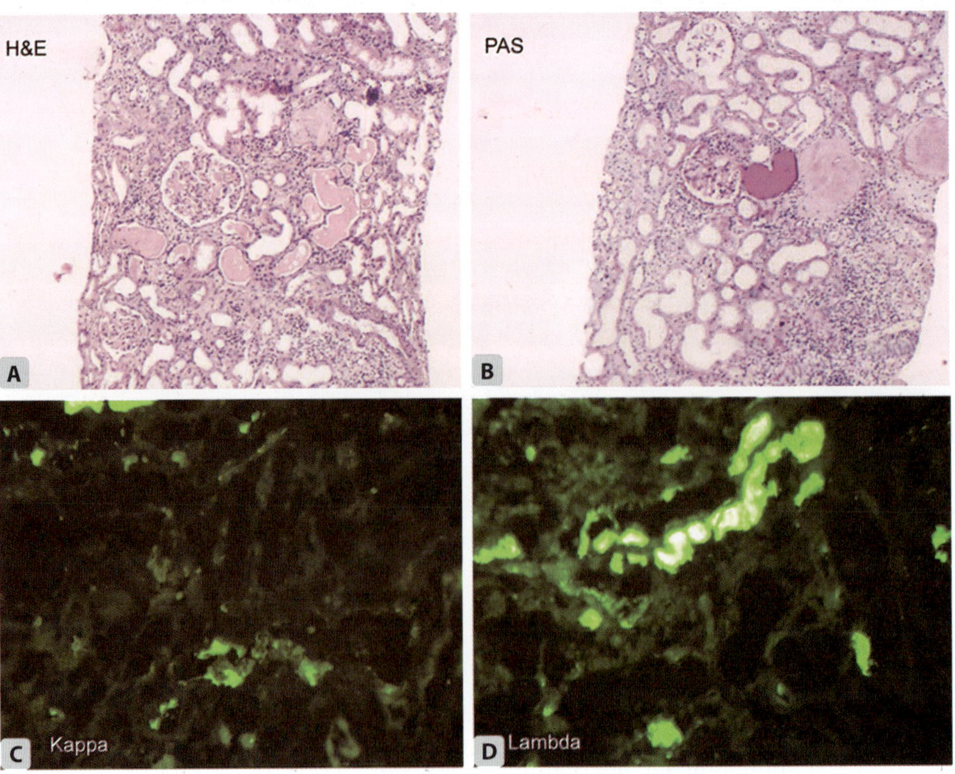

(H&E: hematoxylin and eosin; PAS: periodic acid–Schiff)

FIGURES 3 A to D: Light chain cast nephropathy. The upper panel shows fractured cast in tubules and tubulointerstitial cell infiltration in light microscopy; where lower panel of immunofluorescence shows restriction of kappa light chain with monotypic staining for lambda.

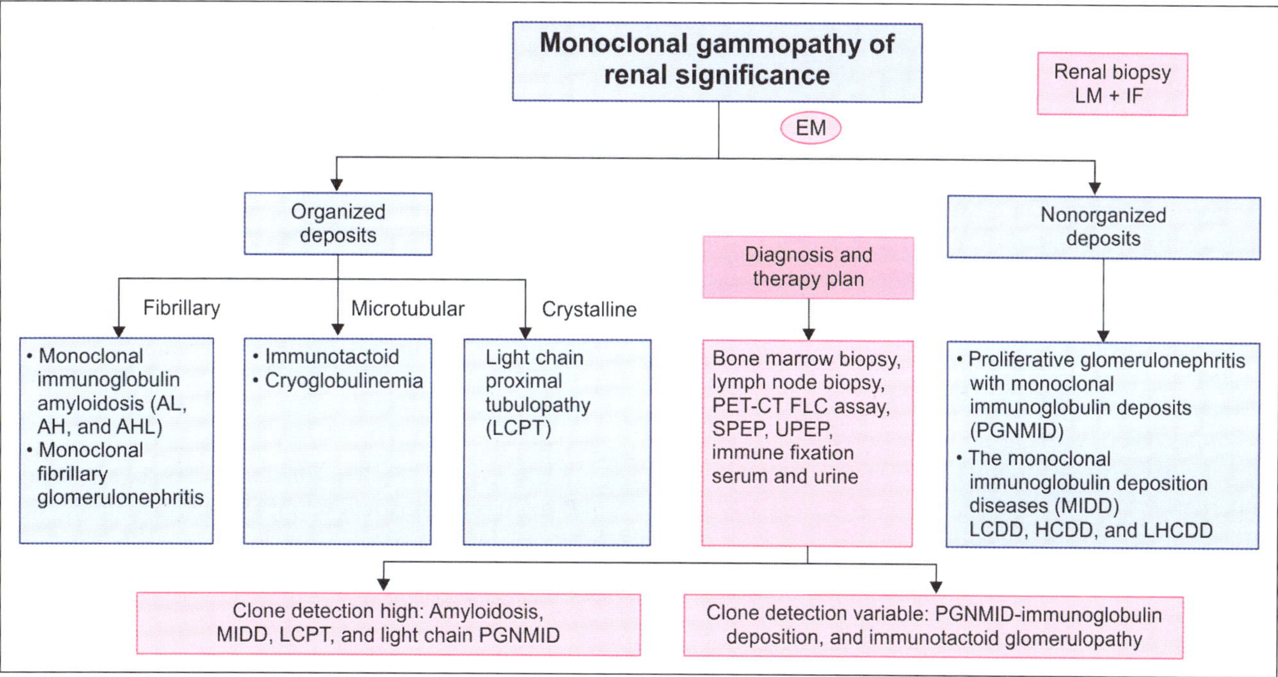

Note:
- Blue box shows International Kidney and Monoclonal Gammopathy Research Group classification of MGRS lesions
- Pink box shows work up and therapy plan

(EM: electron microscopy; FLC: free light chain; IF: immunofluorescence; HCDD: heavy chain deposition disease; LCDD: light chain deposition disease; LHCDD: light and heavy chain deposition disease; LM: light microscopy; SPEP: serum protein electrophoresis; UPEP: urine protein electrophoresis)

FLOWCHART 4: International Kidney and Monoclonal Gammopathy Research Group classification of MGRS lesions.

TABLE 7 The three common deposition diseases with dysproteinemia.

Disease	Syndromic renal involvement	Extrarenal signs	Diagnosis	Renal biopsy
Light chain cast nephropathy	• Acute kidney injury and nonalbumin proteinuria • In few, slowly progressive CKD	• Myeloma defining condition Coexistent anemia bone pain Mimicker of CKD	• SPEP, serum and urine immunofixation, and FLC assay • Bone marrow and renal biopsy	• Brightly eosinophilic fracture cast in distal tubule associated tubulointerstitial nephritis
Amyloidosis due to immunoglobulin deposit	• Nephrotic syndrome with or without renal dysfunction	• Purpura and anemia, organomegaly, and macroglossia	• SPEP, serum and urine immunofixation, and FLC assay • Bone marrow and renal biopsy and fat pad biopsy	• Eosinophilic deposits that stains poorly with PAS and silver • Congo red positive and apple green birefringence on polarized microscopy EM may identify typical amyloid fibril
Monoclonal immune deposition disease	• Subnephrotic nephrotic proteinuria, decreased renal function, progression to renal failure, 60–80% have monoclonal gammopathy of renal significance (MGRS), bone marrow fails to show >10% plasma cells	• 20% may have overt myeloma	• As mostly renal limited, renal biopsy is the key pointer. SPEP, serum and urine immunofixation, and FLC assay • Bone marrow	• Immunofluorescence showing monoclonal light chain restriction is the diagnostic feature. EM shows

(FLC: free light chain; PAS: periodic acid–Schiff; SPEP: serum protein electrophoresis) been attempted to immediately lower FLC level such as high-cutoff hemodialysis and plasmapheresis, but none have been able to gain universal recommendation. While bortezomib along with other drugs remain an option of therapy for plasma cell clone, for lymphoid clone rituximab remains the preferred choice. Standard initial antiplasma cell therapy is three-drug therapy, usually including a proteasome inhibitor (bortezomib or carfilzomib), high-dose steroids (usually dexamethasone), and a third agent CYC, thalidomide, lenalidomide, or the anti-CD38 antibody daratumumab).

MYELOMA AND KIDNEY (TABLE 8)

Myeloma is characterized by neoplastic proliferation of plasma cells producing monoclonal immunoglobulin, which in 95% cases includes an excess of light chain component, which can be nephrotoxic. Various causes and manifestations of AKI may happen with myeloma, but the most common is light chain cast nephropathy. The other causes are given in **Table 7**. Detailed discussion is beyond the scope of this article, but two important issues: (1) Presence of bone pain and anemia, which are two cardinal features of myeloma are also present in chronic kidney disease (CKD) sometimes with coexistent background of diabetes, hypertension (as it is a disease of elderly myeloma may mimic CKD, so a high index of suspicion is required; and (2) Light chain cast nephropathy or hypercalcemia is acute medical emergency which if intervened rightly may prevent CKD progression with bortezomib-based triple drug therapy outcome is much better than before. So early diagnosis and appropriate intervention remains determine patient and organ survival.

RHEUMATIC DISEASES ASSOCIATED WITH RENAL INVOLVEMENT

Many collagen disorders may be complicated with renal involvement. Awareness about these may be useful in diagnosis, in guidance of drug choice, and for treating complications of disease itself and therapy. The diseases are:

- Systemic lupus erythematosus (SLE)
- *Rheumatoid arthritis (RA)*: Both disease and therapy may cause renal injury
- *Mixed connective tissue disease*: Membranous and mesangioproliferative glomerulonephritis (MesPGN)
- *Rheumatic fever*: Renal infarct and diffuse PGN
- Ankylosing spondylitis and seronegative arthropathy
- *Scleroderma*: Vascular injury
- *Sjögren's syndrome*: Tubulointerstitial injury

SYSTEMIC LUPUS ERYTHEMATOSUS

Systemic lupus erythematosus is the prototypic autoimmune disease that has potential to involve multiple organ systems of the body with kidneys being one of the most common to get affected. Though the exact prevalence of SLE in India is not known, studies have reported that the prevalence varies from 30 to 50 in Asians to 200 in Blacks per 100,000 population. The incidence of renal involvement is also highly variable depending on the population studied (Asians 33–55%; African-Americans 34–51%; Hispanics 31–43%; and Caucasians 14–23%) and the criteria used for diagnosis. As much as 60% subjects can have overt renal manifestations at the time of diagnosis of SLE, while about 20% cases present with only renal involvement. The glomerular compartment is the most frequently involved, though the disease can involve the tubulointerstitium and blood vessels as well. Just like the pathogenesis of SLE, the exact causation of lupus nephritis (LN) is not clearly established. Majority of researchers implicate the role of autoantibodies and subsequent formation of immune complexes against a number of antigens [e.g., double-stranded deoxyribonucleic acid (ds-DNA)]. The immune complexes can be formed either in the circulation or inside the glomeruli. These immune complexes subsequently cause complement-mediated damage to the kidneys. Various other mechanisms have also been proposed, however the immune complex-mediated damage is the widely accepted pathogenetic mechanism.

Clinical manifestations: The clinical manifestations of LN are quite variable. Various clinical manifestations of LN include asymptomatic urinary abnormalities, subnephrotic proteinuria, nephrotic-range proteinuria, nephritis syndrome, and rapidly progressive renal failure. A high index of suspicion is required to identify the renal involvement

TABLE 8 Causes of renal injury and clinical manifestations in myeloma.

	Mechanism	Causes	Clinical manifestations
Prerenal	• Volume depletion Hemodynamic Others	• Hypercalcemia • Nausea • Vomiting • Sepsis • Drugs • Hyperviscosity • Hyperuricemia	• Altered sensorium • Nausea vomiting • Polyuria and polydipsia • Hypertension and oliguria, hyperkalemia • Tumor lysis syndrome
Renal	• Tubulointerstitial	• Light chain cast nephropathy	• Acute kidney injury (AKI)
	• Proximal tubule	• Light chain proximal tubulopathy	• Fanconi syndrome and tubular proteinuria, crystalluria
	• Glomerulus	• Light chain deposition disease • Amyloid	• Nephrotic range proteinuria and hematuria

at early stage. It is recommended that all patients of SLE should undergo a urine examination and renal function test at the onset and subsequently at frequent interval.

Renal biopsy: Due to a highly variable clinical course and an imperfect clinicopathological correlation, a kidney biopsy is essential in majority of patients who presents with any of the above renal manifestations. The American College of Rheumatology guidelines suggest that a kidney biopsy should be performed in all patients presenting with either a high serum creatinine without an alternative cause or have proteinuria > 1 g/day with or without active sediments or > 0.5 g/day with active sediments. The recent classification criteria proposed by Systemic Lupus International Collaborating Clinics (SLICC) as well the American College of Rheumatology-European League Against Rheumatism (ACR-EULAR) criteria have given importance to the renal biopsy findings of LN in classifying the patient as a case of SLE. Certain findings in kidney biopsy are considered relatively specific for LN, which include (1) on LM—pleomorphicity, wire loop lesions, hyaline thrombi, and karyorrhexis; (2) on IF—full-house pattern, i.e., deposition of all the immunoglobulins along with complement factors C3, C4, and C1q; and (3) on electron microscopy—tubuloreticular inclusions. The histopathological classification of LN is extremely useful in guiding therapy, prognostication, and follow-up. The most up to date classification is by International Society of Nephrology/Renal Pathology Society (ISN/RPS), which divides the LN into six classes (**Table 1**), with class IV being most common.

Treatment: The treatment of LN is guided by the clinical presentation and the histological class. Not all patients may require immunosuppressive treatment. However, nonimmunosuppressive therapy is required in most subjects and will include hydroxychloroquine (HCQ) and renin-angiotensin system blockers. HCQ has been shown to decrease the risk of renal and extrarenal relapse and is recommended for all patients. Ocular toxicity needs to be monitored in patients on long-term HCQ. In addition, most patients with proteinuria should receive angiotensin-converting enzyme (ACE) inhibitor or angiotensin receptor blocker (ARB) therapy. In addition, statins may be required for cholesterol lowering.

The therapy for class I and II LN is determined primarily by the severity of extrarenal manifestations, except for few patients of class II LN with nephrotic range proteinuria. These subjects have associated podocytopathy and are treated with a course of oral steroids or calcineurin inhibitors (CNIs) as for minimal change disease (MCD). Class III LN with <25% involved glomeruli and absence of severe proliferative or necrotizing lesions is generally treated with oral steroids alone, while other cases are treated like class IV. As the class IV LN is the most common form, its treatment has been studied well in large and randomized trials. The treatment for such patients is usually divided into induction and maintenance. Induction therapy denotes the initial phase, usually comprising 3–6 months, aimed to induce remission, either complete or partial. Treatment is initiated with IV pulse steroids followed by high-dose oral steroids. The key factors which determine the additional immunosuppressive therapy for induction include severity of renal histology (like presence of extracapillary proliferation or crescents), extent of proteinuria and serum creatinine, age and desire to preserve fertility, response to previous therapy, finances, and patient's preference. The most commonly used induction agents for proliferative LN in the current era are IV CYC and oral MMF combined with corticosteroids. These agents are used in three protocols, namely:

1. Monthly IV CYC [National Institute of Health (NIH) regimen]
2. Low-dose IV CYC [Euro-Lupus Nephritis Trial (ELNT) regimen]
3. Oral MMF

Cyclophosphamide is usually administered for six doses either as monthly, high dose (0.75–1 g/m^2) pulses (NIH regimen) or as low, fixed dose (500 mg) fortnightly regimen (Euro-Lupus regimen).

Common side effects observed with high-dose IV CYC were bone marrow suppression, premature gonadal failure, and malignancy. Urinary tract malignancy was increased by 5-fold. Gonadal toxicity is dose-dependent in male patients and has an age- and dose-dependent effect on female patients. Although shown to be similar in efficacy, inclusion of less severe proliferative LN in most trials on low-dose IV CYC limits any conclusion for its use in all categories of patients with proliferative LN.

Oral MMF was observed to be useful in patients with resistant/relapsing LN first in 1999. It has been the standard of care treatment in patients with proliferative LN after the ALMS (Aspreva Lupus Nephritis Management Study) trial showed its noninferiority as compared to IV CYC and a safer side effect profile.

The dose and tapering schedule of corticosteroids is not specified and usually ranges between 0.5 and 1 mg/kg/day of oral prednisolone with tapering after 4–6 weeks of therapy to a maintenance dose of 5–10 mg/day. We found low dose (0.5 mg/kg/day) of prednisolone to be inferior to standard dose (1 mg/kg/day) of prednisolone in inducing remission in patients with proliferative LN at our center.

The induction therapy is usually followed by a prolonged low-dose immunosuppressive therapy, commonly labeled as maintenance therapy. The maintenance therapy is usually with MMF or azathioprine, with the former being proven superior in recent trials. The optimal duration of maintenance therapy is debatable. However, most guidelines recommend using the maintenance therapy for at least 3 years after achieving a complete remission (CR). Recent reports suggest role of performing protocol renal biopsies before deciding to stop the maintenance therapy in cases of LN.

The therapy for patients with class V LN is not well defined. Those with nephrotic range proteinuria are usually treated with combination of oral steroids and one of the following agents: MMF, CYC, CNI, or azathioprine. Evidence to support one agent over the other is weak. Unlike patients with idiopathic membranous nephropathy, who frequently remit spontaneously on follow-up, patients with class V LN seldom do so. Since persistent nephrotic state leads to adverse renal and cardiovascular outcomes, patients are generally treated with immunosuppressive drugs at presentation.

Response to induction therapy is classified as CR, partial remission (PR), and resistant disease. These terms have been defined differently in trials as a result of which the overall (CR + PR) response rates have been reported quite variably (30–80%). Other potential factors which contribute to this variability are the duration of follow-up and racial composition of the study participants. Options for resistant disease include switching from CYC to MMF or vice versa, rituximab, CNI, intravenous immunoglobulin (IVIG), immunoadsorption, plasmapheresis, or immunoablation with stem cell transplantation.

Patients with LN may relapse on follow-up. Treatment for relapse is similar to initial therapy; depending on the response to initial therapy, side effects, and the cumulative dose of the CYC. The overall survival of LN patients has increased from 51% to over 90% from 1950 to 2000 owing to the use of aggressive induction agents for management of LN.

SYSTEMIC SCLEROSIS

Systemic sclerosis (SSc) is another important systemic disease that has potential to involve kidneys and can lead to rapid and permanent loss of kidney function. Though the clinical involvement of kidneys is less common, in autopsy series, kidneys are involved in 60–80% of cases. The severity of renal disease varies from mild subclinical reduction in the renal blood flow to malignant hypertension and rapidly progressive renal failure [scleroderma renal crisis (SRC)]. The SRC occurs early in the course of disease (80% within first 4 years) and is more common with the diffuse cutaneous variety, in subjects with ribonucleic acid polymerase III antibodies and treatment with high-dose steroids. It has been shown that SRC is more common in Caucasians than in Asians. Although the patients usually have an uncontrolled hypertension, absence of hypertension has been noted in about 10% of patients. Pathologically, the SRC is characterized by intimal and medial proliferation with luminal narrowing that typically involves the arcuate and interlobular arteries. In addition, there may be nonspecific changes of malignant hypertension and ischemic nephropathy (**Box 1**).

The prognosis of SRC has improved significantly with the introduction of renin-angiotensin system blockers; however, still about 40% of patients end up with end-stage renal disease. These patients should continue to take these drugs, as renal recovery has been reported to occur even after months of being on dialysis. Other drugs shown to be beneficial are endothelin receptor antagonists. Plasma exchange may improve patient and renal survival and has been used in selected cases.

BOX 1 Renal involvement in scleroderma.

- Acute kidney injury with low-grade proteinuria, renal dysfunction, and mild MesPGN
- *Scleroderma renal crisis*: Malignant hypertension with TMA involving kidney with TMA involving arcuate and interlobular arteries and ischemic glomerular changes
- Other systemic features include hypertensive emergency with heart failure and convulsions, schistocytes in peripheral blood, and elevated LDH. Responds well to use of ACEI-ARB which controls BP and even to be continued on dialysis patients with expectation of renal recovery

(MesPGN: mesangioproliferative glomerulonephritis; TMA: thrombotic microangiopathy)

RHEUMATOID ARTHRITIS

Renal involvement in RA can be either due to the disease itself, as a complication of therapy, or secondary to the long-standing inflammatory nature of the disease. The direct involvement of the kidneys is less common and usually is in the form MesPGN or membranous glomerulopathy, and rarely focal or diffuse PGN. MesPGN in RA may have either IgM (more frequent) or IgA predominant pattern on IF. In cases of membranous nephropathy, antibody to phospholipase A2 receptor is usually negative and spontaneous remissions are less common. The more common causes of renal involvement are the complication of therapy like toxicity to nonsteroidal anti-inflammatory drugs or methotrexate. Another complication of a chronic inflammatory process is development of secondary amyloidosis affecting kidneys, that can present as nephrotic syndrome or CKD (**Box 2**).

MIXED CONNECTIVE TISSUE DISORDER

The term mixed connective tissue disorder (MCTD) is used to describe a disease that have constellation of clinical features of different autoimmune disorders such as SLE, SSc, polymyositis, or RA along with the presence of a specific autoantibody, called anti-U1-RNP. Over a period, these patients may evolve into defined diseases such as SLE, SSc, or less commonly RA. The renal involvement occurs in about 25–50% of patients. The renal lesions are variable and can have either predominant glomerular involvement (as in LN) or vascular involvement (as in SSc). The common patterns of glomerular involvement are membranous nephropathy, MesPGN, or focal PGN. However, severe proliferative lesions are less common. A predominant interstitial or vascular involvement may be seen in about 15–25% patients. The treatment depends on the underlying pathology and its severity and the use of immunosuppression is similar as in the underlying predominant autoimmune component.

PRIMARY SJÖGREN'S SYNDROME

Primary Sjögren's syndrome (pSS) predominantly affects the salivary and lacrimal glands. The renal involvement is mainly in the form of functional tubular defects such as distal renal tubular acidosis (dRTA),

BOX 2 Renal disease in rheumatoid arthritis.

Glomerular involvement due to disease:

- Membranous nephropathy
- Mesangial proliferative GN with IgA or IgM deposits
- Diffuse proliferative GN
- Necrotizing crescentic GN (rheumatoid vasculitis)
- Amyloidosis

Renal complications due to drugs:

- *Gold*: Minimal change disease, membranous nephropathy, and acute tubular necrosis
- *Penicillamine*: Membranous nephropathy, minimal change disease, and crescentic GN
- *NSAIDs*: Acute tubule interstitial nephritis and minimal change disease
- *Cyclosporine*: Vasculopathy and tubule interstitial nephritis
- *Pamidronate*: Idiopathic focal segmental glomerulosclerosis
- *TNF-α inhibitors*: Lupus-like GN and crescentic GN

hypercalciuria, impaired concentrating defects, and rarely proximal RTA. dRTA is reported in 5–70% cases, while impaired concentration defect has been reported in up to 4–28% cases. The main histopathological finding is tubulointerstitial nephritis (TIN), characterized by either acute or chronic inflammatory infiltrate admixed with plasma cells and variable degrees of interstitial fibrosis and tubular atrophy. The glomerular involvement in pSS is distinctly uncommon. Another rare manifestation of pSS includes infiltration of the kidneys by lymphoma. The treatment is usually supportive. Those with TIN usually respond to steroids; however, the RTA is usually unresponsive to immunosuppressive therapy and these patients require a long-term alkali and potassium supplementation.

SARCOIDOSIS

Renal involvement in sarcoidosis is variably reported in 1–50% cases depending on the criteria used. The common renal manifestations include hypercalcemia, hypercalciuria, and medullary nephrocalcinosis with or without granulomatous interstitial nephritis (GIN). The vascular involvement has been reported rarely due to compression of renal vessels by enlarged lymph nodes. Similarly, obstructive uropathy can develop due to compression of ureter by enlarged lymph nodes or secondary to nephrolithiasis. The renal sarcoidosis is more commonly associated with extrarenal involvement though rarely it can be in isolation.

Sarcoid granuloma has an excessive expression of 1-α-hydroxylase enzyme which results in increased formation of activated vitamin D. This leads to excessive absorption of calcium from the gut and the bone, resulting in hypercalcemia and hypercalciuria. The hypercalciuria secondary to excessive filtration of calcium can lead to medullary nephrocalcinosis causing progressive renal failure.

Granulomatous interstitial nephritis has been reported in about 7–23% of patients and can manifest as either acute, rapidly progressive, or a chronic renal failure. Most patients will develop subnephrotic proteinuria, microscopic hematuria, and sterile pyuria. A high index of suspicion, early renal biopsy, and timely institution of therapy with steroids goes a long way in preserving the renal functions. Glomerular diseases, particularly membranous nephropathy have been rarely reported.

ANTIPHOSPHOLIPID SYNDROME

Antiphospholipid syndrome (APLS) can be either primary or secondary to other autoimmune disorders. The renal involvement is similar in both types and reported in about 9–25% cases. Both arteries and veins and vessels of any size can be involved with thrombosis.

INFLAMMATORY MYOPATHIES

The inflammatory myopathies (polymyositis, dermatomyositis, and inclusion body myositis) are a group of autoimmune disorders characterized by inflammation and destruction of the skeletal muscles. The renal involvement occurs in 20–25% cases and presents either as acute kidney disease or CKD. AKI can be seen in about 10% cases and is secondary to rhabdomyolysis. It usually has a poor outcome with over 80% of patients progressing to CKD. Nephrotic syndrome has rarely been reported with inflammatory myopathy.

RECOMMENDED READINGS

1. Catran DC. (2020). Primary and secondary glomerular diseases. [online] Available from https://nephsap.org/view/journals/nephsap/19/2/nephsap.19.issue-2.xml.
2. Kitching AR, Anders HJ, Basu N, Brouwer E, Gordon J, Jayne DR, et al. ANCA-associated vasculitis. Nat Rev Dis Primers. 2020;6:71.
3. McAdoo SP, Pusey CD. Anti-Glomerular Basement Membrane disease. Clin J Am Soc Nephrol. 2017;12(7):1162-72.
4. Leung N, Bridoux F, Batuman V, Chaidos A, Cockwell P, D'Agati VD, et al. The evaluation of monoclonal gammopathy of renal significance: a consensus report of the International Kidney and Monoclonal Gammopathy Research Group. Nat Rev Nephrol. 2019;15:45-59.
5. Jain A, Haynes R, Kothari J, Khera A, Soares M, Ramasamy K. Pathophysiology and management of monoclonal gammopathy of renal significance. Blood Adv. 2019;3(15):2409-23.
6. KDIGO. (2020). KDIGO Clinical Practice Guideline on Glomerular Diseases. [online] Available from https://kdigo.org/wp-content/uploads/2017/02/KDIGO-GN-GL-Public-Review-Draft_1-June-2020.pdf.

CHAPTER

172 Pregnancy and Kidneys

S Shiri, Arpana Iyengar

ABSTRACT

Pregnancy is a dynamic physiological state that sustains a delicate balance between maternal and fetal health. With regard to maternal kidney health, the occurrence of specific kidney diseases related to pregnancy and manifestations of a pre-existing renal disease needs recognition. Pregnancy-related acute kidney injury (P-AKI) is associated with significant morbidity and demands early recognition and prompt management. Pre-eclampsia (PE), thrombotic microangiopathy (TMA), and acute cortical necrosis are the salient causes of AKI. Pre-existing renal diseases like diabetic nephropathy (DN) and lupus nephritis (LN) are known to manifest during pregnancy. Severe renal involvement can lead to consequences such as persistent proteinuria and progression to chronic kidney disease (CKD).

The growing fetal kidney is vulnerable to insults that occur due to maternal, genetic, or environmental factors. Nephrogenesis is an ongoing process that results in new nephron formation until 36 weeks of gestation. Impaired nephrogenesis can result in a spectrum of disorders that are collectively termed as congenital anomalies of the kidney and urinary tract. These anomalies lead to a spectrum of renal sequelae, from mild disease to life-threatening disorders. Antenatal diagnosis of fetal renal anomalies is critical through appropriate imaging techniques. This chapter provides an overview of the physiological adaptation, diagnosis, and management of both maternal and fetal kidney diseases associated with pregnancy.

"A good decision is based on knowledge and not on numbers"

—Plato

PHYSIOLOGICAL ADAPTATIONS IN PREGNANCY

Pregnancy results in specific physiological hemodynamic changes due to an interplay of cardiovascular, renal, and endocrine functions that are protective to the mother and the growing fetus. Hemodynamic changes in the form of decline in blood pressure and increasing cardiac output begin as early as 6 weeks of gestation. The predominant renal changes include increase in renal blood flow and glomerular filtration rate (GFR). These physiological cross talks are illustrated in **Figure 1**.

Pregnancy is a state of generalized vasodilatation. Early in the first trimester, there is a decline in peripheral vascular resistance (PVR) and systemic vascular resistance (SVR) that reaches a nadir in the second trimester. This has downstream effects on the cardiac function resulting in a 40% increase in cardiac output and reduction of mean arterial pressure by 10 mm Hg. As a consequence of this, there is renal vasodilatation thereby increasing the renal plasma flow (RPF) by 45–50% and GFR by 55–60%. The changes in specific cardiovascular and renal parameters across gestational age are depicted in **Figures 2 A** and **B**, respectively.

FACTORS RESPONSIBLE

- *Changes in the renin-angiotensin system*: Pregnancy results in the activation of renin-angiotensin system. The level of renin correlates with the rise in beta-human chorionic gonadotropin (β-hCG). The role of specific hormones in the renal physiology of pregnancy is listed in **Table 1**. Despite the hyperreninemic state, there is resistance to the peripheral actions of angiotensin II due to the inhibition of angiotensin AT_1 and AT_2 receptors by progesterone and vascular endothelial growth factor (VEGF) that leads to a state of low renal vascular resistance.
- *Role of relaxin*: Relaxin increases endothelin levels by activating nitric oxide synthase resulting in renal vasodilatation, decline in SVR, and increase in CO. Secreted by corpus luteum, it increases postconception, peaks at the end of first trimester to reach nadir by mid of second trimester, and thereafter maintains stable levels throughout pregnancy.
- *Changes in renal structure and function*: There is an increase in the length and volume of kidneys that is noted during pregnancy secondary to increase in RPF. By the end of first trimester, the length of the kidneys is noted to increase by 1 cm and volume by 30%. At around 6 weeks of gestation, an increase in diameter of pelvis by 0.5 mm per week until 26 weeks is observed followed by increase by 0.3 mm until full term.
- *Altered tubular function*: Pregnancy results in altered proximal tubule functions that result in urinary wasting of glucose, amino acids, proteins, and uric acid. Renal glucosuria is seen in normal pregnancy with normal

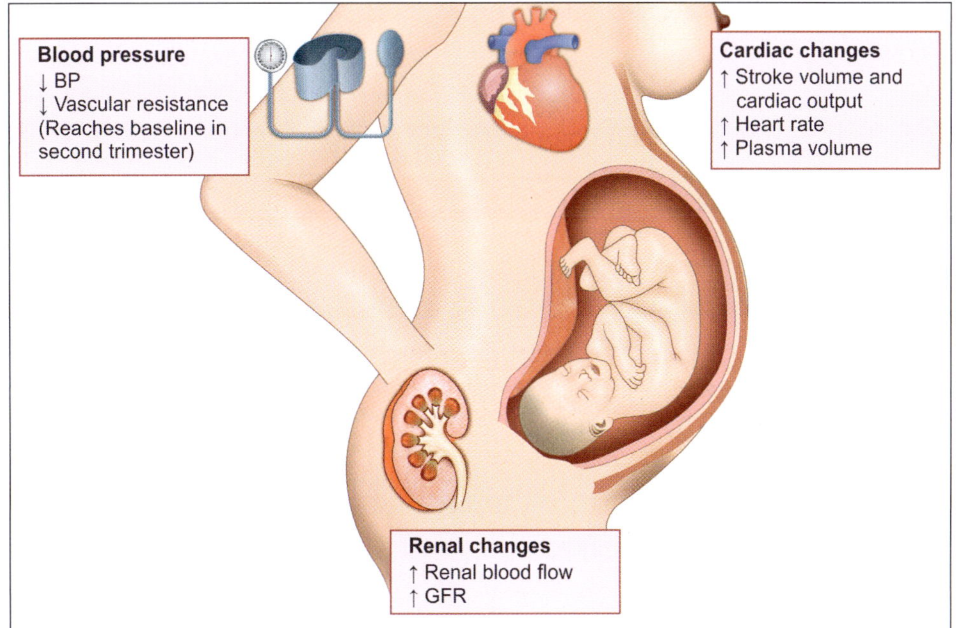

(BP: blood pressure; GFR: glomerular filtration rate)

FIGURE 1: Interplay between cardiovascular and renal functions in pregnancy.

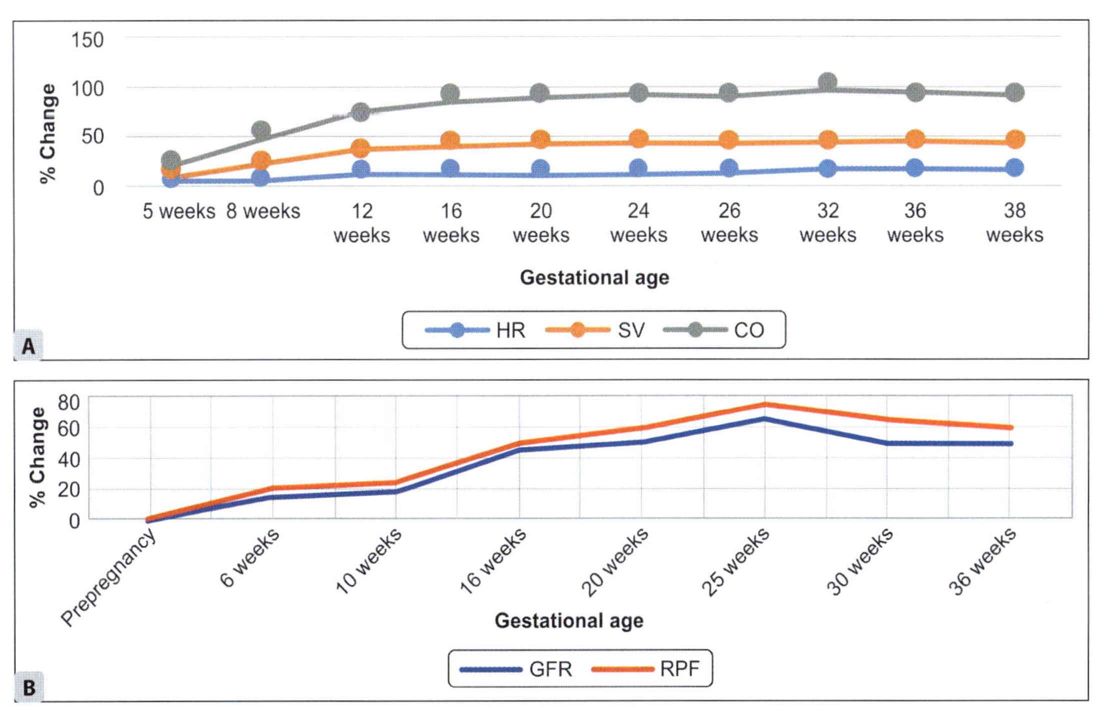

(CO: cardiac output; GFR: glomerular filtration rate; HR: heart rate; RPF: renal plasma flow; SV: stroke volume)

FIGURES 2 A & B: **(A)** Cardiovascular changes across gestational age; **(B)** Changes in GFR and RPF with gestational age.

plasma glucose levels. Proteinuria can be seen within 300 mg/dL in a 24-hour urine sample.

- *Changes in body water and mineral metabolism*: Due to low peripheral and SVR, there is an activation of the baroreceptors and sympathetic activity resulting in release of arginine vasopressin, increase in total body water by 50% and total plasma volume by 40–50%. Renal-related changes and changes in body composition during pregnancy are depicted in **Figure 3**.

MATERNAL KIDNEY INVOLVEMENT IN PREGNANCY

Kidney diseases in pregnancy can be classified as follows:

- *Kidney diseases specific to pregnancy*: P-AKI, PE-related kidney disease, acute fatty liver of pregnancy (AFLP), TMA, and acute cortical necrosis
- *Chronic pre-existing kidney disease*: DN, LN, GN, CKD, and polycystic kidney disease

TABLE 1 Hormonal changes in pregnancy and renal effects.

Hormone	Gestational age	Effects on the kidney
β-hCG	4–6 weeks	• 10 times release of prorenin • Increase in relaxin
Estrogen	6–8 weeks	• Increase in levels of plasma renin
Progesterone	4–6 weeks	• Reduced actions of angiotensin II • Natriuretic
Relaxin	8–12 weeks	Decrease in angiotensin II/VEGF Natriuresis
Aldosterone	8–12 weeks	Salt and water retention
Angiotensin II	8–10 weeks	• Reduced sensitivity at AT1 receptor • State of vasodilatation
Atrial natriuretic peptides	6–10 weeks	Natriuretic

(β-hCG: beta-human chorionic gonadotropin; VEGF: vascular endothelial growth factor)

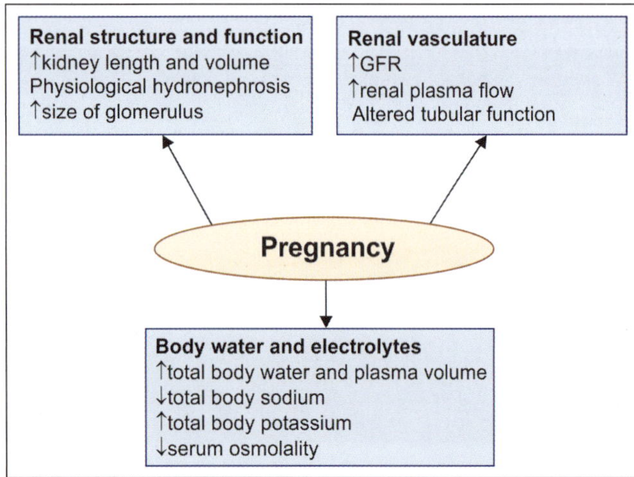

FIGURE 3: Renal adaptations with regard to structure and function during pregnancy.

Pregnancy-related acute kidney injury: Pregnancy-related acute kidney injury is an important cause of fetomaternal morbidity and mortality. In recent years, early recognition and treatment of the underlying kidney disease during pregnancy have resulted in a decline in the burden of P-AKI in developing countries from 65–70% to 5–20%. In India, P-AKI accounts for 3–7% of all causes of AKI. Among Indian studies, P-AKI is most commonly seen due to postpartum causes (60%) with sepsis and PE being the most common causes (55%) with 20% maternal mortality. P-AKI can be classified based on the traditional approach of prerenal, intrinsic renal, and postrenal AKI or according to time of gestation and etiology (**Tables 2** and **3**). Some of the causes have been discussed in detail here.

Preeclampsia: Preeclampsia is an important disorder that is specific to pregnancy with multisystem involvement causing severe adverse outcomes both in the mother and the fetus. It often presents as new onset hypertension of >140/90 mm Hg and proteinuria of >300 mg/dL seen after 20 weeks of gestation. PE can lead to acute pulmonary edema, acute liver cell failure, and neurological and hematological consequences.

Acute kidney injury secondary to PE is mainly a consequence of impaired renal perfusion due to high renal and SVR. AKI secondary to PE is seen in 18–20% of the pregnancies. It can range from mild-to-severe form of AKI requiring renal replacement therapy (RRT) and progress to CKD and end-stage kidney disease (ESKD).The pathophysiology and risk factors of PE-induced AKI are depicted in **Figures 4** and **5**, respectively.

Newer concepts of renal dysfunction secondary to PE:

- Antiangiogenic factors: Abnormal VEGF and transforming growth factor (TGF) beta levels cause endothelial dysfunction leading to hypertension and proteinuria.
- Oxidative stress: The hypoxic placenta is found to release soluble fms-like tyrosine kinase-1 (sflT-1) [fms is a proto-oncogene that codes for macrophage colony-stimulating factor (m-CSF)] that causes renal vasoconstriction and ischemia.
- Role of relaxin: A state of excess relaxin along with abnormal VEGF causes impaired renal vasodilatation and hypoperfusion.

Management: Aggressive and symptomatic control of blood pressure is the foremost important step in controlling PE. In case of severe AKI, early initiation of dialysis is crucial to prevent life-threatening complications like pulmonary edema and hypertensive encephalopathy. In most situations, early termination of pregnancy is indicated to prevent maternal mortality. Many studies have shown that renal involvement in severe PE is common and there is a risk to progression to ESKD (**Table 4**).

Thrombotic microangiopathy: Thrombotic microangiopathies during pregnancy can be secondary to atypical hemolytic-uremic syndrome (HUS) or thrombotic thrombocytopenic purpura (TTP) characterized by microangiopathic hemolytic anemia, thrombocytopenia, and AKI. TTP includes neurologic manifestations and fever in addition to the above three features. The clinical and biochemical effects of TMA and its outcomes closely resemble severe PE and hemolysis, elevated liver enzymes, and low platelet count (HELLP) syndrome making it difficult to differentiate them. However, the presence of microangiopathic hemolytic anemia with low serum haptoglobin favors the diagnosis of TMA.

Thrombotic microangiopathy can cause severe renal dysfunction that results in life-threatening consequences

TABLE 2 Causes of pregnancy related-AKI based on timing of gestation.			
Time of gestation	**Prerenal AKI**	**Intrinsic renal AKI**	**Postrenal AKI**
Early	• Hyperemesis gravidarum	• Hemorrhage • Sepsis, APLA • CKD progression GN, TTP	• Stones
Late	• Placenta previa • Abruptio	• CKD progression • Drug induced	• Uterine obstruction
	• Acute fatty liver of pregnancy	• HELLP syndrome • APLA, GN	• Stones
Postpartum	• Hemorrhage • Drug-induced	• HUS • Severe PE/HELLP • ATN • CKD progression	• Retained clots

(APLA: antiphospholipid antibody syndrome; ATN: acute tubular necrosis; CKD: chronic kidney disease; GN: glomerulonephritis; HELLP: hemolysis elevated liver enzymes low platelet; HUS: hemolytic uremic syndrome; PPH: postpartum hemorrhage; PE: preeclampsia)

Source: Adapted from Hussein W, Lafayette RA. Renal function in normal and disordered pregnancy. Curr Opin Nephrol Hypertens. 2014;23:46-53.

TABLE 3 Etiology of pregnancy related-AKI.		
Obstetrical complication	**Pregnancy-specific risk**	**Pre-existing renal disease**
1. Septic abortion	1. Severe preeclampsia	1. Chronic kidney disease
2. Antenatal hemorrhage	2. Acute fatty liver of pregnancy	2. IgA nephropathy
◦ Placenta previa	3. HELLP syndrome	3. Diabetic nephropathy
◦ Abruptio	4. Acquired TTP	4. Lupus nephritis
3. Sepsis		5. Vasculitis
4. Intrauterine fetal death		6. Pyelonephritis

(HELLP: hemolysis elevated liver enzyme low platelet; IgA: Immunoglobulin A; TTP: thrombotic thrombocytopenic purpura)

Source: Adapted from Gonzalez Suarez M, Kattah A, Grande JP, Garovic V. Renal disorders in pregnancy: core curriculum 2019. Am J Kidney Dis. 2019;73(1):119-30.

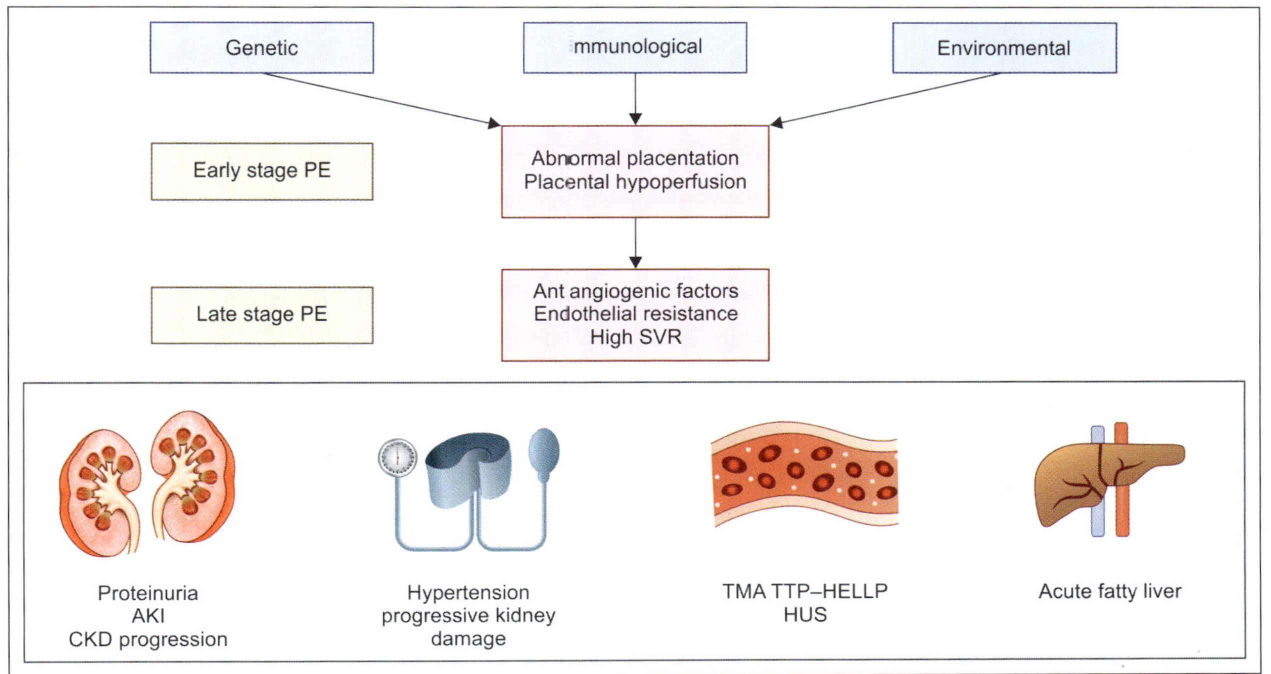

(HUS: hemolytic-uremic syndrome; TMA: thrombotic microangiopathy; TTP: thrombotic thrombocytopenic purpura; PE: preeclampsia)

FIGURE 4: Pathophysiology of preeclampsia and impaired renal and cardiovascular physiology along with its downstream effects.

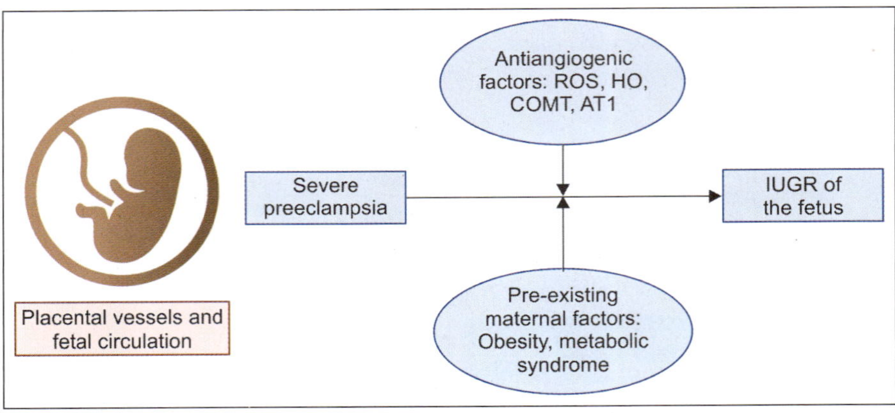

(AT1: angiotensin I receptor; COMT: catechol-o-methyltransferase; HO: heme oxygenase; IUGR: intrauterine growth restriction; ROS: reactive oxygen species)

FIGURE 5: **Risk factors of placental insufficiency in severe preeclampsia.**

TABLE 4 Risk of progression to CKD in mothers with severe preeclampsia.

Study	Cohort	Outcomes
Khashan et al. 2019	Swedish registry *n* = 1,366,441 singleton pregnancies	• Preeclampsia in 5% of pregnancies • Incidence rate of ESKD in PE 1.86 per 100,000 person years. Significant association of PE with ESKD [HR = 4.96 (3.89,6.32) $p < 0.001$]
Tanwar et al. 2018	• *n* = 68 • P-AKI	• Among P-AKI 35% had severe PE • eGFR of <60 mL/min/1.73 m^2 in 51% at end of 3 months
Vikse et al. 2012	*n* = 582 severe PE	• Progression to ESKD in 13% with severe PE after 4 years. The relative risk of ESKD was 1.1 (95% CI 0.63–2.4) in those women who were diagnosed with severe PE in first half of gestation

(P-AKI: pregnancy-related acute kidney injury; PE: preeclampsia)

like pulmonary edema and hypertensive encephalopathy. Hence, early diagnosis and management is important. In case of atypical HUS in addition to RRT, initiation of plasma exchange should also be considered. In severe cases, immunosuppression, such as intravenous methylprednisolone and rituximab, is indicated. The use of eculizumab can result in clinical and hematological remission with protective effects on the fetus. In case of TTP, apart from RRT, control of blood pressure and seizures are critical. Evaluation with ADAMTS13 antibodies level for TTP should be considered. In pregnancy-related TMA (atypical HUS or TTP) risk of progression to ESKD has been reported to be 75%.

Acute fatty liver of pregnancy: Acute fatty liver of pregnancy is one of the rare complications postulated to be secondary to impaired mitochondrial functions and disorder of beta-oxidation of fat. AFLP can present as P-AKI or as an overlap of clinical manifestations with HELLP syndrome.

It is one of the rarest causes of P-AKI presenting in later half of the gestation with varying degree of renal failure in 50–75%. AFLP resembles HELLP syndrome in terms of clinical and biochemical parameters like anemia, thrombocytopenia hypofibrinogenemia, and severe liver dysfunction. Management is supportive care with early termination of pregnancy in severe cases.

Acute cortical necrosis: Acute cortical necrosis during pregnancy is an irreversible cause of AKI with poor prognosis. The mortality is around 18–20% and risk of progression to ESKD is almost 50%. Certain causes of acute cortical necrosis are septic abortion and hemorrhage, fetoplacental hemorrhage, abruptio placenta or placenta previa, disseminated intravascular coagulation (DIC), HELLP syndrome, and HUS. The histopathological features of acute cortical necrosis after renal biopsy undertaken in the postpartum period are shown in **Figure 6**. Management is supportive care with continuation of RRT. Termination of pregnancy and maternal safety is priority.

PRE-EXISTING CHRONIC DISEASES

Diabetic nephropathy: Diabetic nephropathy is one of the rare renal complications encountered during pregnancy. It has a slow indolent course with worsening of proteinuria, hypertension, and progression to CKD and ESKD. A tight glycemic control with glycated hemoglobin (HbA1c) <6.5% is necessary. In pregnancy, DN can result in progression to ESKD, drug toxicity, and adverse consequences on the embryo.

Serum creatinine >1.4 mg/dL and presence of significant proteinuria >3 g/day have risk of worsening renal function and progression to ESKD during pregnancy. Diabetes itself has effect on the developing fetus resulting

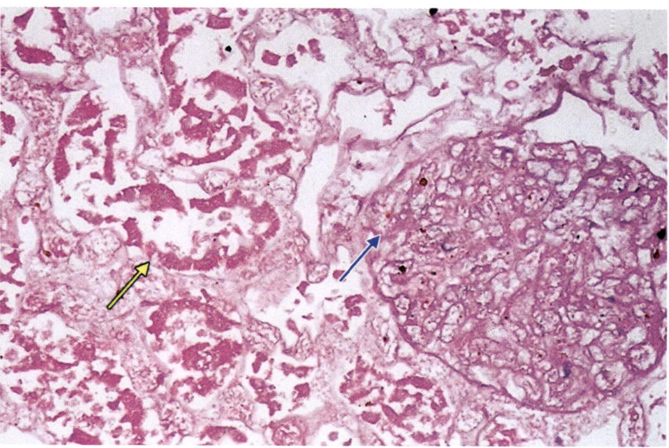

FIGURE 6: H & E stain showing features of acute cortical necrosis in pregnancy-related acute kidney injury. Blue arrow indicates coagulative necrosis of the glomerulus with pyknotic appearance of the nuclei. Yellow arrow shows pale and necrotic tubules with distorted architecture.

Courtesy: Dr Anila Abraham, Renopath, Center for Renal and Urological Pathology Pvt., Chennai, India. (Figs 6 & 7)

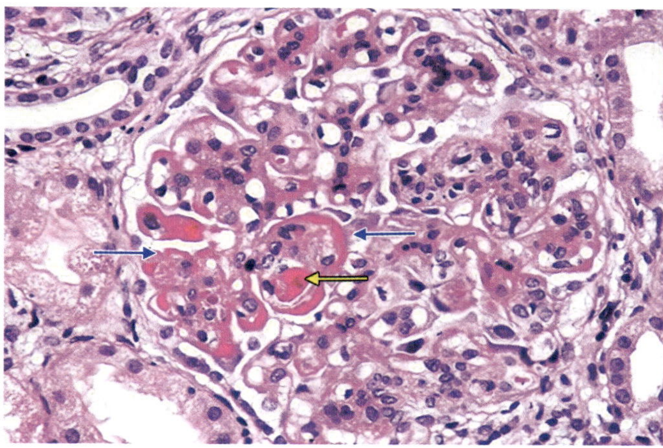

FIGURE 7: Histopathology of lupus nephritis in pregnancy. Wire-loop lesion (blue arrows) and pseudothrombus (yellow arrow) with endocapillary and mesangial hypercellularity are seen in this H & E stained slide.

in macrosomia, sacral agenesis, hirsutism, and ear and eye anomalies. It also causes various complications like respiratory distress syndrome, congenital heart disease, gastrointestinal anomalies, and most importantly congenital anomalies of kidney and urinary tract (CAKUT). These severe manifestations are due to poor glycemic control with accumulation of advanced end glycosylation products.

Management: Angiotensin-converting enzyme (ACE) inhibitors and angiotensin receptor blocker (ARB) antagonists that are used for proteinuria and hypertension can result in AKI in the mother with teratogenic effects on the growing fetus. Hence, they are contraindicated in pregnancy. Oral hypoglycemic agents can also result in adverse consequences on the embryo making the use insulin with sliding scale more appropriate during pregnancy. Low-dose aspirin has been suggested to prevent fetoplacental insufficiency.

Lupus nephritis: Lupus nephritis is one of the common systemic disorders observed in pregnancy. Management is challenging due to the underlying multisystemic nature of disease and the need for long-term immunosuppression that can have detrimental effects in both the mother and the fetus. It is of utmost importance to have a state of remission for at least 6 months (both clinical and biochemically) before conception. Most common form of LN seen in pregnancy is a combination of class IV and class V. A postpartum renal biopsy image of a 30-year-old female with LN (class IV+ class V) that presented as proteinuria during pregnancy is shown in **Figure 7**.

Managing LN in pregnancy has the following challenges:

- *Long-term immunosuppression*: Mycophenolate mofetil (MMF) and cyclophosphamide have known detrimental risks of teratogenicity in the fetus. Hence they should be discontinued during pregnancy. Corticosteroids, calcineurin inhibitors, and azathioprine have their own risks and the use of these agents should clearly outweigh potential complications. Hydroxychloroquine is found to be safe and has to be continued due to decreased risk of flare and adverse outcomes. As pregnancy itself is a prothrombotic state, initiation of oral aspirin becomes important during second week of gestation. Class V LN is also known to be associated with thrombotic tendencies.
- *Risk of flares*: There is an increased risk of life-threatening flares during pregnancy and it closely resembles PE. Lupus is an important trigger for PE as well. Aggressive immunosuppression becomes important with sessions of plasma exchange in severe cases. In case of irreversible severe consequences, termination of the pregnancy remains the only option for maternal safety.

Diseases like CKD, urinary tract infection, GN, and polycystic kidney disease could manifest during pregnancy and are listed in **Table 5**.

Dialysis and transplantation: In case of patients with ESKD, diagnosis of pregnancy may be difficult in view of secondary amenorrhea and anuria. Hence serum hCG along with ultrasonography has been suggested for confirmation of pregnancy. Intensive hemodialysis with optimization of CKD comorbidities is important for optimal health of the mother and fetal well-being.

Patients in ESKD are usually advised to undergo renal transplantation before pregnancy. In case of those willing to donate or receive a kidney, guidelines recommend a waiting period for 1 year after delivery. In case of previously transplanted patients, a combination of prednisolone, azathioprine, and tacrolimus is considered safe. Kidney donors have risk of PE and preterm birth during pregnancy.

TABLE 5 Chronic diseases of maternal kidney and their salient features during pregnancy.

Disorder	Time line	Clinical features	Diagnosis	Outcomes
Chronic kidney disease	• Early-to-late gestation • Postpartum period	• Pulmonary edema • Uremia • Hypertension	• Pre-existing • Newly detected • Staging as per KDIGO	• RRT, risk of PE • Preterm birth • Miscarriages • IUGR
UTI and pyelonephritis	First and third trimester	• Asymptomatic miscarriages • Febrile UTI and AKI	• Significant pyuria and CFU (>10^5) of organism	• Risk of stones • Reflux nephropathy • CKD progression
Chronic GN	Any time of gestation	• Edema, new onset HTN, and hematuria	• Urine RE/PCR • C3, C4, CBC, ANA • Renal biopsy	• Risk of progression to ESRD
Polycystic kidney disease	Any time of gestation	• Pre-existing HTN • Renal dysfunction • UTI	• Renal imaging • USG and MRI	• Inheritance to fetus • Progression to CKD/ESRD

(CFU: colony forming unit; IUGR: intrauterine growth restriction; KDIGO: kidney disease improving the global outcome; PCR: protein creatinine ratio; PE: preeclampsia; RRT: renal replacement therapy; USG: ultrasonogram)

GUIDELINES FOR PREGNANCY AND KIDNEY DISEASES

Clinical practice guidelines on pregnancy and renal disease have proposed recommendations on pregnancy care (assessment of renal function and antenatal care, PE, and thromboembolism prophylaxis, management of blood pressure, anemia, bone health, renal biopsy, perinatal, and postnatal care) and management of associated systemic diseases like lupus, DM, UTI, and CAKUT. The risk of deterioration of renal function and underlying disease during pregnancy depends on the mother and her comorbidities. Prepregnancy stratification of the risks has been laid out that help in the planning for subsequent pregnancy.

FETAL RENAL DEVELOPMENT AND DISORDERS

The human kidney develops from the intermediate mesoderm that forms three embryonic kidneys—(1) pronephros, (2) mesonephros, and (3) metanephros. Understanding the phases of nephrogenesis is important to know the developmental pathway defects that lead to CAKUT. Human nephrogenesis takes place until 36–38 weeks of gestation after which no new nephrons are formed. This makes nephron number during development a critical step that determines nephron mass. A congenital reduction in nephron number predisposes to a greater likelihood of developing adult hypertension and CKD—this is Brenner hypothesis.

NEPHROGENESIS AND NEPHRON ENDOWMENT

Pronephros is not functional in mammals, mesonephros degenerates with only the distal part forming the efferent ducts, epididymis, vas deferens, and seminal vesicles. The human kidney in its mature form is formed by metanephric mesenchyme and the ureteric bud. At around 5th week of gestation, reciprocal inductive signals result in ureteric bud branching from the distal end of the mesonephric duct. Metanephric mesenchyme then condenses around this outpouching to form the primitive progenitors of nephrogenesis. The metanephric mesenchyme differentiates to form a nephron consisting of the glomerulus, proximal tubule, distal tubule, and loop of Henle. The vascular smooth muscle cells, mesangium, and peritubular endothelial cells are formed by the stromal part of metanephric mesenchyme. The phases of nephrogenesis and factors regulating nephron development are shown in **Figure 8** and **Table 6**.

Fetal urine formation begins as early as in the 9th week of gestation. The average number of nephrons in each kidney is 1,000,000 and this number varies widely across populations. Variations in the number, function, and structure of the developing nephron under the influence of risk and regulatory factors are known as nephron endowment. Factors affecting endowment are gestational age, birth weight, maternal drug intake, nutritional status, environmental toxins, race, ethnicity and genetic, and epigenetic factors. These factors influencing the nephron endowment are depicted in **Figure 9**.

Fetal renal function: Fetal creatinine reflects maternal creatinine. Amniotic fluid represents fetal urine output. The normal composition of amniotic fluid that reflects fetal urine should be as follows—sodium <100 mg/dL, calcium <8 mg/dL, osmolality <200 mOsm/kg, β2-microglobulin <4 mg/dL, and protein <20 mg/dL. The analysis of fetal urine composition is useful in the prognosis of fetal renal function in conditions like posterior urethral valve (PUV).

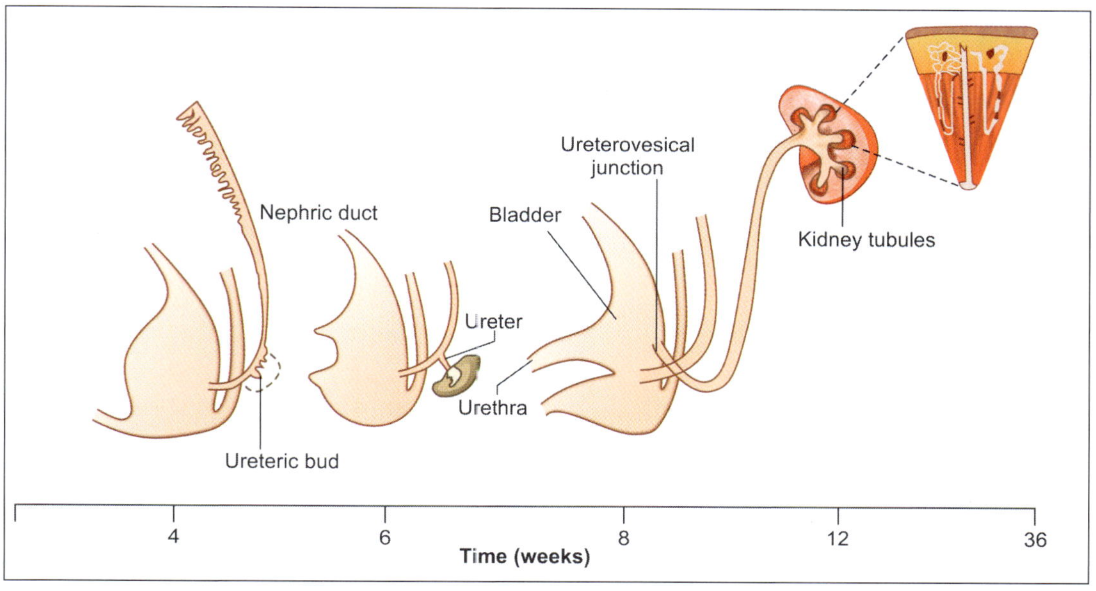

FIGURE 8: Phases of nephrogenesis.

Source: Adapted from Minuth WW. Shaping of the nephron—a complex, vulnerable, and poorly explored backdrop for noxae impairing nephrogenesis in the fetal human kidney. Mol Cell Pediatr. 2020;7:2.

TABLE 6 Stages of nephrogenesis and factors affecting it.

Stages of nephron formation	Gestational age	Regulatory factors
Outer border of nephrogenic zone		
Nephrogenic niche	4–5 weeks	Sal-like 1 (sall 1), sine oculis homeobox homolog (six 1)
Pretubular aggregate	5–6 weeks	Eyes absent homolog 1 (eya 1) GDNF
Renal vesicle	6–8 weeks	WT 1, six2, PAX2, and sall 1
S-shaped vesicle	7–8 weeks	WNT, FGFR, and TGF beta 2
Inner border of nephrogenic zone-maturation zone		
Maturation of glomeruli	10 weeks	WT 1, Pod 1, lim homeobox 1b, and Mafb
Nephron elongation	10 weeks	GDNF RET
Functional differentiation	12 weeks	Fox d1, RAR alpha, and FGF 7

(GDNF: glial cell-derived neurotrophic factor; FGFR: fibroblast growth factor receptor; FGF 7: Fibroblast growth factor 7; PAX2: paired box gene 2; TGF beta: transforming growth factor beta; Pod1: transcription factor 21; RET: rearranged during transfection; RAR: retinoic acid receptor; WT1: Wilms tumor 1; WNT: wingless-related integration site)

ANTENATAL RISK FACTORS

Antenatal risk factors for fetal diseases could be classified as maternal, placental, and fetal factors. Maternal risk factors include obesity, malnutrition, and systemic illness like diabetes mellitus, multivitamin deficiency, and maternal habits as shown in **Table 7**. Uteroplacental insufficiency results in impaired nephrogenesis and poor nephron endowment. The uteroplacental insufficiency could be due to PE, placenta previa, or abruption placenta leading to impaired nephrogenesis and underlying CAKUT.

DRUG INTAKE

Maternal drug intake influences fetal nephrogenesis in various ways. Drugs known to cause nephrotoxicity and those with specific effects on growing fetal kidneys are discussed here—nonsteroidal anti-inflammatory drugs (NSAIDs), ACE inhibitors, and aminoglycosides. The effect of various drugs on the fetal kidneys has been summarized in **Table 8**.

Nonsteroidal anti-inflammatory drugs: The initial nephrotoxicity by NSAIDs was reported in the 1970s when administering indomethacin as a tocolytic resulted in severe adverse consequences on the fetus. Besides, neonates were noted to have renal failure in the early days of life. NSAIDs are known to affect the anatomical structure, function, nephrogenesis, and vascular hemodynamics of the developing kidneys. Severe forms of renal hypoperfusion induced by NSAIDs results from inhibition of prostaglandin synthesis of COX-1 and -2 with irreversible changes. Selective COX-2 inhibitors are also known to cause AKI in the neonate. Renal manifestations specific to this group of drugs include irreversible tubular interstitial fibrosis, tubular atrophy with impaired glomerular differentiation, and tubular dysgenesis.

Angiotensin-converting enzyme inhibitors: Angiotensin-converting enzyme inhibitors block the conversion of

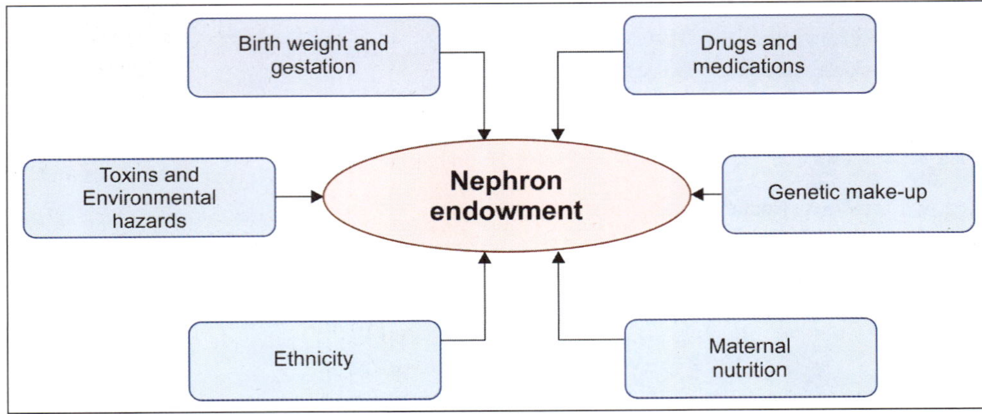

FIGURE 9: Factors affecting nephron endowment.

Source: Adapted from Gurusinghe S, Tambay A, Sethna C. Developmental origins and nephron endowment in hypertension. Front Pediatr. 2017;5:151.

TABLE 7 Maternal risk factors and their specific effect on fetal kidney development.

Maternal risk factors	Effect on fetal kidneys
Obesity	VUR, duplex collecting system
Diabetes mellitus	Hypodysplastic kidneys, cystic dysplastic kidneys
Malnutrition	Low nephron endowment
Folic acid deficiency	Duplex collecting system PUJO
Vitamin A deficiency	Renal hypodysplasia, VUR
Maternal smoking and alcohol intake	• Fetal alcohol syndrome • Renal hypodysplasia • Low nephron endowment

(PUJO: pelviureteric junction obstruction; VUR: vesicoureteric reflux)

TABLE 8 Effect of various medications on renal development during pregnancy.

Medication	Gestational age	Effects on fetal kidneys
Aminoglycosides	Second and third trimesters	Tubular damage and low nephron number
Calcineurin inhibitors	Second and third trimesters	• Ischemic injury of tubules • Low nephron endowment
ACE inhibitors	First to third trimesters	• Impaired nephrogenesis • Atrophy of renal papilla • Tubular dysgenesis
Mycophenolate mofetil	First to third trimesters	• Renal agenesis • Ectopic kidney
Cyclophosphamide	Second to third trimesters	• Renal hypodysplasia • VUR
• **Anticonvulsants** • **Phenytoin** • **Valproate**	First to third trimesters	• Spinal dysraphism with neurogenic bladder • MCDK

(MCDK: multicystic dysplastic kidneys; VUR: vesicoureteric reflux)

angiotensin I to angiotensin II thereby reducing the levels of angiotensin II and aldosterone. The effects on fetal nephrogenesis are mainly by lowering the effective arteriolar resistance resulting in reduction in GFR and RPF. They easily cross the placental barrier to result in elevated levels in maternal and umbilical cord blood. The teratogenic effect of ACE inhibitors is termed as ACE inhibitor fetopathy which includes intrauterine growth retardation, fetal and neonatal hypotension, oligohydramnios, renal failure, limb deformities, and pulmonary hypoplasia.

Certain structural and functional changes of developing nephrons are seen in the form of dilatation of tubules and bowman spaces, absent differentiation of proximal tubules, increased medullary mesenchyme, and ischemic necrosis.

Prenatal corticosteroids: Prolonged corticosteroids in the mother can affect fetal growth causing intrauterine growth restriction resulting in poor nephron endowment. There is impaired cell differentiation and proliferation, altered ureteric bud outpouching, altered genetic pathways for nephrogenesis, and accumulation of advanced glycosylated end products in the event of gestational diabetes.

Aminoglycosides: This group of drugs can affect nephrogenesis in various ways. Reduction in nephron number, reduced ureteric bud branching, and progressive glomerulosclerosis are seen in the fetus.

ANTENATAL DIAGNOSIS OF FETAL KIDNEY DISEASE

Antenatal ultrasonography is an important prenatal diagnostic tool for detection of common kidney diseases like PUVs, pelviureteric junction obstruction, multicystic dysplastic kidneys, and autosomal recessive kidney diseases (**Table 9**). Extrarenal features that suggest an underlying kidney disease are absence of nasal bones and nuchal translucency, single umbilical artery, congenital heart disease, ambiguous genitalia, and spinal defects. Chorionic villus sampling and amniocentesis are important to diagnose certain genetic diseases for the purpose of prenatal counseling and continuation of pregnancy. A magnetic resonance imaging (MRI) of the uterus has higher sensitivity to detect CAKUT along with extrarenal anomalies when compared to ultrasonogram (USG). Renal parenchymal changes on MRI are predictor outcomes in conditions like PUV.

TABLE 9 Antenatal findings of fetal kidney disease.

Antenatal ultrasound	Findings	Imaging
Normal	Bilateral renal echogenicity is normal in second trimester. Fetal kidney length in mm corresponds to the gestational age	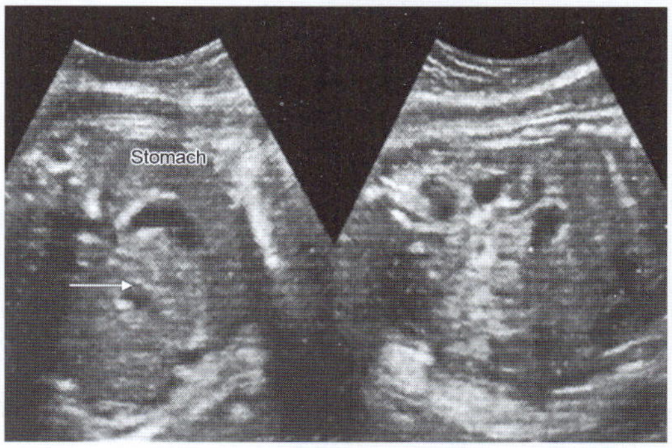 Stomach
Hydronephrosis	Severity is classified based on the stage of gestation In the third trimester: • Mild: APD 7–9 mm • Moderate: APD 10–15 mm • Severe: APD >15 mm	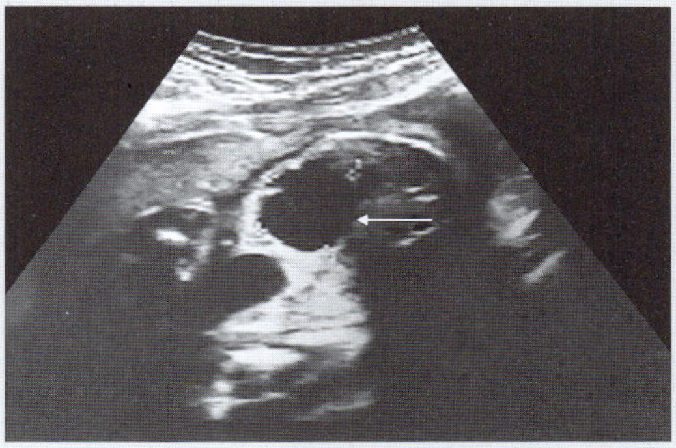
PUJO	Severe hydronephrosis Renal parenchymal thinning PUJ narrowing	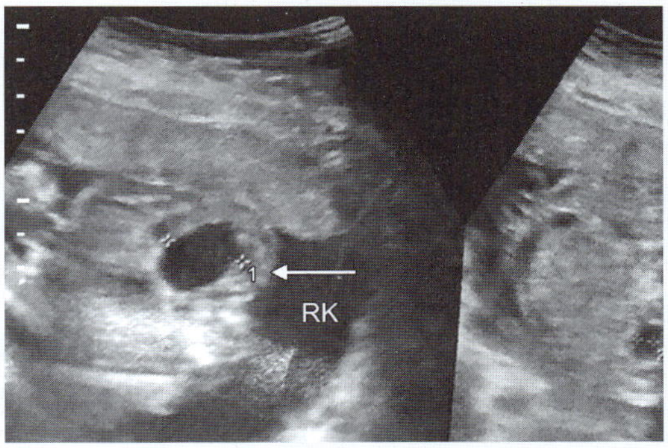 RK
PUV	PUV with severe bilateral HDN can have increased renal parenchyma echogenicity bladder wall thickening and dilated posterior urethra—the key hole sign (arrow)	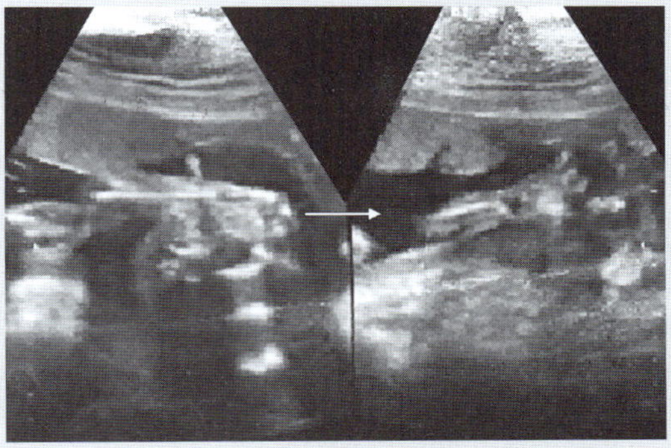

(APD: anteroposterior diameter; PUJO: pelviureteric junction obstruction; PUV: posterior urethral valve)

TABLE 10 Single gene defects and associated fetal kidney diseases.

Kidney disease	Genetic defect	Antenatal ultrasound	Postnatal presentation
Nephronophthisis	NPHS genetic mutations	Echogenic kidneys with accentuated CMD	Normal-sized kidneys with hypodysplasia
• Congenital • Infantile • Childhood • Adolescent	• NPHS1 NPHS2 WT1 • NPHS1-2 WT1 PLCE1	• Bilateral enlarged kidneys Placentomegaly Oligohydramnios	Clinical presentation depends on genetic mutation
CAKUT	• PAX 2 • HNF beta • EYA1/SALL1	• Severe oligohydramnios • Increased echogenicity • Cystic changes • Small kidneys • Hydronephrosis	• Hypodysplasia • Renal cysts • Branchiootorenal syndrome • Towne–Brocks syndrome
PKD	PKD1, PKD2, and PKHD1	• Severe oligohydramnios • Bilateral enlarged kidneys • Accentuated CMD	• ADPKD-PKD1/PKD2 • ARPKD-PKHD1

(EYA1: eyes absent homolog 1; HNF: hepatocyte nuclear factor beta; NPHS 1: nephrin mutation; NPHS 2: podocin mutation; PLCE1: 1-phosphatidylinositol-4,5-bisphosphate phosphodiesterase epsilon-1; PAX2: paired box gene 2; PKD1: polycystin 1 gene; PKD2: polycystin 2 gene; PKHD1: fibrocystin; SALL1: sall restricting enzyme; WT 1: Wilms tumor suppressor 1 gene)

FETAL INTERVENTIONS

Fetal interventions are not routinely carried out even in the best of centers. Vesicoamniotic shunt is an option for conditions like PUV in the presence of severe oligohydramnios and pulmonary hypoplasia. The PLUTO trial (stopped prematurely) showed that vesicoamniotic shunt resulted in lower incidence of pulmonary hypoplasia and need for mechanical ventilation but no benefit was observed with renal outcomes on long-term follow-up.

PRENATAL COUNSELING AND GENETIC DIAGNOSIS

Methods of preimplantation genetic diagnosis include invasive genetic diagnosis (chorionic villus sampling, amniocentesis, and cordocentesis) and noninvasive genetic diagnosis (ultrasound, maternal serum markers, and fetal cell-free DNA in the maternal serum). The various single gene renal disorders with corresponding antenatal and postnatal findings are summarized in **Table 10**.

To summarize, understanding the physiological adaptations and links governing maternal and kidney health during pregnancy is important. Kidneys of both mother and fetus are vulnerable to specific insults that are unique to the state of pregnancy. Prepregnancy risk stratification, diagnosis of renal disease, antenatal screening, and counseling are essential components of pregnancy-related maternal-fetal kidney health.

RECOMMENDED READINGS

1. Odutayo A, Hladunewich M. Obstetric nephrology: renal hemodynamic and metabolic physiology in normal pregnancy. Clin J Am Soc Nephrol. 2012;7:2073-80.
2. Soma-Pillay P, Nelson-Piercy C, Tolppanen H, Mebazaa A. Physiological changes in pregnancy. Cardiovasc J Afr. 2016;27:89-94.
3. Dutta DC. Physiological changes during pregnancy. In: Hiralal Konar (Ed). DC Dutta's Textbook of Obstetrics, 8th edition. New Delhi: Jaypee Brothers Medical Publishers (P) Ltd; 2015. pp. 52-64.
4. Gonzalez Suarez ML, Kattah A, Grande JP, Garovic V. Renal disorders in pregnancy: core curriculum 2019. Am J Kidney Dis. 2019;73(1):119-30.
5. Mahesh E, Puri S, Varma V, Madhyastha PR, Bande S, Gurudev KC. Pregnancy-related acute kidney injury: An analysis of 165 cases. Indian J Nephrol. 2017;27(2):113-7.
6. Prakash J, Ganiger VC. Acute kidney injury in pregnancy-specific disorders. Indian J Nephrol. 2017;27(4):258-70.
7. Ali SK, Marie E, Marius K, Fergus PM, Louise CK, Stenvinkel P, et al. Preeclampsia and risk of end stage kidney disease: A Swedish nationwide cohort study. PLoS Med. 2019;16(7):e1002875.
8. Tanwar RS, Agarwal D, Gupta RK, Rathore V, Beniwal P, Joshi P, et al. Characteristics and outcome of post-partum acute kidney injury requiring dialysis: A single-center experience from North India. Saudi J Kidney Dis Transpl. 2018;29(4):837-45.
9. Wiles K, Chappell L, Clark K, Elman L, Hall M, Lightstone L, et al. Clinical practice guideline on pregnancy and renal disease. BMC Nephrol. 2019;20:401.
10. Kidney Disease: Improving Global Outcomes Transplant Work Group. KDIGO clinical practice guideline for the care of kidney transplant recipients. Am J Transplant. 2009;9:S1-155.
11. Gurusinghe S, Tambay A, Sethna CB. Developmental origins and nephron endowment in hypertension. Front Pediatr. 2017;5:151.
12. Dötsch J, Plank C, Amann K. Fetal programming of renal functions. Pediatr Nephrol. 2012;27:513-20.
13. Woroniecki R, Gaikwad AB, Susztak K. Fetal environment, epigenetics, and pediatric renal disease. Pediatr Nephrol. 2011;26:705-11.

14. Schreuder MF, Bueters RR, Huigen MC, Russel FG, Masereeuw R, van den Heuvel LP. Effect of Drugs on Renal Development. Clin J Am Soc Nephrol. 2011;6:212-7.
15. Kastl JT. Renal function in fetus and neonate. The creatinine enigma. Semin Fetal Neonatal Med. 2017;22:33-9.
16. Brennan S, Schneider M, Watson D, Kandasamy Y, Rudd D. The renal parenchyma—evaluation of a novel ultrasound measurement to assess fetal renal development protocol for an observational longitudinal study. BMJ Open. 2017;7:e019369.
17. Snoek R, Stokman MF, Lichtenbelt KD, van Tilborg TC, Simcox CE, Paulussen ADC, et al. Preimplantation genetic testing for monogenic kidney disease. Clin J Am Soc Nephrol. 2020;15:1279-86.

CHAPTER

173

Drugs and Kidneys

Vivek Kumar, Ashwani Kumar, Ritambhra Nada

ABSTRACT

Kidney is a site for metabolism and excretion of many commonly used drugs. Dialysis and other extracorporeal therapies enhance clearance of some drugs. Therefore, the need of modifying dosage of drugs commonly arises in patients with impaired kidney function. These are important to recognize as errors in dosing of drugs may lead to higher incidence of drug-related adverse events or lack of efficacy. Glomerular filtration rate (GFR) or creatinine clearance calculated as mL/min is used to guide drug dosage in patients with impaired kidney function. On the other hand, kidneys are susceptible to adverse effects of drugs because of various factors related to characteristics of drug or patient. Drug-induced kidney disease (DIKD) is common in hospitalized patients and frequently missed in the early stages. Though commonly acute, it may also present as chronic kidney disease (CKD). Withdrawal of the suspected or offending drug is the first step in management. Drug-induced autoimmune or hypersensitivity-related kidney disease like drug-induced acute interstitial nephritis may need early institution of specific immunosuppressive therapy to prevent chronic damage. An understanding of interactions between drugs and kidney function is important to ensure rational use of drugs and management of DIKD.

"To raise new questions, new possibilities, to regard old problems from a new angle, requires creative imagination and marks real advance in science"

—Albert Einstein

INTRODUCTION

Drugs and kidney function are important considerations during clinical assessment and decision making in medicine. Kidney is a common site of action, metabolism, and excretion of drugs. Conversely, the pharmacokinetic (PK) and pharmacodynamic (PD) aspects of drug metabolism and action are incomplete without assessment of impact of impaired kidney function.

Kidneys are metabolically highly active organs that receive almost 25% of the cardiac output. In addition to excretion of waste products filtered from circulation, kidneys play important role in erythropoiesis, activation of vitamin D, maintenance of fluid and electrolyte balance and between organ cross talk to maintain systemic homeostasis. In clinical practice, kidney function is usually assessed by estimating GFR from serum creatinine and abnormal excretion of protein or albumin in urine. Tubular defects leading to impaired reabsorption and hence, abnormal excretion of filtered substances in urine, are other manifestations of abnormal kidney function. Drugs are designed to interfere with physiologic or pathologic mechanisms that underlie disease manifestations. However, their actions may not be organ-specific.

Drug-induced disease usually results from toxic pharmacological effects of the drug. As drugs are extraneous agents, drug-induced hypersensitivity reactions can also occur in susceptible individuals. Broadly, a drug can affect kidneys either by systemic disturbances or through interference with various local cellular mechanisms that maintain normal glomerular and tubular functions. When kidney function is impaired, drugs that are metabolized or excreted through kidneys need dose adjustments so that toxic accumulation of such drugs can be avoided. In addition, when patients are being treated by dialysis or other forms of extracorporeal therapies, nonrenal dialytic clearances of drug need to be factored in while prescribing and administering drugs.

It is not uncommon for patients to take over-the-counter or indigenous/local drugs, especially in resource-poor settings. This presents a unique challenge as such drugs are frequently used in an unregulated manner and kidney disease due to these is common. It is important to note that drug-induced changes in kidney function may be acute or chronic. As the changes may not be clinically apparent, a high degree of suspicion is required whenever compatible clinical circumstances are present.

Impaired kidney function is common in sick hospitalized patients and prevalence of chronic kidney disease (CKD) has risen markedly over last few decades. Now, the clinicians commonly find themselves in situations where it becomes important to understand interactions between drug use and impaired kidney function. Approach to interaction between drugs and kidney function in clinical practice can be divided into two distinct parts: Effects of impaired kidney function on drug dosing and adverse effects of drugs that lead to impaired kidney function.

DRUG DOSING IN PATIENTS WITH REDUCED KIDNEY FUNCTION

Inappropriate dosing of a drug in relation to patient's clinical status is a medication error. It can potentially harm the patient either by not achieving desired effect or by producing adverse effects. Failure to change the dose or administration schedule of a drug that requires dose modification or stopping in the setting of impaired kidney function are such errors. In a cross sectional study of 79 hospitalized patients with calculated creatinine clearance ≤59 mL/min, inappropriate dosing for the level of kidney function were noted in 73.6% of the instances. Recent studies have reported dosing errors ranging between 28.6% and 58.2% in drug prescriptions for hospitalized patients with CKD. These data show that errors in drug dosing in patients with reduced kidney function continue to be common.

Clinically, impaired kidney function in a patient is categorized as acute kidney injury (AKI), acute kidney disease (AKD), or CKD based on onset, rapidity of progression, and potential of reversibility. Glomerular filtration rate (GFR) is the primary determinant of clearance of a drug that is excreted in urine. Estimated GFR (eGFR) or creatinine clearance are used as surrogates of filtration function of kidneys.

Administration of a drug that is primarily cleared by kidneys in a patient with reduced kidney function will lead to higher steady state concentrations with usual recommended doses for that drug. This in turn will lead to exaggerated effects of the drug which may rapidly tilt the balance in favor of risk. It is important to note that in addition to aforementioned PK and PD changes, patients with reduced kidney function may be more susceptible to effects of drug due to risk conferred by underlying disease status.

Hospitalized patients with severely reduced kidney function may frequently have other complications like decreased serum albumin and volume overload that can affect distribution of drugs and circulating drug levels. There is emerging evidence to suggest that severely impaired kidney function might also interfere with metabolism of some drugs in liver and gut. The risk of drug interactions is also high in such patients as they frequently receive multiple drugs for various complications.

GENERAL CONSIDERATIONS

Measuring GFR by urinary or plasma clearance of an exogenous marker like inulin, iohexol, or iothalamate is impractical in routine clinical settings. Hence, GFR is estimated using serum creatinine-based estimating GFR equations. eGFR, as calculated using commonly used Modification of Diet in Renal Disease (MDRD) and Chronic Kidney Disease Epidemiology Collaboration (CKD-EPI) equations, is expressed as mL/min/1.73 m^2. However, drug clearances are expressed as volume per unit of time (mL/min). Drug dosing recommendations for patients with impaired kidney function have traditionally used measured creatinine clearance or Cockcroft and Gault (CG) equation to estimate creatinine clearance. Both of these are expressed as mL/min and used as surrogates of GFR. eGFR should be re-expressed as mL/min whenever it is calculated as mL/min/1.73 m^2 to prevent drug dosing errors. This is especially important in situations like extremes of body size where the difference between eGFR standardized to body surface area and absolute eGFR would be high.

The methods for measuring and reporting serum creatinine and eGFR have been standardized to ensure uniformity over last 2–3 decades. Formal guidance documents to guide assessment of relationship between PK/PD of drugs and kidney function were first issued in the United States (US) by US Food and Drug Administration (USFDA) in 1998 and in Europe by European Medicines Agency (EMA) in 2004. The USFDA has recently put out a draft of revised guidance document for public comments in September 2020 which is likely to be finalized soon. It is impossible to repeat PK/PD studies for all drugs as per new guidelines and standardizations. In such cases, manufacturer's recommendations about drug dosing adjustments in the product labels are reasonable and should continue to be used.

The National Institute of Diabetes and Digestive and Kidney Diseases (NIDDK) Laboratory Working Group for "Estimation of Kidney Function for Prescription Medication Dosage in Adults" recommends that, for the purpose of drug dosing, the eGFR equation that is validated for staging of CKD in that population, may be used. At present, CKD-EPI_{Cr} is the most widely used eGFR equation. In Indian context, it is important to realize that cystatin C-based CKD-EPI_{Cys} equation has been shown to be more accurate as compared to CKD-EPI_{Cr}. However, these observations need to be verified on a larger scale. As measurement of cystatin C is expensive and not widely available, CKD-EPI_{Cr} still seems to be the most reasonable choice in Indian population.

The therapeutic index, degree of renal clearance, and fraction of active drug that is excreted unchanged in urine are important *drug-specific characteristics* that determine drug dose modification in the setting of reduced kidney function. Drugs with narrow therapeutic index can lose efficacy or cause toxicity even with a small change in drug concentration. Such drugs are usually monitored through some functional biomarker (e.g., prothrombin time in case of warfarin) or circulating drug concentration (e.g., lithium and tacrolimus). When metabolized or excreted through kidneys, the doses of such drugs are titrated downward as per drug or biomarker levels. Conversely, drugs with wide therapeutic index may not need dose modification across a broad range of kidney function. Drugs which are only partially cleared or metabolized in the kidneys need proportionally lesser dose adjustment as compared to drugs that are almost exclusively cleared or metabolized in the kidneys. On similar lines, drugs with more than 50% fractional excretion of active drug through kidneys would need dose reduction in the setting of reduced kidney function.

SPECIAL CONSIDERATIONS

Chronic kidney disease not on dialysis: The PK/PD data and eGFR equations are derived from populations that consist of clinically stable patients. Therefore, the abovementioned general considerations apply for clinically stable patients with CKD who are not on dialysis (**Flowchart 1**). Drug dose adjustment is done as recommended for the level of eGFR. Therapeutic drug monitoring should be done for drugs with narrow therapeutic index. In the presence of hypoalbuminemia, total drug levels may be low but the active unbound drug levels may be in therapeutic range. Loading doses, if required, are not contraindicated and maintenance with usual dose but prolongation of the dosing interval may be preferred.

AKI or AKD not on dialysis: Patients with rapidly deteriorating kidney function as in AKI or AKD are often critically ill and clinically complex with numerous complications. eGFR equations are not valid in such clinically unstable situations. Also, the PK/PD data cannot be extrapolated as these are usually derived from studies in stable patients with CKD. Presence of multi-organ dysfunction syndrome in critically ill patients further compounds the interpretation of data. Measuring urinary clearance of creatinine is an acceptable surrogate of GFR in these situations. This can be done in 24-hour or shorter-timed urine samples. In case of volume overload, higher loading doses (increase by 25–50%) of hydrophilic drugs may be needed to account for increased volume of distribution.

Dialysis and related extracorporeal therapies: When patients with kidney failure are started on dialysis, an additional factor of dialytic clearance of drug warrants careful consideration. Characteristics of drug (e.g., molecular weight, degree of protein binding, and volume of distribution), dialysis membrane (e.g., type of membrane, surface area, and pore size), type of clearance (diffusive, convective, or both), and treatment parameters (e.g., duration of dialysis, blood flow, dialysate and ultrafiltration rates, and mode of delivery of replacement fluid) affect dialytic clearance of a drug. Dialysis prescription parameters are often tailored to clinical condition of the patient especially in unstable patients with AKI. Hence, achieved drug clearances may vary with each dialysis prescription in such patients.

PK/PD data for guiding dose adjustment in stable end-stage kidney disease (ESKD) patients on hemodialysis

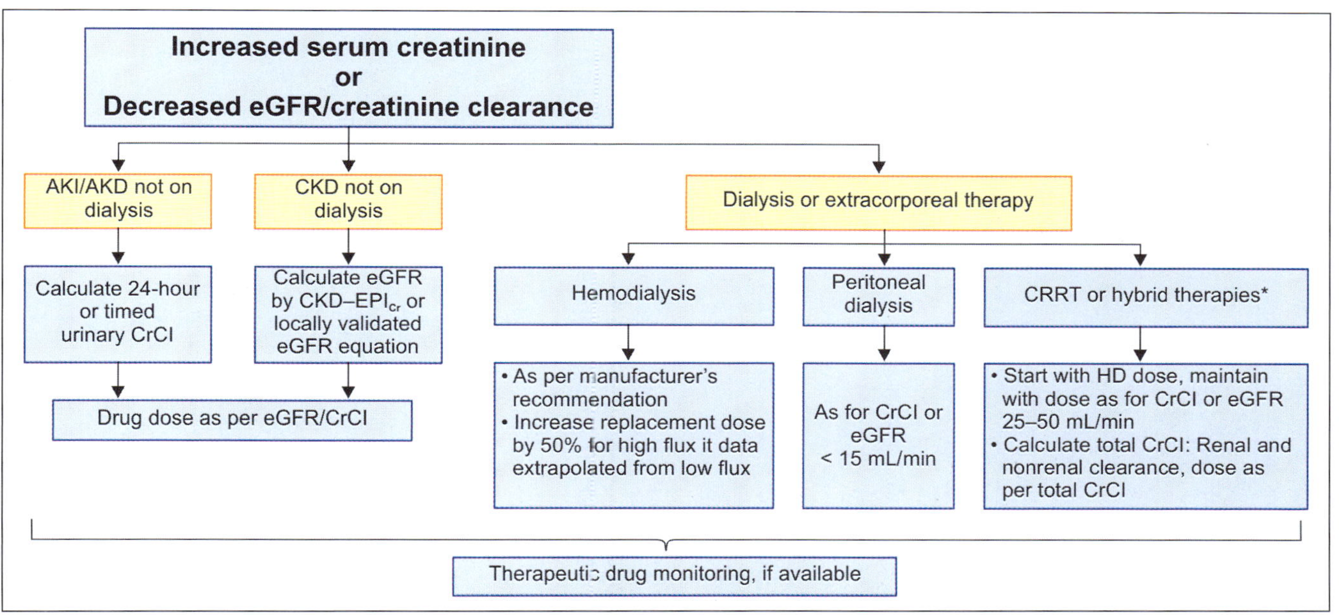

(AKD: acute kidney disease; CKD-EPICr: creatinine-based chronic kidney disease epidemiology collaboration eGFR equation; CrCl: creatinine clearance; CRRT: continuous renal replacement therapy; HD: hemodialysis)

FLOWCHART 1: Drug dosing in kidney failure.

(HD) are available for many drugs. However, these do not simulate all the conditions that clinicians encounter in clinical practice. In addition to dose adjustment for kidney failure, a supplementary dose may be needed after dialysis to replace the fraction lost due to dialytic clearance. Whenever data from low flux dialysis membranes is extrapolated to high flux dialysis membranes, it is advisable to increase the replacement dose by 50%. Similarly, extended dialysis session may warrant higher replacement dose as drug clearance would increase. Whenever possible, the dose of a dialysable drug should be given after HD.

In *patients who receive hybrid dialysis therapies* (e.g., sustained low efficiency daily dialysis or SLEDD etc.) or continuous renal replacement therapies (CRRT), achieved drug clearances can be high. As PK/PD data is not available in such situations for most of the drugs, dosing recommendations for ESKD patients on HD may be used as an initial guide. Whenever available, therapeutic drug monitoring should be used to guide dose adjustment. Total creatinine clearance, calculated as sum of native kidney clearance and extracorporeal clearance, may be used for dose adjustment. This can be extrapolated to eGFR category for dose adjustment. Using this method, most of the drugs would be dosed as for creatinine clearances or eGFRs in the range of 25–50 mL/min. If facilities are available, calculations based on drug's extracorporeal clearance, fraction removed, effluent rate, and filter characteristics can also be used to guide dose adjustment.

The *drug doses for patients on peritoneal dialysis (PD)* are adjusted as for patients with eGFR or creatinine clearance <15 mL/min. This is because of the fact that typical PD prescriptions do not significantly enhance clearance of drugs. For patients with PD-related peritonitis, guidelines for intraperitoneal administration of antibiotics as recommended by International Society of Peritoneal Dialysis (ISPD) should be followed.

Kidney transplant recipients and pediatric patients: Appropriate and validated eGFR equations should be used for calculation of eGFR in kidney transplant recipients and children. Chronic Kidney Disease in Children (CKiD) 2009 (updated bedside Schwartz) equation may be used in children whereas MDRD or CKD-EPI$_{Cr}$ may be used in kidney transplant recipients. Clinicians should always check for drug interactions between immunosuppressants and other drugs in kidney transplant recipients.

DRUG-INDUCED KIDNEY DISEASE

Drug-induced kidney disease is an important cause of reduced kidney function in hospitalized patients. Though commonly identified as AKI, it can present with protracted subacute or chronic presentations. Repetitive subtle insults due to continuous or repeated drug exposures that do not manifest with clinical symptoms or incomplete recovery after substantial acute insult, most likely, lead to subacute or chronic presentations. In studies of critically ill patients from India, the incidence of AKI has been reported to be 6.8–45.9%. In hospitalized patients with AKI, various studies have reported drug-induced nephrotoxicity as cause of AKI in 14–26% of patients.

In the *Acute Kidney Injury Epidemiologic Prospective Investigation (AKI-EPI) study* that evaluated AKI in critically ill patients during first week of intensive care unit (ICU) admission in 97 centers across the world, AKI as defined by Kidney Disease: Improving Global Outcomes (KDIGO) criteria was observed in 57.3% patients. In those with AKI, drug-related causes were present in 14.4%. Treatment with diuretics, nonsteroidal anti-inflammatory drugs (NSAIDs), aminoglycosides, glycopeptides, and radiocontrast agents were noted as predisposing factors for AKI. In the International Society of Nephrology's AKI 0by25 global snapshot study, nephrotoxic agents were identified as

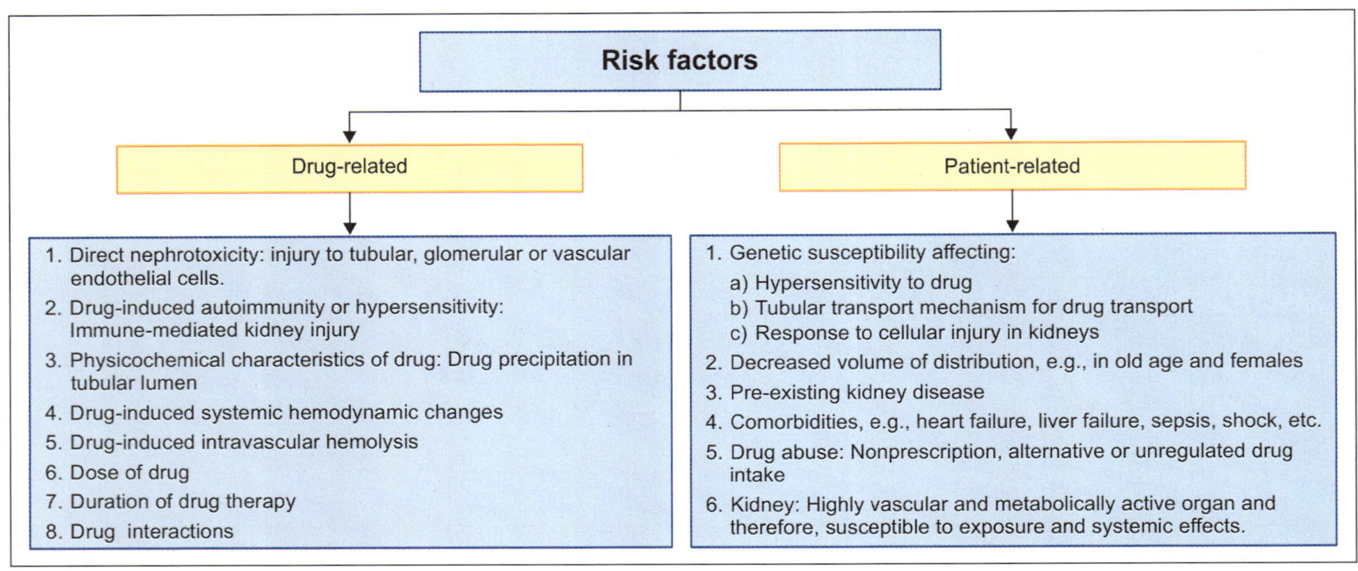

FLOWCHART 2: Risk factors for drug-induced kidney disease.

etiological risk factor in 24% of 4,015 patients enrolled across the world. It is worth noting that this was common (>20%) across high, middle, and low-income countries.

RISK FACTORS FOR DIKD

High incidence of drug-induced kidney disease (DIKD) amongst hospitalized patients is not unusual as such patients would often have multiple comorbidities like diabetes mellitus, hypertension, or acute complications like shock or sepsis that increase the risk of developing kidney dysfunction. Drugs, including those with nephrotoxic potential, are inevitable part of management in such patients. Hence, the risk of interactions between use of drug and development of kidney impairment is very high. However, not all patients with risk factors go on to develop DIKD. Identification of risk factors is important so that drugs can be judiciously selected and appropriate monitoring of kidney function can be instituted right from the beginning. Broadly, these risk factors can be categorized as drug or patient related (**Flowchart 2**).

In kidneys, drugs are either excreted by filtration and/or tubular secretion in urine or metabolized. *Pharmacologic action of drug conferring direct nephrotoxicity* by its action on tubular cells (e.g., aminoglycosides, amphotericin B, and tenofovir) or glomerular/peritubular capillary endothelial cells (e.g., monoclonal antibodies against vascular endothelial growth factor), drug-induced hypersensitivity reactions (e.g., beta-lactam antibiotics, NSAIDs, proton pump inhibitors) leading to inflammatory tubulointerstitial injury, and precipitation of drug within the tubular lumen leading to obstruction by casts and rarely formation of stones (e.g. indinavir, acyclovir) are dominant drug-specific factors. In addition, higher dose of drug and longer duration of therapy amplify the risk of developing DIKD. The risk increases when multiple potentially nephrotoxic drugs are used in combination.

It is important to note that *drug-induced hypersensitivity* may occur even after single dose. Some drugs like diuretics can induce hypovolemia leading to renal hypoperfusion and AKI. Drugs like angiotensin-converting enzyme (ACE) inhibitors or angiotensin II receptor blockers (ARB) change hemodynamics within the kidney and can precipitate AKI in susceptible individuals. Some drugs may induce intravascular hemolysis in susceptible individuals (e.g., those with glucose-6-phosphate dehydrogenase deficiency) and lead to acute tubular necrosis (ATN) due to pigment cast nephropathy. Ethylene glycol as adulterant in cough syrups and acute phosphate intoxication after administration of phosphate-based enemas have been associated with AKI due to tubular deposition of oxalate crystals and calcium phosphate crystals, respectively.

Patient-related factors increase the susceptibility of DIKD when patients are exposed to potentially nephrotoxic drugs. Genetic determinants affecting metabolism, tubular transport (e.g., tenofovir), response to cellular injury (e.g., cisplatin) and allergic immune responses (e.g. acute interstitial nephritis due to many drugs), old age, female sex, pre-existing AKI or CKD, and comorbid conditions like diabetes mellitus, hypertension, urinary tract obstruction, liver failure, heart failure, sepsis, shock etc., are patient-related factors that enhance risk of DIKD. Kidneys are unusually susceptible to risk of DIKD because of high systemic drug exposure due to high vascularity (25% of cardiac output), high susceptibility of medullary regions to injury, and highly active cellular transport mechanisms.

Outside of hospitals and prescriptions in outpatient clinics, a vast number of *over-the-counter drugs* (e.g., dietary supplements and herbal products) and unregulated drugs from alternative systems of medicine are easily available with often, false unverified claims. These drugs frequently use a cocktail of heavy metals, allopathic drugs, natural products, or harmful chemicals. Therefore, it is not surprising to find these drugs as an important cause of DIKD, especially in underprivileged regions in Asia and Africa. In fact, this is an important cause of community-acquired AKI in these regions and should be actively sought during clinical assessment.

CLINICAL PRESENTATION AND DIAGNOSIS

Drug-induced kidney disease can present as AKI, AKD, or CKD. The *most common presentation in hospitalized patients is AKI*. This presents with either progressive increase in serum creatinine or fall in urine output or both. Though AKI is easily picked up in hospitalized patients who are being intensively monitored, it becomes difficult to attribute it to specific drug especially early during the course. This is because of the fact that AKI is usually multifactorial in these circumstances and initial management is directed toward correction of common factors like hypovolemia, sepsis, or primary disease. The suspicion of DIKD becomes high only when the trend of change in kidney function is discordant with the change in overall clinical status. As patients frequently receive multiple drugs, careful history and examination of records are needed to establish temporal association of initiation of drug with onset of impairment in kidney function. However, the trend may not be always apparent. In such case, drugs with known nephrotoxic potential are withdrawn or replaced first.

The diagnosis of AKI due to DIKD in cases of drug-induced hypersensitivity may be picked up early when patients simultaneously develop other hypersensitivity features like new onset fever, rash, pruritus, liver dysfunction, or eosinophilia. Urinalysis may show proteinuria <1 g/day or equivalent, sterile pyuria, white blood cell (WBC) casts, or microscopic hematuria. Presence of eosinophils in urine has not been shown to be of much value in narrowing down differential diagnosis. A diagnosis of *drug-induced acute interstitial nephritis* is likely in these circumstances. However, one must note that this can happen even without any systemic manifestation. It is worth noting that in some cases protracted deterioration in kidney function can occur over weeks, thus qualifying for a diagnosis of AKD or clinical syndrome of rapidly progressive renal failure (RPRF).

Drug-induced kidney disease as cause of CKD is a diagnosis of exclusion when circumstantial association of nephrotoxic drug exposure and CKD due to likely chronic tubulointerstitial injury is present without any obvious cause or risk factors of CKD. Patients with incomplete recovery from AKI/AKD due to drugs would also qualify for diagnosis of CKD after 3 months. Epidemiologically, this may be an important cause of CKD in some regions where widespread use of over-the-counter or alternative drugs are present. In the Indian Chronic Kidney Disease (ICKD) study, a multicentric, prospective cohort study of approximately 4,000 patients with early stage CKD in India, the cause of CKD could not be ascertained in 19.5% of the cohort. The use of alternative drugs and NSAIDs was reported by 22.9% and 15.6% of participants, respectively. As the prevalence of these risk factors is high, this will need further investigation.

Glomerular disease presenting as nephrotic syndrome (secondary to drugs like pamidronate, NSAIDs) or rarely rapidly progressive glomerulonephritis (RPGN) (lupus-like immune complex-mediated glomerulonephritis after hydralazine, procainamide etc., or ANCA-associated pauci-immune glomerulonephritis after rifampicin) are uncommon manifestations of DIKD. These are either due to direct toxic effect on podocytes/other glomerular cells or immune damage secondary to drug-induced auto-immunity. Such patients would have proteinuria >1 g/day or equivalent. In addition, patients with RPGN may show microscopic hematuria with dysmorphic red blood cells (RBCs) or RBC casts on urine examination. Depending on age and clinical course of disease, other common causes of glomerular involvement need to be ruled out. Some drugs like tacrolimus or cyclosporine can lead to glomerular or vascular thrombotic microangiopathy (TMA). Drug-induced TMA involving kidneys clinically presents as RPRF.

Tubular dysfunction leading to renal tubular acidosis, Fanconi syndrome, and diabetes insipidus-like state can also occur due nephrotoxic drug use. Usually, these are dose related and seen with chronic use. Crystalluria with intratubular obstruction due to casts composed of precipitated drug crystals can occur with drugs like indinavir. Rarely, nephrolithiasis can also occur with long-term use of such drugs.

Based on above clinical manifestations, a *classification system* based on clinical phenotype of DIKD has been proposed (**Table 1**). This system provides an initial framework for standardization of DIKD so that systematic assessment of DIKD and its outcomes can be done by ensuring uniformity and comparability across centers. These clinical phenotypes are not mutually exclusive and combinations may occur together or in succession in one patient. Detailed objective criteria have been proposed in this classification system which will allow integration with electronic health records and facilitate early alerts for the treating clinicians.

Suspicion of underlying glomerular disease, acute interstitial nephritis, and persistent or worsening kidney dysfunction despite withdrawal of possible offending drugs are indications for doing *kidney biopsy in a patient with suspected DIKD.* Renal biopsy in such cases has both diagnostic and therapeutic implications. In addition to ruling out other clinical differential diagnoses for AKI or AKD/RPRF, the renal biopsy provides objective evidence for starting immunosuppression (e.g., steroids in acute interstitial nephritis) and prognostic information by demonstrating extent of damage and degree of chronicity. ATN, acute interstitial nephritis, granulomatous interstitial nephritis, crystal-induced nephropathy, osmotic nephrosis, TMA, minimal change disease (MCD), collapsing glomerulopathy, membranous nephropathy, and pauci-immune crescentic glomerulonephritis are some of the morphologic diagnoses on histopathology that have been described in relation to drug-induced nephrotoxicity (**Table 2**).

TABLE 1 Classification of clinical phenotypes in drug-induced kidney disease.

Phenotype	Representative clinical/histological diagnosis
Acute kidney injury	• Acute tubular necrosis • Acute tubulointerstitial nephritis • Osmotic nephrosis
Glomerular disorder	• Nephrotic syndrome • Rapidly progressive glomerulonephritis • Thrombotic microangiopathy
Tubular dysfunction	• Renal tubular acidosis • Fanconi syndrome • Diabetes insipidus
Nephrolithiasis	• Crystalluria • Crystal-induced cast nephropathy • Nephrolithiasis

Drug-induced *acute interstitial nephritis* deserves special mention as it is a common finding in kidney biopsies where index of clinical suspicion is high. Out of 7,308 kidney biopsies that have been done at our center over last 5 years, approximately 0.6% have had a diagnosis of drug-induced acute interstitial nephritis. Typically, interstitial infiltration by eosinophils is found (**Figs. 1 A** to **F**). This is important for pathologists to recognize and clinicians to act upon as immediate therapy with corticosteroids is indicated in addition to withdrawal of offending drug. In organ transplant recipients or other patients who are receiving calcineurin inhibitors like cyclosporine or tacrolimus, calcineurin-induced acute and chronic nephrotoxicity need to be considered.

THERAPEUTIC CONSIDERATIONS

The management of DIKD starts with withdrawal of the offending drug. Based on the clinical situation and judgment, *one or more drugs may be withdrawn or replaced.* This is concurrent with all other strategies that are aimed at other risk factors for AKI. Drug withdrawal may not be needed for just functional tubular defects in acute settings until it becomes difficult to manage resulting complications.

TABLE 2 Morphology of kidney histopathology in drug-induced nephrotoxicity.

Morphology	Drugs associated
Glomerular	
Normal (minimal change disease morphology)	NSAIDs, lithium, and interferon
FSGS: Collapsing type and noncollapsing type	Pamidronate, androgenic anabolic steroids
Membranous nephropathy	Penicillamine, gold salts, and captopril
Lupus-like immune complex glomerulonephritis	Procainamide and hydralazine
Pauci-immune glomerulonephritis	Hydralazine, propylthiouracil, and rifampicin
Thrombotic microangiopathy	Tacrolimus, cyclosporine
Tubulointerstitial	
Acute tubular necrosis	Aminoglycosides, glycopeptides amphotericin B, and cisplatin
Osmotic nephrosis	Radiocontrast agents, plasma expanders, and immunoglobulins
Acute interstitial nephritis	Penicillins, fluoroquinolones, proton pump inhibitors, sulfonamides, NSAIDs, and alternative drugs
Granulomatous interstitial nephritis	Allopurinol
Crystal-induced nephropathy	Indinavir, acyclovir, and sodium phosphate-based enema
Pigment cast nephropathy (secondary to hemolysis)	Primaquine, rifampicin
Vascular	
Thrombotic microangiopathy	Tacrolimus and cyclosporine

(FSGS: focal segmental glomerulosclerosis; NSAIDs: nonsteroidal anti-inflammatory drugs)

Note: A combination of various patterns may be present in one individual.

The benefit of continuing drug may overshadow the risks in such situations, e.g., hypokalemia due to amphotericin B therapy in a patient with disseminated fungal infection. Drugs with dose-related innate nephrotoxic potential, e.g., aminoglycosides, cisplatin, glycopeptides, amphotericin B etc., can be restarted later when the kidney function improves. However, these are always restarted at a lower dose and intensive monitoring of kidney function is warranted. In case of aminoglycosides, single daily dose may be preferred over divided daily doses to prevent nephrotoxicity.

As mentioned previously, *drug-induced acute interstitial nephritis* (including granulomatous interstitial nephritis) warrants immediate immunosuppression with corticosteroids unless contraindicated. The practice is based on immunological nature of insult and data from observational studies that support early recovery with use of steroids. Unfortunately, there are no randomized controlled trials which show that use of steroids or any other immunosuppressive strategy improves the rate of recovery as compared to usual management. The usual strategy is to start prednisolone at 1 mg/kg/day and continue for 2–4 weeks followed by rapid taper over next 4 weeks. There are reports of using pulse therapy of intravenous methylprednisolone up to 500 mg at initiation of therapy. However, this is not the rule. In patients who cannot receive corticosteroids but are candidates for immunosuppression, mycophenolic acid has been used.

In case of *drug-induced glomerular disease*, immunosuppression is initiated early when the underlying mechanism is drug-induced autoimmunity and impairment of kidney function is present as in cases with RPGN. Such patients are usually treated with a combination of corticosteroids and cyclophosphamide. In patients with nephrotic syndrome [MCD or focal segmental glomerulosclerosis (FSGS)], usual course of corticosteroids is given. In patients with drug-induced TMA involving the kidneys, plasma exchange has been used but the role is not clear.

In *patients who already have kidney disease* or are at risk of kidney disease, it is preferable to avoid nephrotoxic drugs. However, this may not be always possible. Therapeutic drug monitoring, if available, should be used for drugs with narrow therapeutic index. If GFR is reduced as a result of DIKD, appropriate drug dose modification should be done for all the prescribed drugs. In case of contrast agents used for imaging, preprocedure hydration should be done. Fear of contrast-induced AKI should not forbid radiocontrast use whenever, it is required for diagnostic or therapeutic purposes.

CONCLUSION

The interaction between drugs and kidneys is inevitable in clinical practice. Kidney disease influences choice of drug, its dose, and dosing schedule. On the other hand, drugs are an important cause of kidney disease. A high degree of suspicion is required to diagnose DIKD as comorbidities and complications frequently confound interpretation in complex clinical situations. In patients with unexplained CKD, history of nephrotoxic drug exposure should be sought.

AKI, the most frequent presentation of DIKD, is one of the most important adverse prognostic factors in hospitalized patients. Preventing drug-induced AKI through judicious use of drugs, withdrawing offending drugs after early recognition of drug-induced AKI and appropriate drug dose modification in patients with reduced kidney function can reduce the burden of DIKD and associated complications. Application of recently proposed classification criteria for DIKD in clinical practice and research are needed to improve its recognition, define outcomes, and identify interventions that can improve outcomes.

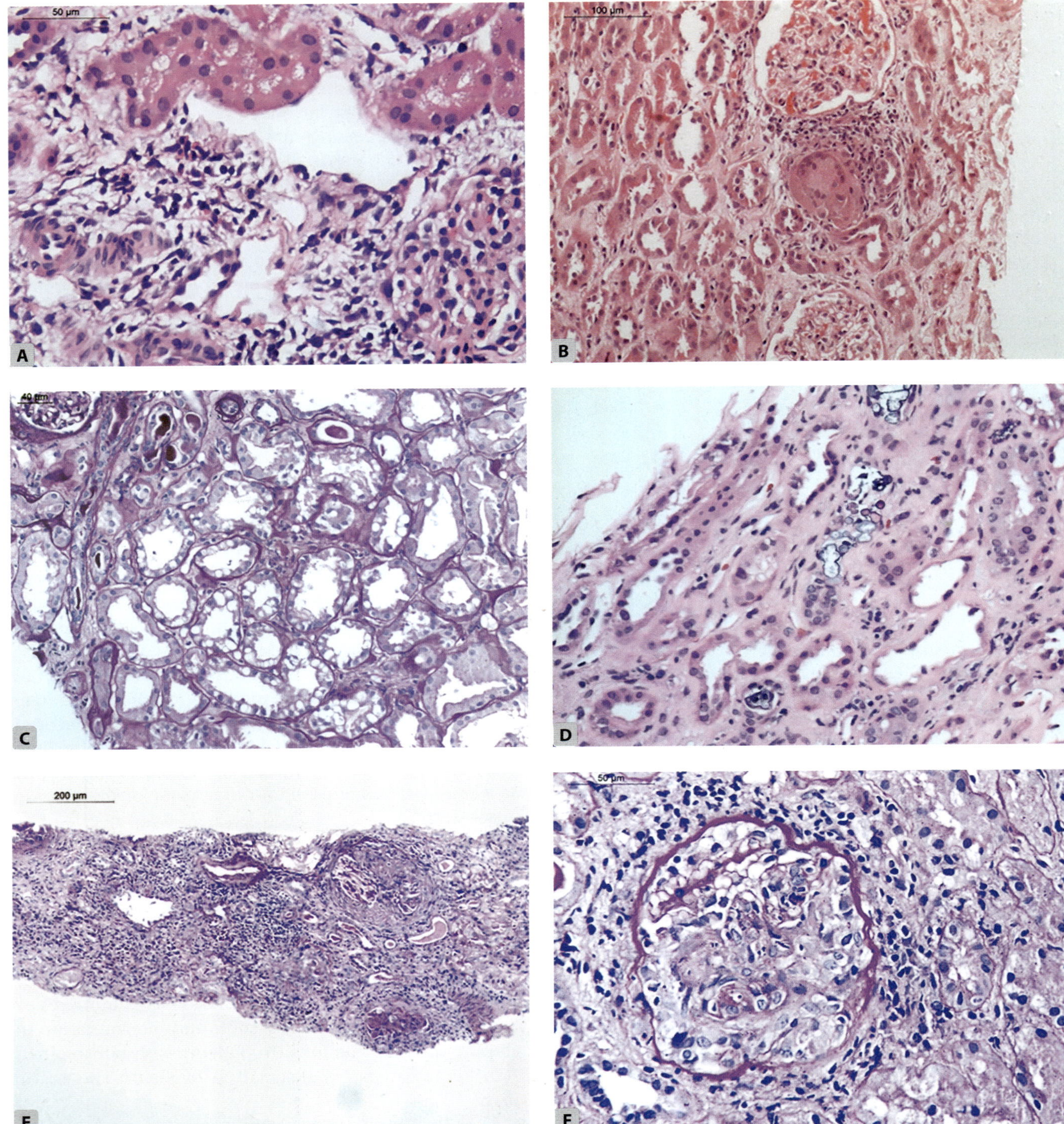

(H&E: hemotoxylin and eosin; PAS: periodic acid-Schiff)

FIGURES 1 A to F: Photomicrographs of kidney biopsies showing **(A)** Acute interstitial nephritis; interstitial inflammation composed of lymphocytes, eosinophils and occasional plasma cell along with interstitial edema in a patients with acute kidney injury who had received alternative drugs; **(B)** Granulomatous tubulointerstitial nephritis; granulomatous inflammation composed of lymphoplasmacytic cells, eosinophils, and foreign body type of giant cell in the interstitium suggestive of drug-induced granulomatous interstitial nephritis [organisms (tuberculosis and fungi) were excluded by special stains] in a patient who took alternative drugs; **(C)** Toxic ATI; proximal tubular cells showing vacuolations in the biopsy with normal distal tubules, glomeruli, and arteries; **(D)** Acute phosphate nephropathy; tubular epithelial cells showing egg-shell type of calcification of individual tubular epithelial cells in a patient with acute kidney injury where it was temporally associated with history of bowel preparation with phosphate-rich bowel preparation formulation; **(E and F)** Rifampicin-associated pauci-immune crescentic glomerulonephritis; kidney biopsy shows cellular crescents without underlying tuft proliferation in patient diagnosed as tuberculosis and started rifampicin (H&E: A to D, PAS: E and F, X400: A, D, and F; X200: B and C; X100-E original magnification: E).

RECOMMENDED READINGS

1. Mehta RL, Awdishu L, Davenport A, Murray PT, Macedo E, Cerda J, et al. Phenotype standardization for drug-induced kidney disease. Kidney Int. 2015;88(2): 226-34.
2. Moledina DG, Perazella MA. Drug-Induced Acute Interstitial Nephritis. Clin J Am Soc Nephrol. 2017;12(12): 2046-9.
3. Perazella MA. Pharmacology behind Common Drug Nephrotoxicities. Clin J Am Soc Nephrol. 2018;13(12): 1897-908.
4. Radhakrishnan J, Perazella MA. Drug-induced glomerular disease: attention required! Clin J Am Soc Nephrol. 2015;10(7):1287-90.
5. NIH. (2015). CKD & Drug Dosing: Information for Providers: National Institute of Diabetes and Digestive and Kidney Diseases. [online] Available from https://www.niddk.nih.gov/health-information/professionals/advanced-search/ckd-drug-dosing-providers
6. Matzke GR, Aronoff GR, Atkinson AJ, Jr., Bennett WM, Decker BS, Eckardt KU, et al. Drug dosing consideration in patients with acute and chronic kidney disease-a clinical update from Kidney Disease: Improving Global Outcomes (KDIGO). Kidney Int. 2011;80(11):1122-37.
7. Doogue MP, Polasek TM. Drug dosing in renal disease. Clin Biochem Rev. 2011;32(2):69-73.
8. Aronson JK. Medication errors: what they are, how they happen, and how to avoid them. QJM. 2009; 102(8):513-21.
9. Bakris GL, Talbert R. Drug dosing in patients with renal insufficiency. A simplified approach. Postgrad Med. 1993;94(8):153-6, 9-60, 63-4.
10. Guidance for Industry: Pharmacokinetics in Patients with Impaired Renal Function - Study Design, Data Analysis, and Impact on Dosing. In: (CDER) CfDEaR (Ed). United States Food and Drug Administration (USFDA); 2020. pp. 1-15.
11. Kulkarni AP, Bhosale SJ. Epidemiology and Pathogenesis of Acute Kidney Injury in the Critically Ill Patients. Indian J Crit Care Med. 2020;24(Suppl 3): S84-9.
12. O'Shaughnessy M, Allen N, O'Regan J, Payne-Danson E, Mentre L, Davin D, et al. Agreement between renal prescribing references and determination of prescribing appropriateness in hospitalized patients with chronic kidney disease. QJM. 2017;110(10):623-8.
13. Saleem A, Masood I. Pattern and Predictors of Medication Dosing Errors in Chronic Kidney Disease Patients in Pakistan: A Single Center Retrospective Analysis. PLoS One. 2016;11(7):e0158677.
14. Mehta RL, Burdmann EA, Cerda J, Feehally J, Finkelstein F, Garcia-Garcia G, et al. Recognition and management of acute kidney injury in the International Society of Nephrology 0by25 Global Snapshot: a multinational cross-sectional study. Lancet. 2016;387(10032):2017-25.
15. Hoste EA, Bagshaw SM, Bellomo R, Cely CM, Colman R, Cruz DN, et al. Epidemiology of acute kidney injury in critically ill patients: the multinational AKI-EPI study. Intensive Care Med. 2015;41(8):1411-23.

CHAPTER 174 Emerging Renal Syndromes: Onconephrology and Cardiorenal Syndrome

R Jayasurya, Sreejith Parameswaran

ABSTRACT

In this chapter, we provide an overview of two emerging areas: "Onconephrology" and "Cardiorenal Syndrome (CRS)." Onconephrology has evolved as a subspeciality in nephrology over the last few years. The relationship between cancer and kidney disease is bidirectional. The diagnosis and treatment of cancer are often complicated by the presence of kidney disease—both acute and chronic. Certain kidney diseases can predispose to malignancy. In the first section, the methods for assessment of kidney function, major causes of acute kidney injury (AKI) in cancer patients, electrolyte and acid–base disturbances, malignancy-associated glomerular diseases, myeloma-related kidney disease, renal adverse effects of chemotherapeutic drugs, and kidney involvement post hematopoietic stem cell transplant (HSCT) are discussed.

In the second part, we have summarized the definition, classification, and complex pathophysiologic mechanisms of CRS. Heart and kidney disease often coexist. The term CRS includes disorders of heart and kidneys where acute or chronic dysfunction of one organ can cause acute or chronic dysfunction of the other organ. The diagnostic approach and treatment options are also described.

"The art of clinical diagnosis lies in the ability to ask the right questions"

—Harriet B Braiker

ONCONEPHROLOGY

INTRODUCTION

Onconephrology is an evolving subspeciality of nephrology dealing with the complex interactions between cancer and kidney disease. Up to 60% of cancer patients can have some form of kidney involvement. Cancer can affect the kidney directly or indirectly. Examples of direct renal involvement by cancer include malignancies, such as multiple myeloma with cast nephropathy, renal amyloidosis, monoclonal immunoglobulin deposition disease (MIDD), genitourinary malignancy with obstructive uropathy, leukemia and lymphoma infiltrating the kidney, and glomerulopathies, such as membranous nephropathy (MN) associated with cancer. Indirect involvement of kidneys can occur secondary to cancer complications such as infections, volume depletion from vomiting, diarrhea, and cardiac and liver involvement with attendant complications.

Drugs used in the treatment of cancer may have nephrotoxicity and cause AKI, chronic kidney disease (CKD), or electrolyte and acid–base abnormalities. Both AKI and CKD are being increasingly recognized in cancer patients. Impaired kidney function can have a significant impact on treatment options and influence the outcome of cancer. Patients with CKD, including those undergoing dialysis and after kidney transplantation, have a higher incidence of cancer compared to those without CKD. Thus, the relationship between cancer and kidney disease is bidirectional.

ASSESSMENT OF KIDNEY FUNCTION

- Estimation of glomerular filtration rate (eGFR) using serum creatinine-based equations is the most convenient way to assess kidney function.
- Modification of Diet in Renal Disease (MDRD) equation and Chronic Kidney Disease Epidemiology Collaboration (CKD-EPI) equation are commonly used for assessment of eGFR.
- Using serum creatinine-based eGFR equations has certain important limitations in cancer patients:
  - Cancer may cause significant loss of muscle mass and the resulting sarcopenia may result in low serum creatinine values. This will lead to overestimation of eGFR resulting in inappropriate dose of chemotherapeutic agents.
  - Serum creatinine values are not reliable when the kidney function is rapidly changing.
- In such instances, more accurate measurement with 24-hour urine creatinine clearance or techniques of radioisotope clearance may have to be used.
- For dosing of drugs, the CKD-EPI equation is the current best method.

ACUTE KIDNEY INJURY IN CANCER

- In a Danish population-based study of 37,267 cancer patients, the 1-year risk of AKI was 17.5% and 5-year risk was 27%.
- Metastatic disease had a higher incidence of AKI.
- The presence of AKI was associated with higher morbidity and mortality.
- Mortality of patients with AKI requiring renal replacement therapy (RRT) was >60%.
- AKI can be due to direct effects of cancer such as tumor infiltration or obstruction, effects of chemotherapeutic drugs, or complications such as sepsis.
- Cancers with the highest risk of AKI include renal cancers, myeloma, and liver cancer. Lymphomas and leukemias undergoing treatment also have a high risk of AKI.

The common causes of AKI in cancer are described in **Box 1**.

ELECTROLYTE AND ACID–BASE DISORDERS

Electrolyte (**Table 1**) and acid–base abnormalities are common in cancer and may be a direct consequence of the cancer or its treatment.

BOX 1	Common causes of acute kidney injury in cancer.
Prerenal causes:	
• Volume depletion due to poor oral intake, vomiting, diarrhea, polyuria, third spacing, insensible losses from skin lesions	
• Fluctuations in hemodynamic stability in sepsis, congestive cardiac failure, hepatorenal syndrome, Budd–Chiari syndrome, inferior vena cava compression or obstruction	
• Intraabdominal compartment syndrome	
Intrinsic renal causes:	
Acute tubular necrosis, acute interstitial nephritis, myeloma-related kidney disease, thrombotic microangiopathy	
Post-renal obstructive causes:	
Bladder outlet obstruction due to prostate, bladder, cervix or uterine tumors, retroperitoneal masses, urethral stricture (BK virus infection or prior radiotherapy), hemorrhagic cystitis (cyclophosphamide, adeno virus or BK virus)	

TABLE 1 Common electrolyte abnormalities in cancer.

Electrolyte abnormality	Cause	Comments
Hyponatremia	• SIADH • Drugs-induced renal loss • GI loss	• The most common abnormality encountered • Pseudohyponatremia may result from very high plasma protein levels in paraproteinemia
Hypernatremia	• Central diabetes insipidus—*leukemic infiltration or primary or metastatic pituitary tumors* • Nephrogenic diabetes insipidus—*hypercalcemia, hypokalemia, obstructive uropathy*	
Hypokalemia	• Usually from poor intake or GI loss • Ifosfamide—renal tubular injury • ACTH-secreting tumors—mineralocorticoid pathway • AML M4 and M5—lysozymuria, tubular injury, and K wasting • Abiraterone—excess mineralocorticoid activity	Urinary K excretion to be assessed
Hypercalcemia	• Direct involvement of bone and osteolytic release of calcium—primary bone cancers, myeloma or metastatic breast and prostate cancer • Humoral hypercalcemia from secretion of PTHrP—squamous cell carcinoma of lung or head and neck • Excess 1,25 (OH)2 vitamin D—lymphoma cells with 1 alpha hydroxylase activity • Primary hyperparathyroidism—cancer of parathyroid, ovaries	• Seen in 20–30% of cancer patients • Treatment strategies include saline hydration, frusemide, bisphosphonates, RANK ligand inhibitor Denosumab, and treatment of underlying malignancy

(PTHrP: parathyroid hormone-related protein; RANK: receptor activator of nuclear factor kappa-B; SIADH: syndrome of inappropriate antidiuretic hormone secretion)

Other common electrolyte imbalances are hypomagnesemia (poor intake, chemotherapeutic drugs such as Cetuximab) and hypophosphatemia (malnutrition or renal tubular wasting due to drugs such as Ifosfamide and Imatinib).

Lactic acidosis (type A and type B): Type A lactic acidosis occurs due to tissue hypoxia in cardiac failure or septic shock and type B lactic acidosis results from anaerobic glycolysis by tumor cells, thiamine deficiency, or the effect of tumor-derived cytokines. *Renal tubular acidosis* can occur due to tubular injury produced by chemotherapeutic drugs, such as Cisplatin, or Fanconi syndrome due to proximal tubular injury in multiple myeloma.

Tumor-induced osteomalacia is a specific syndrome causing hypophosphatemia in tumors such as hemangiopericytoma, giant cell tumor, and osteoblastoma. This occurs due to excessive production of phosphatonin [fibroblast growth factor-23 (FGF-23)]. Metabolic alkalosis can occur in rare renin-producing tumor.

Tumor lysis syndrome is a group of metabolic abnormalities occurring due to spontaneous or chemotherapy-induced tumor cell lysis (**Table 2**). TLS is often encountered in non-Hodgkin's lymphoma, particularly Burkitt cell lymphoma, followed by acute lymphocytic and lymphoblastic lymphoma, in acute myeloid leukemia, and less commonly in chronic leukemia and myeloma.

Prevention of TLS begins with adequate hydration in high-risk patients, use of xanthine oxidase inhibitors and rasburicase to treat hyperuricemia, and close monitoring of TLS parameters. Rarely patients may require RRT when there is oliguric AKI or refractory hyperkalemia.

TABLE 2 Cairo–Bishop definition of laboratory tumor lysis syndrome (TLS) and clinical TLS.

Metabolite/ Electrolyte	Criteria
	Laboratory TLS (LTLS)
Uric acid	≥8 mg/dL or 25% increase from baseline
Potassium	≥6 mEq/L or 25% increase from baseline
Phosphorus	≥6.5 mg/dL (children) or ≥4.5 mg/dL (adults) or 25% increase from baseline
Calcium	<7 mg/dL or >25% reduction from baseline
	Clinical TLS
LTLS with one or more of the following: Serum creatinine >1.5 times the upper limit of normal (≥12 years of age or age adjusted), cardiac arrhythmias or sudden death, seizures	

GLOMERULAR DISEASES AND CANCER

Glomerular diseases may develop as a paraneoplastic manifestation, as an effect of chemotherapeutic drugs, or associated with HSCT. *MN is the most common glomerular disease* associated with malignancy. The prevalence of malignancy in MN is reported as 10%; among patients older than 60 years, the prevalence may be up to 22%. Only 50% of malignancies are evidenced at the time of diagnosis of MN. The most common malignancies associated with MN are pulmonary and gastric carcinomas followed by renal cell carcinoma, prostatic cancers, and thymoma. Absence of anti-PLAR2R antibody, presence of more than eight inflammatory cells per glomerulus, and predominance of immunoglobulin G1 (Ig G1)/Ig G2 glomerular deposits are some of the features which should prompt suspicion of secondary MN. Age- and sex-appropriate screening for malignancy should be done when secondary MN is suspected.

Minimal change disease (MCD) is associated with solid tumors including lung, colorectal, renal cell carcinomas, and thymomas. Focal segmental glomerulosclerosis (FSGS) is reported with renal cell carcinoma, thymoma, lung, breast, and esophageal cancers. The membranoproliferative glomerulonephritis (MPGN) pattern is associated with solid tumors of lung, kidney, stomach, melanoma, breast cancer, and thymoma. IgA nephropathy is seen with solid tumors of the respiratory tract, buccal mucosa, nasopharynx, and renal cell carcinoma. Both solid tumors and hematologic malignancies have been associated with adult Henoch–Schonlein purpura. Gastric, lung, and renal cancers are described with crescentic glomerulonephritis (CGN). Thrombotic microangiopathy (TMA) is linked with mucin-producing gastric lung and breast cancers. Malignancy-associated TMA responds poorly to plasmapheresis. *AA amyloidosis* is described with hepatic adenoma, Castleman disease, and renal cell carcinoma.

In Hodgkin's lymphoma, the most commonly described pathology is MCD. Chronic lymphocytic lymphoma (CLL), hairy cell leukemia, and non-Hodgkin's lymphoma often present with the MN or MPGN pattern. Immunotactoid glomerulopathy, followed by fibrillary glomerulonephritis, is associated with paraproteinemias and CLL. Thymoma is associated with MCD, MN, FSGS, CGN, and lupus-like nephritis.

MYELOMA AND KIDNEY

More than 50% of multiple myeloma can develop AKI and 10% may require RRT at presentation. Major renal manifestations include cast nephropathy, light chain deposition disease, and amyloid light chains (AL) amyloidosis. Hypercalcemia and infections are also common causes of AKI in myeloma.

Cast nephropathy is seen in 41% patients with renal involvement. It occurs when excess light chains precipitate with Tamm–Horsfall protein secreted by the thick ascending limb of loop of Henle and form casts in the distal tubule. Factors which can accelerate cast formation include volume depletion, diuretics, hypercalcemia, and nonsteroidal anti-inflammatory drugs. Free light chains can produce direct toxic effects on proximal tubules leading to tubular injury even in the absence of cast formation.

Light chain deposition disease is the second most common cause of renal involvement in myeloma seen in 19% of cases. Clinically, patients present with proteinuria and renal insufficiency. Renal biopsy shows a nodular glomerulosclerosis picture. Immunofluorescence demonstrates linear staining of the basement membrane with monotypic light chains, most commonly kappa restricted. Electron microscopy demonstrates granular deposits within mesangium, glomerular, and tubular basement membranes.

Amyloid light chain amyloidosis is seen in 15% of patients in autopsy studies of myeloma. AL amyloidosis develops when pathogenic light chains deposit in tissues as insoluble fibrils. The clinical presentation is usually with nephrotic syndrome. Light microscopy of renal biopsy reveals amorphous hyaline material deposited in mesangium, glomerular basement membrane, and vessel walls, with Congo red positivity and apple green birefringence in polarized light. Immunofluorescence demonstrates light chain restriction. Electron microscopy demonstrates deposits of nonbranching randomly oriented fibrils of 8–10-nm diameter.

Other renal manifestations of myeloma include heavy-chain deposition disease, fibrillary glomerulonephritis, immunotactoid glomerulopathy, Fanconi syndrome, cryoglobulinemia, membranous glomerulopathy, and MPGN.

Treatment of cast nephropathy includes adequate hydration, correction of hypercalcemia, and RRT if indicated. Diuretics should be avoided unless there is volume overload. Reduction in free light chain levels by successful chemotherapy is the key treatment. Reduction in light chain clone by 60% by day 21 of diagnosis is associated with renal recovery in 80% cases with severe AKI. Bortezomib, thalidomide, and lenalidomide are commonly used chemotherapeutic agents. In selected patients, HSCT is potentially curative.

CHEMOTHERAPEUTIC DRUGS AND KIDNEY

ANTIANGIOGENIC DRUGS

Angiogenesis is important for tumor growth and metastases. Vascular endothelial growth factor (VEGF) binds to a receptor (VEGFR) which has tyrosine kinase activity. This triggers intracytoplasmic signaling pathways leading to angiogenesis.

Drugs which affect VEGF pathways include Bevacizumab, Ramucirumab, and small-molecule multi-target tyrosine kinase inhibitors (m-TKI)—sunitinib, sorafenib, axitinib, and pazopanib. All the drugs are known to produce hypertension, proteinuria, and TMA. Patients should be assessed for cardiovascular risk factors prior to starting anti-VEGF therapy. They should be carefully monitored for the development of hypertension. In those with hypertension and concomitant proteinuria, angiotensin-converting enzyme (ACE) inhibitors or angiotensin receptor blockers (ARBs) should be started. In patients with hypertension or proteinuria, controlled with medical treatment, anticancer treatment can be continued. Development of nephrotic syndrome, microangiopathic hemolytic anemia, or progressive renal insufficiency should prompt termination of anti-VEGF therapy (**Table 3**).

TABLE 3 Chemotherapeutic drugs and kidney.

Drug	Mechanism of injury	Clinical manifestation	Comments
Cisplatin	Tubular injury is most common though can affect glomeruli and vessels	• Proximal tubulopathy with ◦ Proteinuria and hypophosphatemia ◦ Fanconi syndrome ◦ Sodium and magnesium wasting ◦ Nephrogenic diabetes insipidus • AKI—tubular injury, TMA	• AKI can recover or lead to tubulointerstitial fibrosis and CKD • Prevention—hydration and forced diuresis • Amifostine—reduce tubular injury • Alternative agents such as oxaliplatin and carboplatin in high-risk patients
Ifosfamide	Proximal tubulopathy	• Fanconi syndrome • Nephrogenic diabetes insipidus • AKI	• Risk factors—CKD, cumulative dose >90 g/m^2, and previous cisplatin exposure
Mitomycin	TMA	AKI	Dose exceeding 40 mg/m^2 is not recommended
Methotrexate	Precipitation of 7-OH-methotrexate in distal tubular lumen and free radical injury	AKI	• Prevention—hydration, appropriate drug dosing, and alkalinization of urine • Leucovorin rescue, glucarpidase (cleaves methotrexate to noncytotoxic metabolites), and high-flux hemodialysis useful in treatment of toxicity and AKI
Pemetrexed	Tubular injury, interstitial nephritis, fibrosis	AKI, diabetes insipidus	
Gemcitabine	TMA	AKI	• Prior treatment with Mitomycin C and high dose are risk factors • Treatment is supportive
Crizotinib		AKI	• Inhibitor of anaplastic lymphoma kinase • Used in non-small cell lung cancer
Cetuximab, panitumumab	Activation of TRPC6 by EGFR blocked	• Hypomagnesemia • Secondary hypocalcemia and hypokalemia	• Monoclonal antibodies against EGFR • treatment of epithelial origin tumors
Interferon	Podocyte injury	Nephrotic syndrome—MCN/FSGS	Multiple malignancies
Androgen deprivation therapy	Unknown	Higher incidence of AKI	Prostatic cancer
Carfilzomib		AKI	Novel proteasome inhibitor used in treatment of relapsed/refractory myeloma
Immune checkpoint inhibitors—ipilimumab, pembrolizumab, nivolumab	Inhibit downregulatory receptors on T cells such as CTLA-4, PD-1 and PD-L1	Pauci-immune GN and renal vasculitis, podocytopathies, C3GN, IgA nephropathy, AIN, AA amyloidosis	

(AIN: acute interstitial nephritis; C3GN: C3 glomerulonephritis; CTLA-4: cytotoxic T-lymphocyte-associated protein 4; EGFR: epidermal growth factor receptor; FSGS: focal segmental glomerulosclerosis; IgA: immunoglobulin A; MCN: minimal change nephropathy; PD-1: programmed death-1; PD-L1: programmed cell death ligand 1; TMA: thrombotic microangiopathy; TRPC6: transient receptor potential cation channel subfamily c member 6)

HEMATOPOIETIC STEM CELL TRANSPLANT AND KIDNEY

Up to 70% of patients may develop some sort of renal abnormality after HSCT. GFR <60 mL/min/1.73 m^2 persisting beyond 3 months (CKD) is reported in up to 48% of post-HSCT patients. CKD can develop in period ranging from 6 months to 10 years and progress to ESRD in 4%.

- *Cause of AKI after HSCT*: Total body irradiation, nephrotoxic agents, infections, graft versus host disease (GVHD), calcineurin inhibitor (CNI) toxicity, transplant-associated TMA, and hepatic sinusoidal obstruction syndrome.
- *Risk factors for AKI after HSCT*: Incomplete human leukocyte antigen (HLA) matching, severe GVHD, use of prophylactic methotrexate for GVHD prophylaxis,

diabetes, use of more than three chemotherapy courses prior to transplant.

- *Causes of TMA after HSCT*: Use of CNI, mechanistic target of rapamycin (mTOR) inhibitors, acute GVHD, use of total body irradiation, presence of infections such as BK virus, use of peripheral blood stem cells.
    - Treatment is supportive; therapeutic plasma exchange is usually not effective.
- *Risk factors for CKD*: Previous AKI, acute and chronic GVHD, age >45 years, baseline GFR <90 mL/min/1.73 m^2, high-dose total body irradiation, and presence of hypertension.

Glomerular diseases including MN, MCD, and FSGS are described post HSCT. When MCD occurs post-transplant, recurrence of primary disease has to be ruled out. Occurrence of chronic GVHD is associated with occurrence of nephrotic syndrome.

To conclude, cancer patients need close monitoring for potential development of renal complications. Cancer patients with underlying kidney disease need special precautions and treatment modifications. With the rapid evolution of drug armamentarium of oncology, a wider spectrum of renal toxicities is evolving. Further research and close interdisciplinary team approach are needed for better patient care.

CARDIORENAL SYNDROME

INTRODUCTION

Kidney disease and heart failure often coexist. CKD is observed in about 30% of patients hospitalized with heart failure. Impaired kidney function is an independent predictor of morbidity and mortality in patients with heart disease. In turn, patients with reduced kidney function (GFR) are at a high risk of death from cardiovascular disease, myocardial infarction, and heart failure. The understanding of this close association between heart disease and kidney disease has led to the use of the term CRS, which is used to describe situations where cardiac and renal dysfunction coexists.

DEFINITION

Cardiorenal syndrome is broadly defined as disorders of the heart and kidneys whereby acute or chronic dysfunction in one organ may induce acute or chronic dysfunction of the other. The definition of CRS has evolved over time with better recognition of the bidirectional relationship between heart and kidney disease.

In 2008, Acute Dialysis Quality Initiative (ADQI) classified CRS into two major groups: CRS and renocardiac syndromes (RCS) based on the organ first involved by the disease process. This was further divided into five groups based on the sequence of organ involvement and the nature of onset (acute vs. chronic) of the disease (**Table 4**) **Flowchart 1**.

However, overlap of clinical phenotypes and evolution of one subtype into another is inevitable. The identification of initial insult and subsequent events resulting in decompensated acute or chronic CRS/RCS is often challenging in clinical practice. Therefore, a classification based on various clinical manifestations irrespective of the sequence of organ involvement was proposed. This classification takes into account factors such as hemodynamic compromise, uremic or vascular manifestations, neurohumoral disturbances, mineral—bone disorders, anemia/iron abnormalities and the malnutrition–inflammation complex (**Table 5**).

PATHOPHYSIOLOGY

Pathogenesis of CRS is complex and involves multiple pathways. The relative role of pathophysiologic pathways varies depending upon the clinical status and the type of CRS (**Table 6** and **Flowchart 2**).

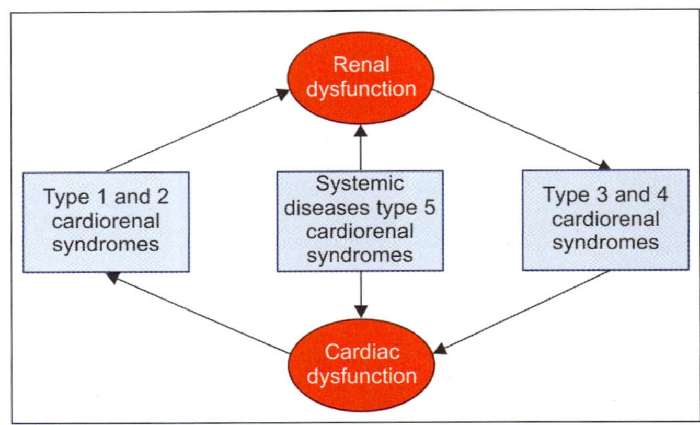

FLOWCHART 1: Subtypes of cardiorenal syndrome.

TABLE 4 Classification of CRS based on ADQI consensus (2008).

Type 1 CRS	Acute CRS	HF resulting in AKI	Acute coronary syndrome resulting in cardiogenic shock and AKI
Type 2 CRS	Chronic CRS	Chronic HF resulting in CKD	Chronic HF
Type 3 CRS	Acute renocardiac syndrome	AKI resulting in HF	HF in the setting of AKI due to volume overload, inflammation, and metabolic changes of uremia
Type 4 CRS	Chronic renocardiac syndrome	CKD resulting in chronic HF	CKD-associated cardiomyopathy
Type 5 CRS	Secondary CRS	Systemic disease resulting renal and cardiac dysfunction	Amyloidosis, sepsis, cirrhosis

TABLE 5 Proposed CRS classification based on putative pathophysiology and clinical applicability at time of patient evaluation.

CRS category	Definition	Comments
Hemodynamic	Hemodynamic compromise is the major clinical manifestation	Can be subclassified as acute (1a) or chronic (1b)
Uremic	Uremic manifestations are the most prominent clinical appearances	Can be subclassified as acute (2a) or chronic (2b)
Vascular	Cardiovascular and/or renovascular manifestations are the most prominent clinical findings	Can be subclassified as acute (3a) or chronic (3b) and as atherosclerotic (as), thromboembolic (te), or endothelial dysfunction (ed)
Neurohumoral	Electrolyte disorders, acid–base disorders, or dysautonomia is the most prominent finding	Can be subcategorized into acute (4a) or chronic (4b) and into electrolyte (el), acid–base (ab), or autonomic dysregulation (ad)
Anemia and/or iron metabolism	Anemia and/or iron metabolism dysregulation are the most prominent clinical manifestations	Can be subcategorized into acute (5a) or chronic (5b)
Mineral metabolism	Dysregulation of calcium and phosphorus and their regulators including vitamin D and FGF-23 are the most prominent clinical manifestations	This category is mostly chronic by nature
Malnutrition–inflammation–cachexia	Malnutrition, cachexia, and inflammatory state are the most prominent clinical manifestation	This category is mostly chronic by nature
Each category shows the most prominent clinical manifestation of the patient that needs to be addressed first. The category of any given patient may vary with time and depends on the current clinical evaluation. The category at any point in time guides the clinician to the main focus of management		

(CRS: cardiorenal syndrome; FGF-23: fibroblast growth factor-23)

TABLE 6 Summary of various pathophysiologic mechanisms of CRS.

Mechanism	Mediator	End organ outcome	
		Heart	Kidney
Increased central venous and intraabdominal pressures	• Increased salt/water retention • Activation of RAAS/SNS	• Acute/chronic HF • Adverse remodeling of heart and lungs	• Renal venous congestion • Reduced GFR
Reduced cardiac output and cardiac index	• Peripheral vasodilation/reduced vascular resistance • Reduced perfusion pressure	• Activation of RAAS/SNS detrimental to heart • Cardiac ischemia from reduced perfusion	• Reduced renal Perfusion • Renal ischemia
• Neurohormonal dysregulation • RAAS activation • SNS activation Adenosine/AVP	• Impaired baroreceptor reflexes • Increased renin secretion • Increased Ang II secretion • Increased aldosterone secretion • Increased ET-1 expression • Oxidative stress	• Myocyte hypertrophy, left ventricular dysfunction • Proinflammation, profibrotic effect • Hypertension	• Arteriolar vasoconstriction • Reduced GFR • Enhanced reabsorption of sodium/water • Proinflammation, profibrotic effect
Oxidative stress	• Increased reactive oxygen species formation • Ang II-enhanced NADPH oxidase activity • Uremic toxin–mediated Cytokine release	• Left ventricular hypertrophy • Accelerated atherosclerosis • Endothelial dysfunction • Inflammation • Fibrosis	• Endothelial dysfunction • Accelerated • Atherosclerosis • Inflammation • Interstitial fibrosis
Inflammatory mediators	• TNF-α • TWEAK • Members of IL-1 family • IL-6 • CRP	• Atherosclerosis • Inflammation • Left ventricular dysfunction • Cardiac hypertrophy • Myocardial cell death • Fibrosis	• Inflammation • Fibrosis • Atherosclerosis • Glomerular damage by mesangial cell apoptosis

Continued...

Continued...

Mechanism	Mediator	End organ outcome	
		Heart	Kidney
Renal failure disturbances	• PBUTs (indoxyl sulfate, p-cresyl sulfate) • Chronic inflammatory cytokines • Oxidative stress • FGF-23 • Calcium/phosphate-mediated inflammation • Anemia	• Endothelial dysfunction • Atherosclerosis • Left ventricular dysfunction • Cardiac hypertrophy	• Atherosclerosis • Inflammation • Increased interstitial and perivascular fibrosis

(Ang II: angiotensin II; AVP: arginine vasopressin; CRS: cardiorenal syndrome; ET-1: endothelin-1; FGF-23: fibroblast growth factor-23; GFR: glomerular filtration rate; IL: interleukin; PBUTs: protein-bound uremic toxins; TNF-α: tumor necrosis factor alpha; TWEAK: tumor necrosis factor alpha–related weak inducer of apoptosis)

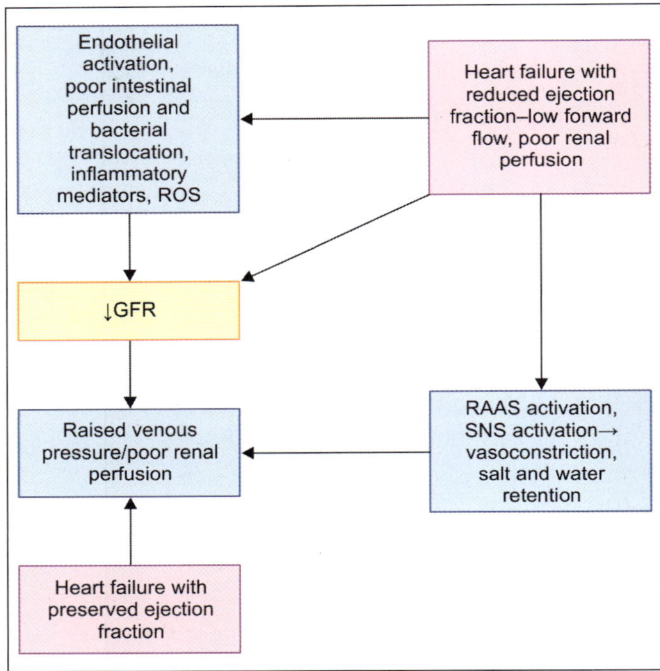

(ROS: reactive oxygen species)

FLOWCHART 2: Pathophysiology of cardiorenal syndrome.

DIAGNOSIS

Diagnostic modalities of CRS include imaging techniques, biomarkers, invasive hemodynamic monitoring, and volume measurement techniques.

Echocardiography is the most used imaging modality which helps to assess hemodynamic parameters including pulmonary capillary wedge pressure/left atrial pressure, cardiac output, and systolic pulmonary artery pressure. Renal ultrasonography and intrarenal venous flow pattern help in assessing the structural abnormalities of kidneys and renal congestion. Cardiac magnetic resonance imaging is another noninvasive method which helps in assessing ventricular dimensions and myocardial fibrosis.

Cardiac biomarkers, brain natriuretic peptide (BNP), and N terminal pro-brain natriuretic peptide (NT-proBNP) are used for diagnosis and prognostication of heart failure. Patients with decreased GFR have higher values of NT-proBNP compared to those with normal kidney function. This is because of impaired renal clearance of NT-proBNP along with the presence of fluid overload in kidney disease patients and CKD-associated left ventricular (LV) hypertrophy or cardiomyopathy. BNP levels are more elevated in CRS compared to heart failure with normal kidney function.

High-sensitivity cardiac troponins T and I are used in the diagnosis of acute myocardial infarction. They are also useful in prognostication of heart failure, even in the absence of myocardial ischemia. When elevated, these markers are associated with higher mortality. The levels of these markers are elevated in those with reduced GFR. But sustained elevation is associated with poor prognosis.

Suppressor of tumorigenicity 2 (ST2) and galectin 3 are other biomarkers which are useful in prognostication of CRS.

Bioimpedance vector analysis, measurement of intra-abdominal pressure, and relative blood volume monitoring devices are some of the methods used for volume assessment, useful in monitoring patients with CRS.

Invasive hemodynamic monitoring is not routinely recommended in heart failure. But it helps to prevent underdiagnosis of pulmonary hypertension prevents underestimation of valvular lesions such as mitral regurgitation and tricuspid regurgitation, and also helps in accurate diagnosis of volume overload and right ventricular failure. Pulmonary artery catheterization helps in situations where there is subclinical congestion and helps to avoid intravascular volume depletion in patients with CRS.

MANAGEMENT

DIURETICS

Diuretics are the most important form of treatment in CRS. Loop diuretics (furosemide, torsemide, bumetanide, and ethacrynic acid) are the most used class of diuretics in CRS. They act by inhibition of Na–K–2Cl cotransporter in the thick ascending limb of the loop of Henle. The duration of action of loop diuretics is 2–3 hours following intravenous and 6 hours following oral administration. Bioavailability of loop diuretics is 50% following oral administration and 100% following intravenous administration.

The goal of diuretic therapy is to eliminate the clinical evidence of fluid retention. Diuretics should be continued though patients may develop mild elevation in renal function. Patients should be monitored for hypokalemia, hypomagnesemia, and metabolic alkalosis. In those who develop reduction in blood pressure, the diuretic therapy should be moderated. Concurrent use of aldosterone antagonist can reduce the risk of hypokalemia. Sodium restriction (<3 g/day) and fluid restriction should be advised along with diuretic therapy.

Diuretic resistance: The major causes of diuretic resistance are inadequate dose, poor compliance to salt and water restriction, hypoalbuminemia, excessive sodium reabsorption from distal parts of nephron, and decreased absorption due to gut mucosal edema. With short-term use, diuretic resistance can be due to "braking phenomenon" and in the long-term, diuretic resistance can be due to distal tubular hypertrophy. The braking phenomenon indicates reduced diuretic efficiency with successive doses. The measures to overcome diuretic resistance include use of higher dose, use of intravenous instead of oral form, use of salt-free albumin, and ensuring salt and fluid restriction in diet. Concomitant use of thiazide diuretics and aldosterone antagonists along with loop diuretics ensures sequential block of sodium reabsorption along the tubule and enhances diuresis.

ULTRAFILTRATION

Ultrafiltration is an alternate method of fluid removal. Several studies including UNLOAD (Ultrafiltration versus Intravenous Diuretics for Patients Hospitalized for Acute Decompensated Congestive Heart Failure), CARRESS HF (Cardiorenal Rescue Study in Acute Decompensated Heart Failure), and AVOID HF (Aquapheresis versus Intravenous Diuretics and Hospitalization for Heart Failure) have compared ultrafiltration and diuretic therapy. Majority of studies showed similar effects with respect to weight loss, whereas some studies have shown higher serious adverse effects with ultrafiltration. Ultrafiltration may be considered as an option for decongestion in patients with diuretic resistance, but further studies are warranted.

RAAS INHIBITORS

As already discussed, RAAS activation in CRS is a major cause of progressive renal and cardiac dysfunction. ACE inhibitors and ARBs have been shown to reduce mortality in heart failure. Up to 30% rise in serum creatinine is acceptable following ACE inhibitor/ARB initiation. Patients should be monitored for hypotension and hyperkalemia. Combination therapy of ACE inhibitor and ARB is not advised because of higher adverse effects.

ANGIOTENSIN RECEPTOR/NEPRILYSIN INHIBITOR

Inhibition of neprilysin (neutral endopeptidase inhibitor) raises the levels of endogenous vasoactive peptides including natriuretic peptides, adrenomedullin, and bradykinin. Two drugs have been evaluated: Omalaprilat and Sacubitril–Valsartan combination. Omalaprilat is withdrawn due to high incidence of angioedema. Sacubitril–Valsartan combination has been shown to successfully improve outcomes in low ejection fraction.

MINERALOCORTICOID RECEPTOR ANTAGONISTS

The long-term effects of ACE inhibitor/ARB are overcome by the phenomenon of aldosterone escape. So, addition of mineralocorticoid antagonists (Aldosterone, Eplerenone, Finerenone) to ACE inhibitors/ARBs produces more consistent suppression of the RAAS axis. Patients on combined therapy should be carefully monitored for hyperkalemia.

BETA-BLOCKERS

Beta-blockers have been shown to reduce symptoms, reduce New York Heart Association (NYHA) class, prolong survival, and reduce hospitalizations. Similar benefits have been demonstrated in patients with lower GFR. Patients should be monitored for bradycardia, hypotension, fluid retention, and fatigue.

VASODILATORS

Vasodilators help to correct elevated filling pressures and LV afterload. They are a part of treatment in refractory heart failure with low cardiac output. In patients who need a rapid reduction in afterload (severe hypertension), vasodilators which reduce arterial tone, such as nitroprusside, may be used. Vasodilators which reduce venous tone, such as nitroglycerin, may be used as an adjunct to diuretic therapy. Blood pressure should be monitored during vasodilator therapy.

INOTROPES

Intravenous inotropes, such as dobutamine or milrinone, will be required in severe LV systolic dysfunction and low perfusion state. Inotropes are required in patients with cardiogenic shock and in those patients awaiting mechanical cardiac device therapy or cardiac transplantation.

CARDIAC RESYNCHRONIZATION THERAPY

Cardiac resynchronization therapy (CRT) uses a biventricular pacemaker which activates both the right ventricle and the left ventricle in a synchronized manner. CRT improves LV ejection fraction and quality of life and reduces mortality. There is limited data on the benefits of CRT in CKD patients. But studies have shown benefits among subgroups of patients with eGFR >90, 60–68, and

30–59 mL/min/1.73 m^2. Improvement of eGFR with the use of CRT was noted in the group with baseline eGFR 30–59 mL/min/1.73 m^2.

CONCLUSION

The presence of renal dysfunction adversely affects the outcomes of HF patients and vice versa. With better understanding of complex pathophysiologic mechanisms of CRS, more therapeutic options are emerging. Early recognition of the various subtypes of CRS and early initiation of appropriate treatment can improve the overall outcome.

RECOMMENDED READINGS

1. Perazella MA. (2016). Onconephrology curriculum. [online] Available from https://www.asn-online.org/education/distancelearning/curricula/onco/
2. Cohen EP, Krzesinski J-M, Launay-Vacher V, Sprangers B. Onco-nephrology: Core Curriculum 2015. Am J Kidney Dis. 2015;66(5):869-83.
3. Porta C, Bamias A, Danesh FR, Dębska-Ślizień A, Gallieni M, Gertz MA, et al. KDIGO Controversies Conference on onco-nephrology: Understanding kidney impairment and solid-organ malignancies and managing kidney cancer. Kidney Int. 2020;98(5):1108-19.
4. Perazella MA. Onco-nephrology: Renal toxicities of chemotherapeutic agents. Clin J Am Soc Nephrol. 2012;7(10):1713-21.
5. Perazella MA, Izzedine H. New drug toxicities in the onco-nephrology world. Kidney Int. 2015;87(5):909-17.
6. Perazella MA, Shirali AC. Immune checkpoint inhibitor nephrotoxicity: what do we know and what should we do? Kidney Int. 2020;97(1):62-74.
7. Hingorani S. Renal complications of hematopoietic-cell transplantation. N Engl J Med. 2016;374(23):2256-67.
8. Rangaswami J, Bhalla V, Blair JEA, Chang TI, Costa S, Lentine KL, et al. Cardiorenal syndrome: Classification, pathophysiology, diagnosis, and treatment strategies: A scientific statement from the American Heart Association. Circulation. 2019;139(16):e840-78.
9. Shah BN, Greaves K. The cardiorenal syndrome: A review. Int J Nephrol. 2011;e920195.
10. Ronco C, Haapio M, House AA, Anavekar N, Bellomo R. Cardiorenal syndrome. J Am Coll Cardiol. 2008;52(19):1527-39.
11. Rangaswami J, Mathew RO. Pathophysiological mechanisms in cardiorenal syndrome. Adv Chronic Kidney Dis. 2018;25(5):400-7.
12. Rubinstein J, Sanford D. Treatment of cardiorenal syndrome. Cardiol Clin. 2019;37(3):267-73.
13. Kiernan MS, Udelson JE, Sarnak M, Konstam M. Cardiorenal syndrome: Prognosis and treatment—UpToDate. [online]. Available from https://www.uptodate.com/contents/cardiorenal-syndrome-prognosis-and-treatment.

CHAPTER 175

Uremic Syndrome: Diagnosis and Management

UK Sharma

ABSTRACT

Chronic kidney disease (CKD) is a clinical spectrum of diseases of the kidney of diverse etiology resulting in pathophysiological processes that progressively compromise multiple renal functions. This results in alteration of *milieu interior* through accumulation of metabolic wastes, toxins, fluid and electrolytes, and nonvolatile acids, and deleterious effects on various endocrine and metabolic functions, producing a set of symptoms and signs called uremic syndrome. Glomerular filtration rate (GFR) is a measure of renal function that shows progressive fall as the disease progresses.

The signs and symptoms of uremic syndrome may be present as early as when GFR declines to <60 mL/min/1.73 m^2 body surface area (BSA) or CKD III. Once GFR declines to <15 mL/min/1.73 m^2 BSA, the renal function is sufficiently depressed to result in accumulation of metabolic wastes and toxins, as well as disruption of various excretory, metabolic, and endocrine functions. This state is not compatible with life. This stage is called CKD V or end-stage renal disease (ESRD), and may result in death unless renal function is replaced through dialysis or renal transplantation. This chapter discusses the diagnosis and management of uremic syndrome. Early detection and effective management can help to slow down the progression of CKD, and prepare the patient for eventual renal replacement therapy (RRT).

"The good-news stories in medicine are early detection, early intervention"

—Thomas R Insel

INTRODUCTION

Uremic syndrome is defined as a set of signs and symptoms resulting from progressive loss of renal function. Though some of these manifestations may be seen in patients of acute kidney injury (AKI), the term is conventionally used to define the clinical presentation resulting from CKD. **Figure 1** provides the Kidney Disease Improving Global Outcome (KDIGO) classification of CKD, based on GFR and albuminuria categories.

ETIOLOGY

Chronic kidney disease can result from diverse etiologies and pathological processes that damage the kidneys. These etiologies may vary with geographical region, race, and age of the patient. An understanding of common etiologies of CKD and a knowledge of etiologies that are prevalent in the geographical region help in knowing when to suspect uremic syndrome. **Box 1** lists the leading or common etiologies of CKD. The list is by no means complete or exhaustive.

EPIDEMIOLOGY

Chronic kidney disease is a common disorder in most populations across the globe. While the prevalence of CKD in USA is estimated to be 15%, there are variations according to age, sex, and race. For instance, prevalence is 38% in adults > 65 years of age as against 13% in adults 45–64 years of age and 7% in adults 18–44 years of age. It is more common in women (15%) than men (12%), more common in non-Hispanic blacks (16%) than non-Hispanic whites (13%) or non-Hispanic Asians (12%), and Hispanics have a prevalence of 14%.

In India, the available data is less than complete and there are wide variations according to geographical regions. The reported prevalence varies from <1% to 13% according to geographical regions. India is a populous country with the world's second highest population. Nearly 17% of global population lives in an area which is <3% of the global landmass. According to a data from International Society of Nephrology's Kidney Disease Data Center Study, the prevalence of CKD is estimated to be as high as 17%.

PATHOPHYSIOLOGY

Urea, creatinine, and uric acid are routinely estimated as part of kidney function tests (KFTs) in patients clinically suspected to have CKD. However, in patients with a GFR

BOX 1 Common etiologies of CKD.

- Diabetic nephropathy
- Glomerulonephritidies
- Hypertension-associated renal disease (including vascular and ischemic kidney disease)
- Autosomal dominant polycystic kidney disease
- Other cystic and tubulointerstitial kidney diseases
- Chronic kidney disease of unknown etiology (CKDu)

Prognosis of CKD by GFR and albuminuria category

Prognosis of CKD by GFR and Albuminuria categories: KDIGO 2012				Persistent albuminuria categories Description and range		
				A1	A2	A3
				Normal to mildly increased	Moderately increased	Severely increased
				<30 mg/g <3 mg/mmol	30–300 mg/g 3–30 mg/mmol	>300 mg/g >30 mg/mmol
GFR Categories (mL/min/1.73m^2) Description and range	G1	Normal or high	≥90	Green	Yellow	Orange
	G2	Mildly decreased	60–89	Green	Yellow	Orange
	G3a	Mildly to moderately decreased	45–59	Yellow	Orange	Red
	G3b	Moderately to severely decreased	30–44	Orange	Red	Red
	G4	Severely decreased	15–29	Red	Red	Red
	G5	Kidney failure	<15	Red	Red	Red

Green: low risk (if no other markers of kidney disease, no CKD);
Yellow: moderately increased risk; Orange: high risk; Red: very high risk

(GFR: glomerular filtration rate)

FIGURE 1: Kidney Disease Improving Global Outcomes (KDIGO) classification of chronic kidney disease (CKD). Gradation of color from green to red corresponds to increasing risk and progression of CKD.

below 60 mL/min/1.73 m^2 BSA (CKD III or worse), there is accumulation of numerous uremic toxins that contribute to clinical manifestations of uremic syndrome. Important ones include Guanidino compounds, hippurates, polyamines, myoinositol, phenols, indoles, and benzoates. Further, accumulation of nitrogenous wastes due to loss of excretory function of the kidneys is not the only contributor to uremic syndrome. Numerous metabolic and endocrine functions subserved by the kidneys are also impaired. These result in anemia of uremia, malnutrition, abnormal metabolism of carbohydrates, fats, and proteins, abnormal levels of hormones such as parathyroid hormone (PTH), fibroblast growth factor-23 (FGF-23), vitamin D, steroid hormones, and many others. There is insulin resistance. Uremia also results in a chronic inflammatory state characterized by malnutrition, protein catabolism, accelerated atherosclerosis, and calcification of blood vessels and soft tissues.

CLINICAL MANIFESTATIONS

Uremia has a profound effect on functioning of all organs and systems due to an abnormal *milieu interior*. This results in protean manifestations that may be variably present in patients with CKD clinical stages III to V depending upon the rate of progression of CKD. **Box 2** gives list of important signs and symptoms of uremic syndrome, classified according to the systems affected. A brief discussion follows.

Renal manifestations include an early increase in nocturnal frequency of urination due to loss of concentrating ability of the kidney. Later, oliguria supervenes due to further loss of GFR. There is expansion of extracellular fluid volume (ECFV) from salt and water retention resulting in peripheral edema and anasarca. Intracellular fluid volume (ICFV) expansion may result in difficult to control hypertension. There may be resistance to action of diuretics administered

BOX 2 Signs and symptoms of uremia.

Renal:
- Nocturia
- Oliguria
- Peripheral edema/anasarca
- Hypertension
- Diuretic resistance

Endocrine and metabolic:
- Hyperkalemia
- Metabolic acidosis
- Hypocalcemia/hyperphosphatemia
- Deficiency of active vitamin D (1,25 dihydroxycholecalciferol)
- Hyperparathyroidism
- Mineral and bone disease of CKD (includes osteitis fibrosa cystica, adynamic bone disease and osteomalacia, pathologic fractures, and calcification of blood vessels and soft tissues)

Continued...

Continued...

- Insulin resistance
- Altered carbohydrate, lipid, and protein metabolism
- Protein–energy malnutrition
- Reduced body temperature
- Reduced resting energy expenditure
- Amenorrhea, fetal losses in pregnancy, and sexual dysfunction in males

Neurological:
- Fatigue
- Peripheral sensory and motor neuropathies
- Altered sense of smell and taste
- Decreased mental acuity and cognitive dysfunction
- Memory loss
- Sleep disturbances
- Restless legs syndrome
- Muscle cramps
- Twitchings, asterixis, and myoclonic seizures
- Drowsiness and coma
- Generalized seizures

Cardiovascular:
- Left ventricular hypertrophy
- Uremic cardiomyopathy
- Chronic heart failure
- Arrhythmias
- Ischemic heart disease
- Valvular and coronary artery calcification
- Pericarditis and pericardial effusion

Hematologic:
- Anemia of uremia
- Granulocyte and lymphocyte dysfunction
- Platelet dysfunction and bleeds
- Coagulation abnormalities

Gastrointestinal:
- Hiccoughs
- Anorexia
- Nausea and vomiting
- Uremic fetor
- Malnutrition and weight loss
- Nutritional deficiencies
- Constipation
- Gastrointestinal bleeds

Dermatologic:
- Pruritus
- Skin pigmentation
- Uremic frost
- Nephrogenic fibrosing dermopathy

(CKD: chronic kidney disease)

to induce clearance of retained fluid. Endocrine and metabolic functions are progressively impaired resulting in a multitude of symptoms and signs. Hyperkalemia usually occurs late in the course of CKD, when GFR has fallen to <25% of normal. It is usually a consequence of unrestricted intake of potassium-rich foods, muscle breakdown and protein catabolism, hemolysis, hemorrhage into gastrointestinal tract and transfusion of stored blood. Certain drugs such as angiotensin-converting enzyme inhibitors (ACEi), angiotensin receptor blockers (ARBs), and potassium-sparing diuretics may also contribute to hyperkalemia.

Metabolic acidosis: Kidney excretes nonvolatile acids. Accumulation results in anion gap metabolic acidosis which may also cause hyperkalemia. Inability of failing kidneys to generate ammonia for excretion of nonvolatile acids in the distal tubules may result in hyporeninemic hypoaldosteronism, and resultant hyperkalemia. This can even be life-threatening. Metabolic acidosis is initially compensated by enhanced removal of volatile acids via respiration causing rapid shallow breathing. Once this compensation fails, severe metabolic acidosis results. This may induce cardiac arrhythmias, poor cardiac contractility, hypotension, and cardiac arrest.

Hyperphosphatemia: Kidney is responsible for excretion of inorganic phosphates. Hyperphosphatemia is a common consequence of CKD. This results in secondary hyperparathyroidism and its consequences on mineral and bone disease (MBD) of CKD. Serum calcium levels are often low due to reduced amounts of active vitamin D leading to reduced absorption from the gut. Elevated PTH and FGF-23 may cause osteitis fibrosa cystica (OFC), bone pains, and pathologic fractures. Low vitamin D levels may cause osteomalacia, whereas uncontrolled treatment with calcium preparations and vitamin D may result in adynamic bone disease and calcification of soft tissues, blood vessels, and heart valves.

General weakness: There is often resistance to action of insulin in uremia. There may be reduced resting energy expenditure, lethargy, malaise, and reduced body temperature. Altered carbohydrate, fat, and protein metabolism are often present. The serum amino acid levels may be reduced. Hypercholesterolemia is another common consequence. The levels of steroid hormones may be altered resulting in amenorrhea and secondary infertility in females and sexual dysfunction in males. Children may show significant growth retardation.

The neuromuscular manifestations of uremia are a legion. Numerous "middle molecules" of nitrogenous substances that are normally excreted by healthy kidneys accumulate. Many act as pseudo-neurotransmitters. Manifestations may vary from chronic fatigue, sensory and motor neuropathies, altered sense of taste and smell, decreased mental acuity, loss of memory, sleep disturbances, drowsiness, restless legs syndrome, muscle cramps, twitching, asterixis, and myoclonic seizures. In advanced uremia, generalized seizures and coma may ensue.

Cardiovascular manifestations of uremia are common. In fact, cardiovascular complications are an important cause of mortality in CKD. Initially, hypertension may result in left ventricular (LV) hypertrophy. Later, LV dilatation and frank heart failure due to uremic cardiomyopathy may occur. Accelerated atherosclerosis and coronary vascular calcification may cause coronary artery disease and resultant myocardial ischemia. Uremic pericarditis marked by a pericardial rub and pericardial effusions may be seen if RRT is not instituted in time.

Hematologic manifestations: Among the hematologic manifestations of uremic syndrome, anemia is the most common manifestation. Kidney is responsible for secretion of erythropoietin. Tubulointerstitial diseases often show anemia out of proportion to the severity of CKD but anemia is eventually seen in all the etiologies of CKD. **Box 3** lists all the important causes of anemia of uremia. Anemia may be normocytic and normochromic to begin with but eventually it is microcytic and hypochromic. Granulocyte and lymphocyte dysfunctions are common, with greater propensity for infections. Platelet dysfunction may also be seen with tendency to bleed, especially in the gastrointestinal (GI) tract. Clotting abnormalities due to disorders of coagulation are yet another common manifestation of uremia.

GI symptoms include hiccoughs, anorexia, nausea, and vomiting. The breath may carry the typical uremic fetor. GI bleeds are often seen. Anorexia results in protein-calorie malnutrition and weight loss. Multiple nutritional deficiencies may be evident.

Dermatologic symptoms include pruritus which may even be refractory to dialysis. The skin complexion may be altered with increased pigmentation due to a combination of anemia, other nutritional deficiencies and deposition of urochromes in the skin. A characteristic thickening of skin called nephrogenic fibrosing dermopathy may be seen in some patients. All in all, many symptoms and signs are seen in a uremic patient due to effects of uremia on virtually all the organs and systems. While some of these respond well to renal replacement with maintenance dialysis, eventual recovery from many may only be seen with successful renal transplantation.

BOX 3 Causes of anemia in chronic kidney disease (CKD).

- Deficiency of erythropoietin
- Diminished red cell survival
- Bleeding diathesis
- Iron deficiency
- Nutritional deficiencies of vitamin B12 and folic acid
- Hyperparathyroidism-related bone marrow fibrosis
- Frequent blood sampling
- Underlying disease

INITIAL EVALUATION

Many of the symptoms and clinical signs of uremia may be very subtle initially. Therefore, a careful history to assess risk factors for kidney disease is very important. History of hypertension, diabetes mellitus, an abnormal urine analysis in the past or a nephrotic syndrome, problems during pregnancy such as preeclampsia or repeated fetal losses, certain autoimmune disorders, and inherited disorders of the kidney should be obtained. A careful drug history should always be obtained to look for administration of nephrotoxic drugs in the past. Past history of episodes of AKI should also be obtained.

A thorough physical examination to search for signs of uremic syndrome should include a careful record of blood pressure and evaluation of target organ damage through detailed cardiovascular and neurological examination as well as examination of fundus.

LABORATORY INVESTIGATIONS

The laboratory work-up of a patient of CKD is listed in **Box 4**, and forms an essential part of assessment of severity and optimal management of uremia, irrespective of the etiology of CKD. Preceding discussion of clinical manifestations guides the need for various basic investigations. In addition, etiology-specific investigations may be required to arrive at correct diagnosis and to plan management strategies. Many of these investigations need judicious repetition during follow-up visits to assess response to treatment and decide on the need for RRT. An *abdominal ultrasound* should be ordered to visualize the kidneys, their sizes, and echotexture and whether corticomedullary distinction is preserved.

Specialized imaging such as Doppler ultrasound of renal vessels, computed tomography (CT) scan or magnetic resonance imaging (MRI) of the abdomen, radionuclide scans of the kidneys, a voiding cystourethrogram to rule out reflux nephropathy may be required if indicated. CKD usually results in contraction of renal sizes and increased echogenicity with loss of corticomedullary distinction. However, renal sizes may be preserved in the face of advanced CKD in diabetes, amyloidosis, and patients of myeloma. The kidneys may even be enlarged in polycystic kidney disease. *Biopsy of the kidney* is seldom required in a patient with uremic syndrome, and advanced uremia may even be a contraindication for carrying out a biopsy. Biopsy of a contracted echogenic kidney may not yield any significant information and may be technically difficult to perform, with a risk of bleeding.

BOX 4	Basic laboratory evaluation in a patient of uremia.

- Urine routine examination
- 24-hours urinary protein excretion or spot urinary protein: Creatinine ratio (PCR)
- Complete blood count
- Prothrombin time (PT/INR) and aPTT
- Peripheral blood smear examination
- Serum iron, total iron-binding capacity (TIBC), transferrin saturation (TSAT), and ferritin
- Kidney function tests—urea, creatinine, uric acid, and electrolytes
- Arterial blood gas (ABG) analysis
- Calcium, phosphorus, alkaline phosphatase, and intact parathyroid hormone (iPTH) assay
- Vitamin D
- Vitamin B12
- Serum proteins, albumin, and globulins
- Serum lipids
- Blood glucose estimation and/or HbA1c
- Chest skiagram
- Echocardiography
- Ultrasonography of the abdomen
- Skeletal survey
- Viral markers of hepatitis B, hepatitis C, and HIV

(aPTT: activated partial thromboplastin time; HbA1c: glycated hemoglobin; HIV: human immunodeficiency virus)

MANAGEMENT

Fluid retention: It may require a judicious restriction of fluid intake and diuretics administration to flush out retained salt and water. Thiazide diuretics are of little help in CKD. Loop diuretics like furosemide and torsemide in higher than usual doses, either alone or in combination with metolazone may be warranted. Moderate salt restriction up to a maximum of 3–4 g of salt in a day is also usually required unless the CKD is due to a salt-losing nephropathy in patients of tubulointerstitial nephritides. In case there is diuretic resistance, dialysis is the only way to get rid of retained fluids. A careful assessment of lean dry weight is necessary to plan fluid removal through ultrafiltration.

Hypertension: It demands a careful evaluation and antihypertensives to maintain the blood pressure at <130/80 mm Hg. In CKD III, ACE inhibitor or ARBs may be employed keeping a close watch on serum potassium levels. However, in later stages of CKD, calcium channel blockers, beta-blockers, alpha-blockers like prazosin, and vasodilators may be used in combination. Potassium homeostasis may be maintained through restriction of foods rich in potassium, use of loop diuretics and potassium-binding resins such as calcium polystyrene sulfonate. RAAS-blocking drugs need to be avoided. Finally, persistent hyperkalemia will require dialysis for removal of excess potassium.

Metabolic acidosis: It can be kept in check by administration of oral sodium bicarbonate which also has a beneficial effect on progression of CKD. However, the additional sodium load will require a careful watch on the volume status.

Hyperphosphatemia: It requires restriction of dietary phosphates but a very restrictive diet may not be possible keeping the requirement of proteins in mind. Phosphate binders are prescribed to bind dietary phosphates in the GI tract for excretion in feces. Initially, calcium-based phosphate binders like calcium carbonate, calcium acetate, and calcium citrate are preferred as there may be hypocalcemia of uremia that also needs correction. In later stages of CKD, sevelamer carbonate and lanthanum are preferred. The aim is to maintain normal serum phosphates and an intact parathyroid hormone (iPTH) level between 150 and 300 pg/mL. Calcitriol may also have a role in combating hyperparathyroidism as well as hypocalcemia and osteomalacia, but once calcium levels return to normal, vitamin D supplementation may have to be restricted to avoid adynamic bone disease. Calcimimetics like cinacalcet may be required in patients with persistent hyperparathyroidism in the face of normal or high serum calcium. Insulin resistance is a prominent feature of uremia.

In patients of diabetes on insulin, the dose may require careful reduction as the disease progresses. Oral hypoglycemic agents are best avoided and ultrashort-acting insulins may be required in view of the anorexia, nausea, and poor dietary intake. Pronounced reduction in amino acid levels may require parenteral administration of amino acids. Hypercholesterolemia will need administration of statins for control.

Dietary protein intake: Restriction to 0.6–0.8 g/kg body weight has been found beneficial in CKD III to retard progression of the disease and avoid neurological complications of uremia due to accumulation of nitrogenous waste products. The proteins should be of high biological value with a good net protein utilization. In patients with high protein catabolism, keto-analogs of essential amino acids have been utilized to balance the need for protein intake against the neurological complications. Once asterixis, myoclonic seizures, or uremic encephalopathy develops, RRT becomes inescapable. There is evidence that peritoneal dialysis is more efficient than hemodialysis for removal of middle molecules of protein catabolism.

To avoid cardiovascular complications: It is essential to keep hypertension under good control through salt and water restriction, and judicious use of diuretics and antihypertensive drugs. Traditional risk factors of coronary artery disease such as smoking, alcohol intake, hyperlipidemia, hyperglycemia, salt intake, and high levels of homocysteine all need attention, though benefits of reduction of these factors are limited. A careful watch on hypercalcemia and hyperphosphatemia helps in reducing vascular and other soft tissue calcification. Pericarditis is best managed with regular dialysis. Massive pericardial effusion may require pericardiocentesis and regular dialysis for amelioration.

Anemia: The most common cause of anemia of uremia is insufficiency of erythropoietin. Regular administration of erythropoiesis stimulating agents (ESA) helps to manage the same. Hemoglobin should be maintained in a narrow range of 10.5–11.5 g/dL. Resistance to stimulation of erythropoiesis requires detailed investigations including iron studies. If serum iron is low, either oral iron supplements or parenteral iron may be required. Blood transfusions are best avoided, especially if the patient plans to undergo a renal transplantation.

Renal replacement therapy: Eventually, CKD progresses over time to reach ESRD. Therefore, planning and counseling for RRT are an important aspect of management. Once CKD III is established, patient should be immunized against hepatitis B and pneumococcal pneumonia. Choice of modality of RRT should rest with the patient after detailed discussion on maintenance hemodialysis (MHD), continuous ambulatory peritoneal dialysis (CAPD), and renal transplantation. If MHD is chosen, a vascular access such as arteriovenous fistula or graft should be fashioned once GFR falls below 30 mL/min (CKD IV). If a suitable donor is available, a preemptive renal transplantation may be carried out as definitive treatment of CKD. Dialysis may help ameliorate a large number of symptoms of uremia, but some symptoms and signs may not be completely reversed by maintenance dialysis. In such patients, dialysis may at best serve as a bridge to renal transplantation. It is important for the physician to remember that a patient of CKD requires a lot of help and support to progress from conservative management of CKD to RRT. The aim is not to merely add years to life of a patient but to attempt complete physical psychological and social well-being through regular patient education, so as to improve the ultimate quality of life.

CONCLUSION

Uremic syndrome is a manifestation of advanced CKD. The signs and symptoms may be subtle in the initial stages of CKD and most patients may be unaware of their kidney disease. Detailed history and diligent clinical examination of the patient at risk may reveal the presence of uremia. Laboratory investigations and imaging studies help to confirm the presence of CKD. Effective conservative measures are available to retard progression of the disease. A multidisciplinary approach is required for optimal management and effective rehabilitation of the patient who eventually progresses to ESRD. A team comprising primary care physician, nephrologist, diet counselor, social worker, dialysis nurse, and transplant coordinator working in unison can render holistic care. New advances in dialysis and renal transplantation have the potential to offer excellent quality of life to a patient of ESRD.

RECOMMENDED READINGS

1. Bergman JM, Skorecki K. Chronic kidney disease. In: Kasper DL, Fauci AS, Hauser SL, Longo DL, Jameson JL, Loscalzo J (Eds). Harrison's Principles of Internal Medicine, 19th edition. McGraw Hill Education, 2015. p 1811-21.

2. Kidney Disease Improving Global Outcomes (KDIGO) Chronic Kidney Disease Work Group. KDIGO Clinical Practice Guideline for the Evaluation and Management of Chronic Kidney Disease. Kidney Intl Suppl 2013; 3:1-150.
3. Meyer TW, Hostetter TH. Uremia. N Engl J Med 2007; 357:1316-1325.
4. Vanholder R, De Smet R, Glorieux G, Argilés A, Baurmeister U, Brunet P, et al. Review on Uremic Toxins: Classification, concentration and interindividual variability. Kidney Intl 2003;63:1934-43.
5. Babb AL, Ahmad S, Bergström J, Scribner EH. The middle molecule hypothesis in perspective. Am J Kidney Dis 1981; 1:46-50.
6. Brouns R, De Deyn PP. Neurological complications in renal failure: a review. Clin Neurol Neurosurg 2004; 107:1-16.

CHAPTER 176

Preventing Chronic Kidney Disease: In Whom, When, and How?

Divya Bajpai, Gopesh K Modi

ABSTRACT

Chronic kidney disease (CKD) is a growing public health concern globally and its increasing burden and high cost of care mandate preventive measures. Primary prevention to mitigate risk factors and prevent the onset of CKD involves public health strategies managing diabetes, hypertension, and obesity and by promoting a healthy lifestyle. Avoidance of nephrotoxic drugs, environmental toxins, acute kidney injury (AKI), and optimum management of infections and kidney stones are other methods of primary prevention. Secondary prevention focuses on early detection of CKD so that timely intervention can prevent progression to advanced stages. Targeted approach of CKD screening should be adopted where "at-risk" individuals are screened for proteinuria and a decrease in the glomerular filtration rate (GFR). Prompt measures to slow down the progression of CKD (improved glycemic and blood pressure control, drugs to reduce proteinuria) will also reduce the burden of cardiovascular diseases which are common in patients with CKD. Effective tertiary prevention relies on the management of advanced CKD including end-stage kidney disease (ESKD). A holistic approach involving strategies at population, institutional, and individual levels is the need of the hour to facilitate the successful prevention of CKD.

"Simplicity of approach is always best"

—C Chaplin

INTRODUCTION

Chronic kidney disease is defined as structural or functional abnormalities of the kidney of >3-month duration (**Fig. 1 of chapter 175**). With an estimated CKD burden of 850 million people worldwide, it is now a major global health issue that affects 1 in 10 adults. The prevalence of CKD in India is reported between 10 and 17%. CKD is projected to become the fifth leading cause of years of life lost in the global burden of diseases. Once kidney disease progresses to end stage, regular dialysis or kidney transplantation become mandatory to sustain life, with enormous clinical impact, social consequences, and healthcare expenditure. CKD is also a strong cardiovascular disease (CVD) risk multiplier. On one hand, the care of ESKD costs 2–3% of healthcare budget for a mere 0.03% of population in developed countries whereas on the other, inequities in access to ESKD care lead to substantial morbidity and premature mortality in low middle income countries. In a developing country like India, these modalities of renal replacement therapies (RRTs) are still out of reach of many patients.

A primary goal of healthcare is to prevent diseases or detect them early enough so that interventions and treatments are more effective. The ever increasing burden of CKD, its associated consequences, and the stress imposed on healthcare systems of societies make a strong case of prevention of CKD. Over the last few decades substantial information has been gathered about prevention of CKD and its progression to ESKD. In this chapter, we provide a broad overview on the prevention of CKD, with a special focus on factors predominant in Indian population.

PREVENTION OF DISEASES: A CONCEPTUAL FRAMEWORK

"An ounce of prevention is worth a pound of cure." This quote from Benjamin Franklin, in AD 1736 captures the essence of prevention of diseases at large. It is imperative that natural affinity to the idea of prevention is weighed against actual delivery of benefits. All interventions aimed at prevention and screening of diseases must be evaluated objectively in terms of net benefit delivered.

In brief, most screening and preventive interventions are done on apparently healthy individuals and those with risk factors and subclinical disease. The interventions have to be safe and easily scalable in case of healthy individuals and in case of those with subclinical disease or risk factors, the interventions have to be balanced against a range of variables—the risk of false diagnosis, chances of unnecessary interventions given the absolute benefit of the intervention, capacity of systems to handle the burden of disease unearthed, and the actual benefits from the efforts invested. The ideal endpoint for such evaluation is reduced incidence or mortality from any disease rather than disease duration bearing in mind the lead time and length time biases. The other commonly used variables are cost-effectiveness ratio, cost per quality-adjusted life years (QALY) or disability-adjusted life year (DALY) added or the number of subjects needed to be screened or treated to prevent disease or death in one individual. For example, the utility of routine prostate-specific antigen (PSA) or mammograms in preventing deaths from respective cancers in population-based efforts is in doubt when analyzed based on above tenets.

With this perspective, we will approach the concept of prevention of CKD. The Center for Disease Control and Prevention (CDC) classifies prevention into primary, secondary, and tertiary prevention based on the natural history of disease and its course (**Fig. 1**).

PRIMARY PREVENTION OF CKD

Case 1: Mrs Asha, a 33-year-old lady, has been recently detected to have diabetes mellitus. She is a banker and overweight. She is worried about developing CKD in the future. She wants to know about the lifestyle changes and other precautions she needs to take. She is also worried about the effects of pregnancy in future on her kidneys.

What is the objective? The objective of primary prevention is to intervene at the level of risk factors and predispositions to prevent the very onset of CKD.

In whom? Primary prevention measures are most useful when carried out at the population level. Interventions for the general population, with a special focus on "at-risk" groups, are beneficial. Risk factors for CKD can be divided into modifiable and nonmodifiable (**Table 1**). The framework of CKD prevention is built around these risk factors and management of these risk factors can avoid or delay the onset of CKD. Although not all the risk factors leading to CKD are modifiable, identification of nonmodifiable risk factors allows identification of high-risk population which benefits the most from preventive measures.

HOW?

Promoting a healthier lifestyle: The essential tenet of primary prevention is lifestyle interventions. These include dietary changes such as low sodium intake, higher intake of complex carbohydrates, three to five servings of fruit and vegetables, less saturated fats, plant-based proteins, and high fiber intake. Regular exercise should be a part of the daily routine. These measures will also help in correcting obesity which is an independent risk factor for CKD and improve cardiovascular risk profile that is associated with CKD. Weight loss has been associated with reduced incidence and better control of diabetes and hypertension. Smoking cessation must be emphasized.

Managing diabetes: Diabetes is the most common cause of CKD and ESKD globally. About 30–40% of patients with diabetes mellitus (DM) develop CKD. Uncontrolled hyperglycemia leads to early onset and rapid progression of diabetic kidney disease (DKD). Glycated hemoglobin (HbA1c) of 7% or less should be targeted. But this goal should be individualized to strike a balance between the risk of DKD with risk of hypoglycemia, which is especially high in type 1 diabetes mellitus (T1DM) and elderly individuals. Lifestyle interventions continue to have a place here as well.

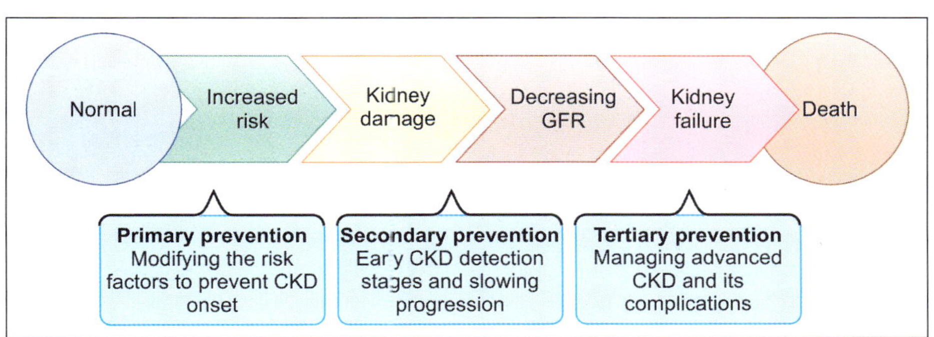

(CKD: chronic kidney disease; GFR: glomerular filtration rate)

FIGURE 1: Kidney disease and levels of prevention.

TABLE 1	Risk factors for chronic kidney disease (CKD).
Nonmodifiable CKD risk factors	
Genetics	• *APOLI* • Uromodulin mutations, *ACE* and *AGTR* genes • Hereditary nephritis/familial causes of CKD
Age	• Kidney function decreases with age • Elderly population is more prone to develop CKD after kidney insults
• Low birth weight	
• Congenital anomalies of kidney and urinary tract	
• Polycystic kidney disease	
• Family history of CKD	
Potentially modifiable risk factors	
Diabetes mellitus (type I and type 2)	
Hypertension	• Essential hypertension • Secondary hypertension
Obesity	
Smoking	
Nephrotoxins	• Nephrotoxic drugs (NSAIDs, PPIs, chemotherapeutic drugs, tenofovir) recreational drugs (cocaine, heroin, methamphetamine) • Herbs and herbal medications • Aminoglycoside lithium • Alternative drugs with heavy metals
Acute kidney injury	
Glomerulonephritis	• Primary glomerular disorders (FSGS, membranous nephropathy, IgA nephropathy etc.) • Systemic vasculitis (lupus nephritis, ANCA associated vasculitis etc.)
Environmental toxins	• Agricultural toxins • Heavy metal exposure • CKD of unknown cause (CKDu)
Nephrolithiasis	
Infections	• Kidney disease associated with HIV, hepatitis B virus, hepatitis C virus • Malaria, Dengue, Bacterial sepsis, TB • Endocarditis
Hematological disease	• Sickle cell disease • Plasma cell dyscrasias • Lymphoma
Liver disease	Hepatorenal syndrome
Cardiac disease	Cardiorenal syndrome
Pregnancy-related AKI	

(ANCA: anti-neutrophil cytoplasmic antibody; FSGS: focal segmental glomerulosclerosis)

Controlling blood pressure: Blood pressure control is essential in preventing the onset and delaying the progression of CKD. Target BP depends upon the presence of underlying diabetes and/or proteinuria. The control of blood pressure should be as per the patient characteristics and the standard guidelines. However, it should be remembered that achieving BP control is more vital than choosing a specific class of drug. Population-level programs to screening for hypertension will help in timely detection and prompt management.

Avoidance and prompt treatment of AKI: Acute kidney injury is a recognized risk factor for future development of CKD. Conditions leading to hypovolemia (vomiting, diarrhea, excessive diuretic use, and bleeding) and hypotension (myocardial dysfunction, sepsis etc.) and tropical infections associated with kidney injury (malaria, Hepatitis B and Hepatitis C, Dengue etc.) must be treated promptly. This is especially crucial in the Indian population where most of cases of tropical AKI can be attributed to reduced kidney perfusion. Similarly, when patients are hospitalized for any reason, they are at risk for AKI and this may go unrecognized. Also, recurrent dehydration associated with work in hot climates (e.g., agricultural work) is now being linked to CKD of unknown cause (CKDu) which is common in parts of Andhra Pradesh (Uddanam nephropathy), parts of Maharashtra, El Salvador, Nicaragua, and Sri Lanka. These inhabitants should maintain adequate hydration, observe caution on hot humid days, and avoid high salt intake.

Avoiding exposure to nephrotoxic drugs: Drugs such as nonsteroidal anti-inflammatory drugs (NSAIDs), angiotensin-converting enzyme (ACE) inhibitors, angiotensin receptor blockers (ARBs), and aminoglycoside can lead to potentially reversible decline in kidney function and they should be used cautiously in patients at high risk for developing CKD. Chronic use of nephrotoxic medications (NSAIDs, tenofovir, lithium, and possibly proton-pump inhibitors) increases the risk of CKD. The dose and duration of the use should be minimized and patients should be regularly screened for CKD. Another peculiarity of CKD in developing countries includes the widespread use of herbal medications that cause chronic interstitial nephritis and AKI. This is compounded by unregulated practice by unqualified practitioners and a high prevalence of fake and counterfeit medicines. Use of over-the-counter medications and unsupervised alternative medications should be discouraged.

Exposure to environmental effects: Exposure to pesticides or agrochemicals has been associated with CKDu. Other environmental nephrotoxins identified are inorganic arsenic, salts present in hard water, and aristolochic acid. Farming communities and worker in hazardous occupations need protective gear and safety education. The exposed individuals must be regularly screened for kidney dysfunction.

It is important to highlight that global warming and air pollution have been linked to increased risk of CKD. While these will need high-level national and social interventions, physicians need to be prepared for changing disease patterns in future.

Antenatal and peripartum management: Pregnancy-related AKI (PRAKI) constitutes 3–7% of total AKI cases in India. It frequently begets residual kidney damage and progressive CKD. Sepsis, pregnancy-induced hypertension (PIH), and peripartum hemorrhage are the common causes of PRAKI in India. PIH is also associated with future risk of hypertension and CKD in mother. Improvement in antenatal and peripartum care (access to universal antenatal care, early detection and prompt management of hypertension in pregnancy, safe delivery, and adequate postpartum monitoring) can prevent PRAKI and subsequent CKD.

Low birth weight: Low nephron dosing related to low birth weight or preterm birth is an established risk factor for CKD in adult life. To some extent, it is a modifiable risk factor as well. In India, up to 16–20% of babies have low birth weight. Improvement in antenatal care, better maternal nutrition, maternal health awareness, and avoidance of preterm birth can lead to a decrease in the incidence of low birth weight babies and a healthier progeny with respect to nephron dosing. Maternal hypertension, diabetes, and obesity are associated with low birth weight of the baby; underscoring the importance of lifestyle modifications in the mother. Healthy mothers give risk to healthy baby girls who become healthy mothers in the future.

Nephrolithiasis: Renal calculus disease is a common cause of CKD in tropical and subtropical areas of the world. The risk of recurrence and injury to kidney warrants sustained lifestyle changes (maintaining adequate hydration, dietary salt restriction, dietary oxalate restriction, reduction of nondairy animal proteins) and prompt medical and surgical management to prevent long-term kidney damage.

Hematological disorders: Sickle cell disease is prevalent in certain parts of India and developing world. These patients are at a significantly higher risk of CKD. Thus, they warrant regular screening and prompt management. Timely medical interventions can prevent kidney damage.

Some common clinical scenarios of interventions preventing CKD seen in Indian context are listed in **Table 2**.

TABLE 2 Examples of common clinical "at-risk" scenarios where CKD can be prevented or its progression can be delayed.

Clinical scenario	Timely intervention to prevent CKD or slow its progression
Secondary HTN in young	Treatment for reversible cause for HTN (e.g., renal artery stenosis, coarctation of aorta, pheochromocytoma, Cushing's syndrome, obstructive sleep apnea, drug induced hypertension)
Nephrolothiasis	Correction of metabolic cause for formation kidney calculus
CAKUT	• Antenatal detection of CAKUT • Correction of posterior urethral valve, meatal stenosis, PUJ obstruction, Vesicoureteric reflux etc. • Patients with anomalies which could not be corrected should be regularly followed up with optimum medical management
Patients on long-term nephrotoxic durgs like tenofovir, NSAIDs/PPI therapies	Regular screening of kidney function and timely discontinuation of drugs
Patients with HIV, HBV, and HCV infecitons	Regular screening of kidney function
Pregnancy-related AKI	Optimum management and long-term follow-up of kidney function and blood pressure
Family members of patients the geneitc diseases	• Preconception genetic testing • Regular screening for kidney disease

(CAKUT: congenital abnormality of kidney and urinary tract; PUJ: pelvic ureteric junction)

SECONDARY PREVENTION OF CKD

Case 2: Mr Shantanu is a 28-year-old gentleman with a family history of polycystic kidney disease in his father and uncle. He is recently detected to have hypertension. He is interested in knowing about screening for CKD in him and methods of secondary prevention of CKD.

What is the objective? The objective of secondary prevention is early detection and prompt treatment of CKD to prevent key adverse outcomes—cardiovascular disease—and to slow its progression to ESKD. The key facet is screening to identify disease early.

In whom? In the prevalence studies for CKD, the majority of patients have early-stage disease [Kidney Disease: Improving Global Outcomes (KDIGO) stage 1 or 2—estimated glomerular filtration rate (eGFR) > 60 mL/min/1.73 m^2] and are asymptomatic. Hence, they are often unaware of the diagnosis. In the United States of America, according to the National Health and Nutrition Examination Survey (NHANES) data (1999–2004), among patients with CKD stage 3 (eGFR 45–59 mL/min/1.73 m^2) only 9.2% of patients were aware of their kidney disease. For the absence of symptoms, most of them do not seek healthcare. This is even more relevant in our country where preventive health awareness is minimal. These patients benefit the most from secondary prevention, which involves screening and early detection of CKD. This early detection often translates to enhanced health awareness leading to lifestyle modifications. Timely therapeutic interventions might delay the progression of CKD. Also, early detection gives adequate time for the preparation of the patient and the family for RRT (dialysis or transplant) in the future, which may improve the outcomes.

Who should be screened for CKD? As explained earlier, case-finding (targeted) approach for CKD screening is better than the population-based approach (**Table 1**). This has been shown in studies and cost-effectiveness analyses as well. It has a high yield and reduces the burden of unnecessary interventions in false-positive individuals. This includes (but is not restricted to) patients with a family history of kidney disease, or with hypertension, diabetes, cardiovascular disease, past AKI, use of nephrotoxic or indigenous drugs, sickle cell trait, urolithiasis, complicated pregnancies, malignancy, and history of kidney disease during childhood. With explosion in omics-based data and correlations, it is likely that secondary prevention will move to genetic or metabolomic risk factor assessment.

In developing countries like ours, as the care of progressive CKD and ESKD remains costly and inaccessible for many patients, this approach will be more cost effective than developed world. Therefore, the screening should also include patients with suboptimal risk like those with prediabetes and prehypertension. The screening should be more widespread in areas where CKDu is prevalent (e.g., parts of Andhra Pradesh and Maharashtra)

How should they be screened for CKD? Patients who are selected for screening should have a urine test for albumin/ protein excretion and sediment for hematuria. This can be effectively done with either with qualitative or quantitative assessment for proteinuria/albuminuria. And, eGFR should be calculated based on serum creatinine value measured by a standardized assay and then employing an eGFR calculation equation, most preferred being CKD EPI equation which is available as a mobile application or online. Patients in whom structural disease is likely should undergo ultrasonography of the urinary tract.

The eGFR and albuminuria assessments need to be reconfirmed within 3 months to establish the diagnosis. Once diagnosed, CKD should be staged according to the latest KDIGO staging (**Fig. 1**).

HOW?

The key objectives here are cardiovascular risk reduction and slowing or ameliorating the progression of CKD. Besides controlling the primary cause for CKD, secondary factors unrelated to primary disease (intraglomerular hypertension, glomerular hypertrophy, and scarring) play an important role in CKD progression. Similarly, conventional and CKD-specific cardiovascular risk factors need attention.

Treatment of underlying cause: Optimum management of underlying etiology [e.g., glomerular disorders, infections such as human immunodeficiency virus (HIV), hepatitis B virus, hepatitis C virus, sickle-cell trait, cardiac, and hepatic disorders] may prevent or slow CKD progression.

Lifestyle measures: Similar to the ones outlined above, these continue to have an important role to play including cessation of tobacco use. Dietary salt restriction is of paramount importance with its benefits being at par with drugs used for treatment of progression.

Glycemic control: Control of blood glucose can slow the development of microalbuminuria, and its progression to overt proteinuria. This helps in GFR preservation in diabetic patients.

Control of hypertension: About 80–85% of patients with CKD have hypertension. Optimum BP control can slow the progression of proteinuric CKD and also reduces the rate of cardiovascular complications in patients. A target clinic BP of 125–130/<80 mm Hg or a home BP/average ambulatory BP of 120–125/<80 mm Hg is recommended. More intensive BP control reduces the risk of CKD progression in proteinuric CKD (but not in nonproteinuric CKD where acceptable BP target is <140/80 mm Hg). But intensive control is also associated with adverse events (hypotensive episodes and AKI). The target BP needs to be individualized (especially in elderly patients) and the benefit of cardiovascular protection needs to be weighed with the risks associated with intensive BP control.

ACE inhibitors or ARBs: Patients with proteinuria (defined as urine protein excretion >500–1,000 mg/day) have a more rapid decline in GFR as compared to nonproteinuric patients. Control of this proteinuria (to <1,000 mg/day) leads to the slowing of CKD progression. High-level evidence suggests the benefit of renin-angiotensin-aldosterone axis (RAAS) suppression using ACE inhibitors or ARBs in both diabetic and nondiabetic proteinuric CKD. The combination therapy of ACE inhibitors + ARB should be avoided. RAAS inhibition for proteinuria reduction is most effective when combined with dietary salt restriction. If a low-salt diet is difficult to achieve, the addition of a diuretic may also enhance the antiproteinuric effect of RAAS inhibitors.

In patients with nonproteinuric CKD, there is no evidence to suggest that ACE inhibitors or ARBs fare better than other drugs. In these patients, it appears that control of BP to target is the most important factor in slowing CKD progression.

Sodium–glucose cotransporter-2 (SGLT-2) inhibitors (e.g., empagliflozin, dapagliflozin): This is a new addition to the CKD treatment paradigms. In patients with proteinuria (with or without diabetes), SGLT-2 inhibitors have beneficial effects on kidney function which are independent of glycemic control. They act by blocking the sodium-glucose cotransporter, resulting in natriuresis, decreased intravascular volume and blood pressure, and normalizing tubuloglomerular feedback. These drugs are also associated with reduction in cardiovascular adverse events. According to the recent DAPA-CKD (Dapagliflozin on Renal Outcomes and Cardiovascular Mortality in Patients with Chronic Kidney Disease) trial, the beneficial effect of dapagliflozin is similar in diabetics and nondiabetics and the drug can be used in patients with eGFR up to 25 mL/min/1.73 m^2.

Vasopressin receptor (V2) antagonist: In the TEMPO (Tolvaptan Efficacy and Safety in Management of Autosomal Dominant Polycystic Kidney Disease and Its Outcomes) and REPRISE (Replicating Evidence of Preserved Renal Function: An Investigation of Tolvaptan Safety and Efficacy in ADPKD) trials, Tolvaptan showed benefit in adult patients of polycystic kidney disease who have a rapidly progressive disease with an eGFR ≥ 25 mL/min/1.73 m^2 by slowing the progression of kidney disease. It should be avoided in patients with liver impairment. The guidelines are based on renal volume and eGFR trajectory. The major prohibitor of its long-term use is the cost of long-term therapy.

- *Dietary protein restriction*: Theoretically, protein restriction may slow CKD progression. But the optimal level of protein restriction is not known. Also, as most of the CKD patients in our country are malnourished, further protein restriction can actually worsen the outcomes once they progress to ESKD. Thus, protein restriction should be advised judiciously under supervision of a nutritionist. It is advisable to prefer or restrict to vegetarian source of protein in the diet.
- *Hyperlipidemia*: All CKD patients should be offered lipid control for secondary prevention of CKD and for cardiovascular benefits as per the calculated cardiac risk.
- *Metabolic acidosis*: Correction of metabolic acidosis by oral sodium bicarbonate has also been shown to reduce the risk of CKD progression and could potentially improve mineral bone disease as well.
- *Vaccinations*: *As per the KDIGO 2012, adults with CKD (any stage) should be given annual influenza vaccine.* Patients with CKD are also advised vaccination for Hepatitis B. Adults with CKD stages 4 and 5 should get polyvalent pneumococcal vaccine.
- *Nephrotoxic drugs and indigenous medications*: Similar to primary prevention, CKD patients are advised to avoid nephrotoxic drugs such as NSAIDs, aminoglycosides, and herbal/indigenous preparations that are not well studied for renal safety. NSAIDs can accelerate the progression of CKD and also increase the risk of ischemic myocardial events.
- *Timely referral to nephrologist*: It is imperative that patients are seen by a nephrologist, especially when eGFR falls <30–45 mL/min/1.73 m^2 to create a long-term plan. This has been shown to improve survival and reduce morbidity over time.

TERTIARY PREVENTION OF CKD

Case 3: Master Ayaan is a 12-year-old male with CKD secondary to reflux nephropathy. His eGFR is progressively declining. His present creatinine is 4.5 mg/dL. His parents ask you about further course of management and when should he be initiated on dialysis?

What is the objective? Tertiary prevention refers to managing advanced CKD to prevent severe complications, to prolong life, and to optimally utilize interventions for care delivery.

In whom? As the longevity of patients with CKD is increasing, the number of patients with advanced CKD (eGFR < 30 mL/min/1.73 m^2) is on a rise. With timely planning and optimum management, patients with advanced CKD can live a long life with minimal morbidity. As kidney function progressively declines (eGFR < 15 mL/min/1.73 m^2), many of these patients will eventually require RRT in form of dialysis or a kidney transplant. However, most of them can be successfully maintained for a long time on conservative management before initiation of RRT.

HOW?

This involves the continued utilization of measures instituted for secondary prevention with close monitoring. More importantly for advanced CKD, it translates into planning future RRT in the form of dialysis or kidney transplantation. Conservative management of advanced CKD comprises holistic care focusing on various pharmacological and nonpharmacological interventions (**Table 3**). Planning for a vascular access (arteriovenous fistula) for dialysis should start early in the course of the disease (at eGFR < 30 mL/min/1.73 m^2). RRT consists of hemodialysis, peritoneal dialysis, and kidney transplant. An informed decision by the patient to choose the optimal mode of RRT should be facilitated. The intricacies of tertiary prevention are beyond the scope of this current text and it is

TABLE 3 Medical management of advanced CKD.

Complication	Management
Volume overload	• Dietary sodium restriction (<2 g/day) • Fluid restriction • Diuretic therapy
Hyperkalemia	• Dietary potassium restriction (<40–60 mEq/day) Withhold drugs (ACE inhibitors, ARBs, NSAIDs, beta-blockers) correction of metabolic acidosis • Potassium binders (patiromer or zirconium cyclosilicate), polystyrene sulfonates
Metabolic acidosis	• Oral bicarbonate supplementation to maintain bicarbonate concentration 23–28 mEq/L
Mineral and bone disorders	• Dietary phosphate restriction, • Phosphate binders (calcium acetate, calcium carbonate, sevelamer, ferric citrate, sucroferric oxyhydroxide) • Cinacalcet • Vitamin D and its analogs • Alterations in dialysate calcium concentrations
Hypertension	• Dietary sodium restriction (<2 g/day) • Fluid restriction • Anti-hypertensive therapy
Anemia	• Iron and vitamin B supplementation • Erythropoieis-stimulating agents • Rule-out other causes like blood loss, hemoglobinopathy

Continued...

Continued...

Complication	Management
Dyslipidemia	• Dietary restriction of calories and fat • Statins ± Ezetimibe
Malnutrition	• Dietary supplementation • Appetite stimulants • Correction of uremia
Uremic bleeding	• Desmopressin, cryoprecipitate, estrogen • Correction of anemia • Correction of uremia
Uremic pruritus	• Correction of metabolic factor. (Ca, P, PTH, thyroid, iron deficiency) • Topical emollients • Oral antihistamines • Gabapentin and pregabalin • Sertraline • Phototherapy • Dikfelikefalin • Correction of uremia
Uremic neuropathy	• Gabapentin, desipramine • Correction of uremia

a domain that is best managed under direct supervision of nephrologist or a kidney center.

Psychosocial support: Patients and their caregivers require extensive psychological support throughout the management of advanced CKD. Burnout is common in caregivers. Patients and families should be made part of "the informed decision-making" process in the care, and therapies need to be individualized as per their needs. This will make them feel empowered and they will have realistic expectations. Such patients are less likely to delay or deny lifesaving interventions in the future

CONCLUSION

In summary, the prevention of CKD is possible. It requires a holistic approach (**Fig. 2**) with efforts on all levels starting from lifestyle modifications in the population, ensuring healthy pregnancies and optimum neonatal care, access to adequate screening for early detection, and timely treatment of risk factors. This is only possible with strengthening of primary care services and integration of CKD prevention with the comprehensive noncommunicable disease prevention programs. Even in patients with advanced CKD, complications can be prevented using a multidisciplinary team approach.

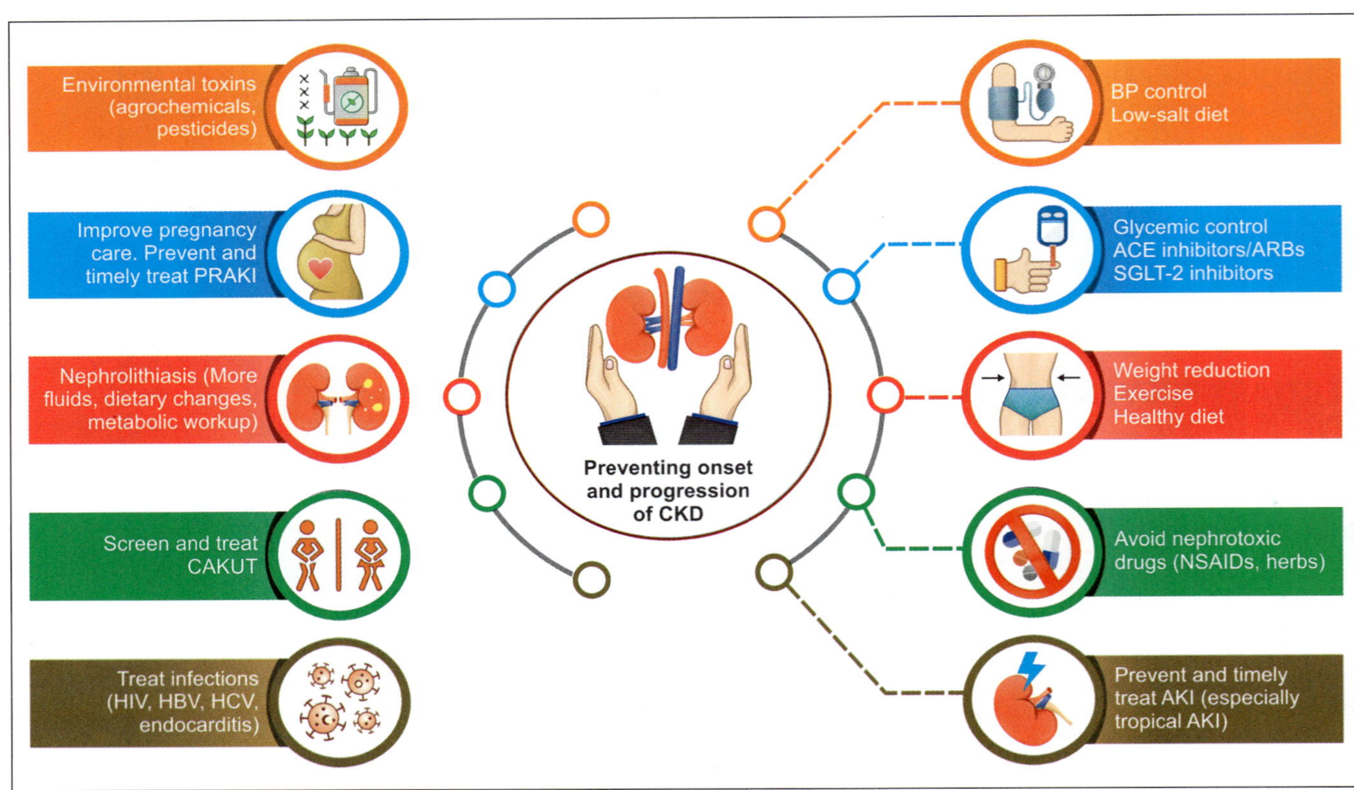

(CAKUT: congenital anomalies of the kidney and urinary tract; PRAKI: pregnancy-related acute kidney injury)

FIGURE 2: Preventing the onset and progression of CKD.

RECOMMENDED READINGS

1. Stevens LA, Bilous PE, Coresh RW, De Francisco J, De Jong AL, P.E., Griffith PE, et al. Kidney Disease: Improving Global Outcomes (KDIGO) CKD Work Group. KDIGO 2012 clinical practice guideline for the evaluation and management of chronic kidney disease. Kidney International Supplements, 2013;3(1): pp.1-150.
2. Ameh OI, Ekrikpo UE, Kengne AP. Preventing CKD in low-and middle-income countries: A Call for urgent action. Kidney International Reports. 2020;5(3): 255-62.
3. Li PK, Garcia-Garcia G, Lui SF, Andreoli S, Fung WW, Hradsky A, et al. Kidney health for everyone everywhere: from prevention to detection and equitable access to care. Clin Nephrol. 2020;93(3):111-22.
4. Bello AK, Nwankwo E, El Nahas AM. Prevention of chronic kidney disease: a global challenge. Kidney International. 2005;68:S11-7.
5. Drawz P, Rahman M. Chronic kidney disease. Annals of internal medicine. 2015;162(11):ITC1-16.
6. Luyckx VA, Cherney DZ, Bello AK. Preventing CKD in developed countries. Kidney International Reports. 2020;5(3):263-77.
7. Rhee JJ, Jardine MJ, Chertow GM, Mahaffey KW. Dedicated kidney disease-focused outcome trials with sodium-glucose cotransporter-2 inhibitors: Lessons from CREDENCE and expectations from DAPA-HF, DAPA-CKD, and EMPA-KIDNEY. Diabetes, Obesity and Metabolism. 2020;22:46-54.
8. Varughese S, Abraham G. Chronic kidney disease in India: a clarion call for change. Clin J Am Soc Nephrol. 2018;13(5):802-4.

CHAPTER

177 Conservative Kidney Care

Ravindra Prabhu Attur, Indu Ramachandra Rao, Shankar Prasad Nagaraju

ABSTRACT

The management of advanced chronic kidney disease (CKD) is complex due to associated comorbidities, high burden of physical, psychological, and social symptoms, high cost of care, and poor prognosis. This necessitates a multidisciplinary approach which aims at retarding progression of disease and focusses on quality of life (QOL) and not only on life sustaining or prolonging therapies. It is increasingly evident that maintenance dialysis has its limitations in relieving symptoms and may be associated with adverse effects especially in elderly, frail, and in those with comorbidities. Conservative care models for kidney disease may fill this gap and are increasingly being used in several developed countries.

Conservative kidney care (CKC) does not imply withdrawal from or denial of dialysis but has a broader scope of holistic approach through domains of minimizing symptom burden, shared decision making, advance care planning, end-of-life care, and psychological and family support. This approach may be achieved through integration of nephrology practice with palliative care principles and a multidisciplinary team. In India, CKD patients face a choice-restricted environment where providing standard nephrology services including renal replacement therapy, i.e., dialysis or kidney transplant is challenging. CKC in this situation will give an added choice and will aid in keeping patients within the health services radar. An organized approach to initiate this service for patients and education of medical personnel at all levels is required.

"Decisions are the frequent fabric of our daily design"

—Don Yaeger

KEY POINTS

- Chronic kidney disease patients have a high burden of symptoms and mortality which increases with stage, age, and associated comorbidities.
- Conservative kidney care is a planned holistic patient-centered care focusing on QOL provided as an alternative to or with life-sustaining therapy.
- Conservative kidney care should begin in CKD stage 4/5.
- Identification of potential candidates for CKC can start with treating nephrologist asking the surprise question: *"Would you be surprised if the patient died in the next 12 months?"* and other tools.
- Conservative kidney care domains include identification of patients who benefit from CKC, shared decision making, active symptom management, advance care

planning, and end-of-life care which may include withdrawal from dialysis.
- Multidisciplinary team approach is required to provide CKC which includes nephrologists, palliative care specialists, and other health professionals.
- Palliative dialysis is an approach where therapy targets symptom relief rather than adequacy.
- Postdeath assessment and bereavement care should also be part of CKC.

INTRODUCTION

Conservative kidney care (CKC) is a concept which aims to improve health-related quality of life (QOL) of patients with chronic kidney disease (CKD) together with or as a substitute for life prolonging therapies. This management strategy derives from high symptom burden; increased mortality these patients face with some being intolerant or developing new symptoms on standard treatment. Consensus for this is building in India on the need to integrate palliative medicine principles and practices to nephrology at all stages of disease. The goal of CKC is to reduce suffering throughout the trajectory of illness, including (but not limited to) the end of life, priority being given to shared decision making, identifying and managing issues important to the patient, treatment of symptoms at physical and psychological level, and advance care planning.

With widespread application and improvement of dialysis therapy since the 1960s, an increasing number of older patients and those with associated comorbidities such as cancer, cardiovascular disease, and dementia are receiving this treatment. It has now become evident that dialysis can relieve only some of the symptoms of CKD, that too in those with relatively less comorbidity. Furthermore, among patients older than 80 years, some observational studies have shown no survival benefit with starting dialysis as compared with active medical management.

Despite advances in predialysis care and dialysis technology, these patients continue to have a shortened life expectancy and poor outcomes, including physical, emotional, and spiritual suffering, and low QOL. Hence dialysis which was initially a bridge to kidney transplant has now become a therapy to prolong life but may not always improve health quality. Present care at end of life focusses on aggressive medical management which may not be in tune with patient preferences. Kidney transplant remains the best option in suitable patients. In others, CKC may be an added choice along with dialysis therapy with freedom of transition between different modalities. This chapter introduces CKC, present concepts, its domains, and its delivery to advanced CKD patients.

COMMON TERMINOLOGIES

Different terms being used for kidney conservative care in the literature are listed in **Box 1**. In this chapter, we use the term "conservative kidney care (CKC)."

BOX 1	Terminology for conservative kidney care.
• "Nondialytic" medical management	
• Conservative kidney management	
• Comprehensive conservative care	
• Kidney supportive care	
• Maximum conservative management	
• Renal palliative care	
• Renal supportive care	
• Residual renal support	
• Palliative renal care	

There are various definitions for CKC. The Kidney Disease: Improving Global Outcomes (KDIGO) Controversies Conference on Supportive Care in Chronic Kidney Disease: Developing a roadmap to improving quality care in its executive summary on renal supportive care in 2013 defines CKC as a planned holistic patient-centered care for advanced CKD patients, which includes:
- Interventions to delay progression of kidney disease and minimize risk of adverse events or complications
- Shared decision making to identify and manage as per priorities important to the patient
- Active assessment and management of symptoms
- Detailed communication with realistic awareness of prognosis and advance care planning
- Psychological/emotional, social, and family support
- Cultural and spiritual domains of care

CONSERVATIVE KIDNEY CARE TEAM

Conservative kidney care is ideally provided through collaboration of nephrologists, palliative care specialists, and a multiprofessional team depending on regional requirements and resources and which should ideally include:
- Nephrologist
- Trained nursing staff
- *Allied health professional*: Psychosocial worker and dietician
- Professional to address spiritual needs
- Professionals to provide community support including family physician/community staff/healthcare volunteers
- Palliative care specialist for consultation to help solve complex situations, refractory symptoms, end-of-life care, and advanced care planning (ACP).

Conservative kidney care discussion: Ideally, the discussion regarding CKC should occur at the time of education on dialysis, i.e., when estimated glomerular filtration rate (eGFR) is <20–30 mL/min/1.73 m^2. However, the timing of initial and subsequent discussions ultimately depends upon the patient's clinical trajectory. The evolving model of conservative care in nephrology is shown in **Figure 1**.

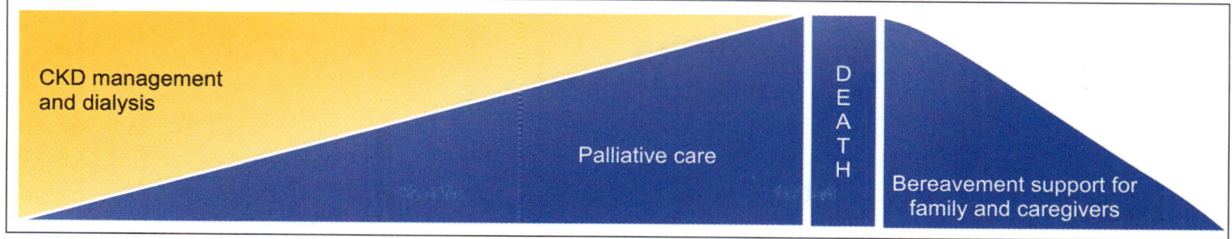

(CKD: chronic kidney disease)

FIGURE 1: Model of palliative care in nephrology.

DOMAINS OF CONSERVATIVE KIDNEY CARE

These represent broad areas of focus applicable to patients across the illness spectrum (**Fig. 2**). These include:

- Delay progression and minimize risk/early identification and treatment of complications of kidney disease
- Identification of patients most likely to benefit from supportive care
- Elicitation of patient preferences, goals, and shared decision making
- Active symptom assessment and management
- Heightened attention to nonphysical dimensions of suffering
- Iterative and patient-centered explorations of prognostic awareness and its communication
- Option of managing advancing disease without dialysis
- Effective use of local palliative medicine and hospice resources

It is important to emphasize that these domains are applicable to patients across the continuum of illness severity and chronicity in nephrology including patients with acute kidney injury (AKI), CKD who are not receiving dialysis and also patients with kidney transplants.

Identifying those who need CKC is a very important step in shared decision making. In advanced kidney disease, those who are unlikely to gain survival or are at risk for hospitalization after initiating dialysis would be candidates for receiving CKC. Identifying these patients is aided by *"surprise question?"* by nephrologist and other criteria. General and specific indicators of decline will aid this process (**Box 2**).

Symptom assessment and management: ESRD patients on dialysis have a high burden of physical and psychological symptoms which remain under reported, under recognized, and undertreated during routine care. Symptoms require to be elicited periodically using validated tools. Symptom burden can be reduced over time using a multidisciplinary team as has been demonstrated from programs in Australia and Canada. Few assessment tools commonly used with their link are listed in **Box 3**. The approach to symptom management should involve evaluation of cause, assessment for reversible factors, and level of distress, interventions both nonpharmacologic and pharmacologic and acknowledgement of limitations of therapy. Common symptoms and their management are shown in **Tables 1** and **2**.

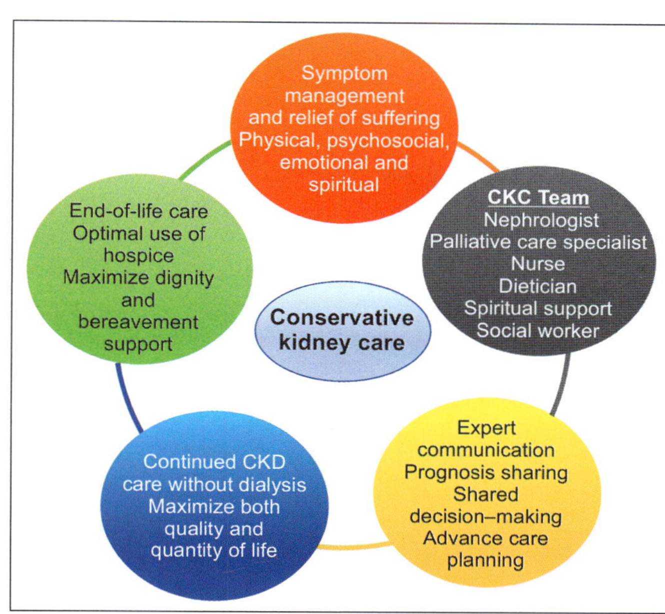

(CKD: chronic kidney disease; CKC: conservative kidney care)

FIGURE 2: Domains of conservative kidney care.

Shared decision making and prognostication: Culturally competent shared decision-making forms the basis of CKC and must be incorporated in nephrology practice. Patient priority may shift from curative intent and prolonging life to improving quality alone toward the end. ACP and shared decision making are a process of detailed discussion between a patient, the family (or other caregiver), and treating staff for the purpose of clarifying preferences in relation to future treatment options, prognosis, and end-of-life care. The focus will be exclusively on QOL rather than survival, with a strong emphasis on emotional, social, and family support. There are tremendous cross-cultural differences in preferences for decision making. Western cultures tend to promote "patient autonomy," where the patient is viewed as the best person to make healthcare decisions. However, many cultures are characterized by strong communal and social bonds where the person is viewed as a "relational-self," where social relationships, rather than individualism, provide the basis for moral judgments. The shared decision making is essential to align treatment with patient and family goals, values, and preferences.

Estimating and communicating prognosis to patients and family, balancing biomedical facts with relevant emotional, social, cultural, and spiritual issues, are required

BOX 2	Advanced CKD patients who are most likely to benefit from CKC.
Surprise question: To identify patients at high risk for death within the next year *"Would you be surprised if the patient died in the next 12 months?"*	
If you answer "no" to the surprise question, then he is right candidate to be considered for CKC	
• Patients who are >80 years old or with significant comorbidities	
• Patients who are frail with functional or cognitive dysfunction with poor quality of life	
• With repeated unplanned admissions	
• Poor tolerance of dialysis with a change in modality	
• High physical or psychosocial symptom burden	
• Patients who have one or more life-shortening comorbidities (e.g., end-stage heart failure or end-stage liver failure)	
• Patients who experience accelerated functional and cognitive decline after starting dialysis	
• Patients who reside in long-term care facilities	
• Patients who view their current and future quality of life as unacceptable, in whom dialysis may prolong life but will also prolong suffering	
• Patients with irreversible mental incapacitation that interferes with their ability to understand the process, risks, and benefits of dialysis in such a way that dialysis cannot be administered safely	

(CKC: conservative kidney care)

BOX 3	Symptom and function assessment tools.
• **Global symptom assessment tools:**	
◦ Edmonton Symptom Assessment Revised: Renal (ESAS Renal) (http://palliative.org/NewPC/_pdfs/tools/ESASr%20Renal.pdf)	
◦ Integrated Palliative Care Outcome Scale Renal (IPOS Renal) (https://pos-pal.org/maix/ipos-renal-in-english.php)	
◦ Dialysis symptom index (DSI) (www.jpsmjournal.com/article/S0885-3924(03)00517-7/fulltext)	
◦ Karnofsky Performance Status (KPS) score (http://www.npcrc.org/files/news/karnofsky_performance_scale.pdf)	
◦ Eastern Cooperative Oncology Group (ECOG), (https://ecog-acrin.org/resources/ecog-performance-status)	
• **Multidimensional pain assessment tool:**	
◦ The Brief Pain Inventory (BPI) (Cleeland CS, Ryan KM. Pain assessment: global use of the Brief Pain Inventory. Ann Acad Med Singapore. 1994;23:129-138)	
• **Quality-of-life assessment tool:**	
◦ 5-level EuroQol 5 dimension (EQ-5D-5L) (Gibbons E, Fitzpatrick R. A Structured Review of Patient-Reported Outcome Measures for People with Chronic Kidney Disease. United Kingdom: University of Oxford; 2009)	

for shared decision making. Studies have shown that despite patients wanting to discuss their prognosis, it is often not done. Prognostication is challenging in CKD given the great variation in individual illness trajectories. Aids such as activity scores, gait speed, frailty indices, activities of daily living, hospitalizations, nutrition scores, and change in weight will help in making this assessment.

It should start with exploring patient knowledge of illness and prognosis through the question "What is your understanding about your current illness?" Additional discussion should ensue to know more about his worries, concerns, hopes, and priorities in the context of his disease. After developing an understanding about priorities, the CKC team should make a treatment plan, which best aligns with the patient's preferences, values, and goals. In situations where prognosis is uncertain, a time-limited trial of dialysis can be given in tune with patient preferences. This serves to avoid conflict of opinion and provides support to patients, family, and treating staff.

Advance care planning: The unpredictable nature of CKD progression and the associated complications make it particularly important for patients and families to plan for end-of-life care needs. ACP is a process that involves understanding, communication, and discussion between a patient, the family (or other caregiver), and healthcare providers, for the purpose of clarifying preferences for end of-life care. It lays out a set of relationships, values, and processes for approaching end-of-life decisions for individual people when they can no longer speak for themselves, including attention to ethical, psychosocial, and spiritual issues relating to starting, continuing, withholding, and stopping dialysis.

The key elements for success of ACP involve the following aspects.

- Ensuring patient understands value of ACP in their situation and agrees to continue the conversation. It is important to identify whom the patient wishes to include in ACP dialogues.
- Advanced care planning should be primarily patient led and includes preferred family members to determine clearly goals of care, including the use of life sustaining treatments.
- They should be made to understand that there is always provision for review of ACP and change as per patient/family member wishes at any time.

Withdrawal from dialysis: Dialysis withdrawal is defined as discontinuation after an active decision to permanently stop dialysis by the patient, family, healthcare power of attorney, or healthcare team. However, there are currently no uniformly accepted definitions of withdrawal of dialysis. The practice of withdrawal from dialysis also differs significantly between countries.

TABLE 1 Management strategies for the most common symptoms in advanced CKD.

Symptom	Identification and treatment of associated factors	Nonpharmacological therapy	Pharmacological therapy
Uremic pruritus	• Xerosis • Drug hypersensitivity • Anemia • Iron deficiency • Hyperphosphatemia • Hypercalcemia • Skin infestations • Contact dermatitis	• Skin care and moisturizers • Avoid dry environment • Avoid scratching—keep fingernails short, wear gloves • Complimentary therapies (benefit doubtful): Trial of phototherapy (UVB) three times weekly for 3 weeks • Acupuncture	Topical: • Topical emollients (glycerol or paraffin based) • Capsaicin 0.025% or 0.03% ± menthol 4% ointment • Pramoxine 1% Systemic: • *First line*: Gabapentin 50–300 mg daily, pregabalin 25–75 mg daily or alternate day (dose based on eGFR) • *Second line*: Tricyclic antidepressant such as doxepin 10 mg daily at night/ sertraline 50 mg/day
Nociceptive pain	Conduct investigations to determine cause	• Physical therapies (e.g., exercise, massage, acupressure, and acupuncture) • Behavioral therapies (e.g., cognitive behavioral therapy, relaxation techniques) • Interventional and surgical therapies (e.g., nerve blocks)	• *Step 1*: Consider topical NSAID for localized pain (e.g., diclofenac gel 5% or 10% 2–3 times daily). Acetaminophen/paracetamol, maximum of 3 g daily • *Step 2*: No safe step 2 analgesics for nociceptive pain • *Step 3*: Add a low dose of strong opioid. Hydromorphone starting at 0.5 mg PO (0.2 mg subcutaneously) every 4–6 h; buprenorphine/fentanyl/ methadone • Preferable to avoid tramadol, codeine, and morphine
Neuropathic pain	Conduct investigations to determine cause	As for nociceptive pain	• *First line*: Gabapentin, pregabalin (dose based on eGFR) • *Second line*: Tricyclic antidepressants, amitriptyline 10–25 mg daily, or doxepin 10 mg daily
Restless legs syndrome	• Iron deficiency • Metabolic acidosis • Hyperphosphatemia • Low PTH • Caffeine, nicotine, alcohol, and certain medications (tricyclic antidepressants, selective serotonin reuptake inhibitors, lithium, dopamine antagonists, calcium channel blockers, and sedative antihistamines)	Regular exercises such as stretching and cycling	• Gabapentin, dopamine agonist (ropinirole and pramipexole) or levodopa/carbidopa • Short-acting benzodiazepines (clonazepam) or clonidine may be tried in those with refractory RLS
Fatigue	• Anemia • Malnutrition • Vitamin D deficiency • Metabolic acidosis • Hypothyroidism • Depression • Sleep disturbances	• Exercise • Nutrition and hydration management • Energy-conservation strategies	Treatment of specific causes

Continued...

Continued...

Symptom	Identification and treatment of associated factors	Nonpharmacological therapy	Pharmacological therapy
Sleep disturbances	• Depression • Sleep apnea • Orthopnea/paroxysmal nocturnal dyspnea due to volume overload or cardiac causes • Restless legs syndrome • Uremic pruritus • Medications	• Good sleep hygiene (e.g., avoid stimulants before bed, avoid napping during the day) • Relaxation therapy • Complementary treatments (e.g., acupressure, massage, and acupuncture)	• *First line*: Gabapentin (50–300 mg at night), especially if the patient has concomitant neuropathic pain, RLS, or uremic pruritus • *Second line*: Doxepin 10 mg at bedtime • *Third line*: Consider mirtazapine 7.5 mg or zopiclone 3.75–5 mg at night or melatonin 2–5 mg at night
Nausea and vomiting	• Uremia or other metabolic abnormalities • Medications (e.g., oral iron and opioids) • Gastrointestinal disturbances (e.g., constipation, delayed gastric emptying)	• Encourage smaller and more frequent meals • Avoid alcohol and greasy, spicy or excessively sweet foods • Minimize exposure to strong odors • Complementary therapies (e.g., relaxation techniques, ginger)	• *First line*: Ondansetron 4–8 mg every 8 h • *Second line*: Metoclopramide 2.5 mg every 4 h • *Third line*: Olanzapine 2.5 mg or haloperidol 0.5 mg given every 8 h
Breathlessness	• Anxiety • Anemia • Infection • Volume overload leading to pulmonary edema	• Salt and fluid restriction • Maintain upright position (e.g., 45°) • Supplemental oxygen • Complementary therapies (e.g., relaxation techniques and music) • Consider palliative dialysis	• If volume overloaded, add a loop diuretic such as furosemide • Metolazone may be added to loop diuretics, if required • Low-dose opioids and benzodiazepines may be advised for symptom relief for those on end-of-life care
Depression	• Fatigue • Insomnia • Poor appetite	• Cognitive behavioral therapy • Exercise	Sertraline 50 mg/day
Anorexia		• Liberalize diet • Low bulk high calorie supplement	Appetite stimulant dronabinol
Dry mouth		• Mouth rinses • Stimulate saliva with candy	Xylitol lozenge

(RLS: restless legs syndrome; UVB: ultraviolet B)

TABLE 2 Chronic kidney disease (CKD) management in patients on conservative care.

Complication	Management
Hypertension	A target blood pressure of <160/90 mm Hg may be reasonable, since more stringent targets may increase risk of falls
Salt restriction	While those with volume overload would require salt restriction and diuretics, a more liberal intake may be advisable for those with anorexia
Anemia	• Treatment with iron supplementation and erythropoietin-stimulating agents (ESAs) may help alleviate symptoms such as fatigue and breathlessness, and improve quality of life • In those on end-of-life care, it may be appropriate to withhold treatment of anemia
Hyperkalemia	• Potassium-restricted diet • Manage acute hyperkalemia if consistent with patient's goals
Metabolic acidosis	Correction of metabolic acidosis with oral sodium bicarbonate therapy prevents fatigue, bone loss, and muscle wasting
Mineral bone disease	• Since restricting dietary phosphorus may lead to protein deprivation and malnutrition, liberalizing diet may be preferable • Phosphorus-restricted diet and phosphate binders may be advised in selected patients • Low-dose vitamin D analogs may improve fatigue, weakness, and prevent muscle loss

Withdrawal from dialysis can happen in following situations:

- Patients with decision-making capacity after receiving complete information decide to refuse or request withdrawal from dialysis voluntarily.
- Patient who has made decision to refuse in the past through appropriate advance care planning, but now no longer possess decision-making capacity.
- Patients without decision-making capacity and withdrawal or refusal of dialysis request are indicated by properly appointed legal agents/surrogates.
- Patients with irreversible, profound neurologic impairment

The process of approaching patients about dialysis withdrawal is not standardized, and the conversation can be emotionally difficult for patient, family member, and nephrologists. For most patients with ESRD, dialysis is considered standard of care. Family members often feel the option of withdrawal as giving up and that it will lead to a painful death. Many a time patients and family members have an unrealistic hope of cure from the illness. In some conditions, ethical dilemmas and legal process make withdrawal decision difficult for the patient. This discussion should be conducted in appropriate setting and involving all decision makers for patients.

Having a multidisciplinary team involving patient's primary care physicians and palliative care team is helpful to initiate a proper discussion. During the conversations, patient's and family members' understanding of disease should be assessed and the physician should help the patient or family members in shared decision-making process. The details of discussion must be documented clearly on patient's medical records and should be informed to the people involved in his care. KDIGO guidelines highlight the process of withdrawal from dialysis as shown in **Box 4**

BOX 4	Stepwise approach for implementation of withdrawal from dialysis.
• Identification of decision maker (patient or family member)	
• **Assessing decision maker's** understanding of the clinical situation and benefit versus burden of disease	
• **Provision of explanation** to the patient/family caregiver for dialysis withdrawal and rationale for it	
• **Reassessing** understanding of decision, ensuring consistency in family caregiver	
• **Introducing palliative care** services and explaining their scope in the management	
• **Documentation** of decision of withdrawal on medical records and informs primary care physician, nephrologist, and palliative care team	
• **Implementation of withdrawal** from dialysis and shifting focus of care to comfort and symptom control of patient and provision of dignified end-of-life care	
• **Exploring conflict** and taking steps toward conflict resolution and review the care process	
• **Provision of bereavement care** for the family members	

End-of-life care and management of terminal days: Historically, uremic death is described as painless. But in reality, patients with advanced CKD have a high symptom burden and special considerations required at the end of life. Surveys of families have shown that 42–75% of patients report pain in terminal part of life. Other important symptoms include weakness, depression, myoclonus or muscle twitching, dyspnea, agitation, and gastrointestinal symptoms.

Contrary to expectations literature shows that symptom burden after dialysis withdrawal remains similar to those on therapy until up to 2 months before death after which it becomes significant and needs active management. Also, patient, family, and caregivers will have significant psychological concerns, anxiety, depressed mood, increased information needs, and practical concerns.

During the terminal phase, symptoms should be anticipated, with arrangement of appropriate prescriptions in place. In addition to specific symptom management, general supportive care should also be emphasized for the dying patient, such as lip balm, mouth swabs, positioning, back rubs, fans, and the elimination of blood draws and dietary restrictions.

Postdeath assessment and bereavement: Postdeath assessment and bereavement care should also be part of kidney supportive care and involve counseling, follow-up phone calls, and due expressions of condolence. As a part of quality assurance, the patient's death should be assessed by CKC team. This helps to ensure establishment of sound ACP, symptom control, and effective communication among interdisciplinary teams, patients, and families during terminal care.

Palliative dialysis: It focusses upon relieving symptoms rather than targeting adequacy and dialysis is done only when symptomatic. This role of palliative dialysis should be conveyed to the patient and family members and should not be perceived as a prelude to dialysis withdrawal. Dialysis patients may transition to a palliative approach to their dialysis care near end of life as their focus shifts to QOL rather than survival.

Conservative kidney care in India: In India, this concept is in a nascent stage. Relative lack of nephrologists and nonavailability/lack of access to dialysis/take up of alternative medicine by patients complicate this already intricate issue. Even in areas where dialysis is state sponsored, there are attrition, mortality, and less take up of transplant services. CKC may be able to partially fulfill these needs. Palliative care in cancer setting has been progressing especially in states of Kerala and in Mumbai. A joint specialty service involving nephrology, palliative care, and emphasis on education and training of CKC at all levels is required.

CONCLUSION

It is well recognized that present model of care in CKD focusses on prolonging life and hence does not address all needs of the patient. CKC may fulfill this unmet need through shared decision making, symptom management, end-of-life care, and address issues such as dialysis withdrawal through advance care planning. CKC must be part of a management model which allows it to integrate with or be an alternative to dialysis therapies with choice to transition between them. This necessarily requires training of nephrologists both early career and mid to senior level with help from palliative specialists, involvement of multidisciplinary teams to provide and improve QOL of patients throughout their illness.

RECOMMENDED READINGS

1. Davison SN, Levin A, Moss AH, Jha V, Brown EA, Brennan F, et al. Kidney Disease: Improving Global Outcomes. Executive summary of the KDIGO Controversies Conference on Supportive Care in Chronic Kidney Disease: developing a roadmap to improving quality care. Kidney Int. 2015;88(3):447-59.
2. Gelfand SL, Scherer JS, Koncicki HM. Kidney supportive care: Core Curriculum 2020. Am J Kidney Dis. 2020;75(5):793-806.
3. Davison SN. Supportive Care in Advanced Chronic Kidney Disease, Chapter 2. In: Yu AS, Chertow GM, Luyckx VA, Marsden PA, Skorecki K, Taal MW (Eds). Brenner and Rector's The Kidney, Volume 2, 11th edition. Philadelphia: Elsevier Inc.; 2020. pp. 2015-35.
4. Burns A, Murtagh FE. Conservative care in advanced chronic kidney disease, Chapter 145. In: Turner NN, Lameire N, Goldsmith DJ, Winearls CG, Himmelfarb J, Remuzzi G (Eds). Oxford Textbook of Clinical Nephrology. United Kingdom: Oxford University Press; 2015. pp. 1165-79.

CHAPTER 178

Hemodialysis

Snehal Gaikwad, Valentine Lobo

ABSTRACT

Hemodialysis is a treatment modality for patients with retention of uremic solutes, electrolyte, and acid-base imbalances due to acute kidney injury or chronic kidney disease. Hemodialysis consists of using the processes of diffusion and convection respectively to remove small and large molecular weight impurities from the patient's blood by running it through a hollow fiber dialyzer countercurrent to a dialysate solution prepared by the dialysis machine from treated water and salts. Anticoagulation is required to keep the blood from clotting in the extracorporeal circuit (ECC) and ensure the process runs uninterrupted. Although several advances have been made in dialyzer and machine technology complications may occur because of the unphysiologic nature of the process. The adequacy of the dialysis process is assessed by measurement of a marker solute, most often urea and the prescription altered based on the delivered dose and presence or absence of residual renal function. Infections, inadequate dialysis, and cardiovascular disease remain the most common causes of lower than acceptable survival in patients on hemodialysis.

"Quietly endure, silently suffer and patiently wait"

—Martin L King Jr

INTRODUCTION

Chronic kidney disease results in retention of organic nitrogenous compounds, electrolyte and acid-base imbalances, alterations in vitamin D metabolism and calcium phosphorous balance, lack of erythropoietin, and myriad manifestations on all organ systems.

Uremic retention solutes are referred to as uremic toxins when they interact with normal biological functions. The term uremic syndrome refers to the clinical picture produced by accumulation in the body of noxious substances which, in health, are eliminated into the urine, The European Uremic Toxin (EUTox) work group listed substances with presumed or proven biological activity, the accumulation of which in the body resulted from end-stage renal failure. **Table 1** lists some of these toxins classified by the work group by molecular weight, protein binding, and removal by dialysis. The purpose of dialysis is removal of solutes and excess fluid, and balancing electrolytes.

Limitations of dialysis, phenomena beyond toxin accumulation, play roles in uremia—oxidative stress, carbamylation, peroxidation, and organ crosstalk. A deficiency rather than excess of specific critical compounds,

TABLE 1 Uremic solutes and their toxicity.

Low-molecular-weight solutes	Middle-molecular-weight molecules	Protein-bound solutes
Molecular weight <500 Daltons	Molecular weight >500 and <60,000 Daltons	Mostly <500 Daltons
Water-soluble and easily removed by all dialysis	Not removed significantly by conventional dialysis	Highly protein bound and therefore difficult to remove by dialysis
Originally 68 members	Around 50 members	Around 25 members
• Asymmetric dimethylarginine (ADMA) • Creatine • Creatinine • Hyaluronic acid • Oxalate • SDMA (symmetric dimethylarginine) • Urea • Uric acid	• Adiponectin • Cystatin C • Leptin • Motilin • 1-microglobulin • Endothelin • Ghrelin • Atrial natriuretic peptide • Prolactin • 2-microglobulin	• Advanced glycation end products (AGEs) • Carboxy methyl propyl furanpropionic acid • Cytokines • Interleukins • Tumor necrosis factor (TNF) • Dimethylguanidines • Hippuric acid • Homocysteine etc.

including natural antioxidants, micronutrients, and certain amino acids which may be worsened by dialysis.

PRINCIPLES OF DIALYSIS

Diffusion is the process by which particles or solutes in solution move from an area of their higher concentration to an area of lower concentration. In dialysis, a two way diffusion occurs across a semipermeable membrane (the dialysis membrane), which separates blood and dialysate. Diffusion follows Fick's laws which state that

$$J_d = -D\ dC/dx \text{ (Fick's first law)}$$

where,

J_d is the diffusive flux or the mass of solute crossing the membrane per unit time
D is the diffusivity which is a function of the membrane surface area, and permeability a function of the size, density, and distribution of pores while
$-dC/dx$ is the concentration gradient.

Thicker membranes will have smaller gradients than thinner ones. Practically in dialysis, the concentration gradient is maximized by counter current flow of blood and dialysis flow. Concentration gradients allow dialysate to remove wastes from a patient's blood and to balance electrolytes in the blood with electrolytes in the dialysate.

Another factor affecting diffusive movement is molecular size, smaller molecules diffuse more rapidly than larger ones.

Since diffusion will cause a change in concentration with time this is given by:

$$dC/dt = D\ d^2C/dt^2 \text{ (Fick's second law)}$$

Ultrafiltration and convection: Movement of fluid through a filter as the result of hydraulic pressure is called filtration. The flow of fluid in any cylindrical tube is given by the:

Hagen–Poiseuille equation:

$$Qv = \pi Pa^4/8l\eta$$

where,

P is the driving pressure
a is the radius of the tube
l its length and
η is the viscosity of the fluid.

This equation is true for all Newtonian fluids, the arterial pressure drives blood through blood vessels, a pump does the same in an extracorporeal circuit (ECC), the dialysate is driven by a flow pump and the transmembrane pressure drives ultrafiltration across cylindrical pores in the dialyzer whose length is infinitesimal. As fluid moves across the membrane, it drags dissolved solutes across with it, a process called solvent drag. The solute transferred in this way by bulk movement of solvent (water) is called convection. The hydraulic permeability Jc of a dialyzer is given by:

$$Jc = Qf\ (Cb \times S)$$

where,

Qf is the ultrafiltration coefficient, and
'S' is the sieving coefficient is the ratio of the solute concentration in dialysate to that in plasma.

This value equals 1 for small solutes and decreases with increasing molecular weight, depending on the pore sizes in the membrane.

Blood and dialysate are two solutions in which the solvent is water, and electrolytes, glucose, and numerous organic nitrogenous compounds are the solutes. The principles of fluid dynamics, diffusion, ultrafiltration, and convection apply to each dialysis treatment. The dialytic process exposes the patient's blood (a solution)—to the dialysate (another solution)—with a semipermeable membrane (dialyzer) between them, with pumps providing the driving forces, and regulators and alarm systems controlling them in the dialysis machine.

Body water and solutes: We know that the human body contains about 60% weight of water (up to 75% in neonates).

This water is distributed in three compartments as shown in **Figure 1**.

1. The intracellular compartment
2. The interstitial compartment and
3. The intravascular (blood) compartment

Differences in the level of sodium and other electrolytes and organic compounds between compartments (gradients) cause water to move. Homeostasis (achieving equilibrium) is an attempt to have the same level of osmotically active solutes in all three compartments, by movement of solutes (diffusion) or water (osmosis). During dialysis, only fluid and solutes from the intravascular compartment, the bloodstream can be removed, while an equilibrium requires to be re-established between the three compartments. **Figure 1** shows how this is established.

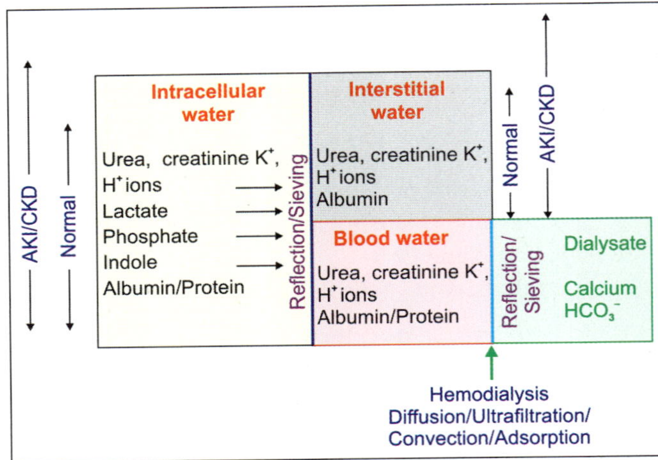

(AKI: acute kidney injury; CKD: chronic kidney disease)

FIGURE 1: Solute pools in AKI and CKD.

INDICATIONS OF DIALYSIS

Potential indications for dialysis can be grouped into two categories: (1) Renal replacement and (2) Renal support. This is particularly true for acute kidney injury as part of multiple organ failure where dialysis primary goal is to provide adequate renal support and permit other organ recovery. **Table 2** shows emergency and nonemergency indications renal and nonrenal for initiating renal replacement therapy.

DIALYZERS

The dialyzer is the artificial kidney, a device in which a large surface area membrane has been spun into thousands of hollow fibers through which blood flow is established by the machine while the dialysate circulates around the fibers. The geometry of the dialyzer allows a large area to be accommodated in a small volume, a cylinder with a length of 20–25 cm and a diameter of around 5 cm.

Dialyzers are classified as high efficiency or high flux depending on their maximal ability to remove small solutes their KoA or the convective removal of high molecular solutes like beta-2 microglobulin. **Table 3** shows the criteria for this classification. The information is provided by the manufacturers in the dialyzer specification sheet and enables a selection of the appropriate dialyzer for a particular treatment. Since solute and fluid transport occurs across the dialyzer membrane, the composition of blood exiting the dialyzer will be very different from that entering the dialyzer. Organic compounds like urea and electrolytes like potassium, present in high concentrations in the blood cross the membrane into the dialysate which does not contain these solutes, while calcium and buffers like

TABLE 2 Strategies for management of renal failure.

	Renal replacement	Renal support
Purpose	Dialysis when there is little to no residual kidney function	Dialysis used as adjunct to enhance kidney function, modify solute control and fluid balance
Application	Renal failure	Renal and nonrenal indications
Indications of HD	**Emergent indications:** • Refractory hyperkalemia (K > 6.5 mEq/L) • Refractory metabolic acidosis (pH < 7.15) • Fluid overload refractory to diuretic therapy and/or pulmonary edema • Uremic complications (symptom/organ dysfunction. Example, encephalopathy, pericarditis etc.)	• Facilitate nutrition • Ultrafiltration in refractory congestive cardiac failure • Poisoning 3 with dialyzable drug or toxin (e.g., ethanol, ethylene glycol, lithium etc.) • Cytokine manipulation in sepsis • Managing fluid balance and treatment of respiratory acidosis due to permissive hypercapnia in ventilated patients in ARDS and MOF • Hyperthermia refractory to regular cooling techniques
	Nonemergent indications: • Regulation of acid base, volume and electrolyte status • Progressive azotemia or oliguria unresponsive to medical management • Uremic bleeding diathesis • Protein energy malnutrition or failure to thrive	

(MOF: multiorgan failure)

TABLE 3 Classification of dialyzers.

Dialyzer characteristic	Conventional	High efficiency	High flux
KoA (urea) (mL/min)	<450	>600	Variable
Urea clearance (mL/min)	<250	>200	Variable
Ultrafiltration coefficient (mL/mm Hg/h)	<12	Variable	>12
Beta-2 microglobulin (B2M) clearance (mL/min)	<10	Variable	>20

bicarbonate present in high concentration in the dialysate are transported in the reverse direction.

The efficiency with which a dialyzer removes a particular solute, thereby lowering its concentration in the blood or "clearing a particular volume of blood of that solute" is called its clearance. The clearance is a function of the blood flow, dialysate flow, concentration gradient, dialyzer membrane composition, size or surface area of the dialyzer, and its pore size and density. The hydraulic permeability of a dialyzer is a function as seen in Poiseuille equation to be a function of the fourth power of the pore radius and the diffusibility is a function of the area of pores and therefore the square of the radius. Thus efficiency of diffusion and convection may be dissociated despite the membrane having the same chemical composition and size. The clearance of small solutes cleared by diffusion is dependent on blood and dialysate flow while that of larger solutes is dependent on the ultrafiltration volume (**Figs. 2** and **3**).

Recently dialyzers with very large pore size allowing passage of molecules having molecular weights >10,000 Daltons and approaching the native kidney have been in use. They are called high cutoff dialyzers or high retention onset dialyzers.

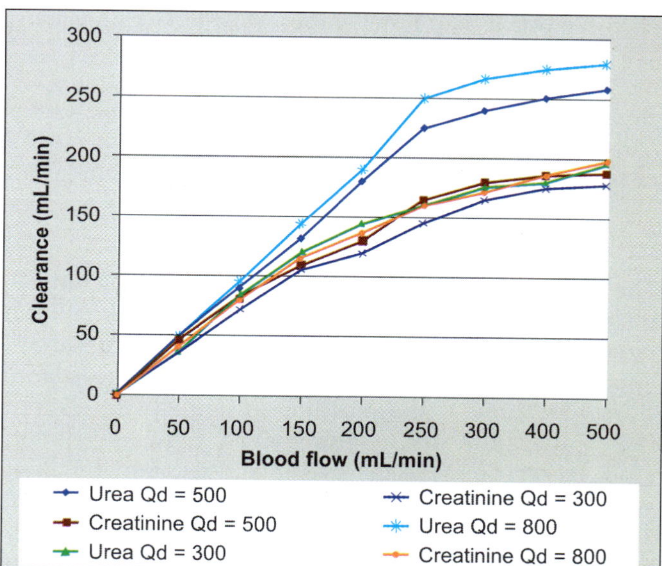

FIGURE 2: Effect of blood and dialysate flow of diffusive clearance.

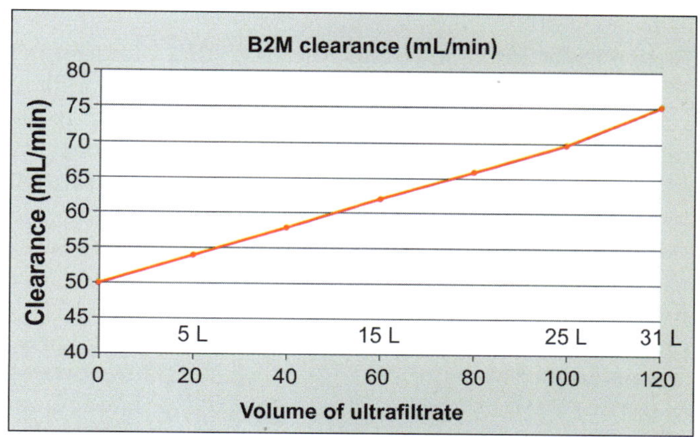

FIGURE 3: Beta-2 microglobulin (B2M) clearance by convection.

Source: Lornoy W, Because I, Billouw JM, Sierens L, Malderen PV, D'Haenems P. On-line haemodiafiltration. Remarkable removal of β2-microglobulin. Long-term clinical observations. Nephrol Dial Transplant. 2000;15:49-54.

DIALYSIS PROCESS AND MACHINES

The dialysis process requires the patient's blood to be exposed to the dialysate separated by a semipermeable membrane the dialyzer. The dialyzer is thus the interface between the patient's milieu intérieur which contains an excess of organic waste compounds, electrolytes like potassium and H^+ ions but deficient in calcium and buffers and the dialysate which should resemble normal extracellular water as closely as possible.

To achieve this we require:

A vascular access which may be:

- Temporary—a catheter placed in the femoral or the internal jugular vein
- Permanent—an arteriovenous fistula either in the forearm or arm
    - The access should be capable of delivering the desired blood flow for dialysis at negative pressures generated by the blood pump. Generally AV fistulae have blood flows in excess of 500 mL/min and this can be obtained in the ECC by 15G needles, while catheters of 12–14 French (F) can deliver the same flow.

The dialysis machine provides the driving force to bring blood to the dialyzer at a designated rate, using a peristaltic pump and tubings, prepares the appropriate dialysate and circulates it at the set rate and utilizes a set of regulatory systems consisting of pressure monitors, sensors, and alarms to ensure patient safety. The dialysis machine also has a highly accurate and precise system for extracting water from the blood passing through the dialyzer with each pass to achieve a weight loss with each treatment. This is based either on flow meters or a volumetric balancing chamber with a membrane pump. Most modern machines are microprocessor based, with analog signals from mechanical, chemical, and electrical sensors amplified and converted to digital inputs which lead to the generation of a digital and analog output. A liquid-crystal display (LCD) or light-emitting diode (LED) display may indicate to the operator the nature of an alarm. A typical dialysis machine is shown in **Figure 4**.

The dialysate solution is prepared by the machine by mixing treated degassed water warmed to normal body temperature, with a set of salts called concentrates in the appropriate proportion to achieve the concentrations shown in **Table 4**. The machine measures and displays the temperature and conductivity (ability to conduct an electric current) of the solution. The conductivity is a surrogate for the electrolytic composition of the solution. **Table 4** shows the appropriate conductivity of a solution having the required concentration of solutes to maintain homeostasis of the extracellular fluid. A solution with an inappropriate composition is bypassed to the drain without entering the dialyzer accompanied by an audible and visual alarm.

Anticoagulation is a system to ensure that blood in the ECC is prevented from clotting and returned to the patient preserving the integrity of the vascular access. During the dialysis procedure, blood is exposed to components of the ECC with variable degree of thrombogenicity, turbulent blood flow and high shear stress, air-blood interaction in the drip chambers, and air detection chambers leading to activation of coagulation cascade and thrombus formation, all of which favor circuit clotting. The risk of bleeding induced by anticoagulation must be balanced against loss of blood, if the circuit is lost. Unfractionated heparin (UFH) is the most widely used anticoagulant followed by use of low molecular weight heparin. Detailed

TABLE 4 Relationship of dialysate ions and conductivity.

Salt	Dialysate concentration cation/anion (mmol/L)	Conductivity (mS/cm)
NaCl	103	10.68
KCl	2.00	0.26
$CaCl_2$	1.5	0.25
$MgCl_2$	0.50	0.09
$NaHCO_3$	34	2.47
CH_3COONa	3.00	0.21
Final Na^+ concentration = 140 mmol/L		13.96

TABLE 5 Different anticoagulation techniques.

Heparin related	Citrate related	Anticoagulant free
Unfractionated heparin (UFH)	Regional citrate anticoagulation (RCA)	No saline flush method
Routine and tight heparinization		
Low molecular weight heparin (LMWH)	Bicarbonate dialysate with low citrate concentration (Citrasate)	Intermittent saline flush method or continuous saline infusion method
Regional heparinization	Not commonly used especially in intermittent dialysis	
Heparin-coated dialyzers	May still require a small dose of anticoagulant	

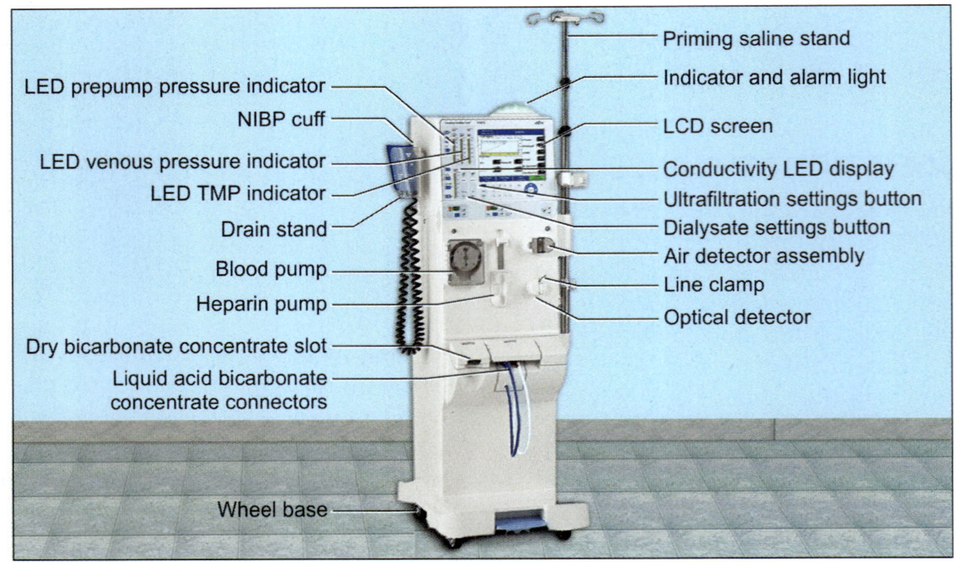

(LED: light-emitting diode; NIBP: noninvasive blood pressure; LCD: liquid-crystal display)

FIGURE 4: **4008S NG machine from Fresenius.**

discussion of rest individual drugs is beyond the scope of present chapter. Listed below in **Table 5** are the different drugs and anticoagulation techniques available.

ISN guidelines for anticoagulation of the dialysis circuit:

- *Intermittent bolus*: Bolus loading dose 35–55 units/kg followed by maintenance dose of 10–20 IU/kg boluses every hour. No heparin to be given during the last half hour of dialysis when using AV fistula as vascular access and continue till the end of dialysis when dialyzing through a catheter.
- *Constant infusion*: Bolus loading dose of 35–55 units/kg followed by constant infusion.
  - *Dose*: Body weight between 50 and 90 kg: No change in dose
  - Body weight outside these limits: Bolus dose 75–100 units/kg; infusion dose 750–1,000 units/h
- *Target clotting times [activated clotting time (ACT) test baseline value 120–150 s]*: During dialysis desired range +80% (200–250 s) and at the end of dialysis +40% (170–190 s)

Patients with intercurrent events such as recent head trauma, pericarditis, recent surgery with bleeding complications or risks of coagulopathy, thrombocytopenia, intracerebral hemorrhage, gastric ulcer, esophageal varices, and active bleeding from any other site are at high risk of bleeding complications. Such patients should be treated with anticoagulant free dialysis. A protocol of tight heparinization is recommended for such patients.

Dose of unfractionated heparin in tight heparinization:

- Bolus dose of 750 units followed by constant infusion of 600 U/h to be continued till the end of dialysis.
- Avoid intermittent UFH bolus technique to prevent sharp rise and fall of ACT during dialysis.
- *Target clotting time (ACT test baseline value 120–150 s)*: During dialysis desired range +40% (170–190 s); at the end of dialysis +40% (170–190 s)

Anticoagulation free dialysis:

- Use of intermittent saline flushes with 100–200 mL 0.9% NS bolus injected predialyzer every 15–30 minutes preferred over continuous saline infusion (post-hoc analysis of HepZero study).
- Blood flow rate as high as clinically permitted (>300 mL/min)
- Ensure complete removal of air from dialyzer and rinse the circuit with heparin saline (3,000 units/L)
- Use of bicarbonate dialysate with low citrate concentration (0.8 mmol/L) (has citrate instead of acetate)
- Avoid blood infusions into dialysate blood lines/ECC
- Use of heparin-coated dialyzers (HeprAN membrane: Polyacrylonitrile membrane with heparin grafted during its dialyzer production) or dialyzer with membranes adsorbing heparin (AN69ST membrane: High flux heparin binding polyacrylonitrile membrane which allows the coating of heparin during priming with heparin solution)

TABLE 6 Complications of hemodialysis.

Complications	Estimated frequency
Hypotension	20–40%
Cramps	5–20%
Nausea and vomiting	5–15%
Headache	5%
Chest and back pain	2%
Pruritus	5%
Fever and chills	<1%
Hemolysis	Unknown very rare
Air embolism	8.5–33/million sessions
Vascular access hemorrhage	Very rare
Vascular needle dislodgment	14–91/million sessions
Cardiac arrest	70/million sessions
Dialyzer reaction	21–170/million sessions

COMPLICATIONS OF DIALYSIS

Because dialysis as a procedure involves exposure of blood to an ECC, rapid fluid shifts, changes in osmolality and the interaction of the patient with a machine, it is inevitable that complications may occur. Machine technology has advanced to the stage where the devices are considered "failsafe" with a complication rate resulting in patient death of 1 per 100 million treatments. Nevertheless many complications arise as a result partially of the unphysiologic nature of the treatment. The frequency of these is shown in **Table 6**.

LONG-TERM OUTCOMES

The goals of providing dialysis are to attempt to replace the function of the native kidneys, as a lifesaving and life-sustaining measure improves patient survivals and quality of life. Hemodialysis, however, can provide only a fraction of the numerous functions of the kidneys. Patients receiving inadequate dialysis develop malnutrition, inflammation, and a poor quality of life and have a shortened life span due to cardiovascular disease and death. In 1981, the **National Cooperative Dialysis Study (NCDS)** first provided evidence of a link between inadequate dialysis and decreased survival, while increasing frequency and duration of dialysis improved survival, quality of life, and medication amounts. No single clinical or laboratory parameter can assess adequacy of dialysis hence it is necessary to develop a comprehensive monitoring system of measuring adequacy of dialysis which is also easy to use and reproducible. The Indian Society of Nephrology Working group has provided some guidelines for assessing and delivering adequate dialysis to patients, which are summarized here.

Patients on maintenance hemodialysis (MHD) must receive three times dialysis in a week for at least 4 hours each time with blood flows of 300 mL/min and dialysate flows of 500 mL/min.

In the presence of residual renal function > 10 mL/min with indication for initiating dialysis, incremental dialysis may be tried initiating with twice weekly sessions. Residual renal function must be monitored every 3 months, by the average of 24 hours urea and creatinine clearance as it may be expected to decrease. As residual renal function facilitates the regulation of fluid and electrolyte balance, and may enhance survival, attempts to preserve it by avoiding hypotensive episodes, and use of nephrotoxic drugs should be made. If malnutrition or fluid overload develops, increase dialysis to three times/week. Those on twice a week dialysis, may be given longer dialysis for 6 hours, i.e., at night.

Following the NCDS study, a measure of adequacy that links dialyzer clearance, and treatment time normalized to total body water Kt/V, a dimensionless constant obtained by measuring pre- and postdialysis blood urea levels or simply the urea reduction ratio (URR) be used as a measure of dialysis prescription. URR should be targeted to >65%. Postdialysis sample should be taken 2 minutes after dialysis or during slowing pump speed to 100 mL/min and sample taken 15 seconds later.

Kt/V of 1.4–1.6 should be achieved in each dialysis. This may be reduced among patients with residual kidney function of greater than 2 mL/min/1.73 m^2.

Dialysis dose in stable hemodialysis patients should be assessed monthly and the cause sought if the above targets are not met. The causes include inadequate treatment duration, technical errors in the method of obtaining BUN samples, low blood flow rates, and hypotensive episodes that require changes in treatment and overestimation of dialyzer clearance. Once identified, the specific condition should be remedied.

Currently many newer dialysis machines have online Kt/V monitors which provide measures of Kt/V delivered. It offers the advantage of monitoring dose of dialysis delivered in each dialysis session, does not require a lag time, and no blood collection is required. Where available, these may be used for more frequent monitoring.

A total of five **studies from India** published between 2012 and 2018 have attempted to identify dialysis practices and the factors affecting survival. These studies have shown that 70–80% of patients receive biweekly dialysis as opposed to the recommended thrice weekly sessions recommended and that consequently mortality is unacceptably high, being about 12.5% at 1 year, 19.6% at 2 years, and almost 80% at 5 years. Infections, cardiovascular disease, and hyperkalemia were identified as the major causes of mortality. The actual mortality may be even higher as these studies only included patients who had survived the initial 3 months.

CONCLUSION

In conclusion, hemodialysis is a treatment in which the filtration function of the native kidneys is mimicked by a machine and an ECC consisting of a dialyzer and tubings. The dialyzer is a compact hollow fiber device where a semipermeable membrane allows diffusion and convection of solutes and water to occur, while the process is controlled by parameters set on the machine. Prescribed doses of dialysis may vary according to the patients residual function and influence survival and quality of life.

RECOMMENDED READINGS

1. Pittard J. Safety Monitors in Dialysis. In: Nissenson A, Fine R (Ed). Handbook of Dialysis Therapy, 4th edition. Philadelphia: Elsevier; 2017.
2. Nalesso F, Ronco C. Selecting a Dialyzer, technical and clinical considerations. In: Nissenson A, Fine R (Ed). Handbook of Dialysis Therapy, 4th edition. Philadelphia: Elsevier; 2017.
3. Young HD, Freedman RA, Ford AL. Fluid Mechanics in Sears and Zemanskys University Physics with Modern Physics, 13th edition. United States: Addison-Wesley; 2011.
4. Lisowska-Myjak B. Uremic toxins and their effects on multiple organ systems. Nephron Clin Pract. 2014;128:303-11.
5. Zawada ET. Initiation of Dialysis. in Daugirdas JT, Blake PG, Ing TS (Eds). Handbook of Dialysis 5th edition. Philadelphia: Wolters Kluwer; 2015.
6. Winchester JF, Harbord NB, Charen E, Ghannoum M. Anticoagulation. In: Daugridas JT, Blake PG, Ing TS (Eds) Handbook of Dialysis. Fifth edition, Philadelphia: Wolters Kluwer; 2015.p. 368-90.
7. ISN Working Group. Minimum hemodialysis Guidelines of Indian Society of Nephrology. 2020;30(7):1-91.
8. Saha M, Allon M. Diagnosis, treatment, and prevention of hemodialysis emergencies. Clin J Am Soc Nephrol. 2017;12:357-69.
9. Lakshminarayana GR, Sheetal LG, Mathew A, Rajesh R, Kurian G, Unni VN. Hemodialysis outcomes and practice patterns in end-stage renal disease: Experience from a Tertiary Care Hospital in Kerala. Indian J Nephrol. 2017;27:51-7.
10. Shaikh M, Woodward M, John O, Bassi A, Jan S, Sahay M, et al. Utilization, costs, and outcomes for patients receiving publicly funded hemodialysis in India. Kidney Int. 2018;94:440-5.

CHAPTER

179

Peritoneal Dialysis

Narayan Prasad, Ruju Gala

ABSTRACT

Peritoneal dialysis (PD) is a modality of renal replacement therapy (RRT), which utilizes the peritoneal membrane as a dialyzer between blood and PD fluid as dialysate. It facilitates the exchanges of solutes and uremic toxins and ultrafiltration (UF) occurs across the osmotic gradient created by the dextrose-rich peritoneal fluid. The vascularity of peritoneal blood supply determines the effective peritoneal surface area which is key for optimal functioning of PD. PD may be formed manually or through a cycler machines called automated PD (APD).

Peritoneal dialysis fluids contain 1.5%, 2.5%, and 4.25% dextrose or icodextrin as the osmotic agent, lactate as buffer, and other electrolytes. After the catheter insertion, PD is started after 10–14 days break-in period. A peritoneal equilibration test (PET) is performed at 4–6 weeks to characterize the peritoneal membrane as high, high-average, low-average, and low transport characteristics do decide the prescription of PD depending on residual renal function and transporter characteristics. Complications may occur in form infectious, mechanical, or metabolic. PD provides a quality dialysis in home environment, particularly become useful in pandemic times, when lockdown kind of restrictions are enforced.

"Part of recovery is relapse. I dust myself off and move forward again"

—Steven Adler

PERITONEAL DIALYSIS

The ultimate treatment for end-stage kidney disease patients is RRT; renal transplantation (RT), or one of the two modes of dialysis, hemodialysis (HD) or PD. All being complementary to each other in integrated care approach in the management of end-stage kidney disease (**Fig. 1**). Each dialysis modality is used to bridge till RT and patients can get back on dialysis again if renal allograft fails. If HD is not possible because of vascular access failure, the patient can be back on PD; if peritoneal membrane fails, HD can be opted in.

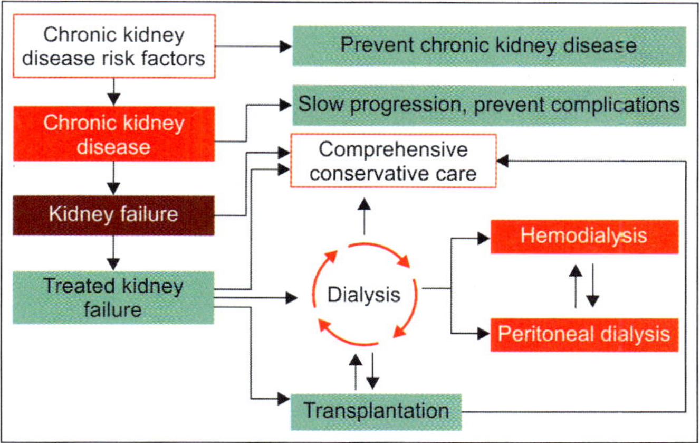

FIGURE 1: Integrated care approach for the management of patients with end-stage kidney diseases.

Hemodialysis is the purification of blood across the hemofilter performed through a dialysis machine, while PD filters out the uremic toxins across the peritoneal membrane in the abdominal cavity. The reasons for choosing one modality over other are multifactorial. PD being simple, convenient, and relatively low or almost similar cost, and done at home itself, weighs in its favor. Blood loss, bloodborne, and vascular access-related complications are not encountered. Moreover, the physician's comfort/expertise with therapy and government reimbursement policies also affects PD as a choice in selecting RRT. PD is used by around 200,000 patients across the globe.

PROCESS OF PERITONEAL DIALYSIS

Peritoneal dialysis PD can be performed manually or with the help of a machine. Continuous ambulatory peritoneal dialysis (CAPD) is the most used modality. The commercially available PD fluid is instilled into the abdominal cavity via Tenckhoff PD catheter connected through transfer set and kept for 4–6 hours, depending on the dwell time. During the exchange time, the uremic solutes are diffused and fluid is ultrafiltered across the peritoneal membrane capillaries into the peritoneal cavity. After that, the used equilibrated fluid with uremic solutes is drained into the drain bag, and the new fluid is replaced for the next exchange. A sketch representing the process of PD is shown in **Figure 2**.

If the fluid is kept throughout the day and night and patients are ambulatory between the exchange procedure, it is called CAPD. In APD, a cycler machine is used that automatically cycles dialysis solution in and out of the abdominal cavity. APD can be continuous cyclic peritoneal dialysis (CCPD), including day and night dwell. Nocturnal intermittent peritoneal dialysis (NIPD), in which dialysis is performed only during night usually through automated cycler machines, keeping the day dry. A sketch representing the three different commonly used modalities is shown in **Figure 3**.

Other uncommon modalities are nightly tidal peritoneal dialysis (NTPD) and continuous flow peritoneal dialysis (CFPD). NIPD is a technique in which, after an initial fill of the peritoneal cavity, only a portion of dialysate is rapidly cycled. In CFPD, continuous circulation of PD fluid is maintained at a high flow rate using two separate catheters or one dual lumen catheter.

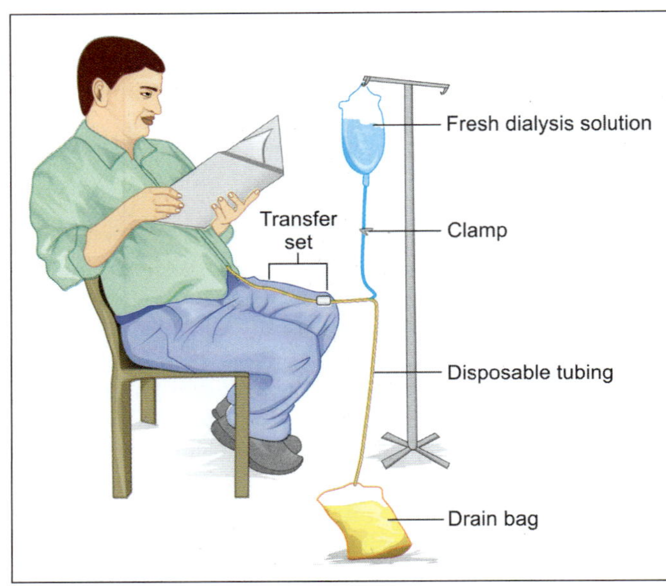

FIGURE 2: Process of peritoneal dialysis.

ANATOMY OF PERITONEAL MEMBRANE

- The peritoneal membrane with a total surface area of 1–2 m^2 is composed of two parts: The parietal peritoneum (10%) covering the diaphragm and the visceral peritoneum (90%) lining the visceral organs.
- The mesothelium is a continuous monolayer of cells secreting surfactant like a lubricant for the peritoneum.
- A basement membrane underlies the mesothelium (**Fig. 4**).
- *Interstitium*: Composed of mucopolysaccharide matrix and glycosaminoglycans, supports the peritoneum, and facilitates the transport of essential nutrients.
- *Blood vessels*: The number of perfused capillaries determines the effective peritoneal surface area, i.e., the functional area of exchange between blood and dialysate compartments.
- *Peritoneal lymphatics*: Aid in the removal of solutes and fluid from the interstitium.

PHYSIOLOGY OF PERITONEAL DIALYSIS

Peritoneal dialysis involves the transport of solutes and water across the peritoneal membrane separating two fluid-filled compartments. Three transport processes occur during PD, namely:

1. *Diffusion*: In PD, the diffusive removal of any solute (blood urea nitrogen and serum creatinine) depends on the "effective" peritoneal membrane surface area, the intrinsic permeability of the membrane, dialysate flow, concentration gradients, and time allowed for transport. Standard PD therapies are therefore limited by dialysate flow.
2. *Ultrafiltration*: Net UF or the removal of fluid is achieved clinically by creating an osmotic pressure gradient (crystalloid or colloid) between blood and dialysate. This also facilitates solute removal, and its contribution to net solute clearance has been termed "solvent drag" or "convection", and
3. *Absorption*: Absorption of fluid occurs through the tissues of the anterior abdominal wall and by the

(CAPD: continuous ambulatory peritoneal dialysis; CCPD: continuous cyclic peritoneal dialysis; NIPD: nocturnal intermittent peritoneal dialysis; PD: peritoneal dialysis)

FIGURE 3: Graphical representations of the three different PD modalities.

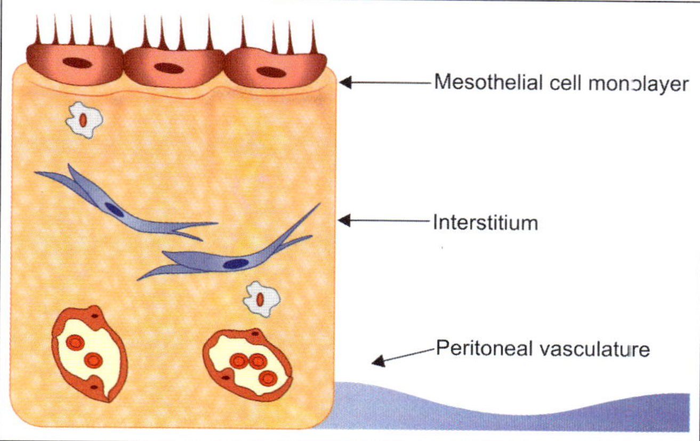

FIGURE 4: Diagrammatic representation of the peritoneal membrane.

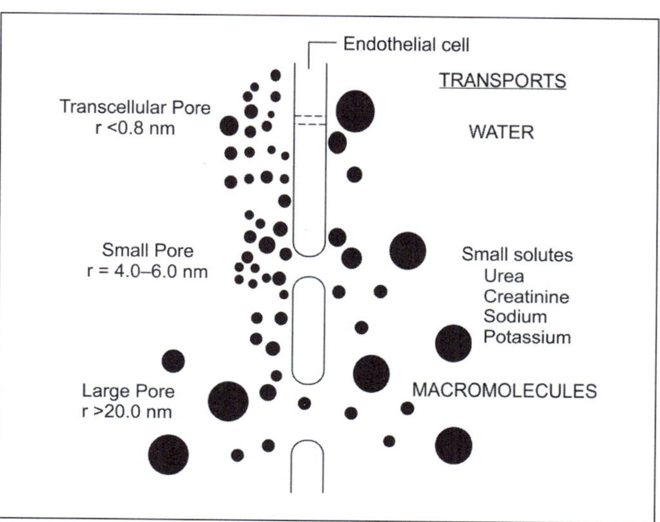

FIGURE 5: Three-pore model of peritoneal transport.

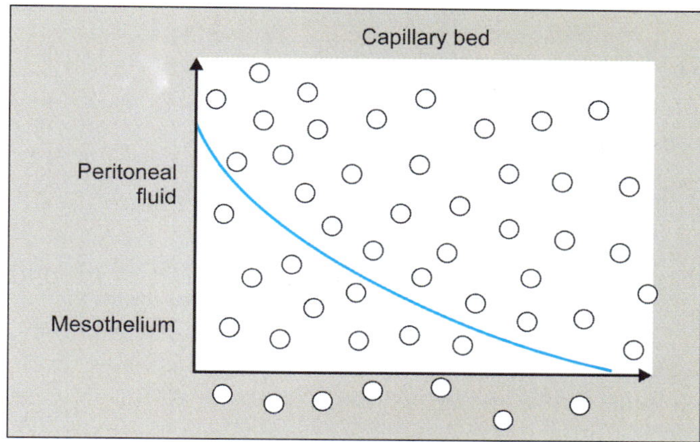

FIGURE 6: Distributed model.

peritoneal lymphatics. Intraperitoneal (IP) volume is thus determined by the relative magnitudes of transcapillary UF and anterior wall plus lymphatic absorption. Measurements of lymphatic absorption rates in CAPD patients using IP dextran as a marker ranged from 0.1 to 3.5 mL/min with a median value of 1.0 mL/min or about 2.2 L/day.

The amount of dialysis achieved and the extent of fluid removed from the abdominal cavity depends on the volume of dialysis solution infused, i.e., dwell volume, how often this solution is exchanged, and the concentration of the crystalloid osmotic or colloid oncotic agent present.

MODELS OF PERITONEAL TRANSPORT

- *The three-pore model*: It states that the peritoneal capillary is the critical barrier to peritoneal transport. The solute and water movement across the peritoneal capillaries is proportional to the relative abundance of pores of three different sizes (**Fig. 5**):
  - i. Large pores: 20–40 nm
  - ii. Small pores: 4–6 nm
  - iii. Ultrapores: <0.8 nm
- *Distributed model*: This concept represents the efficiency of transport from a given capillary to the peritoneal space, maximum for the capillaries closest to the mesothelial boundary (**Fig. 6**).

COMPONENTS OF THE PERITONEAL DIALYSIS SYSTEM

Renal replacement therapy with PD comprises of three important components:

1. The PD catheter,
2. PD solutions, and
3. The peritoneal membrane with its associated vascular supply.

Elaborating these components:

PD CATHETERS

- Catheters inserted for the purpose of PD can be acute or chronic.
  - *Acute use catheters*: Straight and relatively rigid catheters about 3 mm in diameter and 25–30 mm in length. Used for a short-term (2–3 days) period. They are easy to insert and can be done at bedside.
  - *Chronic use catheters*: Used as a standard chronic indwelling PD catheter. Various soft materials are used such as silicone rubber or polyurethane.
- *Silicone rubber catheters*: Most commonly used material is silicone rubber. Advantages being its relatively biocompatible and inert nature.
- *Polyurethane catheters*: Characterized by a better tensile strength, thinner wall resulting in a larger lumen, and faster flow rates.

Peritoneal dialysis catheters consist of three segments: (1) IP, (2) tunneled, and (3) extraperitoneal segment, with one or two polyester cuffs.

Design modifications:

- *Most common*: Straight double-cuff Tenckhoff catheter: 42/47 cm in length
- *Swan neck*: Preform 180° bend between two cuffs, reducing risk of catheter migration and external cuff extrusion
- Coiled tip catheter

Others such as Toronto-Western and presternal catheters for obese patients and Moncrief–Popovich (or embedded) catheters are also available.

Insertion techniques:

Catheter can be inserted by surgical or nonsurgical techniques.

- Bedside by Seldinger method
- Peritoneoscopic-assisted placement
- Surgical placement via laparoscopic or minilaparotomy.

Break-in period: Immediate postcatheter insertion, flush with 0.5–1.5 L of dialysate till clear fluid returns. Ideally, PD should not be initiated until 10–14 days after insertion of catheter, which allows the tunnel, entry, and exit sites to heal.

Urgent start peritoneal dialysis: If a patient needs RRT before 2 weeks, intermittent PD can be started with low-volume dialysate (<1.5 L) in supine position, with gradual optimization of PD.

PERITONEAL DIALYSIS SOLUTIONS

The dialysate used in PD comprises of three key components:

1. Osmotic agent to induce UF
2. Buffer to correct metabolic acidosis, commonly used is lactate
3. Electrolytes such as sodium, calcium, magnesium, and chloride to ensure optimal diffusive solute removal

Most conventional PD solutions use dextrose (1.5%, 2.5%, or 4.25% glucose) as osmotic agent. The major shortcomings being the absorption of glucose, which reduces the osmotic force driving UF over the course of PD. There is formation of toxic glucose degradation products (GDPs), leading to structural and functional changes in the peritoneal membrane due to accumulation of advanced glycosylation end-products.

Glucose-sparing peritoneal dialysis solutions: To mitigate glucose-mediated toxicity locally on the peritoneal membrane as well as systemic side effects of hyperglycemia, PD solutions use:

- Icodextrin, a carbohydrate polymer, or
- Amino acids

Icodextrin peritoneal dialysis solution: About 7.5% solution, high-molecular-weight polymer of glucose, isosmotic to plasma and exerts oncotic pressure driving UF. It is slowly removed from the peritoneal cavity via lymphatics, ensures steady UF over a long dwell time. Side effects include skin rash and sterile peritonitis.

Biocompatible peritoneal dialysis solutions: Biocompatible PD solutions are newer PD solutions with neutral pH and low in toxic GDPs, use a two- or three-compartment bag. In one compartment, the glucose is heat sterilized at a very low pH, which reduces the formation of GDPs, while buffer is present in the other compartment at an alkaline pH, resulting in a neutral pH on mixing of the two compartments. Advantages of these newer solutions are claimed to be prolonged peritoneal membrane life, relatively preserved residual renal function, and lesser peritonitis rates.

PERITONEAL MEMBRANE FUNCTION

A measurement of creatinine clearance is a measurement of the intrinsic transport properties of the peritoneal membrane, specifically a function of peritoneal diffusive permeability (cm/min) and effective peritoneal surface area (in cm^2). To clinically characterize peritoneal transport characteristics, standard PET, developed by Zbylut Twardowski in 1987, is widely used bedside. However, several modifications in the test such as mini-PET and double mini-PET have also been done.

Peritoneal equilibration test:

- After draining off the night dwell, 2 L of 2.5% dextrose-based PD solution is instilled into the abdominal cavity.
- Baseline blood and dialysate samples for urea, sodium, creatinine, and glucose are taken. Same samples are repeated at 2 and 4 hours.
- With these values, we plot the dialysate-to-plasma (D/P) ratios for creatinine and urea and the ratio of glucose in the dialysate compared to its baseline concentration (D/D0) at times 2 and 4 hours on the standard PET graph.

Interpretation of the test: As shown in **Figure 7**, peritoneal membrane transport is divided into four categories: (1) high, (2) high-average, (3) low-average, and (4) low.

High transporters: They most rapidly equilibrate creatinine, thus have excellent solute clearance. Also, because of early glucose absorption, the osmotic gradient also dissipates rapidly causing lesser UF. These patients benefit by performing CAPD with frequent exchanges and shorter dwell times, or ideal for APD.

Low transporters: Conversely, they have poor solute clearance due to slow creatinine exchange. Also, as their osmotic gradient is maintained longer due to slower glucose absorption, they ultrafilter well. These patients ideally should have longer dwell times with lesser exchanges.

Patients in the two average groups tend to perform well with both good solute clearance and UF.

PERITONEAL DIALYSIS PRESCRIPTION

The choice between CAPD versus APD is decided by the patient and caregivers. Then, the selection of a specific prescription is based on clearance, UF, and metabolic requirements of the patient. Initial prescription may be written keeping in mind the patient's weight, residual renal function, and any lifestyle constraints that may need consideration. APD may be preferred in high transporter where frequent exchanges are required to achieve target UF.

Further, a PET test can be performed at 4 weeks of initiating PD, and as per patients' transport characteristics, the initial prescription can be accordingly modified. A decreasing residual renal function should be kept in mind. Clinical and experimental adequacy testing should be repeated to ensure clearances as per the recommended target.

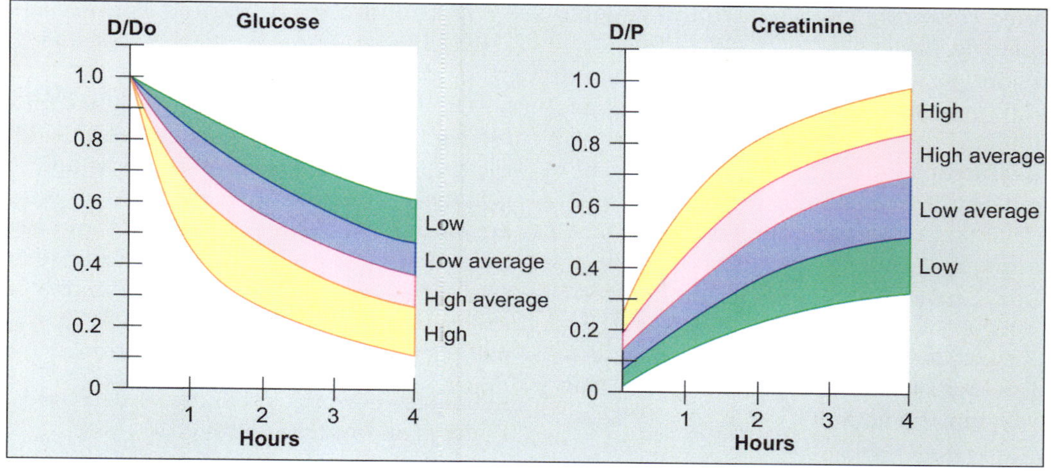

FIGURE 7: A graph plot showing four different categories (high, high-average, low-average, and low) based on dialysate-to-plasma (D/P) creatinine and glucose ratio.

ADEQUACY OF PERITONEAL DIALYSIS

Peritoneal dialysis adequacy is usually estimated by parameters based on the kinetics of small solutes such as total Kt/V_{urea} and total weekly creatinine clearance. Rather than achieving the target number, UF, and other aspects (blood pressure, anemia, nutrition, inflammation, mineral metabolism, and prevention of cardiovascular events) and, in particular, residual renal function must be taken into account. Patient reported outcome measures, person's symptoms; impact of the dialysis regimen on the person's life, mental health and social circumstances; and nutrition status should be assessed regularly through evaluation of the patient's appetite, clinical examination, body weight measurements, and blood tests (potassium, bicarbonate, phosphate, and albumin).

Dietary intake of potassium, phosphate, sodium, protein, carbohydrate, and fat may need to be assessed and adjusted as well. The high-quality goal-directed PD is recommended by International Society of Peritoneal Dialysis (ISPD). At present, for a CAPD patient, a minimum delivered PD dose of total weekly Kt/V_{urea} (peritoneal plus residual kidney) should be at least 1.7. There is no strong evidence to suggest numerical value for the UF volume; however, the Canadian society nephrology work group suggests ensuring a minimal net peritoneal UF volume 750 mL in anuric patient to avoid volume overload state.

COMPLICATIONS

Patients undergoing PD may encounter infectious or noninfectious complications.

INFECTIOUS COMPLICATIONS

Major infectious complications are peritonitis and exit-site or tunnel infections.

Peritonitis: It is the most common infectious complication of PD. The frequency averages one episode every 20–30 patient months, responsible for 16% of deaths.

Definition: Diagnosis is made when at least two of the three conditions are met:

- Symptoms and signs of peritoneal inflammation (pain and rebound tenderness)
- Cloudy dialysis effluent with white blood cell count >100 cells/mm^3 with 50% polymorphonuclear neutrophils response
- Isolation of the organism on smear or growth in peritoneal effluent cultures

Microbiology:

- Most caused by gram-positive cocci seen in 60–75% cases, most commonly *Staphylococcus epidermidis* or *aureus*.
- Gram-negative bacilli account for 15–25%
- Fungi in 2–3%, (in India, reported up to 14% of all episodes)
- *Mycobacterium* in 1%
- In approximately 15–20% of episodes, there is no organism grown, called culture negative peritonitis.
- The finding of anaerobic and/or polymicrobial peritonitis in <10% of patients should raise the concern of an intra-abdominal abscess or perforation and warrants a surgical evaluation.
- Elevated amylase in the peritoneal effluent may suggest intra-abdominal perforation or pancreatitis.

In many centers from India, gram-negative organisms *Escherichia coli* were reported as the most common organism causing PD-related peritonitis.

Management: Peritoneal effluent is checked for cell count with a differential, and Gram staining and culture testing performed. Empirical treatment with IP antibiotics initiated based on Gram staining.

- Empiric antibiotic regimens should be center specific and should include both gram-positive and gram-negative organisms.
- *Gram-positive coverage*: First-generation cephalosporin or vancomycin.

- *Gram-negative coverage*: Third-generation cephalosporin or aminoglycoside.
- Adjuvant treatment with antifungal prophylaxis + IP heparin and fibrinolytic enzymes like streptokinase for clearing of biofilm.
- Antibiotic treatment should target rapid resolution of inflammation and also maintain optimal peritoneal membrane function, preferred route being antibiotic. The recommended dosage of antibiotics for the treatment of PD-related peritonitis is summarized in **Table 1**.
- IP antibiotics can be given as continuous (in all the exchanges) or intermittent dosing (i.e., once daily) allowing dwell time of 6 hours.
  - *Gram-positive organisms*:
    - *Coagulase negative Staphylococcus and Enterococcus*: 14 days
    - *Staphylococcus aureus*: 21 days + oral rifampicin to prevent relapse, 300 mg bd for 5 days every 3 months
    - *Staphylococcus aureus* with concurrent exit site or tunnel infection: Needs catheter removal.
  - *Gram-negative organisms*:
    - Single non-*Pseudomonas* species: 14 days
    - *Pseudomonas* species: Needs two antibiotics with antipseudomonal coverage with catheter removal, continuing antibiotics for 2 weeks after removal.
  - *Fungal peritonitis*: Prompt removal of the catheter with 10–14 days treatment with antifungal.

Automated peritoneal dialysis-related peritonitis: Intermittent IP dosing with rapid exchanges in APD may lead to subtherapeutic levels due to higher peritoneal clearance in APD than in CAPD. Patients on APD with peritonitis may be:
- Temporarily shifted to CAPD modality, or
- Resetting the cycler to permit a longer exchange time

TABLE 1 Intraperitoneal antibiotic dosing recommendations.

	Intermittent (one exchange daily)	Continuous (all exchanges)
Cefazolin	15–20 mg/kg/daily	LD 500 mg/L, MD 125 mg/L
Ceftazidime	1,000–1,500 mg/day	LD 500 mg/L, MD 125 mg/L
Amikacin	2 mg/kg/daily	LD 25 mg/L, MD 12 mg/L
Gentamicin	0.6 mg/kg/day	LD 8 mg/L, MD 4 mg/L
Vancomycin	15–30 mg/kg every 5–7 days	LD 30 mg/kg, MD 1.5 mg/kg/bag
Antifungals		
Fluconazole	IP 200 mg every 24–48 h	No data
Voriconazole	IP 2.5 mg/kg/day	No data

(IP: intraperitoneal; LD: loading dose in mg; MD: maintenance dose in mg)

- Once culture results and sensitivities are known, antibiotic regimens can be adjusted to appropriate narrow-spectrum agents.

Other novel diagnostic techniques may be explored for the early diagnosis of peritonitis like biomarker assays [matrix metalloproteinase-8 and -9, neutrophil gelatinase-associated lipocalin (NGAL), and procalcitonin], polymerase chain reaction (PCR) for bacterial-derived deoxyribonucleic acid (DNA), 16S ribosomal ribonucleic acid (rRNA) gene sequencing, matrix-assisted laser desorption ionization time-of-flight (MALDI-TOF), and pathogen specific-immune fingerprints.

Refractory peritonitis: Failure of peritonitis to clear after 5 days of appropriate antibiotics.

Relapsing peritonitis: Peritonitis with the same causative organism within 4 weeks of discontinuation of antibiotics.

Recurrent peritonitis: Peritonitis due to a different organism within 4 weeks of stopping antimicrobial therapy.

Repeat peritonitis: Fresh episode of peritonitis after 4 weeks of holding antimicrobial therapy.

Prevention of peritonitis:
- Administration of systemic prophylactic antibiotics immediately prior to catheter insertion.
- Disconnect systems with a "flush before fill" design for CAPD.
- Daily topical antibiotic application to the catheter exit site.
- Antibiotic prophylaxis to be given prior to colonoscopy and invasive gynecological procedures.

Exit-site and tunnel infection: Complicate nearly 20% of all episodes of peritonitis in PD patients.
- Incidence being one episode every 24–48 months
- *Causative organisms*: *S. aureus* and *P. aeruginosa*
- Exit-site infection is characterized by redness, swelling, and tenderness at the exit site. With tunnel involvement, these signs extend along the subcutaneous course of the catheter and needs ultrasonography for its diagnosis.
- *Treatment*:
  - For erythema alone, topical application of hypertonic saline or 2% mupirocin is advised.
  - Erythema with purulent drainage should warrant Gram stain and culture to guide appropriate antimicrobial therapy.
  - *Gram-positive organism*: Cephalosporin ± rifampicin. If no response occurs in 2 weeks, catheter removal should be done.
  - *Gram-negative organisms*: Third-generation cephalosporin or aminoglycoside for 2 weeks, while *Pseudomonas* needs 3 weeks duration of therapy, with prompt catheter removal and simultaneous replacement at a different site may be done.
- Prophylactic use of antibiotic creams like mupirocin or gentamicin helps decrease rates of exit-site and tunnel infections.

NONINFECTIOUS COMPLICATIONS

They are divided majorly into mechanical and metabolic complications.

Mechanical complications: They are further subdivided as:

- *Catheter malfunction*:
  - *Obstruction*: Can occur in PD catheters either during infusion or draining of PD effluent during an exchange.
    - *Inflow failure*: May be due to intraluminal fibrin or blood clot. Flushing with heparinized saline or thrombolytic therapy helps. Kinking in the catheter can be diagnosed with an X-ray of the abdomen and needs minimally invasive manipulation of the catheter.
    - *Outflow failure*: Constipation should be ruled out. Distended bowel loops block the distal ends of the catheter, causing outflow failure. Laxatives help relieve obstruction. Intra-abdominal adhesions due to previous abdominal or gynecological surgeries or prior episodes of peritonitis may also be a cause, needing surgical adhesiolysis.
    - *Omental wrap*: Free-flowing inflow with obstructed outflow may be due to wrapping of the distal end of the catheter by a flap of omentum, like a one-way valve mechanism. Omentectomy is the definitive treatment.
    - Rarely fungal peritonitis may cause outflow failure.
  - *Malposition*: Upward migration of the PD catheter to the upper abdomen may cause decreased and delayed outflow. This poor drainage may be improved by positioning of the patient towards the catheter site. If spontaneous repositioning does not occur, mechanical intervention is warranted and intraluminal manipulation of the catheter by a stiff guide wire may be done, last option being laparoscopic repositioning.
  - *Inflow pain*: Jet effect of the dialysate emitting from the distal end of the catheter irritating the surrounding tissues, low pH (5.0–5.2) of the dialysate may be the causes of transient abdominal pain during inflow of exchange, when initiating PD. Use of bicarbonate/lactate buffered neutral pH (7.0–7.4), instillation of 2% lidocaine may help alleviate this inflow pain.
  - *Drain pain*: Pain during outflow of the dialysate, during early days of starting PD may occur due to:
    - Catheter bumping against sensitive parietal peritoneum
    - In APD, hydraulic suction on the peritoneal lining This can be alleviated by tidal PD, by incomplete drainage of the dialysate, or by catheter repositioning.
  - Back pain
  - Shoulder pain

Peritoneal membrane defects:

- *Hernia*: Seen in 10–20% of patients on PD
  - Risk factors include large dialysate volume, congenital anatomical defects, and sitting posture which increase the intra-abdominal pressure.
  - Indirect inguinal hernia occurs due to the out pouching of dialysate through the patent processus vaginalis or along the anterior abdominal wall.
  - Imaging studies using radiographic contrast help in diagnosing hernias.
  - Surgical correction of the hernias followed by supine low-volume dialysis or switching to APD to ensure low intra-abdominal pressure.
- *Abdominal wall and pericatheter leak*:
  - Pericatheter leaks cause wetness due to dialysate on the exit site dressing. Imaging studies help diagnosis. Rest to the peritoneum helps seal the leak spontaneously.
  - Abdominal wall leak occurs due to defect in the abdominal wall integrity. Transient course of day dry APD helps heal the defect and resumption of CAPD.
- *Hydrothorax*: Dialysate travelling from peritoneal to pleural cavity via defects in hemidiaphragm, due to raised intra-abdominal pressure. Pleural effusion composed of dialysis effluent, rich in glucose. Treatment is repair of defects or pleurodesis.
- *Membrane-related complications*:
  - Ultrafiltration failure is the condition of volume overload associated with UF volume <400 mL in a modified PET using a 4.25% dialysate dwell for 4 hours. The diagnosis should be made only after exclusion of the above causes.

UFF has four types:

1. *High transporter with UFF type I*: Increased effective peritoneal surface area in episodes of peritonitis leads to decreased UF. Treatment is adding a dwell with icodextrin or temporarily resting the peritoneum.
2. *Low transporter (type II)*: Decreased effective peritoneal surface area in adhesions and scarring lead to loss of UF. The only way is to shift to HD.
3. *Type III*: Increased lymphatic absorption of PD fluid.
4. *Type IV*: Aquaporin deficiency. Change in dialysate sodium concentration <5 mmol/L in 30–60 minutes with 4.25% dextrose dwell compared to 1.5% dextrose dwell.
   - *Encapsulated peritoneal sclerosis*: Seen rarely in 1–3% of patients.

Early inflammatory changes followed by sclerotic changes in the peritoneal membranes in patients on long-term PD. Computed tomography (CT) scan is diagnostic with features such as cocooning of the bowel with thickening, tethering, enhancement, and calcification of the peritoneal membrane. Corticosteroids and antifibrotic agents like tamoxifen may alleviate symptoms. Surgery is needed in recurrent bowel obstruction.

Metabolic complications:

- *Hypoalbuminemia*: Patients on PD lose 6–8 g of proteins/day, with increased losses during the episodes of peritonitis, predisposing to hypoalbuminemia in these patients.

- *Hyperglycemia*: Around 8% of nondiabetic patients develop new-onset diabetes, due to supraphysiological concentrations of glucose in PD solutions. Use of icodextrin and amino acid dialysate improve glycemic control.
- *Lipid abnormalities*: Obligatory carbohydrate absorption and protein losses in PD, cause increase in cholesterol, triglycerides, and lipoproteins.

RECOMMENDED READINGS

1. Blake PG, Daugirdas JT. Physiology of peritoneal dialysis. In: Daugirdas JT, Blake PG, Ing TS (Eds). Handbook of Dialysis, 5th edition. Philadelphia, Wolters Kluwer Health; 2016. pp. 392-8.
2. Rippe B, Venturoli D, Simonsen O, de Arteaga J. Fluid and electrolyte transport across the peritoneal membrane during CAPD according to the three-pore model. Perit Dial Int. 2004;24:10-27.
3. Lye WC, Kour NW, van der Straaten JC, Leong SO, Lee EJ. A prospective randomized comparison of the swan neck, coiled and straight Tenckhoff catheters in patients on CAPD. Perit Dial Int. 1996;16:S333-5.
4. Arramreddy R, Zheng S, Saxena AB, Liebman SE, Wong L. Urgent start peritoneal dialysis: a chance for a new beginning. Am J Kidney Dis. 2014;63:390-5.
5. Gokal R. Newer peritoneal dialysis solutions. Adv Ren Replace Ther. 2000;7:302-9.
6. Twardowski ZJ, Nolph KD, Khanna R. Prowant BF, Ryan LP, Moore HL, et al. Peritoneal equilibration test. Peritoneal Dial Bull. 1987;7:138-47.
7. Brown EA, Blake PG, Boudville N, Davies S, de Arteaga J, Dong J, et al. International Society for Peritoneal Dialysis practice recommendations: Prescribing high-quality goal-directed peritoneal dialysis. Perit Dial Int. 2020;40(3):244-53.
8. Blake PG, Bargman JM, Brimble KS, Davison SN, Hirsch D, McCormick BB, et al. CSN Workgroup on Peritoneal Dialysis Adequacy. Clinical practice guidelines and recommendations on peritoneal dialysis adequacy 2011. Perit Dial Int. 2011;31:218-39.
9. Woodrow G, Fan SL, Reid C, Denning J, Pyrah AN. Renal Association Clinical Practice Guideline on peritoneal dialysis in adults and children. BMC Nephrol. 2017;18:333.
10. Li PK, Szeto CC, Piraino B, de Arteaga J, Fan S, Figueiredo AE, et al. ISPD peritonitis recommendations: 2016 update on prevention and treatment. Perit Dial Int. 2016;36:481-508.
11. Manley HJ, Bailie GR. Treatment of peritonitis in APD: pharmacokinetic principles. Semin Dial. 2002;15: 418-21.
12. Prasad N, Gupta A. Fungal peritonitis in peritoneal dialysis patients. Perit Dial Int. 2005;25(3):207-22.
13. Prasad N, Gupta A, Sharma RK, Prasad KN, Gulati S, Sharma AP. Outcome of gram-positive and gram-negative peritonitis in patients on continuous ambulatory peritoneal dialysis: a single-center experience. Perit Dial Int. 2003;23 Suppl 2:S144-7.
14. Prasad N, Gupta A, Mathew M, Abraham G. Access-related complications in peritoneal dialysis in developing countries. Adv Ren Replace Ther. 2002;9(2): 144-8.
15. Pennell P, Rojas C, Asif A, Rossini E. Managing metabolic complications of peritoneal dialysis. Clin Nephrol. 2004;62(1):35-43.
16. McCormick BB, Bargman JM. Noninfectious complications of peritoneal dialysis: implications for patient and technique survival. J Am Soc Nephrol. 2007;18(12):3023-5.

CHAPTER

180

Kidney Transplantation

Pranaw Kumar Jha, Ashwini Balasaheb Gadde, Vijay Kher

ABSTRACT

Kidney transplant is the best form of kidney replacement therapy (KRT) for patients with end-stage kidney disease (ESKD). It increases the life expectancy of ESKD patients and gives them a better quality of life than being on the dialysis. Donor and recipient require extensive pretransplant evaluation which includes immunological tests for assessing the compatibility. For patients with immunological barriers such as blood group or human leucocyte antigen incompatibility, options of paired kidney exchange (PKE) or an incompatible transplant with appropriate preconditioning protocol should be explored. Advancement in immunosuppressive medications over the past few decades has led to an improvement in short-term graft survival although improving the long-term graft survival remains a challenge.

"The idea is not to live forever, but maybe to help another live a little longer"

—Anonymous

INTRODUCTION

Chronic kidney disease (CKD) is a major cause of morbidity and mortality worldwide. There were roughly 700 million cases of CKD worldwide in 2017 as per the global burden of disease collaboration report, of which an estimated 115 million were in India. CKD is the 12th leading cause of death globally. ESKD prevalence in India has been reported to be between 151 and 232 per million population. A patient reaching CKD stage 5 or ESKD needs KRT. The options include hemodialysis, peritoneal dialysis, and kidney transplantation. Kidney transplantation is the best form of KRT which increases patient survival and improves the quality of life. The 10-year patient survival in patients undergoing kidney transplant is about 80% while the 5-year survival for patients on hemodialysis is 42%. There is a huge demand and supply mismatch for transplantation. In India, only 2% of ESKD patients receive kidney transplantation every year.

The earliest attempt at human-to-human transplantation was done in 1933 by Yuriy Vorony in Ukraine using a deceased donor kidney. The graft was rejected due to the immunological incompatibilities. It was not until 1954 when the first successful living donor kidney transplantation was done in Boston by Joseph Murray and his team. The donor and recipient were identical twins, and the transplant was done without any immunosuppression. Advances in tissue typing and immunosuppression led to the successful evolution of kidney transplantation over coming decades. First living donor kidney transplantation in India was done in 1971 by Dr Mohan Rao and Dr KV Johny at Christian Medical College, Vellore. It has come a long way since then and about 10,000 kidney transplantations are being done in India every year, although the number is not accurate due to the unavailability of a comprehensive national registry data.

DONOR EVALUATION

Donor kidney in a kidney transplant can come from a deceased donor or a voluntary living donor. While majority of the transplants in western countries are done with a deceased donor, in India it is mostly from living donors. Deceased donor transplant in India accounts for approximately 10% of the total numbers. This too, is unevenly distributed with majority of them being in the southern and western states such as Tamil Nadu, Karnataka, Telangana, Maharashtra, and Gujarat.

There are two types of deceased donor transplants—(1) donation after cardiac death (DCD) and (2) donation after brain death (DBD). In DCD, donation takes place after declaration of death based on the cardiorespiratory criteria while in DBD death declaration is done by the neurological criteria. A DCD kidney has higher chances of warm ischemic damage (warm ischemia time—the time for which kidney remains at body temperature after cessation of its blood supply before cooling starts) and subsequent delayed graft function. Deceased donor from whom the kidney is obtained should be free from any malignancy or transmissible infections. Compromised kidney function and other chronic organ failure are notable contraindications.

A potential living donor should be healthy and should not have any significant medical and surgical risks postkidney donation. He/she should be of sound mental health and should not have any transmissible infections or malignancy. Evaluation of a donor includes a detailed history and physical examination. After this, the various laboratory tests are done including biochemical tests such as kidney function test, liver function test, fasting blood sugar, complete hemogram, urinalysis, proteinuria estimation, and viral serologies. This is followed by diethylenetriaminepentaacetic acid (DTPA) renogram and kidney imaging by computed tomography (CT) angiogram to determine the donor kidney anatomy including the number of kidney vessels on each side.

If found suitable, postevaluation human leukocyte antigen (HLA) typing, and crossmatch test is done. HLA antigens usually checked are A, B, and DRB1. A full repertoire of all the HLA classes I (A, B, and C) and II (DP, DQ, and DR) antigens may be required in case of a sensitized recipient. A sensitized patient is the one who has developed anti-HLA antibodies—secondary to either pregnancies, blood transfusions, or failed kidney/organ transplants. A history of such events needs to be carefully evaluated. Kidney Disease: Improving Global Outcomes (KDIGO) published clinical practice guideline on the evaluation and care of living kidney donors in 2017.

RECIPIENT EVALUATION

Any ESKD patient who has a life expectancy of more than 5 years is a candidate for kidney transplantation as the life expectancy is higher for a transplanted patient when compared to a risk matched patient on dialysis. A suitable blood group matched donor is the prerequisite. Preemptive transplantation is the transplantation done in a patient with late-stage CKD who has not yet been initiated on dialysis. This can be done once the glomerular filtration rate is ≤20 mL/min.

Despite being the best treatment modality for ESKD, there are few contraindications to kidney transplantation. These may be relative or absolute (**Table 1**). A recipient undergoes extensive evaluation which includes basic workup including biochemical tests and complete hemogram. Viral serologies for hepatitis B, C, and human immunodeficiency virus (HIV) are done to rule out any active infection. If the recipient is found to be infected with one of these, he needs to be treated pretransplant. Cytomegalovirus (CMV) serology is done in donor and recipient for assessing CMV risk and the need for prophylaxis posttransplant. Imaging such as chest X-ray and ultrasound abdomen is done. Any active infection and malignancy

TABLE 1 Kidney transplant contraindications.

Absolute contraindications	Relative contraindications
• Active malignancy • Short life expectancy—variable • Primary oxalosis—combined kidney and liver transplant advised • Overt AIDS (however, HIV infection per se is not a contraindication) • Active substance abuse	• Active infections • Active systemic disease • Morbid obesity • Poor psychosocial status, behavioral abnormalities • Treatment nonadherence • Decompensated liver disease (combined kidney-liver transplant required)

should be excluded before transplantation. Patients having history of malignancy require malignancy free period of 2–5 years (depending upon the type of malignancy) before getting transplanted. A thorough cardiac evaluation is needed to rule out any correctable coronary artery disease. This usually includes a 2D ECHO or stress test. In patients symptomatic for angina or with high risk of coronary artery disease, a coronary angiogram is required.

After completing the workup, the patient undergoes immunological evaluation which includes testing for major HLA antigens especially A, B, and DRB1. A crossmatch is done with the intended donor to look for the HLA compatibility. The crossmatch is of two types—complement-dependent cytotoxicity (CDC) which is less sensitive than a flow cytometric crossmatch. A positive CDC entails very high risk of hyperacute rejection and graft loss due to the presence of preformed anti-HLA antibodies and hence, such a transplant is avoided. Patients with a positive flow cytometry, crossmatch can undergo kidney transplant after appropriate desensitization. In patients with a positive crossmatch, a single antigen-bead assay test is done to identify the specific culprit anti-HLA antibodies and to know the overall sensitization status of the recipient. A virtual crossmatch can be done if the details of anti-HLA antibodies are available in the recipient and the donor antigens are known.

IMMUNOSUPPRESSION IN KIDNEY TRANSPLANT

Recipient of a kidney allograft needs lifelong immunosuppressive medications to prevent the transplanted kidney from getting rejected on detection of foreign HLA antigens by the immune system of the recipient. Initially, total body irradiation in sublethal dose was employed in the early 1960s. Soon, use of medications such as prednisone and azathioprine started and over the next two decades this was the maintenance immunosuppressant. Introduction of cyclosporine in 1980s dramatically improved the short-term graft survival.

Immunosuppressive medication in kidney transplant consists of initial induction given during the perioperative period and maintenance immunosuppression which must be continued lifelong

- *Induction*: Induction therapy is given at the time of kidney transplant to reduce the future risk of acute rejection. It is recommended for all the kidney transplant recipients except for very low risk patients such as recipients of HLA identical living related donor kidney. Induction consists predominantly of two types.
  1. Lymphocyte depleting agents—this includes rabbit-antithymocyte globulin (ATG) thymoglobulin which is the most commonly used agent. Other agents in this category include alemtuzumab (used infrequently) and muromonab (no longer in use).
  2. Examples of nondepleting agent include interleukin-2 (IL-2) receptor antagonist. Basiliximab is the commonly used IL-2 receptor antagonist while daclizumab is no longer used.
- *Maintenance immunosuppression*: This consists of immunosuppressants, which has to be continued lifelong. It includes a combination of the following medications:
  1. A calcineurin inhibitor (CNI)—tacrolimus or cyclosporine
  2. An antiproliferative agent—mycophenolate mofetil (MMF) or azathioprine
  3. Oral steroid—usually prednisolone.

Most commonly used maintenance immunosuppressive combination is tacrolimus, MMF, and prednisolone. Some centers practice steroid free protocol for transplantation where only a CNI and an antiproliferative agent are used as maintenance immunosuppression. Drug level of CNI is monitored and the dose is adjusted accordingly depending upon the duration post-transplant and other factors such as history of rejection or infection. Mammalian target of rapamycin (m-TOR) inhibitors like sirolimus and everolimus are used in special circumstances.

Table 2 summarizes the mechanism of actions and adverse effects of commonly used maintenance immunosuppressants medications in kidney transplantation.

POST-TRANSPLANT MANAGEMENT

The kidney transplant surgery (donor and recipient) takes 3–4 hours. The immediate postoperative period in a living donor transplant is characterized by brisk diuresis. This happens due to the solute load in the recipient as well as the inability of an ischemic kidney to regulate sodium and water excretion. The electrolytes need to be monitored very closely to avoid dyselectrolytemia and the fluid loss needs to be replenished to avoid dehydration and graft dysfunction. A deceased donor kidney may function slowly in view of prolonged ischemia time and acute tubular injury. Such patients might require dialysis in postoperative period due to delayed graft function. Recovery might take days to weeks. Patient may have a superimposed rejection, and this can be diagnosed by a graft kidney biopsy. Delayed graft function is rare in a living donor kidney transplant.

TABLE 2 Maintenance immunosuppressants in kidney transplantation.

Drug	Mechanism of action	Adverse effects
Tacrolimus	Forms complex with FKBP. The complex inhibits calcineurin and impairs cytokines gene expression	Nephrotoxicity, hypertension, glucose intolerance, and neurotoxicity
Cyclosporine	Forms complex with cyclophilin. The complex inhibits calcineurin and impairs cytokines gene expression	Same as tacrolimus. Also causes hirsutism and gum hypertrophy
Mycophenolate mofetil	Inhibits IMPDH and blocks de novo purine synthesis pathways	Bone marrow suppression, diarrhea
Azathioprine	Acts as purine analogue and inhibits purine nucleotide synthesis and ultimately RNA synthesis	Bone marrow suppression, hepatitis, and pancreatitis
Prednisolone	Blocks T-cell derived and APC derived cytokines and their receptor expression	Glucose intolerance, weight gain, hyperlipidemia, and hypertension
m-TOR inhibitor	Binds FKBP and the complex inhibits TOR thereby preventing G1 to S phase of cell division	Nephrotoxicity, impaired wound healing, and hyperlipidemia

(APC: antigen presenting cell; FKBP: FK binding protein; IMPDH: inosine-5′-monophosphate dehydrogenase; mTOR: mammalian target of rapamycin; RNA: ribonucleic acid)

Kidney function is monitored closely in the posttransplant period. There may be multiple reasons for graft dysfunction in a kidney transplant recipient. This includes obstruction, dehydration, acute rejection, acute tubular injury, infection, and vascular thrombosis.

Apart from the regular immunosuppressants as discussed above, transplant patients also receive various other medications. Trimethoprim-sulfamethoxazole prophylaxis is given to prevent *Pneumocystis jiroveci* pneumonia while valganciclovir is used as an anti-cytomegalovirus prophylaxis. Clotrimazole is used as antifungal prophylaxis. Antihypertensives may be required for adequate blood pressure control, although the requirement for antihypertensive medications mostly reduces post-transplant. Patients might develop new onset diabetes post-transplant, thereby requiring insulin and oral hypoglycemic agents.

COMPLICATIONS IN A RECIPIENT

Despite being the best form of KRT, the course of a patient undergoing kidney transplant may be complicated by the following issues:

Rejection: It can be of different types such as hyperacute, acute, and chronic rejections. Hyperacute rejection occurs because of preformed anti-HLA antibodies. Patients having blood group incompatibility can also get hyperacute rejection due to the naturally occurring antiblood group antibodies. Although both anti-HLA and blood group incompatible transplants can be done successfully with appropriate preconditioning protocol, this needs more intense immunosuppression and has higher rates of infective complications. Acute cellular rejections occur in 10–15% transplant recipients mostly during first year and respond to high dose methylprednisolone and thymoglobulin. Inappropriate iatrogenic reduction or non-adherence to immunosuppressive drugs leads to development of donor specific antibodies, which can cause antibody mediated rejection—a common cause of graft loss.

Infections: It is an important cause of morbidity and mortality in kidney transplant recipients. It could be donor or recipient derived or could be related to perioperative factors. The type of infection varies according to the phase of the post-transplant period. Infection in the first month post-transplant is usually nosocomial while from second to sixth month it is an opportunistic infection with reactivation of latent infection and after 6 months, it is usually a community acquired infection. **Table 3** shows common post-transplant infections by duration since transplant.

Cardiovascular disease: This remains the most common cause of mortality in kidney transplant recipients. Both traditional risk factors such as diabetes, hypertension as well as transplant-related risk factors such as immunosuppressive medications are responsible.

Malignancy: Long-term use of immunosuppression predisposes kidney transplant recipient to the development of malignancy. Malignancy is almost twofold to fourfold higher in kidney transplant recipients compared to the general population. Common cancers with high incidence in kidney transplant recipients include lymphoma, colon cancer, lung cancer, melanoma, and nonmelanomatous skin cancer. Most common amongst these being skin cancers. Although many of these skin cancers are found predominantly in patients from Australia and New Zealand. The cancers not increased by kidney transplant include that of breast, prostate, ovarian, cervical, and brain.

A close follow-up of kidney transplant recipient is required to detect above mentioned complications at the earliest stage to take appropriate corrective measures. Common cause of death in kidney transplant recipients is infections and cardiovascular disease. Common cause of graft loss is chronic antibody-mediated rejections and death with functioning grafts.

PAIRED KIDNEY EXCHANGE

Blood group and HLA compatibilities are essential prerequisites for a successful transplant. In a regular transplant, blood group compatibility is as shown in

TABLE 3 Infections in kidney transplant recipients.

<1 months	1–6 months	>6 months
• Postoperative complications—wound and catheter-related infection • Donor-derived infections (rare) • Urinary tract infection	• BK viremia • CMV infection—in absence of prophylaxis • PJP—in absence of prophylaxis • Community acquired pneumonia • Fungal infection • Urinary tract infection • Tuberculosis	• Opportunistic fungal infections—mucormycosis and aspergillosis • Pneumonia—community acquired • Nocardiosis • Late CMV—after stopping prophylaxis • Urinary tract infection

(CMV: cytomegalovirus; PJP: *Pneumocystis jiroveci* pneumonia)

TABLE 4 Conventional blood group compatible transplants.

Donor group	Recipient group
A, O	A
B, O	B
O	O
A, B, O, AB	AB

TABLE 5 Blood group incompatible transplant (ABO incompatible transplant).

Donor group	Recipient group
B, AB	A
A, AB	B
A, B, AB	O

Table 4. Matching of the rhesus system is not important as it is not expressed on the vascular endothelium of graft unlike major blood group antigens. In case, the donor does not have a compatible blood group, the options of PKE or ABO incompatible kidney transplant can be undertaken. In an ABO incompatible kidney transplant, the antiblood group antibody is removed by plasmapheresis or immunoadsorption technique and the transplantation is done once a desired antiblood group antibody titer is achieved. ABO incompatible transplant increased in popularity initially in Japan in 1990s. Later, it picked up in Europe and USA and now the numbers are increasing even in India. **Tables 4** and **5** show recipient and donor blood groups in conventional blood group compatible and an ABO incompatible kidney transplant, respectively. In a PKE transplant, the donor of an incompatible pair (say pair A) donates to a recipient of another incompatible pair (say pair B) with whom the donor of pair A is blood group compatible while the donor of pair B donates to the compatible recipient from pair A (**Fig. 1**). This is the simplest form of PKE also known as a two-way exchange.

Similarly, in patients who have a positive crossmatch due to HLA incompatibility, a PKE may be done, or an HLA incompatible transplant may be done after plasmapheresis. The long-term outcome of such transplants is relatively poor

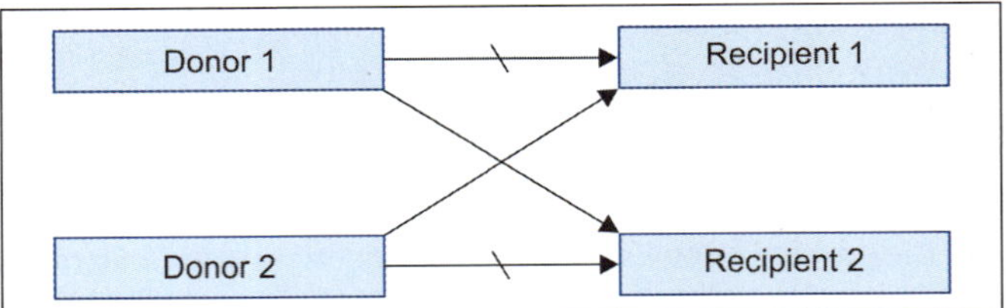

FIGURE 1: A two-way paired kidney exchange transplant.

due to higher incidences of acute and chronic antibody mediated rejection.

CONCLUSION

Kidney transplantation is the best form of KRT. There is a significant improvement in patient survival as well as the quality of life of transplant recipient when compared to dialysis. An extensive evaluation is required for optimal recipient and donor selection. A close follow-up is required to detect post-transplant complications at an early stage for appropriate management. In recipient with immunological barriers of blood group or HLA incompatibility, a PKE or incompatible transplant after appropriate preconditioning protocol is the available option.

RECOMMENDED READINGS

1. Cockwell P, Fisher LA. The global burden of chronic kidney disease. Lancet. 2020;395(10225):662-4.
2. Modi GK, Jha V. The incidence of end-stage Kidney disease in India: a population-based study. Kidney Int. 2006;70(12):2131-3.
3. Rajapurkar MM, John GT, Kirpalani AL, Abraham G, Agarwal SK, Almeida AF, et al. What do we know about chronic kidney disease in India: first report of the Indian CKD registry. BMC Nephrol. 2012;13:10.
4. Goodship TH, Cook HT, Fakhouri F, Fervenza FC, Fremeaux-Bacchi V, Kavanagh D, et al. Atypical hemolytic uremic syndrome and C3 glomerulopathy: conclusions from a "Kidney Disease: Improving Global Outcomes" (KDIGO) Controversies Conference. Kidney Int. 2017;91(3):539-51.
5. Kidney Disease: Improving Global Outcomes (KDIGO) Transplant Work Group. KDIGO clinical practice guideline for the care of kidney transplant recipients. Am J Transplant. 2009;9 Suppl 3:S1-155.

6. Fishman JA. Infection in solid-organ transplant recipients. N Engl J Med. 2007;357(25):2601-14.
7. Engels EA, Pfeiffer RM, Fraumeni JF, Kasiske BL, Israni AK, Snyder JJ, et al. Spectrum of cancer risk among US solid organ transplant recipients. JAMA. 2011;306(17):1891-901.
8. Jha PK, Bansal SB, Sethi SK, Jain M, Sharma R, Nandwani A, et al. ABO-incompatible Kidney transplantation in developing world - crossing the immunological (and mental) barrier. Indian J Nephrol. 2016;26(2):113-8.
9. Kute VB, Patel HV, Shah PR, Modi PR, Shah VR, Rizvi SJ, et al. Impact of single centre kidney paired donation transplantation to increase donor pool in India: a cohort study. Transpl Int. 2017;30(7):679-88.

CHAPTER

181

COVID-19 and Kidneys

Mayuri Trivedi, Raja Ramachandran

ABSTRACT

Besides the lung, kidney involvement seems to be a significant determinant of outcomes in patients with coronavirus disease-2019 (COVID-19) infection. Underlying kidney disease apart from predisposing to a heightened risk for severe disease and poor outcomes also creates unique hurdle in the diagnosis and treatment of the infection. Acute kidney injury (AKI) is seen in a significant proportion of patients, especially the critically ill and is multifactorial. Patients on long-term immunosuppression like those with renal transplantations or glomerular disease prove to be diagnostic and treatment dilemmas. Data regarding the effective treatment of this infection in patients with kidney dysfunction is scarce and further complicates the treatment and care.

"The oldest and strongest emotion of mankind is fear, and the oldest and strongest kind of fear is fear of the unknown"

—HP Lovecraft

INTRODUCTION

Severe acute respiratory syndrome-coronavirus-2 (SARS-COV-2) apart from causing a devastating acute respiratory illness also has significant crosstalk with other organs, especially the kidney. Not only has it shown to cause acute kidney injury (AKI), but also has led to worsening outcomes in patients with pre-existing chronic kidney disease (CKD) and postrenal transplantation. Besides, the patients with underlying kidney disease are at a higher risk for contracting the infection, including a more severe disease at presentation and higher mortality. The sequelae of the COVID-19 pandemic impact both short- and long-term nephrology care.

PATHOPHYSIOLOGY OF KIDNEY INJURY

Analysis of the existing literature points toward a multifactorial mechanism for kidney injury in patients with COVID-19. It is still primarily debated whether the kidney injury is a direct consequence of viral infection of the kidney epithelial cells or the result of complications arising outside the kidney. The SARS-COV-2 virus is known to enter the cell via the angiotensin-converting enzyme-2 (ACE-2) receptor, which is expressed in large numbers in the lung and the proximal tubular epithelium of the kidney and bladder urothelium, apart from other organs. However, there are points which argue against the *direct injury of the renal tissue* by the virus itself.

Urine examination of the patients with COVID-19 infection commonly reveals proteinuria and hematuria, which is transient and resolves with the resolution of the infection. Transient urine abnormalities are consequent to the release of *various proinflammatory cytokines* which affect the glomerular filtration barrier creating a loss of its integrity. Several studies, reporting on postmortem biopsy on critically ill patients with COVID-19 infection and AKI reveal severe acute tubular injury along with positive viral antigen staining of the tubules with lymphocytes/macrophage aggregates. However, there are many factors which can induce acute tubular injury in a critically ill patient with COVID-19, thus making the direct causal relationship between viral infection and tubular injury debatable. Despite the evidence of distinct viral inclusion on electron microscopy (postmortem biopsy), indicating a direct entry and replication in the renal tubular epithelium, the absence of the viral cytopathic effect (cell detachment and death), once again argues against a causal relationship between the infection and subsequent renal injury. Thus, in conclusion, there is no reproducible proof of viral tropism with active COVID-19 infection, which would require concurrent kidney cell infection together with viral replication.

ACUTE KIDNEY INJURY AND COVID-19

There has been a vast body of literature reporting AKI from all over the globe, yet the exact incidence is unknown. There is *heterogeneity in the reporting of AKI* with regards the population size, the locations, the available healthcare resources, and the efficiency of the existing healthcare system in coping with the pandemic and definition of AKI besides the severity of the disease. The incidence of AKI ranges from 1% to 46%. There is a sizeable difference in the incidence of AKI (in critically ill) as well as those who required some form of renal replacement therapy (RRT). The incidence of patients requiring RRT ranges from 0% to 23%. Apart from the efficiency of the local healthcare system and medical infrastructure in coping with the increased patient burden, local policies with regards to the timing of RRT, use of RRT as extracorporeal therapy beyond the classical indications, the incidence of comorbidities and the severity of the illness at presentation play a critical role in elucidating the varying incidence. Patients who developed AKI have a mortality rate as high as 32–35% with around 90% of those who expired requiring RRT.

Apart from alterations secondary to altered gas exchange in the lungs leading to *various hemodynamic instabilities, fluid overload, sepsis leading to a cytokine storm*, volume depletion, use of nephrotoxic drugs including alternative medicines, myalgia and muscle injury leading to rhabdomyolysis, and direct cellular damage due to binding of the virus to the renal tubular epithelial cells are the probable mechanisms leading to AKI (**Box 1**) in COVID-19. *Renal biopsy reports* from critically ill patients with COVID-19 infections and AKI (acute tubular injury) additionally reveal a variety of glomerular and tubulointerstitial findings, including collapsing glomerulopathy and various immune-mediated glomerular diseases. Despite the exact mechanism of renal injury still being elusive, its presence portends a poor prognosis.

BOX 1 Proposed causes of AKI in COVID-19.

- **Prerenal causes:**
  - Volume depletion
  - Febrile state
  - Diarrheal illness
  - Anorexia and poor intake
  - Restricted access to fluids in critical care unit
  - Hemodynamic instability
- **Intrinsic renal causes:**
  - Nephrotoxic agents including NSAIDs, alternative drugs
  - Direct renal injury
  - Sepsis
  - Cytokine storm
  - Hypotension
  - Coagulation defects
  - Acute muscle injury/rhabdomyolysis
- **Postrenal causes:**

Not specifically defined for COVID-19

CHRONIC KIDNEY DISEASE AND COVID-19

The presence of underlying CKD including end-stage kidney disease (ESKD) in patients is a significant risk factor for severe COVID-19 infections at presentation, with a 14–16 times higher mortality as compared to the general population. Admittedly, one-third of the CKD patients succumb to the disease with mortality ranging from 30% to 38%. The mortality is higher in CKD stage-G5D compared to other stages.

BOX 2 Proposed causes for high risk for severe disease and poor outcomes in CKD with COVID-19.

- Preexisting proinflammatory state associated with CKD
- Maladapted innate and acquired immunity
- Malnutrition
- Frequent visits to healthcare facilities including dialysis centers
- Exposure to HCWs (especially ESRD patients)
- Delayed diagnosis due to overlap of clinical and radiological features with complications of CKD/ESRD
- Coexisting comorbidities (DM and HTN)
- Chronic immunosuppression therapy (posttransplantation, glomerular disease)
- Inadequate dedicated infrastructure and dialysis facilities for COVID-19 patients
- Nonavailability of immunosuppressive drugs, dialysis consumables etc., due to nationwide lockdown

Though speculative, the possible reasons for poor outcomes in the CKD population are numerous and mentioned in **Box 2**. Additionally, the clinical and radiological features of severe COVID-19 infection can masquerade complications of CKD/end-stage renal disease (ESRD), including volume overload and pulmonary edema and thus delay timely diagnosis and initiation of appropriate therapy, including dialysis.

RENAL TRANSPLANTATION & COVID-19

Coronavirus disease-2019 infection has a dismal outcome in the elderly and those with various comorbidities. Owing to the comorbidity and the detrimental effect of immunosuppressive drugs, recipients of solid organs, including kidneys, have an unsatisfactory outcome with higher mortality as compared to the rest of the population. These patients have a rapid clinical deterioration and mortality as high as 30% as compared to the 1–5% mortality in the general population. Another unique issue is the lack of the classic symptoms of fever, cough, and sore throat in the post-transplant patients. Features like diarrhea, thrombocytopenia, or pancytopenia may be mistaken for opportunistic infections or drug-related complications, thus delaying the diagnosis and optimal management of COVID-19. They may also develop AKI or in more severe cases cause graft loss and eventually require RRT for the worsening renal functions. There is limited knowledge on the optimal management of the immunosuppressive regimen during an active COVID-19.

Nevertheless, the consensus is to *withdraw the anti-metabolite drugs* (mycophenolate mofetil or azathioprine) universally, and calcineurin inhibitors in severe disease, to tide over the acute period temporarily. The patients may require a concomitant increase in the dose of steroids (up to 20–25 mg) that was being administered regularly as a part of the standard triple immunosuppression regimen commonly prescribed in renal transplantation. In patients with severe disease, intravenous dexamethasone may replace oral prednisolone for the management of acute respiratory distress syndrome (ARDS).

MANAGEMENT

The treatment of COVID-19 infection remains elusive in patients with underlying renal involvement owing to the scarcity of data of various treatment options in kidney disease patients. Most treatments advocated in kidney disease patients till date are on compassionate grounds as adapted from nonrenal failure cases.

The results of the RECOVERY trial establish the therapeutic potential of a moderate dose of dexamethasone (6 mg daily for 10 days), which modulates inflammation-induced acute lung injury, reduced mortality at 28 days in hospitalized patients with COVID-19 and respiratory failure requiring supplemental oxygen or mechanical ventilation. *Dexamethasone* may be safely used in patients with renal dysfunction and requires no dose modifications. Tocilizumab (interleukin-6 antagonist) is an anti-inflammatory monoclonal antibody expected to alleviate the acute cytokine storm in patients with moderate to severe COVID-19 infections. Admittedly, the data regarding the effectiveness of tocilizumab remains controversial. There is no randomized control trial (RCT) testing the drug specifically in COVID-19 patients with preexisting renal involvement or postrenal transplantation. Subgroup analysis and small observational studies advise close monitoring (as per manufacturer's advice) during its use in patients with impaired renal functions, though no dose modification or specific adverse effects reported in patients with renal dysfunction.

Remdesivir, an antiviral drug, is a nucleotide analog that inhibits RNA-dependent RNA polymerase and has shown some benefit in the treatment of hospitalized patients with COVID-19 infection. The ACTT-1 trial revealed remdesivir helps in reducing the median time of recovery in hospitalized patients with lower respiratory involvement due to COVID-19 infections. Sulfobutylether-b-cyclodextrin (SBECD), the vehicle used for the intravenous preparation of the drug has limited water solubility and is associated with renal tubular obstruction on prolonged use. Continuous dialysis eliminates the drug. Also, the limited duration (5–10 days) and a relatively low dose of 100 mg/day of the drug used in COVID-19 infections suggest that the benefit may outweigh the risk even in patients with estimated glomerular filtration rate (eGFR) < 30 mL/min/1.73 m^2. Thus, patients who are on continuous or intermittent dialysis or those with AKI (with an eGFR < 30 mL/min/1.73 m^2) expected to be transient may be given remdesivir if indicated.

Favipiravir is a novel antiviral drug used in mild-moderate stable nonhypoxic patients. The absence of substantiating RCTs for the same posits the dubiety of the recommendation. Though this drug is eliminated via the kidney with plasma levels three to five times higher in patients with eGFR < 50 mL/min/1.73 m^2, the range does not appear to be nephrotoxic and hence may be given in kidney patients without serious adverse effects or dose modifications on compassionate grounds after explicit consent, if indicated.

While the effectiveness of plasma therapy in severe COVID-19 infections is controversial, the available data on the use of convalescent plasma therapy has shown no increased adverse events in patients with kidney diseases and may be safely prescribed.

The other drugs of questionable benefit in the treatment of COVID-19 include azithromycin, hydroxychloroquine lopinavir/ritonavir, ivermectin, and doxycycline. All these may be safely used in patients with impaired renal functions with no specific adverse events.

Recommendations for the use of *anticoagulation therapy in patients with COVID-19* and renal involvement are similar to those without the infection. Conventional (unfractionated) heparin as compared to low-molecular weight heparin (LMWH) is the preferred agent during the acute hospitalized phase as it requires no specialized dose modification for impaired renal function. Patients treated with LMWH may need antifactor Xa monitoring. Similarly, warfarin is the preferred oral anticoagulation drug as compared to the newer oral anticoagulants (NOACs). Amongst the NOACs, dabigatran may be used at lower doses (75 mg twice daily) in patients with a creatinine clearance of up to 15–30 mL/min/1.73 m^2. Rivaroxaban is contraindicated in patients with a creatinine clearance of less than 15 mL/min/1.73 m^2. Apixaban may be used in patients with serum creatinine ≥ 1.5 mg/dL at a reduced dose of 2.5 mg twice daily.

HURDLES IN THE MANAGEMENT

Patients with underlying kidney disease (CKD and ESRD) or those at risk for the same (AKI) are a specialized population who require differential care and targeted treatment plans apart from problems related to the diagnosis of COVID-19 in these patients.

The infection predominantly affects the lower respiratory tract where patients present with ARDS. The ARDS may mimic volume overload and pulmonary edema, especially in the later stages of CKD or patients with ESKD on dialysis, thus delaying diagnosis. The presence of elevated inflammatory markers like C-reactive protein (CRP), ferritin, and lactate dehydrogenase (LDH) is common in patients with kidney dysfunction. It may not help diagnose the severity of the COVID-19 infection.

However, another unique problem faced by the ESRD population is the inability of the peripheral or stand-alone dialysis units to provide regular maintenance hemodialysis due to the *social stigma of the infection*, lack of personal protective equipment, and appropriate isolation practices and infrastructure, the severe shortage of healthcare workers including dialysis technicians and nurses to cater to COVID-19 positive patients.

The onset of the pandemic in India in March 2020 saw a rapid closure of many dialysis units due to the reasons as mentioned above. The closure of the units resulted in skipped dialysis sessions by the ESRD patients. The ensuing chaos resulted in an increased load of emergency presentations of the CKD/ESRD patients especially the dialysis-dependent population to various public sector hospitals with fluid overload, lung shadows mimicking COVID-19, metabolic emergencies compounded with a delay in offering treatment due to the need for COVID-19 testing to avoid the *inadvertent mixing of COVID-19 and non-COVID-19 cases.* Apart from this, the decision to treat the kidney dysfunction with dialysis is complicated by associated hemodynamic instability due to the associated multi-organ dysfunction syndrome (MODS), especially in patients with severe COVID-19 and AKI.

Lastly, the nationwide lockdown in a few countries led to a significant *shortage of various lifesaving drugs* including immunosuppressant and dialysis consumables, overwhelming of the existing healthcare facilities and infrastructure, lack of transportation facilities to hospital and dialysis centers, *shortage of healthcare workers*, and a widespread social stigma of the disease.

Cumulatively, all these factors led to a negative impact on the diagnosis and treatment strategies for patients with COVID-19 and kidney disease. However, over time, we grew wiser, and the various task force groups lead by experts along with the assistance from the state and the central government led to protocoled guidelines drawn with specialized diagnostic and therapeutic algorithms along with dedicated dialysis units for COVID-19 patients set up across the country. The measures, as mentioned above, addressed the few hassles faced in the care of COVID-19 patients with kidney disease.

THE LESSONS LEARNT

The onset of this devastating pandemic was unexpected and caught both the patient and the medical professional completely unawares. The nationwide closure of dialysis centers due to the various reasons already discussed, shortage of dialysis disposables, and overwhelming of the existing medical infrastructure lead to skipped dialysis sessions amongst the ESRD patients with the resultant complications and higher mortality amongst this subgroup. The routine care of other patients on long-term care including CKD, glomerular disease, and transplantation patients also suffered.

The preparedness for the pandemic involved a *team-based approach* that combined various competencies including doctors, paramedics, nursing staff, and the administration. The guiding principles for the crisis team included uncompromised patient care, staff safety, regular communications, and flexibility in patient care policy based on incoming data and changing experience.

Regular nonemergent patient care shifted from in-person consultation with doctors and experts to *tele-consultations and virtual meetings.* Home-based therapies like home dialysis and peritoneal dialysis were encouraged in suitable patients to avoid frequent exposures to the hospital and dialysis centers. These measures compensated for the lack of transportation facilities due to the nationwide lockdown and prevented the caretaker exposure to the hospital environment also. As the pandemic continues to rage a war, we have learnt the *importance of preparedness* that is required for taking care of patients with kidney diseases and these lessons may be successfully extrapolated to other crisis situations in the future like natural calamities, war like situations etc.

A PEEK INTO THE FUTURE

We are several months into the pandemic of COVID-19, which has impacted the way we will care for our patients in the future. We have grown wiser over time. However, there exist lacunae in our understanding. The etiopathology and cellular mechanism of AKI in COVID-19 continue to elude us. Details on the contribution of direct viral cytopathic effects, the role of cytokine storm, hypercoagulability, and endothelial damage to the kidney injury are lacking. While the ACE-2 receptor seems to play a significant role in the entry of the virus into the cell and the kidney is second only to the lung in the concentration of ACE-2. We are yet to appreciate the *natural history of this infection* in patients with kidney involvement and the ability of the kidneys to recover fully or progress to ESRD in the long-term, similar to the increased incidence of lung fibrosis in patients with ARDS. As we move forward, we must try and understand the pathophysiology of COVID-19 infection and kidney injury, which will aid in finding possible (targeted) therapies and influence the long-term care of infected patients with kidney involvement.

CONCLUSION

COVID-19 pandemic has shown an internationally variable but a concerning effect on patients with or at risk of kidney disease. Though lung injury is the overwhelming manifestation in most patients, kidney injury seems to be a significant determinant of the outcome of the infection. The presence of an underlying CKD or ESRD proves to be a risk factor as well as portends a poor outcome in the patient with a high mortality rate.

Acute kidney injury seems to be multifactorial and also defines a worse outcome with higher rates of mortality early in the disease course. Limited data suggest a controversial role of antivirals and immunomodulators, and the decision to use the medications may be made on a case-to-case basis or compassionate grounds after seeking explicit consent.

The presence of underlying kidney disease has proved to be a significant hurdle in seeking medical and dialysis care as well as delayed diagnosis, thus worsening outcomes in this subset of patients. Unique and ingenious methods may overcome the difficulties faced by these patients during the pandemic and decrease the hassle of diagnosis and to seek treatment. Acknowledging the need to recognize, evaluate, and effectively treat the patients with COVID-19 and kidney injury may increase the chances of improving the prognosis of these patients.

RECOMMENDED READINGS

1. Hamilton P, Hanumapura P, Castelino L, Henney R, Parker K, Kumar M, et al. Characteristics and outcomes of hospitalised patients with acute kidney injury and COVID-19. PLoS One. 2020;15(11):e0241544.
2. Valeri AM, Robbins-Juarez SY, Stevens JS, Ahn W, Rao MK, Radhakrishnan J, et al. Presentation and Outcomes of Patients with ESKD and COVID-19. J Am Soc Nephrol. 2020;31(7):1409-15.
3. Trivedi M, Shingada A, Shah M, Khanna U, Karnik ND, Ramachandran R. Impact of COVID-19 on maintenance haemodialysis patients: The Indian scenario. Nephrology (Carlton). 2020;25(12):929-32.
4. Ramachandran R, Jha V. Adding insult to injury: kidney replacement therapy during COVID-19 in India. Kidney Int. 2020;98(1):238-9.
5. Naicker S, Yang CW, Hwang SJ, Liu BC, Chen JH, Jha V. The Novel Coronavirus 2019 epidemic and kidneys. Kidney Int. 2020;97(5):824-8.
6. Rossi GM, Delsante M, Pilato FP, Gnetti L, Gabrielli L, Rossini G, et al. Kidney Biopsy Findings in a Critically Ill COVID-19 Patient With Dialysis-Dependent Acute Kidney Injury: A Case Against "SARS-CoV-2 Nephropathy". Kidney Int Rep. 2020;5(7):1100-5.
7. RECOVERY Collaborative Group, Horby P, Lim WS, Emberson JR, Mafham M, Bell JL, et al. Dexamethasone in Hospitalized Patients with Covid-19. N Engl J Med. 2021;384(8):693-704.
8. Guaraldi G, Meschiari M, Cozzi-Lepri A, Milic J, Tonelli R, Menozzi M, et al. Tocilizumab in patients with severe COVID-19: a retrospective cohort study. Lancet Rheumatol. 2020;2(8):e474-84.
9. Adamsick ML, Gandhi RG, Bidell MR, Elshaboury RH, Bhattacharyya RP, Kim AY, et al. Remdesivir in Patients with Acute or Chronic Kidney Disease and COVID-19. J Am Soc Nephrol. 2020;31(7):1384-6.
10. Beigel JH, Tomashek KM, Dodd LE, Mehta AK, Zingman BS, Kalil AC, et al. Remdesivir for the Treatment of Covid-19 - Final Report. N Engl J Med. 2020;383(19):1813-26.
11. Cai Q, Yang M, Liu D, Chen J, Shu D, Xia J, et al. Experimental Treatment with Favipiravir for COVID-19: An Open-Label Control Study. Engineering (Beijing). 2020;6(10):1192-8.

MULTIPLE CHOICE QUESTIONS

To access the multiple choice questions of this Section online, kindly scan the QR code.

CHAPTER 182

Neurological Disorders: Basic Considerations and Clinical Approach

Lakshmi Narasimhan Ranganathan, Karthika Ajit, Guhan Ramamurthy

ABSTRACT

The importance of meticulous history taking and relevant clinical examination cannot be overemphasized. Detailed history of symptoms and clinical examination are essential to arrive at a diagnosis. Accurate neurological diagnosis can be achieved by the end of skillful history taking. General physical examination is an essential component to neurologic examination. It provides important clues which aids in the diagnosis of neurological diseases. Observation of the patient during history taking begins the examination. The neurologic examination can be challenging, but can be mastered by repeated organized and focused examination of patients. This chapter provides an overview of clinical approach to neurology.

"Turn the mental blocks into building blocks"

—D Roopleen

INTRODUCTION

Neurological disorders are very common in day-to-day practice. Approaching the complex intricacies in the diagnosis of neurological illness poses a great challenge for primary care physicians. There is a perception among the majority of general practitioners that neurological history taking and clinical examination is a tedious process. However, meticulous history taking and relevant clinical examination often reveals the correct diagnosis. This chapter focuses on simplifying the approach to a patient with neurological illness.

NEUROLOGIC HISTORY

In all branches of medicine, detailed history of symptoms and clinical examination are essential to arrive at a diagnosis. Accurate neurological diagnosis can be achieved by the end of skillful history taking. Conversely, many diagnostic errors happen because of an incomplete history. Attentive listening, observation of manners of the patient and understanding the patient as an individual as well as his view about the illness are paramount in patient assessment. Some symptoms such as recurrent headache, dizziness, and sleep disorders rely solely on accurate description by the patient, as they lack corresponding demonstrable physical findings.

When it comes to neurological illness, empathetic demeanor is crucial for patient-physician interactions. History taking is an art. It may require more skill and experience than performing examination. Standard practice is to document the patient's chief complaint and history of development of symptoms in chronological order, followed by the past medical and surgical history, the family history, and personal and social history. All this information helps in formulating a hypothesis to achieve the anatomical and etiological diagnoses. By analyzing the presence or absence of specific clinical symptoms, the formal examination by an experienced physician adds to the previous data. This leads to the generation of possible differential diagnoses. Based on the above conclusion, carrying out relevant laboratory and imaging studies will establish the final diagnosis as shown in **Flowchart 1**.

The unique aspect to neurology is the significance of localization and phenomenology. A patient who presents with a weak leg may have a lesion in muscles,

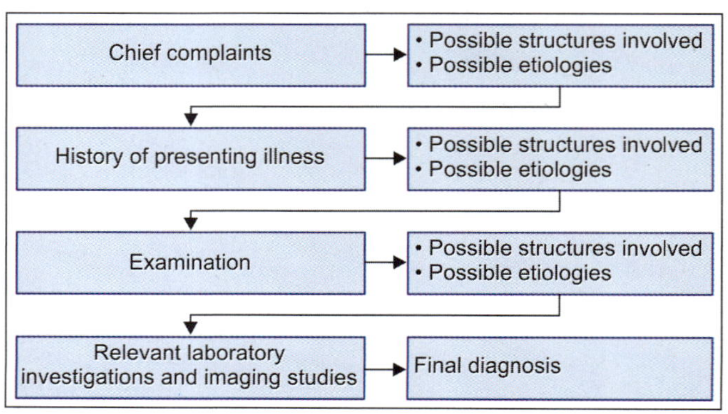

FLOWCHART 1: A neurologist's approach to reach a diagnosis.

neuromuscular junction, peripheral nerves, lumbar plexus, spinal roots, spinal cord, brainstem, or cerebral cortex. A detailed and organized examination allows localization of the lesion. Recognizing phenomenology is important for physicians to differentiate similar looking events, like tics, chorea, and myoclonus.

Although history should be taken in patients' own words, active questioning is necessary to elicit the symptoms ignored by the patient as insignificant and to confirm the absence of important localizing symptoms. At each step, the physician should focus on the possible structural localizations and etiologies.

CHIEF COMPLAINTS

The neurologic history starts with collecting demographic data and handedness. The chief complaints (or the main complaints) are the first clue to the diagnosis. They help to focus on the relevant questions to be asked further. The duration of the symptoms also aids to form an etiological diagnosis.

HISTORY OF PRESENTING ILLNESS

It addresses the *mode of onset and course of the symptomatology* (**Box 1**). Mode of onset is important as sudden onset may indicate a stroke. The temporal profile of every symptom is significant. For example, gradual onset headache and slowly progressive one-sided weakness could suggest a mass lesion, while rapid onset headache with maximal weakness at the onset might be a presentation of intracerebral hemorrhage. Thus, temporal profile provides an idea regarding the etiology though the symptoms, signs, and severity of presentation are similar. The history should include details regarding the onset of symptoms, whether symptoms are present intermittently or constantly, what is the severity of each symptom, whether there is progression or regression of symptoms, whether there is seasonal or diurnal variation, and whether there is response to earlier treatment.

BOX 1	Important symptoms to be enquired pertaining to the present illness.
• History of seizures	
• History of loss of consciousness	
• History of vertigo	
• History of headache	
• History of reduced vision	
• History of double vision	
• History of hearing loss or tinnitus	
• History of speech difficulty	
• History of swallowing difficulty	
• History of weakness	
• History of abnormal movements	
• History of numbness or tingling sensation	
• History of gait abnormality	
• History of incoordination	
• History of sexual dysfunction	
• History of difficulty with sphincter control	
• History of memory disturbances	
• History of sleep disturbances'	
• History of frequent falls	
• History of depression	

The history pertaining to the time course of the illness is often instrumental in determining etiology. Sudden onset followed by variable degrees of improvement is characteristic of trauma and vascular events. A gradual onset and slow progression may indicate neurodegeneration. Gradual onset of symptoms and steady progression is characteristic of a tumor. Spontaneous hemorrhage in a tumor may present with sudden worsening. Though relapses and remissions with variable progression of severity of symptoms are characteristic of multiple sclerosis, chronic progressive forms may also be seen. Paroxysmal episodes may be indicative of migraine, seizures, periodic paralysis, or episodic ataxia. Skillful history taking requires *documenting major milestones of the present illness*: When was the last time patient considered himself to be in a state of well-being; when did he stop going to job due the symptoms; since when has he started using the assistance of others for day-to-day activities; and how severe does he consider his illness to have progressed?

The antecedent events during the recent time period before the symptom onset may uncover the diagnosis, e.g., diarrheal illness precipitating Guillain-Barré syndrome (GBS), or a camping trip which may have caused a tick bite. Patients have the tendency to assume that recent events are responsible for the present illness. It is prudent to avoid the trap that temporal relationship implies etiological relationship in all cases (the *post hoc ergo propter hoc* fallacy).

Sir William Osler said, "*give the patient's own words in the complaint.*" At the same time, one should be aware that the language of the physician and the patient may be different for the same symptom. The patient may describe a paralyzed limb as "numb." Patients use the word "dizziness" to describe confusion, lightheadedness or weakness rather than vertigo as the physician would expect. "Blackouts" may mean loss of vision, syncope or loss of consciousness. The description of "blurred vision" may indicate underlying diplopia. It is common to hear the descriptions such as "throbbing headache", but it might not be a pulsating headache. Thus, physician must be vigilant about the description of each symptom, mode of onset, nature of progression, relation of one finding to another and aggravating factors and relieving factors. In children, temporal profile should also incorporate birth history and developmental milestones. Active questioning may bring out significant past events, which patient might have thought them to be trivial or unrelated. Past history of trauma, vascular events, or demyelination may give new insights to the present complaints. In a patient presenting with symptoms suggestive of myelopathy, past history of vision loss may give clue to the diagnosis.

OTHER ASPECTS OF HISTORY

The physician should also obtain *medication history* and history of allergies. *Past history* of inflammatory bowel disease, malabsorption syndromes, gastric surgery, or a vegetarian diet may be risk factors for the development of vitamin B12 deficiency. History of thyroid disease, diabetes or connective tissue diseases may indicate that the presenting illness may be a manifestation of these systemic problems. History of cancer may suggest that the present symptoms may be a result of metastases or a paraneoplastic syndrome. History of myocardial infarction or valvular heart disease may be a contributing factor in a case of cerebrovascular disease. A detailed inquiry into patient's *birth history, developmental history* and *scholastic performance* may give clues to the etiology. Many drugs have neurologic side effects—nonsteroidal anti-inflammatory drugs may cause aseptic meningitis, proton pump inhibitors can cause headaches, chemotherapeutic drugs can cause neuropathy, and antiepileptic drugs can cause dizziness or ataxia. Patients often conceal details of taking alternative medicines. Such medications are found to have neurologic side effects.

Family history can give clues regarding heredofamilial disorders. History of consanguinity may be an indicator of a genetic disorder. Some diseases may have minimal manifestations in other family members. For example, in a patient with Charcot-Marie-Tooth disease, family members may not consider *pes cavus* as abnormal. Chronic neurologic symptoms may be attributed to "arthritis" by family members.

The physician should also take *social history*, which includes educational status, personal habits, occupational history, and marital status. These may uncover any history of toxin exposure, tobacco, alcohol, and substance abuse. CAGE questionnaire, BUMP questionnaire, and HALT questionnaire are helpful in assessing the impact of alcohol consumption on the patient's life (**Table 1**). Tactful questioning is necessary to establish drug abuse as very often patients hide drug habits. Use of vernacular terms or street terms helps in eliciting better history.

Review of the *history pertaining to other systems* is paramount in diagnosis of certain neurologic diseases. A few such relevant histories are given in **Box 2**.

It is important to *assess the reliability of the history*. Reliability depends on patient's educational status, social status, intelligence, memory, language functions, attention, and secondary gains such as obtaining a disability certificate. Though it is necessary sometimes, to ask direct questions, some patients have tendency to give positive nods for all the questions to an authoritative figure. A reliable bystander will be helpful in such instances. Taking history from bystanders is also important in cases of seizures and dementia.

The physician may have to take history more than once. Whenever there is doubt in the diagnosis, retaking the history may give clues. With experience, the physician will be able to generate more hypotheses for the patient's symptoms and ask relevant questions to include or exclude a particular condition.

TABLE 1 Questionnaires to assess alcohol abuse.

CAGE	• Have you ever thought of **C**utting down on drinking habit? • Have you ever got **A**nnoyed by others because of your drinking? • Have you ever felt **G**uilty because of your drinking? • Have you ever had "**E**ye opener" drink to overcome hangover, in the morning?
BUMP	• Have you experienced **B**lackouts? • Have you ever consumed alcohol more than intended way? (**U**nplanned) • Have you ever consumed alcohol for **M**edicinal reasons? • Have you ever tried **P**rotecting your supply of alcohol?
HALT	• Do you consume alcohol to get **H**igh? • Do you consume alcohol **A**lone? • Do you **L**ook forward an occasion to drink? • Are you becoming more **T**olerant to alcohol?

BOX 2 Review of important histories pertaining to systems in diagnosis of neurologic diseases.

- **General:**
  - Weight loss (cancer, depression)
  - Fever (infection)
  - Trauma
- **Eyes:**
  - Episodic visual loss (amaurosis fugax)
  - Progressive visual loss (optic neuropathy)
  - Eye pain (optic neuritis)
  - Double vision (third nerve palsy)
  - Ptosis (myasthenia gravis)
  - Dry eyes (Sjögren's syndrome)
- **Ears:**
  - Tinnitus (Ménière's disease)
  - Hearing loss (vestibular schwannoma)
  - Ear vesicles (herpes zoster)
- **Nose:**
  - Loss of smell (olfactory groove meningioma, parkinsonism)
  - Discharge from nose [cerebrospinal fluid (CSF) rhinorrhea]
- **Mouth:**
  - Ulcers (Behcet syndrome)
  - Sore tongue (nutritional causes)
- **Neck:**
  - Stiffness (meningitis)
  - Pain (radiculopathy)

Continued...

Continued...

- **Cardiovascular:**
    - Hypertension, valvular heart disease, myocardial infarction (stroke)
- **Respiratory:**
    - Difficulty in breathing (neuromuscular disease)
    - Tuberculosis (meningitis)
- **Gastrointestinal:**
    - Vomiting (raised ICT)
    - Diarrhea (malabsorption syndromes)
    - Constipation (dysautonomia)
    - Dysphagia (neuromuscular disease)
- **Genitourinary:**
    - Urinary incontinence/urinary retention (neurogenic bladder)
    - Sexual dysfunction (dysautonomia)
- **Menstrual history/obstetric history:**
    - Repeated abortions [antiphospholipid antibody (APLA) syndrome]
    - Oral contraceptives [stroke, idiopathic intracranial hypertension (IIH)]
    - Hormone replacement therapy (migraine)
- **Endocrine:**
    - Weight gain, constipation, dry skin, and menstrual irregularities (hypothyroidism)
    - Large hands and feet (acromegaly)
    - Amenorrhea (pituitary insufficiency)
- **Musculoskeletal:**
    - Muscle pain (myositis)
    - Muscle cramps [amyotrophic lateral sclerosis (ALS)]
    - Joint pains (connective tissue disease)
- **Hematopoietic:**
    - Fatigability—anemia (vitamin B12 deficiency)

The physician should always pay close attention to the history to identify augenblickdiagnose (diagnoses made after hearing a fragment of key, essential information). Some classic histories include headache during sexual intercourse (suggestive of subarachnoid hemorrhage), and nocturnal hand paresthesia (suggestive of carpal tunnel syndrome).

NEUROLOGIC EXAMINATION

GENERAL PHYSICAL EXAMINATION

General physical examination is an essential component to neurologic examination. It provides important clues which aids in the diagnosis of neurological diseases. The examination commences from the observation of the patient during history taking.

Vital signs: Pulse rate, rhythm and character are vital in the neurological examination. Sinus bradycardia occurs in setting of raised intracranial pressure. Arrhythmias predispose to cerebral hypoperfusion. It is important to identify the irregular pulse in atrial fibrillation which predisposes to cardioembolic stroke. Low volume pulse is observed in aortic stenosis and bounding pulses are observed in hyperthyroidism or aortic regurgitation.

Measurement of blood pressure (BP) must be done in supine, seated, and upright position. Orthostatic hypotension is defined as fall in systolic BP and diastolic BP by >20 and 10 mm Hg respectively. It occurs in the setting of peripheral conditions as in diabetic neuropathy as well as central causes like multiple system atrophy. Significant asymmetries in the BP between the two limbs point to extracranial cardiovascular occlusive disease. High BP occurs in patients with acute stroke or subarachnoid hemorrhage.

Respiratory rate abnormalities have been noted in neurological patients. Respiratory rate, rhythm, depth, character, and single breath count must be noted. Usage of accessory muscles of respiration and in GBS and amyotrophic lateral sclerosis (ALS) patients denote impending respiratory failure. Abnormal patterns of respiration, Cheyne-Stokes, Biot's, or Kussmaul's breathing may be seen in various neurological diseases.

General appearance: General appearance of the patient provides multiple clues to the presence of systemic illness (**Table 2**). It reveals evidence of acute or chronic systemic illness. In common neurological conditions such as stroke, specific abnormal posture in spastic hemiparesis causes flexion of upper limb with flexion and adduction at the shoulder, flexion at the elbow and wrist, and flexion and adduction of the fingers. The posture adopted by the lower limb in spastic hemiparesis is extension at the hip, knee, and ankle with an equinus deformity at the foot. In Parkinson's disease, there is flexion of the trunk with stooping, rigidity, masking, tremors, and slowness of movement. In myopathies, lordosis with waddling gait and hypertrophied calves are observed.

GENERAL OUTLINE OF NEUROLOGICAL EXAMINATION

Neurologic examination can be challenging, but can be mastered by repeated organized and focused examination of patients. The American Academy of Neurology (AAN) has published a curriculum to provide basic knowledge and skills to ensure that all medical students who graduate are able to identify common neurological disorders and manage neurologic emergencies.

Neurology and sherlock holmes: Dr Joseph Bell, an Edinburgh surgeon, was reported to have legendary observational skills and acted as an inspiration for his pupils and friends (Sir Arthur Conan Doyle), and fictional detective (Sherlock Holmes). Through Sherlock Holmes, Dr Joseph Bell's words "my method is based on the observation of trifles". An astute neurologist carefully looks for the most subtle findings to clinch the diagnosis. Dr Wadia's astute observation of the workers in the ferromanganese plants lead to identification of manganese toxicity in these workers.

TABLE 2	Important general examination findings in patients with neurologic disease.
General appearance	• Malnutrition ∘ Hyperthyroidism ∘ Tuberculosis ∘ Alzheimers dementia ∘ Amyotrophic lateral sclerosis ∘ Whipples disease ∘ Celiac disease ∘ Amyloidosis • Overweight ∘ Idiopathic intracranial hypertension ∘ Endocrinopathies • Short stature ∘ Endocrinopathies ∘ Mitochondrial diseases ∘ Refsum's disease ∘ Niemann–Picks disease • Excessive height ∘ Marfans syndrome ∘ Homocystinuria ∘ Klinefelter's syndrome ∘ Sotos syndrome
Skin	• Neurocutaneous markers ∘ Café au lait spot (**Fig. 1**) ∘ Shagreen patch ∘ Ash-leaf macule ∘ Adenoma sebaceum ∘ Port-wine stain • Erythema chronicum migrans ∘ Lyme disease • Purpura, petechiae ∘ Meningococcemia ∘ Rocky Mountain spotted fever ∘ Thrombotic thrombocytopenic purpura • Eschar ∘ Scrub typhus • Vesicular eruption ∘ Herpes zoster • Livedo reticularis ∘ Antiphospholipid antibody (APLA) syndrome ∘ Cryoglobulinemia • Spider angiomas ∘ Alcohol abuse • Hyperpigmentation ∘ Vitamin B12 deficiency ∘ Addison's disease ∘ Carotenemia • Angiokeratoma ∘ Fabry disease • Painless nonhealing ulcers ∘ Syringomyelia ∘ Hereditary sensory neuropathy • Scars, needle marks ∘ Substance abuse

Continued...

Continued...

	• Shawl sign, heliotrope rash ∘ Dermatomyositis • Trophic changes ∘ Peripheral nerve disease ∘ Tabes dorsalis ∘ Myelopathy
Head	• Microcephaly ∘ Craniosynostosis ∘ Chromosomal abnormalities ∘ Phenylketonuria ∘ TORCH infections ∘ Zika virus infection • Macrocephaly ∘ Obstructive hydrocephalus ∘ Megalencephaly • Bulging anterior fontanelle ∘ Raised intracranial pressure (ICP) • Port-wine angioma ∘ Sturge–Weber syndrome • Battles sign ∘ Head trauma • Racoon sign ∘ Basilar skull fracture • Palpable skull defect ∘ Meningocele ∘ Encephalocele • Frontal bossing ∘ Hydrocephalus • Temporal artery tenderness ∘ Giant cell arteritis • Transillumination ∘ Hydranencephaly • McEwan's sign ∘ Hydrocephalus (in infants and children)
Face	• Hatchet facies ∘ Myotonic dystrophy (**Fig. 2**) • Masked faces ∘ Parkinson's disease • Procerus sign ∘ Progressive supranuclear palsy
Eyes	• Ptosis ∘ Myasthenia gravis ∘ Myotonic dystrophy • Exophthalmos ∘ Thyroid disease • Unilateral arcus senilis ∘ Carotid stenosis • Lens dislocation ∘ Marfans syndrome • Kayser–Fleischer ring ∘ Wilson disease (**Fig. 3**) • Lisch nodules ∘ Neurofibromatosis • Brushfield spots ∘ Down's syndrome

Continued...

Continued...

Ears, nose, mouth, throat	• Bulging tympanic membrane 　○ Basilar skull fracture • Saddle nose 　○ Congenital syphilis • Watery rhinorrhea 　○ CSF rhinorrhea • Bacterial infection in dangerous area of face 　○ Cavernous sinus thrombosis • Atrophic glossitis 　○ Vitamin B12 deficiency • Smooth, shiny, atrophic, red tongue 　○ Vitamin B1 deficiency • Trident tongue 　○ Myasthenia gravis • Macroglossia 　○ Amyloidosis 　○ Myxedema 　○ Down syndrome • Tongue bite marks 　○ Seizures 　○ Neuroacanthocytosis 　○ Lesch–Nyhan syndrome • Xerostomia 　○ Sjögren syndrome • Lead lines 　○ Lead toxicity • Mucosal ulceration 　○ Behçet's disease • Hutchinson's teeth 　○ Congenital syphilis
Neck	• Short neck 　○ Klippel–Feil syndrome 　○ Syringomyelia 　○ Platybasia 　○ Chiari malformation • Posture 　○ Cervical dystonia • Lymphadenopathy 　○ Lymphoma 　○ Mononucleosis 　○ HIV 　○ Lyme disease 　○ Phenytoin pseudolymphoma 　○ Sarcoidosis • Restricted neck movements 　○ Cervical spondylosis 　○ Craniovertebral junction (CVJ) anomalies 　○ Cervical dystonia

Continued...

Continued...

Extremities	• Palmar erythema 　○ Alcohol abuse • Skeletal deformity (hammer toes, pes cavus) 　○ Friedreich's ataxia (**Fig. 4**) • Hypermobile joints 　○ Marfans syndrome 　○ Ehlers syndrome • Arthropathy 　○ Connective tissue disease
Hair and nails	• Alopecia 　○ Myotonic dystrophy 　○ Hypothyroidism 　○ Secondary syphilis 　○ SLE 　○ Leigh's disease • Hypertrichosis 　○ POEMS syndrome 　○ Porphyria • Poliosis 　○ Waardenburg syndrome • Kinky hair 　○ Menkes disease 　○ Giant axonal neuropathy • Mees' lines 　○ Arsenic poisoning • Clubbing of nails 　○ Bronchogenic carcinoma 　○ Cyanotic congenital heart disease • Periungual fibroma 　○ Tuberous sclerosis (**Fig. 5**)
Genitalia and rectum	• Genital ulcers 　○ Behcets disease • Scrotal angioma 　○ Fabry disease • Lax anal sphincter 　○ Myelopathy
Spine	• Gibbus 　○ TB spine • Lumbar lordosis 　○ Muscular dystrophy • Scoliosis 　○ Friedreich's ataxia • Spinal tenderness 　○ Spinal epidural abscess • Dimpling of skin 　○ Spinal dysraphism 　○ Tethered cord 　○ Diastematomyelia

(ICP: intracranial pressure; POEMS: polyneuropathy, organomegaly, endocrinopathy, monoclonal gammopathy, and skin changes; TB: tuberculosis; TORCH: Toxoplasmosis, Other, Rubella, Cytomegalovirus, and Herpes)

Similarly, the observations by Dr Meenakshisundaram and colleagues lead to identification of Madras-motor neuron disease, which is associated with hearing impairment and occurs in younger age.

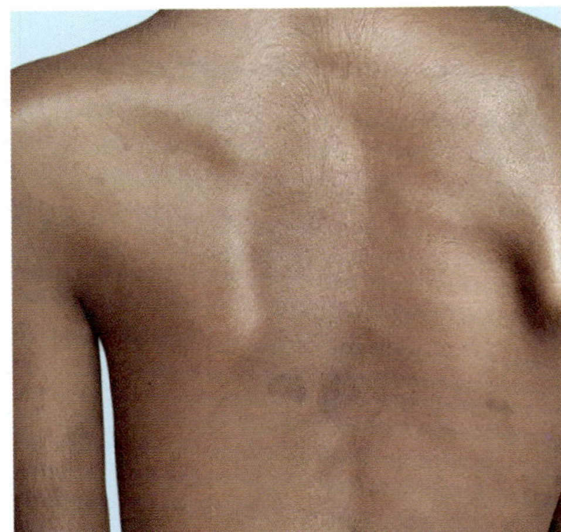

FIGURE 1: Café au lait spot.

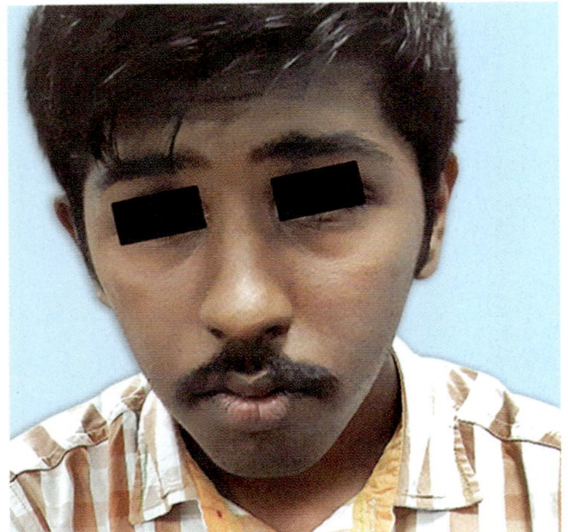

FIGURE 2: Hatchet facies of myotonic dystrophy.

Neurological assessment of a patient should start from the time patient enters the clinic and waits for his or her consultation. A look at a patient in the waiting room might be sufficient to make a diagnosis in the blink of an eye (*augenblickdiagnose*). Some common neurological disorders that can be diagnosed in such a manner are listed in **Box 3**.

The components of neurological examination (**Box 4**) include assessment of mental state followed by cranial nerves, motor system, reflexes, sensory system, coordination, and gait examinations.

MENTAL STATUS EXAMINATION

The mental status examination ensues by observing and speaking with the patient. The Mini-Mental State Examination (MMSE) is a useful tool to assess cognitive function and takes <10 minutes to complete. The test is 85% sensitive and specific for making the diagnosis of dementia, especially in educated patients. Core elements of the mental status examination can be divided into level of consciousness, orientation, speech and language, memory, fund of information, insight and judgment, abstract thought, and calculations.

Level of consciousness is described as the state of awareness of the self and the environment. The response

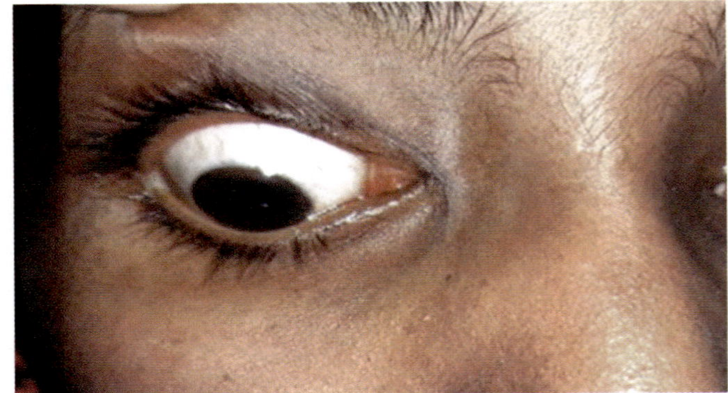

FIGURE 3: Kayser–Fleischer ring in Wilson disease.

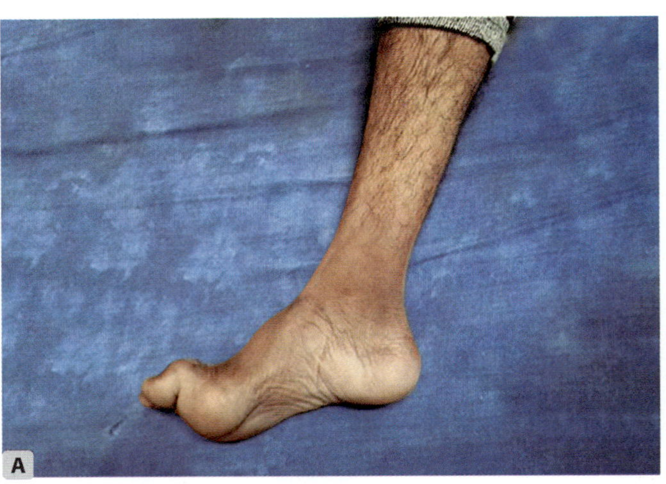

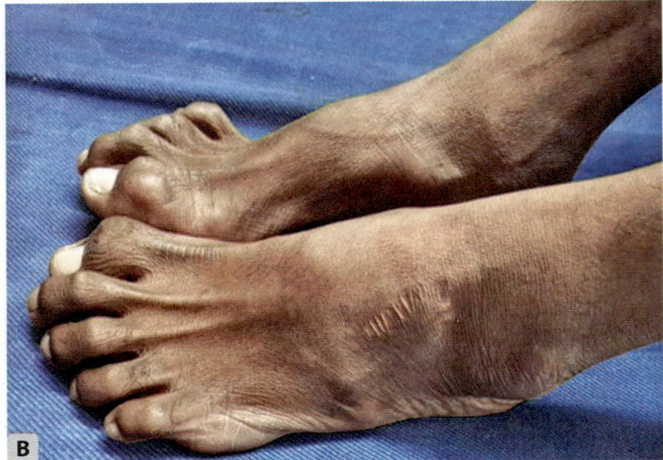

FIGURES 4 A & B: A patient with Friedreich's ataxia having (A) Pes cavus and **(B)** hammer toes deformities.

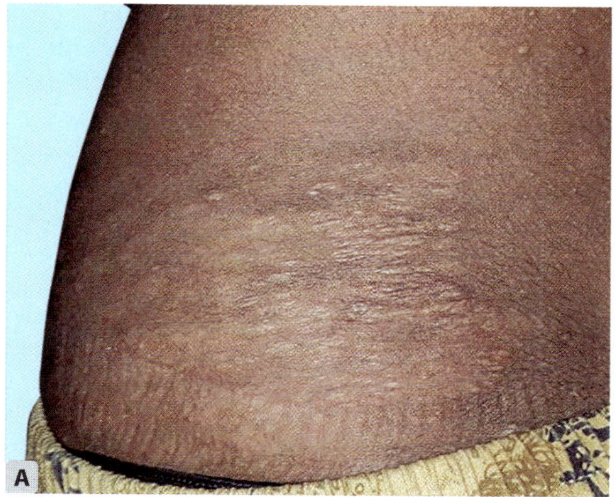

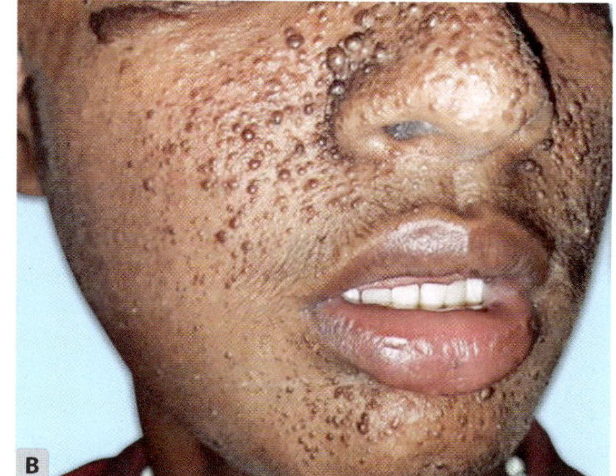

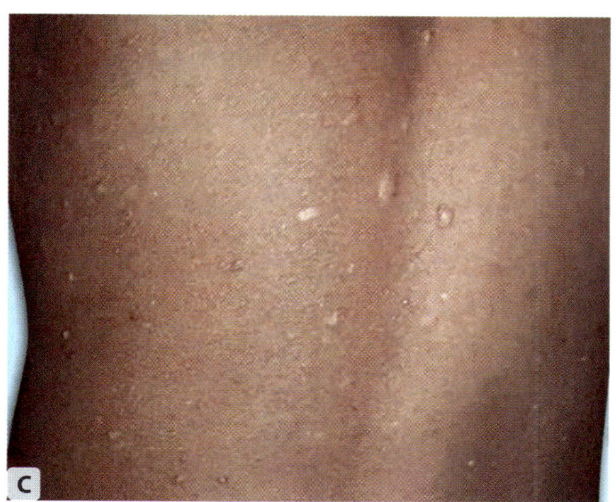

FIGURES 5 A to C: A patient with tuberous sclerosis having (A) Shagreen patch, **(B)** Adenoma sebaceum, and **(C)** Ash-leaf macule.

BOX 3	Neurological disorders susceptible to augenblickdiagnose.
	• Parkinson's disease
	• Neurocutaneous syndromes
	• Bell's palsy
	• Hydrocephalus
	• Charcot–Marie–Tooth disease
	• Essential tremor
	• Cervical dystonia
	• Carotid-cavernous fistula
	• Facioscapulohumeral muscular dystrophy
	• Myotonic dystrophy
	• Complete third cranial nerve palsy
	• Craniosynostosis syndromes
	• Spastic hemiplegia/diplegia

to the minimum stimulus necessary to elicit a reaction is noted when the patient is not fully awake.

Orientation is tested by asking the person to state his or her name, location, and time (day of the week and date); time is usually the first to be affected in a variety of pathologies.

BOX 4	Components of neurologic examination.
	• Mental status
	• Cranial nerves
	• Motor
	• Sensory
	• Reflexes
	• Cerebellar function, coordination
	• Gait and station

Speech assessment is done by observing articulation, rate, rhythm, and prosody.

Language assessment is done by observing the spontaneous speech which comprises fluency, comprehension, repetition, naming, reading, and writing. Patient is asked to name a watch or a pen, repeat the phrase "No ifs, ands, or buts"; follow a three step, verbal command; write a sentence; and read and respond to a written command.

Memory is assessed with three main time scales: (1) immediate memory—immediate repetition of three items which the examiner has listed out; (2) short-term memory—ask the patient to recall the same three items 5 and 15 minutes later; and (3) long-term memory—ask the patient about personal events.

Fund of information is assessed by asking questions about major historic or current events, according to educational level.

Insight and judgment is assessed by asking the patient to describe his or her response to situations (e.g., "What would you do if you found a wallet on the road?").

Abstract thinking is assessed by asking the patient to describe similarities between various objects or concepts (e.g., apple and orange, desk and chair).

Calculation ability is assessed by having the patient perform serial subtraction of 7 from 100.

CRANIAL NERVE EXAMINATION

CN I (olfactory): With eyes closed, patient is asked to sniff a mild stimulus such as coffee and identify the odorant.

CN II (optic): Check visual acuity (with corrected refraction) using a Snellen chart. Test the visual fields by confrontation, i.e., by comparing the patient's visual fields to your own. Patient must be seated at a distance of approximately 1 m and examiner places his hands at the periphery of his visual fields such that it is equidistant between examiner and the patient. The patient is asked to look at the center of your face and to indicate when he or she sees fingers moving. Optic fundi are examined with an ophthalmoscope, and the color, size, and degree of swelling or elevation of the optic disk noted, vessels and appearance of the retina.

CN III, IV, VI (oculomotor, trochlear, abducens): Size and shape of pupils and reaction to light and accommodation should be assessed. To check extraocular movements, patient is instructed to keep his or her head still while tracking the movement of the tip of your finger slowly in the horizontal and vertical planes. Horizontal nystagmus is best assessed at 45° and not at extreme lateral gaze.

CN V (trigeminal): Examine ophthalmic, maxillary, and mandibular sensation on each side of the face. The corneal reflex is tested by lightly touching the cornea with a wisp of cotton. The motor component of trigeminal nerve is tested by asking the patient to open the jaw, move it sideways and close the jaw while palpating for the muscles.

CN VII (facial): Look for facial asymmetry at rest by assessing nasolabial fold. Test eyebrow elevation, forehead wrinkling, eye closure, smiling, and cheek puff. Weakness of the lower two-thirds of the face with preservation of the upper third suggests an upper motor neuron (UMN) lesion, whereas weakness of an entire side suggests a lower motor neuron lesion.

CN VIII (vestibulocochlear): Testing for air versus mastoid bone conduction (Rinne) and lateralization of a 512-Hz tuning fork placed at the center of the forehead (Weber) should be done. Vestibular function tests include vestibule-ocular reflex, dynamic visual acuity, star walking test, and Fukuda tests.

CN IX, X (glossopharyngeal, vagus): Position and symmetry of the palate and uvula at rest and with phonation ("aah") must be observed. The gag reflex is evaluated by stimulating the posterior pharyngeal wall on each side with a sterile and blunt object.

CN XI (spinal accessory): Check shoulder shrug (trapezius muscle) and rotation of head to either side (sternocleidomastoid) against resistance.

CN XII (hypoglossal): Inspect the tongue for atrophy or fasciculations, position with protrusion, and strength when extended against the inner surface of the cheeks on each side.

MOTOR EXAMINATION

The motor examination is done by observations of muscle appearance, tone, and strength.

Appearance: Inspection and palpation of muscle groups must be done under good light. Muscle bulk—atrophy or hypertrophy, fasciculations, and tenderness must be checked for.

Tone: Muscle tone is tested by measuring the resistance to passive movement of a relaxed limb. In the upper limbs, tone is examined by rapid pronation and supination of the forearm and flexion and extension at the wrist. Examination of tone in the lower limbs is done by placing the examiner's hands behind the knees and raising it quickly; there is an immediate lift of the heel off the surface in case of increased tone. Increased tone may be either spasticity (velocity dependent: Corticospinal tract disease), rigidity (similar resistance in all angles of motion; extrapyramidal disease), or paratonia (variable changes in resistance; frontal lobe pathways).

Strength: Pronator drift can be used to assess subtle upper limb weakness. With eyes closed, patient is asked to hold both arms fully extended and parallel to the ground for approximately 10 seconds; any asymmetric flexion at the elbow or fingers or pronation of the forearm is a sign of weakness. The grading of muscle strength is provided in **Box 5**.

REFLEX EXAMINATION

Muscle stretch reflexes: Jaw jerk is elicited with the examiner placing his thumb or index finger on the middle

BOX 5	Grading of muscle power.
0	= No movement
1	= Flicker or trace of muscle contraction
2	= Movement with elimination of gravity
3	= Movement against gravity but not against resistance
4–	= Movement against a mild degree of resistance
4	= Movement against moderate resistance
4+	= Movement against strong resistance
5	= Full power

of patient's chin, with mouth midway open with jaw relaxed and then striking with knee hammer. Upward jerk of the mandible is the normal response.

Biceps (C5, C6), brachioradialis (C5, C6), and triceps (C7, C8) reflexes in the upper limbs and the patellar or quadriceps (L3, L4) and Achilles (S1, S2) reflexes in the lower limbs are assessed. Reflexes may be enhanced by asking the patient to voluntarily contract other, distant muscle groups. Upper limb reflexes may be reinforced by voluntary teeth-clenching, and the lower limb reflexes by hooking the flexed fingers and attempting to pull them apart. The grading of MRS is provided in **Box 6**.

Superficial reflexes: The plantar reflex is elicited by stroking the lateral surface of the sole of the foot. The normal reflex consists of plantar flexion. In UMN lesions, there is a paradoxical extension of the toe is observed associated with fanning and extension of the other toes (termed an *extensor plantar response*, or *Babinski sign*). Superficial abdominal reflexes are elicited by lightly stroking the abdominal surface near the umbilicus in a diagonal fashion with a sharp object and observing the movement of the umbilicus. Normally, the umbilicus will pull toward the stimulated quadrant. These reflexes are absent in UMN lesions. Cremasteric reflex consists of stroking the medial thigh with ipsilateral elevation of the testicle which is mediated by L1. Anal reflex consists of contraction of the anal sphincter when the perianal skin is scratched and mediated by S2, S3, and S4 reflexes.

Primitive reflexes: Primitive reflexes appear with disease of the frontal lobe pathways. The grasp reflex consists of involuntary flexion of the fingers and hands following stimulation of the palmar surface of the hand elicited by touching the palmar surface of the hand. The palmomental response consists of contraction of the mentalis muscle (chin) ipsilateral to a scratch stimulus diagonally applied to the palm.

SENSORY EXAMINATION

The *primary sensory modalities—light touch, pain, temperature, vibration, and joint position*—are tested in all four limbs. Assessment of light touch by stimulation of the skin with single, very gentle touches of a wisp of cotton. Pain is tested using a new pin and temperature by using test tubes containing warm or cold water (e.g., 41–50°F for testing warmth, 5–10°C for testing cold). Testing of vibration is done by using a 128-Hz tuning fork applied to the distal phalanx of the great toe or index finger. Joint position testing is done by the examiner holding the digit laterally and distal to the joint being assessed and performs small 1- to 2-mm excursions. The *Romberg's test* is done by patient standing with the feet as close together as possible to maintain balance keeping the eyes open, and then with closed eyes. Swaying with the eyes closed is an abnormal response. Two point discrimination (discrimination of two closely placed stimuli as separate), stereognosis (identification of an object by touch) and graphesthesia (the identification of numbers or letters written on the skin surface) comprise cortical sensations.

BOX 6	Grading of deep tendon reflexes.
0	= Absent
1	= Present but diminished
2	= Normoactive
3	= Exaggerated
4	= Clonus

COORDINATION

Finger-to-nose testing is a test of cerebellar function; the patient is asked to touch his or her index finger repetitively to the nose and then to the examiner's outstretched finger, similarly in the lower limbs, test is performed by asking the patient to raise the leg to touch the examiners finger with the great toe. Heel-knee-shin testing is done for assessing coordination in the lower limbs by asking the patient, who is in supine position to slide the heel of each foot from the knee down the shin of the other leg. Testing for dysdiadochokinesia is performed by asking the patient to perform rapid alternating movements of supination and pronation of the upper limbs quickly as possible. Accuracy, speed, and rhythm are noted for all the above movements.

GAIT

The patient should be observed from the point of getting up from sitting position, walking and turning normally, walking on the heels, walking on the toes, and walking heel-to-toe along a straight line.

DIAGNOSIS

After obtaining a thorough history and performing a focused examination, clinical data must be interpreted to arrive at an anatomic localization (**Table 3**) that best explains the clinical findings, so that diagnostic possibilities can be narrowed down and appropriate selection of laboratory tests can be done. Integration of the anatomic localization, mode of onset and course of illness, other medical data, and laboratory findings are then done to establish an etiologic diagnosis. It is important to understand that not all pathological signs are of localizing value. Some neurological signs suggest involvement of more than one site in the central nervous system while some signs can be observed in both central as well as peripheral disorders (**Table 4**).

A detailed understanding of neuroanatomy is essential to localize and lateralize the lesion. Understanding the presence and the level of decussations (and double decussations) are crucial to localize the lesion.

A heuristic refers to a simple decision strategy which ignores part of the available information and instead focuses on a few relevant predictors to achieve a rapid diagnosis. They aid in early diagnosis of certain disorders based on the presence of a combination of certain key findings (**Table 5**). However, an over-reliance on heuristics need to be avoided

TABLE 3	Localization within nervous system.
Cortical (cerebrum)	• Altered mental status • Cognitive impairment • Seizures • Unilateral pyramidal pattern of weakness and sensory abnormalities including head and limbs • Language abnormalities • Visual field abnormalities • Movement abnormalities
Brainstem	• Cranial nerve involvement (single or multiple) • "Crossed" weakness • Sensory abnormalities of head and limbs • Internuclear ophthalmoplegia
Spinal cord	• Back pain or tenderness • Weakness and sensory abnormalities sparing the head • Horizontal sensory level • Bowel and bladder involvement
Spinal roots	• Radicular limb pain • Weakness or sensory abnormalities following root distribution • Loss of reflexes
Peripheral nerve	• Distal weakness • Mid or distal limb pain • Weakness or sensory abnormalities following nerve distribution • "Stocking or glove" distribution of sensory loss • Loss of reflexes
Neuromuscular junction	• Fatigability • Bilateral weakness including face (ptosis, diplopia, dysphagia) and proximal limbs • No sensory involvement
Muscle	• Bilateral proximal or distal weakness • No sensory involvement

TABLE 4	Localizing value of common neurological signs.
Signs with localizing value	• Dementia, aphasia, apraxia, alexia (cortex) • Abnormalities of mood, behavior (cortex) • Crossed findings—ipsilateral cranial nerve signs and contralateral long tract signs (brainstem) • Sensory level (spinal cord, rarely brainstem)
Signs with non-localizing value indicating CNS disease	• Hemiparesis • Hemisensory loss • Hemiataxia • Supranuclear eye movement abnormalities
Signs with nonlocalizing value indicating CNS or PNS disease	• Monoparesis, hemiparesis, paraparesis, quadriparesis • Dysarthria, dysphagia • Gait abnormalities • Positive Romberg sign • Extensor plantar response

TABLE 5 Examples of heuristics to diagnose neurological disorders.

Clinical scenario	Diagnosis
Scoliosis with absent abdominal reflex	**Syringomyelia**
Muscle disease with Beevor's sign	• **Facioscapulohumeral muscular dystrophy** • **Nonaka myopathy**
• Bilateral trigeminal neuralgia • Internuclear ophthalmoplegia	**Multiple sclerosis**
Elbow and neck contractures in a patient with atrial fibrillation	**Emery–Dreifuss muscular dystrophy**
Spontaneous, unprovoked, and unwelcome erections in an elderly person when walking	**Lumbar spinal stenosis (neurogenic claudication and spontaneous priapism)**
Cavernous sinus lesion in a patient with poorly controlled diabetes mellitus	**Invasive rhino-orbital mucormycosis**
Seizures with subcutaneous skin nodules	**Neurocysticercosis**

as they can be misleading and result in incorrect diagnosis and management.

The process of neurological diagnosis requires the careful analysis of all available information to reach a diagnosis. The physician needs to remember that diagnosis does not end with the identification of the biological disease alone and requires a holistic understanding of the patients' prevalent emotional and social factors. Physicians often fail to recognize the absence of a sign which may be as important as its presence and might provide valuable information regarding the diagnosis (similar to looking at a half full glass, where the empty half may be as revealing). Also, when a past diagnosis is encountered we need to think in terms of Robbins Pathology Textbook (Backward—what caused it? Forward—what it causes? and Present—how it is being treated?). The art of diagnosis needs to be a lifetime learning endeavor and the physician needs to always "look it up" as early and as often, as a habit, before arriving at a final decision. Access to online resources, textbooks or discussion with resource persons/experienced consultants help to improve the process of diagnosis. The authors feel that the commentary which includes the 24 principles by Schattner, *"Teaching clinical medicine: the key principles"* is worth reading to improve the art of clinical reasoning and diagnosis.

MANAGEMENT PLAN

The next step after the detailed history and examination is to obtain the necessary laboratory and imaging studies. It is observed that ordering unnecessary investigations may lead to confusion, instead of giving clarity to the physician and causing increased financial burden for the patient. Hence, relevant investigations, when carried out for the appropriate clinical context, are pivotal in reaching the final diagnosis and to initiate timely treatment.

CONCLUSION

Neurological history should be taken in an organized manner. General examination gives clues to the presence of systemic illness. Detailed neurological examination helps in anatomical localization. All these, when combined with the relevant laboratory studies, help to reach a final diagnosis.

ACKNOWLEDGMENT

We are thankful to Dr Deepa Avadhani and Dr Shrivarthan R, Residents, Institute of Neurology, Madras Medical College, Chennai for helping us prepare this chapter.

RECOMMENDED READINGS

1. Daroff RB, Jankovic J, Mazziotta JC, Pomeroy SL, (Eds). Bradley's Neurology in Clinical Practice, 7th edition. London: Elsevier; 2015.
2. Campbell WW, Barohn RJ, Ranganathan LN, (Eds). Dejong's The Neurologic Examination, South Asian edition. New Delhi: Wolters Kluwer Pvt Ltd; 2019.
3. Alpert JN. The Neurologic Diagnosis, 2nd edition. Cham, Switzerland: Switzerland AG Springer Nature; 2019.
4. Marvel K, Major G, Jones K, Pfaffly C. Dialogues in the exam room: medical interviewing by resident family physicians. Fam Med. 2000;32:628-32.
5. Campbell WW. Augenblickdiagnose. Semin Neurol. 1998;18(2):169-76.
6. Brazis PW, Masdeu JC, Biller J, Ranganathan LN, (Eds). Localization in Clinical Neurology, South Asian edition. India: Wolters Kluwer Pvt Ltd; 2020.
7. Safdieh JE, Govindarajan R, Gelb DJ, Odia Y, Soni M. Core curriculum guidelines for a required clinical neurology experience. Neurology. 2019;92(13):619-26.
8. Peschel RE, Peschel E. What physicians have in common with Sherlock Holmes: discussion paper. J R Soc Med. 1989;82:33-6.
9. Kishore B. The Toxic Effects of Heavy Metals on the Nervous System (Neurology India 12, 29-41, 1964). J Neurol Sci. 1965;2:203-12.
10. Meenakshisundaram E, Jagannathan K, Ramamurthi B. Clinical pattern of motor neuron disease seen in younger age groups in Madras. Neurol India. 1970;18 (Suppl 1):109+.
11. Araújo R, van de Warrenburg B, Lang A, Lees A, Bloem B. The Waiting Room: neurological observations made outside the movement disorder specialist's consulting office. Pract Neurol. 2019;19(4):295-301.
12. Lowenstein D, Martin J, Hauser L. Introduction to Neurology: Harrisons Neurology in Clinical Medicine, 4th edition, New York: Mc GrawHill; 2017.
13. Vickrey BG, Samuels MA, Ropper AH. How neurologists think: a cognitive psychology perspective on missed diagnoses. Ann Neurol. 2010;67(4):425-33.
14. Schattner A. Teaching clinical medicine: the key principals. QJM: An International Journal of Medicine. 2015;108(6):435-42.

CHAPTER

183

Migraine and Other Headaches

Sanjay Cheema, Salwa Kamourieh, Manjit Matharu

ABSTRACT

Headache is one of the most common reasons for a person to consult with a doctor. In any patient with headache a diagnosis can usually be made on the basis of the history, taking into account the onset, location, severity, quality, duration, exacerbating and relieving factors, and associated symptoms of the headache. The majority of headache in the population is due to primary headache disorders such as migraine, tension-type headache, and cluster headache. It is also essential to recognize secondary causes of headache which may threaten life or vision, such as subarachnoid hemorrhage, giant cell arteritis, and headaches caused by raised intracranial pressure.

Migraine, which affects 15% of the population, is the most likely headache disorder to present to medical professionals and causes a high degree of disability. Migraine is characterized by recurrent headache attacks lasting 4–72 hours, which typically have a unilateral location, throbbing quality, moderate-to-severe pain intensity, association with nausea and/or vomiting, sensitivity to light, sound, and motion. Treatment of migraine includes lifestyle measures, acute treatments such as nonsteroidal anti-inflammatory drugs (NSAIDs) and triptans, and preventive treatments such as beta blockers, antiepileptics, and tricyclic antidepressants.

"I opened my eyes to the brightness of the sun. I groaned, feeling the migraine take over"

—Sylvie Raven

INTRODUCTION

Headache is one of the most frequent presenting symptoms to primary care practitioners and is the most common presenting symptom to neurologists. Almost everyone will experience headache at least once in their lifetime, and the fact that in the majority of the population headache is an infrequent transient experience which may explain why headache disorders are often overlooked as a cause of disability. Headache disorders such as migraine can in fact be extremely disabling—the World Health Organization (WHO) considers a day spent with severe migraine as being equivalent in disability to a day spent with dementia, quadriplegia or psychosis, and has found migraine to be the largest cause of disability worldwide in people under the age of 50 years.

"Secondary" causes of headache are rare as a cause of headache overall, but understandably raise concern from the patient and doctor, and their features must be recognized due to the risk of morbidity and mortality. "Primary" headache disorders on the other hand are disorders which cause recurrent headaches in the absence of an identifiable structural cause and are not life-threatening but are common and cause recognizable symptoms. Differentiation between primary and secondary headaches as well as between the primary headache syndromes predominantly relies on accurate history taking. Secondary headaches require treatment of their underlying cause. Migraine and other primary headache disorders once correctly recognized are usually manageable with a variety of lifestyle measures, pharmacological, and injectable treatments.

CLINICAL ASSESSMENT

HISTORY

The following features should be asked about specifically when assessing a patient with headache.

Onset: Headache with sudden "thunderclap" onset has a number of medically serious secondary causes which must be investigated for, whereas a headache with a gradual progressive onset is far more likely to be due to a primary headache disorder; a new onset persistent headache after the age of 50 years is more concerning of a secondary cause such as giant cell arteritis, compared to the onset of headaches in a person in their teenage years or 20s, which is typical in migraine and tension-type headache.

Location of the pain: Migraine does not have a consistent location in the head but usually starts unilaterally; tension type headache is typically a bilateral headache; cluster headache is a strictly unilateral headache; trigeminal neuralgia is unilateral and felt in the face, especially in the second and third divisions of the trigeminal nerve.

Severity of the pain: Tension-type headache causes mild or moderate pain severity, while cluster headache causes severe or excruciating pain, migraine has a varying severity which is usually in-between that of tension-type headache and cluster headache.

Quality of the pain: The pain of migraine is usually described as throbbing, tension-type headache as pressing or tightening, cluster headache as stabbing or boring, and neuralgiform headache and facial pain disorders as electric shock-like.

Duration of attacks: Migraine attacks typically last 4–72 hours, cluster headache attacks typically last 15–180 minutes, trigeminal neuralgia, and other neuralgiform disorders last seconds.

Triggers for attacks: A postural relationship or predictable diurnal relationship suggests a cerebrospinal fluid (CSF) pressure disorder; headache which is triggered by coughing, sneezing, or other Valsalva maneuvers suggest raised intracranial pressure; a variety of triggers may be reported in migraine including sleep deprivation, stress, menstruation, and dehydration; cutaneous triggers such as cold, wind, or touch are common triggers of trigeminal neuralgia.

Associated symptoms: Migraine is typically associated with nausea and/or vomiting, photophobia, phonophobia, and motion sensitivity; tension-type headache is typically featureless with no associated symptoms; cluster headache is associated with cranial autonomic symptoms and agitation or restlessness during attacks.

A number of "red flag" features should be considered specifically as they may suggest an underlying secondary cause for the headache (see **Table 1**).

EXAMINATION

Neurological examination should be performed in all patients at the time of first presentation with headache and should be targeted at identifying signs which require further investigation for a secondary cause. Examination should include fundoscopy, assessment of visual fields and eye movements which may show abnormalities in patients with raised intracranial pressure, and in a patient over the age of 50 years examination should include

TABLE 1 SNOOP4 mnemonic of important red flags for secondary causes of headache.

	Clinical feature	Possible secondary cause
S	Systemic symptoms: Fever and weight loss	Infection, malignancy, and giant cell arteritis
N	(Focal) Neurological symptoms or signs	Any secondary cause, especially stroke, mass, abscess, and encephalitis
O	Onset: Thunderclap	Subarachnoid hemorrhage, and other vascular disorders
O	Older age: Onset > 50	Giant cell arteritis
P	Papilloedema	Raised intracranial pressure
P	Positional	Low intracranial pressure
P	Precipitated by Valsalva maneuvers	Raised or low intracranial pressure
P	Progressive or pattern change	Many secondary causes

palpation of the temporal arteries looking for tenderness, thickening, or absent pulsation, which may suggest giant cell arteritis.

INVESTIGATIONS

Investigations are not necessary in a patient with recurrent headache attacks in keeping with a primary headache disorder, but targeted investigation should be performed if a secondary cause is suspected. This may include erythrocyte sedimentation rate (ESR) and C-reactive protein (CRP) where giant cell arteritis is a concern, and other blood tests if a systemic disease is suspected. Computed tomography (CT) of the head should be performed acutely to identify subarachnoid hemorrhage in the patient presenting with thunderclap headache. Magnetic resonance imaging (MRI) of the brain should be performed in patients when there is a suspicion of neoplastic disease, other focal brain lesion, or spontaneous intracranial hypotension secondary to a CSF leak. Lumbar puncture should be performed if an infectious or neuroinflammatory disease is suspected, or to measure CSF pressure in the diagnosis of idiopathic intracranial hypertension.

Brain imaging may in some cases be performed in patients with a suspected primary headache in the absence of "red flag features" for reasons of reassurance to the patient. This decision should be balanced against the chance of finding incidental abnormalities which are unrelated to the headache which occurs in approximately 2% of MRI brain scans.

SECONDARY HEADACHES

THUNDERCLAP HEADACHE

Subarachnoid hemorrhage is the archetypal cause of a thunderclap headache, which is excruciating from onset, reaching peak severity within a few seconds, and typically described as the "worst headache of one's life". After a subarachnoid hemorrhage signs of meningeal irritation such as neck stiffness and photophobia, delirium, and reduced consciousness are common but not necessarily present.

Subarachnoid hemorrhage has a high mortality rate so a first episode of thunderclap headache should always be investigated. Noncontrast CT should be performed, which has a sensitivity of >99% within 6 hours of headache onset. The sensitivity reduces over time, so after a delayed presentation following thunderclap headache a lumbar puncture must be performed to look for presence of xanthochromia-breakdown products of blood in the CSF. Approximately, 80% of subarachnoid hemorrhages are caused by a bleeding aneurysm in the circle of Willis. Management includes supportive care, nimodipine to prevent ischemic complications due to vasospasm, and surgical clipping or coiling of the aneurysm to prevent further bleeding.

Thunderclap headache can occur due to other causes including arterial dissection, cerebral venous sinus thrombosis, ischemic stroke, reversible cerebral vasoconstriction syndrome, and pituitary apoplexy.

GIANT CELL ARTERITIS

Giant cell arteritis is a form of vasculitis which carries a risk of visual loss due to anterior ischaemic neuropathy and is also a risk for other ischemic complications. It should be considered in any patient over the age of 50 years with new onset headache and should especially be suspected in those with scalp tenderness, prominence or absence of pulsation of the temporal arteries, jaw claudication, or visual symptoms. ESR and CRP are usually elevated. Definitive diagnosis requires temporal artery biopsy and can be aided by temporal artery ultrasound imaging. Prompt treatment with high-dose corticosteroids is required due to the risk of visual loss and should be started based on a clinical diagnosis rather than waiting for results of biopsy.

INTRACRANIAL HYPERTENSION

Features suggesting raised intracranial pressure include headache which is triggered by coughing, sneezing, or other Valsalva maneuvers; headache which is worst on waking in the morning; persistent vomiting; transient visual obscurations; pulsatile tinnitus; and the presence of papilloedema. Raised intracranial pressure may be caused by a space occupying lesion such as metastasis, primary brain tumor, or abscess; cerebral edema following traumatic brain injury or stroke; obstructed venous flow secondary to a cerebral venous sinus thrombosis; or obstruction to CSF flow such as from Chiari malformation or meningeal disease. It may also occur without a structural cause in the condition idiopathic intracranial hypertension. Any headache with features of raised intracranial hypertension requires imaging to exclude structural causes. Assessment of vision and visualization of the optic disk is also essential due to the risk of visual loss secondary to papilloedema. Treatment is targeted at the underlying condition causing raised intracranial pressure, and CSF diversion procedure if necessary.

PRIMARY HEADACHES

MIGRAINE

Migraine is a primary headache syndrome characterized by recurrent headache attacks, typically occurring in phases as demonstrated in **Figure 1**. Attacks are commonly preceded by a premonitory phase including symptoms such as fatigue, yawning, food cravings, thirst, mood change, and neck stiffness. Approximately, 30% of patients experience transient neurological symptoms as an aura before the headache develops. Migraine aura typically involves "positive" symptoms (as opposed to the "negative" symptoms of a transient ischemic attack). The most common type of aura is visual, often described as a fortification spectrum or scintillating scotoma. It may also take the form of a spreading sensory disturbance, speech disturbance, brainstem-related symptoms or focal weakness.

The headache phase then follows and lasts 4–72 hours. Not every migraine is typical, but the headache in migraine is typically unilateral in location, pulsating in quality, and has a moderate or severe pain intensity. Attacks are usually associated with nausea and/or vomiting, sensitivity to light, sound, strong smells, and motion. A "postdrome" period usually follows for up to 48 hours, with features including fatigue, difficulty concentrating, neck stiffness, and/or mood changes.

Many people with migraine will recognize triggers, which may include sleep deprivation, psychological stress, overexertion, dehydration, alcohol, and dietary factors or hunger. In women, migraine is often associated with the menstrual cycle.

In the majority of people with migraine it is an episodic disorder. Approximately, 10–15% of people have chronic migraine, meaning they have a headache on more days than not. Chronic migraine usually occurs and follows a period of gradual increase in headache severity over months to years, often in association with regular use of acute analgesics.

Diagnosis: Migraine is a clinical diagnosis based on the history. The diagnosis of migraine and other primary headache syndromes can be made according to International Classification of Headache Disorders criteria (see **Table 2**). Usually, the diagnosis is straightforward. In patients with headache attacks lasting <4 hours cluster headache should be considered. In patients with strictly unilateral continuous headache a trial of indomethacin should be considered to rule out hemicrania continua.

Epidemiology and risk factors: Migraine affects approximately 15% of the population worldwide (approximately one billion people), a rate which is similar in most countries studied. In a cross-sectional study in Karnatka, south India, the 1-year prevalence of migraine was 25.2%.

Migraine is 2–3 times more common in women. In women, migraine is associated with fluctuation in estrogen levels, and often starts after the age of menarche, worsens in the days preceding or during menstruation, improves during pregnancy, and improves after the menopause.

Many of those with migraine have other relatives with the disorder and twin studies suggest a genetic heritability of between 30 and 60%. Migraine rarely occurs due to a single gene defect, except in familial hemiplegic migraine,

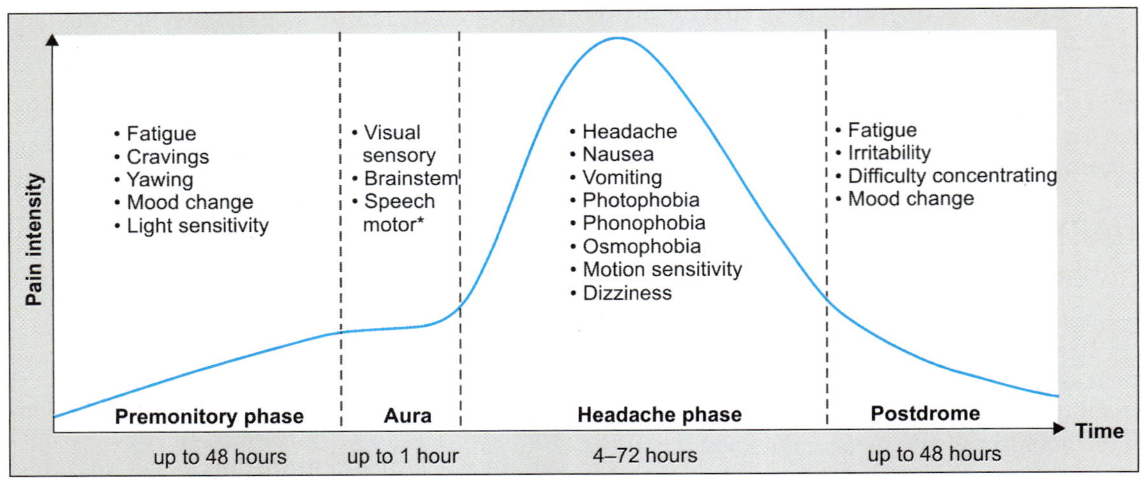

*Motor weakness in hemiplegic migraine may continue through the headache phase and up to 72 hours.

FIGURE 1: Typical phases of a migraine attack.

TABLE 2 International Classification of Headache Disorders 3rd edition criteria for migraine.

ICHD-3 criteria for migraine without aura	ICHD-3 criteria for migraine with aura
A. At least five attacks fulfilling criteria B and D **B.** Headache attacks lasting 4–72 hours (untreated or unsuccessfully treated) **C.** Headache has at least two of the following four characteristics: 1. Unilateral location 2. Pulsating quality 3. Moderate or severe pain intensity 4. Aggravation by or causing avoidance of routine physical activity (e.g., walking or climbing stairs) **D.** During headache at least one of the following: 1. Nausea and/or vomiting 2. Photophobia and phonophobia **E.** Not better accounted for by another ICHD-3 diagnosis	**A.** At least two attacks fulfilling criteria B and C **B.** One or more of the following fully reversible aura symptoms: 1. Visual 2. Sensory 3. Speech and/or language 4. Motor 5. Brainstem 6. Retinal **C.** At least three of the following six characteristics: 1. At least one aura symptom spreads gradually over ≥5 minutes 2. Two or more aura symptoms occur in succession 3. Each individual aura symptom lasts 5–60 minutes 4. At least one aura symptom is unilateral 5. At least one aura symptom is positive 6. The aura is accompanied, or followed within 60 minutes, by headache **D.** Not better accounted for by another ICHD-3 diagnosis

which is inherited in an autosomal dominant manner, most cases linked to the *CACNA1A*, *ATP1A2*, and *SCN1A* genes.

Management:

Nonpharmacological management: People with migraine are often more sensitive to disruption in regularity of their daily life. Optimization of certain lifestyle factors as far as possible will benefit most patients including regular exercise, regular sleep, and good hydration, avoidance of excessive caffeine or alcohol, intake and stress reduction. In patients who have identified reliable triggers or their headaches then these should be avoided as far as possible. Relaxation, biofeedback, mindfulness, and cognitive behavioral therapy can be effective in reducing the impact of migraine on quality of life and disability.

Acute treatments: Acute treatments are medications taken during a migraine attack in order to reduce pain severity or terminate the attack (see **Table 3**). This includes paracetamol, aspirin, NSAIDs, and triptans. High-doses of aspirin such as 900 mg and ibuprofen 600–800 mg are usually more effective than lower ones. Triptans are a class

TABLE 3 Acute treatments for migraine.

	Dose range
Paracetamol	1 g
Aspirin	600–900 mg
NSAIDs	
Ibuprofen	400–800 mg
Naproxen	500 mg
Triptans	
Sumatriptan	50–100 mg
Zolmitriptan	2.5–5 mg
Rizatriptan	10 mg
Almotriptan	12.5 mg
Eletriptan	40–80 mg
Frovatriptan	2.5 mg
Naratriptan	2.5 mg

of serotonin 5-$HT_{1B}/_{1D}$ agonists, which are specifically effective for headaches rather than other causes of pain and are usually highly effective in migraine. A combination of a triptan with aspirin or an NSAID is often more effective than either taken alone. Prokinetic antiemetics such as metoclopramide or domperidone are a helpful addition even in the absence of nausea or vomiting, as gastroparesis frequently occurs during migraine attacks, therefore they can aid the absorption of acute medications. Opioid including medications should not usually be used due to the high risk of dependence and development of medication overuse headache.

Preventive treatments: Preventive treatments are taken on a daily basis in order to reduce the frequency of the headaches and usually do not have their full effect for a number of weeks after being started. Preventive medication should be considered if migraine occurs >1 day/week or is otherwise having an adverse effect on quality of life.

A large number of oral medications have been shown to be effective in the preventive treatment of migraine (see **Table 4**). The majority of these medications were originally developed for other conditions including hypertension, epilepsy, and depression. All have shown relatively similar efficacy rates over placebo in trials therefore choice should be based on patient choice and comorbidity, as well as cost and availability. For example, topiramate has a good evidence base, but should not be used in patients with a history of renal stones or glaucoma and should be used with caution in women of child-bearing age, its potential for weight loss may be seen as a benefit in some patients who are overweight.

OnabotulinumtoxinA is an injectable neurotoxin which is effective for the treatment of chronic migraine when given as a series of injections into the superficial muscles of the head and neck. Monoclonal antibodies targeting the calcitonin gene-related peptide (CGRP), a protein

TABLE 4 Pharmaceutical preventive treatments for migraine.

	Medication class	Dose range (total daily dose)	Potential side-effects/contraindications
Amitriptyline	TCA	10–75 mg	Drowsiness, dry mouth, and constipation
Nortriptyline	TCA	10–75 mg	As above
Dosulepin	TCA	25–75 mg	As above
Propranolol	BB	40–160 mg	Fatigue, postural hypotension, erectile dysfunction, and contraindicated in asthma
Metoprolol	BB	100–200 mg	As above
Topiramate	AED	25–200 mg	Cognitive dysfunction, weight loss, paresthesia, renal stones, glaucoma, teratogenicity, and reduced efficacy of combined oral contraceptive pill
Sodium valproate	AED	400–2000 mg	Nausea, weight gain, tremor, hair loss, and teratogenicity
Flunarizine	CCB	5–10 mg	Lethargy, weight gain, and depression
Candesartan	ARB	8–32 mg	Renal dysfunction, and hyperkalemia
Pizotifen	Serotonergic	0.5–3 mg	Weight gain
Riboflavin	Nutraceutical	400 mg	
Magnesium	Nutraceutical	600 mg	Diarrhea
Co-enzyme Q10	Nutraceutical	600 mg	

(AED: antiepileptic drug; ARB: angiotensin receptor blocker; BB: beta blocker; CCB: calcium-channel blocker; TCA: tricyclic antidepressant)

which is thought to be involved in migraine pathophysiology have recently been shown in large randomized controlled trials to be effective for preventive treatment of episodic and chronic migraine. These are given as subcutaneous or intravenous injection at 1-3 monthly intervals. Currently, due to cost and need for trained personnel to give these treatments, onabotulinumtoxinA and CGRP monoclonal antibodies are mainly reserved for patients who are intractable to a number of oral preventive medications.

Medication overuse headache: If acute treatments are taken more frequently than 10 days per month then this can lead to worsening or chronification of migraine as a phenomenon called medication overuse headache. To prevent medication overuse headache from developing, it is usually recommended to take acute treatments on no >10 days per month. The number of days when medication is taken is thought to be more important than dose strength or total doses taken. Once medication overuse has developed, it can be beneficial to attempt a "medication withdrawal" for a period of at least 2 weeks during which time no acute treatments are used. This can worsen the headaches in the short-term but following this some patients will revert to having less frequent headaches.

TENSION-TYPE HEADACHE

Tension-type headache is at least as common or more so than migraine, with a prevalence of approximately 30%, but is less likely to present to medical professionals due to its milder severity.

Episodes of tension-type headache are typically bilateral, with pressing or tightening (nonthrobbing) quality, mild-to-moderate intensity, and duration between 30 minutes and 7 days. There is no associated nausea, although one of photophobia or phonophobia may be present.

Tension-type headache has previously been attributed to either psychological or muscular "tension", however like migraine it is now thought of as a neurological disorder. The relationship between tension-type headache and migraine is debated with some experts considering them variants of the same disorder. Many patients with migraine will at times also have headaches with a tension-type phenotype.

Most people with tension-type headache have infrequent attacks and will self-manage with lifestyle measures and over-the-counter analgesics. Paracetamol, aspirin, or NSAIDs can be used as acute treatments. Lifestyle measures including regular exercise, stress management, good hydration, and improvement in sleep are also likely to benefit most patients. Medication overuse should be managed if present. Tricyclic antidepressants, most commonly amitriptyline, can be used as preventive treatment in those with frequent attacks.

CLUSTER HEADACHE

Cluster headache is a primary headache syndrome which causes unilateral attacks which are shorter in duration than migraine but of excruciating severity. Attacks usually occur in "clusters" (also called bouts or periods) lasting from a few weeks to a few months, often predictably at certain times of the year. During bouts attacks occur with a frequency between one every other day and eight per day, often at the same time(s) each day. Attacks of cluster headache last between 15 minutes and 3 hours if untreated, are strictly unilateral in the orbital, supraorbital or temporal region. Attacks are associated with unilateral cranial autonomic symptoms on the same side as the headache, which may include any of conjunctival injection, lacrimation, nasal congestion, rhinorrhea, forehead and facial sweating, miosis, ptosis, and/or eyelid edema. In contrast with migraine, where people usually prefer to be still during attacks, cluster headache attacks are usually accompanied by restlessness or agitation.

Cluster headache is far rarer than migraine, affecting approximately 0.1% of the population. In contrast with migraine, cluster headache is approximately four times more common in men. Cigarette smoking is extremely common in people with cluster headache. Imaging studies as well as the circadian and circannual association of attacks have suggested that the hypothalamus is key in the pathophysiology of cluster headache.

Parenteral acute treatments should ideally be used in cluster headache due to the faster onset and shorter duration of attacks, compared with migraine where oral treatments are preferred. Subcutaneous sumatriptan is usually effective within a few minutes and can be used up to twice daily. If patients are not able to use the injectable form, alternatives are intranasal sumatriptan and intranasal zolmitriptan. Inhaled high flow 100% oxygen given at 7–15 L/min can also be used as an acute treatment.

Both greater occipital nerve block injections and short courses of oral corticosteroids (for example prednisolone 60 mg for 1 week then reduced by 10 mg every 3 days until stopped) are often effective for a period of few weeks, and can be used as transitional treatments, either while a preventive treatment is being uptitrated or to cover a bout in patients with short and infrequent bouts. Oral steroids should not be used frequently or as a preventive treatment due to the potential long-term side-effects.

Verapamil is the most widely used preventive treatment. It is sometimes only effective once high doses are reached. Electrocardiogram (ECG) monitoring is required prior to each dose increase due to the risk of bradycardia and heart block. Alternative preventive options with lower degrees of evidence include lithium, topiramate, gabapentin, and melatonin.

OTHER TRIGEMINAL AUTONOMIC CEPHALALGIAS

Cluster headache is one of a family of primary headache disorders called trigeminal autonomic cephalalgias. All share the features of unilateral head pain and association with cranial autonomic symptoms. The other disorders in this group are short-lasting unilateral neuralgiform headache attacks, which cause neuralgiform pain lasting 1–600 seconds and usually respond to sodium channel-blocking drugs carbamazepine and lamotrigine; paroxysmal hemicrania, which causes attacks lasting 2–30 minutes and responds absolutely to the NSAIDs indomethacin; and hemicrania continua, which causes a persistent headache of fluctuating severity and also responds absolutely to indomethacin.

OTHER PRIMARY HEADACHE DISORDERS

There are a variety of other miscellaneous primary headache disorders which are individually rare. All are benign but can mimic secondary causes, which must be excluded before making the diagnosis of a primary headache disorder.

Primary cough headache, primary exercise headache, and primary headache associated with sexual activity are brought on and occur only in association with coughing or other Valsalva maneuver, exercise, or sexual activity respectively.

Cold stimulus headache is a headache resulting from cold stimulus applied externally to the head or ingested or inhaled.

External-pressure headache is a headache resulting from sustained compression of or traction on the scalp.

Primary thunderclap headache is characterized by benign recurrent thunderclap headaches. This is a diagnosis of exclusion and secondary causes must be ruled out before making the diagnosis.

Primary stabbing headache (may also be called ice-pick headache, jabs and jolts syndrome, opthalmodynia periodica) is characterized by transient localized stabs of pain in the head lasting a few seconds.

Nummular headache is a head pain felt exclusively in a small 1–6 cm in diameter, well-circumscribed, round or elliptical region of the scalp, occurring the absence of any local structural or dermatological lesion.

Hypnic headache is characterized by recurrent headache attacks which develop during sleep and cause awaking, which are not better accounted for by another diagnosis.

New daily persistent headache describes a headache which is daily and persistent for at least 3 months from the time of onset, often developing after a precipitant such as a systemic infection, stressful life event, or extracranial surgery.

RECOMMENDED READINGS

1. Headache Classification Committee of the International Headache Society (IHS) The International Classification of Headache Disorders, 3rd edition. Cephalalgia. 2018;38(1):1-211.
2. National Institute for Health and Care Excellence. (2012). Headaches in over 12s: diagnosis and management: Clinical Guideline [CG150] [online]. Available from: https://www.nice.org.uk/guidance/cg150.
3. Ravishankar K, Chakravarty A, Chowdhury D, Shukla R, Singh S. Guidelines on the diagnosis and the current management of headache and related disorders. Ann Indian Acad Neurol. 2011;14 (Suppl 1):S40-59.
4. Kulkarni GB, Rao GN, Gururaj G, Stovner LJ, Steiner TJ. Headache disorders and public ill-health in India: prevalence estimates in Karnataka State. J Headache Pain. 2015;16:67.

5. Ray BK, Paul N, Hazra A, Das S, Ghosal MK, Misra AK, et al. Prevalence, burden, and risk factors of migraine: a community-based study from Eastern India. Neurol India. 2017;65(6):1280-8.
6. Ashina M. Migraine. N Eng J Med. 2020;383(19): 1866-76.
7. Sinclair AJ, Sturrock A, Davies B, Matharu M. Headache management: pharmacological approaches. Pract Neurol. 2015;15(6):411-23.
8. Chowdhury D. Tension type headache. Ann Indian Acad Neurol. 2012;15(Suppl 1):S83-8.
9. Cheema S, Matharu M. Cluster headache: what's new? Neurol India. 2021;69(Supplement):S124-S134.

CHAPTER 184

Raised Intracranial Pressure and Hydrocephalus

Vedantam Rajshekhar

ABSTRACT

Intracranial pressure (ICP) is increased (>20 cm of water) when there is an increase in the volume of tissue (due to tumors, brain edema, or a blood clot) or cerebrospinal fluid (CSF) (as in hydrocephalus) within the cranial cavity. Diagnosis of raised ICP is based on clinical examination but brain imaging [computed tomography or magnetic resonance imagining (CT or MR)] is required in most instances to identify the cause. In some instances, the cause might not be evident in spite of imaging as in an entity known as idiopathic intracranial hypertension (IIH). Both medical and surgical treatments might be required depending on the etiology of raised ICP.

Hydrocephalus is one of the causes of raised ICP. Obstructive hydrocephalus occurs when there is an obstruction to the ventricular pathways or at the fourth ventricular outlet. Communicating hydrocephalus occurs when there is increased CSF production, blockage of CSF pathways in the subarachnoid space around the brain or when the absorption of CSF in the venous sinuses is reduced. While most patients with hydrocephalus have raised ICP, in some instances, especially in the elderly, hydrocephalus may be associated with normal CSF pressure which is termed as normal pressure hydrocephalus (NPH). Ventriculoperitoneal (VP) shunt is the most common surgical procedure used to treat hydrocephalus but endoscopic third ventriculostomy (ETV) might help to avoid a shunt in selected patients. Raised ICP due to any etiology should be treated promptly as it can result in loss of vision or mortality if left untreated.

"Symptoms, they are in reality nothing but the cry from suffering organs"

—JM Charcot

RAISED INTRACRANIAL PRESSURE

INTRACRANIAL PRESSURE

Intracranial pressure is the pressure within the cranial cavity. The contents of this closed compartment include the brain, CSF, and the blood within the blood vessels (veins, arteries, and venous sinuses). While the ICP varies with age, the normal range of ICP in an adult is between 8 and 20 cm of water or 5–15 mm Hg. ICP of >20 cm of water is generally considered to be raised ICP.

The volume of the contents of the cranial cavity is governed by the Monro–Kellie doctrine (**Fig. 1**) which states that the sum of the volumes of the brain, CSF, and blood within the cranial cavity is a constant. The approximate volumes of the brain, CSF, and blood in an adult are 1,400 mL, 150 mL, and 150 mL, respectively.

PATHOPHYSIOLOGY

Pressure-volume curve (Fig. 2): Intracranial pressure does not initially rise, if a mass lesion (e.g., tumor or blood clot) grows gradually or if the mass lesion is small. This is because of compensatory mechanisms whereby the CSF and blood are pushed out of the cranial cavity by the mass lesion. This is represented by the flat portion of the pressure-volume (PV) curve. The compensatory mechanisms can usually accommodate up to 120 mL additional volume. However, once these compensatory mechanisms are exhausted then

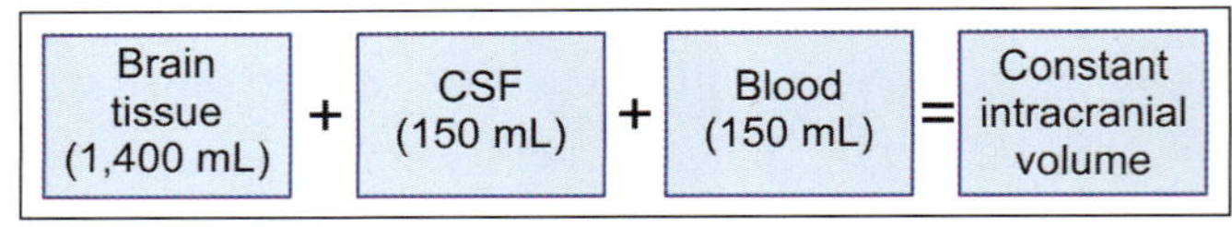

FIGURE 1: Monro–Kellie doctrine.

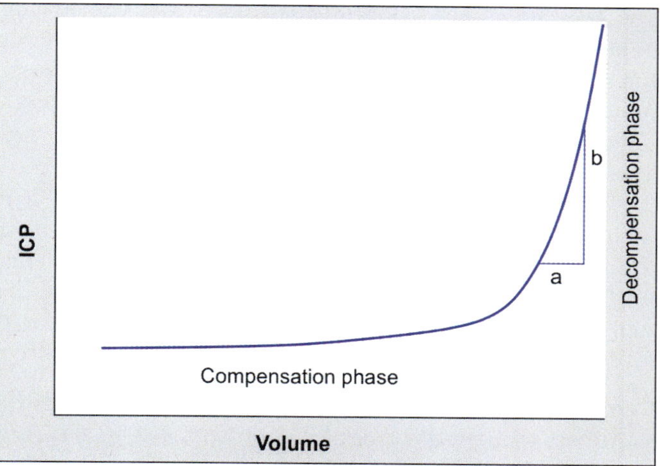

FIGURE 2: Pressure-volume relationship. Note the sharp rise in ICP (b) for a small rise in intracranial volume (a) in the decompensation phase of the curve.

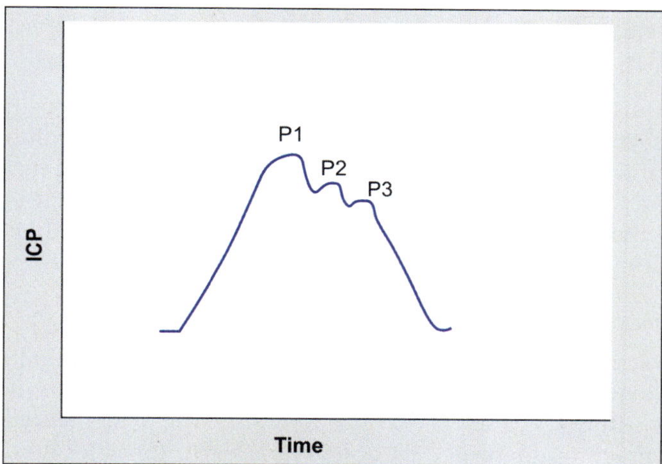

FIGURE 3: Normal intracranial pressure (ICP) wave.

even a small rise in volume of the lesion will result in a large increase in ICP. This is represented by the steep rising limb of the PV curve. Patients who are in this part of the PV curve will manifest clinical features of raised ICP and at the height of the curve will have features of brain herniation.

Intracranial pressure waves: It is important to recognize that ICP is not a static number that remains steady in time. ICP is dynamic which varies with every respiratory and cardiac cycle. The normal ICP has a waveform (**Fig. 3**) with three upstrokes. P1 (percussion wave) represents the arterial pulsation, P2 (tidal wave) represents the intracranial compliance, and P3 (dicrotic wave) represents the venous pulsation. Normally, P1 > P2 > P3. If P2 > P1 then it suggests that there is intracranial hypertension. Abnormal waveforms occur in patients with raised ICP. Lundberg described three types of waves. Type A waves (plateau waves) are the most significant and have pressures of >50 mm Hg. They last from 5 to 20 minutes and are seen in the decompensated phase of the PV curve. Type A waves should prompt urgent action to lower the ICP. Type B waves have a pressure of 20–30 mm Hg and last <3 minutes. They have been attributed to normal fluctuations in respiration and cerebral blood flow and may be seen in sleep and in ventilated patients. They also indicate early intracranial decompensation. Type C waves correspond to the Traube–Hering–Mayer fluctuations in systolic blood pressure and are the least significant of the ICP waves.

BOX 1	Causes of raised ICP.
Increase in CSF volume (common):	
• Hydrocephalus due to various causes (see **Box 2**)	
Increase in brain/tissue volume (common):	
• Brain tumor/abscess/cyst	
• Brain edema due to any cause (tumor, infection, ischemia, metabolic, and head injury)	
• Hematomas in any intracranial compartment (intracerebral, subdural, or epidural)	
Increase in blood volume (uncommon):	
• Hypercarbia	
• Cardiac failure causing increase in central venous pressure	
Decrease in cranial volume (uncommon):	
• Craniosynostosis	

(CSF: cerebrospinal fluid; ICP: intracranial pressure)

CAUSES

Transient elevation of ICP occurs with physiological events such as straining, coughing, and sneezing. There are several pathological causes of raised ICP which can be broadly categorized as those due to increase in volume of the brain parenchyma (edema, abnormal growths, and hematoma), CSF, or blood. In a young child, the growing brain has to be accommodated by corresponding increase in the volume of the skull. If the growth of the skull is prevented by premature closure of the cranial vault sutures (craniosynostosis), then the ICP will rise. **Box 1** shows the pathological causes of sustained increased ICP.

SYMPTOMS AND SIGNS (TABLE 1)

Patients with raised ICP usually present with headache, vomiting, blurring of vision, and diplopia with or without alteration of sensorium. Symptoms and signs in a young child (<2 years of age) consist of enlarging head, bulging anterior fontanel, sun-setting sign (upgaze paresis), dilated scalp veins, and failure to acquire milestones. Severely raised ICP in later stages might present with decerebrate and decorticate posturing. A preterminal event of raised ICP is the development of bradycardia and hypertension (Cushing reflex) caused by herniation of the cerebellar tonsils through the foramen magnum and compression of the medullary cardiovascular centers.

The headache is typically present early in the morning and might wake up the patient. It is holocranial and is associated with vomiting. The vomiting is projectile in nature and is not associated with nausea unlike vomiting associated with abdominal or other systemic causes.

TABLE 1 Symptoms and signs of raised intracranial pressure (ICP).

Symptom/Sign	Feature	Pathophysiology
Common		
Headache	Usually early morning and holocranial	Stretching of dura and increase in $PaCO_2$ during sleep which increases ICP
Vomiting	Early morning, projectile, without nausea	Pressure on the chemoreceptor trigger zone in the medulla
Blurring of vision/visual loss	Intermittent at the peak of headache or persistent	Reduction in the perfusion of the retina
Diplopia	Intermittent at the peak of headache or persistent (*false localizing sign*)	Stretching of the sixth cranial nerve (abducens) and compression against the clivus
Altered sensorium	See the **Table 2** on herniation syndromes for details	Ischemia of the ascending reticular activating system (ARAS) in the midbrain
Infrequent		
Tinnitus	Unilateral or bilateral (*false localizing sign*)	Stretching/ischemia of the cochlear nerve
Hearing loss	Unilateral or bilateral (*false localizing sign*)	Stretching/ischemia of the cochlear nerve
In children only		
Upgaze palsy	Also known as the "sun-setting" sign seen often in young children with severe hydrocephalus	Compression of the tectal region by the enlarged suprapineal recess of third ventricle
Enlarged head ± frontal bossing	Increased head circumference associated with a large anterior fontanel	Sutures which are not fused allow the skull to expand due to increased ICP
Enlarged scalp veins	Large veins especially in the frontal regions	Increased ICP blocks the normal venous channels and blood is diverted into the scalp veins through the emissary veins

Blurring of vision can be present at the peak of the headache or may be constant and is due to the transmission of the raised ICP through the optic nerve sheath which results in venous congestion in the retina. Ultimately, papilledema develops, which can lead to optic atrophy in time and permanent diminution of visual acuity and enlargement of blind spot. Other explanations for blurred vision or transient blindness at the peak of the headache (also known as visual obscurations) are reversible herniation of the parahippocampal gyrus and obstruction of the posterior cerebral arteries supplying the primary visual cortex in the occipital lobes. Diplopia can also be intermittent being present at the peak of the headache and is due to the stretching of the sixth nerve and compression of the nerve against the clivus. Sixth nerve paresis or palsy can be unilateral or bilateral and can be persistent in patients with severely raised ICP.

In a patient with the typical symptoms of raised ICP mentioned above, the optic fundus should be examined for papilledema. It must be remembered that papilledema might not be present in patients in whom the rise in ICP was rapid. It usually takes about 1 week of persistent raised ICP for papilledema to develop.

Cerebellar fits: In patients with raised ICP (particularly, in those with hydrocephalus), episodes of posturing ("cerebellar fits") (that are transient with return of consciousness levels to normal within a few minutes) are often misdiagnosed as seizures and treatment is directed toward seizure control. One should be extremely cautious in making a diagnosis of seizure in a patient with raised ICP without a supratentorial lesion or if the episodes persist despite adequate dosages of anticonvulsant medications.

Herniation syndromes: Altered sensorium is a sign of severely raised ICP and is a consequence of herniation of the temporal lobe or lobes through the tentorial hiatus and compression of the reticular activating system in the midbrain. The types of herniation syndromes and their common clinical features are shown in **Tables 2** and **3**.

INVESTIGATIONS

Measuring intracranial pressure: While papilledema denotes the presence of raised ICP, it cannot quantify it. Bedside tests which can measure the ICP include lumbar puncture (LP) and manometric measurement of the CSF pressure or cranial invasive devices such as ventricular catheters, subdural and extradural bolts, and pressure transducers inserted in the brain parenchyma. Ultrasonographic measurement of optic nerve sheath diameter is also a validated surrogate marker for real-time changes in ICP. It is less invasive and easy to perform at the bedside.

In most clinical situations, measurement of the ICP is not necessary to manage the patient. Continuous ICP monitoring is typically used in the management of patients with head injury where the ICP can change rapidly and urgent interventions might be needed in a patient who is sedated or paralyzed and ventilated and therefore, clinical monitoring is not feasible.

Avoiding lumbar puncture: As a general rule, LP should be avoided in any patient who presents with clinical features of raised ICP with or without papilledema. If there is a clinical indication to obtain CSF sample or check the ICP, then LP can be performed after cranial imaging has ruled out an intracranial mass lesion or hydrocephalus. One such situation is in patients with IIH in which it is as perfectly safe to perform on LP.

The risks of LP in a patient with an intracranial mass lesion include acute transtentorial or transforamen

TABLE 2 Herniation syndromes.

Syndrome	Location of mass	Features
Subfalcine herniation	Supratentorial, unilateral frontal, or parietal lobes	• Usually no specific symptoms except those of raised ICP; late stage—contralateral lower limb weakness due to anterior cerebral artery territory infarction
Uncal herniation	Supratentorial, one cerebral hemisphere	• Altered sensorium • Ipsilateral pupil dilated and nonreactive to light; finally both pupils will be dilated and nonreactive • Contralateral hemiparesis • Ipsilateral hemiparesis can occur due to the Kernohan's notch • Side of dilated pupil is the side of lesion • Do not use side of hemiparesis for lateralization of lesion
Central transtentorial herniation	Supratentorial, bilateral frontal/parietal or callosal or diffuse both hemispheres	See **Table 3** for stages
Tonsillar herniation	• End stage of all herniation syndromes • Posterior fossa	• Cardiorespiratory changes • Bradycardia and hypertension (Cushing reflex) • Finally respiratory arrest precedes cardiac arrest
Upward transtentorial	Posterior fossa	• Upgaze palsy due to tectal compression by the herniating anterosuperior part of the vermis • Altered sensorium

(ICP: intracranial pressure)

TABLE 3 Stages of central herniation.

Stage	Sensorium	Pupils/Eye movements	Respiration	Motor response
Early diencephalic	• Drowsy but arousable • Sighs and yawns	• Small, reacting • Roving	Normal	Localizes pain
Late diencephalic	Not arousable	Small, reacting	Cheyne–Stokes	Decorticate posturing
Midbrain	Comatose	Midpoint, nonreactive	Regular or shallow and rapid	Decerebrate posturing
Pontine	Comatose	Pinpoint, nonreactive	Central neurogenic hyperventilation	Flaccid, flexor response
Medullary	Comatose	Dilated, nonreactive	Ataxic/apnea	Flaccid limbs; no deep tendon reflexes

magnum herniation and death. This may occur over a period of hours after the LP but can also occur several days after the LP as the CSF continues to leak into the subcutaneous tissue from LP needle puncture site in the lumbar dura. Hence, the concept of a "guarded" LP is flawed.

Imaging: A patient with clinical features of raised ICP should undergo cranial imaging, either a contrast-enhanced CT or MR. The pathology being sought is a mass lesion or hydrocephalus. Infrequently, diffuse or focal edema of the brain might be present due to a metabolic or infective cause. An entity where imaging might not reveal any obvious cause for the raised ICP is IIH. This is frequently seen in middle aged, obese women, and may be associated with intake of certain drugs such as oral contraceptives or stenosis of the junction of the transverse and sigmoid sinuses. However, most often an etiology cannot be identified.

MANAGEMENT

The management of raised ICP should be directed at the cause that is identified on brain imaging. For example, in patient with a brain tumor causing raised ICP, the tumor must be excised to provide relief.

The urgency for management of raised ICP depends on the patient's clinical condition. In a patient who complains of headache only and has no other symptoms or signs, the treatment of the cause for the raised ICP can be done some days or even weeks later depending on the natural history of the cause. However, in a patient who presents with one of the herniation syndromes, the raised ICP must be reversed within minutes.

Medical management: Medical management of raised ICP is usually offered as a temporizing measure while preparing for definitive treatment of the cause. Most medical treatments are not effective after a period of few days. Medical management is directed at reducing the volume of one or more of contents of the intracranial compartment. **Table 4** lists the commonly used measures in the intensive care unit (ICU) to treat patients with raised ICP.

Avoid hypercarbia: Carbon dioxide is a potent vasodilator of the intracranial arteries and will lead to an increase in intracranial blood volume. Hence, hypercarbia should be avoided. The partial pressure of carbon dioxide ($PaCO_2$) should be maintained around 40 mm Hg.

Avoid hypotonic intravenous solutions: Hypotonic intravenous solutions such as 5% dextrose should be avoided as they will lead to hypo-osmolality of the blood and increase

TABLE 4 ICU management of raised ICP.

Medication/Intervention	Mechanism/Comments	Route of administration and uses
Reducing CSF volume		
Acetazolamide	Decreases CSF production by inhibiting carbonic anhydrase	• Oral • Mainly used in patients with IIH
External ventricular drainage	Decreases CSF volume by intermittently draining CSF through a ventricular catheter that is also used to measure the ICP	Frequently used in patients with head injury and hydrocephalus
Reducing brain tissue volume		
Dexamethasone	Membrane stabilizer and reduces brain edema	• Oral or IV • Frequently used in neurosurgical patients with tumor-related brain edema and after most brain surgeries
Mannitol	• Osmotic agent which increases plasma osmolality and does not cross the blood brain barrier. It increases flow of water from the brain tissues into the blood • Also improves circulation by altering rheology of RBCs and decreasing blood viscosity	• IV • Frequently used during brain surgery and after as boluses for 48–72 h in patients with brain edema including head injury
Oral glycerol	Osmotic agent which increases plasma osmolality and does not cross the blood brain barrier	• Oral • Can be used for several days or weeks • Frequently used in patients with tumor-related brain edema
Hypertonic saline	Osmotic agent which increases plasma osmolality and flow of water from the brain tissues into the blood	• IV • Used in patients with head injury and during brain surgery
Furosemide	A loop diuretic which lowers ICP by increasing the plasma osmolality due to diuresis and possibly inhibiting CSF secretion	• Oral or IV • Often used with mannitol for synergetic effect
Urea	Osmotic agent but has many side effects and therefore not used presently	• IV • Not presently used
Reducing blood volume		
Head elevation	Increases venous return	Very often used in all patients with raised ICP in the operating room and ICU. The head should be elevated by 15°–30° for optimal effect on ICP without reducing cerebral perfusion pressure
Hyperventilation	By decreasing the $PaCO_2$ it induces vasoconstriction and reduces the blood volume in the cranial cavity	• Very often used in patients with head injury targeting a $PaCO_2$ of around 30 mm Hg. Should be used for brief periods of around 15–30 min • Mild hyperventilation is also used during brain surgery
Barbiturate coma	Reduces cerebral blood volume by decreasing cerebral metabolism	Rarely used in patients with refractory raised ICP, due to high complication rates

Adjunct measures:
- Ensure adequate hydration, oxygenation, and normal mean arterial pressure
- Aggressive steps to maintain normal serum sodium levels
- Antiseizure prophylaxis if there is a supratentorial lesion

(CSF: cerebrospinal fluid)

in brain edema if present. Hypertonic or isotonic solutions such as 5% dextrose saline or Ringer's lactate should be used.

Surgical management: Surgical management of raised ICP is ideally directed to the causative pathology. However, in the case of IIH where a causative pathology is often not discernible, surgery is done to reduce the ICP by diverting the CSF from the intracranial cavity. A thecoperitoneal/VP shunt and endoscopic fenestration of the optic nerve sheath are the two commonly performed procedures.

Decompressive craniectomy is a procedure which provides space for the swollen brain by removing part of the skull and expanding the dural covering. This surgery is most often performed in patients with severe head injury, malignant middle cerebral artery (MCA) territory stroke, and cerebral venous thrombosis (CVT), as there is brain swelling, which is refractory to medical therapy. It can also be offered to patients with metabolic or infective causes for diffuse brain swelling causing raised ICP.

HYDROCEPHALUS

DEFINITION

Hydrocephalus refers to the enlargement of part or whole of the ventricular system in the brain often associated with raised ICP. When both lateral and third ventricles are enlarged with a normal fourth ventricle, it is referred to as triventricular hydrocephalus. Ventricles are generally larger (ventriculomegaly) in older persons as a result of cortical atrophy without a rise in the ICP.

Normal pressure hydrocephalus is a condition affecting older people where there is ventriculomegaly but the measured ICP is within the normal range.

Hydrocephalus *ex vacuo* is a condition in which part or whole of the lateral ventricle can be dilated due to loss of volume of the adjacent brain. This can happen following injury or infarct of a large part of the cerebral hemisphere. Again there is no rise in the ICP in this form of hydrocephalus.

In patients who develop hydrocephalus following ventriculitis, meningitis, or intraventricular hemorrhage, the lateral ventricles may develop septations with separate loculi of CSF. This type of hydrocephalus is termed multiloculated hydrocephalus.

PHYSIOLOGY OF CEREBROSPINAL FLUID

A brief understanding of the production, circulation, and absorption of CSF is important for the management of hydrocephalus.

Production: Cerebrospinal fluid is secreted through an active energy consuming process mainly by the choroid plexus in the lateral and fourth ventricle. There may be other sources such as the ependymal lining of the ventricles.

The volume of CSF in an adult is around 150 mL of which 125 mL is in the subarachnoid spaces and 25 mL in the ventricles. About 500–600 mL of CSF is produced daily. Therefore, the entire CSF in the brain is replaced about 4–5 times every day.

Circulation: The CSF produced in the lateral ventricles flows through the interventricular foramen (foramen of Monro) into the third ventricle and then through the aqueduct to the fourth ventricle. It exits the fourth ventricle through three foramen—midline foramen of Magendie and two lateral foramen of Luschka. The CSF thus enters the large cisterns, cisterna magna, and cerebellopontine angle cisterns and flows into the spinal subarachnoid space and also into the other basal cisterns of the brain.

Absorption: The CSF finally flows over the cerebral hemispheres and is absorbed through the arachnoid granulations in the superior sagittal sinus and other dural sinuses.

Obstructive and communicating hydrocephalus: Hydrocephalus can result from increased production, blockage to the ventricular pathways, or decreased absorption.

Dandy introduced the terms "Obstructive" and "Communicating" hydrocephalus, in the early 1900s while working on a hydrocephalus model in dogs. If a dye introduced into the CSF in the lateral ventricles could be seen in the lumbar CSF obtained through LP, then the hydrocephalus was "communicating," whereas if the lumbar CSF did not contain the dye then the hydrocephalus was "obstructive."

Unilateral or parts of the ventricular system can be enlarged when there is obstruction to the CSF pathway between the different ventricles. However, all four ventricles can be enlarged when there is obstruction at the fourth ventricular outlets or when there is a block in subarachnoid spaces in the brain which prevent the CSF from reaching the arachnoid granulations in the superior sagittal sinus and getting absorbed. Obstruction along the ventricular pathway (foramen of Monro, aqueduct, or the fourth ventricular outlet) causes *obstructive hydrocephalus.* Blockage of CSF flow in the subarachnoid spaces (cisterns) results in *communicating hydrocephalus.* Less frequently, overproduction of CSF such as by a choroid plexus papilloma, can lead to *communicating hydrocephalus.*

CAUSES

The causes of hydrocephalus are numerous. Understandably, the causes of obstructive and communicating hydrocephalus are quite distinct.

Obstructive hydrocephalus (Figs. 4 A and B): The narrowest parts of the ventricular pathways are most prone to obstruction. These are the aqueduct, foramen of Monro, and the fourth ventricular outlets. There can be a congenital obstruction of the aqueduct known as aqueductal stenosis which is the most common form of congenital hydrocephalus. A mass lesion such as a neoplasm or an infective granuloma can obstruct the ventricular pathways from within the ventricle or from outside.

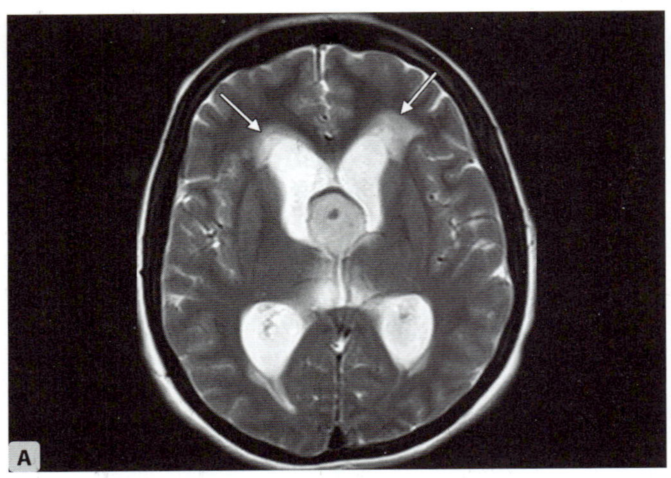

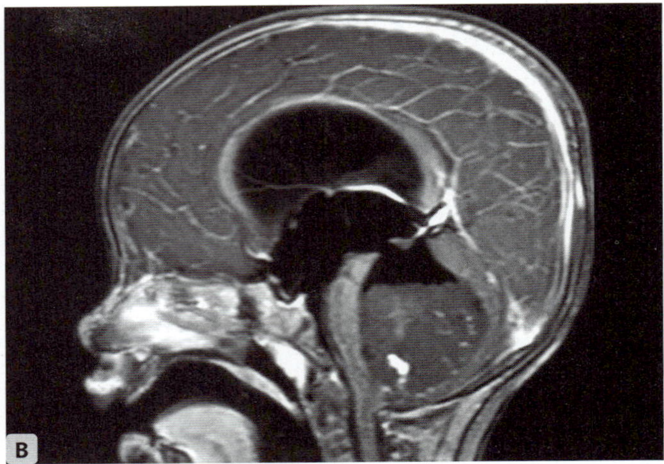

FIGURES 4 A & B: Obstructive hydrocephalus. (A) Axial T2W MR image showing obstructive hydrocephalus due to a colloid cyst in the anterior third ventricle. Note the presence of transependymal seepage of CSF anterior to the frontal horns (arrows). **(B)** Sagittal T1W gadolinium enhanced MR image in a child showing a large tumor in the fourth ventricle with enlargement of the superior part of the fourth ventricle, aqueduct, third and the lateral ventricles.

Communicating hydrocephalus (Figs. 5 A to D): One of the most common causes of communicating hydrocephalus in India is tuberculous meningitis (TBM). Pyogenic meningitis in neonates and infants also is frequent cause of hydrocephalus in children. Hydrocephalus can also be seen in adults several weeks or months following aneurysmal subarachnoid hemorrhage. An infrequent cause of communicating hydrocephalus is Froin's syndrome where the high quantity of protein in the CSF reduces absorption. This is seen with tumors such as small vestibular schwannomas and even spinal cord schwannomas.

Common causes of obstructive and communicating hydrocephalus are listed in **Box 2**.

DIAGNOSIS

A diagnosis of hydrocephalus is suspected in patients presenting with clinical features of raised ICP. CT or MRI is diagnostic procedure of choice. In fetuses and young children (usually <18 months of age) with an open anterior fontanel, ultrasound can be used to image the ventricles.

Although, most clinicians recognize dilatation of the ventricular system on CT or MRI, without actually measuring the size of the ventricles, there are quantitative methods which can objectively confirm the diagnosis.

Evan's ratio (Fig. 6): Evan's ratio or index is calculated by dividing the maximal width of the frontal horns by the maximum internal diameter of the skull in the same axial CT or MR image. While this ratio varies with age and sex, a ratio of >0.3 is considered as ventriculomegaly.

Periventricular lucency (Fig. 7): Another feature to look for in the CT or MR is the presence of hypodensity (on CT) around the frontal horns or occipital horns in the presence of ventriculomegaly. This finding is considered to be diagnostic of raised ICP and is reversible following appropriate therapy. It occurs due to the transependymal seepage of CSF when the intraventricular pressure is elevated.

Contrast imaging (Fig. 8): Contrast imaging is recommended in patients suspected to have hydrocephalus to detect mass lesions which are contrast enhancing and also in patients in whom there is a history suggestive of intracranial infection. In the latter situation, contrast imaging might demonstrate the presence of enhancement of the ependymal lining of the ventricular wall which is diagnostic of ventriculitis.

Obstructive or communicating?

It is difficult if not impossible to distinguish obstructive from communicating hydrocephalus when all the four ventricles are enlarged. A large communication between the fourth ventricle and the cisterna magna might provide a clue to the diagnosis of communicating hydrocephalus but in the absence of this finding, the hydrocephalus might be of either type.

TREATMENT

The treatment of hydrocephalus should be directed toward the cause of the hydrocephalus. For example, in patients with obstructive hydrocephalus due to a cerebellar tumor, excision of the tumor will often relieve the hydrocephalus. But in several instances, the cause of the hydrocephalus might not be amenable to therapy or there if there is delay in the resolution of the etiology, it could lead to irreversible harm to the patient. In such situations, the hydrocephalus itself has to be treated.

Temporary measures: In situations where there could be delay in the treatment or resolution of the cause of the hydrocephalus, temporary procedures can be utilized to relieve the raised ICP caused by the hydrocephalus. Temporary procedures are usually performed in an emergency situation to save the patient's life while preparing for a more permanent treatment.

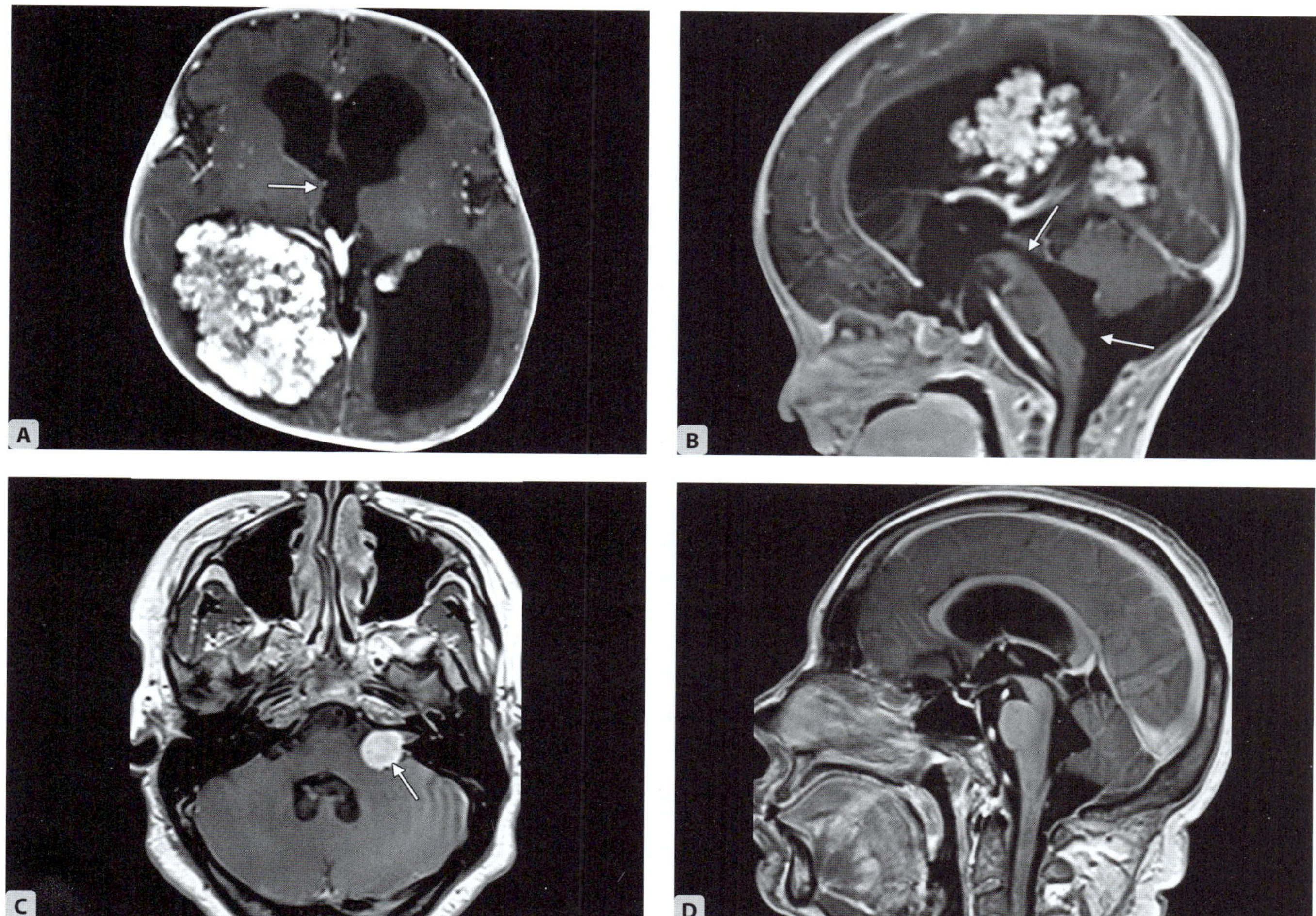

FIGURES 5 A to D: **(A and B) Communicating hydrocephalus in an infant** with a right lateral ventricular choroid plexus. Gadolinium enhanced axial MR image shows the enhancing tumor in the right atrium. Note the open foramen of Monro bilaterally (arrow). **(B)** Sagittal image shows the enlarged aqueduct and open fourth ventricular outlet (arrows). **(C and D) Small vestibular schwannoma with communicating hydrocephalus. (C)** Axial T1W gadolinium enhanced MR image showing a small left vestibular schwannoma (arrow). **(D)** Sagittal T1W gadolinium enhanced MR image showing open fourth ventricle and aqueduct.

Ventricular puncture: This procedure is usually an emergency bedside procedure performed using a twist drill. The drill is used to make a small opening in the skull (usually in the frontal region). A VP needle which is blunt tipped and graduated is then inserted into the frontal horn to tap the ventricle and let out CSF which will be under pressure. However, the needle cannot be left in situ and therefore, the CSF pressure will rise again over a period of few hours. A common indication for this procedure is not for treatment of hydrocephalus but to obtain CSF for diagnosis of leptomeningeal infections when there is an obstructive hydrocephalus and to rule out infection prior to insertion of a shunt in a patient with suspected postmeningitic hydrocephalus.

External ventricular drain: For more prolonged drainage, an external ventricular drain (EVD) is inserted after the VP to continue to drain CSF from the lateral ventricle (usually the frontal horn). It is brought out through a short subcutaneous tunnel in the scalp to drain into a closed drainage system. An EVD can be maintained for a maximum duration of about 5 days as a longer duration increases the risk of infection.

When an EVD has to be in place for a longer duration (such as hydrocephalus associated with active meningitis), then the length of the subcutaneous tunnel is increased and the drain is brought out through the abdominal wall—long-tunnel EVD. This can be maintained for several weeks as the risk of infection is less than the traditional EVD.

Definitive surgery: A shunt from the lateral ventricle to the peritoneal cavity (VP shunt) is most frequently employed shunt in the treatment of hydrocephalus (**Fig. 9**). The CSF which is drained into the peritoneal cavity is absorbed there. The earliest indwelling shunt systems introduced in the 1960s were ventriculoatrial (VA) shunts which were placed in the right atrium. However, VP shunts are safer and have less risk of infection and almost completely replaced VA shunts. VA shunts were also sometimes associated with a complication known as shunt nephritis. Shunts being foreign bodies can be associated with several complications including infection, extrusion, and erosion of skin over the

BOX 2	Common causes of hydrocephalus.
Children	
• Obstructive:	
∘ Aqueductal stenosis	
∘ Dandy–Walker malformation	
∘ Craniopharyngiomas	
∘ Opticochiasmatic hypothalamic glioma	
∘ Arachnoid cysts	
∘ Intraventricular tumors (glioma)	
∘ Tectal glioma	
∘ Cerebellar tumors (medulloblastoma, pilocytic astrocytoma, and ependymoma)	
∘ Cerebellar tuberculoma	
• Communicating:	
∘ Posthemorrhagic	
∘ Postpyogenic meningitis	
∘ TBM hydrocephalus	
∘ Choroid plexus papilloma	
Adults	
• Obstructive:	
∘ Colloid cyst of third ventricle	
∘ Intraventricular tumors (glioma, central neurocytomas, and meningioma)	
∘ Pineal region tumors (pineal parenchymal tumor, epidermoid, and teratoma)	
∘ Tectal glioma	
∘ Posterior fossa tumors (vestibular schwannoma, meningioma, epidermoid, and hemangioblastoma)	
∘ Neurocysticercosis (intraventricular and subarachnoid)	
∘ Cerebellar tuberculoma	
• Communicating:	
∘ TBM hydrocephalus	
∘ Postaneurysmal SAH	
∘ Posthead injury	
Elderly	
• Communicating:	
∘ Normal pressure hydrocephalus	
∘ Carcinomatous meningitis	

(TBM: tuberculous meningitis; SAH: subarachnoid hemorrhage)

shunt components, blockage and migration which can occur even several years after the surgery. Overdrainage leading to subdural hygromas or hematomas and the slit ventricle syndrome are other possible shunt-related complications.

In order to avoid the placement of a foreign body, ETV was introduced in the 1990s. However, ETV is not a panacea for patients suffering from hydrocephalus. It can only be used when the obstruction is distal to the posterior third ventricle. It is most useful in patients with obstruction at the level of the aqueduct.

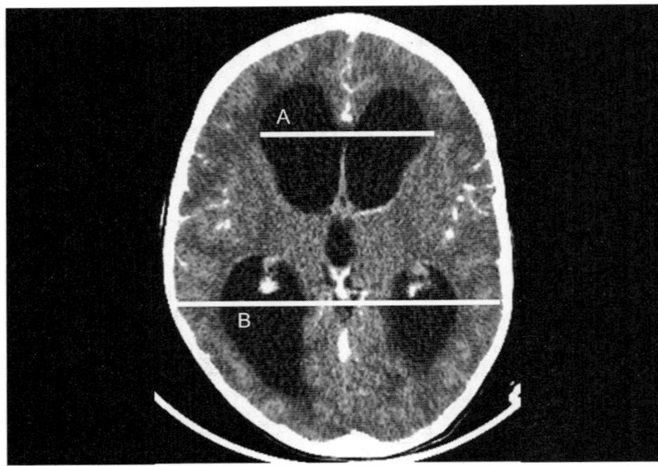

FIGURE 6: Evan's ratio. Axial CT image showing measurement of the Evan's ratio. **A** is the widest diameter of the frontal horns (59 mm). **B** is the widest diameter of the cranial cavity in the same axial plane (115 mm). **A/B** > 0.3 is diagnostic of hydrocephalus. Evan's ratio in this patient is 0.51.

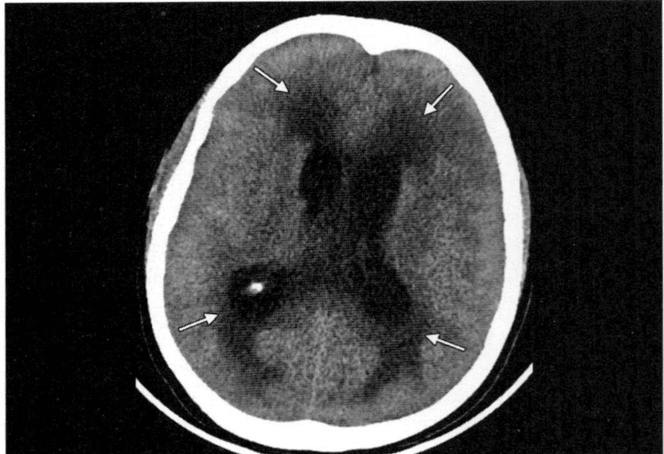

FIGURE 7: Periventricular lucency (PVL). Computed tomography (CT) scan showing PVL around the frontal horns and atria (arrows).

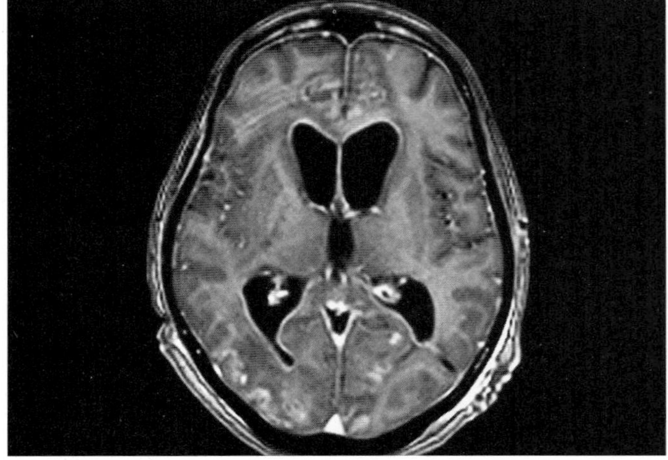

FIGURE 8: Contrast enhanced magnetic resonance (MR) showing ependymitis seen as enhancement of the ependymal lining of the ventricles.

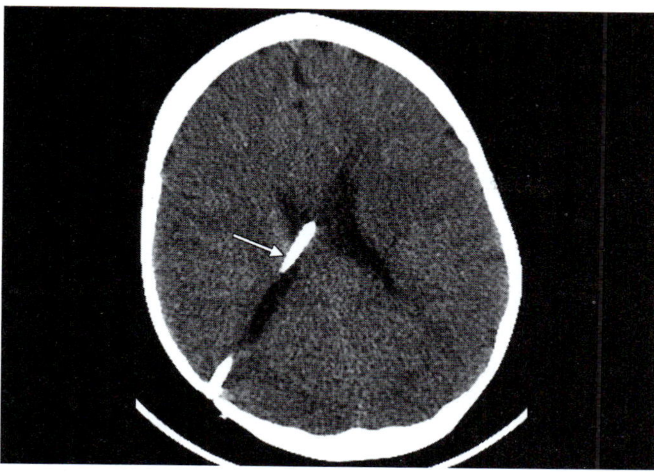

FIGURE 9: Follow-up image after a right-sided VP shunt. CT scan of the patient shown in Figure 6 showing collapsed ventricles suggesting a well-functioning shunt (arrow).

TUBERCULOUS MENINGITIS WITH HYDROCEPHALUS

Tuberculous meningitis with hydrocephalus (TBMH) is a very common cause of hydrocephalus in India. The management of TBMH has been rationalized since the 1990s but there are still some unanswered questions especially regarding the utility of shunts in patients in poor grade TBM. The Vellore grading of TBMH is a useful grading system (**Table 5**) for guiding the management and prognostication in these patients.

TABLE 5 Vellore grading of TBMH.

Grade	Features
I	GCS 15; no neurological deficit
II	GCS 15; neurological deficit present
III	GCS 9–14; with or without neurological deficit
IV	GCS 3–8; with or without neurological deficit

(TBMH: tuberculous meningitis with hydrocephalus; GCS: Glasgow Coma Scale score)

ACKNOWLEDGMENT

I am grateful to Dr Ranjith K Moorthy, Professor of Neurosurgery, for his suggestions.

RECOMMENDED READINGS

1. Dunn LT. Raised intracranial pressure. J Neurol Neurosurg Psychiatry. 2002;73(suppl 1):i23-7
2. Lundberg N. Continuous recording and control of ventricular fluid pressure in neurosurgical practice. Acta Psychiatr Scand Suppl. 1960;36(149):1-193.
3. Posner JB, Saper CB, Schiff ND, Claassen J. Plum and Posner's Diagnosis and Treatment of Stupor and Coma, 5th edition). Oxford: Oxford University Press; 2019.
4. Gallia GL, Rigamonti D, Williams MA. The diagnosis and treatment of idiopathic normal pressure hydrocephalus. Nat Clin Pract Neurol. 2006;2:375-81.
5. Rajshekhar V. Management of hydrocephalus in patients with tuberculous meningitis. Neurol India. 2009;57:368-74.

CHAPTER

185

Seizures and Epilepsy

Gagandeep Singh

ABSTRACT

The occurrence of two or more unprovoked seizures is no longer considered as a correct definition of epilepsy. Epilepsy is a disorder of the brain that is characterized by a long-lasting predisposition to generate epileptic seizures and by its neurobiologic, cognitive, psychological, and social consequences. Clinically either of the condition must occur in epilepsy; at least two unprovoked seizures with a gap of >24 hours; one unprovoked seizure and a probability of further seizures similar to the general recurrence risk that is at least 60% after two unprovoked seizures, occurring over the next 10 years or, diagnosis of an epilepsy syndrome. Seizures are mainly classified into two types; provoked also known as acute symptomatic seizures that result due to some sort of injury to the central nervous system (CNS) or unprovoked seizures.

The epileptic seizure could be of several types based on the signs and symptoms during the event. A detailed history and semiology are crucial for the correct diagnosis. Sometimes, ancillary data, such as electroencephalographic (EEG), magnetic resonance imaging (MRI), and genetic tests are also used to support the diagnosis of seizure types. MRI is considered as the investigation of choice for epilepsy as it shows epileptogenic substrates with high levels of sensitivity and specificity. Treatment of epilepsy and choice of antiseizure medicines (ASMs) depend on the group of symptoms and signs usually occurring together. Moreover, prompt management is critical in cases of status epilepticus.

"The human brain has 100 billion neurons, each neuron connected to 10 thousand other neurons. Sitting on your shoulders is the most complicated object in the known universe"

—Michio Kaku

DEFINITION

Epilepsy is a brain disorder characterized by an *enduring* predisposition to generate *epileptic seizures* and by its neurobiologic, cognitive, psychological, and social consequences. This new and currently followed definition represents a departure from the traditional definition of epilepsy, i.e., the occurrence of two or more unprovoked seizures. From a practical standpoint, the conceptual definition translates to (1) at least two unprovoked (or reflex) seizures occurring >24 hours apart; (2) one unprovoked (or reflex) seizure and a probability of further seizures similar to the general recurrence risk (at least 60%) after two unprovoked seizures, occurring over the next 10 years; (3) diagnosis of an epilepsy syndrome. Epilepsy can be diagnosed under any of three conditions specified above. It is easy to understand the first condition—the application of the 24 hours time period between two unprovoked seizures, although arbitrary, is easy to understand inasmuch as seizures occurring within the close time window of 24 hours are likely to represent seizure clusters. The second and third conditions perhaps require some explanation.

Epilepsy can also be diagnosed when only a single (or first) isolated seizure occurs and the treating physician estimates the risk of seizure recurrence to be high (>60%). Estimating seizure recurrence is undoubtedly difficult. However, some clinical, EEG or imaging findings suggest that the risk of recurrence following a single seizure might be high. Examples of these conditions include but are not limited to evidence of definite epileptogenic abnormality on EEG, the identification of brain tumors or other structural lesions on MRI, the occurrence of antecedent neurological illnesses, e.g., traumatic brain injury. On the contrary, there might be a clinical situation in which an individual has an isolated generalized tonic-clonic seizure with no known epileptogenic antecedents and a normal EEG and MRI. If one were to estimate the risk of recurrence of seizure, this might be <25%. This is based on the risk of recurrence estimated from studies of follow-up of people with a single unprovoked seizures. The last of three conditions refers to epilepsy syndromes. The latter are a set of clinical manifestations with specific age or gender characteristics.

SEIZURES: ACUTE SYMPTOMATIC AND UNPROVOKED

Besides the number of seizures, the presence or not of a provocative factor for seizures is also highly relevant to the diagnosis of epilepsy. Seizures might be classified to provoked (also known as acute symptomatic seizures) or unprovoked. The propensity to recurrent unprovoked seizures constitutes epilepsy. Provoked or acute symptomatic seizures are defined as clinical seizures occurring in close temporal relationship with acute CNS insults, which may be metabolic, toxic, structural, infectious, or inflammatory. Examples of acute symptomatic seizures include post-traumatic and poststroke seizures, seizures during the active phase of neurological infections such as meningitis, encephalitis and neurocysticercosis, and seizures associated with electrolyte imbalance, e.g., hyponatremia and alcohol withdrawal seizures.

The duration between the cerebral insult and acute symptomatic seizure is variable and depends on the underlying insult. In acute stroke and traumatic brain injury, this time period is 7 days. Thus, immediate post-traumatic and immediate poststroke seizures are good examples of provoked seizures. The risk of subsequent or late unprovoked seizures is relatively negligible. Thus individuals with immediate post-traumatic and poststroke seizures perhaps do not require long-term ASMs for two reasons: (1) The risk of late unprovoked seizures is relatively low and (2) None of the currently available ASMs is antiepileptogenic, i.e., these do not prevent the development of epilepsy. Nonetheless, the distinction between provoked and unprovoked seizures is critical, especially from the standpoint of diagnosis of epilepsy.

CLASSIFICATION OF SEIZURES

The next step after a diagnosis of epilepsy is established is to classify the type of seizures. The classification of seizures has also evolved over time and currently, the use of the term, partial seizures is best avoided. Instead, the term, focal seizures may be used (see **Table 1** for complete list of changes in new classification of epilepsy). Focal seizures may remain "focal" without impairment of consciousness or awareness or might be followed by impaired awareness or bilateral tonic-clonic seizures (**Fig. 1**).

In classifying seizures, most experts attempt to elicit the symptoms (**Table 2**) and signs during the paroxysmal event through a perceptive history both from the individual who had the seizure/e and one or more witnesses. The patient's account is of prime importance as it will undoubtedly provide information on the type and sequence of events that take place during a focal seizure in which the patient

TABLE 1 Wording changes.

Old term	New term
Unconscious (still used, not in name)	Impaired awareness (surrogate)
Partial	Focal
Simple partial	Focal aware
Complex partial	Focal impaired awareness
Dyscognitive (word discontinued)	Focal impaired awareness
Psychic	Cognitive
Secondarily generalized tonic-clonic	Focal to bilateral tonic-c onic
Arrest, freeze, pause, and interruption	Behavior arrest

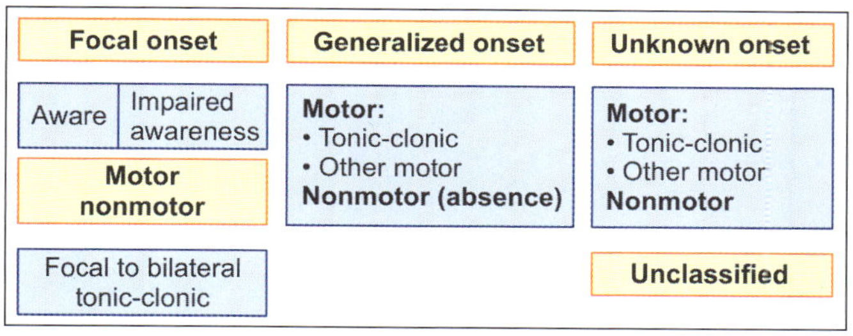

Focal onset		Generalized onset	Unknown onset
Aware	Impaired awareness	**Motor:** • Tonic-clonic • Other motor **Nonmotor (absence)**	**Motor:** • Tonic-clonic • Other motor **Nonmotor**
Motor nonmotor			
Focal to bilateral tonic-clonic			Unclassified

(ILAE: International League Against Epilepsy)

FIGURE 1: Current ILAE seizure classification.

TABLE 2 Common symptoms during seizures.

Symptoms	Medical term
Automatic behaviors	Automatisms
Emotions or appearance of emotions	Emotions
Extension or flexion postures	Tonic
Flushing/sweating/piloerection	Autonomic
Jerking arrhythmically	Myoclonus
Jerking rhythmically	Clonus
Language or thinking problems, déjà vu	Cognitive
Lid jerks	Eyelid myoclcnia
Limp	Atonic
Numb/tingling, sounds, smells, tastes visions, vertigo	Sensations
Pausing, freezing, activity arrest	Behavior arrest
Thrashing/pedaling	Hyperkinetic
Trunk flexion	Spasm

does not loose consciousness or awareness of self and environment.

Obtaining a historical account from the patient also helps in characterizing *the "aura,"* which refers to conscious recollection of perceptual sensation usually at the beginning of the seizure. The aura is not only a warning but also provides important localization information about the cortical region from which the seizure originates or first becomes symptomatic. For instance, a seizure originating from the left primary sensory cortex might produce an abnormal sensation in the right hand, constituting a somatosensory aura while another arising from the right occipital cortex might manifest with a sensation of twinkling stars in the left visual hemifield, thereby constituting a visual aura. It is clear that these phenomena at the beginning of the seizure provide immensely useful information on the localization of the structural lesion that underpins epilepsy. Thus, an aura is basically a focal seizure and information about this can only be obtained from the patient alone. However, as alluded earlier, it is also important to obtain an account of events that take place during the seizure from an eyewitness because the patient most often is unaware or unconscious or is unable to recount the events because of episode amnesia.

Lastly, the elucidation of signs during the seizure can be deduced from observation during video-EEG monitoring or perhaps more conveniently by mobile phone video recordings of the seizures by the witness. Given the widespread availability of video cameras on mobile phones, people with epilepsy should be encouraged to bring in video recordings of their seizures during consultation in clinics. These often might serve the distinguish between epileptic seizures and other conditions such as psychogenic nonepileptic seizures but in addition, the several signs observed in the recordings render information on the unambiguous lateralization and localization of seizures. A list of such signs and their lateralizing and localizing significance is presented in **Table 3** (see also **Videos 1** to **3** with explanations).

Together the symptoms and signs of a seizure are referred to as semiology. Seizures are thus classified according to semiology. While classifying seizures, the clinician looks for familiar patterns of the symptoms and signs (**Tables 2** to **4**) and the sequence thereof (**Fig. 1**). The clinician, however, can make use of ancillary data, e.g., EEG, MRI, and genetic tests to support the diagnosis of seizure types.

Once the necessary semiological information is derived, the next step is to classify seizures. Accordingly, seizures may be classified on a two-step process. The first step is to decide whether, seizures are of the generalized, focal, and unknown variety (**Box 1**). The second step is to decide whether seizures are associated with impaired awareness of self or environment or loss of consciousness. Elements that constitute the assessment of awareness or consciousness are listed in **Box 2**. If awareness is judged to be impaired during the seizure, the latter is classified accordingly, e.g., focal seizures with awareness impaired or otherwise, e.g., focal seizures without impaired awareness (this is simply the occurrence of an aura alone).

The earlier term for focal seizures with awareness impaired was complex partial seizures; the latter term has now been discarded by the International League Against Epilepsy and should not be used. Awareness is always impaired in generalized seizures. Of note, impaired

TABLE 3 Lateralizing signs of focal seizures.

Ictal sign	Subtype	Symptomatogenic zone or mechanism	Lateralization
Motor signs in complex motor seizures	Dystonic limb posturing	Activation of basal ganglia	Contralateral
	Tonic posturing	Activation of SSMA, basal ganglia, cingulum, and primary motor cortex	Contralateral
	Immobile limb	Activation of negative motor areas or exhaustion of primary motor or premotor cortex	Contralateral
	Head turning	Exhaustion of epileptogenic hemisphere, seizure propagate to basal ganglia, or neglect of contralateral space	Ipsilateral
	Facial alterations	Activation of emotional network (amygdala, prefrontal cortex, hypothalamus, orbitofrontal region, insula) or emotional facial movements in cingulum	Contralateral (if facial weakness)
	Eye version	Frontal eye fields (area 8) and extrastriate cortex (area 19)	Contralateral
	Unilateral eye blinking	Mesial temporal structures	Ipsilateral
	Nose wiping	Ictal olfactory hallucinations, increased nasal secretions, or contralateral postictal immobile limb	Ipsilateral
Nondominant temporal signs	Automatisms with preserved responsiveness	Nonspeech-dominant temporal lob and anterior cingulum	Nondominant
	Ictal vomiting	Mesial temporal structures, insula, and mesial frontal regions	Nondominant
	Ictal splitting	Complex automatisms, excessive salivation, or bad mouth sensations	Nondominant
	Ictal urinary urge	Activation of central bladder control	Nondominant
	Peri-ictal water drinking	Hypothalamic involvement	Nondominant
	Ictal/postictal cough	Increased secretions or direct activation of central autonomic system	Nondominant
	Unilateral ear plugging	Superior temporal gyrus	Contralateral
Signs during secondary generalized tonic-clonic seizures	Head version	Premotor area (areas 6 and 8)	Contralateral
	Asymmetric tonic limb posturing	SSMA and precentral area	Contralateral
	Asymmetric ending of clonic jerks	Exhaustion of hemisphere of seizure onset	Ipsilateral
Language manifestation	Ictal/postictal aphasia	Anterior or posterior language areas	Dominant
	Ictal speech	Inhibition of D hemisphere or overexcitement of nondominant hemisphere	Nondominant

awareness generally implies the involvement of neural networks involving both hemispheres. On a different note, focal seizures, which progress to generalized tonic-clonic seizures, are referred to as focal seizures evolving to bilateral tonic-clonic seizures. By another example, a seizure witnessed by someone who enters the bedroom and finds the spouse to be having a tonic-clonic seizure while asleep would be classified as an unknown onset seizure as it cannot be determined whether the seizure began as a focal seizure and evolved to a bilateral tonic-clonic seizure or was generalized from the beginning. Using all the information and scheme described above, it is conveniently possible to classify seizures according to **Figure 1** (see **Table 5**). Lastly, a given individual may have multiple types of seizures, e.g., generalized tonic-clonic, myoclonic, and absence.

CLASSIFICATION OF EPILEPSY

Once, the type/s of seizures are clearly elucidated, the next steps are to expound the epilepsy syndrome and etiology. An *epilepsy syndrome* is *characterized* by a group of symptoms and signs usually occurring together. The features in a *syndrome* may include types of *seizures* commonly seen, age when *seizures* commonly begin, part of the brain involved, usual course, genetic information, EEG, and MRI findings. Examples of epilepsy syndromes are provided in **Flowchart 1**. An attempt must be made to fit in an epilepsy syndrome in every case. However, specific syndromes can be assigned in roughly 10–50% cases only.

Following the diagnosis of an epilepsy syndrome, what remains is to commit to a putative etiology for epilepsy. There is long list of etiological conditions associated with

TABLE 4 Common descriptors of other symptoms and signs during seizures.	
Cognitive	**Automatisms**
Acalculia	Aggression
Aphasia	Eye-blinking
Attention impairment	Head-nodding
Déjà vu or jamais vu	Manual
Dissociation	Oral-facial
Dysphasia	Pedaling
Hallucinations	Pelvic thrusting
Illusions	Perseveration
Memory impairment	Running (cursive)
Neglect	Sexual
Forced thinking	Undressing
Responsiveness impairment	Vocalization/speech
Emotional affective	Walking
Agitation	**Motor**
Anger	Dysarthria
Anxiety	Dystonic
Crying (dacrystic)	Fencer's posture
Fear	Incoordination
Laughing (gelastic)	Jacksonian
Paranola	Paralysis
Pleasure	Paresis
Autonomic	Versive
Asystole	**Sensory**
Bradycardia	Auditory
Erection	Gustatory
Flushing	Hot-cold sensations
Gastrointestinal	Olfactory
Hyper/hypoventilation	Somatosensory
Nausea or vomiting	Vestibular
Pallor	Visual
Palpitations	**Laterality**
Piloerection	Left
Respiratory changes	Right
Tachycardia	Bilateral

These are not seizure types, just suggested descriptive words. A free text description is also highly encouraged.

BOX 1 Focal and generalized seizures: Current conceptual definitions.

- **Focal seizures:** Seizures arising from networks limited to one hemisphere or portions within one hemisphere
- **Generalized seizures:** Seizures arising at some point within and rapidly engaging bilaterally distributed networks
- **Unknown seizures:** Seizures, which cannot be classified with a high degree of confidence as focal or generalized based on available information

BOX 2 Elements of awareness or consciousness used in classification of seizures.

- Awareness of environment around and of ongoing activities
- Awareness of self as being distinct from others
- Responsiveness to verbal and nonverbal stimuli during seizures
- Recall of events that take place during a seizure

epilepsy (**Table 6**). The etiology may be deduced from clinical and demographic data but more often requires elaborate and sophisticated investigations. Epilepsy is just a clinical disorder. It is of crucial importance to determine the underlying etiological condition not only to complete the diagnosis but also from the prognostic standpoint. The prognosis for seizure control (or not) is to a large extent determined by the underlying etiological condition. For instance, there are pathological substrates such as hippocampal sclerosis or cortical developmental malformations, which are inherently highly epileptogenic and often associated with high seizure burdens with poor response to ASMs. Consideration of and work-up for surgical treatments are important considerations in both etiological conditions.

INVESTIGATIONS

Several different investigations may be performed in the work-up of epilepsy but these might be mainly of *three types: Imaging, EEG, and blood tests.* Although both computed tomography and MRI are available for the work-up of epilepsy, the latter, i.e., MRI is the investigation of choice for epilepsy. It demonstrates epileptogenic substrates such as hippocampal sclerosis and cortical developmental malformations with high levels of sensitivity and specificity. MRI should ideally be undertaken on a 3-Tesla scanner using specialized epilepsy protocols, which essentially entail the performance of volume acquired images acquired coronally in a plane perpendicular to the long-axis of the hippocampus. EEG is another investigation, exquisitely useful in the work-up of epilepsy. It is helpful in establishing a diagnosis of epilepsy, which happens when it is unequivocally abnormal and in classifying epilepsies from the syndromic standpoint. The EEG is unequivocally abnormal in 40% of cases of epilepsy and demonstrates nonspecific abnormalities in another 40%. The EEG is normal in 20% cases of epilepsy. A normal EEG does not rule out epilepsy. Contrariwise, about 1% of the general population might demonstrate clearly epileptogenic abnormalities on EEG in the absence of seizures. Epilepsy is a clinical diagnosis and an abnormal EEG does not imply a diagnosis of epilepsy. The yield of EEG improves with the length of recording and also with the use of provocative techniques such as hyperventilation and photic stimulation. The EEG is also helpful in distinguishing between focal and generalized epilepsies. Besides MRI and EEG, a range of blood (or serum) tests might help provide clues to the etiology of epilepsy. Most often, these include genetic blood tests to establish genetic etiologies. Next-generation

TABLE 5 Examples of seizure types.

Word	Definition
Absence, typical	A sudden onset, interruption of ongoing activities, a blank stare, possibly a brief upward deviation of the eyes. Usually, the patient will be unresponsive when spoken to. Duration is a few seconds to half a minute with very rapid recovery. Although not always available, an EEG would show generalized epileptiform discharges during the event. An absence seizure is by definition a seizure of generalized onset. The word is not synonymous with a blank stare, which can also be encountered with focal onset seizures
Absence, atypical	An absence seizure with changes in tone that are more pronounced than in typical absence or the onset and/or cessation is not abrupt, often associated with slow, irregular, generalized spike-wave activity
Arrest	See behavioral arrest
Atonic	Sudden loss or diminution of muscle tone without apparent preceding myoclonic or tonic event lasting approximately 1–2 seconds, involving head, trunk, jaw, or limb musculature
Automatism	A more or less coordinated motor activity usually occurring when cognition is impaired and for which the subject is usually (but not always) amnesic afterward. This often resembles a voluntary movement and may consist of an inappropriate continuation of preictal motor activity

Interventions for emergency department, in-patient setting, or prehospital setting with trained paramedics

↓

Stabilization phase—(0–5 min)

- Stabilize patient (airway, breathing, circulation, disability—neurologic examination)
- Time seizure from its onset, monitor vital signs
- Assess oxygenation, give oxygen via nasal cannula/mask, consider intubation if respiratory assistance needed
- Initiate electrocardiogram monitoring
- Collect finger stick blood glucose. If glucose <60 mg/dL then:
  - Adults: 100 mg thiamine intravenous (IV) then 50 mL D50W IV
  - Children ≥2 years: 2 mL/kg D25W IV Children <2 years: 4 mL/kg D12.5W IV
- Attempt IV access and collect electrolytes, hematology, toxicology screen, (if appropriate) anticonvulsant drug levels

↓

Initial therapy phase—(5–20 min)

A benzodiazepine is the initial therapy of choice (Level A):

- Choose one of the following three equivalent first-line options with dosing and frequency:
  (i) Intramuscular midazolam (10 mg for >40 kg, 5 mg for 13–40 kg, single dose, level A) OR
  (ii) IV lorazepam (0.1 mg/kg/dose, maximum: 4 mg/dose, may repeat dose once, level A) OR
  (iii) IV diazepam (0.15–0.2 mg/kg/dose, maximum: 10 mg/dose, may repeat dose once, level A
- If none of the three options above are available, choose one of the following:
  - IV phenobarbital (15 mg/kg/dose, single dose, level A) OR
  - Rectal diazepam (0.2–0.5 mg/kg, maximum: 20 mg/dose, single dose, level B OR
  - Intranasal midazolam (level B), buccal midazolam (level B)

↓

Second therapy phase—(20–40 min)

There is no evidence based preferred second therapy of choice (Level U):

- Choose one of the following second-line options and give as a single dose:
  - IV fosphenytoin (20 mg PE/kg, maximum: 1,500 mg PE/dose, single dose, level U) OR
  - IV valproic acid (40 mg/kg, maximum: 3,000 mg/dose, single dose, level B) OR
  - IV levetiracetam (60 mg/kg, maximum: 4,500 mg/dose, single dose, level U)
- If none of the options above are available, choose one of the following (if not given already)
  - Intravenous phenobarbital (15 mg/kg, single dose, level B)

↓

Third therapy phase—(40–60 min)

There is no clear evidence to guide therapy in this phase (Level U):

Choices include: Repeat second-line therapy or anesthetic doses of either thiopental, midazolam, phenobarbital, or propofol (all with continuous electroencephalogram monitoring)

FLOWCHART 1: Proposed algorithm for management of convulsive status epilepticus.

TABLE 6 Suggested scheme for an etiological classification of epilepsy.

Main category	Subcategory
Idiopathic epilepsy	Pure epilepsies due to single gene disorders
	Pure epilepsies with complex inheritance
Symptomatic epilepsy	
Predominately genetic or developmental causation	Childhood epilepsy syndrome
	Progressive myoclonic epilepsies
	Neurocutaneous syndromes
	Other neurologic single gene disorders
	Disorders of chromosome function
	Developmental anomalies of cerebral structures
Predominately acquired causation	Hippocampal sclerosis
	Perinatal or infantile causes
	Cerebral trauma
	Cerebral tumor
	Cerebral infection
	Cerebrovascular disorders
	Cerebral immunologic disorders
	Degenerative and other neurologic conditions
Provoked epilepsy	Provoking factors
	Reflex epilepsies
Cryptogenic epilepsies	

sequencing is being used increasingly in order to provide a genetic diagnosis in epilepsy.

DIFFERENTIAL DIAGNOSIS

Several paroxysmal disorders may be confused with epileptic seizures. These include but are not limited to syncope, breath-holding spells, psychogenic nonepileptic seizures, and parasomnias. **Tables 5** and **6** depict the salient differences between epileptic seizures and syncope and psychogenic nonepileptic attacks. Parasomnias, e.g., nightmares, night terrors, and rapid eye movement (REM) sleep behavior disorders also can be confused with nocturnal seizures but there are reliable scales to differentiate between the two conditions.

TREATMENT

A range of ASMs, some traditional and other newer agents are available for the treatment of epilepsy. The choice of ASM and duration of treatment depend on the epilepsy syndrome. For instance, there are conditions such as juvenile myoclonic epilepsy, which are easily controlled with ASMs but require long-term, often life-long treatment. Another epilepsy syndrome, benign epilepsy with centrotemporal spikes, onsets at 5–7 years and remits around 12–14 years and hence requires treatment for this period of time.

Certain ASMs are more effective for focal seizures, e.g., phenytoin and carbamazepine. Other ASMs, e.g., valproate are effective in generalized epilepsies. Many ASMs, particularly newer ones, e.g., topiramate and levetiracetam, are broad spectrum. Certain ASMs may paradoxically worsen seizures, the typical example being carbamazepine, which exacerbates myoclonic and absence seizures.

While treating new-onset epilepsy, monotherapy, i.e., use of a single ASM, should be the rule. Resort to polytherapy is required only when maximally tolerated doses of a single ASM do not control seizures. In choosing ASMs, the side-effect profile and tolerability are also important issues.

DRUG-RESISTANT EPILEPSY

Drug-resistant epilepsy is defined as failure of adequate trials of two tolerated, appropriately chosen and used ASM schedules (whether as monotherapies or in combination) to achieve sustained seizure freedom. A diagnosis of drug-resistant epilepsy leads to consideration of surgical and alternative therapies, e.g., the use of ketogenic diet in children. Drug-resistant epilepsy entails the performance of several sophisticated investigations including MRI with more advanced protocols, long-term video-EEG, positron emission tomography (PET), and single-photon emission computed tomography (SPECT) scans and sometimes intracranial (or stereo-) EEG. These investigations are costly and labor intensive and essentially establish the epileptogenic cortex and the suitability of surgical resection of the epileptogenic lesion. Given appropriate work-up, surgical treatments have a high rate of success in ensuring seizure freedom in drug-resistant focal epilepsies.

STATUS EPILEPTICUS

This is the most serious expression of epilepsy and is defined as the continued occurrence of seizures beyond a time limit of 5 minutes. It should be treated with utmost urgency because any time lost leads not only to failure to control seizures but also to irreversible brain damage. Status epilepticus lasting beyond 30 minutes despite optimal treatment is referred to as refractory status epilepticus and beyond 24 hours as super refractory status epilepticus. Prompt management using a standard protocol is required for the treatment of these conditions.

RECOMMENDED READINGS

1. Scheffer IE, Berkovic S, Capovilla G, Connolly MB, French J, Guilhoto L, et al. ILAE classification of the epilepsies: Position paper of the ILAE commission for classification and terminology. Epilepsia. 2017; 58(4):512-21.

2. Commission on classification and terminology of the International League Against Epilepsy. Proposal for revised classification of epilepsies and epileptic syndromes. Epilepsia. 1989;30:389-99.
3. Fisher RS, Cross H, French JA, Higurashi N, Hirsch E, Jansen FE, et al. Operational classification of seizure types by the International League Against Epilepsy: Position paper of the ILAE commission for classification and terminology. Epilepsia. 2017;58:522-30.
4. Shorvon SD. The etiologic classification of epilepsy. Epilepsia. 2011;52:1052-7.
5. Kwan P, Arzimanoglou A, Berg AT, Brodie MJ, Allen Hauser W, Mathern G, et al. Definition of drug resistant epilepsy: Consensus proposal by the adhoc task force of the ILAE commission on therapeutic strategies. Epilepsia. 2010;51:1069-77.
6. Foldvary-Schaefer N, Unnwongse K. Localizing and lateralizing features of auras and seizures. Epilepsy Behav. 2011;20:160-6.
7. Beghi E, Carpio A, Forsgren L, Hesdorffer DC, Malmgren K, Sander JW, et al. Recommendation for a definition of acute symptomatic seizure. Epilepsia. 2010;51:671-5.

CHAPTER 186

Acute Ischemic Stroke: A Recent Update

Jeyaraj Durai Pandian, Ivy Anne Sebastian

ABSTRACT

Stroke is one of the leading causes of disability and death globally. About 87% of all strokes are ischemic strokes in which the blood supply to one part of the brain is decreased or occluded. With each minute that is delayed to treatment, millions of neurons are damaged irreversibly. Newer advents in stroke care have emerged in acute stroke management, care after stroke, and rehabilitation, which has greatly improved patient outcomes after stroke. Time is brain—Early recognition of stroke and timely reperfusion treatment are crucial for decreasing the morbidity and mortality associated with stroke.

"The brain is the last and grandest biological frontier, the most complex thing we have yet discovered in our universe. It contains hundreds of billions of cells interlinked through trillions of connections. The brain boggles the mind"

—James D Watson

INTRODUCTION

Stroke is an important global health problem and is now the third leading cause of death and disability worldwide. The burden of stroke is higher in low-income and middle-income countries than in high-income countries and is rising. The cumulative incidence of stroke in India ranged from 105 to 152/100,000 persons per year during the past two decades in different parts of the country. Pooled data incorporating multiple studies reveal that ischemic stroke occurs in 68–80% and hemorrhagic stroke in 20–32% in India.

Stroke characterizes an abrupt onset of focal neurological deficit which is attributable to a vascular cause. Based on the causative mechanism, stroke can be broadly classified into two types: Hemorrhagic or ischemic.

Acute ischemic stroke is caused by thrombotic or embolic occlusion of a cerebral artery, whereas hemorrhagic stroke occurs due to rupture of a cerebral artery and subsequent leak of blood into the cerebral parenchyma.

In this chapter, we will be dealing with *acute ischemic stroke*, its classification, mechanisms, and management.

DEFINITIONS

The newer definition of ischemic stroke is, "An episode of neurological dysfunction caused by focal cerebral, spinal, or retinal infarction." Central nervous system infarction includes brain, spinal cord, or retinal cell death attributable to ischemia, based on:

- Pathological, imaging, or other objective evidence of cerebral, spinal cord, or retinal focal ischemic injury in a defined vascular distribution; or
- Clinical evidence of cerebral, spinal cord, or retinal focal ischemic injury based on symptoms persisting ≥24 hours or until death, and other etiologies excluded.

TRANSIENT ISCHEMIC ATTACK

This is defined as "A transient episode of neurological dysfunction caused by focal brain, spinal cord or retinal ischemia without infarction." The current definition of transient ischemic attack (TIA) is based on tissue pathophysiology rather than symptom duration.

PATHOPHYSIOLOGY

Ischemic stroke results from mechanisms that diminish or stop cerebral blood flow (CBF). Thrombosis in situ, thrombotic embolism, or relative hypoperfusion can cause decrease in CBF, with subsequent cell hypoxia and neuronal death.

ISCHEMIC CORE AND PENUMBRA

When a sudden vascular occlusion occurs, as in the case of an ischemic stroke, the affected vascular territory has heterogeneous involvement of ischemia. The magnitude of ischemia depends upon the individual vascular anatomy, site of occlusion, collateral blood supply of the area, and systemic blood pressure. Regions with CBF rates below 10 mL/100 g of tissue/min undergo rapid cell death within minutes of stroke onset, and are referred to as the core. Surrounding the core is a zone of reversible dysfunction with decreased perfusion (<22 mL/100 g of tissue/min), collectively called the ischemic penumbra. The tissue in the penumbra can remain viable for several hours owing to the marginal perfusion; however, if left untreated, it will proceed to infarction. The zone of oligemia is an area of hypoperfusion that correlates with CBF values <60 mL/100 g/min but more than the ischemic threshold of 22 mL/100 g/min. The oligemic zone is usually asymptomatic and recovers without the need for reperfusion treatment. The main objective behind all the reperfusion strategies is to salvage the penumbra (**Fig. 1**).

THE ISCHEMIC CASCADE

At the cellular level, cerebral infarction occurs via two well-defined pathways:

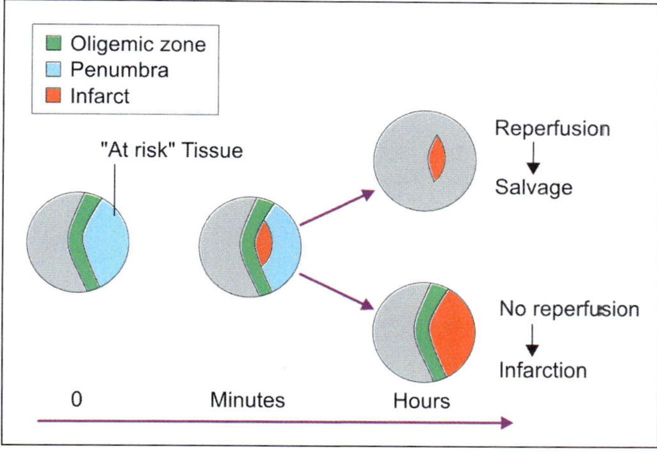

FIGURE 1: Depicting the heterogeneous tissue involvement after ischemia. Lack of reperfusion leads to complete infarction.

1. A necrotic pathway primarily due to depletion of neuronal adenosine triphosphate (ATP) and energy failure.
2. An apoptotic pathway where programmed cell death occurs (**Flowchart 1**).

Over time, usually over weeks to months following infarction, this damaged tissue undergoes liquefaction necrosis, with volume loss leaving behind an area of encephalomalacia and cystic change.

In around 5% of ischemic strokes, spontaneous hemorrhagic transformation of the infarct may occur. Seen more often in large strokes or those of cardioembolic origin, it occurs due to reperfusion injury either from recanalization of the occluded vessel or from collateral blood supply.

RISK FACTORS

Risk factors for ischemic stroke include modifiable and nonmodifiable conditions (**Box 1**). The INTERSTROKE study identified ten potentially modifiable risk factors which collectively were associated with around 90% of stroke globally.

Genetic factors: Substantial evidence now exists that shows that genetic factors contribute to the development of atherosclerosis and other inflammatory mechanisms attributable to stroke. It is now postulated that apart from conventional risk factors such as low-density cholesterol (LDL) and smoking, infections also can contribute to endothelial injury which is the primary inciting event for atherosclerosis. Although inherited risk for stroke is likely polygenic, number of host genetic factors can modify response to these stimuli.

Some of the common gene mutations which increase susceptibility to stroke are:

- *F2* and *F5* gene: Increased risk of thrombosis
- *NOS3*: Involved in vascular relaxation
- *ALOX5AP*: Involved in arachidonic acid metabolism
- *PRKCH*: Involved in major signal transduction systems
- *MTHFR*: Involved in homocysteine metabolism
- *CST3*: Amyloid angiopathy with diffuse amyloid deposition
- *NOTCH 3*: Results in *CADASIL* (Cerebral autosomal dominant arteriopathy with subcortical infarcts and leukoencephalopathy)

Other mutations involving genes *HDAC9, PITX2,* and *ZFHX3* are associated with large-vessel strokes.

CLASSIFICATION OF ISCHEMIC STROKE

TOAST CLASSIFICATION

The system of categorizing stroke mainly based on etiology was developed in the multicenter TOAST (Trial of ORG 10,172 in Acute Stroke Treatment) which denotes the five subtypes of ischemic stroke mechanisms (**Table 1**).

The various etiological subtypes have quintessential findings which can help the clinician to classify the stroke syndrome as "Possible" or "Probable" with an acceptable

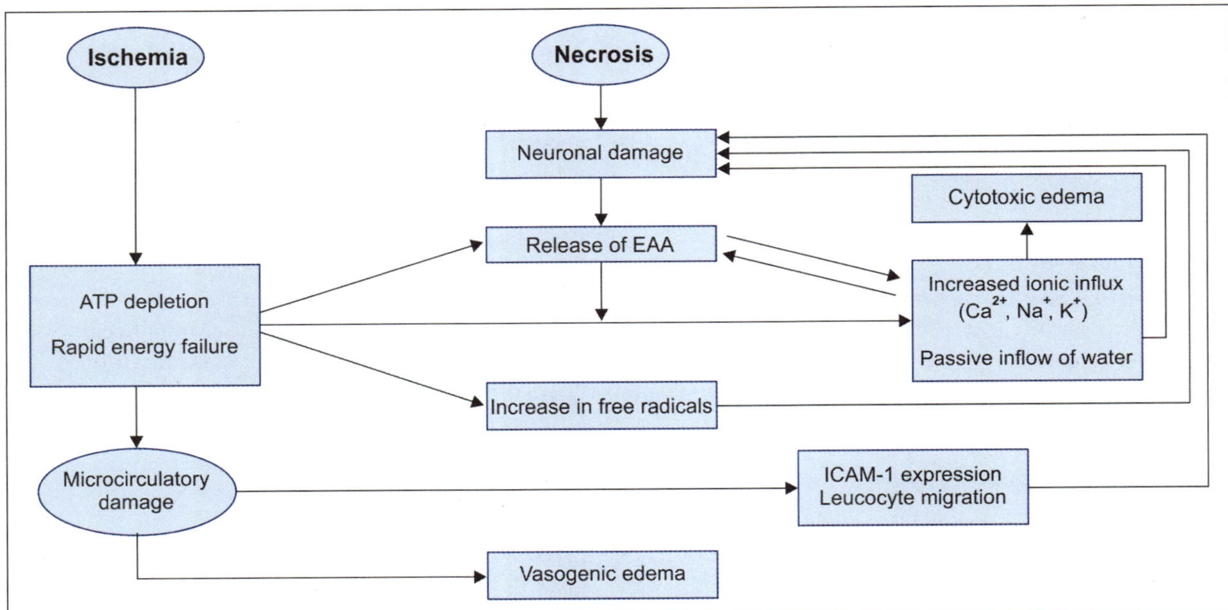

FLOWCHART 1: Even mild reduction in cerebral blood flow (CBF), results in depletion of neuronal ATP and rapid energy failure. The ability to maintain the ionic gradient across cell membrane is lost; influx of sodium (Na^+), calcium (Ca^{2+}), and potassium (K^+) ions occurs, with passive inflow of water leading to cytotoxic edema. Simultaneously, excitatory amino acids (EAA) such as glutamate are released causing more calcium influx, free radical production, and neurotoxicity. Increased expression of intercellular adhesion molecule-1 (ICAM-1) leads to blood–brain barrier breakdown with resultant vasogenic edema.

BOX 1	Risk factors of stroke.
Nonmodifiable risk factors	
• Age	
• Race/ethnicity (African Americans and Hispanics more than whites)	
• Gender (men > women)	
• Family history of stroke/TIA	
Modifiable risk factors	
• Hypertension	
• Diabetes mellitus	
• Cardiac causes:	
◦ Mechanical prosthetic valve	
◦ Valvular disease (mitral stenosis with atrial fibrillation)	
◦ Atrial fibrillation (other than lone atrial fibrillation)	
◦ Left atrial/atrial appendage thrombus Sick sinus syndrome	
◦ Recent myocardial infarction (<4 weeks), left ventricular thrombus, dilated cardiomyopathy, akinetic left ventricular segment, atrial myxoma, infective endocarditis	
◦ Patent foramen ovale, atrial septal aneurysm	
• Dyslipidemia	
◦ Hypercoagulable states: Factor V Leiden deficiency, protein C/protein S deficiency, hyperhomocysteinemia, antithrombin III deficiency, Sickle cell disease	
◦ Oral contraceptive use	
◦ Current smoking/tobacco use	
◦ Alcohol consumption	

Continued...

Continued...

• Dyslipidemia
◦ Illicit drug abuse (e.g., cocaine, LSD)
◦ Physical inactivity, waist-to-hip ratio
◦ Apolipoprotein B/A1 ratio
◦ Chiropractic handling/neck trauma
◦ Migraines

(LSD: lysergic acid diethylamide)

degree of certainty, based on the clinical features, brain imaging computed tomography (CT)/MRI findings, cardiac imaging (echocardiography), Doppler imaging for extracranial [common carotid artery and internal carotid artery (ICA)] and laboratory reports.

- *Probable diagnosis*: Clinical findings, brain imaging, and results of diagnostic tests are consonant with one subtype and other etiologies have been excluded.
- *Possible diagnosis*: Clinical and neuroimaging findings suggest one subtype but other investigations are yet to be done (**Table 2**).

OXFORDSHIRE CLASSIFICATION

The Oxfordshire classification system, also known as the *Bamford classification* system, categorizes stroke based on the initial presenting symptoms and clinical signs. This system does not require imaging to classify the stroke (**Table 3**).

TABLE 1 Etiological classification of stroke according to the TOAST classification.

Large artery atherosclerosis*	• Due to embolization of atherosclerotic fragments in carotid vertebrobasilar and cerebral arteries, typically proximal to major branches • In situ thrombosis and plaque ulceration also can occur
Cardioembolism*	• 20% of acute ischemic strokes • Originate from aortic arch and heart (valvular and mural thrombi) • "Paradoxical embolization" through patent foramen ovale
Small-vessel occlusion*	• Obstruction of deep penetrating branches of major arteries • Represent around 13–20% of all ischemic strokes • Related to hypertension, usually • Microatheroma formation, lipohyalinosis, and hyaline arteriosclerosis are pathological hallmarks
Stroke of other determined etiology*	• Rare causes such as hypercoagulable states, hematological disorders, and vasculopathies • Detailed evaluation to identify etiology and exclude other causes
Stroke of undetermined etiology	• Negative evaluation • Incomplete evaluation • Unidentified stroke etiology • Sometimes multiple etiologies may be found causing inability to determine causative etiology with certainty

*Possible or probable depending on results of ancillary studies.

(TOAST: Trial of ORG 10,172 in Acute Stroke Treatment)

CLINICAL APPROACH

"Neurology is learned "stroke by stroke."

—Charles Miller Fisher

Stroke is the prototype of a focal, well-circumscribed brain lesion. Any patient who presents with a sudden onset of a focal neurological deficit, headache, or alteration in sensorium, should be evaluated for stroke.

CLINICAL PRESENTATION

While almost all stroke patients will present with an abrupt onset of focal neurological deficit such as motor weakness, sensory loss, and speech or language deficits, the clinical presentation may vary depending upon the blood vessel affected. An intimate understanding of the cerebral anatomy and vasculature is therefore essential to determine stroke localization.

Simplistically, the blood supply of the brain can be divided into *anterior (carotid) and posterior (vertebrobasilar)* circulations. The various blood vessels, the structures they supply, and their clinical manifestations are given in **Table 4**.

PHYSICAL EXAMINATION

The aim of the physical examination is to have an objective assessment of the baseline deficit to monitor the temporal course, and to establish the stroke severity for prognostication and management of the patient. The examination must include examination of level of consciousness and vital signs, and neurological examination given in **Table 5**.

No clinical feature distinguishes ischemic from hemorrhagic stroke, although some points may tip the balance in favor of one over the other. Headache, nausea, vomiting, alteration in sensorium, and raised blood pressure are more often seen in hemorrhagic strokes as compared to ischemic strokes; however, a brain imaging in the form of CT/MRI scan is ultimately needed to confirm diagnosis.

TABLE 2 Clinical and other distinguishing features between the etiological subtypes of stroke.

Features	Large-artery atherosclerosis	Cardioembolism	Small-artery occlusion	Other causes
Clinical				
• Cortical or cerebellar involvement	Yes	Yes	No	May be seen
• Lacunar syndrome	No	No	Yes	May be seen
Neuroimaging				
• Cortical, cerebellar, brainstem, or subcortical infarct >1.5 cm	Yes	Yes	No	May be seen
• Subcortical or brainstem infarct <1.5 cm	No	No	May be seen	May be seen
• Multiple, scattered infarcts in bilateral hemispheres involving different vascular territories	No	Yes	No	May be seen
• Extracranial ICA stenosis	Yes	No	No	No
• Cardiac source of emboli	No	Yes	No	No
• Other abnormality on tests	No	No	No	Yes

(ICA: internal carotid artery)

TABLE 3	Oxfordshire classification of stroke.
Syndrome	**Definition**
Total anterior circulation syndrome (TACS) Total anterior circulation is involved	All the following three need to be present: • Unilateral weakness (and/or sensory deficit) of the face, arm and leg • Homonymous hemianopia • Higher cerebral dysfunction (dysphasia, visuospatial disorder)
Partial anterior circulation stroke (PACS) Only part of anterior circulation is involved	Two of the following need to be present: • Unilateral weakness (and/or sensory deficit) of the face, arm and leg • Homonymous hemianopia • Higher cerebral dysfunction (dysphasia, visuospatial disorder)
Lacunar stroke (LACS) Subcortical stroke secondary to small vessel disease	One of the following needs to be present: • Pure sensory stroke • Pure motor stroke • Sensorimotor stroke • Ataxic hemiparesis
Posterior circulation syndrome (POCS) Involvement of posterior circulation	One of the following need to be present: • Cranial nerve palsy and a contralateral motor/sensory deficit • Bilateral motor/sensory deficit • Conjugate eye movement disorder (e.g., horizontal gaze palsy) • Cerebellar dysfunction (e.g., vertigo, nystagmus, ataxia) • Isolated homonymous hemianopia

TABLE 4	Blood supply of the brain and its applied anatomy.	
	Structures supplied	**Clinical manifestations**
Anterior cerebral artery (ACA)	• **Cortical branches:** Medial frontal and parietal lobe • **Medial lenticulostriate branches:** Caudate head, globus pallidus, anterior limb of internal capsule	• Disinhibition and speech perseveration • Primitive reflexes (grasping, sucking reflexes) • Altered mental status • Impaired judgment • C/L weakness (legs > arms) • C/L cortical sensory deficits • Gait apraxia • Urinary incontinence
Middle cerebral artery (MCA)	• **Cortical branches:** Lateral frontal and parietal lobes, lateral and anterior temporal lobe • **Lateral lenticulostriate branches:** Globus pallidus and putamen, internal capsule	• C/L hemiparesis (face, arm > leg) • C/L hypesthesia • I/L hemianopia • Gaze preference toward side of lesion • Agnosia • Motor and/or sensory aphasia (if involving dominant hemisphere) • Neglect, inattention, and extinction of double simultaneous stimulation (nondominant hemisphere usually)
Anterior choroidal artery (AChA)	Optic tracts, medial temporal lobe, ventrolateral thalamus, corona radiata, posterior limb of the internal capsule	
Posterior cerebral artery (PCA)	• **Cortical branches:** Occipital lobes, medial and posterior temporal and parietal lobes • **Perforating branches:** Brainstem, posterior thalamus, and midbrain	• C/L homonymous hemianopsia • Cortical blindness • Visual agnosia • Altered mental status • Impaired memory

Continued...

Continued...

	Structures supplied	Clinical manifestations
Posterior inferior cerebellar artery (PICA)	Inferior vermis, and posterior and inferior cerebellar hemispheres	• Vertigo • Nystagmus • Diplopia, Visual field deficits • Dysphagia • Dysarthria • Facial hypesthesia • Syncope • Ataxia
Anterior inferior cerebellar artery (AICA)	Anterolateral cerebellum	
Superior cerebellar artery (SCA)	Superior vermis; superior cerebellum	

TABLE 5 Approach to physical examination in a suspected stroke patient.

	Assess	To look for
Level of consciousness	Airway, breathing, and circulation	Whether patient is able to maintain airway or not
Vital signs	Heart rate, pulse rate	Irregular rhythm, unequal pulses, absent pulses in extremities, carotid bruit
	Blood pressure (BP)	Hypertension, hypotension, unequal BP in extremities
	Respiratory rate, saturation	Tachypnea, hypoxemia
	Ocular fundus	Retinopathy, emboli, hemorrhage
Neurological examination	Rapid but complete examination of the neuraxis including cranial nerves, speech, and language deficit, motor or sensory deficit, and cerebellar involvement	Focal neurological deficit

STROKE MIMICS

Conditions which may present with symptoms similar to a stroke, however, are not due to a vascular cause. Up to 19% patients diagnosed as strokes, prior to brain imaging, were stroke mimics in one study.

Most common causes:

- Hypoglycemia
- Seizure
- Systemic infection
- Brain tumor
- Toxic-metabolic disorders such as hyponatremia and hypoglycemia
- Positional vertigo
- Conversion disorder

EVALUATION

APPROACH IN THE EMERGENCY ROOM

As soon as a patient with suspected stroke reaches the emergency room, the stroke-on-call team is immediately alerted. Meanwhile, the emergency doctor and emergency staff nurse should quickly stabilize the patient.

Time is brain—With each minute of delay in treatment, 1.9 million neurons are lost. This is equivalent to 12 km (7.5 miles) of myelinated fibers being destroyed. The ischemic brain ages 3.6 years with each hour of delay in treatment. With the advent of reperfusion therapies in stroke, the main intent while approaching a patient with stroke is to salvage penumbra. Therefore, history and examination while accurate should also be rapid and brief. Key points to be kept in mind while approaching a patient with stroke are summarized in **Box 2**.

LABORATORY STUDIES

Extensive laboratory testing is not routinely required before deciding for fibrinolysis. However, detailed laboratory tests should be done at a later stage to avoid missing pertinent findings (**Table 6**).

IMAGING STUDIES

Every patient with a suspected stroke should undergo emergent brain imaging within 30 minutes of arrival to hospital so as to:

- Confirm the diagnosis of stroke.
- Establish mechanism of stroke.
- Rule out mimics (subarachnoid hemorrhage and subdural hemorrhage).

Computed tomography scanning:

- Noncontrast CT scanning is the most used modality of imaging in the acute stroke setting.
- Multimodal CT imaging and CT perfusion (CTP) with vessel imaging techniques such as CT angiography (CTA) help to identify large-vessel occlusions (LVO) and areas of salvageable tissue.
- Ease of accessibility, rapid acquisition, shorter period of imaging, and lower cost are some of its benefits.
- In addition, it can be performed in patients who are unable to tolerate or have contraindications for an MRI examination.

Magnetic resonance imaging (MRI): Magnetic resonance imaging with magnetic resonance angiography (MRA) provides a more detailed imaging of the brain parenchyma. Diffusion-weighted imaging (DWI) sequence is highly sensitive to early cellular edema, and can detect ischemia much earlier than standard CT scan. It has proved to be sensitive for detection of intracranial hemorrhage as well. However, it is more time consuming and not as easily available as CT scanning. Some patients may be unable to tolerate or may have contraindication to an MRI (pacemaker implantation and aneurysmal coiling).

Brain imaging findings in acute ischemic stroke: Computed tomography and MRI findings in acute ischemic stroke vary, depending upon the time from stroke onset to imaging. For ease of remembering, they have been classified according to the different times given in **Table 7** and shown in **Figures 2** to **7**.

Magnetic resonance imaging findings: Within minutes of arterial occlusion DWI sequences on MRI reflect hyperintensity with a corresponding low-signal/hypo-intensity on apparent diffusion coefficient (ADC) sequences. This is known as DWI restriction and is one of the first changes to be visible on MRI in acute ischemic stroke. After around 5–6 hours, T2 weighted (T2W) and T2 fluid-attenuated inversion recovery (FLAIR) images show hyperintensity which continues to increase over the next few days, whereas T1 weighted (T1W) images reflect a hypointensity in the corresponding areas. Gradually over

BOX 2 Approach to a patient with stroke.

- Check vitals (blood pressure, pulse rate, and saturation); Stabilize ABC
- Confirm the presence of stroke syndrome
- Distinguish stroke from stroke mimics
- Establish two intravenous (IV) lines and IV fluids
- Clearly establish the time of onset of stroke, or last-seen-well time
- Focused medical history to identify etiology, risk factors, and any concomitant conditions
- Objective assessment of stroke severity
- Identify conditions that may influence treatment decisions (e.g., recent surgery or trauma, active bleeding, active infection, and use of oral anticoagulant drugs)

TABLE 7 Chronological evolution of Ischemic stroke on computed tomography (CT).

Stages	CT
Immediate	• Hyperdense sign and dot sign • Earliest visible sign • Direct visualization of intravascular thrombus/embolus • Most commonly seen in middle cerebral artery
Early hyperacute (0–6 h)	• Loss of gray-white matter differentiation • Insular ribbon sign • Hypoattenuation of deep nuclei • Cortical hypodensity, associated parenchymal swelling, gyral effacement
Acute (24 h to 1 week)	• Marked hypoattenuation and swelling • Mass effect (especially in large infarcts)
Subacute (1–3 weeks)	• Swelling starts to subside • CT fogging phenomenon: Small cortical petechial hemorrhages result in elevation of the attenuation of the cortex
Chronic (>3 weeks)	• Swelling decreases • Gliosis appears as a region of low density and negative mass effect • Cortical mineralization can sometimes occur, and is seen as hyperdensity

TABLE 6 Blood investigations in a stroke patient.

Urgent tests	• Random blood sugar	• Rule out hypoglycemia/hyperglycemia
	• Coagulation studies	• If patient is on oral anticoagulants
	• Complete blood count	• Thrombocytopenia, anemia, polycythemia, thrombocytosis, thrombocytopenia, leukemia
Routine blood tests	• Renal and liver profile	• Hyponatremia, hypokalemia, renal or hepatic insufficiency
	• Fasting lipid profile	• Dyslipidemia
	• Thyroid profile	• Hypothyroidism, thyrotoxicosis
	• Glycosylated hemoglobin (HbA1c)	• Diabetes mellitus, impaired glucose levels
	• Cardiac biomarkers	• Concomitant myocardial infarction (MI)
	• Vasculitic workup	• Vasculitis
Additional tests	• Homocysteine level	• Hyperhomocysteinemia
	• Toxicology screen	• Drug overdose
	• Pregnancy test	
	• Rapid plasma reagent (RPR)	

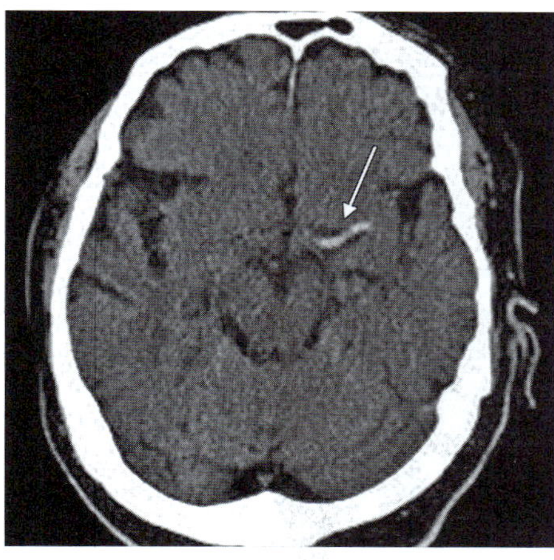

FIGURE 2: Hyperdense left middle cerebral artery (MCA) sign.

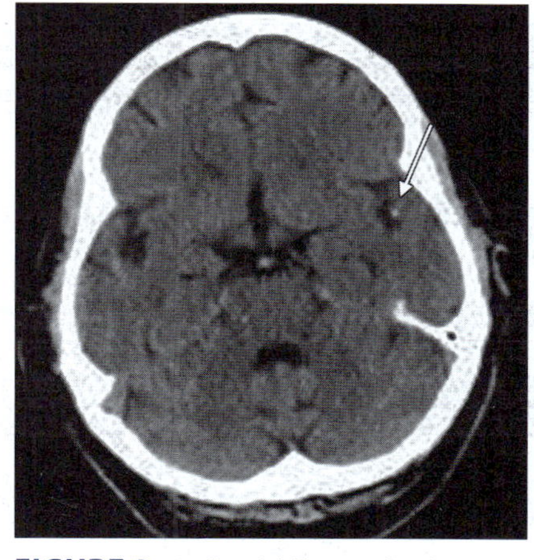

FIGURE 3: Left middle cerebral artery (MCA) dot sign. [Represents thromboembolism within a segmental branch of the MCA located within Sylvian fissure (M2 segment, when MCA is viewed in axial section)].

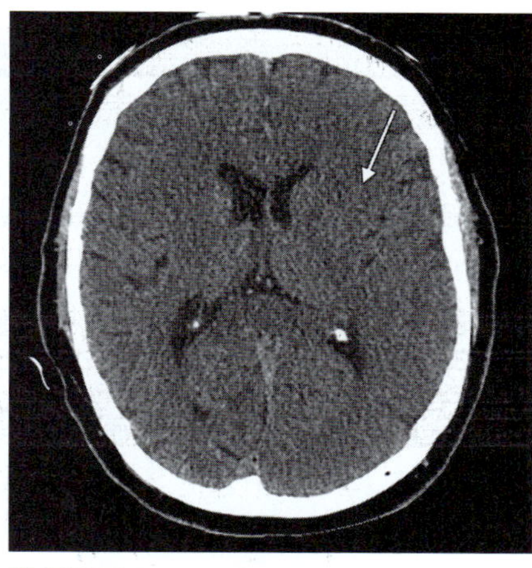

FIGURE 4: Loss of gray-white differentiation in the left (arrow).

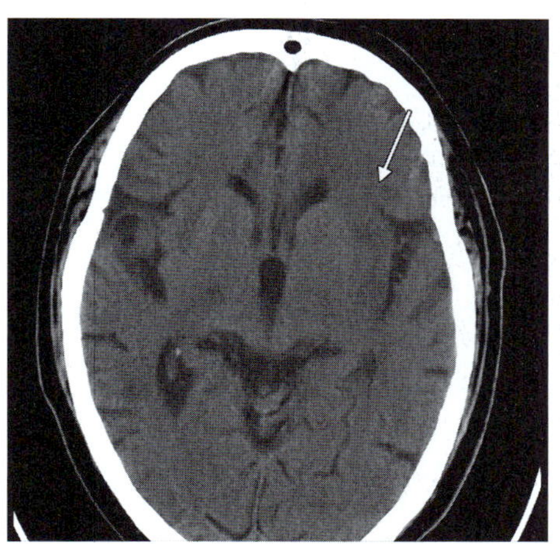

FIGURE 5: Insular ribbon sign—loss of the normal insular cortex gray-white differentiation.

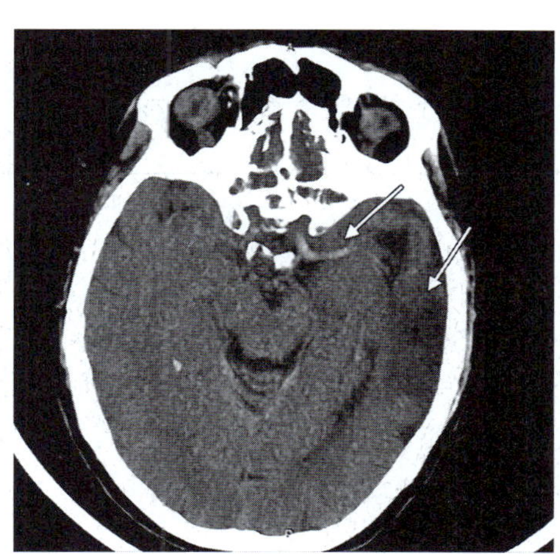

FIGURE 6: Established left middle cerebral artery (MCA) territory infarct with left MCA hyperdense sign.

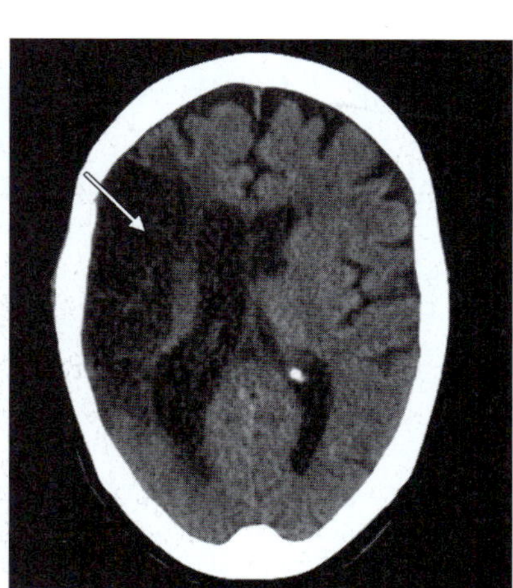

FIGURE 7: Chronic right middle cerebral artery (MCA) territory infarct.

days, low signals on ADC get brighter and this is known as "pseudonormalization." As the stroke becomes subacute to chronic, the DWI restriction disappears and only the T1W hypointensity remains (**Figs. 8** and **9**).

Other imaging studies: Carotid Doppler scanning is a valuable test and is increasingly being done in the acute stroke setting. It not only helps identify the etiology of stroke but also helps classify patients for either medical management or carotid intervention if they have carotid stenoses.

Transcranial Doppler ultrasonography is useful for evaluating more proximal vascular anatomy—including the middle cerebral artery (MCA), intracranial ICA, and vertebrobasilar artery—through the infratemporal fossa.

Digital subtraction angiography (DSA) is the definitive method for evaluating vessel pathology including occlusions, stenoses, dissections, and aneurysms involving aortic arch as well as large vessels of the neck (**Figs. 10** to **12**).

Echocardiography is obtained in all patients with acute ischemic stroke in whom cardiogenic embolism is suspected.

Chest radiography should be done in acute stroke; however, it should not delay the administration of thrombolysis as decision-making in most cases would not be affected.

HYPERACUTE MANAGEMENT OF STROKE

As soon as the CT scan is done, both radiologist and stroke physician/neurologist must report the scan and rule out any signs of hemorrhage.

What is the window period?

Window period refers to the window of time during which ischemic strokes should be treated for better outcomes. Studies have shown that fibrinolytics when given within 3–4.5 hours of acute ischemic stroke onset, are most effective and result in improved outcomes, thereby known as the WINDOW PERIOD.

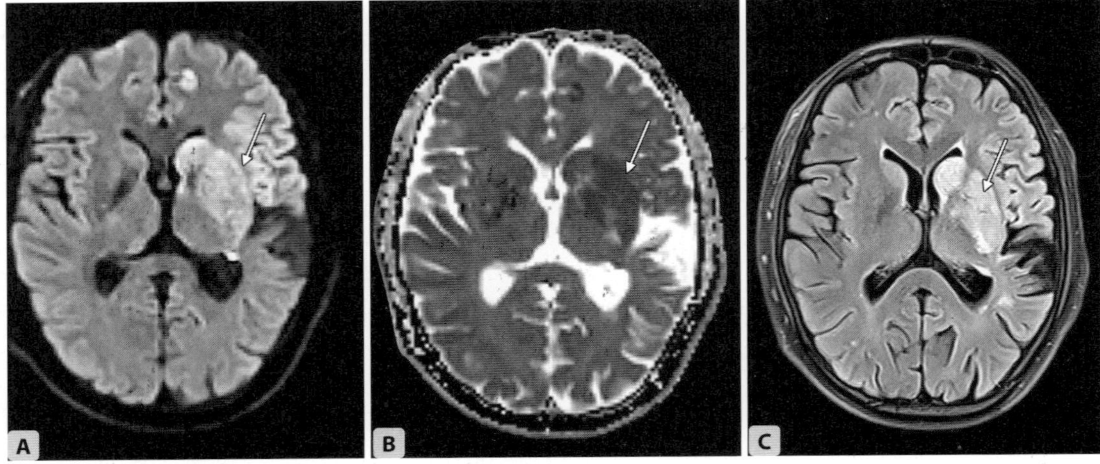

(FLAIR: fluid-attenuated inversion recovery; MCA: middle cerebral artery)

FIGURES 8 A to C: (A) Diffusion-weighted imaging (DWI) hyperintensity seen in left MCA territory; **(B)** Corresponding ADC drop (reduced signal); **(C)** T2 FLAIR image showing hyperintense lesion in corresponding region.

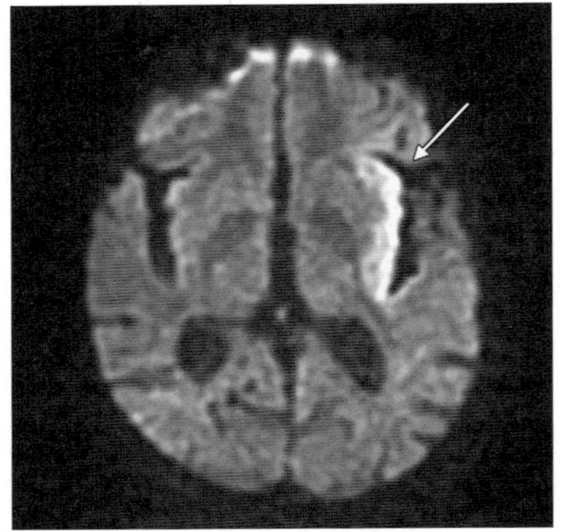

(MRI: magnetic resonance imaging)

FIGURE 9: Loss of insular ribbon on MRI.

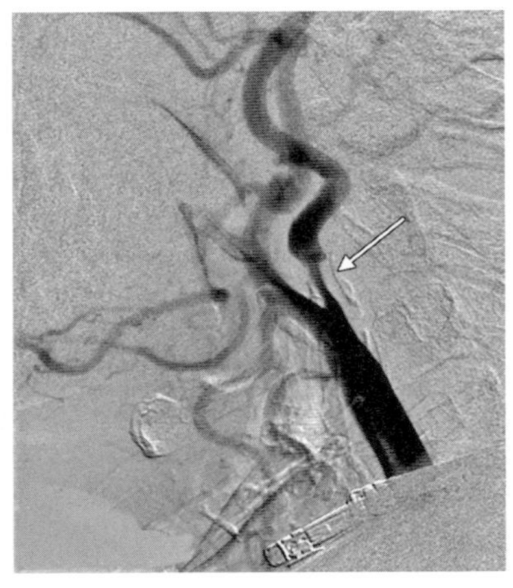

(DSA: digital subtraction angiography; ICA: internal carotid artery)

FIGURE 10: DSA image showing stenosis of the ICA.

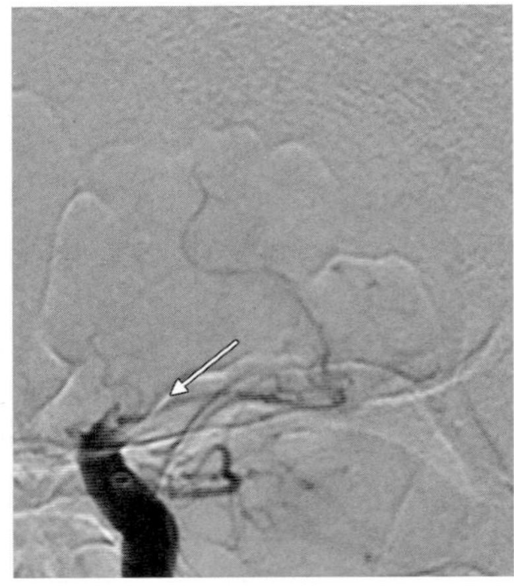

(DSA: digital subtraction angiography; ICA: internal carotid artery)

FIGURE 11: DSA image showing left distal occlusion of the intracranial ICA.

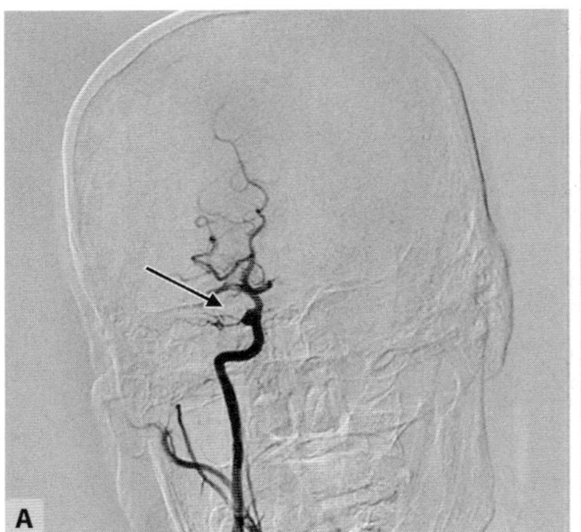

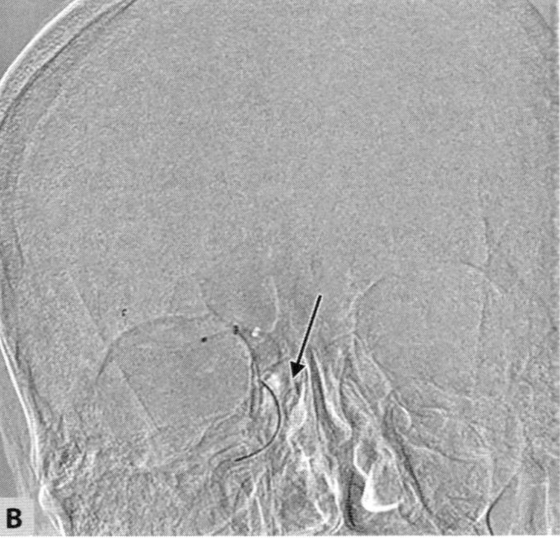

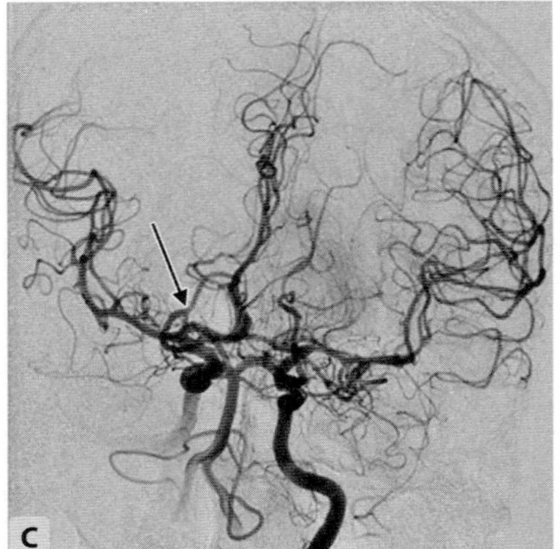

(DSA: digital subtraction angiography; MCA: middle carotid artery)

FIGURES 12 A to C: (A) DSA image showing occlusion of the right MCA; **(B)** Presence of stent in right MCA; **(C)** DSA images showing recanalization of right MCA after removal of clot using stent retriever.

If the patient is within the window period for thrombolysis, an informed consent must be taken after excluding all contraindications for the same.

Patient should immediately be shifted to stroke unit and proceeded with thrombolysis.

If patient is out of window period, then patient should be managed with antiplatelets and/or anticoagulants as required.

FIBRINOLYTIC THERAPY

Tissue plasminogen activator (tPA) or actilyse, as the name itself indicates, specifically targets fibrin clots and breaks them up by activating plasminogen, thereby restoring blood flow in the affected vessels. However, it does increase the risk of hemorrhage and therefore should be given in carefully selected patients.

How to administer?

Actilyse is given at a total dose of 0.9 mg/kg body weight. 10% of this calculated dose is given as an IV bolus while the remaining 90% is given as a slow IV infusion.

Inclusion criteria:

- Patients >18 years of age
- Symptoms and signs of clinically definite acute stroke
- Clearly established time of stroke onset that will allow thrombolysis to be given within 4.5 hours
- Intracranial or subarachnoid hemorrhage excluded by CT/MR brain scanning
- Independent prior to stroke

Exclusion criteria for thrombolysis are given in **Table 8**.

Complications of IV actilyse:

- Spontaneous intracerebral hemorrhage (ICH) (6.4%) (**Fig. 13**)
- Orolingual angioedema (5.1%)
- Bleeding from other sites

Performance indicators for hyperacute stroke management are given in **Box 3**.

Tenecteplase is a new type of tissue plasminogen activator of increasing interest for treatment in acute ischemic stroke. It has higher fibrin specificity and longer half-life than alteplase, thereby providing ease of single-bolus administration. It has a lower bleeding risk compared to alteplase. It is currently being studied in several trials and has been found noninferior to alteplase, with few studies having shown higher reperfusion and better functional outcomes with tenecteplase. There is moderate-quality evidence to choose tenecteplase (dose 0.25 mg/kg) over alteplase in patients eligible to undergo mechanical thrombectomy. Future trials are needed to further evaluate the efficacy and safety of tenecteplase in patients who are ineligible for alteplase.

ENDOVASCULAR TREATMENT

Endovascular treatment (EVT) or mechanical thrombectomy refers to the procedure in which the blood clot causing occlusion is removed from the blood vessel. Microcatheters are inserted from the groin or arm and directed toward the large vessel which is occluded, and

TABLE 8 Exclusion criteria for thrombolysis.

Absolute exclusion criteria	• Stroke or significant head trauma within 3 months
	• Major surgery or serious trauma within 14 days
	• GI or GU (genitourinary) hemorrhage within 21 days
	• Arterial puncture at a noncompressible site within 7 days
	• History of ICH, intracranial neoplasm, AVM, or aneurysm
	• Active internal bleeding
	• Clear and large hypodensity on CT scan, Malignant MCA infarction
	• Serum glucose <50 (If symptoms persist after correction, or infarct is verified, consider IV rtPA)
	• Current bleeding diathesis
	  ○ INR ≥1.7
	  ○ Heparin within 48 h with abnormal PTT
	  ○ Platelets <100,000/mm^3
	  ○ NOACs use within 48 h
	  ○ On warfarin (regardless of INR)

Relative contraindications	• Minor deficit (NIHSS <5)* • MI in the past 3 months • Seizure at presentation • Pregnancy: Weigh risks and benefits in individual context

**Exclusions to the rule*: Complete hemianopia, aphasia, visual or sensory extinction, motor weakness limiting sustained effort against gravity. Rapidly improving deficits are not a contraindication unless remaining deficit is minor.

(GU: genitourinary; IV rtPA: intravenous recombinant tissue plasminogen activator; MI: myocardial infarction; NOACs: non-vitamin K oral anticoagulants; NIHSS: National Institutes of Health Stroke Scale)

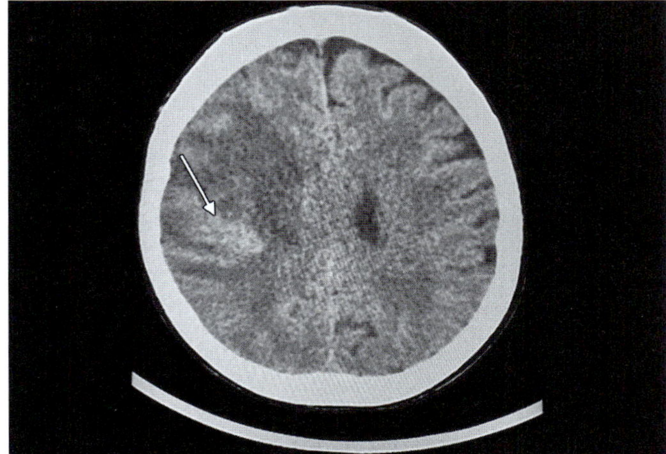

(MCA: middle carotid artery; NIHSS: National Institutes of Health Stroke Scale)

FIGURE 13: CT head of a patient with diabetes, hypertension, and atrial fibrillation with large right MCA infarction (NIHSS 29), post thrombolysis showing confluent regions of homogenous hyperdensities within the infarct tissue with no/minimal mass effect suggestive of hemorrhagic transformation.

BOX 3	Performance indicators for hyperacute stroke management
• Door to physician ≤10 min	
• Door to stroke team ≤*15 min*	
• Door to computed tomography (CT) initiation ≤*25 min*	
• Door to CT interpretation ≤45 min	
• Door to IV tPA ≤*60 min*	
• Door to stroke unit admission ≤3 h	
• The presence of an acute stroke team, primed and prepared for the arrival of any stroke patients recommended as part of MDT stroke system of care	

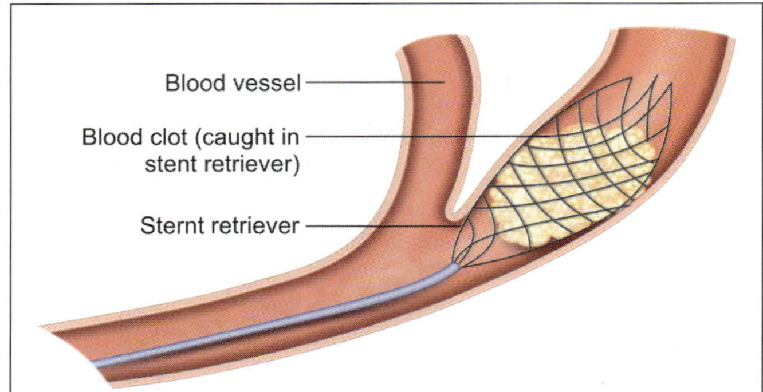

FIGURE 14: Pictorial representation of stent retriever being used to remove blood clot from lumen of blood vessel.

through aspiration devices or stent retrievers, the clot is suctioned or pulled out (**Fig. 14**). Sometimes a thrombolytic agent can directly be given into the artery which is occluded; this is known as intra-arterial thrombolysis.

Endovascular treatment has become the main treatment in ischemic stroke due to large-vessel occlusion [LVO, i.e., MCA (M1, M2 segments), anterior cerebral artery (ACA), ICA-terminus occlusion, and basilar artery]. It can be offered in patients who are even out of the window period for thrombolysis. The current indications for EVT are given below:

- LVO: Symptom onset <6 hours, National Institutes of Health Stroke Scale (NIHSS) of ≥6, Alberta Stroke Program Early CT score (ASPECTS) >6;
- LVO in the anterior circulation: Symptom onset—6–16 hours, and meeting the **DAWN**[1] or **DEFUSE-3**[2] eligibility criteria.
- LVO in anterior circulation: Symptom onset—16–24 hours, and meeting other DAWN eligibility criteria. (Level IIa)

[1] **DAWN criteria** were based on clinical imaging mismatch. Patients were further classified into three groups:
1. Age <80 years, with NIHSS ≥10 and core volume—0–30 mL
2. Age <80, NIHSS ≥20, core volume—31–50
3. Age ≥80, NIHSS ≥10, core volume—0–20 (**Figs. 15** to **18**).

[2] **DEFUSE 3 criteria** were based on CT or MR perfusion imaging determined by an automated processing system and included patients ≥18 years of age, with NIHSS >6, with LVO (ICA and/or M1), with core volume <70 mL and penumbra/core mismatch ratio >1.8.

STROKE UNIT CARE

A stroke unit is a designated area within the hospital which is exclusive for the management of stroke patients, where a coordinated multidisciplinary team specializing in stroke management attends to the patient.

Stroke patients who received organized inpatient care in a stroke unit were more likely to be alive, independent, and living at home 1 year after the stroke.

STRUCTURE AND FUNCTIONING OF A STROKE UNIT

Structure and functioning of a Stroke unit is given in **Table 9**.

STROKE UNIT CARE PROTOCOLS

Management of hypertension: Patients with ischemic stroke may often have high blood pressure, and require careful management (**Table 10**).

Intravenous fluids: IV Fluids preferably *normal saline* should be given to maintain hydration. Continue for longer if the patient is kept nil per orally. Avoid dextrose solutions due to potential risk of worsening cerebral edema.

Oxygen replacement: Oxygen supplementation should be considered in stroke patients if they are drowsy, hypoxemic or hypotensive, and has shown outcome benefits.

FeSS protocol: Management of simple physiological abnormalities such as *F*ever, *S*ugar and *S*wallow in patients with stroke translates to better outcomes.

Fever causes release of excitotoxic aminoacids and increased inflammatory response. Source of infection should be sought and treated. Regular paracetamol administration to maintain temperatures <37°C is recommended.

Hyperglycemia is associated with poor outcome in stroke, regardless of diabetic status. Blood sugar should be controlled and maintained between 90 and 200 mg/dL.

Every stroke patient must undergo a formal swallow assessment before receiving anything orally including medications. If patient fails swallow assessment, early nasogastric (NG) feeds should be initiated.

Management of complications: Stroke patients, especially those with large strokes are prone to various complications.

Pneumonia is one of the most common complications and occurs due to aspiration, or ill-timed oral feeding. Broad-spectrum antibiotics, frequent suctioning, chest physiotherapy, and nebulization should be used as required.

Prolonged immobilization can lead to formation of deep vein thrombosis (DVT). Prophylaxis with low molecular weight heparin or unfractionated heparin is the treatment

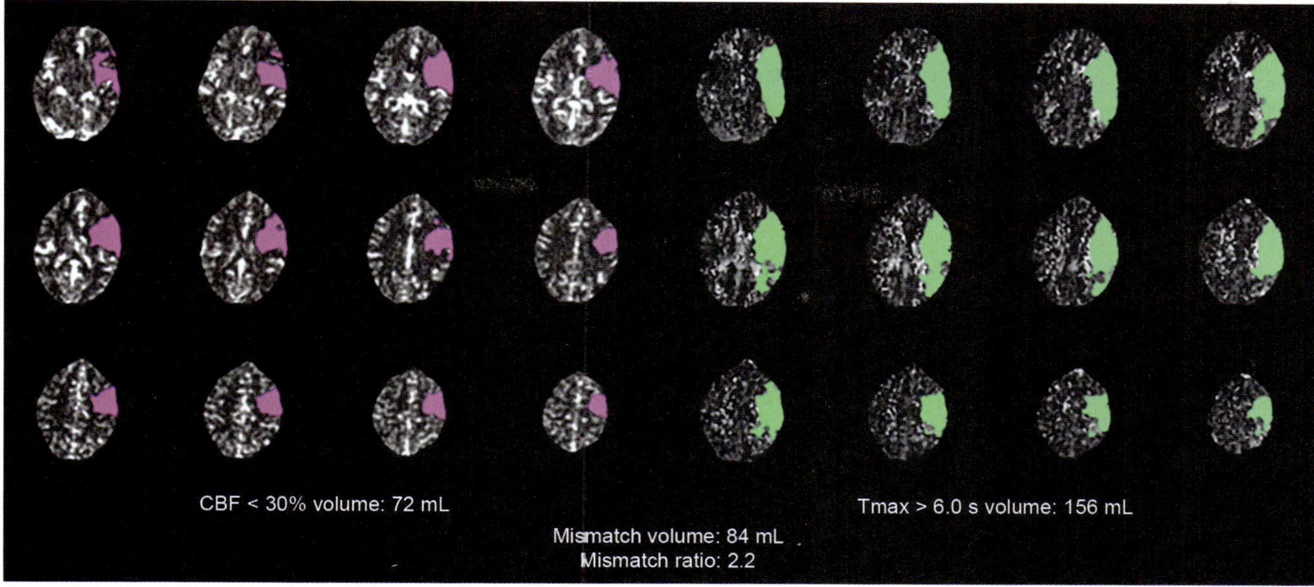

(CBF: cerebral blood flow; CTP: computed tomography perfusion)

FIGURE 15: Color-coded CTP images with CBF and time to maximum (Tmax) maps. Infarct core is represented by CBF map (pink color, CBF < 30%; volume: 72 mL) and ischemic tissue (infarct core and ischemic salvageable penumbra) is represented by Tmax map (green color, Tmax > 6 s; volume: 156 mL). Mismatch volume (Tmax/CBF)represents ischemic but salvageable penumbra, 84 mL. Mismatch ratio (Tmax/CBF) > 1.8 is significant.

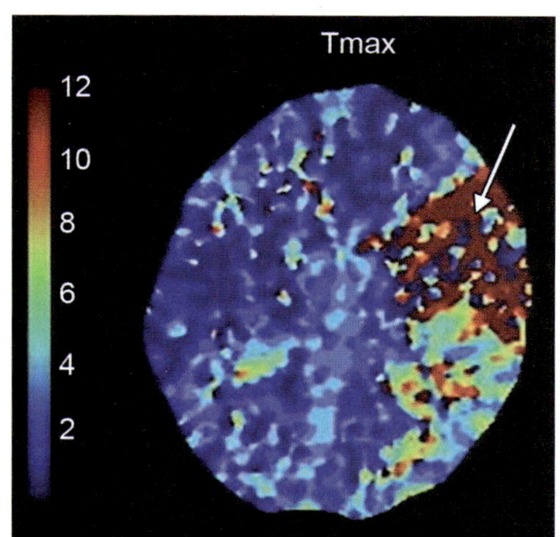

(CTP: computed tomography perfusion; Tmax: time to maximum)

FIGURE 16: Color-coded Tmax CTP map with scale on the right side shows infarct core (Tmax >10 s, red color) and ischemic tissue (Tmax >2 s, green–yellow color).

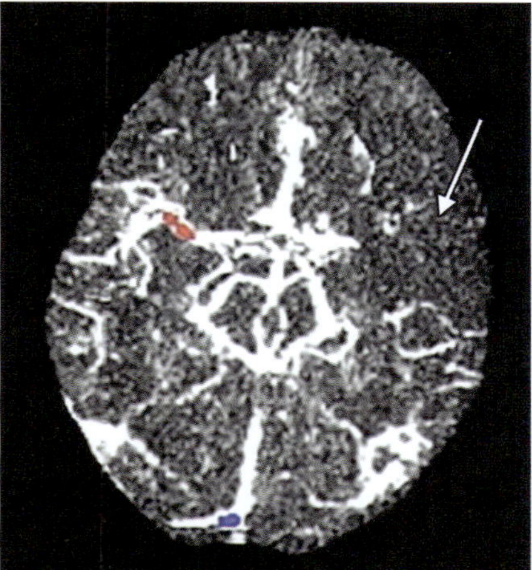

(CTP: computed tomography perfusion)

FIGURE 17: Maximum intensity projection (MIP) image of CTA shows occlusion of left M1 MCA with some flow in the posterior temporal region through leptomeningeal collaterals.

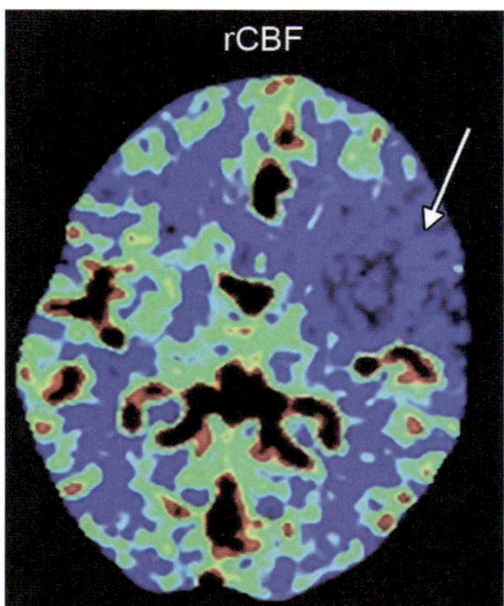

(CBF: cerebral blood flow)

FIGURE 18: Color-coded relative CBF CTP map shows wedge-shaped area of infarct (CBF < 30%, blue color) in left frontotemporal region.

of choice; however, risk of hemorrhage must be considered. Intermittent pneumatic compression devices are also effective.

Raised intracranial pressure (ICP) can occur in large strokes with edema and mass effect. Anti-edema measures such as mannitol (0.25–0.5 g/kg/4–6 hourly), Lasix or hypertonic saline (3% saline) infusion, and head elevation should be done. Intubated patients can be hyperventilated to reduce ICP.

Rehabilitation after stroke: Early rehabilitation after stroke is important and helps improve outcomes. The caregiver for the patient should be identified early and patient and caregiver should be involved in identifying short-term and long-term recovery goals. Early discharge planning is recommended and family should be involved in the decision-making. Arrangements for the stroke patient at home for rehabilitation should be planned for to help in expedited recovery.

TABLE 9	Structure and functioning of a stroke unit.
Infrastructure	• At least **four to six** designated "stroke beds" • Monitoring facilities for ECG, BP, and saturation, and access to ICU • Rehabilitation area
Personnel	• Multidisciplinary team (MDT) of stroke physician, nurses, physiotherapist, occupational therapist, speech and language pathologist and social worker
Stroke unit care*	• Hypertension management • FeSS protocol • Prevention of ***DVT*** and PE • Management of stroke complications
Early rehabilitation and discharge planning	• Identification of caregiver • Involvement of patient and family in recovery goal setting and discharge planning
Secondary prevention	• Antiplatelets and statins • Anticoagulation (documented AF) • Control of risk factors • Carotid endarterectomy and stenting in selected cases

* Protocols of stroke management are explained in the following text. (Also, see **Table 11**).

(FeSS: fever, sugar and swallow)

TABLE 10	Protocols of stroke management.			
Patients eligible for thrombolysis				
Pre-thrombolysis	If blood pressure (BP) ≥185/110 mm Hg	Injection labetalol bolus 10–20 mg; Repeat once if required	Nicardipine infusion 5 mg/h. Increase by 2.5 mg/h at 5–15-min intervals (maximum dose of 15 mg/h)	If BP still ≥185/110 mm Hg, defer thrombolysis
During and post thrombolysis	If BP ≥180/105 mm Hg	Injection labetalol bolus 10–20 mg; repeat every 10–20 min (maximum dose 300 mg) or Labetalol infusion at 2–8 mg/min	Nicardipine infusion at 5 mg/h; Increase by 2.5 mg/h every 5–15 min intervals	If BP still uncontrolled, consider sodium nitroprusside
Aggressive BP monitoring: Check BP Q15 min during thrombolysis and for another 2 h, Q30 min for 6 h, then Q1 h for next 16 h				
Patients not eligible for thrombolysis				
• Permissive hypertension is recommended in ischemic stroke not eligible for reperfusion				
• Lower BP only if ≥220/120 mm Hg; lower by 15% over first 24 h				
• Labetalol 10–20 mg IV bolus can be given; it can be repeated				
• Monitor BP Q2H in all stroke patients				
• Avoid calcium channel blockers (can cause sudden hypotension)				

SURGICAL MANAGEMENT

Despite acute interventions such as intravenous thrombolysis and EVT, up to 10% of strokes result in large areas of infarction.

Malignant MCA infarction is associated with significant edema, raised ICP, secondary brain injury, transtentorial herniation, and high (80%) mortality rates. Such patients may require urgent surgical intervention in the form of decompressive hemicraniectomy to combat life-threatening raised ICP and limit extensive tissue damage (**Fig. 19**).

Indications for surgery:

- Malignant MCA infarction
- CT evidence of infarction of at least 50% of MCA territory
- Perfusion deficit of >66% on CT
- Infarct volume > 82 mL within 6 hours of onset (on MRI)
- Or infarct volume > 145 mL within 14 hours on DWI

Advantages:

- Decreasing ICP and prevent transtentorial herniation
- Improve penumbra perfusion
- Decrease mortality

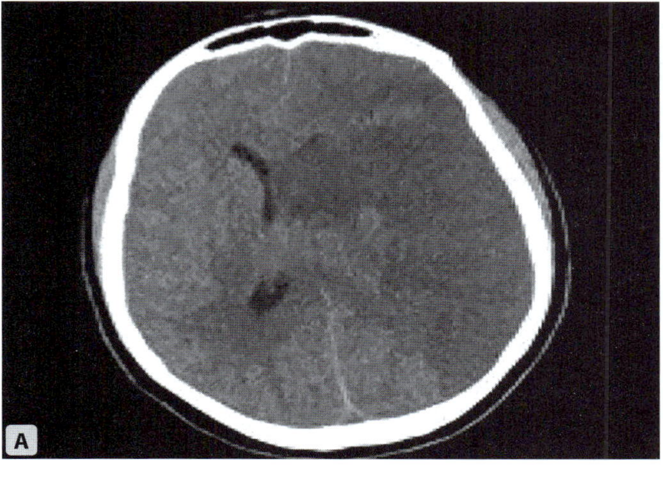

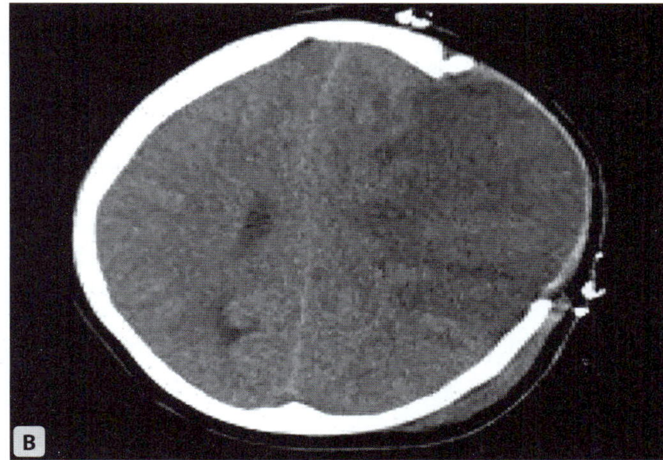

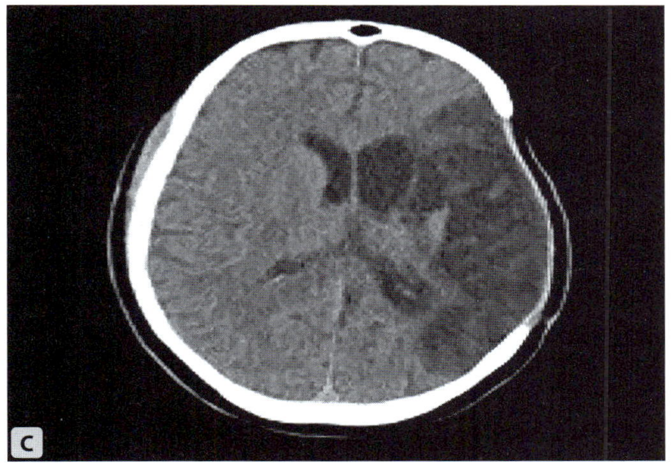

(CT: computed tomography; MCA: middle cerebral artery)

FIGURES 19 A to C: (A) Preoperative CT scan of a patient with left-sided malignant MCA infarction. **(B)** CT head status-post decompressive hemicraniectomy (Day 1). **(C)** Post-operative, 3rd week CT head showing no midline shift.

Disadvantages:

- Highly invasive procedure
- Resource intensive (monetary cost, neurosurgeons, OT, ICU care)

Cerebellar infarction is another entity which requires close monitoring. Cerebral edema secondary to infarction in the posterior fossa can rapidly result in fourth ventricle obstruction, brainstem compression, or fatal herniation of cerebellar tonsils through foramen magnum, all of which are urgent indications for surgery.

In the presence of any clinical neurological deterioration or worsening of sensorium, the above should be suspected and suboccipital decompressive craniotomy should be considered.

CONCLUSION

Time is brain. Every minute conserved is millions of neurons saved. With the advent of newer treatment pathways and widening indications for EVT, the window for offering treatment to patients with stroke has expanded largely, potentially reversing the significant disability associated with the disease. However, it also implies a need for improving our systems of care and the efficiency of delivering them. Early detection and timely referral to a stroke-ready center is vital for optimal outcomes. Stroke unit care is a cost-effective intervention which can decrease mortality and improve outcomes even in patients presenting beyond the window period, which can be effectively applied even in resource-poor settings. Timely swallow assessment; appropriate management of blood pressure, sugar, and body temperature; initiation of antiplatelets within 48 hours; and prevention of complications are essential. Promoting early rehabilitation measures, control of other risk factors, and encouraging an early supported discharge are crucial to favorable outcomes. A protocoled approach that involves the entire continuum of stroke care can result in significant transformation in stroke morbidity and mortality.

ACKNOWLEDGMENTS

We acknowledge Dr Vivek Agarwal, Assistant Professor, Division of Neuro and Vascular Intervention, Christian Medical College and Hospital, Ludhiana, for providing neuroimaging and digital subtraction angiography images.

RECOMMENDED READINGS

1. Kim J, Thayabaranathan T, Donnan GA, Howard G, Howard VJ, Rothwell PM, Feigin V, et al. Global stroke statistics 2019. Int J Stroke. 202015(8):819-38.

2. Zerna C, Thomalla G, Campbell BC, Rha JH, Hill MD. Current practice and future directions in the diagnosis and acute treatment of ischaemic stroke. The Lancet. 2018;392(10154):1247-56.
3. Pandian JD, Kalkonde Y, Sebastian IA, Felix C, Urimubenshi G, Bosch J. Stroke systems of care in low-income and middle-income countries: challenges and opportunities. The Lancet. 2020;396(10260):1443-51.
4. Pandian JD, William AG, Kate MP, Norrving B, Mensah GA, Davis S, et al. Strategies to improve stroke care services in low-and middle-income countries: a systematic review. Neuroepidemiology. 2017;49(1-2): 45-61.
5. Langhorne P, de Villiers L, Pandian JD. Applicability of stroke-unit care to low-income and middle-income countries. The Lancet Neurology. 2012;11(4):341-8.
6. Bernhardt J, Urimubenshi G, Gandhi DB, Eng JJ. Stroke rehabilitation in low-income and middle-income countries: a call to action. The Lancet. 2020;396(10260):1452-62.
7. Winstein CJ, Stein J, Arena R, Bates B, Cherney LR, Cramer SC, et al. Guidelines for adult stroke rehabilitation and recovery: a guideline for healthcare professionals from the American Heart Association/ American Stroke Association. Stroke. 2016;47(6): e98-169.

CHAPTER 187

Hemorrhagic Cerebrovascular Diseases

MV Padma Srivastava, Ajay Garg

ABSTRACT

Hemorrhagic stroke [intracerebral hemorrhage (ICH)] accounts for 10–15% of all strokes worldwide although there exists stroke belts with increased percentage of ICH (40–45%) in parts of India (Northeast and East) and is far eastern countries (China and Japan). ICH carries a high mortality and morbidity, the rates of which have not changed much over last several decades: Immediate mortality in first 48 hours is the highest (50%). Disability assessment at 6 months shows a mere 20% to be independent after a major ICH. The focal signs and symptoms accompanying ICH reflect the location of the hemorrhage and are indistinguishable from ischemia occurring in the same vascular territory.

Plain CT scan of the brain remains the mainstay of diagnosis of ICH. Hematoma volume and presence of intraventricular hemorrhage (IVH) are the two most significant predictors of early neurological deterioration; however, factors such as glucose concentration, levels of fibrinogen, and increased BP should also be taken into consideration. Hematoma expansion is considered to be an independent indicator of poor outcome as well as mortality. For improving functional outcome, early after ICH presenting with systolic blood pressure (SBP) between 150 and 220 mm Hg, acute reduction of SBP to 140 mm Hg is safe (Class I, Level A) as well as effective. For evacuating an ICH, the four identified surgical procedures include the following: 1. Simple aspiration, 2. Craniotomy with open surgery, 3. Endoscopic evacuation, and 4. Stereotactic aspiration. The improvement of the standardization of clinical treatment protocols as well as clinical research studies in ICH can be done by using scale such as ICH score.

"The secret of change is to focus all of your energy not on fighting the old, but on building the new"

—Socrates

INTRODUCTION

Spontaneous ICH is the deadliest most disabling and least treatable form of stroke. Following a major hemorrhage, 35–52% are dead within a month and <20% were living independently after 6 months. The hospital mortality rates of ICH who are comatose and mechanically ventilated is 60%. ICH constitutes 15% of all strokes in the West and 20–30% in Asian populations. The lack of proven medical or surgical treatment for ICH leads to great variation among physicians concerning both surgical and medical treatment. Although guidelines based on scant data from randomized trials are uncertain at best and may be wrong at worst, they can provide a reasonable treatment approach at present while outlining questions for future study.

Nearly 15–20% of strokes are due to ICH, in which there is arterial bleeding directly into the brain substance with the formation of a localized hematoma. The percentage of hemorrhagic strokes may vary between different regions

BOX 1	Causes of intracerebral hemorrhage.
• **Abnormal blood vessels:**	
◦ *Vascular malformations*:	
– Arteriovenous malformations	
– Saccular aneurysms	
– Cavernous angiomas	
– Septic and mycotic aneurysms	
◦ Lipohyalinosis and microaneurysms	
◦ Amyloid angiopathy	
◦ Cerebral tumors	
◦ Cerebral venous thrombosis	
◦ Vasculitis	
◦ Moyamoya syndrome	
◦ Hemorrhagic transformation	
• **Systemic bleeding tendency:**	
◦ Hemophilia	
◦ Leukemia	
◦ Thrombocytopenia	
◦ Anticoagulants	
◦ Antiplatelet agents	
◦ Thrombolytic agents	
• **Illicit drugs:**	
◦ Amphetamines	
◦ Cocaine	
• **Hyperperfusion syndrome**	
• **Trauma**	

within India and there is increasing literature suggesting higher percentage of hemorrhagic strokes (30–40% of all strokes), in Northeastern regions including Calcutta. Death at 1 year for ICH varies by location of ICH, 50% for deep hemorrhage; 57% for lobar; 42% for cerebellar and 65% for brainstem bleeds. Of the major strokes <25% are independent at the end of 6 months. The most important risk factor for ICH is poorly controlled chronic hypertension. Long-term adequate treatment of chronic hypertension significantly reduces the risk of ICH. Advanced age is an additional risk factor for ICH, with the rate doubling with each decade of life until 80, when the incidence plateaus at nearly 25 times that of previous decade.

Etiology of nontraumatic, nonaneurysmal intracerebral hemorrhage: The various etiological factors for ICH are listed in **Box 1**.

ETIOLOGY

CHRONIC HYPERTENSION

The most common sites of hypertensive hemorrhage are deep gray matter (putamen, globus pallidus, and thalamus) (65%), subcortical white matter (10–20%), pons (10–15%), and cerebellum (8–10%) (**Fig. 1**). Hemorrhages have been associated with microscopic changes in blood vessels, but the exact mechanism is debated. Miliary aneurysms (Charcot–Bouchard aneurysms) are found on the lenticulostriate branches of the middle cerebral artery and paramedian branches of the basilar artery in nearly 50% of hypertensive patients over 66 years of age. Destruction of the tunica media through a process variably described as lipohyalinosis and fibrinoid necrosis on the other hand is found in vessels within the area of ICH. An anatomic factor that may contribute to hypertensive ICH is that perforating vessels are small perpendicular branches directly off major arteries that are subject to much higher shear stress than cortical feeders, which reside at the end of the circulatory tree. It is likely that hypertension-induced ICH is the result of some combination of altered flow dynamics and histopathologic changes within the vasculature.

VASCULAR MALFORMATIONS

Up to 25% of ICH are attributable to bleeding from rupture of aneurysms and arteriovenous malformations (AVMs). Rupture of an aneurysm produces ICH is 5–25% of cases. If the aneurysm is adherent to the brain parenchyma, hemorrhage may be directed into the substance of the brain rather than purely into the subarachnoid space. In some cases, the bleeding is actually limited to the parenchymal component, and no subarachnoid blood is found on CT scan. Anterior communicating aneurysms may produce flame-shaped hemorrhages in the base of the frontal lobes.

Over half of patients with AVMs present with some type of hemorrhage; 60% of which are parenchymal in location. Lesions are found throughout the cerebrum, brainstem, or cerebellum. AVMs characteristically rupture during the second to fourth decades of life. Symptoms of AVM-induced ICH depend on location. Multiple calcified vascular channels may be seen within a hematoma on CT scan, suggesting the presence of an underlying AVM. MRI and four-vessel cerebral angiography are useful adjuncts in diagnosis and planning management (**Fig. 2**).

CEREBRAL AMYLOID ANGIOPATHY

This is characterized pathologically by the deposition of amyloid in cerebral vessels, primarily small and medium-sized arteries of the cortex and leptomeninges. The classical birefringent amyloid material is seen on histological examination in the media and adventitia, which stains positive for Congo red. The incidence of these histopathological changes at postmortem increases steadily with age, occurring in as many 60% of unselected autopsies of individuals older than 90 years. The incidence of hemorrhage secondary to amyloid angiopathy also increases with age and is rare before age 55 years. The mechanism of rupture of affected arteries is thought to be either a weakening of the vessel wall or the formation of microaneurysms at the sites of amyloid deposition. It is strikingly restricted to vessels of the leptomeninges and gray matter, and usually stops abruptly when a penetrating

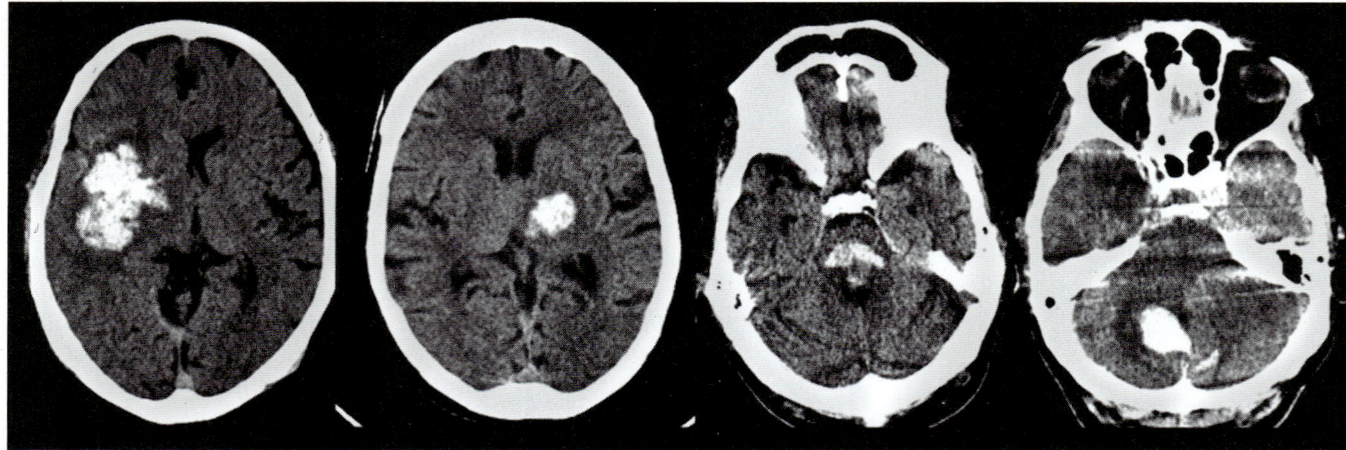

FIGURE 1: Hypertensive hematoma.

vessel reaches a junction of cortex and subcortical white matter. Hemorrhages in cerebral amyloid angiopathy (CAA) are almost exclusively lobar and often superficially close to the surface, with the site of rupture usually being at the gray-white matter junction.

CAVERNOUS ANGIOMAS (CAVERNOMAS)

These are of unknown etiology, but it has been suggested that at least part of the lesion forms as a localized reaction to small hemorrhages. They are mainly diagnosed from the characteristic magnetic resonance imaging (MRI) appearance of a central nidus of irregular bright signal intensity on T2-weighted imaging, surrounded by a peripheral hypointense ring resulting from hemosiderin deposition due to previous episodes of bleeding. No abnormalities are seen on angiography. Cavernous angiomas are predominantly supratentorial, most commonly affecting the temporal, frontal, and parietal lobes. The most frequent infratentorial site is the pons. Cavernous angiomas may present with seizures, ICH or progressive neurological deficit. The last of these is more likely to occur in brainstem cavernous angioma. The majority of cavernous angiomas are asymptomatic and are frequently found on MRI performed for other reasons. The outlook in the vast majority of asymptomatic cases is benign.

OTHER CAUSES

Approximately 10% of ICHs are attributable to coagulopathies, resulting from anticoagulation, platelet inhibition, thrombolytic therapy, or underlying systemic disease. Warfarin, heparin, aspirin, dipyridamole, tissue plasminogen activator (tPA), streptokinase, and urokinase have all been implicated as causes of ICH. Additionally, ICH occurs in 1–2% of patients receiving anticoagulants for systemic indications. Systemic disease such as renal and hepatic failure, thrombocytopenia and the leukemias produce coagulopathic states that may also result in ICH.

Hemorrhage from an underlying neoplasm is rare. This occasionally appears in malignant tumors, including glioblastoma multiforme, lymphoma, and metastatic tumors such as malignant melanoma, choriocarcinoma, renal cell, and bronchogenic carcinoma. Benign tumors are almost never associated with ICH.

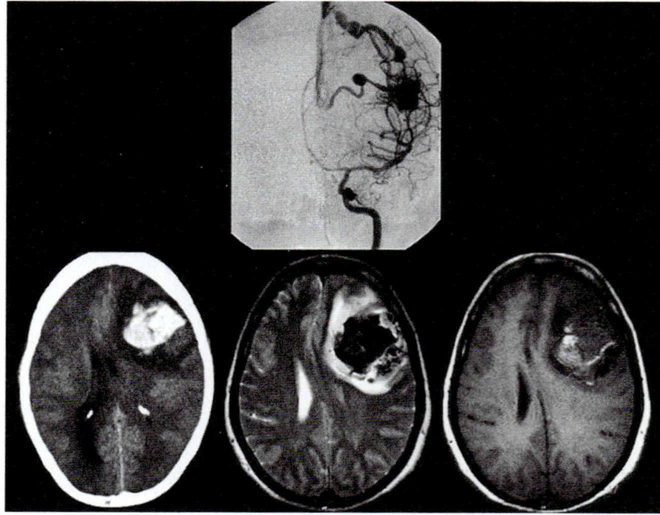

FIGURE 2: Arteriovenous malformation.

Infections may also result in ICH. Fungal infections predispose to cortical and subcortical hemorrhage by direct infiltration of the vessel wall by the organism. In its extreme form, herpes simplex may produce acute, necrotizing encephalitis that preferentially affects the temporal and frontal lobes.

ICH may occur following reperfusion (e.g., following carotid endarterectomy or acute thrombolysis), 1 or 2 days after head trauma as a result of venous sinus occlusion, and consequent to the use of drugs such as cocaine, amphetamines, pseudoephedrine, and phenylpropanolamine. Sinus thrombosis is associated with a variety of medical conditions, including pregnancy, dehydration, local or systemic infection, sickle cell trait, oral contraceptive use, and hypercoagulable states.

CLINICAL FEATURES

The focal signs and symptoms associated with the ICH indicate the hemorrhage location; these clinical features are identical to that of ischemia that occur in the same vascular territory. Generally, lobar hemorrhage result in sensory loss or contralateral weakness, language disturbance, parietal lobe signs, and lesser field disorders or hemianopia. Their association with the cortex renders it more possibly that seizures complicate them. In ICH, seizures are more common, taking place in about a quarter of patients; however, they are also observed in approximately 5% of patients who have ischemia, specifically early after onset.

Very small hematomas sometimes present with symptoms that are different from transient ischemic attacks (TIAs). Though, complete stroke is caused by most of the ICHs.

Putaminal hemorrhages characteristically result in contralateral hemiparesis along with varying degrees of sensory loss, ataxia as well as with large-sized hematomas (i.e., a homonymous hemianopia).

Contralateral sensory loss and weakness is caused by the thalamic hemorrhages; whereas when extension or compression of the superior midbrain is caused by the thalamic hemorrhages, they may lead to depressed signs. Usually, pontine hemorrhages lead to pinpoint pupils, reduction in consciousness, bilateral weakness, and dysfunction of pontine cranial nerve; these can be severely disabling.

It is significant to clinically recognize cerebellar hemorrhages because surgical intervention may be needed, that can be save life. The onset can mislead because of initial nonspecific brainstem symptoms such as double vision or vertigo; this is followed a few hours or even days later by progressive clinical features may follow few hours or even days later, which include headache, nystagmus, gait, trunk or limb ataxia, vomiting, and coma due to compression of brainstem. Rarely, hemiparesis may be observed. At the time of onset, it is difficult to predict the clinical course of cerebellar hemorrhage. Following a period of clinical stability, there may be an abrupt deterioration. Poor outcome is predicted by the moderate degrees of quadrigeminal cisternal compression unless there is evacuation of the hematoma early in the course. Severe mass effect on the cistern is reported to have a poor prognosis.

INVESTIGATIONS

PLAIN CT SCAN

CT of the brain remains the mainstay of diagnosis of ICH. Blood is easily seen and appears hyperdense on noncontrast-enhanced CT scans. Magnetic resonance imaging is also very sensitive to ICH provided the appropriate sequences are used. However, interpretation of hemorrhage on images is more complicated than with CT. Following hemorrhage, a series of events occurs that can be detected using MRI; these include initial deoxygenation of the blood within the hemorrhage; its subsequent chemical breakdown from hemoglobin into methemoglobin, and finally the formation of iron-containing hemosiderin deposits. MRI can therefore be used to distinguish between previous cerebral infarction and hemorrhage at a time when the appearances on CT are identical.

Certain radiological features characterize particular underlying causes of ICH. An AVM may be seen on MRI as a cluster of vascular channels with flow voids. Cavernous angiomas appear as small areas of high signal on T2-weighted images surrounded by a ring of low intensity due to hemosiderin deposition. Hemorrhage secondary to tumors can contain complex mixtures of increased and decreased signal related to the presence of viable tumor, necrotic tissue, calcification and hemorrhage occurring at various time points. Cerebral vasculitis may be suggested by the concurrent appearance of both ischemic and hemorrhagic lesions. Angiography [conventional four vessel; magnetic resonance angiography (MRA) or CT angiography] will be required to exclude a treatable source of recurrence such as aneurysm, AVM etc.

Plain CT of head [noncontrast computed tomography (NCCT)] remains the "work-force" of investigation in the triage area in a patient with acute stroke. The most common form of hemorrhage in patients with acute stroke is ICH. Hemorrhages may be classified based on their anatomic location; intracerebral (superficial vs. deep); intraventricular, subarachnoid, subdural, or extradural (**Figs. 3** and **4**).

ICH volume, IVH, and hematoma location: The volume of ICH can be determined with the *ABC/2 formula*, where A represents the greatest diameter of hemorrhage on the CT; B is the diameter aligned at 90° angle to A, and C is the approximate number of CT slices with hemorrhage multiplied by the slice thickness. A hematoma volume of 30 mL represents the cut-off point for increased mortality.

The presence and ongoing expansion of IVH are considered to be the powerful as well as independent predictors of functional outcomes after ICH.

In the recent times, recognized markers of poor prognosis with ICH observed on NCCT head are:

- *Black hole sign*: This is a hypodense region that is surrounded by a hyperdense region not attached with the adjoining brain tissue.
- *Island sign*: This includes minimum three scattered small hemorrhages distinct from the main hemorrhage.
- *Blend sign*: This is a hemorrhage with hyperdense as well as hypodense regions.

COMPUTED TOMOGRAPHY ANGIOGRAPHY

Since blood vessels are imaged with the help of computed tomography angiography (CTA), it is considered to be a powerful tool for understanding the etiology as well as pathophysiology of any ICH. A routine head CTA should be done to detect pathologies such as dural arteriovenous (AV) fistulas, AVMs, intracranial aneurysms, and other vascular malformations.

In adults, the probability of finding such secondary causes of ICH is in the range of 15%, and in patients

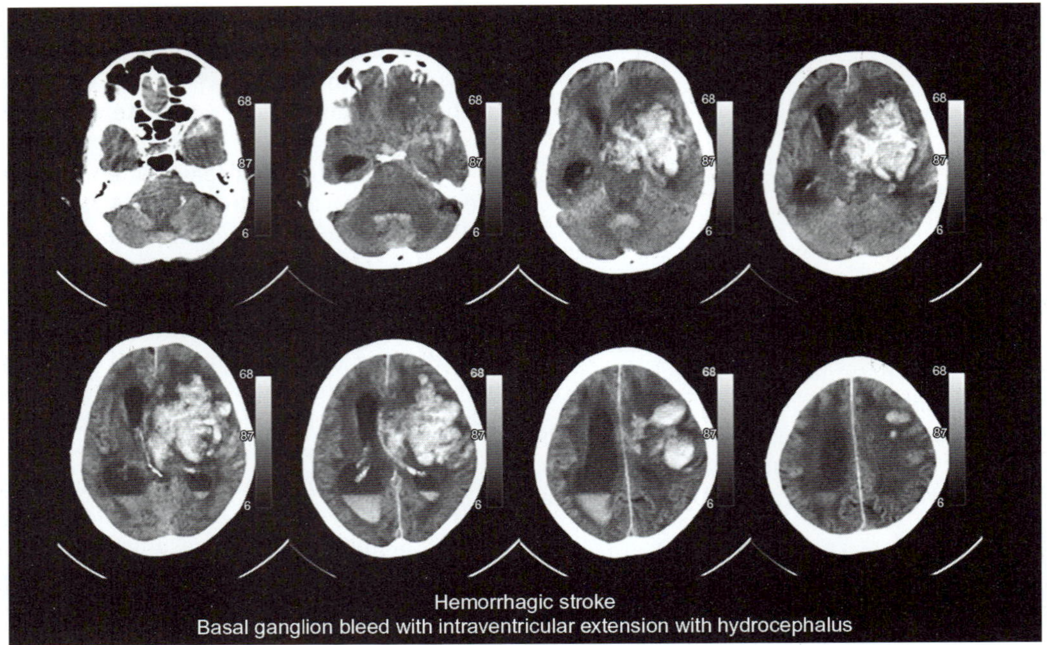

FIGURE 3: A 79-year-old man, had loss of consciousness for last 5 hours.

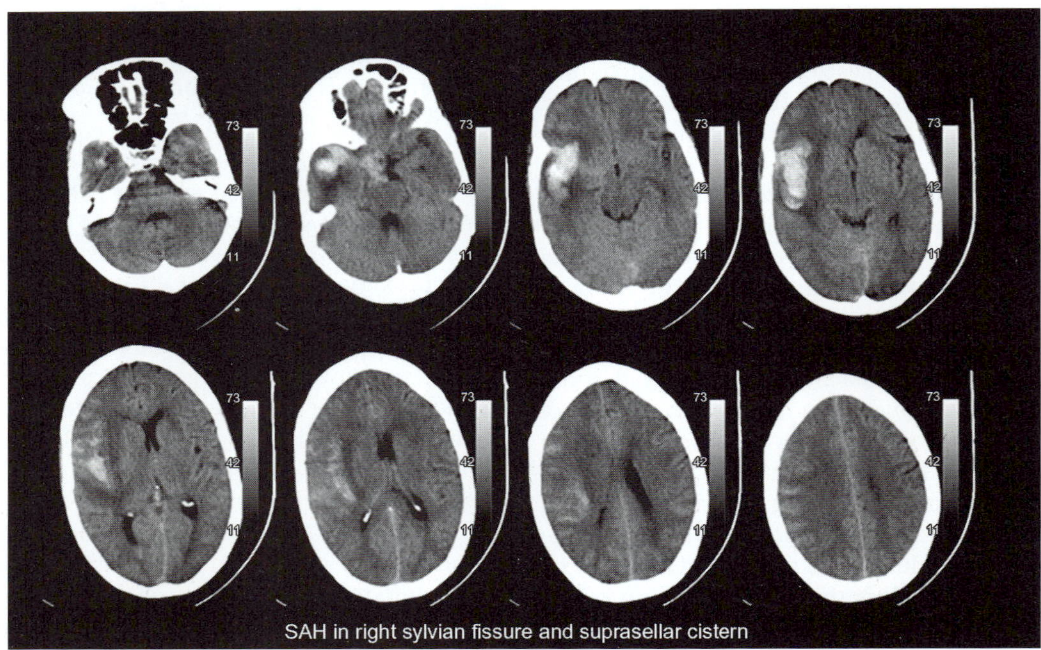

FIGURE 4: Subarachnoid hemorrhage: F60, presented with vomiting followed by loss of consciousness 1 day prior.

<40 years this is nearly 65%. Thus, it is recommended to perform a head CTA in the case of patients having ICH who are of young age, have hemorrhage located at infratentorial or lobar location, and do not have impaired coagulation or hypertension.

Computed tomography angiography is useful for clinicians in predicting the risk of hemorrhage growth over time in the case of patients who have primary ICH, which is possibly caused because of hypertension.

A serpiginous or linear contrast density, which is situated within the parenchymal hemorrhage, is the spot sign. There should not be anatomic continuity of spot sign with any adjacent blood vessels. If these criteria are not fulfilled, the spot sign mimics, as these other contrast densities are known as, may be markers of different pathologies such as aneurysms, moyamoya disease, microarteriovenous malformations, choroidal calcifications, and tumors.

Early neurological deterioration and hematoma expansion: The term early neurological deterioration is usually used to indicate a decline from the initial neurological examination or progression to death. Though the two most important predictors of early neurological deterioration are the hematoma volume and presence of IVH, other factors such as glucose concentration, fibrinogen levels, and elevated BP also need to be considered. Hematoma expansion is an independent indicator of poor outcome and mortality.

Hematoma expansion: Majority of patients develop varying degrees of hematoma expansion most significant during the first few hours of ictus. The degree of hematoma growth is an independent predictor of eventual outcomes in terms of death and disability. The mass effect of hematoma has a direct bearing on the adjacent structures as well as dissection into the ventricles causing IVH. The size, location, IVH, and edema have a direct effect on degree of raised intracranial hypertension. The perihematoma edema is said to be maximum between 48 hours to 7 days postictus following which there is gradual diminution of the pressure effect. Thrombin within the hematoma plays a pivotal role in promoting perihematomal edema. Hemoglobin and its products—heme, iron are potent mitochondrial toxins leading to cell death.

Predictors of hematoma expansion: The risk of hematoma expansion ranges from 3.4 to 7.1% in patients with zero risk factors to a whopping 70–85% in patients obtaining the maximum score.

Prediction scores share several common factors:

- Shorter time from ICH onset to CT
- Warfarin use
- Evidence of spot sign on CTA

Studies are enrolling spot sign-positive patients for treatment with recombinant factor VIIa:

- STOP-IT: Spot Sign for Predicting and Treating ICH Growth Study
- SPOTLIGHT: "Spot Sign" Selection of Intracerebral Hemorrhage to Guide Hemostatic Therapy
- SCORE-IT: SPOT for aggressive antihypertensive treatment

TREATMENT

TREATMENT OF ACUTE ICH

- Potential treatments of ICH include stopping or slowing the initial bleeding during the first hours after the onset
- Removing blood from the parenchyma or ventricles;
- Management of raised intracranial pressure (ICP) and decreased cerebral perfusion;
- Good general supportive management.

Immediate general care: Paying significant attention to the ABCs of resuscitation as well as rapid correcting deranged parameters are needed in patients with ICH. Mechanical ventilation may be needed in nearly 50% of such patients. As indicated by recent evidence, over the first few hours, several hematomas enlarge; this suggests that aggressively correcting coagulopathies might be useful.

Airway and respiratory management: Airway obstruction may occur either because of a diminished level of consciousness which results in relaxation of the pharyngeal musculature and tongue and suppress cough and gag reflexes or because of a complete loss of pharyngeal tone and absent cough, swallow and gag reflexes in posterior fossa ICH. The initial airway management includes proper positioning, frequent suctioning, and placement of an oral or nasal airway. Frequent assessments for sonorous respirations, difficulty managing oral secretions or decreased oxygen saturation are necessary. If conservative measures are ineffective, intubation is necessary. Although not all patients need intubation, airway protection, and appropriate ventilation are essential. For aggressive airway management, the candidates include patients who display signs of brainstem dysfunction or reducing level of consciousness. Instead of an arbitrary cut-off such as a particular Glasgow Coma Scale (GCS) score, intubation should be guided by imminent respiratory insufficiency. Indication of intubation is for insufficient ventilation as indicated by hypoxia ($pO_2 < 60$ mm Hg or $PCO_2 > 50$ mm Hg), or evident risk of aspiration. For preventing aspiration, patients who have endotracheal tubes receive.

Orogastric or nasogastric tubes: Intubated patients are at a high risk for pneumonia. Factors that contribute to pneumonia include colonization of the oropharynx, sinuses, trachea and gastrointestinal tract, and contamination through hospital personnel or equipment. Appropriate measures should be taken to minimize this risk.

TREATMENT OF HYPERTENSION

Most patients with ICH are hypertensive on presentation. Blood pressure tends to decline to prehemorrhage levels during the first week. In chronically hypertensive patients the blood pressure on presentation is usually higher than the patient's baseline. Several arguments exist for treatment of acute hypertension in ICH. Some suggest that high blood pressure might enhance hematoma expansion. Very high blood pressure might conceivably exacerbate vasogenic edema by increasing capillary hydrostatic pressure, especially when there is already damage to the blood–brain barrier.

Patients with moderate to severe hypertension are also at risk for systemic complications of elevated blood pressure including myocardial ischemia, congestive heart failure, and acute renal failure. Monitoring for end organ dysfunction is necessary.

It should be noted that several reasons argue that hypertension should not be treated. Chronic hypertension shifts the cerebral autoregulatory curve so that higher cerebral perfusion pressures (CPPs) are required to maintain adequate cerebral blood flow. Lowering the blood pressure to "normal" levels might lead to inadequate cerebral blood flow in these patients. Acute lowering of the mean arterial pressure (MAP) by 15% in hypertensive patients with acute ICH did not reduce cerebral blood flow around the hematoma.

Consensus: Early after ICH, there appears to be no compelling need to treat hypertension aggressively unless there are signs of systemic complications, especially in the setting of large bleeds with raised ICP. However new data suggest that modest (15%) reduction of blood pressure does not lower cerebral blood flow (CBF) in patients within 24 hours of ICH. Thus modest reduction in blood pressure of very hypertensive patients (MAP >130 mm Hg) is indicated.

Aggressive management of BP: Early lowering of SBP to <140 mm Hg produced no significant adversary effect in two large phase III multicenter, prospective randomized controlled trials (RCTs).

The INTERACT II trial compared early lowering of SBP at two levels namely <140 mm Hg and 180 mm Hg. Intensive lowering of BP was found to improve functional outcomes as shown by an ordinal analysis of modified Rankin scores.

The ATTCH – II trial using intravenous nicardipine within 3 hours of ICH onset to target SBP < 140 mm Hg versus SBP < 180 mm Hg reported no significant difference in the primary endpoints of death and disability at 3 months although the intensive treatment was associated with a higher incidence of adverse renal events (9% vs. 4%).

- For ICH patients presenting with SBP between 150 and 220 mm Hg, acute lowering of SBP to 140 mm Hg is safe (Class I, Level A) and can be effective for improving functional outcome (Class IIa, Level B) (revised).
- For ICH patients presenting with SBP >220 mm Hg, it may be reasonable to consider aggressive reduction of BP with a continuous intravenous infusion and frequent BP monitoring (Class IIb, Level C) (new).

Choice of antihypertensives: The most appropriate antihypertensive agent to use in ICH patients is one that has a short half-life and moderate efficacy with minimal cerebrovascular effects. Drugs should be administered so as to avoid sudden large drops in blood pressure. Vasodilators, especially those that dilate veins, can raise ICP by increasing cerebral blood volume and should be avoided. Sodium nitroprusside and nitroglycerin increase ICP and lower CBF in patients with reduced intracranial compliance. Labetalol, a combined α-blocker and β-blocker, alters neither ICP nor CBF thus making it a popular agent. However, large doses may be required to counteract the sympathetic nervous system stimulation associated with ICH. Other useful agents include hydralazine, the calcium-channel blockers nicardipine, and angiotensin-converting enzyme inhibitors, enalapril.

MANAGEMENT OF INCREASED INTRACRANIAL PRESSURE

Intracranial pressure is considered a major contributor to mortality after ICH. ICP may be managed through osmotherapy, controlled hypertension, and barbiturate coma. Elevated ICP is defined as ICP ≥20 mm Hg for >5 minutes. A therapeutic goal for all treatment of raised ICP is ICP <20 mm Hg and CPP of >70 mm Hg. Patients with suspected elevated ICP and deteriorating level of consciousness are candidates for invasive ICP monitoring (level of evidence V, grade C recommendation). Intraventricular ICP monitors and intraparenchymal fiberoptic ICP devices are two commonly used methods of monitoring ICP.

The CPP-guided therapy focuses on maintaining a CPP of >70 mm Hg to minimize reflex vasodilation or ischemia. Despite long-standing debates, no controlled trial has demonstrated the superiority of approaches.

A balanced approach begins with simple and less aggressive measures, such as head positioning, analgesia, and sedation and then progresses to more aggressive measures.

Head of bed elevation: Elevation of the head of the bed to 30° improves jugular venous outflow and lowers ICP.

Osmotic therapy: The most commonly used agent is mannitol, an intravascular osmotic agent that can draw fluid from both edematous and nonedematous brain tissue. It also decreases ICP through cerebral autoregulation. Mannitol decreases blood viscosity which results in reflex vasoconstriction and decreased cerebrovascular volume. Osmotherapy is considered to be the first medical line of defense. However, prophylactic use should be avoided. Use of mannitol 20% (0.25–0.5 g/kg every 4 h) is held in reserve for patients who have type B ICP waves, progressively enhancing levels of ICP, or clinical deterioration related with mass effect (level of evidence V, grade C recommendation). Due to rebound phenomenon, recommendation of mannitol is only for few days to a week. Furosemide (10 mg, 2–8 hourly) may be given along with osmotherapy for maintaining an osmotic gradient. In patients receiving osmotherapy, measurement of serum osmolarity should be done twice daily and targeted to 310 mOsm/L or less.

Hypertonic saline solutions have been shown to reduce ICP in some cases of refractory raised ICP to mannitol and hyperventilation. Exact dose, concentration, and mode are not clarified.

Cerebrospinal fluid drainage: When an intraventricular catheter is used to monitor ICP, CSF drainage is an effective method for lowering ICP, particularly in the setting of hydrocephalus. The principal risks associated with ventriculostomy are infection and hemorrhage. In addition to the mass effect of the hematomas, secondary hydrocephalus may contribute to elevated ICP. Ventricular drains should be used in patients with or at risk for hydrocephalus. Because of infectious complications, external drainage devices must be checked regularly and duration of placement ideally should not exceed 7 days (level of evidence V and grade C recommendation). Use of anti-infectious prophylaxis is recommended (level of evidence V, grade C recommendation).

Neuromuscular blockade: Muscle activity may further raise ICP by increasing intrathoracic pressure and obstructing cerebral venous outflow. If the patient is not responsive to analgesia and sedation alone neuromuscular blockade is considered.

Hyperventilation: Hyperventilation is one of the most effective methods to reduce raised ICP. However, it has fallen out of favor primarily because of the simultaneous effect of lowering CBF. And it is also transient in its effect. In fact, after a patient has been hyperventilated for >6 hours, rapid normalization of arterial PCO_2 can cause a significant rebound increase in ICP. The target levels of CO_2 for hyperventilation are 30–35 mm Hg. The beneficial effect of sustained hyperventilation ceases when the pH of CSF reaches equilibrium. As with osmotherapy, rebound effects can occur if normal ventilation is resumed too quickly.

Barbiturate coma: High-dose barbiturate treatment acts by depressing cerebral metabolic activity. This results in reduction in CBF, which is coupled to metabolism, and a fall in ICP. The use of barbiturates in the treatment of refractory ICP requires intensive monitoring and is associated with a significant risk of complications.

MANAGEMENT OF GLUCOSE LEVELS

As indicated by evidence, there is an association between persistent hyperglycemia (>140 mg/dL) during the first 24 hours following stroke and poor outcomes; therefore, this is widely accepted that in patients with acute stroke, treatment of hyperglycemia should be done. According to the guidelines for ischemic stroke, increased concentrations of glucose, i.e., >185 mg/dL and probably >140 mg/dL, possibly should trigger insulin administration. It is also reasonable to use these guidelines for ICH also.

FLUID MANAGEMENT

The goal is euvolemia. If hypovolemia is thought to contribute to hypotension, central venous pressure (CVP) should be maintained between 5 and 12 mm Hg. Electrolytes should be checked and substituted; acidosis and alkalosis should be corrected according to blood gas analysis.

PREVENTION OF SEIZURES

Seizure activity can result in neuronal injury and destabilization of an already critically ill patient and must be treated aggressively. Additionally, nonconvulsive seizures may contribute to coma in ≤10% of neurocritical care patients. In patients with ICH, prophylactic antiepileptic drug (AED) may be considered for a month and then tapered and discontinued if no seizure activity occurs during treatment (level of evidence is V, grade of recommendation C).

MANAGEMENT OF BODY TEMPERATURE

Normothermia should be maintained. Acetaminophen or cooling blankets may be used to treat hyperthermia. Appropriated cultures and smears (tracheal, urine, blood) should be obtained and antibiotics given.

SURGICAL THERAPY

The four recognized surgical procedures to evacuate an ICH are simple aspiration, craniotomy with open surgery, endoscopic evacuation and stereotactic aspiration. Their use in clinical practice is inconsistent. In some countries, e.g., the Netherlands, they are rarely performed; in others, e.g., in USA, they are undertaken in about 20% of patients with ICH and in others, e.g., some centers in Germany and Japan, they are offered to 50% or more of patients. Such wide variation in practice reflects uncertainty about the effectiveness and risks of surgery due to a lack of appropriate evidence.

Stereotactic aspiration: Despite reports of stereotactic aspiration without endoscopy, usually combined with installation of fibrinolytic agents, in >500 patients with supratentorial intraparenchymal or IVH, this technique has not been evaluated by RCTs.

CONSENSUS GUIDELINES

Recommendations for initial medical therapy:

Class I evidence:

- Monitoring and management of patients with an ICH should take place in an intensive care unit setting because of the acuity of the condition, frequent elevations in ICP and blood pressure, frequent need for intubation and assisted ventilation, and multiple complicating medical issues.
- Appropriate antiepileptic therapy should be used for treatment of clinical seizures in patients with ICH.
- Sources of fever should be treated and antipyretic medications should be administered to lower temperature in febrile patients with stroke.
- Early mobilization and rehabilitation are recommended in patients with ICH who are clinically stable.

Class II evidence:

- Treatment of elevated ICP should include a balanced and graded approach that begins with simple measures such as elevation of the head of the bed and analgesia and sedation. More aggressive therapies to decrease elevated ICP such as osmotic diuretics, drainage of CSF via ventricular catheter, neuromuscular blockade and hyperventilation require concomitant monitoring of ICP, and blood pressure with a goal to maintain CPP >70 mm Hg.
- Evidence indicates that persistent hyperglycemia (>140 mg/dL) during the first 24 hours after stroke is associated with poor outcomes and thus it is generally agreed that hyperglycemia should be treated in patients with acute stroke.
- A brief period of prophylactic antiepileptic therapy soon after ICH onset may reduce the risk of early seizures in patients with lobar hemorrhage.

Recommendations for prevention of deep vein thrombosis:

Class I:

- Patients with acute primary ICH and hemiparesis should have intermittent pneumatic compression for prevention of venous thromboembolism.
- Treatment of hypertension should always be part of long-term therapy because such therapy decreases the risk of recurrent ICH.

Class II:

- After documentation of cessation of bleeding, low-dose subcutaneous low-molecular weight heparin or unfractionated heparin may be considered in patients with hemiplegia after 3–4 days from onset.
- Patients with an ICH who develop an acute proximal venous thrombosis, particularly those with clinical or subclinical pulmonary emboli, should be considered for acute placement of a vena cava filter.
- The decision to add long-term antithrombotic therapy several weeks or more after placement of a vena cava filter must take into consideration the likely cause of the hemorrhage, associated conditions with increased arterial thrombotic risk and the overall health and mobility of the patient.

Rationale for ultra-early hemostatic therapy for ICH:

Recombinant factor VIIa:
Recombinant factor VIIa is available and approved for treating bleeding related to hemophilia in patients who have antibodies to factors VIII or IX, Glanzmann's thrombasthenia and factor VII deficiency. Could it also control bleeding in ICH?

Trials of recombinant activated factor VII: Recombinant activated factor VIIa (rFVIIa) is approved to treat bleeding in patients with hemophilia who have antibodies to factor VIII or IX and it has been reported to reduce bleeding in patients without coagulopathy as well. Interaction of rFVIIa and tissue factor stimulates thrombin generation. rFVIIa also activated factor X on the surface of activated platelets which leads to an enhanced thrombin burst at the site of injury. Thrombin converts fibrinogen into fibrin which produces a stable clot. rFVIIa has a half-life of 2.6 hours.

Two small dose ranging pilot safety studies and a larger dose finding phase II study focusing on decreasing with growth of ICHs have been published. In the small dose-ranging studies the overall thromboembolic and serious adverse event rate in the 88 patients tested at escalating doses from 5 to 160 μg/kg was low enough to encourage further testing.

In the moderate sized phase II trial, treatment with rFVIIa within 4 hours after the onset of ICH limited the growth of the hematoma, reduced the mortality rate and improved functional outcome at 90 days despite a small increase in the frequency of thromboembolic adverse events.

However, a larger phase III randomized trial of rFVIIa largely was negative with no definitive evidence in favor of using rFVIIa in primary ICH.

Class II recommendation: Treatment with rFVIIa within the first 3–4 hours after onset to slow progression of bleeding, has shown promise in one moderate sized phase II trial and a negative phase III trial. The efficacy and safety of this treatment must be confirmed in further trials before its use in patients with ICH can be recommended outside of a clinical trial.

ICH-related to antithrombotic or fibrinolytic therapy: *ICH-related to intravenous heparin* requires rapid normalization of activated partial thromboplastin time (aPTT) by protamine sulfate with adjustment of dose according to time elapsed since the last heparin dose (for <30 min: 1 mg; 30–60 min: 0.5–0.75 mg; for 60–120 min: 0.375–0.5 mg, for >120 min 0.25–0.3 mg/100 units of heparin). Protamine sulfate is given by slow intravenous not to exceed 5 mg/min (maximum of 50 mg). Protamine sulfate may also be used for ICH related to use of subcutaneous low-molecular weight heparin.

- Monitor for signs of anaphylaxis; the risk is higher in diabetics who have received insulin.
- Follow-up with STAT aPTT every 1 hour for the next 4 hours, then every 4 hours through 12 hours of hospitalization.

Patients with acenocoumarol/warfarin-related ICH should be managed with vitamin K, fresh frozen plasma (FFP), and wherever available prothrombin complex concentrate (PCC).

Vitamin K (10 mg IV) should not be used alone because it takes at least 6 hours to normalize the international normalized ratio (INR).

Fresh frozen plasma (15–20 mL/kg) is an effective way of correcting INR, but there is risk of volume overload and heart failure. Both PCC and factor IX complex concentrate require smaller volumes of infusion than FFP (and correct the coagulopathy faster but with greater risk of thromboembolism).

For symptomatic hemorrhage *after thrombolysis*, administration of IV alteplase should be stopped if still infusing until NCCT head has been done. (If CT shows no evidence of bleeding, then infusion can be resumed).

If the CT shows hemorrhage, then immediately check values of: Complete blood count (CBC), prothrombin time (PT), aPTT, platelets, fibrinogen, and D-dimer. If fibrinogen is <100 mg/dL, then give cryoprecipitate 0.15 units/kg rounded to the nearest integer. Give four units of platelet-rich plasma if platelet dysfunction is suspected.

If heparin has been administered in the past 3 hours, then follow the above paragraph on ICH related to heparin use.

Serious extracranial hemorrhage should be treated in a similar manner. In addition, compressible sites of bleeding should be manually compressed.

Neurosurgery or vascular surgery may be consulted as needed for intracranial or extracranial bleeding respectively as needed.

Restarting vitamin K antagonists: Patients with a very high risk of thromboembolism (those with mechanical prosthetic heart valves), vitamin K antagonist (VKA) therapy may be restarted at 7–10 days after onset of the index intracranial hemorrhage. Those with lower risk may be restarted on antiplatelet therapy.

Recommendations for surgical approaches:

Class I: Patients with cerebellar hemorrhage >3 cm who are deteriorating neurologically or who have brainstem compression and/or hydrocephalus from ventricular obstruction should have surgical removal of the hemorrhage as soon as possible.

Class II:

- Although stereotactic infusion of urokinase into the clot cavity within 72 hours of ictus apparently reduces the clot burden and risk of death, re-bleeding is more common, and functional outcome is not improved; therefore, its usefulness is unknown.
- Although theoretically attractive, the usefulness of minimally invasive clot evacuation utilizing a variety of mechanical devices and/or endoscopy awaits further testing in clinical testing; therefore, its current usefulness is unknown.
- For patients presenting with lobar clots within 1 cm of the surface, evacuation of supratentorial ICH by standard craniotomy might be considered.

Class III: The routine evacuation of supratentorial ICH by standard craniotomy within 96 hours of ictus is not recommended. Possible exception is for patients presenting with lobar clots within 1 cm of the surface.

Recommendations for timing of surgery:

Class II: No clear evidence at present indicates that ultra-early craniotomy improves functional outcome or mortality rate. Operative removal, within 12 hours particularly when performed by less-invasive methods, has the most supportive evidence, but the number of subjects treated within this window is very small.

Class III: Delayed evacuation by craniotomy appears to offer little if any benefit with a fairly high degree of certainty. In those patients presenting in coma with deep hemorrhages, removal of ICH by craniotomy may actually worsen outcome and is not recommended.

Recommendation for decompressive craniectomy:

Class II: Too few data currently exist to comment on the potential of decompressive craniectomy (DC) to improve outcome in ICH.

Interventions:

- *Intracranial pressure monitoring*:
  - *Recommendations*:
    - Ventricular drainage as treatment for hydrocephalus is reasonable, especially in patients with decreased level of consciousness (Class IIa, level of evidence B) (revised).
    - Patients with a GCS score <8, those with clinical evidence of transtentorial herniation or those with significant IVH or hydrocephalus might be considered for ICP monitoring and treatment. A CPP of 50–70 mm Hg may be reasonable to maintain depending on the status of cerebral autoregulation (Class IIb, level of evidence C).
    - Corticosteroids should not be administered for treatment of elevated ICP in ICH (Class III, level of evidence B) (new).
- *Intraventricular hemorrhage*: The largest trial of intraventricular fibrinolysis to date is the CLEAR-IVH trial, which included 100 patients and showed clinical benefit with tPA. The phase III randomized CLEAR III trial is in progress.

Alternative procedures for IVH include:

- Endoscopic surgical evacuation and ventriculostomy
- Early ventriculoperitoneal shunting
- Endoscopic third ventriculostomy
- Lumbar drainage

Recommendations for other surgical modalities:

- Patients with cerebellar hemorrhage who are deteriorating neurologically or who have brainstem compression and/or hydrocephalus from ventricular obstruction should undergo surgical removal of the hemorrhage as soon as possible (Class I, level of evidence B). Initial treatment of these patients with ventricular drainage rather than surgical evacuation is not recommended (Class II, level of evidence C).
- For most patients with supratentorial ICH, the usefulness of surgery is not well established (Class IIb, level of evidence A) (revised).
- A policy of early hematoma evacuation is not clearly beneficial compared with hematoma evacuation when patients deteriorate (Class IIb, level of evidence A) (new).
- Supratentorial hematoma evacuation in deteriorating patients might be considered as a lifesaving measure (Class IIb, level of evidence C) (new).
- Decompressive craniotomy with or without hematoma evacuation might reduce mortality for patients with supratentorial ICH who are in coma, have large hematomas with significant midline shift, or have elevated ICP refractory to medical management (Class IIb, level of evidence C) (new).
- The effectiveness of minimally invasive clot evacuation with stereotactic or endoscopic aspiration with or without thrombolytic usage is uncertain (Class IIb, level of evidence B) (revised).

ICH SCORE

In an attempt to develop a standard clinical grading scale for ICH analogs to those for traumatic brain injury, subarachnoid hemorrhage (SAH) or ischemic stroke, Hemphill et al. developed the ICH score. The factors included for ICH score were:

- GCS score 3–4 (2 points), 5–12 (1 point), 13–15 (0 point); age >80 years—yes (1 point), no (0 point); infratentorial origin of ICH, yes (1 point), no (0 point); ICH volume, 30 cm^3 (1 point), <30 cm^3 (0 point); and intraventricular extension, yes (1 point), no (0 point). All 26 patients with an ICH score of 0 survived and all 6 patients with an ICH score of 5 died. 30 days mortality increased steadily with ICH score ($p < 0.005$). The ICH score is a simple clinical grading scale that allows risk stratification on presentation with ICH. The use of a scale such as the ICH score could improve standardization of clinical treatment protocols and clinical research studies in ICH.

The time is nearing when ICH will join ischemic stroke and SAH as a cerebrovascular disease with scientifically proven therapies.

RECOMMENDED READINGS

1. Broderick JP, Brott T, Tomsick T, Miller R, Huster G. Intracerebral hemorrhage more than twice as common as subarachnoid hemorrhage. J Neurosurg. 1993;78:188-91.
2. Das SK, Banerjee TK, Biswas A, Roy T, Raut DK, Mukherjee CS, et al. A prospective community-based study of stroke in Kolkata, India. Stroke. 2007;38:906-10.
3. Qureshi AI, Tuhrim S, Broderick JP, Batjer HH, Hondo H, Hanley DF. Spontaneous intracerebral hemorrhage. N Engl J Med. 2001;344:1450-60.
4. Challa VR, Moody DM, Bell MA. The Charcot-Bouchard aneurysm controversy: impact of a new histologic technique. J Neuropathol Exp Neurol. 1992;51:264-71.
5. Lammie GA. Hypertensive cerebral small vessel disease and stroke. Brain Pathol. 2002;12:358-70.
6. Ruiz-Sandovall JL, Cantu C, Barinagarrementeria F. Intracerebral hemorrhage in young people: analysis of risk factors, location, causes and prognosis. Stroke. 1999;30:537-41.
7. Stapf C, Labovitz DL, Sciacca RR, Mast H, Mohr JP, Sacco RL. Incidence of adult brain arteriovenous malformation hemorrhage in a prospective population -based stroke survey. Cerebrovasc Dis. 2002;13:43-6.
8. Yamada M. Cerebral amyloid angiopathy: an overview. Neuropathology. 2000;20:8-22.
9. Sjalander A, Engstrom G, Bernstorp E, Svensson P. Risk of hemorrhagic stroke in patients with oral anti-coagulation compared with the general population. J Intern Med. 2003;254:434-8.
10. Palareti G, Leali N, Poggi M, Manotti C, D'Angelo A Coccheri S, et al. Bleeding complications of oral anti-coagulant treatment: an inception-cohort, prospective collaborative study (ISCOAT). Lancet. 1996;348:423-8.
11. Antithrombotic Trialists' Collaboration. Collaborative meta-analysis of randomized trials of antiplatelet therapy for prevention of death, myocardial infarction, and stroke in high risk patients. BMJ. 2002;324:71-86.
12. Diener HC, Bogousslavsky J, Brass LM, Cimminiello C, Csiba L, Kaste M, et al. Aspirin and clopidogrel compared with clopidogrel alone after recent ischaemic stroke or transient ischaemic attack in high-risk patients (MATCH): randomised, double-blind, placebo-controlled trial. Lancet. 2004;364:331-7.
13. Larrue V, von Kummer R, Müller A, Blumki E. Risk factors for severe hemorrhagic transformation in ischemic stroke patients treated with recombinant tissue plasminogen activator: a secondary analysis of the European-Australasian Acute Stroke Study (ECASS II). Stroke. 2001;32:438-41.
14. Intracerebral hemorrhage after intravenous t-PA therapy for ischemic stroke. The NINDS t-PA Stroke Study Group. Stroke. 1997;28:2109-18.
15. McCabe DJ, Brown MM, Clifton A. Fatal cerebral reperfusion hemorrhages after carotid stenting. Stroke. 1999;30:2483-6.
16. Broderick JP, Adams HP Jr, Barsan W, Feinberg W, Feldmann E, Grotta J, et al. Guidelines for the management of spontaneous intracerebral hemorrhage: A statement for healthcare professionals from a special writing group of the Stroke Council, American Heart Association. Stroke. 1999;30:905-15.
17. Mayer SA, Brun NC, Begtrup K, Broderick J, Davis S, Diringer MN, et al. Recombinant activated factor VII for acute intracerebral hemorrhage. N Engl J Med. 2005;352:777-85.
18. Zazulia AR, Diringer MN, Derdeyn CP, Powers WJ. Progression of mass effect after intracerebral hemorrhage. Stroke. 1999;30:1167-73.
19. Mendelow AD, Gregson BA, Fernandes HM, Murray GD, Teasdale GM, Hope DT, et al. Early surgery versus initial conservative treatment in patients with spontaneous supratentorial intracerebral haematomas in the International Surgical Trial in Intracerebral Haemorrhage (STICH): a randomised trial. Lancet. 2005;365:387-97.
20. Hemphill JC, Bonovich DC, Besmertis L, Manley GT, Johnston C. The ICH score: A simple, reliable, grading scale for intracerebral hemorrhage. Stroke. 2001;32:891-7.

CHAPTER
188
Acute Bacterial Meningitis

Neeraj Balani, Amol Nanak Singh, Manish Modi

ABSTRACT

Acute bacterial meningitis and brain abscess are neurological emergencies. Acute bacterial meningitis can be community acquired or nosocomial. *Streptococcus pneumoniae, Neisseria meningitidis,* and *Haemophilus influenzae* are most common pathogens causing bacterial meningitis. Bacteria gain entry into subarachnoid space and brain through bloodstream through different mechanisms causing neuronal injury. Classic triad of meningitis consists of fever, neck stiffness, and change in mental status. The triad is present in 41–51% of patients. Bacterial meningitis can have systemic and neurologic complications. Neurological complications include seizures, hearing loss, hydrocephalus, and cerebrovascular complications such as ischemic stroke, hemorrhagic stroke, subdural empyema, cerebral venous thrombosis, and cerebral edema.

Cerebrospinal fluid (CSF) examination is the key for establishing diagnosis and determining etiology. CSF culture is gold standard for diagnosis of bacterial meningitis. CSF culture is positive in 80–90% cases of bacterial meningitis patients who are treatment naïve. Empirical treatment of suspected bacterial meningitis should be started as soon as possible in emergency along with steroids. Brain abscess is a focal collection of pus in brain tissue surrounded by capsule. *Streptococcus* species are the most common cause of brain abscess in different case series and *Streptococcus milleri* group was most commonly identified bacteria among *Streptococcus* species. Infection can reach the brain through direct extension from neighboring structures, hematogenous spread, or direct inoculation from trauma. Development of brain abscess can be divided into early cerebritis, late cerebritis, early capsule, and late capsule formation. Diagnosis of brain abscess is based on clinical suspicion and neuroimaging. Brain abscess patient should be actively managed with neurosurgical intervention and antibiotics.

"In all chaos there is a cosmos, in all disorder a secret order"

—Carl Jung

ACUTE BACTERIAL MENINGITIS

Acute bacterial meningitis is purulent infection of membranes covering the brain, i.e., meninges leading to severe inflammation of meninges and frequently brain parenchyma and/or cerebral vasculature. It is a neurological emergency and can have significant mortality and morbidity if left untreated. In this chapter, we will discuss about epidemiology, etiopathogenesis, clinical features, approach, and management of bacterial meningitis. We have divided acute bacterial meningitis into community-acquired bacterial meningitis and nosocomial meningitis. Nosocomial meningitis results from invasive procedures, complicated head trauma, and rarely dissemination of bacteria through hospital-acquired bacteraemia.

EPIDEMIOLOGY

Globally, 2.82 million cases of meningitis were documented in 2016. Meningitis incidence rates were highest in sub-Saharan African countries, also called meningitis belt (stretching from Senegal through Ethiopia and South Sudan). Nearly 0.6% of deaths in all age groups were due to bacterial meningitis in 2016. In India, 504,959 cases of meningitis were documented in 2016 which is an underestimation, although incidence in India has decreased by around 36% as compared to meningitis cases in 1990. Out of 504,959 cases 63,001 died (12.48%) in India. Neonatal period is peak age for incidence of meningitis. Death due to meningitis is highest in children <5 years and among those who survive, rates of disability are highest in younger children. In 2018, an Indian study found that out of 19,670 children below 5 years of age admitted in different hospitals across the country, 3,104 (15.78%) were suspected to have meningitis clinically and 257 (8.28%) cases were found to have confirmed meningitis with laboratory confirmation for causative organism by CSF culture and/or blood culture or by latex agglutination or polymerase chain reaction (PCR).

ETIOLOGY

COMMUNITY-ACQUIRED

Streptococcus pneumoniae, N. meningitidis, and *H. influenzae* are most common pathogens causing bacterial meningitis. The reported mean frequency ranges from 9.6 to 75.2%, 3.2 to 47%, and 0.2 to 15.5%, respectively. *S. pneumoniae* is the most common cause in meningitis in all age groups. Earlier *H. influenzae* type b (Hib) was the most common cause of bacterial meningitis, but after introduction of Hib vaccination it is the third most common cause of meningitis. Government of India introduced pentavalent vaccine [diphtheria, tetanus, pertussis (DPT) + hepatitis B (HBV) + Hib] in universal immunization program since 2012 in a phased manner. Causative microorganisms differ in specific age groups (neonates, children, adults, and elderly) as described in **Table 1**. In immunodeficiency states such as diabetes, malignancy, and immunosuppressive drugs *Listeria monocytogenes* is more often found. Splenectomy, alcoholism, human immunodeficiency virus (HIV) infection, diabetes mellitus, and hypogammaglobulinemia predispose to pneumococcal and *H. influenzae* meningitis.

NOSOCOMIAL

Etiological organisms in nosocomial meningitis are different from community-acquired meningitis. The predisposing factors and causative organisms are discussed in **Table 2**.

TABLE 1 Common etiology of bacterial meningitis in different age groups.

Age group	Organisms (descending order of frequency)
Neonates	• *Streptococcus agalactiae* • *Escherichia coli* • *Streptococcus pneumoniae*
Children up to 5 years	• *Neisseria meningitidis* • *Streptococcus pneumoniae* • *Haemophilus influenzae*
Children after 5 years and adults	• *Streptococcus pneumoniae* • *Neisseria meningitidis* • *Haemophilus influenzae* • *Listeria monocytogenes* (especially in elderly and immunocompromised)

PATHOGENESIS

Mechanism by which bacteria reaches brain and produce bacterial meningitis is a continuous process, but it can be divided into following processes for the purpose of understanding.

- Colonization
- Entry into bloodstream
- Invasion of subarachnoid space
- Neurological inflammation and damage

COLONIZATION

Neisseria meningitidis, S. pneumoniae, and H. influenzae initially colonize the upper respiratory tract and avoid host defense mechanisms. They are transmitted through inhalation of large droplets or through nasal or oral secretions. These bacteria possess pili that help in attachment with epithelial cells and entry into cell. Pili of *N. meningitidis* attach to various receptors such as PAFR, CD147, and beta-2 adrenergic receptors, while laminin receptors PIgR and PAFR receptors are used by pneumococcus for adhesion. *L. monocytogenes* attach to intestinal mucosa after eating contaminated vegetables, unpasteurized milk, or milk products, especially cheese.

ENTRY INTO BLOODSTREAM

After attachment to mucosa, entry of bacteria into bloodstream occurs between cells (pericellularly) or through the cells (transcellularly) (**Fig. 1**). Meningococci enter bloodstream transcellularly using phagocytic vacuoles while pneumococci pass into bloodstream using both pathways. After entry into bloodstream, to survive, bacteria evade the immune mechanisms in host body. Bacterial capsules of *S. pneumoniae, N. meningitidis,* and *H. influenzae* help them to evade macrophagocytosis. Microorganisms can also produce dysregulation of complement pathway and evade host body's immune system.

However, it is possible that bacteria colonizing the upper respiratory tract enter the central nervous system

TABLE 2 Predisposing factors and common pathogens in nosocomial meningitis.

Predisposing factors	Common pathogens	Remarks
Postneurosurgery, e.g., craniotomy	• Gram-negative bacilli, *Staphylococcus aureus* • Coagulase-negative staphylococci	• Occurs in 0.8–1.5% cases undergoing craniotomy • One-third cases occur in first week, further one-third occur in second week of surgery
Ventricular or lumbar catheter	• Coagulase-negative staphylococci • *Staphylococcus aureus* • Facultative and aerobic gram-negative bacilli	• Incidence ranges from 4 to 17% • Most infections present within 1 month of surgery
Penetrating trauma	*Staphylococcus aureus*, coagulase-negative staphylococci, gram-negative bacilli including *Pseudomonas aeruginosa*	• Incidence 1.4% after moderate-to-severe head injury • 5% after compound cranial fractures
Basilar skull fracture	• *Streptococcus pneumoniae* • *Haemophilus pneumoniae* • Group A beta-hemolytic streptococci	Meningitis rate is quite high up to 25% cases occurs within 10–12 days of fracture

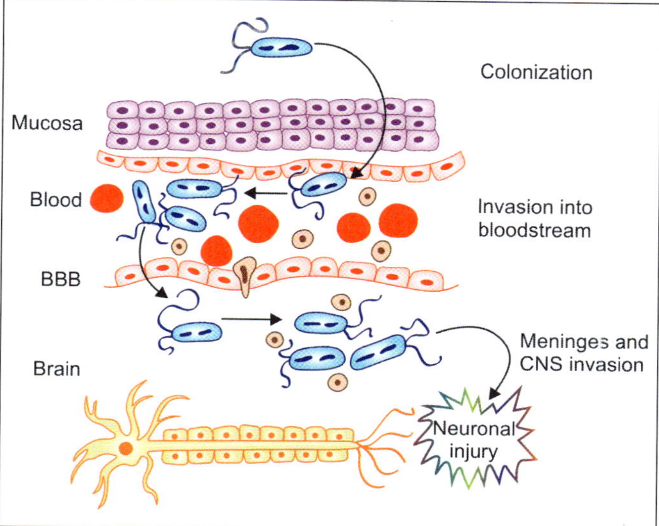

FIGURE 1: Pathogenesis of bacterial meningitis. Different steps include: (1) Colonization of mucosa; (2) Invasion into bloodstream; (3) Brain and meningeal invasion; and (4) Neurological inflammation and damage due to inflammatory response.

(CNS) from nose through dural defects or spread from paranasal sinuses or ear cavities directly to brain as seen in some cases after sinusitis or otitis media.

INVASION OF SUBARACHNOID SPACE

Once the pathogen gains entry into bloodstream, they gain access to CSF space through transcytosis or through the choroid plexus of lateral ventricles or if blood–brain barrier (BBB) is already disrupted due to prior inflammation, bacteria can gain entry directly into subarachnoid space. Once in CSF space, bacteria multiply relatively faster because of lacking host defenses in subarachnoid space.

NEUROLOGICAL INFLAMMATION AND DAMAGE

Macrophages and dendritic cells are present in leptomeninges, choroid plexus, and perivascular spaces. The bacterial cell wall products and bacterial deoxyribonucleic acid (DNA) then induce an inflammatory response after interaction with toll-like receptor 2 (TLR2) on macrophages, dendritic cells, and microglia leading to production of chemokines and inflammatory cytokines. Tumor necrosis factor-α, interleukin 1β (IL-1β), and IL-6 are some important cytokines involved in pathogenesis of bacterial meningitis. Chemokines recruits more cells, especially neutrophils to subarachnoid space and inflammatory cytokines alters BBB permeability allowing leakage of serum proteins and other molecules into CSF resulting in vasogenic edema and formation of purulent exudate. The purulent exudate is responsible for many symptoms and complications in bacterial meningitis. Exudates can block the CSF absorption from arachnoid villi leading to hydrocephalus. Cranial nerve deficits can arise due to exudates surrounding cranial nerves. Inflammatory cells may infiltrate the arterial wall causing vasculitis. Cerebral blood flow decreases due to loss of autoregulation after initial increase in blood flow. Systemic hypoperfusion also leads to cerebral hypoperfusion. Combination of vasculitis and cerebral hypoperfusion leads to cerebral ischemia leading to cytotoxic edema. Raised intracranial pressure (ICP) and coma are produced due to combination of interstitial, vasogenic, and cerebral edema. The inflammatory cytokines also induce the formation of free radicles and other products which induce massive apoptosis and contribute to vasospasm and vasculitis.

GENETIC PREDISPOSITION

Genetic factors of host determine the susceptibility to infections due to microorganisms. Single base pair variations in genes known as single-nucleotide polymorphism are responsible for variability in host response to pathogens. Such mutations in genes encoding for proteins in complement system and TLR pathways can cause increased chances of infection due to bacteria causing meningitis. Examples of such genetic causes leading to increased chances of meningitis are C2 deficiency, factor D deficiency, and polymorphisms in mannose-binding lectin. Single nucleotide polymorphisms (SNPs) in C3 (complement factor 3) are associated with decreased susceptibility to bacterial meningitis. Similarly, genetic variations in some genes are associated with decreased response to treatment, e.g., SNP in GLCCT1 (glucocorticoid-induced transcript 1 gene).

RISK FACTORS

Various risk factors predispose to acute bacterial meningitis in different age groups (**Table 3**) and should be investigated.

CLINICAL FEATURES

Classic triad of meningitis consists of fever, neck stiffness, and change in mental status. The triad is present in 41–51% of patients of meningitis. At least two of the following four signs are present in 95% of patients: (1) fever, (2) headache, (3) neck stiffness, and (4) altered mental sensorium. Individually, fever, headache, neck rigidity, and altered sensorium are present in 77%, 87%, 83%, and 69% of patients, respectively.

Sensitivity of neck stiffness, Kernig's sign, and Brudziński's sign vary from 9 to 31% though specificity is up to 95%. Thus, these clinical findings in adults have low sensitivity meaning that absence of these signs cannot be used to exclude possibility of bacterial meningitis.

Clinical characteristics at extremes of ages can vary. In neonates, bacterial meningitis presents with nonspecific symptoms such as poor feeding, irritability, respiratory distress, or hypo/hypertonia. Fever is less commonly seen in neonates. In general, more younger the patient of bacterial meningitis more subtle and atypical are the symptoms. In elderly and immunocompromised patients, also bacterial meningitis can have atypical presentation and classic signs like neck rigidity may be absent.

Classic triad is more often present in pneumococcal meningitis. Pneumococcal meningitis is more severe having higher frequency of seizures, focal neurological deficits, and lower level of sensorium of patients as compared to other causes. Rash may be seen in 26% of patients which is usually petechial (89%). One should suspect meningococcal meningitis if rash is present along with meningitis.

About 33% patients have focal neurological deficit at admission. Papilledema is found in around 3% patients of acute bacterial meningitis.

TABLE 3 Risk factors for developing bacterial meningitis in different age groups.

Age group	Risk factors
Neonates and infants	• Low birth weight • Preterm birth • Maternal infections such as chorioamnionitis, endometritis, or group B streptococci colonization • Prolonged labor and traumatic delivery • Fetal hypoxia • Down syndrome • Congenital heart disease
Children	• Malnutrition • Primary immunodeficiency • HIV infection • Asplenia • Sickle cell anemia • Cochlear implant • CNS shunt or leak • Lack of immunizations • Dermal sinus of spine • Recent exposure to meningococcal or *Haemophilus influenzae* meningitis
Adults and elderly	• Living in groups or retirement homes • Concurrent pulmonary disease: Pneumonia, asthma, and COPD • Smoking • Malignancy and chemotherapy • Chronic sinusitis or middle ear disease • Autoimmune diseases such as rheumatoid arthritis and SLE • Immune deficiency: HIV, primary immunodeficiency, and asplenia • Alcoholism • Severe anemia • CKD and CLD • Indwelling catheters, especially into CSF spaces

COMPLICATIONS

Bacterial meningitis can have systemic and neurologic complications. Systemic complications which can occur in acute bacterial meningitis are sepsis (15%) with or without septic shock, hypothermia, oliguria, acute respiratory distress syndrome (ARDS), disseminated intravascular coagulation (8%), cardiorespiratory failure (29%), hyponatremia (30% patients), and hypernatremia (7%). Arthritis can co-occur with bacterial meningitis in 7% patients. It can be due to hematogenous dissemination of bacteria to joints or due to deposition of immune complex in joints.

Neurological complications include seizures (17%), hearing loss (17–22%), hydrocephalus (3–5%), and cerebrovascular complications—ischemic stroke (14–25%), hemorrhagic stroke (3%), subdural empyema (3%) (**Fig. 2**), brain abscess (2%), cerebral venous thrombosis (1%), and cerebral edema (**Fig. 3**) often leading to increased ICP. Cognitive deficits occur in around 41% children and 32–37% adults who survive.

DIFFERENTIAL DIAGNOSIS

Differential diagnosis of bacterial meningitis can be other infective meningitis or noninfectious inflammation of meninges. Infectious meningitis in differential of bacterial meningitis includes viral, fungal, tubercular meningitis, or rickettsial meningitis. Noninfectious causes that can be considered in differentials of bacterial meningitis are subarachnoid hemorrhage, carcinomatous or lymphomatous meningitis, or neuroinflammatory diseases like neurosarcoidosis.

INVESTIGATIONS

On suspicion of bacterial meningitis clinically, CSF examination is the key for establishing diagnosis and determine etiology. But before discussing lumbar puncture, let us discuss some other investigations that are to be done simultaneously in a patient of bacterial meningitis.

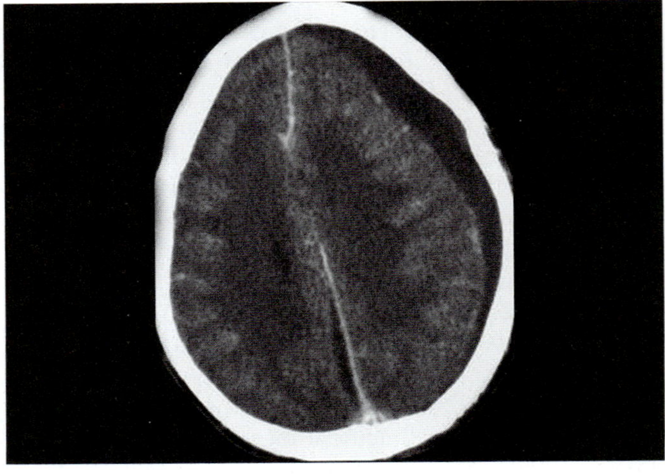

FIGURE 2: Noncontrast computed tomography (NCCT) head showing subdural empyema.

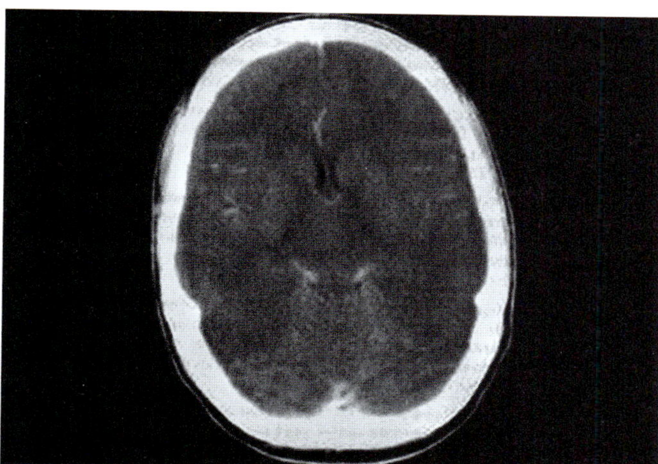

FIGURE 3: Computed tomography (CT) head of a bacterial meningitis patient showing cerebral edema.

BLOOD INVESTIGATIONS

Complete blood count, renal functional tests/liver function tests, and electrolytes are although not helpful in diagnosis of bacterial meningitis, but they can rule out other possible etiologies, e.g., presence of malarial parasite in a febrile and altered sensorium patient will lead us towards cerebral malaria. Dyselectrolytemia can complicate acute bacterial meningitis. Blood glucose concentration should be documented whenever feasible in patients presenting to emergency as that will contribute in interpreting CSF analysis besides ruling out hypoglycemia in a sick patient.

BLOOD CULTURE

Blood culture is positive in one-third to two-thirds patients of bacterial meningitis. Therefore, it is a good practice to take blood cultures in suspected bacterial meningitis patients before starting antibiotics. The results of blood culture are not available immediately but it can contribute, especially if CSF examination is delayed due to some reasons or empirical therapy fails in a patient of bacterial meningitis.

CSF EXAMINATION

CSF examination is important in establishing or refuting diagnosis of bacterial meningitis and determining etiology.

Brain imaging first or lumbar puncture: Brain imaging in form of computed tomography (CT) head or magnetic resonance imaging (MRI) brain in patient of suspected meningoencephalitis has become a routine practice in emergency setting. A retrospective study showed that getting CT head in patients before lumbar puncture delayed treatment in about 63% patients (15 out of 24 patients) by >6 hours and in patients with suspected bacterial meningitis, around 5% have lesions that can cause brain shift/herniation. Therefore, to avoid diagnostic and treatment delays, patients who should undergo brain imaging before CSF examination should be actively selected by using clinical examination. Patients having features tabulated in **Box 1** should undergo CT head before lumbar puncture.

BOX 1	Indications of brain imaging before lumbar puncture.
• Focal neurologic deficits	
• Altered sensorium (GCS < 10)	
• Dilated and fixed pupils or fixed deviation of eyes	
• New-onset seizures	
• Papilledema	
• Immunocompromised state and elderly patients	

(GCS: Glasgow Coma Scale)

CSF pressure: CSF opening pressures of >200 mm CSF are present typically, ranging between 200 and 500 mm CSF and CSF pressure continue to elevate for first 24–36 hours before subsiding.

Gross appearance of CSF: Turbid appearance of CSF signifies presence of inflammatory cells or microorganisms, but turbidity may not be always present. Turbid CSF predicted bacterial meningitis (probable or proven) in <40% cases and in 1% cases CSF may be turbid even in absence of bacterial meningitis according to Kenyan studies.

CSF cytological and biochemical analysis: Typical CSF findings for bacterial meningitis are polymorphonuclear pleocytosis, raised CSF proteins, and reduced CSF sugars. A white blood cell count of >1,000 per µL is found in 90% patients with bacterial meningitis. CSF cell count can be low in immunocompromised patients or children with bacterial meningitis. In neonates, even in culture proven bacterial meningitis, CSF cell count can be fewer than 3 cells. The abnormalities in CSF also depend on etiological organism. In a cohort of 62 patients with *L. monocytogenes* meningitis, 26% had CSF abnormalities not typical for bacterial meningitis. Neutrophilic CSF examination can be found in initial stages of tubercular meningitis and in some viruses causing meningitis. However, neutrophils rarely exceed >80% in these cases. CSF protein concentration is elevated usually >100 mg/dL. CSF glucose concentration is usually <40 mg/dL. Normal CSF glucose is about two-thirds of serum level. Typical CSF features in different etiologies of meningitis is tabulated in **Table 4**.

- **CSF Gram stain,** *culture, latex agglutination tests, and PCR*: CSF Gram stain is a rapid and inexpensive method for diagnosis of bacterial meningitis. Bacteria can be seen on Gram staining in 69-93% in *S. pneumoniae* meningitis, 30–89% in *N. meningitidis* meningitis, and 23–35% in *L. monocytogenes*. CSF Gram stain specificity is high (97%).

CSF culture is gold standard for diagnosis of bacterial meningitis. CSF culture is positive in 80–90% cases of bacterial meningitis patients who are treatment naïve. But after starting oral antibiotics these figures fall down to 67% and 65% after giving parenteral antibiotics.

TABLE 4 Typical cerebrospinal fluid (CSF) findings in different types of meningitis.

Findings	Normal	Acute bacterial meningitis	Tuberculous meningitis	Fungal meningitis	Viral meningoencephalitis
CSF opening pressure	10–20 cm CSF	High	High	High-very high	Normal-high
Color	Clear	Cloudy	Cloudy/Straw colored	Clear/Cloudy	Clear
Total cells/mm^3	<5, lymphocytes	100–50,000, neutrophils	25–500, lymphocytes	Up to 1,000, lymphocytes	Up to 1,000, lymphocytes
Proteins (mg/dL)	15–45	>100	100–500 or more	50–100	50–100
CSF/Plasma glucose ratio	66%	Low	Low-very low <30%	Normal-low	Normal

CSF PCR is helpful when patient has received antibiotics already and Gram staining and cultures are negative for CSF. The reported sensitivities and specificities of PCR vary from 67 to 100% and 91 to 100%, respectively. Latex agglutination test sensitivity varies from 22 to 100% depending on causative organism. However, CSF PCR is not available everywhere and high cost is a limiting factor in our country. PCR cannot provide antimicrobial sensitivity data and PCR can be negative in 5% culture proven cases. CSF latex agglutination tests have limited value in clinical settings. The sensitivity of latex agglutination decreases from 60 to 9% if the patient has received antibiotics.

Some contraindications to lumbar puncture are coagulopathy, local skin infection at puncture site, and septic shock. In patients of acute respiratory failure and septic shock, management of these conditions takes precedence over lumbar puncture that can be done once patient is stable.

One of dreaded complication of lumbar puncture is brain herniation. Risk of brain herniation after lumbar puncture is 1–5% in children and adults with suspected bacterial meningitis. It is difficult to distinguish herniation due to acute bacterial meningitis versus lumbar puncture as acute bacterial meningitis itself can cause brain herniation.

BRAIN IMAGING

CT head, MRI brain, and ultrasonography: CT head and MRI brain help in excluding etiologies which can present like acute bacterial meningitis and also help in assessing the complications of bacterial meningitis such as hydrocephalus, ventriculitis, subdural empyema, or stroke (**Fig. 4**). In a study of 136 patients of CSF proven bacterial meningitis, 75 patients underwent MRI brain. MRI brain was abnormal in 82.7% showing altered signal intensities at intraventricular, sulcal, cortical, and white matter (54.7%, 29.3%, 20%, and 26.7%, respectively). Leptomeningeal enhancement was seen in 27% (**Fig. 5 A**), while dural enhancement was seen in 9.5% patients (**Fig. 5 B**). Brain imaging also helps in identifying conditions predisposing to meningitis. In the above study 125 patients underwent CT head, acute sinusitis and acute mastoiditis was seen in 23.2 and 28% patients, respectively and skull base fracture in 0.8% patients. Ultrasonography can be used in infants through transfontanel approach to see for complications of meningitis.

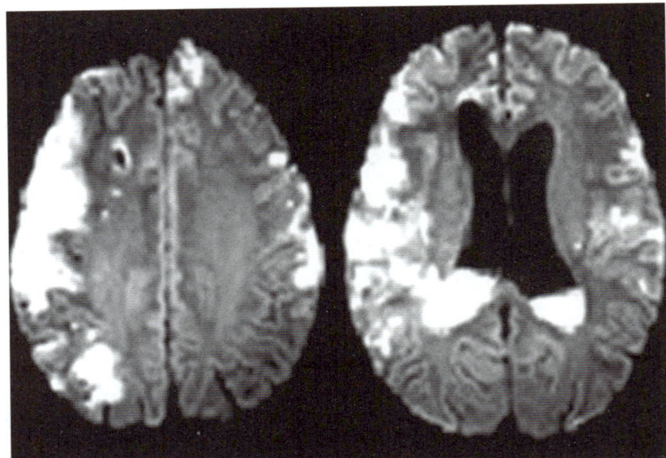

FIGURE 4: Diffusion-weighted magnetic resonance image showing cortical infarcts in a patient of bacterial meningitis.

TREATMENT

ANTIBIOTICS

Treatment of suspected bacterial meningitis should be started as soon as possible in emergency, ideally after taking both blood and CSF culture. Empiric antibiotic treatment is first started and later on based on identification of etiology-specific antibiotic should be given.

Empiric antibiotic treatment: Empiric antibiotic choice should be based on age of the patient, drug susceptibility patterns in etiologic organisms, and availability and CSF penetration of antibiotics. Suggested empirical antibiotics in bacterial meningitis are given in **Table 5**.

Reason for third-generation cephalosporins in first choice is that they are effective against the most common pathogens and their good CSF penetration even in uninflamed meninges. If penicillin resistance is suspected, especially in *S. pneumoniae* meningitis vancomycin or rifampicin is added. There is no national data from India regarding penicillin resistance in *S. pneumoniae* but according to the World Health Organization (WHO) report

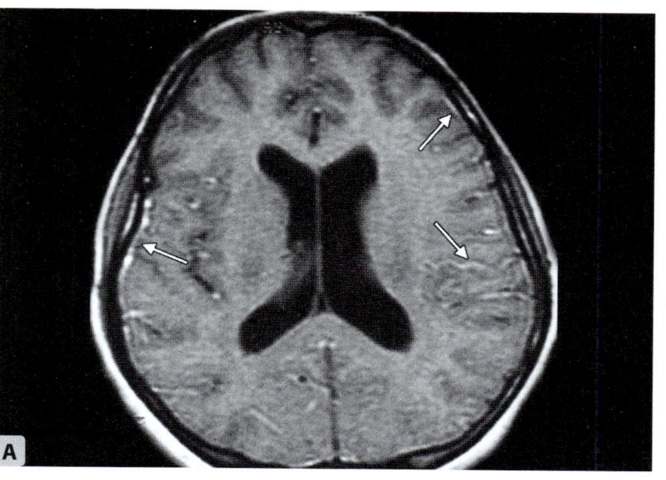

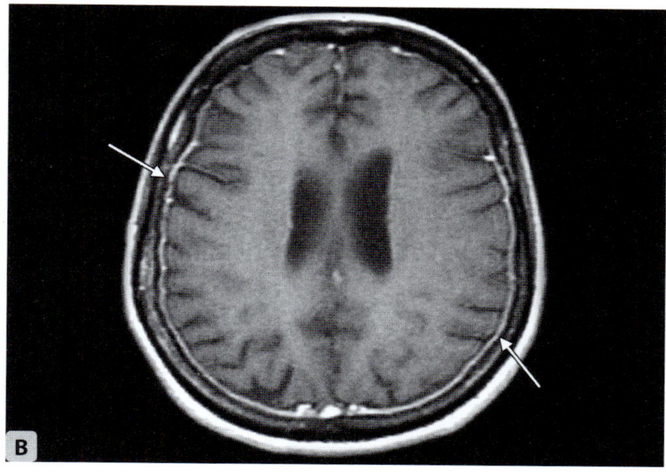

FIGURES 5 A & B: **(A)** Contrast-enhanced T1-weighted axial magnetic resonance image showing leptomeningeal enhancement; **(B)** Contrast-enhanced T1-weighted axial magnetic resonance image shows diffuse dural enhancement in a patient of bacterial meningitis.

TABLE 5 Treatment of bacterial meningitis in different age groups.

Age group	Preferred choice		Alternative if anaphylaxis to beta lactams	
	Standard treatment	Treatment in areas of high prevalence of penicillin resistance	Standard treatment	Treatment in areas of high prevalence of penicillin resistance
Neonates	Amoxicillin/ampicillin/ penicillin plus cefotaxime or amoxicillin/ampicillin plus an aminoglycoside			
Age 1 month to 18 years	Cefotaxime 75 mg/kg q6–8h, ceftriaxone 50 mg/kg q12h	Cefotaxime or ceftriaxone plus vancomycin 10–15 mg/kg q6h	Chloramphenicol. 25 mg/kg IV q6h	Vancomycin 15–20 mg/kg IV q8–12h plus moxifloxacin 400 mg IV q24h
18–50 years	Cefotaxime 2 g in q4–6h or ceftriaxone 2 g IV q12h	Cefotaxime or ceftriaxone plus vancomycin 15–20 mg/kg IV q8–12h	Chloramphenicol 25 mg/kg IV q6h	Vancomycin 15–20 mg/kg IV q8–12h plus moxifloxacin 400 mg IV q24h
>50 years or risk factors for listeria meningitis	As above plus amoxicillin or ampicillin 2 g q4h	As above plus amoxicillin or ampicillin	As above plus co-trimoxazole 5 mg/kg IV q6–12h	As above plus co-trimoxazole 5 mg/kg IV q6–12h

(IV: intravenous)

on surveillance of antimicrobial report 2014 mentions around 5% rate of penicillin resistance based on scattered publications from India. If resistance rate is >3% then it is considered better to give vancomycin to standard treatment regimen. If patient is elderly and immunocompromised, ampicillin should be added to treatment regimen to cover *L. monocytogenes* meningitis.

Fluoroquinolones are good alternatives in case of penicillin-resistant pneumococci, but in country like India where tuberculosis is so rampant, we avoid using fluoroquinolones and rifampicin to prevent development of resistance in mycobacterium tuberculosis. Antibiotic resistance is rare in meningococci.

Duration of treatment: Antibiotics should be given for 10–14 days in meningitis based on expert recommendations. There are insufficient studies to approve or refute the duration. It is seen that meningococcal meningitis can be treated with shorter duration of antibiotics 5–7 days in children if patient is clinically stable after 3 days of treatment, but pneumococcal meningitis requires treatment for longer duration (10–14 days). However, in developing countries, the etiologic agent is frequently not identified and thus if empiric treatment is continued it should be given for 10–14 days. Meningitis due to listeria should be treated for 21 days.

Treatment of nosocomial meningitis consists of vancomycin plus cefepime, ceftazidime, or meropenem. If ventricular or lumbar catheters are infected, removal of catheter is associated with more cure rates than using intravenous (IV) antibiotics only (65% vs. 35%). In case of basilar skull fracture, vancomycin plus third-generation cephalosporin (ceftriaxone or cefotaxime) is treatment of choice.

ADJUNCTIVE DEXAMETHASONE TREATMENT

The recommended dose of dexamethasone is 0.15 mg/kg every 6 hours in children and 10 mg every

6 hours in adults for duration of 4 days. Dexamethasone should be started before antibiotics or with first dose on antibiotics. A 2013 Cochrane review found that corticosteroids reduced short-term neurological sequelae and overall hearing loss, but had no effect on mortality. Subgroup analysis showed that patients in high-income countries were benefitted more than low-income countries and mortality is reduced in pneumococcal meningitis, but not in other causes of meningitis. However, presently dexamethasone is recommended in every patient of bacterial meningitis except in neonates where steroids are not recommended with antibiotics because of lack of studies on effect of steroids in neonatal meningitis.

PROPHYLACTIC USE

No role of prophylactic use of mannitol, glycerol, hypertonic saline, or antiepileptics. They can be given as per indication, but should not be given prophylactically.

BRAIN ABSCESS

Brain abscess is a focal collection of pus in brain tissue surrounded by capsule. Brain abscess is a fatal neuro-infection if treatment is delayed. Brain abscess can be caused by bacteria (most common >85% cases), fungi, mycobacteria, and helminths. In some Indian studies, tubercular abscess (60% tubercular and 40% bacterial) were found to be more common than pyogenic abscess. We will focus on bacterial causes of brain abscess in this chapter. Mortality rate is around 10%. A multidisciplinary approach is needed for management of brain abscess including neurologist, neurosurgeon, neuroradiologist, and microbiologist.

EPIDEMIOLOGY

The incidence of brain abscess is around 8% in developing countries and 2% in developed countries. It is more commonly s een in male patients with male to female ratio of 1.3:1 to 3.0:1. Brain abscess is more common in younger age group, most of them present in first two decades. In a study from NIMHANS Bangalore, median age of presentation was 22 years and ranged from 1 to 70 years.

ETIOLOGY

Streptococcus species are the most common cause of brain abscess in different case series and *Streptococcus milleri* group were most commonly identified bacteria among *Streptococcus* species *Staphylococcus* species is second most common bacteria isolated from patients of brain abscess. Around 23% cases have anaerobic bacteria as causative agent in brain abscess. Commonly isolated anaerobes are *Peptostreptococcus*, *Bacteroides* species, and *Fusarium*. In 14–25% cases, brain abscess is polymicrobial in origin and gram-negative bacteria are frequently cultured in polymicrobial cases are *Proteus, Klebsiella, Escherichia coli,* and Enterobacteriaceae. No etiological organism can be identified in 19–42% cases in different studies and possibly due to use of antibiotics prior to aspiration of abscess.

PATHOPHYSIOLOGY

Abscess arises due to inflammatory response of brain tissue to local infection. Infection reaches brain through following processes:

- Direct extension from neighboring structures such as sinusitis (found in 10% cases), otitis or mastoiditis (33%), meningitis (6%), and dental infections (5%)
- Hematogenous spread from a distant site (found in 33% cases) such as pneumonia, infective endocarditis, or other source of hematogenous spread
- Direct inoculation from trauma (found in 14% patients) or preceding neurosurgery (present in 9% patients)

  Most of the cases (86%) can have these predisposing conditions (**Table 6**), if examined carefully. After focal infection of brain, further development of brain abscess can be divided into following stages based on serial CT and MRI scan studies.
- *The early cerebritis stage*: Occurs from 1 to 3 days and characterized by neutrophil recruitment, tissue necrosis, and edema. Initially pyogenic bacteria induce damage to brain parenchyma leading to a localized suppurative lesion causing direct damage to CNS. TLR2 helps in recognizing the bacteria and causes microglial and astrocyte activation that occur at this stage and continues throughout the process of abscess development.
- The intermediate, or late cerebritis stage, occurs from 4 to 9 days and characterized by predominant macrophage and lymphocyte infiltration.
- The early capsule formation (11–14 days) characterized by capsule formation which tends to be thinner on the medial or ventricular side of the abscess and prone to rupture in this direction.
- The late capsule formation stage occurs from 14 days onward. The capsule formed becomes thick with gliotic, collagenous, and granulation layers.

The last two stages of capsule formation are associated with the formation of a well-vascularized abscess wall, thus sequestering the lesion and protecting the surrounding normal brain parenchyma from additional damage.

The mature abscess has an inner core of necrosis, surrounded by layer of inflammatory cells just inside thick collagen capsule. The capsule is surrounded by an area of marked gliosis with large number of reactive astrocytes.

CLINICAL FEATURES

Mean duration after onset of symptoms to presentation is 8.3 days in a systemic review. An abscess causes symptoms and signs due to following reasons:

- Focal/diffuse destruction
- Focal mass expansion
- Intracranial hypertension

Patient of brain abscess can present with nonspecific symptoms and signs. Classic triad of headache fever

TABLE 6 Predisposing conditions, abscess site and causative organisms.

Source of infection/ Predisposing conditions	Site of abscess	Causative organism
Paranasal sinusitis	Frontal lobe	• *Streptococcus* species (usually *Streptococcus milleri*) • *Staphylococcus aureus* • *Bacteroides* species • Enterobacteriaceae (*Escherichia coli, Klebsiella, Proteus,* and *Salmonella*)
Otitis media	Temporal lobe, cerebellum	• *Streptococcus* species • *Haemophilus* species • Enterobacteriaceae • *Bacteroides* species
Hematogenous spread	Frequently multiple abscesses; any lobe may be involved	• Depends on source • Endocarditis: *Streptococcus aureus* and *Streptococcus* species • Lung abscess: *Streptococcus* species, *Actinomyces*, and *Fusobacterium* • Congenital heart disease: *Streptococcus* and *Haemophilus* species • Urinary tract—Enterobacteriaceae and Pseudomonadaceae • Dental infection: Mixed infection with *Fusobacterium, Prevotella, Actinomyces, Bacteroides*, and *Streptococcus* species
Penetrating trauma	At site of trauma	• *Staphylococcus aureus* • *Clostridium* species • Enterobacteriaceae
Postoperative	At site of surgery	• *Staphylococcus epidermidis* • *Staphylococcus aureus* • Enterobacteriaceae • Pseudomonadaceae
Immunocompromised		• HIV infection: *Toxoplasma gondii, Nocardia, Mycobacterium, Listeria monocytogenes*, and *Cryptococcus neoformans* • Neutropenia: Aerobic gram-negative bacilli, *Aspergillus* species, *Mucorales, Candida*, and *Scedosporium* species • Transplantation: *Aspergillus* and *Candida* species, *Mucorales, Scedosporium* species, Enterobacteriaceae, and *Nocardia* species

and focal neurologic deficit is seen in 20% patients. But individually headache is present in 69% cases, fever in 53%, and focal neurologic deficit in 48%. Seizure occurs in 25–34% at presentation. Decreased sensorium is present in up to 50% patients. Nausea, vomiting, malaise, and photophobia are some nonspecific symptoms which can be present in patients of brain abscess. The clinical picture is an interplay of host organism interaction, number, size, and location of abscess. The most common sites of brain abscesses are frontal, temporal, parietal, cerebellar, and occipital lobes in descending order. Abscesses can be multiple in 5–50% patients.

INVESTIGATIONS

NEUROIMAGING

Diagnosis of brain abscess is primarily based on neuroimaging. CT head is frequently the first modality to be used while imaging a patient of brain abscess as it is easily available around the clock in most institutes as well cheaper and less time consuming than MRI brain. CT head is less sensitive than MRI in picking brain abscess during early cerebritis stage but usually patient presents after >3 days thus increasing the yield of CT head. MRI brain can differentiate between brain abscess and other intracranial pathologies reliably. CT and MRI findings in different stages of brain abscess are given in **Table 7**.

ASPIRATION OF BACTERIAL ABSCESS

Exact etiology causing bacterial abscess is determined by Gram stain and culture of purulent material from brain abscess. Etiology can be identified in 58–81% cases in different series. Frequently brain abscess is drained after giving IV antibiotics thus lowering the diagnostic yield. Obtaining blood culture is therefore important in patients of brain abscess before stating antibiotics as it can help in identification of etiological organism.

If bacterial brain abscess cultures are negative then PCR-based 16S ribosomal sequencing of DNA can be helpful in providing an etiological diagnosis.

TABLE 7 MRI findings in brain abscess.

MRI sequences	Early cerebritis stage (Fig. 6)	Late cerebritis stage (Fig. 7)	Early capsule stage (Fig. 8)	Late capsule stage (Fig. 9)
T1W MRI	Hypointense	• Hypointense at centre • Hyperintense periphery • Hypointense surrounding edema	Same as in previous stage	Same as in previous stage
T2W MRI	Hyperintense	• Iso- to hyperintense centre • Iso- to hypointense rim • Hyperintense edema	• Hyperintense centre • Hypointense rim • Hyperintense edema	Loss of hypointense rim
FLAIR MRI	Hyperintense	• Iso- to hyperintense central zone • Iso- to hypointense rim • Hyperintense edema	• Hyperintense centre • Hypointense rim • Hyperintense edema	Same as early abscess
DWI/ADC MRI	T2 shine through can be present, no diffusion restriction	Patchy diffusion restriction at central zone	Uniform diffusion restriction at centre	Same as early abscess
T1W contrast	Nodular or no enhancement	Partial or complete enhancement of rim with some enhancement extending into central zone	Smooth and thin rim enhancement without extension to central part	Same as early abscess
MRS	MRS shows cytosolic amino acid along with lactate or lipid + lactate peak			

(ADC: apparent diffusion coefficient; DWI: diffusion-weighted imaging; FLAIR: fluid-attenuated inversion recovery; MRI: magnetic resonance imaging; MRS: magnetic resonance spectroscopy; T1W: T1-weighted; T2W: T2-weighted)

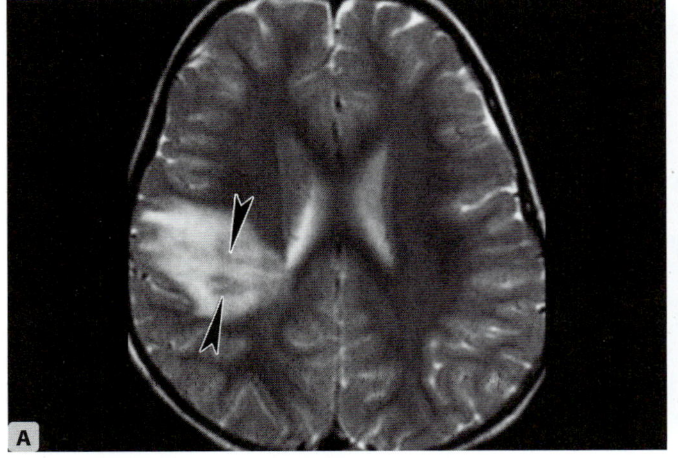

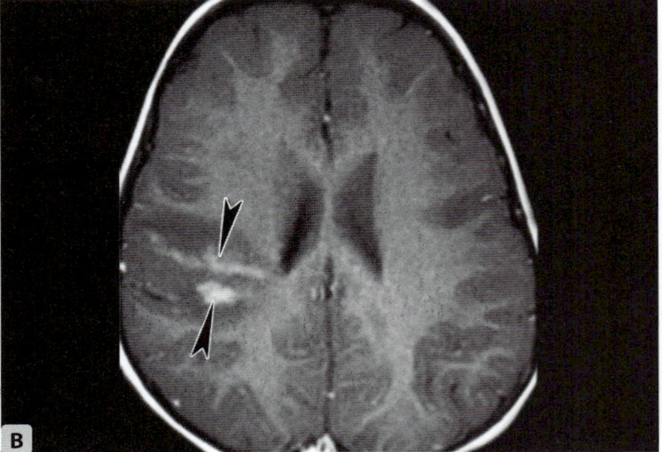

FIGURES 6 A & B: **(A)** T2-weighted (T2W) and **(B)** T1 contrast magnetic resonance imaging (MRI) brain image showing **brain abscess in early cerebritis stage** with hyperintense lesion on T2 and contrast enhancement on T1 contrast image.

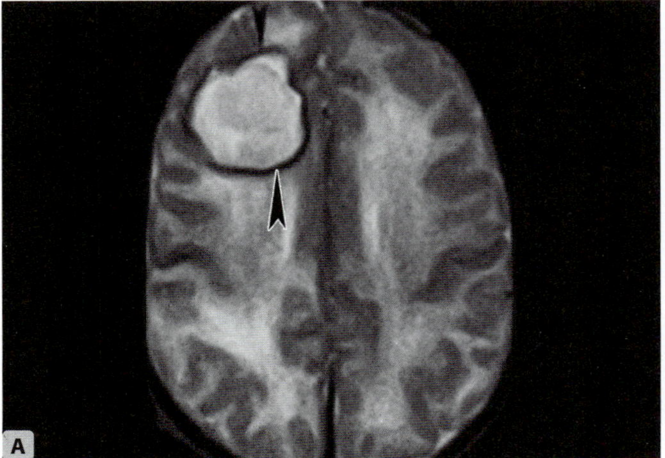

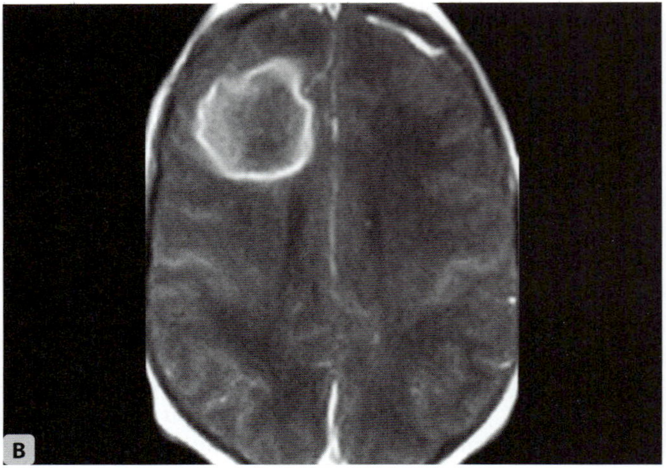

FIGURES 7 A & B: **(A)** T2-weighted (T2W) and **(B)** T1 contrast magnetic resonance imaging (MRI) brain showing **brain abscess in late cerebritis stage**.

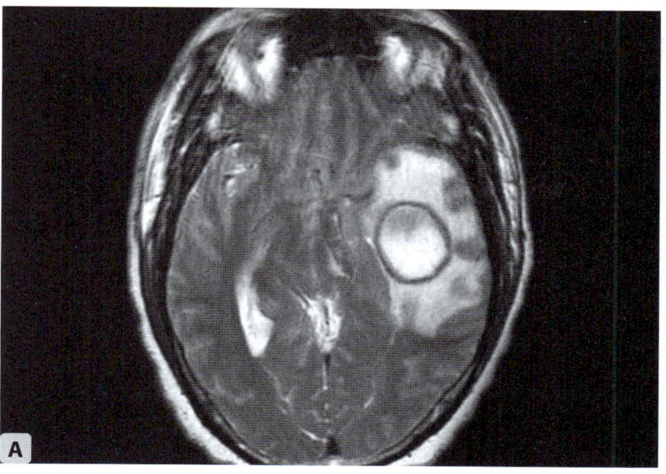

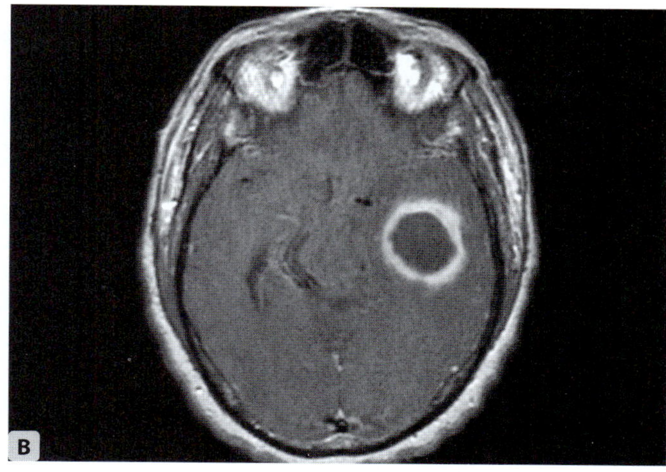

FIGURES 8 A & B: Magnetic resonance imaging (MRI) brain T2-weighted (T2W) and T1 contrast image showing **brain abscess in early capsule stage**. Notice only peripheral rim contrast enhancement in early capsule stage as compared to enhancement extending to center of abscess in late cerebritis stage.

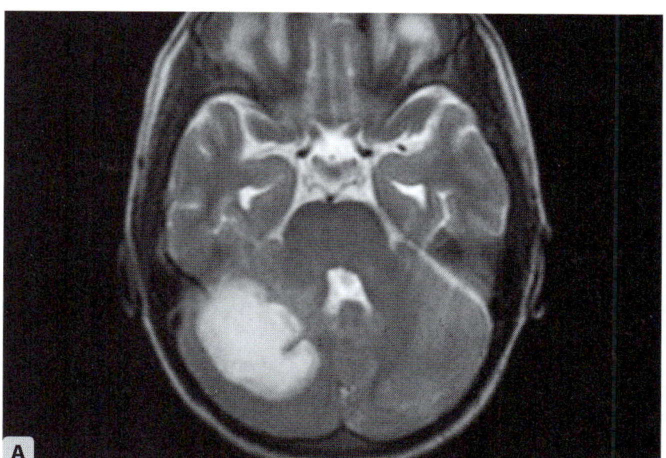

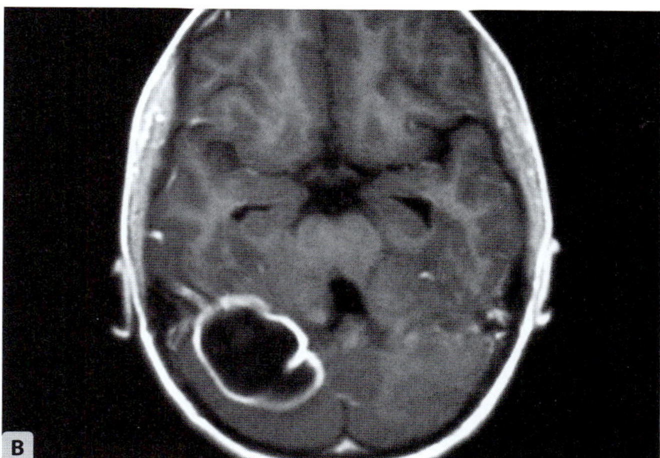

FIGURES 9 A & B: Brain abscess late capsule stage. Notice loss of hypointense rim in T2-weighted (T2W) images.

TREATMENT

Neurosurgery is required for identification of etiology and for reducing the size of abscess in some patients. Using modern stereotactic techniques, brain abscess of at least 1 cm in size is amenable for aspiration. Trajectory planning can be done in advance to avoid eloquent areas of brain. It is recommended that stereotactic aspiration should be done for diagnosis and decompression unless contraindicated. Contraindications for aspiration are no definite central cavity of abscess as seen in early cerebritis stage. poor general health, and coexisting risk factors making surgery high risk. In HIV/acquired immunodeficiency syndrome (AIDS) patients, if toxoplasmosis is suspected and immunoglobulin G (IgG) antitoxoplasma antibodies are positive, empiric therapy is justified prior to aspiration.

During diagnostic aspiration, maximal drainage of abscess should be achieved. Resection was advised for brain abscess rather than aspiration in older case series, but with modern techniques and potent antibiotics, resection of abscess may not be needed unless the abscess is superficial, located in noneloquent areas of brain or suspicion of fungal or tubercular abscess or nocardiosis.

If the etiology is already known, the decision of aspiration of abscess depends on its size and location. Any abscess >2.5 cm in diameter is considered an indication for neurosurgical intervention. Patients in whom brain abscess is leading to brain shift and herniation, neurosurgical intervention should be sought regardless of size of abscess. Similarly, in an abscess abutting ventricular system, drainage should be considered to prevent ventriculitis. In patients with multiple small brain abscesses, the abscess with largest diameter should be aspirated.

Antibiotics: The choice of initial empiric antibiotics are based on likely etiology. The empirical antibiotics used in brain abscess patients are listed in **Table 8**.

- *Bacteroides* species, *Actinomyces* species, *Fusobacterium* species, Enterobacteriaceae, and *Haemophilus* species may be part of mixed bacterial infection and combination therapy may be considered.

TABLE 8 Antibiotic treatment in brain abscess.

Empirical treatment		Based on isolated pathogen	
Etiology	**Antibiotics**	**Etiology**	**Antibiotics**
Etiology unknown/no known risk factor	Ceftriaxone (2 g q12h) or cefotaxime (2 g q4h) plus metronidazole (500 mg q6h) plus vancomycin (45–60 mg/kg/day) intravenous	*Streptococcus* species	Penicillin G or ceftriaxone or cefotaxime
Sinusitis associated	Metronidazole plus ceftriaxone or cefotaxime. Vancomycin if methicillin-resistant *Staphylococcus aureus* suspected	• *Staphylococcus aureus*	
		• Methicillin-sensitive	• Nafcillin or oxacillin (2 g q4h)
		• Methicillin-resistant	• Vancomycin
Otitis associated	Metronidazole plus ceftriaxone or cefotaxime plus penicillin G (3–4 million units q4h)	*Bacteroides fragilis*	Metronidazole
Penetrating head trauma	Ceftriaxone or cefotaxime plus vancomycin	Enterobacteriaceae	Ceftriaxone or cefotaxime or cefepime or meropenem
Postneurosurgery	Vancomycin plus meropenem (2 g q8h) or ceftazidime (2 g q8h)	*Fusobacterium* species	Metronidazole
Transplant recipient	Cefotaxime or ceftriaxone plus metronidazole, voriconazole and trimethoprim-sulfamethoxazole or sulfadiazine	*Haemophilus* species	Cefotaxime or ceftriaxone
Human immunodeficiency virus (HIV) infection	Cefotaxime or ceftriaxone plus metronidazole, pyrimethamine and sulfadiazine	*Listeria monocytogenes*	Ampicillin
		Nocardia species	Trimethoprim-sulfamethoxazole or sulfadiazine
		Pseudomonas aeruginosa	Ceftazidime or cefepime

Once the infecting pathogen is isolated, specific antibiotics can be given. Duration of IV antibiotics is 6–8 weeks, but can be prolonged if recovery is delayed. Brain imaging should be repeated if patient deteriorates clinically or not improving after 1–2 weeks of appropriate antibiotics and should be considered for neurosurgical intervention if size of abscess is increasing.

Corticosteroids should be avoided if possible in brain abscess patients as they can decrease antibiotic penetration into the abscess. However, in patients with mass effect or significant edema, raised ICP dexamethasone is recommended intravenously 10 mg every 6 hours for 3–7 days.

There are two schools of thought for prophylactic antiepileptics, some recommend antiepileptics to all patients for at least 1 year and subsequent tapering if electroencephalogram (EEG) is normal while others are not favoring prophylactic antiepileptics. The decision to start antiepileptics can be individualized in a given patient.

COMPLICATIONS

Abscess near to ventricular system, especially in posterior fossa can compress ventricular system leading to hydrocephalus. Rupture into ventricles can cause ventriculitis which is associated with high mortality (27–85%). Brain herniation and raised ICP can occur due to expanding brain abscess and edema. Long-term sequelae include risk of seizures and cognitive dysfunction. Seizures occur in 30–50% patients after a latent period of as long as 5 years.

CONCLUSION

In conclusion, pyogenic brain infections including bacterial meningitis and brain abscess should be treated promptly on suspicion and antibiotic administration should not be delayed for want of investigations in emergency settings.

Some practical questions which arise during management of patients of acute bacterial meningitis and brain abscess are given below.

RECOMMENDED READINGS

1. Zunt JR, Kassebaum NJ, Blake N, Glennie L, Wright C, Nichols E, et al. Global, regional, and national burden of meningitis, 1990–2016: a systematic analysis for the Global Burden of Disease Study 2016. Lancet Neurol. 2018;17(12):1061-82.
2. Jayaraman Y, Veeraraghavan B, Chethrapilly Purushothaman GK, Sukumar B, Kangusamy B, Kapoor AN, et al. Burden of bacterial meningitis in India: Preliminary data from a hospital based sentinel surveillance network. PLoS One. 2018;13(5):e0197198.
3. Oordt-Speets AM, Bolijn R, van Hoorn RC, Bhavsar A, Kyaw MH. Global etiology of bacterial meningitis: A systematic review and meta-analysis. PLoS One. 2018;13(6):e0198772.
4. Van de Beek D, Cabellos C, Dzupova O, Esposito S, Klein M, Kloek AT, et al. ESCMID guideline: diagnosis and treatment of acute bacterial meningitis. Clin Microbiol Infect. 2016;22:S37-62.

5. van de Beek D, Drake JM, Tunkel AR. Nosocomial bacterial meningitis. N Engl J Med. 2010;362(2): 146-54.
6. McGill F, Heyderman RS, Panagiotou S, Tunkel AR, Solomon T. Acute bacterial meningitis in adults. Lancet. 2016;388(10063):3036-47.
7. Kasanmoentalib ES, Brouwer MC, van de Beek D. Update on bacterial meningitis: epidemiology, trials and genetic association studies. Curr Opin Neurol. 2013;26(3):282-8.
8. Heckenberg SG, Brouwer MC, van de Beek D. Bacterial meningitis. Handb Clin Neurol. 2014;121:1361-75.
9. Brouwer MC, Thwaites GE, Tunkel AR, Van De Beek D. Dilemmas in the diagnosis of acute community-acquired bacterial meningitis. Lancet. 2012;380: 1684-92.
10. van de Beek D, de Gans J, Spanjaard L, Weisfelt M, Reitsma JB, Vermeulen M. Clinical features and prognostic factors in adults with bacterial meningitis. N Engl J Med. 2004;351(18):1849-59.
11. Scarborough M, Thwaites GE. The diagnosis and management of acute bacterial meningitis in resource-poor settings. Lancet Neurol. 2008;7(7):637-48.
12. Davis LE. Acute bacterial meningitis. Continuum (Minneap Minn). 2018;24(5):1264-83.
13. Soloman T, Hart I, Beeching N. Viral encephalitis: a clinician's guide. Pract Neurol. 2007;7:288-305.
14. Lummel N, Koch M, Klein M, Pfister HW, Brückmann H, Linn J. Spectrum and Prevalence of Pathological Intracranial Magnetic Resonance Imaging Findings in Acute Bacterial Meningitis. Clin Neuroradiol. 2016;26(2):159-67.
15. WHO. (2014). Antimicrobial resistance: Global Report on Surveillance. [online] Available from https://apps.who.int/iris/bitstream/handle/10665/112642/9789241564748_eng.pdf;jsessionid=AB1ED33FD0D163A88420371ACAABD38B?sequence=1.
16. Muzumdar D, Jhawar S, Goel A. Brain abscess: an overview. Int J Surg. 2011;9(2):136-44.
17. Shruthi U, Prabhu Raj AR, Kumari HBV, Nagarathna C. Anaerobic bacteriological profile of brain abscess in a tertiary care center in southern India. Anaerobe. 2019;59:68-71.
18. King N. Brain abscess. Handb Clin Neurol. 2010;96: 65-74.
19. Brouwer MC, Coutinho JM, van de Beek D. Clinical characteristics and outcome of brain abscess: systematic review and meta-analysis. Neurology. 2014;82(9):806-13.
20. Brouwer MC, Tunkel AR, McKhann GM 2nd, van de Beek D. Brain abscess. N Engl J Med. 2014;371:447-56.

CHAPTER 189

Tuberculous Meningitis

Jayantee Kalita, Usha K Misra

ABSTRACT

Tuberculosis (TB) is a leading health problem in Southeast Asia and Africa leading to 1.5 million deaths per year. TB primarily is a disease of lung but about 10% may have extrapulmonary TB, of whom tuberculosis meningitis (TBM) is the most devastating. Central nervous system (CNS) spread of *Mycobacterium tuberculosis* occurs through hematogenous spreading forms Rich focus in subpial and subependymal regions. Rupture of these Rich focus in to the subarachnoid or ventricular system results in meningitis. TBM is a subacute or chronic meningitis and manifests with low grade fever, headache, vomiting, and meningeal signs. There may be altered sensorium, seizures, focal weakness, and cranial nerve palsy.

Cerebrospinal fluid (CSF) reveals lymphocytic pleocytosis and in 20–40% patients *M. tuberculosis* may be detected in smear or culture. Nucleic acid amplification tests (NAATs) of CSF although have higher sensitivity than smear and culture, but about 30% patients may not be confirmed by these tests. Diagnosis of TBM in this group therefore is based on clinical, CSF, and computed tomography/magnetic resonance imaging (CT/MRI) findings. Cranial CT/MRI reveals basal exudates infarcts in basal ganglia, granuloma, and hydrocephalous in various combinations. GeneXpert helps in diagnosing TBM and drug sensitivity.

Combination of isoniazid (INH), rifampicin, ethambutol, and pyrazinamide is used during intensive phase followed by rifampicin and INH during continuation phase for a period of 12 months. In INH resistance, levofloxacin should be added. Rifampicin- and INH-resistant TBM is treated with four or more second-line drug along with pyrazinamide and ethambutol for ≥18 months. Corticosteroid and aspirin are helpful in reducing mortality. Treatment of complications such as hyponatremia, hydrocephalous, and seizure are important.

"The brain is a world consisting of a number of unexplored continents and great stretches of unknown territory"

—S J Cajal

INTRODUCTION

Tuberculosis is a global health problem especially in Southeast Asia and Africa. In 2018, about 1.7 billion people globally were infected with *M. tuberculosis*, and 10 million developed the disease. About 1.5 million people die of TB annually, and 95% deaths occur in the developing countries. TB primarily affects lung, but about 10% patients may have extrapulmonary TB and 5% may have tuberculous meningitis. Incidence of CNS TB is higher in high TB burden areas compared to low TB burden areas. Among those aged 5 years or more, TB kills more people than acquired immunodeficiency syndrome (AIDS), malaria, diarrhea, leprosy, and all of the tropical diseases combined. Treating TB is the most efficient and cost-effective of all health interventions. The burden of TB is increased because AIDS, migration, poverty, unhygienic living conditions, malnutrition, drug abuse, immunosuppressants, and anticancer drugs. In the population with lower TB prevalence, TBM occurs mostly in adults, whereas in populations with a higher TB prevalence, the peak incidence is in 2–4 years of age.

ETIOLOGY AND PATHOGENESIS

Nearly all the CNS TB is due to human tubercle bacillus *M. tuberculosis* which is a nonmotile, rod-shaped, nonspore-forming bacterium, measuring 0.5 µm by 3 µm. *M. tuberculosis* does not stain on Gram staining; however, once stained the bacillus cannot be decolorized by acid or alcohol; therefore, it is known as acid fast bacillus (AFB). *M. tuberculosis* grows slowly. Its generation time is 15–20 hours as opposed to <1 hour for pyogenic bacteria. The mycobacterial cell wall has complex proteins, peptides, lipids, and glycolipids with specific immunologic properties. Other antigens are present in the cytoplasm.

Mycobacterium tuberculosis enters the lung through droplet infection and activates alveolar macrophage, dendritic cells, and neutrophils, which release cytokines, chemokines, and antimicrobial peptides. Bacilli may be killed or some infected dendritic cells may migrate to draining lymph nodes, activates helper T cells, and cytokine release leading to killing of *M. tuberculosis* or formation of granuloma.

CNS involvement occurs by hematogenous spread: (1) During the primary infection, some infected dendritic cells may reach the brain through hematogenous route; and (2) Progression of latent to active pulmonary TB in adult and young children during immunocompromised state may break the alveolar epithelium with the help of early secretory antigenic target 6, culture filtrate protein 10 KDA, and heparin-binding hemagglutinin adhesion. This leads to hematogenous spread of bacilli or through the infected monocytes. These infected materials cross blood–brain barrier and blood–CSF barrier to infect CNS by two mechanisms: (1) "Trojan horse" in which bacilli cross these barriers via infected macrophages and neutrophils; and (2) Bacilli invade endothelium with the help of *M. tuberculosis* pknD (Rvo931c). These bacilli in the brain form Rich focus in subpial or subependymal regions.

There may be granuloma formation due to focal inflammation or may rupture into the subarachnoid space of ventricular system leading to meningitis. Rarely the source of TBM is adjacent extraneural infection such as vertebrae, ear, mastoid sinuses etc. In a relatively immuno-incompetent host, especially infants or children below 5 years of age, the "Rich" focus may rupture during the primary infection resulting in concomitant meningeal and pulmonary or meningeal and miliary infection.

PATHOLOGY

In TBM, the meninges, brain parenchyma, and blood vessels are affected; hence it is more appropriately called a meningoencephalitis. There are exudate, vasculitis, hydrocephalus, border-zone encephalitis or infarction, tubercular encephalopathy, tuberculoma, and tubercular abscess. The main pathology is thick gelatinous or nodular exudates within the subarachnoid space especially at base of brain, around interpeduncular fossa, enveloping optic nerves at the chiasma and extending into the Sylvian fissure, cerebral hemispheres, pons, and cerebellum. The exudate often covers the choroid plexus in the lateral ventricle. Exudate contains polymorphonuclear leukocytes, red blood cells, macrophages, and lymphocytes within a fibrin network with variable number of mycobacteria. As the disease progresses, lymphocytes predominate along with fibroblasts and connective tissue.

Typical tubercles may develop into the exudate and areas of caseation necrosis are formed. The blood vessels traversing tubercular exudate reveal characteristic inflammation. Small arteries may be obliterated by exudates or vasculitis. *Ischemic arterial infarction* resulting from tubercular arteritis is a common complication primarily in the distribution of middle cerebral arteries and deep perforating vessels. *Hydrocephalus* is more common in children compared to adults. Nearly all the children with TBM exceeding 6 weeks may have hydrocephalus. Generally, hydrocephalous is communicating and is attributed to the blockade of basal cisterns and arachnoid villi by exudate impeding CSF absorption. Obstruction in the ventricular system, i.e., foramen of Monro or aqueduct, is responsible for obstructive hydrocephalus in a small proportion of TBM. Border-zone encephalitis is a tissue reaction adjacent to thick adherent exudate. *Tubercular encephalopathy* is probably due to allergic phenomenon and is associated with cerebral edema, perivascular demyelination, or hemorrhagic leukoencephalopathy. It affects young children with progressive primary TB. *Tubercular abscesses* may be single or multiple, and are more commonly found in elderly or immunocompromised patients. There are numerous AFB in the pus and evidence of granuloma formation in the wall. Streptomycin-treated patients have marked organization and fibrosis of the basal exudates. Much of the exudate is replaced by hyalinized connective tissue if the duration of treatment exceeds 2 years.

CLINICAL FEATURES

The clinical manifestations of neurotuberculosis depend on the predominant pathology.

TBM classically a subacute or chronic meningitis, but rarely may present within a week. The clinical feature of TBM has been divided into prodrome, stage of meningeal irritation, and stage of diffuse or focal cerebral involvement.

Prodrome: The prodrome generally lasts for 2–3 weeks, and occasionally 2–3 months. In children, it manifests with vague ill health, apathy, lack of appetite, vomiting, and pain in the abdomen.

Stage of meningeal irritation: There is headache, vomiting and fever, apathy, irritability, photophobia, and varying degrees of neck stiffness which may progress to opisthotonus in young children. In infants, a tense fontanelle and vomiting are more frequent than headaches and neck stiffness. A comparison of clinical features of TBM in adults and children is shown in **Table 1**. Seizures, cranial nerve palsy, and hemiparesis may precede, accompany or follow the meningeal symptoms. Sometimes TBM is diagnosed in a patient being investigated for hydrocephalus or brain tumor.

Stage of focal or diffuse cerebral involvement: As TBM progresses, stupor and coma replace apathy and irritability. Features of raised intracranial tension become obvious; enlarging head, tense fontanelle in young children and sutural diastasis in older children, hyperventilation, extensor posturing, and occasionally papilledema. Cranial neuropathy, seizures, and focal deficit occur in 20–50% patients. Rarely abnormal movement disorders such as chorea, hemiballismus, or tremor may be present.

During the course of illness, spread of inflammation and exudate to spinal meninges result in radiculomyelopathy leading to paraplegia or quadriplegia. Acute onset paraparesis may be due to tubercular vasculitis or tubercular myelitis. Rarely intracranial meningitis may be secondary to spinal TB.

TABLE 1 Clinical presentation of tuberculous meningitis (Zugar 2004).

Parameters	Children	Adults
Fever	50–100%	60–100%
Headache	20–50%	50–60%
Nausea/Vomiting	50–75%	8–40%
Behavioral changes	30–70%	30–70%
Seizures	10–20%	0–15%
Past history of tuberculosis	55%	8–12%
Neck stiffness	70–100%	60–70%
Cranial nerve palsy	15–30%	15–40%
Altered sensorium	30–45%	20–30%

The terminal illness in TBM is characterized by deep coma, decerebration or decortication, extensor rigidity, and convulsions. Pupils may be dilated and fixed. Respiration becomes irregular Cheyne–Stoke's or Biot's type. Direct infiltration of the diencephalon may be responsible for irreversible coma.

SEVERITY OF TUBERCULOSIS MENINGITIS

The clinical severity of TBM can be graded as:

- Stage I: Alert and orientated without focal neurological deficit.
- Stage II: Glasgow Coma Score 14–11 with or without focal neurological deficit or Glasgow Coma Scale score 15 with focal neurological deficit
- Stage III: Glasgow Coma Scale score <11 with or without focal neurological deficit.

The patients in any of the above stage needing intubation and mechanical ventilation suggest grave outcome, and may be categorized separately as stage IV.

INVESTIGATIONS

CRANIAL CT SCAN AND MRI

Contrast CT scan is adequate for routine management of neurotuberculosis but MRI reveals more parenchymal changes especially stroke. Cranial imaging reveals enhancing basal exudates, hydrocephalous, infarction, or tuberculoma in various combinations (**Figs. 1 A** to **D**). Communicating hydrocephalus is characterized by dilated ventricles, including the fourth ventricle with periventricular lucency. Sometime there may be obstructive hydrocephalus, in such situation only the lateral and third ventricles, or only one lateral ventricle may be dilated due to block in the aqueduct or foramen of Monro, respectively.

Infarctions in TBM occurs in half the patients and are usually small, multiple, and commonly located in the basal ganglia involving caudate nucleus, anterolateral thalamus, genu, and anterior limb of internal capsule (tubercular zone) (**Figs. 2 A** to **C**). Ependymitis is seen as a linear enhancement along the margin of the ventricles. Tuberculoma may be solitary or multiple; round, oval, or lobular shaped and iso- or hyperdense on CT scan. These are located commonly in the frontal and parietal regions; however, tuberculoma may also be seen in the infratentorial region.

On contrast administration, immature tuberculoma enhances as small ring or disks with massive edema and mature tuberculoma are seen as a large ring or lobulated mass. The margin of ring is irregular, unlike cysticercosis. En plaque meningeal tuberculoma are demonstrated as lenticular enhancing lesions. Calvarial TB is rarely associated with TBM which may be a circumscribed, single calvarial defect with or without sclerosis or expanding lytic lesions with well-defined margins that may be surrounded by a faint zone of osteoporosis. These lesions can spread across the suture line. Tubercular otomastoiditis may be seen in children. In the early stage, CT scan reveals soft tissue in

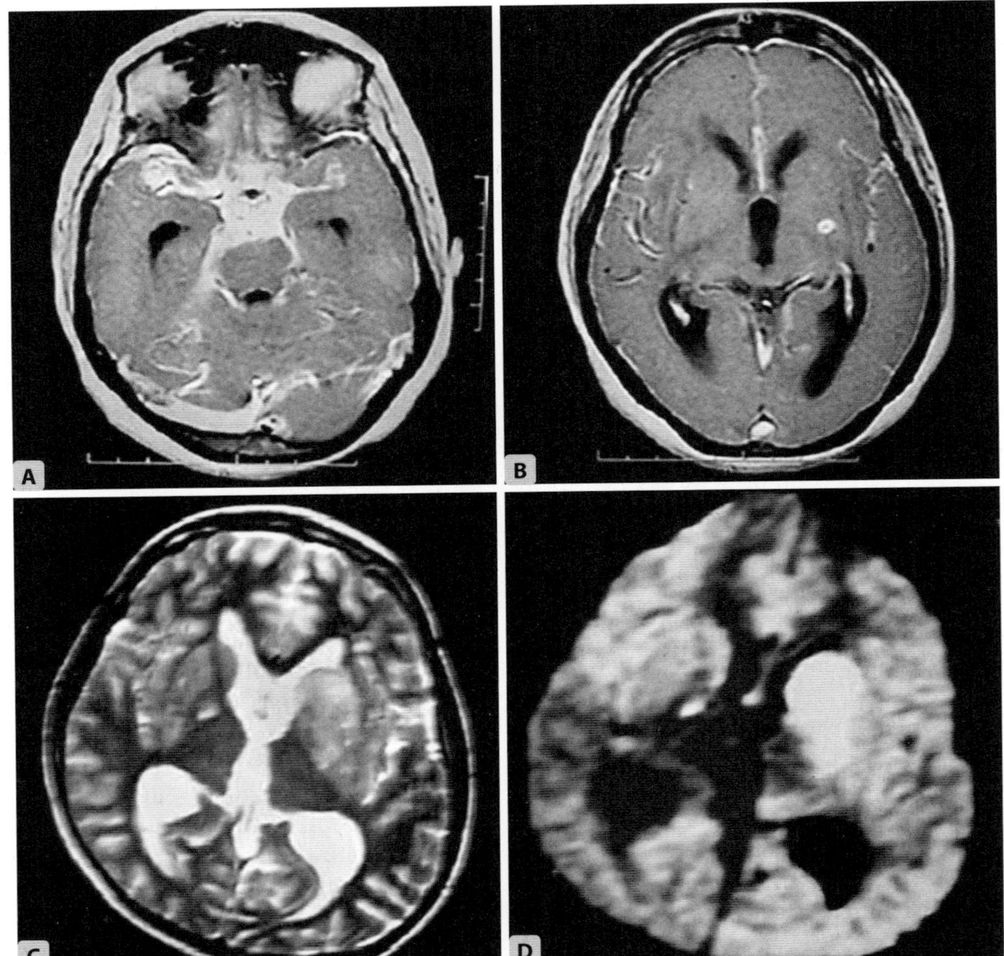

FIGURES 1 A to D: MRI in tuberculous meningitis showing exudate, granuloma, hydrocephalous, and infarction. **(A)** Basal exudates and dilated temporal horn of lateral ventricle in T1 contrast image; **(B)** Enhancing granuloma in left basal ganglia and hydrocephalus in T1 contrast image; **(C)** Hydrocephalous with left caudate infarct in T2 sequence; and **(D)** Hyperintese on DWI in left caudate suggesting infarction.

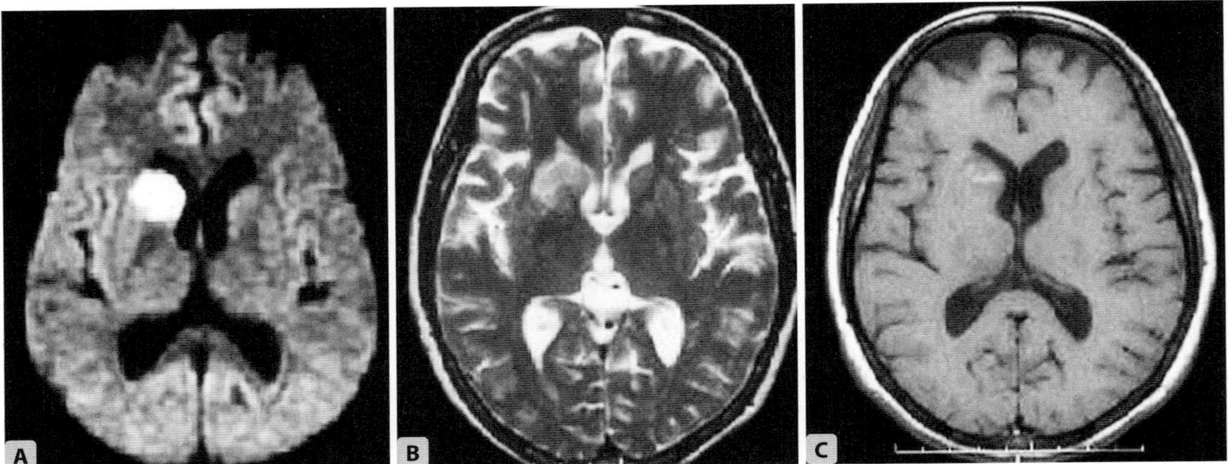

FIGURES 2 A to C: Infarction in tubercular zone in tuberculous meningitis.

Source: With permission from Kalita J, Misra UK, Nair PP. Predictors of stroke and its significance in the outcome of tuberculous meningitis. J Stroke Cerebrovasc Dis. 2009;18(4):251-8.

the tympanic cavity and later destruction of middle ear structures, signs of mastoiditis, and retroauricular or epidural abscess. Abnormal enhancement of the choroid plexus and lining of the ventricular system may also be seen.

Infarctions are reported in 41% of autopsy specimens, 20.5% and 38% in CT scan, and up to 60% in MRI. The MRI features of tuberculoma depend on whether the granuloma is noncaseating with a solid center or caseating with a liquid center. Miliary tubercules are <2 mm and are either not visible on conventional spin echo MR or are seen as tiny foci of hyperintensity on T2-weighted acquisition or on contrast (**Figs. 3 A** to **C**). Nonenhancing residual encephalomalacia with or without calcification is also a sign of healing.

Magnetic resonance features of spinal tubercular meningitis include CSF loculation and obliteration of CSF subarachnoid space with loss of outline of the spinal cord in the cervicothoracic region and walling of nerve roots in the lumbar region. Gadolinium-enhanced MR images reveal thick linear intradural enhancement often completely filling the subarachnoid space. This may be noted when unenhanced images appear normal. In the chronic stage, gadolinium enhancement may not be present and even unenhanced images may show signs of arachnoiditis.

The vascular changes can be noninvasively studied employing *MR angiography* which reveals irregular narrowing of middle, anterior, and posterior cerebral arteries. There may be narrowing of supraclinoid carotid arteries or narrowing or occlusion of vertebral or basilar artery. Vasculitis is evidenced by enhancement of arterial wall (**Figs. 4 A** to **F**). Cerebral venous system involvement usually does not occur. Single-photon emission computed tomography (SPECT) studies have confirmed hypoperfusion in the basal ganglia, cerebral cortex, or both. Positron emission tomography (PET) scan in TBM reveals extra CNS involvement in the majority. The main limitations to these brain imaging techniques are: CT scans are normal in about 30% of individuals at an early stage of TBM, while MRI scans are normal in about 15%, and these facilities are not available in primary healthcare setting.

CEREBROSPINAL FLUID ANALYSIS

Characteristic CSF findings in TBM are protein >100 mg/dL and cells >20/dL, mostly lymphocytic. CSF may be rarely normal. A wide variety of CSF changes have been reported in TBM which are classified as serous, pseudopyogenic, encephalitic, or block patterns.

Bacteriological diagnosis: Demonstration of *M. tuberculosis in* CSF smear or culture is the gold standard for the diagnosis of TBM. For smear positivity in Ziehl–Neelsen

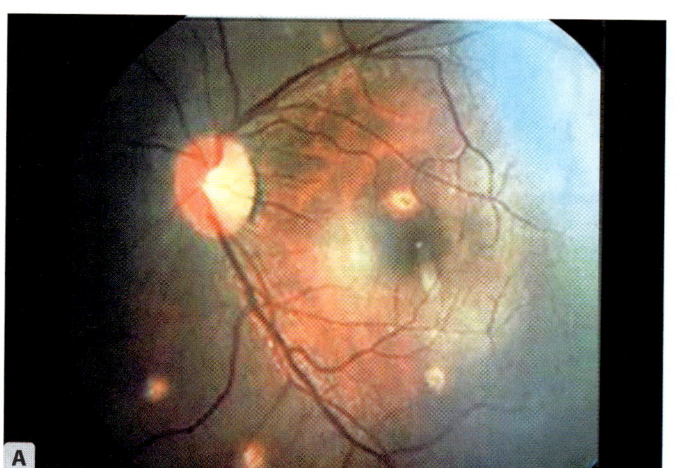

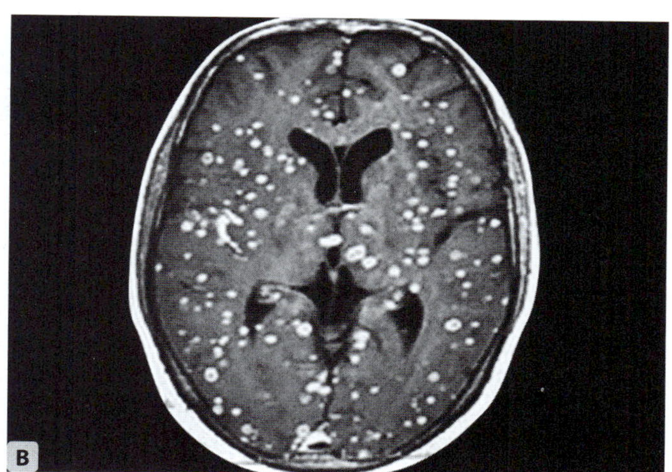

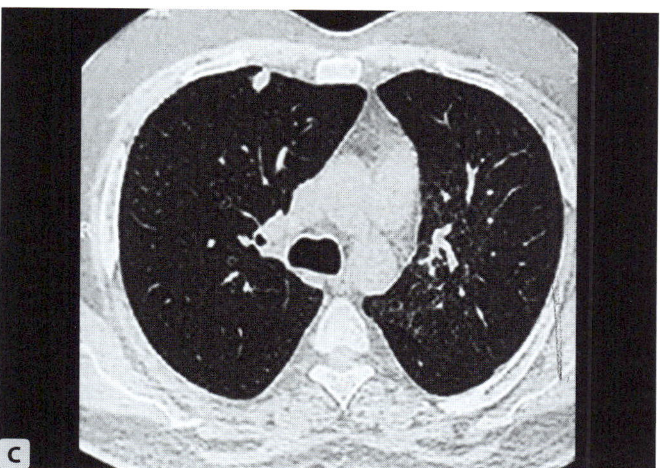

FIGURES 3 A to C: (A) Fundus photograph shows multiple choroid tubercles; **(B)** Cranial MRI shows enhancing numerous miliary tuberculoma looking like a starry sky; and **(C)** CT thorax shows miliary tuberculoma in both the lung fields.

Source: With permission from Kalita J, Pandey PC, Misra UK. Starry Sky in Disseminated Tuberculosis. Am J Med. 2020:S0002-9343(20)30937-2.

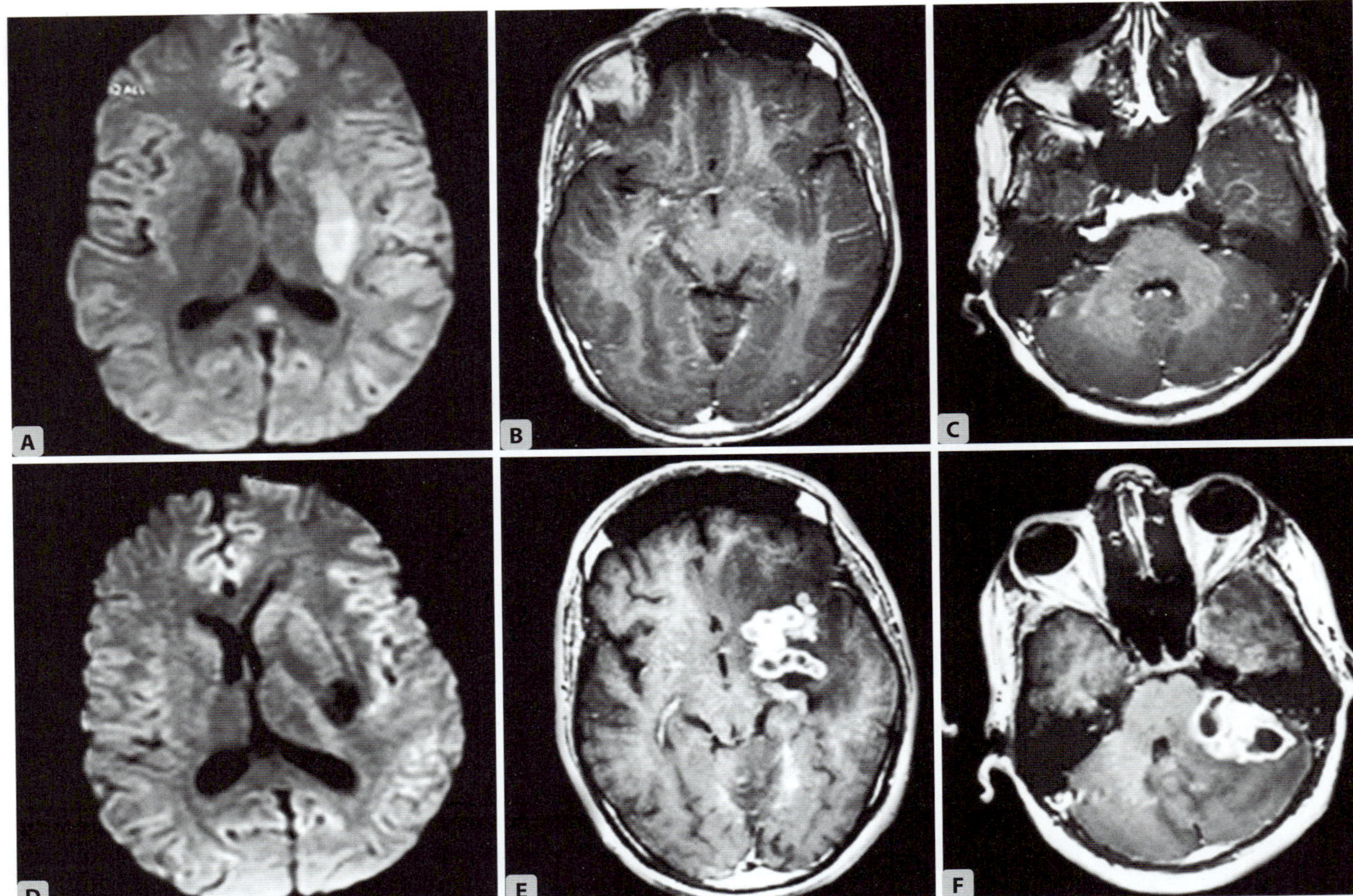

FIGURES 4 A to F: Paradoxical response in a patient with definite tuberculous meningitis. The baseline MRI pictures **(A to C)** show left basal ganglia acute infarct in diffusion-weighted imaging **(A)** and mild basal exudates **(B and C)**. A follow up MRI at 3 months after antitubercular treatment reveals old infarct in left basal ganglia **(D)**, enhancing granuloma in left insular **(E)** and cerebellar region **(F)**.

Source: With permission from Kalita J, Prasad S, Misra UK. Predictors of paradoxical tuberculoma in tuberculous meningitis. Int J Tuberc Lung Dis. 2014;18(4):486-91.

staining, a bacterial load of 10×10^4 AFB/mL is required and conventional cultures in Lowenstein–Jensen media are positive at a concentration of 10–100 AFB/mL. In most patients with TBM, the bacterial load of such magnitude is uncommon. The following measures may improve the yield: (1) staining the cobweb coagulum, (2) examining the centrifuge deposit of a large volume of CSF, and (3) repeated CSF examination; testing second, third, or even fourth sample.

Cerebrospinal fluid culture in Lowenstein–Jensen takes up to 8 weeks for detectable colonies to appear whereas BACTEC culture takes 18 days. AFB detection rate in CSF ranges between 10% and 15%, and in culture 40% and 60%.

Molecular tests: To overcome the limitations of microbiological diagnosis, commercial NAATs are available. Sensitivity of NAATs is better in pulmonary samples than CSF; therefore, these tests are not reliable for ruling out TB from extrapulmonary specimens. A number of meta-analyses have reported sensitivity of 64–82% and specificity of 98–99% against CSF for commercial NAATs.

The Xpert MTB/RIF test is an automated closed-cartridge system that allows the rapid (within 2 h) detection of both *M. tuberculosis nucleic acid* and rifampin (RIF) resistance simultaneously. The World Health Organization (WHO) recommends the GeneXpert test for the diagnosis of TBM with CSF specimen in adults and children. Its sensitivity in TBM is 8–72%. Xpert MTB/RIF Ultra (Xpert Ultra) has been developed to overcome the inadequate sensitivity and has 70% sensitivity for probable or definite TBM compared with 43% obtained by either Xpert or culture. Loop-mediated isothermal amplification (LAMP) test is another NAAT which may be useful in resource-poor settings, as it does not require expensive instruments or expertise, and result could be obtained in 60 minutes. Another NAAT that is commercially available (the Amplicor TB PCR test) has a sensitivity of 40% and specificity of 90–100% in the diagnosis of TBM, but requirements of skilled staff and high cost are the limiting factors.

The Gen-Probe amplified M. tuberculosis direct (MTD) test and Genotype MTBDRplus are other molecular tests that target specific genes for *M. tuberculosis* complex detection, as well as RIF and INH susceptibility. While most NAATs have shown potential as diagnostic tests for TBM, more data on the performance of the tests are still required. Overall, commercial NAATs have demonstrated high specificity but have suboptimal sensitivity for TBM, whereas Xpert Ultra, although promising, can still miss up to 30% of TBM patients. Although NAATs are a major diagnostic advance, these are still inadequate to replace culture methods. The CRISPR-*M. tuberculosis* and metagenomic next-generation sequencing (mNGS) may improve the detection of *M. tuberculosis* in CSF samples with low AFB load.

Immune response-based diagnosis: Immunodiagnostic tests, such as interferon gamma release assays (IGRAs), cannot differentiate latent TB infection (LTBI) from active TB disease; therefore, are not recommended. Adenosine deaminase (ADA) is released by lymphocytes and plays an important role in the proliferation and differentiation of T cells. Evidence about the clinical usefulness of CSF ADA is contradictory and has high false positivity.

TUBERCULIN TEST

The tuberculin test is done by a subcutaneous injection of 0.1 mL of 5T4 of PPD-5 (purified protein derivative) or 1 unit of PPD-RT23 into the volar aspect of the forearm. The response is assessed after 48–72 hours. The maximum diameter of induration is measured by palpation and interpreted as: >15 mm or ulceration—strongly positive; >10 mm—positive; 5–9 mm—intermediate; and <5 mm—negative. This test has a limited value because of low sensitivity and specificity, more so in the endemic area. False negative results are common in immunosuppressed patients and false positive in subjects with latent *M. tuberculosis infection* or BCG vaccination.

SEARCH FOR EXTRA CNS TUBERCULOSIS

Effort should be made to collect evidence of extra CNS TB by investigations such as radiograph of the chest, fine needle aspiration cytology of the enlarged lymph node, abdominal ultrasound, or CT scan. About 77% of TBM patients with human immunodeficiency virus (HIV) have extrameningeal TB compared to only 9% without HIV.

None of the currently available methods is adequate for use as a stand-alone test for the diagnosis of TBM. Therefore a combination of meningitis symptoms with characteristic CT/MRI and CSF changes, and evidence of extra CNS TB is considered in the diagnosis of TBM. Presence of AFB in smear, culture or NAATs is considered as definite TBM, clinical with two supportive features (CSF, CT/MRI, and therapeutic response) as probable and one supportive feature as possible TBM.

DIFFERENTIAL DIAGNOSIS

The differential diagnosis of subacute or chronic meningitis is difficult because of diverse clinical picture and multiplicity of etiological considerations including infectious and noninfectious etiologies.

Chronic neutrophilic meningitis—with hypoglycorrhachia is attributed to bacteria (*Nocardia, Actinomyces*, and *Brucella*) and fungi. In exceptional cases, noninfectious causes such as endogenous chemical meningitis due to release of contents of epidermoid tumor or craniopharyngioma, exogenous chemical meningitis due to intrathecally administered drugs, or contrast agents and systemic lupus erythematosus should be considered.

Chronic lymphocytic meningitis—includes spirochetal (*Treponema pallidum, Borrelia*, and lyme disease) and bacterial meningitis (*Brucella, Actinomyces israelii, M. tuberculosis*). Fungi are an important cause of chronic lymphocytic meningitis and need specific antifungal therapy. The important fungi producing chronic lymphocytic meningitis include *Cryptococcus neoformans, Candida, Coccidioides immitis, Histoplasma capsulatum*, and *Blastomyces dermatitidis*. CSF glucose is reduced in fungal meningitis, particularly in cryptococcal. India ink preparation is positive in 50% of patients with cryptococcal meningitis and cryptococcal polysaccharide antigen in 90%. Certain other conditions such as parameningeal infection, brain abscess, cysticercosis, toxoplasmosis, and viral meningitis (mumps meningoencephalitis, lymphocytic choriomeningitis, and persistent CNS echo virus infection in patients with agammaglobulinemia) occasionally have a prolonged course.

Noninfectious causes—include carcinomatous meningitis, primary or secondary neoplasms, meningeal sarcoidosis, cerebral granulomatous arteritis, and multiple sclerosis. The salient causes of chronic meningitis are mentioned in **Box 1**. Chronic meningitic syndrome remains a challenge to the physician's skill in differential diagnosis.

MANAGEMENT

Management of TBM includes antitubercular drugs, host-directed therapy, and management of complications such as hydrocephalus, stroke, seizure, and hyponatremia.

BOX 1	Differential diagnosis of chronic meningitis.
• Tuberculous meningitis	
• Partially treated pyogenic meningitis	
• *Fungal*: Cryptococcal, *Candida, Coccidioides, Histoplasma, Blastomyces*, and parameningeal infection	
• *Viral*: Mumps, Japanese encephalitis, lymphocytic choriomeningitis, HIV, persistent CNS echovirus infection in agammaglobulinemia	
• Sarcoidosis	
• Cerebral granulomatous meningitis	
• IgG4-related disease	
• Carcinomatous meningitis	

ANTITUBERCULAR DRUGS

Streptomycin came as a first antitubercular treatment (ATT) in 1948 followed by INH in 1952 and rifampicin and pyrazinamide in 1971. Thereafter a number of drugs have been used which are not primarily designed as an antibiotic. The ideal antitubercular drug in TBM should have good CSF penetration and be effective against both intracellular and extracellular organisms. Combination of drugs is used for better efficacy and to prevent drug resistance. The WHO recommended ATT, and their dose, duration, and CSF penetration are mentioned in **Table 2**. The antitubercular drugs are divided on the basis of efficacy and toxicity into first- and second-line drugs. The first-line drugs are INH, rifampicin, pyrazinamide, and ethambutol, and remaining are second-line drugs.

Isoniazid: INH is active against both intracellular and extracellular organisms in both the growing and resting stage of AFB. Peak plasma concentration after the oral dose generally ranges between 3 and 5 µg/mL and *M. tuberculosis* strains are inhibited in vitro by 0.025–0.05 µg/mL of the drug. INH is well absorbed orally and the recommended oral dose is 10 mg/kg/day in children and 300 mg daily in adults. Parenteral formulation of INH is also available. The side effects are hepatotoxicity ranging from asymptomatic enzyme elevation to fulminant hepatic failure and peripheral neuropathy if pyridoxine is not supplemented. INH overdose may manifest with psychosis, seizures, and coma; moreover, it interferes with metabolism of phenytoin resulting in phenytoin toxicity.

Rifampicin: Rifampicin is bactericidal to both intracellular and extracellular mycobacteria with a minimum inhibitory concentration ranging from 0.005 to 0.2 µg/mL. Uncertainty surrounds its penetration into the CSF, 80% is protein bound leaving only 20% to penetrate into the CSF. Rifampicin is well absorbed orally and recommended dose is 8–12 mg/kg/day. Side effects of rifampicin are hepatic, renal, and hematologic. A flu-like syndrome and hypersensitivity reactions have also been reported with intermittent treatment regimen. Up to 30–60% patients receiving INH, rifampicin and pyrazinamide develop drug-induced hepatitis, which is 10 times more frequent than those receiving one of these drugs. Rifabutin may be substituted in the patients with HIV or in drug-induced hepatitis because of its lesser drug–drug interaction. Its role in TBM is doubtful due to poor CSF penetration.

Pyrazinamide: Pyrazinamide inhibits the growth of mycobacteria within the cytoplasm of phagocytes as it can act in acid pH. A 1 g oral dose produces a plasma concentration of about 45 µg/mL which exceeds the bactericidal concentration of 12.5 µg/mL. Pyrazinamide has excellent CSF penetration. Pyrazinamide in a dose of 50 mg/kg/day produces hepatotoxicity in 15% of recipients; therefore, a 20–30 mg/kg/day dose is recommended.

TABLE 2 Antituberculous drugs in tuberculous meningitis and drug-resistant tuberculosis.

Drug	CSF penetrance (CSF: Plasma concentration	WHO recommended daily dose	WHO recommended duration
First-line treatment in drug sensitive TBM in adults			
Rifampicin	10–20%	10 mg/kg (8–12 mg/kg); maximum 600 mg	12 months
Isoniazid	80–90%	5 mg/kg (4–6 mg/kg); maximum 300 mg	12 months
Pyrazinamide	90–100%	25 mg/kg (20–30 mg/kg)	2 months
Ethambutol	20–30%	15 mg/kg (15–20 mg/kg)	2 months
Second-line drugs in TBM in adults			
Levofloxacin	70–80%	10–15 mg/kg	Throughout treatment
Moxifloxacin	70–80%	400 mg	Throughout treatment
Linezolid	30–70%	600 mg	Throughout treatment
Amikacin	10–20%	15 mg/kg; maximum 1 g IV or IM	Intensive phase
Kanamycin	10–20%	15 mg/kg; maximum 1 g IV or IM	Intensive phase
Capreomycin	very low	15 mg/kg; maximum 1 g IV or IM	Intensive phase
Ethionamide or prothionamide	80–90%	15–20 mg/kg; maximum 1 g	Throughout treatment
Cycloserine	80–90%	10–15 mg/kg; maximum 1 g	Throughout treatment
Other drugs used in treatment of multidrug-resistant TB but of uncertain benefit in TBM			
Clofazimine	low	100 mg	No recommended duration
p-aminosalicylic acid	very low	200–300 mg/kg	No recommended duration
Bedaquiline	very low	Not determined	
Delamanid	No data	Not determined	

Ethambutol: Ethambutol is a bacteriostatic drug and most of *M. tuberculosis* strains are inhibited at 1–5 μg/mL concentration. Following a dose of 25 mg/kg, peak serum concentrations ranges between 1 and 8 μg/mL with a mean of 4 μg/mL. With a dose of 15 mg/kg, average concentrations range between 1.8 and 1.9 μg/mL. Ethambutol has good CSF penetration and CSF concentration usually above 1 μg/dL in the presence of meningeal inflammation; however, in the absence of meningeal inflammation it has minimal CSF penetration. Ethambutol is orally administered in a dose of 15–20 mg/kg/day. At higher dose, nearly 5% patients develop optic neuropathy heralded by diminished visual equity and green color vision defect.

Streptomycin: In vitro, streptomycin is bactericidal but in vivo it appears to be bacteriostatic against extracellular organisms only. Following 1 g intramuscular injection in an adult and 20–40 mg/kg in children, the serum concentration of 20 μg/mL persists for 24 hours. It has minimal CSF penetration in the absence of meningeal inflammation, but in meningitis, the CSF concentration may be up to 25% of serum concentration. The most important side effect of streptomycin is irreversible ototoxicity, and dependent on total dose and excessively high serum concentration. Adults are more prone and less able to compensate for vestibular toxicity of streptomycin. The drug is administered daily in the 1st week, subsequently the frequency may be reduced to 2–3 times/week. Intrathecal therapy is not recommended.

Second-line antitubercular drugs: A number of antitubercular drugs because of their toxicity, limited efficacy, or difficulty in administration are regarded as second-line drugs. Multidrug-resistant (MDR) TB or intolerance to first-line drugs may require second-line ATT. Quinolones and linezolid are core second-line drugs because of good CSF penetration and bactericidal effect. The details are mentioned in **Box 2**.

Treatment regimen: For drug-sensitive TBM, a 4-drug ATT including INH, rifampicin, pyrazinamide, and ethambutol has been recommended by WHO. All four drugs are given for 2 months followed by INH and rifampicin for another 10 months. The duration of treatment may be adjusted on the basis of the severity of meningitis. In India and many developing countries, the patients are often brought late with incomplete and irregular treatment; therefore, long duration treatment has been recommended. Authors prefer 18 months of antitubercular therapy in TBM with initial intensive phase of 4–6months.

Baseline and subsequent evaluation: All the patients at baseline should be investigated for HIV and if positive, CD4 count should be carried out. High-risk individuals for hepatitis (drug abusers, HIV patients, and Asians or Africans) should undergo serology for hepatitis B and C, baseline liver enzymes, serum bilirubin, serum creatinine, and platelet counts. The patients on ethambutol therapy should undergo vision testing and red-green color discrimination test. On subsequent follow up, routine liver and kidney function testing are not required unless patient has baseline abnormality or has high risk of hepatotoxicity (alcoholism). On monthly follow up, the patient should be enquired about visual disturbance such as blurring or scotoma. Red-green discrimination is tested if patient is on ethambutol therapy for >2 months.

Drug resistance: Among patients with prior treatment for >1 month, the prevalence of resistance to any drug ranged from 5.3 to 100% and the prevalence of multidrug resistance to both INH and rifampicin was 0 to 54%. The problem of drug resistance has been increasing over the years; it was 2% in 1960 and 9% in 1990. About 50% patients of MDR TB are in India, China, and Russia. Asians, undernourished people, AIDS patients, drug addicts, and those in contact with drug-resistant tubercular patients have a high prevalence of drug resistance. It is now possible to detect drug-resistant strains of *M. tuberculosis* employing GeneXpert. The best combination of drugs and the desired duration of treatment of MDR TBM are unclear. MDR TBM should be treated on the same principles as MDR pulmonary tuberculosis. In INH monoresistance, fluoroquinolone is added with rifampicin, pyrazinamide, and ethambutol for 12 months. Rifampicin and both INH and rifampicin-resistant TBM are treated with adding 4 or more drugs from the second line for at least 18 months (8 months intensive phase). The treatment of drug-resistant TBM is summarized in **Box 2**.

HOST IMMUNE-DIRECTED THERAPY

Evidence-based data are suggestive that *adjunctive corticosteroid decreases mortality in TBM* but its role in long-term sequelae is not well established. The largest randomized controlled trial in TBM has used dexamethasone in TBM patients having Glasgow Coma Scale score below 15 or those with focal neurological

BOX 2	Antitubercular treatment in drug-resistant tuberculous meningitis.
A. Isoniazid monoresistance:	
1.	Levofloxacin 10–15 mg/kg/day or moxifloxacin 400 mg/day with rifampicin, pyrazinamide, and ethambutol
2.	Treatment duration 12 months
B. Isoniazid and rifampicin resistance:	
Selected first-line drugs with:	
1.	Intensive phase 8 months with >4 second-line drugs (levofloxacin, amikacin/capreomycin/kanamycin, ethionamide/prothionamide, linezolid, clofazimine, and cycloserine)
2.	Continuation phase >12 months—with >3 second-line drugs mentioned in B1
3.	Total treatment duration >18 months
C. Rifampicin monoresistance:	
1.	As mentioned in B with substituting ethionamide with isoniazid
2.	Duration of treatment 18 months

deficits, in a dose of intravenous (IV) dexamethasone (0.4 mg/kg/day in week 1, 0.3 mg/kg in week 2, 0.2 mg/kg in week 3, and 0.1 mg/kg in week 4) for 4 weeks followed by oral taper of dexamethasone (4 mg/day, 3 mg/day, 2 mg/day, and 1 mg/day each for a period of 1 week). Thus the patient receives 2 months of dexamethasone. The patient with normal mental status without any neurological sign receives IV dexamethasone for 2 weeks (0.2 mg/kg and 0.1 mg/kg/day for 1 week each) followed by oral taper as described above. We however use oral prednisolone 0.75–1 mg/kg daily for a month, then tapering off in the next month.

In the early stage, the diagnosis of TBM is seldom certain in majority of patients due to low diagnostic sensitivity, associated HIV, pneumonia, septicemia, bed sore, and MDR TB especially in developing countries. The decision about adjuvant corticosteroid therapy therefore should be individualized based on their comorbidities. Corticosteroids have a definite role in patients with TBM associated with adrenal or pituitary hypofunction, which manifest with persistent hyponatremia and hypotension. In TBM patients with HIV, the role of steroid is not established. The benefit of steroid in LTA4H homozygous mutation has been reported. Thalidomide in children has resulted in increased mortality. Tumor necrosis factor alpha (TNFα) blocker in tuberculoma not responding to traditional treatment has been tried but needs further studies because of higher incidence of TB reactivation with these drugs in rheumatoid arthritis. Aspirin 150 mg daily has shown to reduce mortality.

WORSENING/PARADOXICAL RESPONSE

In pulmonary and lymph node TB, enlargement or deterioration after ATT has been referred as paradoxical response and attributed to immunological reaction. Similar deterioration has been reported in TBM (**Figs. 5 A** to **C**), more frequently with HIV coinfection. Radiological worsening has been noted in 30–60% patients and 50% of them have clinical worsening in the form of altered sensorium, focal deficit, seizure or raised intracranial pressure. The diagnosis of paradoxical response should be made after exclusion of an alternative cause such as pyogenic, fungal or parasitic infection, or drug resistance. After confirming the paradoxical response, the patient may be treated with anti-inflammatory drugs—corticosteroids (prednisolone 1–2 mg/kg) for 1–2 weeks followed by oral taper. In HIV, paradoxical response is attributed to immune reconstitution syndrome as a consequence of effective antiretroviral therapy.

TBM IN SPECIAL SITUATIONS

The hepatotoxic drugs should be stopped in the presence of drug-induced hepatitis [three times elevation in aspartate transaminase (AST) in symptomatic and five times in asymptomatic patients]. The patient should be investigated for hepatitis A, B, C, and alcohol consumption. The patient should receive two or more nonhepatotoxic drugs (ethambutol, streptomycin/amikacin, or quinolone) till the cause of hepatitis is established. As the AST levels decline to two times of the normal, the first-line antitubercular drugs are introduced one by one in a sequential manner (INH followed by rifampicin then pyrazinamide) monitoring clinical symptoms and liver enzymes.

In a patient with established liver disease, the first-line antitubercular drugs such as INH, rifampicin, and pyrazinamide are avoided or used in isolation with ethambutol or quinolone. In a randomized controlled trial sequential ATT resulted in fewer drug-induced hepatitis, lower hospital mortality and better 6 months outcome. In renal failure, streptomycin and ethambutol are avoided or

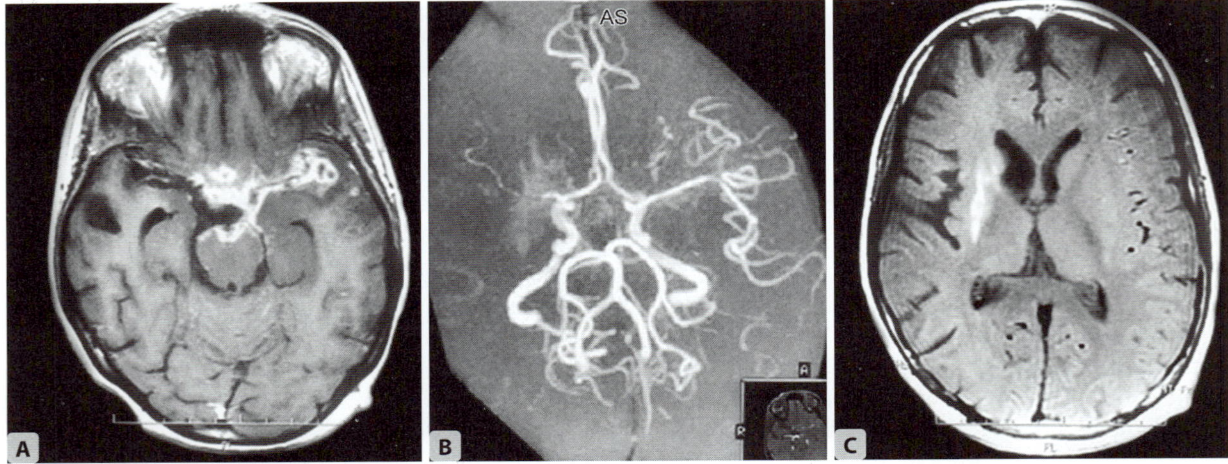

FIGURES 5 A TO C: Vasculitis leading to infarct in tuberculous meningitis. Cranial MRI and MRA of a 26-year-old lady with stage II tuberculous meningitis. **(A)** T1 contrast image shows basal exudates and enhancement of arterial wall of the circle of Willis and proximal portion of middle cerebral arteries; **(B)** MRA shows occlusion of right middle cerebral artery; **(C)** FLAIR sequence shows hyperintensity of right basal ganglia with dilatation of ipsilateral frontal horn of lateral ventricle.

Source: Kalita J, Singh RK, Misra UK, Kumar S. Evaluation of cerebral arterial and venous system in tuberculous meningitis. J Neuroradiol. 2018;45(2):130-5.

their dose and frequency should be reduced. In pregnancy streptomycin is avoided as it results in congenital deafness. Breastfeeding should be encouraged. In children, ethambutol is avoided lest it produces visual toxicity.

MANAGEMENT OF COMPLICATIONS

Hydrocephalous and raised intracranial pressure: To overcome the raised intracranial pressure temporarily intravenous mannitol or frusemide may be used.

Surgical therapy: Surgery has a limited but definite place in the management of CNS TB for secondary complications or when the diagnosis is not clear. In the patients with hydrocephalus with raised intracranial pressure (altered sensorium) and whose consciousness improves after CSF drainage are the appropriate candidate for ventriculoperitoneal shunt. The results of shunt surgery, however, are poor in patients who are deeply comatose and decerebrating. Lumboperitoneal shunt and third ventriculostomy are not encouraged because of adhesive arachnoiditis and blockade of CSF flow at absorptive sites.

Seizure: The patients with seizure should receive nonenzyme-inducing antiepileptic drugs such as levetiracetam, lacosamide, lamotrigine, or clobazam. Status epilepticus should be treated as in other acute symptomatic status epilepticus. How long antiepileptic should be continued is not clear, but at least 1 year may be appropriate if there is no breakthrough seizure.

Stroke: Aspirin with corticosteroid may be useful in preventing stroke in TBM although there is paucity of evidence. TBM may also increase the risk of stroke in the survivors; therefore, aspirin at least for 18 months may be prescribed. Other antiplatelet drugs may also be useful, but aspirin is cheap and time-tested drug.

Hyponatremia: Hyponatremia (serum sodium < 135 mg/dL) may occur in 40–50% TBM. Hyponatremia may be due to vomiting, poor intake, natriuretic drugs, hypothyroidism, adrenal failure, pituitary dysfunction, cerebral salt wasting (CSW), or syndrome of inappropriate secretion of antidiuretic hormone (SIADH). The offending drugs and modifiable risk factors should be managed. Polyuria, high urinary sodium excretion, and intravascular volume contraction suggest CSW syndrome. CSW patients should receive saline and oral salt 10 g/day, and in refractory cases fludrocortisone (0.4–1 mg/daily in two divided doses) may be tried. In SIADH which is rare complication of TBM, there is intravascular volume expansion and hypo-osmolality. Fluid restriction with or without V2 receptor antagonist (tolvaptan, conivaptan, lixivaptan, and satavaptan) may be tried but may not be helpful. Patients with asymptomatic and mild hyponatremia (130–134 mEq/L) may be managed by normal saline and oral salt (10–12 g/day in four divided doses). Symptomatic patients (seizure, altered sensorium, and vomiting) and those with severe hyponatremia (<120 mEq/L) should receive 3% saline (0.5–2 mL/kg/h) till the symptoms improve; thereafter normal saline and oral salt. Sodium should not be corrected >10 mEq/L in first 24 hour and 8 mEq/L in the next 24 hours to prevent osmotic demyelination. In resource-poor countries, repeated serum sodium measurement may not be possible; therefore, in severe hyponatremia 150 mL of 3% saline followed by normal saline and oral salt has been suggested till the serum sodium is normal.

Intracranial tuberculoma: At times, tuberculoma is difficult to distinguish from tumor, fungal granuloma, or abscess on the basis of clinical and radiological findings. Consensus statement suggests 18 months ATT in tuberculoma. Corticosteroid may reduce perilesional edema. Some authorities, therefore, advocate biopsy or excision and deny any role for empirical therapy. Biopsy, however, may not always be successful, or without risk; therefore, a therapeutic trial under careful monitoring is practiced. Surgery for tuberculoma is indicated in the following situations: Tuberculoma producing visual loss and life-threatening raised intracranial pressure, lack of clinical or radiological improvement, and doubtful diagnosis. In selected patients with sequelae of meningitis, such as chiasmal arachnoiditis or a focal spinal arachnoiditis, surgery has a role. Some case series suggest that thalidomide could help to alleviate these problems. Case reports have revealed success with anti-TNF biological agents (such as infliximab) and interferon-gamma (IFN-γ) treatment.

PROGNOSIS AND SEQUELAE

The decline in mortality in TBM has been associated with a corresponding rise in varying degrees of neurologic sequelae in the survivors. Mortality in TBM is 20–30%. The prognosis is related to the stage of meningitis and depth of coma at the time of presentation and need of mechanical ventilation. A number of clinical, radiological, and laboratory findings such as age, BCG (Bacillus Calmette–Guérin) vaccination, extrameningeal TB, signs of raised intracranial tension, focal neurologic deficit, hydrocephalus, infarction, and CSF changes have been reported in various studies. In the post-INH era, neurologic and psychiatric sequelae have been reported in 25–50% of the survivors.

The neurologic sequelae include spastic hemiparesis, seizures, ataxia, and cranial nerve palsy in decreasing order. Adult survivors are commonly left with organic brain syndrome, cranial nerve palsy, paraplegia, hemiplegia, and visual impairment. Eighth nerve dysfunction has been reduced due to lesser use of streptomycin. Syringomyelia, myelopathy, and endocrine disturbance due to hypothalamopituitary adrenal dysfunctions have also been reported following TBM.

CNS TUBERCULOSIS AND AIDS

Human immunodeficiency virus patients are at a higher risk for reactivation of TB or exogenous reinfection. Reduced Th1 response in HIV-infected patients contributes to their susceptibility to TB. Clinical studies have shown detrimental effects of TB on the course of HIV infection. The risk of death in HIV-infected patients with TB was reported to be twice that in HIV patients without TB, independent of CD4 cell count. The high mortality rate among HIV patients with TB appears to be due to progressive HIV infection rather than TB.

The clinical presentation of TBM is similar in HIV and immunocompetent patients, except intracranial mass lesions are more common in HIV patients. The CSF may occasionally be acellular and AFB positivity may be higher in TBM patients with HIV infection. In patients with AIDS, coinfection with multiple pathogens such as *M. tuberculosis, Toxoplasma,* and cryptococci has been reported.

Antitubercular drugs are effective, although these patients may succumb to other opportunistic infection. In patients with CNS TB and HIV coinfection, the treatment protocol is similar to the patient without HIV infection. However, the duration of treatment is longer due to poorer bacteriological clearance and drug resistance in HIV patients.

Highly active antiretroviral therapy (HAART) regimens have dramatically improved the prognosis of HIV-infected patients but have complicated the management of TB. HAART should be started 4–6 weeks after the ATT to prevent immune reconstitution syndrome. Rifampicin induces the activity of cytochrome P450 CYP3A, which lowers the concentration of HIV protease inhibitors and non-nucleoside reverse transcryptase inhibitors to subtherapeutic level.

Previous guidelines from Centers for Disease Control and Prevention (CDC) specifically stated that rifampicin was contraindicated in patients who were taking any protease inhibitor or non-nucleoside reverse transcriptase inhibitor (NNRTI). However, new data indicate that rifampicin can be used for the treatment of TB with certain combinations of antiretroviral agents. Intensive rifampicin treatment (oral 750–1,350 mg/day and 600 mg infusion) compared conventional 450 mg/day has shown improved survival, but more studies are needed because of high incidence of drug-induced hepatitis in India. Rifabutin, another antitubercular drug, is less potent inducer of CYP3A and may be preferred with indinavir or nelfinavir, but not with saquinavir. Rifabutin in a dose of 150–300 mg is well-tolerated and is as effective as rifampicin in a standard antitubercular regimen. It has been suggested that INH, ethambutol, and pyrazinamide for 18–24 months may be preferable in HIV patients with TB.

PREVENTION

Prevention of CNS TB is related to overall prevention of TB. In developing countries where TB is rampant, the strategies for prevention have been identified and are different from those in the developed countries. BCG vaccine has been extensively used since 1921 but its contribution to TB control has been limited for two reasons: (1) Its protective efficiency varies considerably (0–80%), and (2) when effective, it offers a high degree of protection against the serious but usually noninfectious forms of primary TB, and gives little or no protection against postprimary forms of TB due to endogenous reactivation or exogenous reactivation. BCG vaccination is indicated in persons not infected by *M. tuberculosis* with a Mantoux response <4 mm. Infants below 3 months may be vaccinated without PPD test. Persons who have received the BCG vaccine should be revaccinated if a PPD test is negative and there is no scar formation at the site of previous vaccination. BCG should not be given in symptomatic AIDS and immunosuppressed patients as it is a live vaccine.

In view of these limitations, search for an alternative vaccine is which can be given to the people already infected to prevent postprimary TB is on. Approaches currently under investigation include modified ways of administering BCG, development of genetically modified live vaccines, and nonviable subunit vaccines including naked DNA. Supervised treatment programs have been successful in controlling outbreaks of AIDS-associated TB in the USA. The principal cause of failed TB control is "noncompliance" for which the patient is usually blamed but generally the fault is of healthcare provider. WHO has recommended directly observed therapy (DOT) that will only work if the attention is given to various social, cultural, and ethnic issues.

RECOMMENDED READINGS

1. Misra UK, Kalita J. Tuberculous Meningitis International Research Consortium. Mechanism, spectrum, consequences and management of hyponatremia in tuberculous meningitis. Wellcome Open Res. 2021;4:189.
2. Wilkinson RJ, Rohlwink U, Misra UK, van Crevel R, Mai NTH, Dooley KE, et al. Tuberculous meningitis. Nat Rev Neurol. 2017;13:581-98.
3. Misra UK, Kalita J, Maurya PK. Stroke in tuberculous meningitis. J Neurol Sci. 2011;303(1-2):22-30.
4. Kalita J, Prasad S, Misra UK. Predictors of paradoxical tuberculoma in tuberculous meningitis. Int J Tuberc Lung Dis. 2014;18(4):486-91.
5. Kalita J, Misra UK. Tuberculous meningitis. In: Kalita J, Misra UK (Eds). Diagnosis and Management of Neurological Disorder, 1st edition. Gurugram, India: Wolters Kluwer India Pvt. Ltd.; 2011. pp. 143-66.

CHAPTER
190

Viral Encephalitis

Dhananjay Duberkar

ABSTRACT

Encephalitis is an inflammation of the brain parenchyma often associated with meningitis. Viral encephalitis is a major public health concern in India because of its high morbidity and mortality. The spectrum of brain involvement and the outcome of the disease depend on the specific pathogen, immunological state of the host, and multiple environmental factors. The tropism of viruses for different cell types within the central nervous system (CNS) may lead to characteristic neurological findings. Diagnostic strategies and technologies are being developed to allow identification of an expanding list of pathogens and to differentiate viral encephalitis from its mimics. Here we will focus on the most relevant agents of clinically important viral encephalitis.

"Take two opposites, connect the dots, and you have a straight line"

—Yahia Lababidi

INTRODUCTION

Encephalitis is a syndrome characterized by altered mental status and various combinations of acute fever, seizures, neurologic deficits, cerebrospinal fluid (CSF) pleocytosis, and neuroimaging and electroencephalographic (EEG) abnormalities. Encephalitis is an inflammation of the brain parenchyma and often associated with meningitis. Viral infection is the most common and important cause of encephalitis, although other organisms may cause an encephalitis. Viruses vary widely in their potential to produce CNS infection.

VIRUSES CAUSING ENCEPHALITIS

- Herpes simplex virus (HSV)* (HSV-1 in 90% and HSV-2 in 10% cases)
- *Other herpes viruses*: Varicella-zoster virus (VZV), cytomegalovirus (CMV), Epstein–Barr virus (EBV), and human herpes virus 6 (HHV6)
- Adenoviruses
- Influenza A
- Enteroviruses*, poliovirus
- Measles*, mumps, and rubella viruses
- Rabies*
- *Arboviruses*:
  - Alphaviruses: Chikungunya*, Eastern, Western, and Venezuelan equine encephalitis virus
  - Flaviviruses: Dengue virus*, Japanese B encephalitis*, Kyasanur forest disease, West Nile encephalitis St Louis encephalitis virus, and Zika virus
  - Coltiviruses: Colorado tick-borne encephalitis viruses
  - Bunyaviruses: La Crosse strain of California virus
  - Reoviruses: For example, Colorado tick fever virus
  - Arenaviruses: For example, lymphocytic choriomeningitis virus

EPIDEMIOLOGY

Incidence of viral encephalitis varies between studies but is generally between 3.5 and 7.4 per 100,000 patient years, and is higher in children. A variety of viruses cause encephalitis, amongst which the Japanese encephalitis virus (JEV) is most prevalent in India. Worldwide HSV accounts for majority of identified viral cases. HSV encephalitis occurs in all age groups and does not have a specific seasonal or geographic pattern. Arbovirus encephalitis has significant seasonal variation. Japanese encephalitis (JE) tends to be endemic; cases occur sporadically throughout the year, with a peak after the start of the rainy season (July to September).

The factors that affect susceptibility of host to encephalitis are poorly understood. Certain viruses like JE involve predominantly children and young adults; viruses, such as West Nile virus (WNV), tend to cause severe disease in the elderly, whereas HSV encephalitis occurs in persons at both ends of the age spectrum.

CLINICAL FEATURES

The history must focus on the season, geographic location, travel and exposure history, contact with animals, health of relatives, immune status, and known causes of encephalitis in the given geographic area. The presence of exanthem or enanthem is helpful in identifying some forms

*Denotes common viruses in India.

of viral encephalitis but does not have high specificity. Patients usually present with headache, fever coupled with altered level of consciousness, confusion, behavioral abnormalities, or a depressed level of consciousness ranging from mild lethargy to coma, and evidence of either focal or diffuse neurologic signs and symptoms. Commonly encountered focal findings include aphasia, ataxia, weakness either upper motor neuron or lower motor neuron type, anterior horn cell involvement (WNV and polio virus), involuntary movements (e.g., myoclonic jerks and tremor), and cranial nerve deficits (e.g., ocular palsies and facial weakness). Involvement of the hypothalamic-pituitary axis may result in temperature dysregulation, diabetes insipidus, or the development of the syndrome of inappropriate secretion of antidiuretic hormone (SIADH) leading to hyponatremia and worsening of sensorium.

HERPES SIMPLEX ENCEPHALITIS

Herpes simplex virus-1 is a double-stranded deoxyribonucleic acid (DNA) virus and it spreads by salivary or respiratory route. HSV-1 infection generally is asymptomatic and herpes simplex encephalitis (HSE) is a rare complication of HSV-1 infection. During the primary infection, virus is transported to the local sensory fibers by retrograde transport and lies dormant in the sensory ganglia. Reactivation of virus can be induced by skin or nerve trauma, by immune suppression and irradiation.

Herpes simplex encephalitis occurs due to primary infection, reactivation, or reinfection. Clinical manifestations are due to orbitofrontal and medial temporal lobe involvement. Along with fever, headaches personality and behavioral changes may be noted before the typical clinical picture manifests. Typically manifests with fear, agitation, olfactory hallucinations, amnesia, bizarre behavior, and sometimes frank psychosis. Seizures are very common and are often focal and almost one-third patients have early onset seizures and may progress to convulsive or nonconvulsive status epilepticus. Hemiparesis, aphasia, superior quadrantanopia, and paraesthesia may occur. Some patients develop rapidly progressive coma and signs of raised intracranial tension. The disease usually follows a monophasic course but rarely patients develop a neurologic relapse within weeks or months after the initial event . In few case the relapse seems to be immune-mediated rather than a viral reactivation. Recently reports of autoimmune encephalitis associated with anti-N-methyl-D-aspartate receptor (NMDAR) antibodies after HSV encephalitis have been published, which supporting the likelihood that central nervous system (CNS) HSV infection may trigger an autoimmune response.

JAPANESE ENCEPHALITIS

Japanese encephalitis is mostly a disease of children and young adults. JE epidemics are related to rainfall, flood, and mosquito breeding which has also been linked with paddy cultivation and pig farming. JE is a zoonosis transmitted by a mosquito bite, and man is the dead-end host. Virus is introduced into the human body by the bite of an infected mosquito. The virus multiplies in the epithelial cells and then virus spreads through the hematogenous route resulting in primary viremia. Further replication occurs in reticuloendothelial system and produces secondary viremia with dissemination of virus to organs, such as brain, kidney, and liver.

Japanese encephalitis typically presents with nonspecific febrile illness, which may include coryza and diarrhea. This is followed by headache, vomiting, and altered sensorium often heralded by a convulsion. In older children and adults, abnormal behavior may be the only presenting feature. Convulsions occur often in JE, and are more common in children. Generalized tonic-clonic seizures occur more often than focal motor seizures. Multiple or prolonged seizures and status epilepticus are associated with a poor outcome.

Focal neurological deficits become apparent as the general condition improves and consciousness returns. The focal signs include hemiplegia, quadriplegia, lower motor neuron, and cerebellar signs. Two major types of movement disorders are a transient form of Parkinsonism and dystonia or dyskinesia. The movement disorders become more apparent as the patient recovers from deep coma. The classic description includes a dull mask-like facies with wide eyes and reduced blinking, tremor, generalized hypertonia, and cogwheel rigidity. Opisthotonus and spasms on stimulation occur less commonly and indicate poor prognosis. Other abnormal movements include head nodding and pill-rolling movements, opsoclonus myoclonus, choreoathetosis, bizarre facial grimacing, and lip smacking.

Changes of respiratory pattern, flexor and extensor posturing, and abnormalities of the pupillary reflexes are poor prognostic signs. About one-third of patients admitted to hospital with JE die, and around half of the survivors have severe neurological sequelae. Learning difficulties and behavioral problems are common in recovered patients. A higher rate of sequelae is reported for children than adults.

DENGUE ENCEPHALITIS

Two main presentations of dengue are referred to as dengue fever and severe dengue. Neurological dengue is classified as a form of severe dengue. Dengue encephalitis (DENV) is a member of the *Flavivirus* genus of the family Flaviviridae. There are four genetically and antigenically distinct serotypes of dengue (DENV 1–4). Cocirculation of multiple serotypes (hyperendemicity), serotype virulence, and hyperimmune responses are risk factors for severe dengue. Following DENV infection, three major changes determine the clinical findings: (1) Increased vascular permeability, (2) Thrombocytopenia, and (3) Coagulopathy.

Dengue encephalopathy is the most common neurological manifestation and is characterized by altered sensorium in whom CSF analysis for cell, protein, and sugar is normal and there is no evidence of CNS invasion by DENV. Shock, hypoxia, hyponatremia, acute liver or kidney failure, intracerebral hemorrhage, and cerebral edema may lead to dengue encephalopathy.

Dengue encephalitis is an infrequent but serious manifestation of dengue virus infection. Patients with DENV may be at risk of developing complications of dengue hemorrhagic but rarely patients with encephalitis may not show other features of the disease. The onset of encephalitis is usually sudden with nonspecific prodromal symptoms like myalgia, malaise, fever, vomiting, and diarrhea. Later headache, disorientation, depressed sensorium, and seizures develop. Seizures are common in encephalitis as compared to dengue encephalopathy. Other features include frontal release signs, abnormal posturing, facial nerve palsy, and quadruparesis.

Acute disseminated encephalomyelitis (ADEM), acute transverse myelitis, acute optic neuritis, Guillain–Barré syndrome, and mononeuropathy involving phrenic, long thoracic, oculomotor nerve are immunological complications of dengue fever. Transient muscle dysfunction characterized by creatine kinase (CK) rise, with or without muscle weakness and rhabdomyolysis may occur in addition to other neurological manifestations.

CHIKUNGUNYA ENCEPHALITIS

Chikungunya is an arboviral disease caused by chikungunya virus (CHIKV) characterized by fever, skin rash, and arthralgia. CHIKV is an alpha virus of Togaviridae family transmitted by the mosquitoes of *Aedes* genus.

Sudden onset of high-grade fever, maculopapular rash, arthralgia, and retrobulbar pain are characteristics of first stage. Chronic stage is characterized by polyarthralgia which can be incapacitating and may last for weeks to years. Neurological manifestations occur early in the course of disease. The neurological manifestations include encephalopathy, seizures, meningoencephalitis, and stimulus sensitive myoclonus. Rarely, Guillain–Barré syndrome, optic neuritis, and ADEM are reported.

RABIES ENCEPHALITIS

In the Latin *rabere* means "to rage or to rave," *rabhas* means "violence" in Sanskrit; and *lyssa* or *lytta* means "madness" in Greek. Rabies is acute, fatal encephalitis caused by a highly neurotropic ribonucleic acid (RNA) virus, taxonomically belonging to genus *Lyssavirus*, family Rhabdoviridae. In India, dogs are the main vectors, accounting for majority of the reported cases.

It is characterized by two distinct well-recognized clinical syndromes in humans: Furious and paralytic (dumb) rabies. The classic clinical presentation of furious rabies is of fever, fluctuating sensorium, and autonomic hyperactivity. Phobic spasms of the larynx, pharynx, neck muscles, and diaphragm can be triggered by attempts to swallow water (*hydrophobia*) or by inspiration (*aerophobia*). The paralytic form presents with ascending paralysis without "hydrophobic" symptoms. Rabies virus antigen in brain tissue or in the neural innervation of hair follicles at the nape of the neck enables the diagnosis. Polymerase chain reaction (PCR) amplification of viral nucleic acid from CSF and saliva or tears may also enable the diagnosis.

MEASLES VIRUS ENCEPHALITIS

In measles virus (MV) infection, CNS involvement can occur early or late after acute measles, causing acute and subacute forms of encephalitis. Acute measles encephalitis generally occurs in immunocompetent children and adolescent during the exanthematic phase and within 8 days after clinical onset. Onset of encephalitis at a later phase results either in measles inclusion body encephalitis (MIBE) or in subacute sclerosing panencephalitis (SSPE). MIBE is a subacute/chronic neurologic disease that may be observed in immunosuppressed children and young adults. SSPE is a demyelinating CNS disease occurring several years (generally 6–8) after acute measles infection. SSPE is characterized by cognitive deterioration, poor school performance, ataxia, behavioral changes, myoclonus (characteristically slow relaxation), seizures, and chorioretinitis with visual deficit. Although progression differs in time death invariably occurs within 1–3 years.

DIFFERENTIAL DIAGNOSIS

METABOLIC ENCEPHALOPATHY

From a practical point of view, a clinician confronted with a patient with fever, headache, and altered mental status must initially distinguish encephalitis from noninfectious causes of brain dysfunction (encephalopathy). Clinical distinction between viral encephalitis and a metabolic encephalopathy may not always be straightforward. The presence of fever is not sufficient to make a diagnosis of infective encephalitis as encephalopathy may be precipitated by systemic infections or sepsis without cerebral inflammation like in septic encephalopathy (**Table 1**).

ACUTE DISSEMINATED ENCEPHALOMYELITIS

Acute disseminated encephalomyelitis is monophasic, with multifocal symptoms appearing within days, or over weeks, either in the presence or absence of fever and meningismus. Focal motor and sensory deficits, optic neuritis, cranial neuropathies, seizures, myoclonus, and ataxia are common neurological manifestations. White matter changes affect the cortical and subcortical grey matter on magnetic resonance imaging (MRI) brain and long segment demyelination on spinal cord MRI.

Autoimmune encephalitis: Autoimmune encephalitis is a difficult clinical diagnosis and has many similarities in the clinical, imaging, and laboratory findings of many forms of autoimmune and infectious encephalitis. Patients generally have impaired memory and cognition over a period of days or weeks. A detailed approach to testing for infectious diseases and various neuronal antibodies can lead to the diagnosis.

TABLE 1 Difference between encephalopathy and encephalitis.

	Encephalopathy	Encephalitis
Clinical features:		
• Headache	Rare	Common
• Focal neurologic signs	Uncommon	Common
• Types of seizures	Generalized	Generalized or focal
Laboratory findings:		
• CSF	Pleocytosis uncommon	Pleocytosis common
• Electroencephalographic	Diffuse slowing, triphasic waves	Diffuse slowing and focal abnormalities like PLEDs
• MRI	Often normal	Focal abnormalities

(PLEDs: periodic lateralizing epileptiform discharges)

EVALUATION

Laboratory evaluation is based on three important investigations:

1. Neuroimaging
2. CSF
3. EEG

NEUROIMAGING

Neuroimaging plays an important role in visualization of typical lesion patterns that contributes to diagnosis. Neuroimaging helps to identify or exclude alternative diagnoses and assists in the differentiation between a focal, as opposed to a diffuse, encephalitic process. Focal findings should always raise the possibility of HSV encephalitis. Examples of focal findings include: (1) Increased signal intensity in the frontotemporal, cingulate, or insular regions of the brain on T2-weighted, fluid-attenuated inversion recovery (FLAIR), or diffusion-weighted MRI; (2) focal areas of low absorption, mass effect, and contrast enhancement on computerized tomography (CT). **Table 2** illustrates characteristics of brain structure involvement seen on MRI brain in different viral encephalitis.

CSF

This is an essential part of the investigation of encephalitis and should be the next logical step after neuroimaging unless contraindicated by severely raised intracranial pressure. CSF opening pressure is increased; CSF typically consists of a lymphocytic pleocytosis, a mildly elevated protein concentration, and a normal glucose concentration. A CSF pleocytosis (>5 cells/μL) occurs in >95% of immunocompetent patients. In rare situation a pleocytosis may be absent on the initial lumbar puncture (LP) but present on subsequent LPs. **Table 3** describes characteristics of CSF finding in bacterial, viral, and tuberculous meningitis.

Polymerase chain reaction and reverse transcriptase PCR: Polymerase chain reaction is for detection of DNA viruses, and reverse transcriptase PCR (RT-PCR) is for detection of RNA viruses. CSF PCR has become the primary diagnostic test for CNS infections caused by HSV, CMV, EBV, HHV-6, and enteroviruses. This technique is exquisitely sensitive for the presence of viral genome in spinal fluid, can be rapidly accomplished (within 6–8 hours), and requires only a very small volume of CSF. The *CSF HSV PCR* test may be negative in the first 72 hours of symptoms of HSV encephalitis. A repeat study should be considered in patients with an initial early negative PCR in whom diagnostic suspicion of HSV encephalitis remains high and no alternative diagnosis has yet been established.

Serological tests: Serologic testing of CSF immunoglobulin M (IgM) may help diagnose encephalitis due to arboviruses, VZV, EBV, measles virus, mumps virus, rubella virus, rabies virus, or other causes. HSV CSF antibody testing is of value in selected patients whose illness is >1 week in duration and who are CSF PCR negative for HSV. In the case of VZV infection, CSF antibody tests may be positive when PCR fails to detect viral DNA. The best test for WNV encephalitis is the *CSF IgM antibody test.*

EEG

Electroencephalographic abnormalities occur commonly in HSV encephalitis; they typically involve the temporal lobes. Few patients have a distinctive EEG pattern consisting of periodic, stereotyped, sharp and slow complexes originating in one or both temporal lobes and repeating at regular intervals of 2–3 seconds known as periodic lateralizing epileptiform discharges (PLEDs). Electroencephalogram may help in diagnosis when other tests are pending and when HSV encephalitis is suspected.

TREATMENT

Specific treatment must be targeted to the suspected or identified etiological agent. In the initial stages of encephalitis patients usually require intensive care unit. Basic vital monitoring and supportive therapy should include careful monitoring of intracranial pressure (ICP), fluid restriction, avoidance of hypotonic intravenous solutions, and management of fever. Seizures should

TABLE 2 Imaging findings on MRI brain and site of involvement.

Temporal lobe	Basal ganglia/ thalamus	Corpus callosum	Brainstem	Diffusion restriction
• HSV-1 • HHV6	• JEV • WNV • Dengue • COVID • Influenza	• Dengue • Influenza	• Enterovirus • Dengue • Rabies • JE • WNV	• Dengue • Chikungunya • Ebola • NIPAH • ZIKA

(HHV6: human herpes virus-6; JEV: Japanese encephalitis virus; WNV: West Nile virus)

Courtesy: Dr Rahul Kulkarni.

TABLE 3 CSF findings in bacterial, viral, and tuberculous meningitis.

	Cells	Proteins	CSF sugar	Other specific tests
Normal CSF	All lymphocytes (0–5 cells/mm^3)	15–40 mg/dL	>50% of blood glucose	None
Bacterial meningitis	Leukocytes (usually PMNs), 100–10,000/mm^3	Elevated 100–500 mg/dL	Extremely low or undetectable	• Gram staining • Bacterial culture • Multiplex PCR panel
Viral meningitis	10–500 cells Lymphocytes (may be mixed; PMNs and lymphocytes during the first 24–48 hours)	Elevated 50–200 mg/dL	Usually normal or mildly reduced	• Multiplex PCR panel/ conventional PCR • IgM for HSV virus
Tuberculous meningitis	50–1,000 cells lymphocyte predominant	Elevated 100–300 mg/dL	<50% of blood glucose (may be extremely low)	• Acid-fast staining • PCR • Culture • CSF gene Xpert

(IgM: immunoglobulin M; PCR: polymerase chain reaction; PMN: polymorphonuclear)

be treated with standard anticonvulsant regimens, and prophylactic therapy should be considered in severe cases of encephalitis. Patients are at risk for aspiration pneumonia, bed sores, contractures, deep venous thrombosis and its complications, and infections of indwelling lines and catheters.

There are several guidelines for empirical and specific antiviral treatment of patients with encephalitis. However, few currently available treatments have been subjects of randomized, controlled clinical trials.

Acyclovir in adults with HSV encephalitis used a regimen of 10–14 days of intravenous therapy (10 mg/kg of body weight every 8 hours for patients with normal renal function). Neither a higher dose of acyclovir, nor longer duration improves outcomes in adults. Ganciclovir or foscarnet for encephalitis related to CMV and HHV-6 and acyclovir for VZV-related encephalitis are suggested based on limited clinical experience. Oral antiviral drugs with efficacy against HSV, VZV, and EBV, including acyclovir, famciclovir, and valacyclovir, have not been evaluated in the treatment of encephalitis either as primary therapy or as supplemental therapy following completion of a course of parenteral acyclovir.

OUTCOMES

The outcome of acute viral encephalitis has significantly improved in recent times. Immunocompromised state, a Glasgow Coma Scale score of 8 or less (on a scale from 3 to 15, with lower scores indicating greater neurologic deficits), the need for admission to an intensive care unit, and an age of >65 years indicate poor prognosis in case with viral encephalitis.

CONCLUSION

Significant advances have been made in our understanding of the natural history and pathogenesis of viral encephalitis. The development of PCR has greatly increased our ability to diagnose viral infections of the CNS. Treatment remains largely empirical with the exception of acyclovir for HSV encephalitis. New therapies to prevent infection and inhibit viral replication are needed.

RECOMMENDED READINGS

1. Hauser SL (Ed). Harrison's Neurology in Clinical Medicine, 3rd edition. Mc Graw Hill Education; 2013.
2. Tyler KL. Acute viral encephalitis. N Engl J Med. 2018;379:557-66.
3. Solomon T. Recent advances in Japanese encephalitis. J Neurovirology. 2003;9(2):274-83.
4. Davis LE. Diagnosis and treatment of acute encephalitis. Neurologist. 2000;6:145-59.
5. Ferrari S, Toniolo A, Monaco S, Luciani F, Cainelli F, Baj A, et al. Viral encephalitis: etiology, clinical features diagnosis and management. Open Infect Dis J. 2009;3:1-12.

CHAPTER 191

Fungal and Parasitic Diseases of the Nervous System

Jagarlapudi MK Murthy, Sundaram Challa

ABSTRACT

Fungal infections of the central nervous system (CNS) are being increasingly diagnosed in India due to the expansion of immunocompromised individuals at risk. The size and morphology of the fungus determine the phenotype of CNS pathology. Small fungi, yeast (*Cryptococcus* species) cause meningitis/meningoencephalitis; intermediate size fungi (*Candida* species) cause microabscesses; and large size fungi, septate (*Aspergillus*) and nonseptate (Mucorales) usually infect juxta-cranial sites (paranasal sinuses, orbit, oral cavity etc.) and then may invade contiguous cranial bones, meninges, and basal cerebral venous sinuses, and intracranial arteries resulting in large infarcts. The resulting cerebral infarct may lead to cerebritis and abscess formation. Sinocranial aspergillosis in otherwise immunocompetent individuals is commonly reported from countries with temperate climate like India.

Parasitic infections are mostly endemic to certain geographical regions for reasons of climate and the availability of intermediate hosts to transmit them to humans. Neurocysticercosis (NCC) is the most common parasitic disease of the human CNS. Malaria, caused by protozoans of the *Plasmodium* genus, is a major public health concern worldwide. The common pathogenic species to humans include *P. falciparum*, *P. vivax*, *P. ovale*, and *P. malaria*. Worldwide, cerebral malaria (CM) occurs in African children and Asian adults. Half of malaria deaths occur in those with CM.

"Look to the nervous system as the key to maximum health"

—Galen

FUNGAL INFECTIONS

In the recent years, fungal infections of the CNS are increasingly being diagnosed. It is mostly due to expansion of immunocompromised population at risk, increased awareness, and availability of better diagnostic facilities. The fungi are ubiquitous in the environment and are inhaled and colonized in the sinuses and also colonized in the external auditory canals. Healthy host is resistant to fungal infections due to effective immunity. However, immunocompromised host becomes vulnerable to these infections. Environmental factors such as hot and humid climate and constant exposure to large inoculum of fungi are implicated for certain geographically specific fungal diseases.

Intracranial extension of infection may occur by contiguous spread from sinuses or ears and by hematogenous spread, mostly from lungs and in intravenous (IV) drug abusers. Directly inoculated fungi into the subarachnoid space or brain parenchyma may result from traumatic brain injury, neurosurgical procedures, or epidural injections. Rarely it is by perineural spread via trigeminal nerve as in the rhinocerebral mucormycosis (**Table 1**). Recently in United States of America, CNS fungal infections caused by epidural injections of a contaminated glucocorticoid product have been described.

The host-pathogen interaction depends on the virulence of the organism, species involved, the immune status of the host, and innate/adaptive immune mechanisms in the brain. Microglia and the perivascular, meningeal, and choroid plexus macrophages along with complement constitute the innate immune system in the CNS.

The size and morphology of the fungus determine the phenotype of CNS pathology. Small (up to 20 μm in diameter; yeast) fungi access the microcirculation and can seed the subarachnoid space. This can cause meningitis/

TABLE 1 Common fungal pathogens, risk factors for infection, route of spread, and pathology.

Common etiologic agent (species)	Risk factor	Route of spread	Pathology
Molds			
Aspergillus species (*A. fumigatus A. flavus**) **Figures 1 A** to **C**	Immunocompromised state, temperate climate, environmental factors, trauma/surgery Immunocompetent host in countries with temperate climate	Hematogenous spread from lung and heart, contiguous spread from sinuses, orbit or otic, direct implantation	Granuloma, abscess, angioinvasion, infarct, mycotic aneurysms
Mucorales (*Rhizopus oryzae Mucor* species, *Rhizomucor*) **Figures 1 D** to **F**	Immunocompromised state diabetes, ketoacidosis, metabolic acidosis, deferoxamine therapy, iron overload, contaminated devices, IV drug abuse, trauma	Rhinocerebral, intravenous drug abuse, hematogenous, perineural along trigeminal nerve	Angioinvasion, infarct, suppurative inflammation, perineural invasion
Dematiaceous (pigmented) fungi (*Cladophialophora bantiana, Exserohilum rostratum*)	No risk factor identified in the majority (immunocompetent), CARD9 deficiency, contaminated drug	Inoculation (minor trauma), contaminated drugs/devices	Abscess, suppurative granuloma, meningitis
Yeast			
Cryptococcus species (*C. neoformans, C. gattii**) **Figures 1 G** to **J**	HIV, SOT, patients on immunosuppression, steroids, chronic liver disease, rarely in healthy hosts	Inhalation and subsequent hematogenous spread	Meningitis/ME, granuloma
Candida species (*C. albicans, C. auris*)	Prematurity, neonates, prolonged ICU stay, broad-spectrum antibiotics, IV drug use/catheter, neurosurgery, shunts/devices, CARD9 deficiency	Hematogenous in disseminated infections, associated with shunts/devices	Abscess, meningitis/ME
Dimorphic			
Blastomyces species (*B. dermatitidis**) *Coccidioides* species (*C. immitis**),	Healthy hosts with environmental exposure due to disruption of soil/vegetation, less frequent in immunosuppressed hosts with HIV, TNF-α inhibitors, steroids	Inhalation, rarely hematogenous in disseminated disease	Meningitis, abscess, vasculitis
Paracoccidioides (*P. brasiliensis*) *Histoplasma* species (*H. capsulatum*)	Uncertain		

*Geographically specific.

(CARD9: caspase recruitment domain family member 9; ME: meningoencephalitis; SOT: solid organ transplant)

meningoencephalitis and subpial ischemic lesions. Intermediate (larger than 20 μm; *Candida*) fungi can occlude the small vessels and produce local tissue necrosis and subsequent microabscess formation. Larger size fungi, septate (*Aspergillus*), and nonseptate (*Mucorales*) usually infect juxta-cranial sites (paranasal sinuses, orbit, oral cavity etc.) and then may invade contiguous cranial bones, meninges, and basal cerebral venous sinuses, and intracranial arteries resulting in large infarcts. The resulting cerebral infarct may lead to cerebritis and abscess formation. Good host immunity may result in granuloma formation (**Table 1**).

Clinical syndromes of CNS fungal infections are varied and depend on the part of the neuraxis involved, type of fungus, and the pathology. These clinical syndromes can occur either alone or in combinations (**Tables 1** and **2**). Of the various clinical syndromes, meningitis/meningoencephalitis and intracranial mass lesions (abscesses and granuloma) are the common syndromes. Meningitis and meningoencephalitis is the most common clinical syndrome with most of the yeasts in the immunocompromised individuals. In India, skull base syndromes due to aspergillosis often in an immunocompetent are the common clinical syndromes. This chapter discusses common fungal infections seen in India.

TABLE 2 Clinical syndromes caused by fungi: Genus/Class.

Clinical syndrome	Species
Meningitis/meningoencephalitis	*Cryptococcus; Coccidioides; Histoplasma*
Meningoencephalitis	*Cryptococcus; Coccidioides*
Brain abscess	*Aspergillus; Candida; Mucorales; Blastomyces; Coccidioides*
Rhinocerebral	*Mucorales (Rhizopus, Absidia, Rhizomucor, Syncephalastrum*
Skull base syndromes	*Aspergillus*
Stroke/infarction	*Mucorales; Aspergillus*

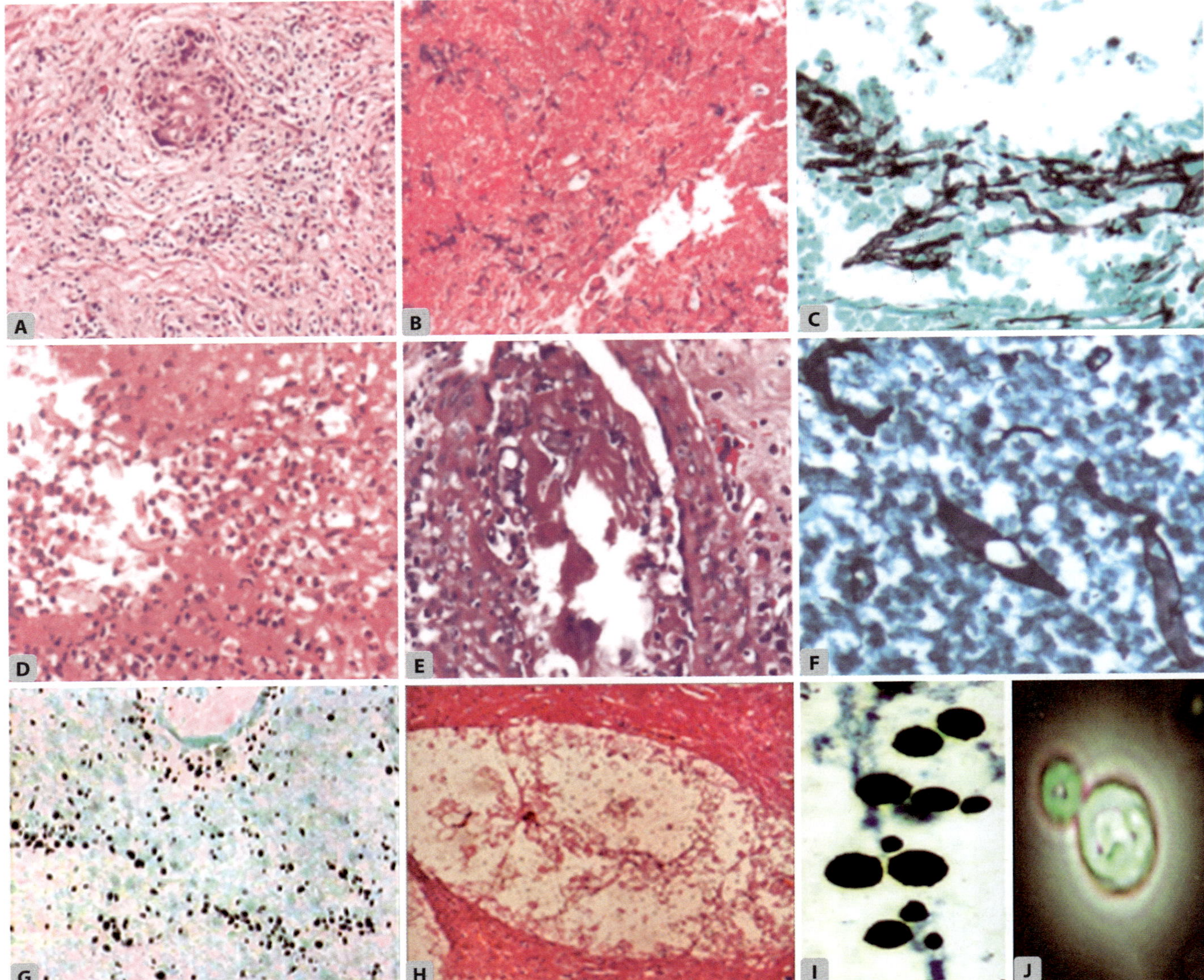

FIGURES 1 A to J: Aspergillosis: (A) Granuloma (H&E × 100); **(B)** Infarct with fungal hyphae seen at the edge (H&E × 10); **(C)** Septate acute angle branching hyphae (GMS × 400). Mucormycosis: **(D)** Suppurative inflammation (H&E × 100); **(E)** Angioinvasion (H&E × 400); **(F)** Broad aseptate hyphae with irregular branching (GMS × 400). Cryptococcosis: **(G)** Meningitis with numerous yeast forms (GMS × 100); **(H)** Capsulated yeasts in the Virchow–Robin space (H&E × 400); **(I)** Narrow-based budding yeasts (GMS × 400); **(J)** India-ink preparation showing budding yeasts.

CRYPTOCOCCAL MENINGITIS

Of the *Cryptococcus* species, *C. neoformans/C. gattii* complex is the most commonly known to cause human disease, *C. neoformans* typically causes disease in immunocompromised patients and *C. gattii* in immunocompetent individuals. The most common risk factor for cryptococcosis is advanced human immunodeficiency virus (HIV) infection followed by solid organ transplant (SOT)-related immunosuppression. Clinically, meningitis/meningoencephalitis (CME) is the main presentation of cryptococcosis. Cryptococcal meningitis is one of the acquired immunodeficiency syndrome (AIDS)-defining illness and typically occurs when the CD4+ cell count is <100–200 cells/mL. Symptoms usually develop over several weeks and the symptoms include headache, nausea, stiff neck, fever, personality changes, seizures, and cranial nerve palsies. Obstructive hydrocephalus due to elevated yeast burden obstructing cerebrospinal fluid (CSF) outflow, leads to increased intracranial pressure (ICP). Cryptococcoma is the other rare neurological presenting clinical syndrome.

Diagnosis: Characteristic CSF findings are raised opening pressure, elevated cell count, predominantly lymphocytes, elevated proteins, and low sugar. Definite diagnosis is by detection of *Cryptococcus* in CSF by microscopy (sensitivity 86%) (**Figs. 1 G and J**), culture (90%), or antigen. Capsular antigen (CrAg) detection by latex agglutination provides sensitivity and specificity of 97–98% and 86–100%, respectively. CrAg, is detectable in blood and CSF of infected patients with point of care lateral flow assays (LFAs), highly sensitive (99.3%), and specific (99.1%) in CSF.

Treatment: Treatment of CME consists of an induction phase followed by consolidation and maintenance phases. The induction phase aims at reducing the CSF fungal burden as much as possible within first 2 weeks. The World Health Organization (WHO) guidelines recommend 7-day amphotericin B (AmB) plus flucytosine, followed by 7-day high-dose fluconazole for induction treatment of HIV-associated CME. Alternate options are: (1) 2 weeks of fluconazole plus flucytosine or (2) 2 weeks of AmB deoxycholate plus fluconazole. The WHO's preferred therapy for the treatment of HIV-related cryptococcal meningitis in low- and middle-income countries (LMICs) is 1 week of AmB plus flucytosine and the alternative therapy is 2 weeks of fluconazole plus flucytosine. Fluconazole (800 mg daily for adults) is recommended for the consolidation phase (for 8 weeks following the induction phase). Fluconazole (200 mg daily for adults) is recommended for the maintenance phase (secondary prophylaxis) (**Box 1**).

Management of raised intracranial pressure (ICP) (>25 cm H_2O) relies mainly on therapeutic lumbar punctures (LPs), shown to be associated with up to 69% improved survival, irrespective of baseline opening pressure. Draining up to 30 mL of CSF each day is safe. Percutaneous lumbar drain is a therapeutic option for patients with persistently high opening pressure.

BOX 1	Management of the fungal infections of central nervous system.
I. Cryptococcal meningitis	
Induction (HIV positive): Liposomal amphotericin B (LAmB 3–6 mg/kg/day; ABLC 5 mg/kg/day; LAmB 0.7 mg/kg/day) + 5-flucytosine 100 mg/kg/day in divided doses for 2 weeks or 14 days of oral combination with flucytosine + high-dose fluconazole	
Consolidation phase: Fluconazole 400–800 mg/day for 8 weeks	
Maintenance phase: Fluconazole 200–400 mg/day for a period of 1 year in patients with HIV infection	
II. Aspergillosis	
First-line: Voriconazole: 6 mg/kg IV every 12 hours for 1 day, followed by 4 mg/kg IV every 12 hours; oral therapy can be used at 200–300 mg every 12 hours, total duration of therapy is not clearly defined	
Alternative: LAmB (3–5 mg/kg/day) IV, ABLC (5 mg/kg/day) or combination therapy with voriconazole (6 mg/kg/day in two divided doses) and caspofungin (50 mg/m²/day)	
III. Mucormycosis	
First-line: Amphotericin B 1.5 mg/kg/day IV by continuous infusion or LAmB (3–5 mg/kg/day) IV for initial 28 days	
Alternative: Isavuconazole 300 mg three times for 2 days followed by 300 QD. IV or PO	
Duration of treatment: At least 6 months (duration of treatment depends on the extent of surgery and the immune status of the patient)	

(ABLC: amphotericin B lipid complex)

Immune reconstitution inflammatory syndrome: Immune reconstitution inflammatory syndrome (IRIS) is common in patients with CM. IRIS is characterized by the onset of new or worsening signs and symptoms including neuroimaging findings after a rapid reversal of immune deficiency. International Network for the Study of HIV-associated IRIS (INSHI) recognized two forms of cryptococcal IRIS (C-IRIS): paradoxical C-IRIS and antiretroviral therapy (ART)-associated cryptococcosis and unmasking C-IRIS (ART-associated cryptococcosis). The definition for paradoxical C-IRIS applies to patients with recognized pre-ART cryptococcal disease who subsequently deteriorate while on ART. The definition of ART-associated cryptococcosis applies to those without recognized cryptococcosis at the time of initiating ART, who develop cryptococcosis on ART. Paradoxical C-IRIS occurs in one-third of patients with cryptococcosis diagnosed pre-ART. IRIS is more frequent when baseline CD4 cell counts are <50 cells/μL.

Infectious Diseases Society of America guideline does not recommend treatment of minor IRIS manifestations; these symptoms usually resolve spontaneously. Currently dexamethasone is the only drug for more severe cases. In cases of severe C-IRIS in SOT recipients, or in case of steroid resistant C-IRIS, adalimumab [a recombinant human monoclonal tumor necrosis factor alpha (TNF-α) antagonist] and thalidomide use has been shown to be beneficial. In ART naïve patients, initiation is usually delayed for 2–4 weeks, because of increased mortality attributed to IRIS.

Cryptococcal meningoencephalitis (CME) is fatal if untreated. Despite optimal treatment, 3-month mortality is about 30% in HIV patients and 20–30% in non-HIV nontransplant patients. Presence of IRIS is associated with increased mortality in both HIV and SOT populations.

ASPERGILLOSIS

Central nervous system aspergillosis primarily occurs in immunocompromised individuals. Of the *Aspergillus* species, *A. fumigatus* is the most frequent species followed by *A. flavus.* In India, sinocranial aspergillosis is the common form. Intracranial spread occurs by direct extension of the infection from sinuses, nose, and ear canal. Hematogenous spread occurs, usually from a pulmonary focus and rarely by direct inoculation after head trauma or surgery. The sinocranial form of aspergillosis is often reported from countries with temperate climate often in otherwise immunocompetent individual.

Patients with sinocranial aspergillosis *present with features* of intracranial focal mass lesions and skull base syndromes which include orbital apex syndrome, cavernous sinus syndrome, proptosis with or without ocular nerve palsies, polyneuritis cranialis, and orbito-cranial syndromes (**Tables 1** and **2**). *Aspergillus* species has predilection for angioinvasion and invasive aspergillosis can present with stroke-like syndromes: Cerebral infarction, hemorrhage and subarachnoid hemorrhage can occur due to mycotic aneurysm. Meningitis/meningoencephalitis can rarely be the presenting feature.

Neuroimaging may help in suspecting the diagnosis of sinocranial aspergillosis. Presence of homogenously enhancing skull base lesions in association with sinus, orbital, and mastoid lesions should suggest the diagnostic possibility of *Aspergillus* infections, more so in countries with temperate climate. On magnetic resonance imaging (MRI), *Aspergillus* sinusitis appears as iso- to hypointense on T1-weighted (T1W) and hypointense on T2-weighted (T2W) images. This T2 shortening is related to the presence of iron, magnesium, as well as increased calcium contents in the lesions (**Fig. 2**). Definite diagnosis of invasive aspergillosis is by culture of the organism. On histological examination of *Aspergillus* species, hyphae are slender, septate, and acute angle branching (**Figs. 1 A** to **C**). However, tissue sections cannot differentiate it from those of other hyaline septate hyphae such as *Fusarium* species and *Scedosporium* species. Serum and bronchoalveolar lavage (BAL) galactomannan (GM) is recommended as an accurate marker for the diagnosis of invasive aspergillosis. Serum assays for (1→3)-β-D-glucan are recommended for diagnosing invasive aspergillosis in high-risk patients [hematologic malignancy and allogeneic hematopoietic stem cell transplant (HSCT)], but are not specific for *Aspergillus.*

Voriconazole is the drug of choice for CNS aspergillosis and lipid formulations of AmB are reserved for those intolerant or refractory to voriconazole (**Box 1**). Duration of therapy should be based on the evidence of disease, probable for the period of resolution of infection. Surgical resection of granuloma or abscesses eliminates areas containing viable fungi. A mortality benefit of surgery has been shown in a retrospective study. Aggressive surgical management of fungal mass lesions including excision of sinus lesions in patients with sinocranial aspergillosis along with voriconazole for the period of resolution of infection is likely to be associated with better outcomes. CNS invasive aspergillosis is a devastating infection with 50–100% mortality. In sinocranial aspergillosis, radical surgical excision of the lesion and treatment with voriconazole might reduce mortality.

MUCORMYCOSIS

Mucormycosis is *caused by* the genera Mucorales. The medically most important pathogenic genera include *Mucor, Rhizopus, Rhizomucor,* and *Absidia.* The specific predisposing factors for mucormycosis include diabetes mellitus (particularly ketoacidosis), deferoxamine therapy, and IV drug abuse. The Mucorales have tropism

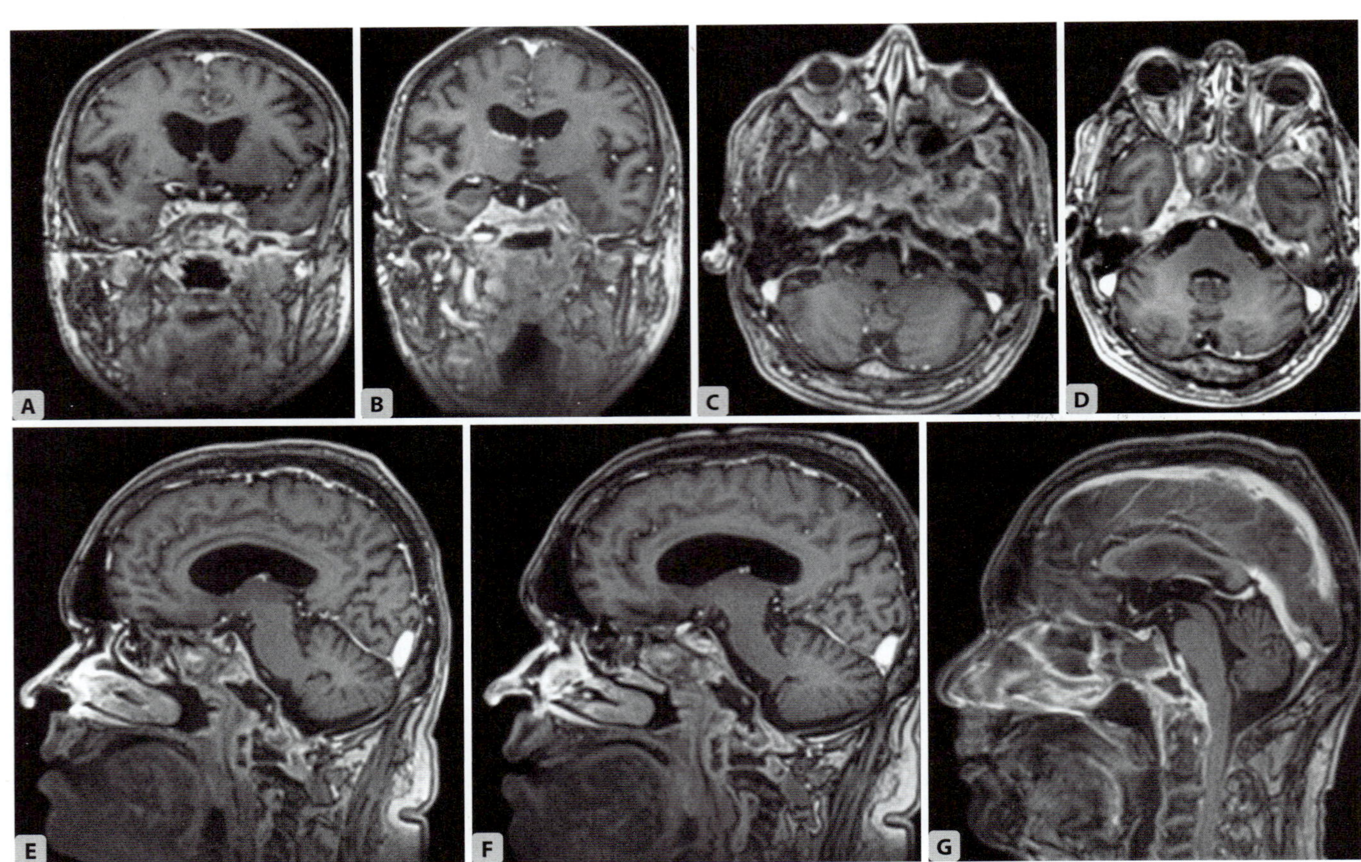

FIGURES 2 A to G: (A to D) Aspergillus sinusitis. Postcontrast T1 coronal and axial showing heterogeneously enhancing lesion filling the sphenoid sinus spreading laterally to cavernous sinus and eroding floor of left middle cranial fossa; **(E and F)** Postcontrast T1 image showing destruction of most anterior portion of clivus with sclerotic changes in the rest of the clivus, enhancing craniovertebral (CV) junction with abscess in prevertebral space; **(G)** Postcontrast T1 image showing partial resolution following treatment.

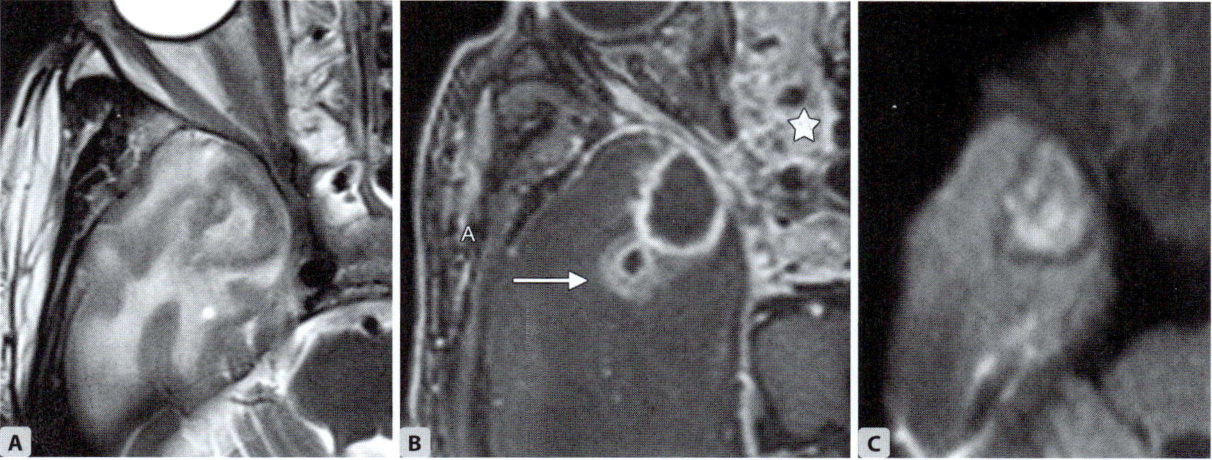

FIGURES 3 A to C: Mucormycosis. Rounded peripherally enhancing lesion in the anterior most portion of the right temporal lobe **(B)**, its walls appear irregular and hypointense on T2-weighted (T2W) images, central hyperintensity and perilesional edema is noted in T2W images **(A)**. A smaller thick-walled peripherally enhancing lesion is seen posterolateral to it (arrow). The lesion shows diffusion restriction within it **(C)**. Also seen in the enhancement within the ethmoidal air cells (star in **B**).

for angioinvasion, resulting in infarction and necrosis. Perineural invasion is frequent. Rhinocerebral form is the most common presenting clinical syndrome. Among injectable drug users, isolated cerebral form is common. Manifestations of the disease may reflect the sequential involvement of the nose, sinuses, eye, and brain. Sinusitis produces necrotic eschars in the nasal mucosa or palate. Clinical features of cavernous sinus thrombosis include loss of vision, internal and external ophthalmoplegia, and contralateral hemiplegia due to thrombosis of the internal carotid artery.

The diagnosis of mucormycosis is by identification of the fungal pathogen in the tissue with culture confirmation Mucorales are broad, aseptate hyphae with irregular or right angle branching (**Figs. 1 D** to **F**). Due to few or no septae, the hyphae are easily damaged during biopsy and hence yield on culture is low (40–70%). Neuroimaging is of help in visualizing the affected area and is also of help in obtaining the tissue for histopathological studies and culture (**Fig. 3**).

Initial antifungal therapy is high-dose IV liposomal AmB (L-AmB); however, the total dose needed for cure has not been determined. For patients who have responded to L-AmB, posaconazole or isavuconazole can be used for oral step-down therapy. For salvage therapy, posaconazole or isavuconazole can be used for patients who do not respond to or cannot tolerate AmB (**Box 1**). Surgical debridement has been a key component of treatment of mucormycosis and survival rates are much better in patients treated with combined medical and surgical therapy than in patients treated with medical therapy only.

The *estimated mortality* associated with cerebral mucormycosis is 79% and for disseminated infection with CNS involvement is 98%, while morality for both localized cerebral and rhinocerebral infection is about 62%. The outcomes may improve with the effective use of newer antifungal agents.

PARASITIC INFECTIONS

Parasitic infections are mostly endemic to certain geographical regions for reasons of climate and the availability of intermediate hosts to transmit them to humans. However, because of the increase in the international travel and migration of people from their native countries, these infections are reported from countries outside the endemic regions. For many of the parasites CNS is one of the systems involved. This chapter discusses common parasitic infections seen in India.

NEUROCYSTICERCOSIS

Neurocysticercosis is the most common parasitic disease of the human CNS and is caused by the larval form of the cestode, *Taenia solium*. Areas endemic to NCC include Latin America, Africa, South East Asia, India, China, and Nepal.

Life cycle and pathology: In the life cycle of *T. solium*, pigs are intermediary host harboring the cystic larvae in their flesh and humans are the definitive host harboring the adult tapeworm in the small intestine. Pigs can access human stool contaminated with tapeworm eggs and get infected with cysticerci. When infected pork is ingested by humans, larvae evaginate and can develop into mature tapeworms that attach to the mucosa of the small intestine. The proglottids of *T. solium* containing thousands of infective eggs are excreted with the stools and infect other pigs, closing the cycle. Humans get NCC by ingesting tapeworm eggs via fecal/oral contamination. It has also been suggested that humans may be able to autoinfect themselves (**Fig. 4**).

Cysticercus cellulosae is the most frequently observed form of cysticercus in patients with NCC. Parenchymal cysticercus is divided into four evolutive stages: (1) Vesicular (active), (2) Colloidal vesicular, (3) Granular nodular, and (4) Fibrocalcific. Colloidal vesicular and granular nodular

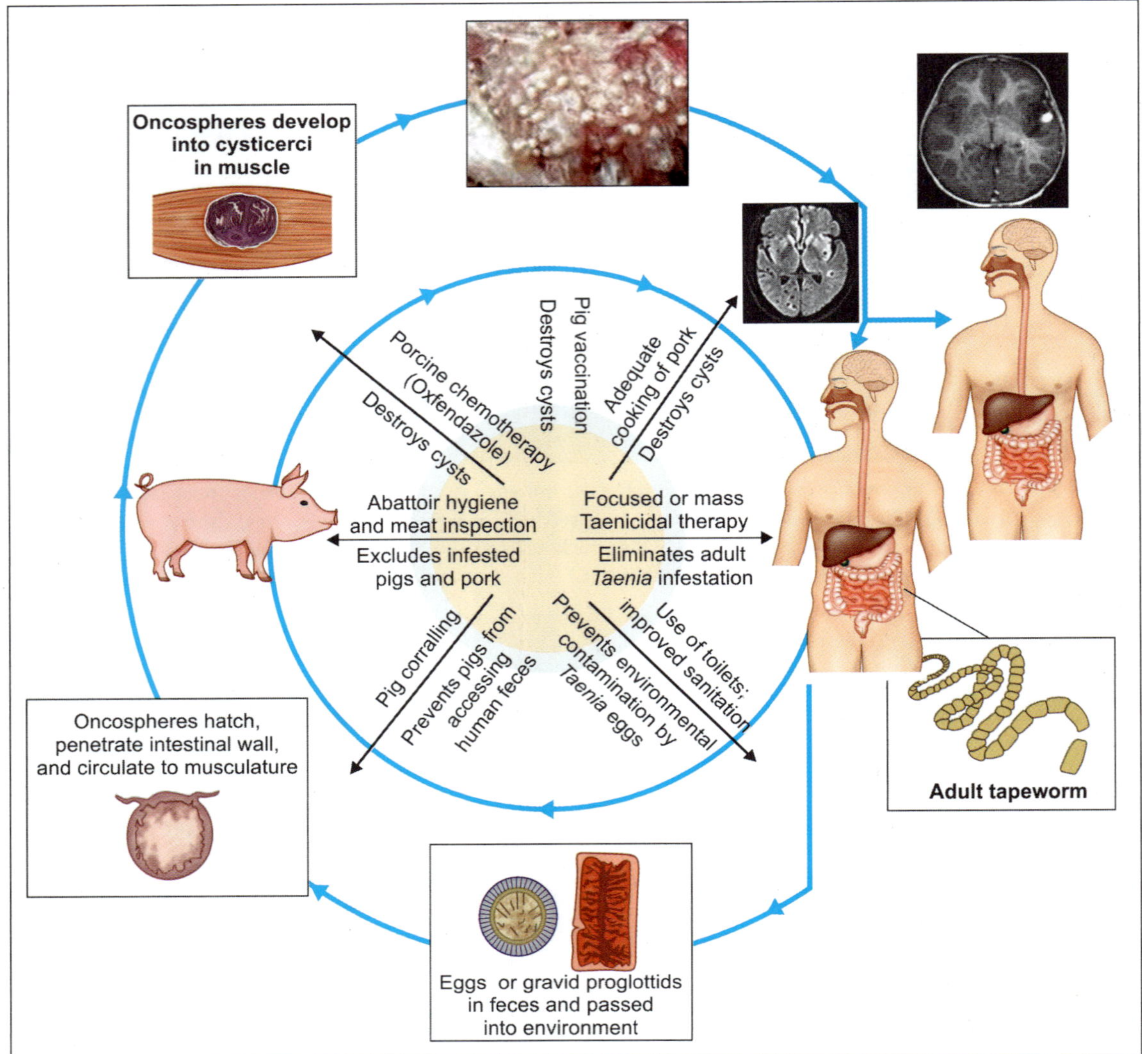

FIGURE 4: Life cycle of *Taenia solium*.

stages represent the degenerative phase of parenchymal cysticerci (**Fig. 5 A**). Infection per se does not typically cause symptoms. The main clinical manifestation, seizures, is caused by the host inflammatory response.

Clinical presentation: The clinical presentation is pleomorphic and dependents on the parasite load, both the size and number of cysticerci and the stage of cysticercus evolution and cyst location (**Table 3**). The parenchymal type is the most common type; corticomedullary junction is the primary location of the parenchymal form. One patient can have lesions in different stages of the disease simultaneously (**Fig. 6 A**). Solitary cysticercus granuloma (SCG), which represents single parenchymal cysticercal cyst in degenerative phase, is the most frequent presenting form in India and in other endemic countries. SCG accounts for about 20% of all cases of active NCC (**Fig. 6 B**).

The two most common clinical presentations are seizures and increased ICP. Seizure(s) is the presenting clinical feature of all the evolutive stages of parenchymal NCC, in about 80% of patients. Patients can present with single seizure, seizure cluster, and very rarely status epilepticus. Initial seizure burden can be high. Seizures due to NCC can be categorized under acute symptomatic seizures and unprovoked seizures. Seizures due to degenerative phase of cysticerci are categorized under acute symptomatic seizures and are attributed to the acute perilesional inflammatory reaction. Whereas seizures due to calcific stage of neurocysticercosis (cNCC) (**Fig. 6 C**) are categorized under unprovoked seizures and are attributed to the perilesional gliosis. There is a robust epidemiological evidence favoring the relationship between cNCC and epilepsy. Focal cNCC is the most common cause of acquired epilepsy in people >20 years of age in the countries endemic to NCC.

Cysticercal encephalitis is a rare form of parenchymal disease with numerous cysticerci and diffuse cerebral edema. This form has been more commonly reported in young females and present with seizures and features of ICH. Disseminated cysticercosis is a rare form and is mostly described from India. Heavy dissemination of larvae in muscles gives an appearance of pseudo-muscular hypertrophy, which in extreme cases imparts a characteristic "Herculean appearance."

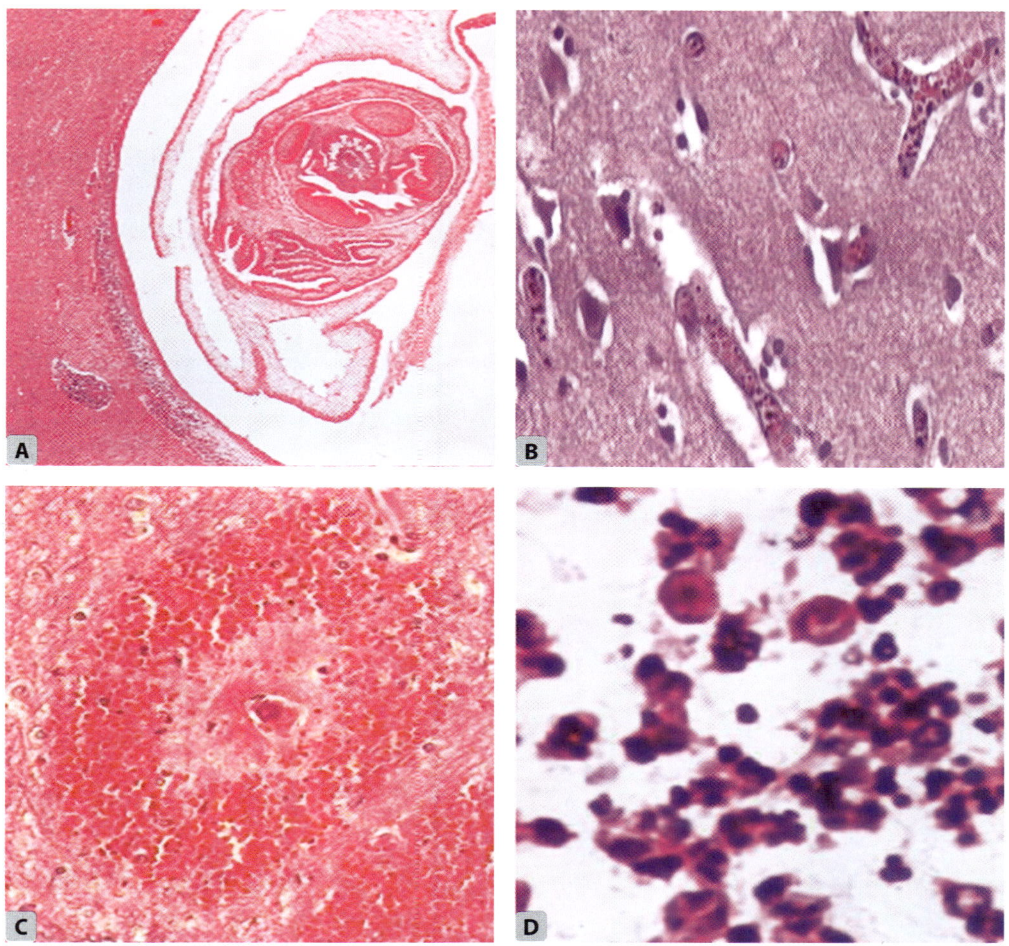

FIGURES 5 A to D: **(A)** Cysticercus larva with scolex (H&E × 400); **(B)** Cerebral malaria sequestration in the capillaries (H&E × 100); **(C)** Ring hemorrhages (H&E × 400); **(D)** Acanthamoeba encephalitis with both trophozoites and cyst forms (H&E × 400).

TABLE 3 NCC forms: Treatment protocols.

NCC: Form	Clinical features	Antiparasitic therapy	Antiseizure medication and corticosteroids
Viable intraparenchymal: 1–2 cysts	Seizures, headache	Monotherapy with albendazole (15 mg/kg/day in two daily doses up to 1,200 mg/day) with food for 10 days	ASM for the period of resolution of the lesion + corticosteroids
Degenerative intraparenchymal: single degenerative cyst (SCG)	Seizures, rarely headache	Monotherapy with albendazole (15 mg/kg/day in two daily doses up to 800 mg/day) for 1–2 weeks	ASM treatment for the period of resolution of the lesion in the follow-up neuroimaging + corticosteroids
Viable intraparenchymal: >2 cysts	Seizures, headache, rarely focal deficits	Albendazole (15 mg/kg/day in two daily doses up to 1,200 mg/day) combined with praziquantel (15 mg/kg/day in three daily doses) for 10 days	ASM and corticosteroids
Degenerative intra-parenchymal: >2 cysts	Seizures, headache, rarely focal deficits	Albendazole (15 mg/kg/day in two daily doses up to 1,200 mg/day) combined with praziquantel (15 mg/kg/day in three daily doses) for 10 days	ASM and corticosteroids
Calcific stage	Seizures	None	To be treated as a case of epilepsy with ASM
Intraventricular	Headache, obstructive hydrocephalus		

Continued...

Continued...

NCC: Form	Clinical features	Antiparasitic therapy	Antiseizure medication and corticosteroids
Subarachnoid	Communicative hydrocephalus, headache, meningitis, stroke	VP shunt followed by chronic corticosteroids and intensive antiparasitic therapy	Corticosteroids for a long period based on the repeat neuroimaging findings
Spinal	Radiculomyelopathy	Surgical removal of cyst	May be considered for a short period
Ocular	Impaired vision, ocular palsy	Surgical removal of cyst	May be considered for a short period

Note: The optimal dose and duration of corticosteroids has not been defined, but doses have included dexamethasone 0.1 mg/kg/day for the duration of therapy or 1–2 mg/kg/day of prednisone or prednisolone have been used.

(ASM: antiseizure medication; NCC: neurocysticercosis; SCG: solitary cysticercus granuloma; VP: ventriculoperitoneal)

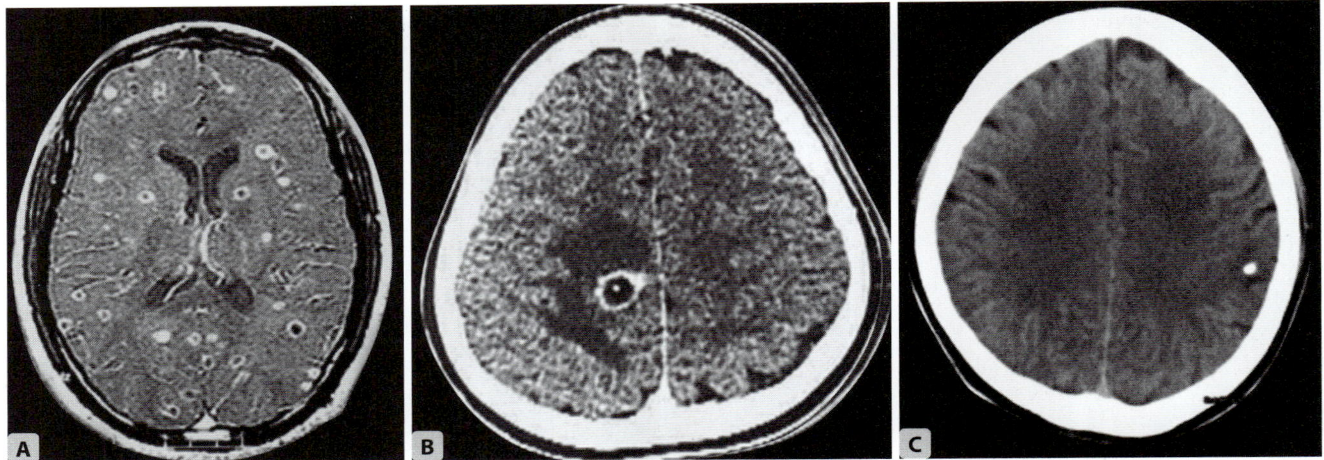

FIGURES 6 A to C: Neurocysticercosis. (A) Contrast magnetic resonance imaging (MRI) showing various evolutive stages of neurocysticercosis; **(B)** Contrast computed tomography (CT) showing solitary cysticercus granuloma with scolex; **(C)** CT showing single calcific neurocysticercosis with perilesional edema.

Diagnosis: Clinical features in patients with NCC are often nonspecific; new-onset convulsive seizure and headache are the two most common presenting clinical features. The diagnosis of NCC relies predominantly on the combination of clinical features and characteristic neuroimaging features. Recently the earlier proposed diagnostic criteria for NCC were revised (**Box 2**). The revised set is structured in absolute, neuroimaging, and clinical/exposure criteria. Direct visualization of the parasite on fundoscopic examination is pathognomonic for NCC. Evaluation of suspected NCC should include neuroimaging with both noncontrast CT and MRI of the brain. Noncontrast CT is highly sensitive for identifying calcific stage of NCC (**Figs. 6 A** to **C**). The neuroimaging appearance of cysts mirrors the pathophysiologic stages of cyst degeneration. The characteristic neuroimaging features of viable cyst are little or no surrounding edema or rim enhancement, cyst fluid isodense with CSF and may show visible scolex which is a strong evidence for NCC. The characteristics of degenerative cysts are uniform-rim enhancement pattern or disc enhancement with surrounding edema. Over time the gliosis that ensues may lead to calcification.

Among the serological tests for detection of *T. solium* antibodies, the test of choice is the enzyme-linked immunoelectrotransfer blot (EITB) assay. EITB test is less sensitive in CSF than in serum. The sensitivity of the immunoblot assay varies with the form of NCC, near 100% sensitive in those with multiple parenchymal cysticerci, subarachnoid or intraventricular lesions and in patients with single lesion the sensitivity is as low as 50–60%. The antibodies can persist in the serum for long periods after the resolution of the lesions.

Treatment: Antiparasitic therapy is important in NCC. Parenchymal form has better outcome if treated with antiparasitic drugs along with corticosteroids (**Table 3**). Both phenytoin and carbamazepine reduce the bioavailability of praziquantel. A high dose of praziquantel (50 mg/kg) instead of the conventional dosage (25 mg/kg) is recommended in people concomitantly receiving enzyme-inducing antiseizure medications (ASMs). In patients with subarachnoid the optimal management may require chronic anti-inflammatory therapy (corticosteroids), intensive antiparasitic therapy, and surgical therapy. Ventricular NCC of the third and lateral ventricles should

BOX 2 Revised diagnostic criteria and degrees of diagnostic certainty for neurocysticercosis.

Absolute criteria:

- Histological demonstration of the parasite from biopsy of a brain or spinal cord lesion
- Visualization of subretinal cysticercus
- Conclusive demonstration of a scolex within a cystic lesion on neuroimaging studies

Neuroimaging criteria:

- Major neuroimaging criteria:
  - Cystic lesions without a discernible scolex
  - Enhancing lesions[a]
  - Multilobulated cystic lesions in the subarachnoid space
  - Typical parenchymal brain calcifications[a]
- Confirmative neuroimaging criteria:
  - Resolution of cystic lesions after cysticidal drug therapy
  - Spontaneous resolution of single small enhancing lesions[b]
  - Migration of ventricular cysts documented on sequential neuroimaging studies[a]
- Minor neuroimaging criteria:
  - Obstructive hydrocephalus (symmetric or asymmetric) or abnormal enhancement of basal leptomeninges

Clinical/Exposure criteria:

- Major clinical/exposure:
  - Detection of specific anticysticercal antibodies or cysticercal antigens by well-standardized immunodiagnostic tests[a]
  - Cysticercosis outside the central nervous system[a]
  - Evidence of a household contact with *Taenia solium* infection
- Minor clinical/exposure:
  - Clinical manifestations suggestive of neurocysticercosis[a]
  - Individuals coming from or living in an area where cysticercosis is endemic[a]

Degrees of diagnostic certainty:

Definitive diagnosis:

- One absolute criterion
- Two major neuroimaging criteria plus any clinical/exposure criteria
- One major and one confirmative neuroimaging criteria plus any clinical/exposure criteria
- One major neuroimaging criteria plus two clinical/exposure criteria (including at least one major clinical/exposure criterion), together with the exclusion of other pathologies producing similar neuroimaging findings

Probable diagnosis:

- One major neuroimaging criteria plus any two clinical/exposure criteria
- One minor neuroimaging criteria plus at least one major clinical/exposure criteria

[a] Operational definitions—***cystic lesions:*** rounded, well-defined lesions with liquid contents of signal similar to that of cerebrospinal fluid (CSF) on computed tomography (CT) or magnetic resonance imaging (MRI); ***enhancing lesions:*** single or multiple, ring- or nodular-enhancing lesions of 10–20 mm in diameter, with or without surrounding edema, but not displacing midline structures; ***typical parenchymal brain calcifications:*** single or multiple, solid, and most usually <10 mm in diameter; migration of ventricular cyst: demonstration of a different location of ventricular cystic lesions on sequential CTs or MRIs; ***well-standardized immunodiagnostic tests:*** so far, antibody detection by enzyme-linked immunoelectrotransfer blot assay using lentil lectin-purified T. solium antigens, and detection of cysticercal antigens by monoclonal antibody-based enzyme-linked immunosorbent assay (ELISA); ***cysticercosis outside the central nervous system:*** demonstration of cysticerci from biopsy of subcutaneous nodules, X-ray films or CT showing cigar-shape calcifications in soft tissues, or visualization of the parasite in the anterior chamber of the eye; **suggestive clinical manifestations:** mainly seizures (often starting in individuals aged 20–49 years; the diagnosis of seizures in this context is not excluded if patients are outside of the typical age range), but other manifestations include chronic headaches, focal neurologic deficits, intracranial hypertension and cognitive decline; ***cysticercosis-endemic area:*** a place where active transmission is documented.

[b] The use of corticosteroids makes this criterion invalid.

Source: De Brutto OH, Nash TE, White Jr AC, Rajshekhar V, Wilkins PP, Singh G, et al. Revised diagnostic criteria for neurocysticercosis. J Neurol Sci. 2017;372: 202-10.

be treated with endoscopic surgery. Open craniotomies are options for fourth ventricular lesions.

The optimal dose and duration of corticosteroids in patients with seizures due to NCC has not been defined. Corticosteroids are used for few days to weeks concomitantly with antiparasitic therapy to prevent or ameliorate any adverse reactions. In patients with features of elevated intracranial, prednisolone (1–2 mg/kg) or dexamethasone (1 mg/kg IV) are used. In patients with cysticercal encephalitis, antiparasitic drugs are avoided and the diffuse cerebral edema is treated with corticosteroids. Dexamethasone reduces serum praziquantel levels by nearly 50%, potentially compromising its efficacy. Enzyme-inducing ASMs induce the metabolism of corticosteroids. These data should be considered in people concomitantly receiving ASMs and praziquantel and corticosteroids.

There are no high quality trials that evaluated individual ASMs in people with NCC. In most patients with seizures due to NCC, seizure remission can be achieved with single ASM. Viable or calcific stage of NCC is associated with enduring predisposition for recurrent seizures. Patients with seizures due to these lesions should be considered to have epilepsy and should be treated with ASM for a long period. For patients presenting with seizure in the setting of patients with seizures due to SCG, ASM should be continued for the period of resolution of the lesion on follow-up neuroimaging.

CEREBRAL MALARIA

Malaria caused by protozoans of the *Plasmodium* genus is a major public health concern worldwide. The common pathogenic species to humans include *P. falciparum, P. vivax, P ovale*, and *P malaria*. Human malaria infection occurs during the blood meal of an infected female mosquito belonging to the *Anopheles* genus (**Fig. 7**). Worldwide, cerebral malaria (CM) occurs in African children and Asian adults. Half of malaria deaths occur in those with CM. It is estimated that around 1% of children infected with *P. falciparum* develop a more severe form of malaria, which may eventually lead to cerebral complications including CM. CM was less frequently reported in adults with *P. vivax* infection.

Definition: Cerebral malaria has been restricted to the "syndrome in which altered consciousness (Glasgow coma score less than 11 in adults or a Blantyre coma score less than three in children) associated with a malarial infection, could not be attributed to convulsions, sedative drugs, or hypoglycemia alone or to a nonmalarial cause". Finding of retinopathy, patch retinal whitening in the macula (perifoveal), and/or in the peripheral retina and white or orange discolouration of retinal vessels, improves the specificity, 95% sensitivity and 90% specificity. Presence of retinopathy is highly suggestive of the presence of intracerebral parasite sequestration a characteristic histopathological feature of fatal CM.

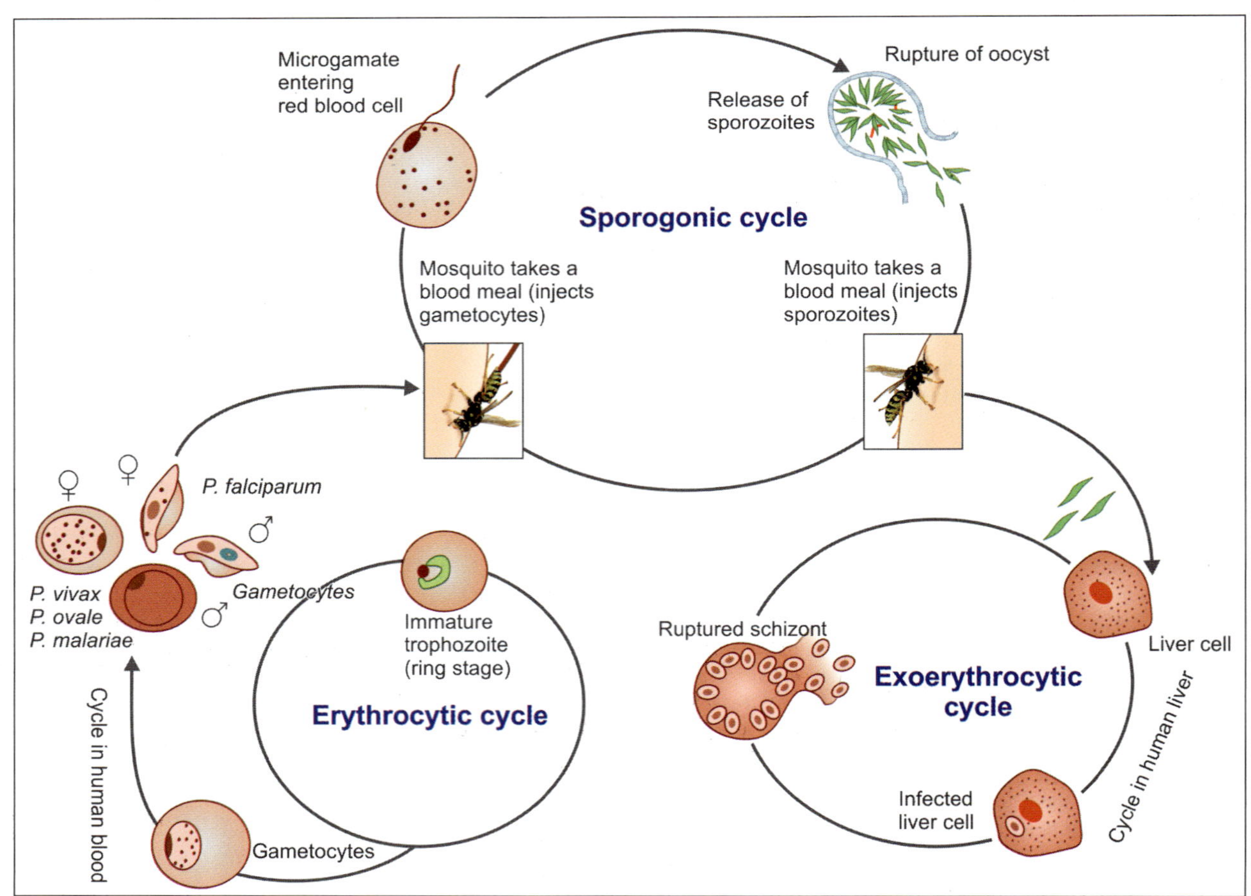

FIGURE 7: Life cycle of *Plasmodium*.

Pathogenesis: The pathogenesis of CM has not yet fully elucidated. The pathology indicates a clear disease of the vascular endothelium. It is characterized by parasite sequestration, inflammatory cytokine production, and vascular leakage, eventually resulting in brain hypoxia. Parasite sequestration in the brain occurs by the adhesion of infected red blood cells (iRBCs) to specific host receptors including endothelial protein C receptor (EPCR) and intercellular adhesion molecule (ICAM)-1. This cytoadherence of iRBCs to endothelial receptors is mediated by *P. falciparum* erythrocyte membrane protein (PfEMP)-1. Brain injury in CM seems to be caused by hypoxia and ischemia resulting from the sequestration of infected erythrocytes in small brain vessels (**Figs. 5 B** and **C**).

Clinical features and diagnosis: Patients with CM (more frequently children) initially present with fever, malaise, vomiting, and neurological symptoms that may include seizures or altered mental status leading to coma. Seizures are more frequently focal onset. CNS involvement in adult patients is usually associated with severe disease and compromise of other body systems (**Table 4**). CM is associated with high mortality, estimated around 20% in the hospital setting, and patients who survive frequently suffer from chronic epilepsy and altered cognition, motor, or sensory deficits. Diagnosis is by demonstration of asexual form of *P. falciparum* in peripheral blood smear in thick and thin blood smear films stained by Giemsa stain. At least three smears 6 hours apart should be examined before excluding CM. Neuroimaging findings associated with CM are best defined on MRI, mostly as focal infarcts and cerebral edema, although thalamic and cerebellar damage as well as brainstem demyelination have also been described.

Treatment: Cerebral malaria is a medical emergency requiring prompt administration of an effective antimalarial and supportive care, ideally in an intensive care unit. Corticosteroids should not be used in these patients. Mannitol administration to reduce ICP is not recommended. A single dose of mannitol in children with CM found no benefit on clinical outcomes compared with placebo. In adults with CM and brain swelling, mannitol prolonged coma recovery time compared with controls not receiving mannitol. The drug therapy and dosages are given in **Box 3**. In patients with nonresolving coma, workup for other associated or concomitant conditions such as nonconvulsive status epilepticus, metabolic abnormalities, or other infections should be done.

TABLE 4 Differences between pediatric and adult cerebral malaria.

	Children	Adults
Clinical variables		
Mortality	18%	30%
Average duration of symptoms before onset of severe disease	3 days	5 days
Time to coma resolution	1–2 days	2–4 days
CNS manifestations		
Convulsions	31%	12%
Coma	34%	40%
Abnormal brainstem reflexes	More common	Rare
CSF pressure	Often raised	Usually normal
Neurocognitive deficits	25%	<5%
Other clinical signs		
Severe anemia	26%	6%
Jaundice	2%	48%
Renal failure	Rare	Common
Retinopathy		
Hemorrhages	40–46%	9–55%
Whitening	44–50%	5–55%
Vessel color changes	20–32%	0
Papilledema	8–15%	5–12%

Source: Hawkes M, Elphinstone RE, Conroy AL, Kain KC. Contrasting pediatric and adult cerebral malaria: role of the endothelial barrier. Virulence. 2013;4(6):543-55.

AMEBIC INFECTIONS

The CNS infection with free-living amoebae of the genus *Acanthamoeba, Balamuthia,* and *Naegleria* has rarely been described from India. Human infection occurs when the trophozoites invade the CNS. *Naegleria fowleri* causes acute meningoencephalitis and primary amebic meningoencephalitis (PAM) in previously healthy children and adults through transnasal spread during swimming in fresh water in summer months. *Acanthamoeba* species and *Balamuthia mandrillaris* cause a more chronic disease, called granulomatous amebic encephalitis (GAE). The spread to brain is possible by hematogenous route.

BOX 3 Severe malaria: Treatment protocols in adults and children.

First-line initial therapy:

- Artesunate intravenously 2.4 mg/kg per dose at hour 0, 12, and 24, then every 24 hours; in patients with weight less than 20 kg: artesunate intravenous 3.0 mg/kg per dose

Alternative initial therapy:

- Quinine dihydrochloride intravenous infusion 20 mg/kg loading dose (over 4 hours) then maintenance dose 10 mg/kg (over 2 hours) every 8 hours (dose requires renal adjustment)
- Artemether intramuscular (anterior thigh) injection 3.2 mg/kg loading dose, then 1.6 mg/kg every 24 hours

After 24 hours and able to eat and drink:

- Artemisinin-based combination therapy orally for 3 days; travel history to countries with artemisinin resistance: Intravenous artesunate plus intravenous quinine (expert opinion, no evidence)
- If intravenous artesunate is not available, use artemether in preference to quinine in adults and children
- Mefloquine is contraindicated in patients with postmalaria epilepsy or neuropsychiatric disorders

Source: World Health Organization. (2015). Guidelines for the treatment of malaria, 3rd edition. [online] Available from https://apps.who.int/iris/bitstream/handle/10665/162441/9789241549127_eng.pdf;jsessionid=BAA10AD49980898E5276FB5D63FB59BC?sequence=1.

Primary amebic meningoencephalitis is a fulminant rapidly progressive disease. The clinical features are acute-onset rhinitis with anosmia or ageusia, fever, severe headache, vomiting, irritability, seizures, and coma rapidly progressing to death within 7–10 days of onset of the disease. Diagnosis is by tissue identification or culture from brain biopsy specimens (**Fig. 5 D**). Neuroimaging shows ring enhancing lesions with perilesional edema and pseudotumor pattern. The ideal treatment regimen for PAM remains unknown and PAM is associated with high mortality despite treatment. The currently used drugs in the treatment of PAM include AmB, azithromycin, fluconazole, rifampin, miltefosine, and dexamethasone. Early diagnosis and treatment as well as aggressive management of cerebral edema were thought to have contributed to the survival of these patients.

Granulomatous amebic encephalitis is characterized by subacute onset and progressive course, low-grade fever, focal signs, seizures, ICH, and behavioral changes. Polymerase chain reaction (PCR) is the preferred diagnostic tool because it is fast, highly sensitive, and species-specific; however, this test is nor freely available in resource poor countries. Demonstration of parasites in the biopsy specimens is confirmatory. Neuroimaging may show cystic or granulomatous lesions with perilesional edema. The optimal treatment of GAE is known. Drugs that have been used successfully in combination to treat *Acanthamoeba* GAE include pentamidine, sulfadiazine, trimethoprim-sulfamethoxazole, flucytosine, fluconazole, and miltefosine-chlorhexidine. The drugs for *Balamuthia* disease include pentamidine, sulfadiazine, flucytosine, fluconazole, azithromycin/clarithromycin, and miltefosine.

RECOMMENDED READINGS

1. Murthy JMK, Dastur FD, Khadilkar SV, Kochar DK. Rabies, tetanus, leprosy, and malaria. In: Biller J, Ferro JM (Eds). Handbook of Clinical Neurology: Systemic Diseases. Amsterdam, Netherlands: Elsevier; 2014.
2. Murthy JMK, Sundaram C. Fungal infections of central nervous system. In: Biller J, Ferro JM (Eds). Handbook of Clinical Neurology: Systemic Diseases. Amsterdam, Netherlands: Elsevier; 2014.
3. Singh G, Rajshekhar V, Murthy JMK, Prabhakar S, Modi M, Khandelwal N, et al. A diagnostic and therapeutic scheme for a solitary cysticercus granuloma. Neurology. 2010;75:2236-45.
4. Del Brutto OH, Nash TE, White AC Jr, Rajshekhar V, Wilkins PP, Sing G, et al. Revised diagnostic criteria for neurocysticercosis. J Neurol Sci. 2017;372:202-10.
5. White Jr AC, Coyle CM, Rajshekhar V, Singh G, Hauser WA, Mohanty A, et al. Diagnosis and Treatment of Neurocysticercosis: 2017 Clinical Practice Guidelines by the Infectious Diseases Society of America (IDSA) and the American Society of Tropical Medicine and Hygiene (ASTMH). Clin Infect Dis. 2018;66:e49-75.

CHAPTER 192

Demyelinating Diseases of the Central Nervous System

Michlene R Passeri, Ram N Narayan

ABSTRACT

Demyelinating diseases are a heterogenous group of disorders that affect both the central nervous system (CNS) and peripheral nervous system. Disorders that cause demyelination in the CNS are numerous and may be classified into inflammatory, infectious, inherited, toxic/metabolic categories. Multiple sclerosis (MS) is considered as a prototype of a CNS inflammatory demyelinating condition. Besides MS, other CNS inflammatory demyelinating disorders include neuromyelitis optica spectrum disorders (NMOSD), myelin-oligodendrocyte associated disorders (MOGAD), transverse myelitis (TM), acute disseminated encephalomyelitis (ADEM), and neurosarcoidosis.

An example of infection leading to demyelination is progressive multifocal leukoencephalopathy. Other conditions include inherited, toxic/metabolic conditions leading to demyelination. Some conditions, such as neuromyelitis optica (NMO), used to be thought of as an MS variant, and it is important to recognize these conditions as a separate entity with accurate diagnosis since prognosis and treatment may differ substantially. Destruction of myelin with relative axonal sparing is considered to be the main pathological features in most of these conditions. Some peripheral nervous system demyelinating disorders include Guillain–Barré syndrome, chronic inflammatory demyelinating neuropathy, anti-MAG neuropathy etc., although these will not be discussed in this chapter.

"God may forgive your sins, but your nervous system won't"

—Alfred Korzybski

MULTIPLE SCLEROSIS

Multiple sclerosis is a chronic inflammatory immune-mediated disease of the CNS characterized by variable degrees of demyelination and axonal injury. It generally presents with recurrent, subacute, and focal neurologic symptoms and signs that affects the optic nerves, brain, and/or spinal cord and improves (at least to some degree) over several weeks to months, and may lead to clinical progression in some cases.

EPIDEMIOLOGY

Multiple sclerosis has a higher prevalence in regions that are further away from the equator. For example, prevalence is <1 per 100,000 in equatorial areas and 30–80 per 100,000 in Canada, northern United States, and northern Europe. The mean age of onset is about 28–31 years in various studies, with most presenting between age 15 and 45. There is a two to three times higher prevalence in women than men.

RISK FACTORS

The specific cause or initiating event leading to MS is still unclear and is thought to result from a combination of genetic, environmental, and probable infectious triggers just like many other autoimmune diseases. There are genetic susceptibilities for MS with over 200 polymorphisms identified and certain alleles such as *HLA-DRB*1501* on Chromosome 6 are thought to increase the risk for MS. On the other hand, certain alleles such as the *HLA-C*05* are thought to protective for MS. Monozygotic twins have a 25–30% concordance rate. Other epigenetic, gene–gene, or gene–environment interactions may also play a role.

Environmental risk factors:

- Epstein–Barr viral infection when young (infectious mononucleosis)
- Adolescent obesity
- Low vitamin D levels
- Low sunlight exposure
- Smoking
- *Geographic location*: Further away from the equator and generally more Northern latitude (first 16 years of life)

PATHOLOGY

It is believed that autoreactive lymphocytes gain access to the CNS and start a pathogenic cascade that results in demyelination, neuroaxonal degeneration, synaptic loss, dying-back oligodendrogliopathy, synaptic loss, and eventually tissue loss and astrogliosis. Both T- and B-cell-mediated mechanisms are equally implicated. Inflammatory T cells, B cells, and macrophages are typically seen on histopathologic examination of MS lesions. At least four histopathologic subtypes of MS demyelinating lesions have been described. The basic pathologic feature in MS is multifocal demyelinating plaques scattered throughout the CNS with a predilection for the periventricular white matter, optic nerves, brainstem, cerebellum, and spinal cord (**Box 1**).

BOX 1	Plaque types in multiple sclerosis (MS).
	• **Active:** Correlates with symptomatic relapse or asymptomatic MRI activity, presence declines with age
	• **Inactive:** Present mainly in inactive progressive MS, limited number of activated microglia, presence increases with age
	• **Shadow:** Have full remyelination capacity, present equally in all phases of MS
	• **Smoldering (slowly expanding):** Seen in progressive forms of MS, have slowly expanding rim of microglia with an inactive center, associated with ongoing axonal injury and neurodegeneration

(MRI: magnetic resonance imaging)

Source: Frischer JM, Weigand SD, Guo Y, Kale N, Parisi JE, Pirko I, et al. Clinical and pathological insights into the dynamic nature of the white matter multiple sclerosis plaque. Ann Neurol. 2015;78(5):710-21.

CLINICAL SYMPTOMS AND SIGNS

There are no clinical signs/symptoms unique to MS. Sensory symptoms are the most common earliest symptoms in MS. Some conditions are highly suggestive and typical of MS-related demyelination:

- *Optic neuritis*: It is a presenting symptom in about 25% and will eventually develop in 50% of patients with MS at some point in course of disease. It typically involves the anterior portion of the optic nerve.
- *Acute myelitis/Transverse myelitis (TM)*: There is a 90% chance of a patient with TM to have MS if there are two or more brain MRI lesions.
- Isolated brainstem syndrome [e.g., vertigo, diplopia, internuclear ophthalmoplegia (INO), trigeminal neuralgia]
- Cerebellar syndromes (e.g., ataxia)

Other common associated symptoms seen in MS are:

- Lhermitte's sign (electric shock-like sensations that run down the back and/or limbs upon flexion of the neck)
- Uhthoff's phenomenon (temporary worsening of neurologic symptom generally when body gets overheated)
- *Pulfrich phenomenon*: Patients with optic neuritis in MS may describe a sensation that oncoming targets or vehicles appear to veer toward them at the last moment. This is due to delayed conduction from the affected eye to the brain.
- *Fatigue*: Most common nonspecific symptom in MS
- Bowel or bladder dysfunction may present as urinary urgency, frequency, nocturia, incontinence, retention, double voiding, and frequent urinary tract infections (UTIs).

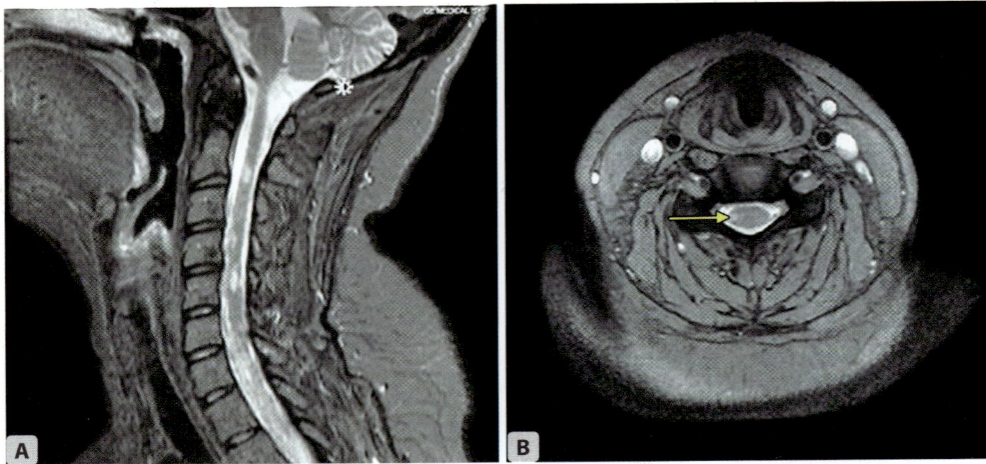

FIGURES 1 A & B: Multiple short-segment cervical spine lesions (skip lesions). An eccentric lateral cord lesion in multiple sclerosis (MS) indicated by the yellow arrow.

Courtesy: Barrow Neurological Institute. (Figs. 2, 3, 5, 8, and 11 also)

- Cognitive impairment and seizures are very rare as presenting symptoms. However, cognitive symptoms can be seen in about 70% of MS patients during the disease course.

Additional common presenting symptoms are highly variable and include focal weakness, numbness, and tight-band sensation around the trunk (MS hug).

IMAGING FINDINGS

Radiologic findings in MS are based on MRI sequences and are based on the concept of dissemination in time and space as stated above. Lesions that are "typical" for MS include typical MS lesions in the following locations:

- Periventricular
- Cortical or juxtacortical (contrast with subcortical lesions)
- Spinal cord (preferentially cervical cord, eccentrically placed, multiple skip lesions may be seen) (**Figs. 1 A** and **B**)
- *Infratentorial*: Brainstem (especially pons) or cerebellar (higher predilection for the middle cerebellar peduncle)
- Optic neuritis [shown as gadolinium enhancement on T1-weighted (T1W) images]

Multiple sclerosis lesions (plaques) usually have an ovoid appearance. Periventricular lesions are characteristically arranged at right angles to the corpus callosum as if radiating from this area; when viewed on sagittal images, they are referred to as "Dawson fingers" (**Figs. 2** and **3**).

Gadolinium-enhanced T1W MR images allow active lesions to be distinguished from inactive lesions, since enhancement occurs as a result of increased blood-brain barrier permeability and corresponds to areas of ongoing inflammation. T2 lesions are also monitored on MRI and expected in MS. Lesions that persistently appear dark on pre- and postcontrast T1W images (lesions also known as "black holes") are associated with more severe tissue damage and in long-standing MS (both demyelination and axonal loss) (**Fig. 4**).

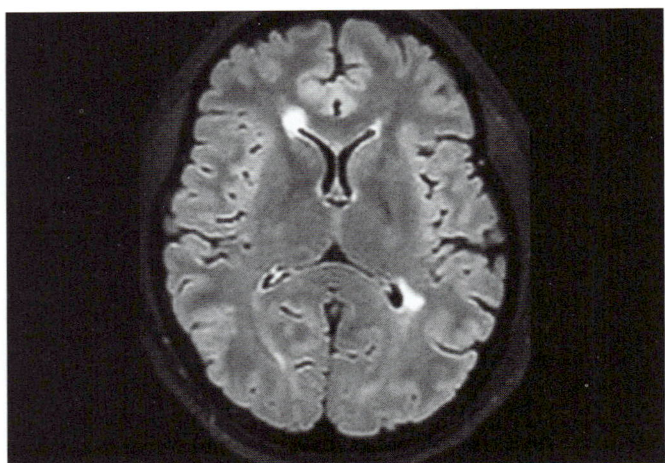

FIGURE 2: Two periventricular lesions typical of multiple sclerosis (MS).

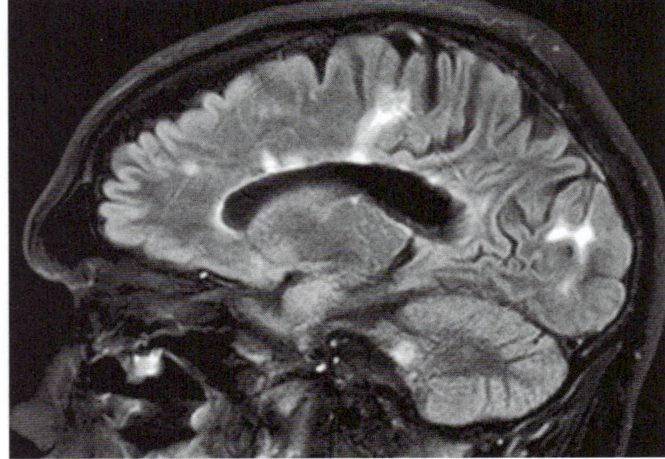

FIGURE 3: "Dawson's Fingers"—lesions are perpendicular to the lateral ventricles.

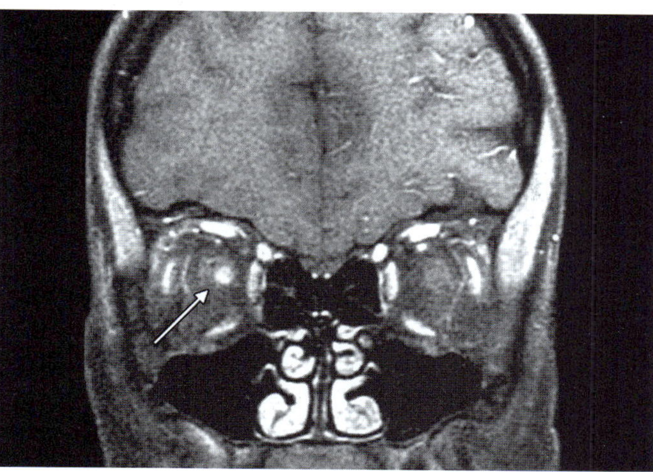

FIGURE 4: Coronal post gadolinium image showing abnormal enhancement of the right optic nerve in a case of optic neuritis.

Source: Ropper AH, Samuels MA, Klein J, Prasad S. Adams and Victor's Principles of Neurology. USA: McGraw-Hill Education; 2014. (Figs. 6 also)

LABORATORY FINDINGS

To date, there are no specific laboratory findings such as a "biomarker" specific for MS; however, some laboratory findings are suggestive.

- *Oligoclonal bands (OCBs)*: They are the most widely used cerebrospinal fluid (CSF) test and included in 2017 McDonald criteria and are a sensitive marker in MS but *not* specific They are seen in up to 90% of cases of adult MS. Gamma-globulin proteins that are produced in the CSF are considered a marker of CNS inflammation.
- *Pleocytosis*: Typically <50 cells/mm^3, rarely up to 100 cells/mm^3. It is seen more with acute exacerbations.
- *CSF gamma globulin (IgG) index*: It is proportion of IgG in reference to total protein in CSF. It is also suggestive of ongoing inflammation but less sensitive than OCBs.
- *Myelin basic protein (MBP)*: It may be elevated in acute attacks more than chronic disease or remission. Suspected MBP reflects destruction of myelin and is nonspecific marker in the CSF that may suggest an inflammatory process in the CNS.
- *CSF protein*: It is increased in 40% of MS patients.

MISCELLANEOUS WORKUP

Optical coherence tomography: Optical coherence tomography (OCT) is an imaging technique that uses low-coherence light to capture images that provide rapid high-resolution reconstruction of retinal anatomy. This detects damage to the afferent visual system (e.g., in optic neuritis) but also is being studied as a marker of neuroaxonal damage in MS and NMOSD. This is evaluated by determining the presence and degree of peripapillary retinal nerve fiber layer (pRNFL) thickness. Atrophy of the ganglion cell-inner plexiform (GCIP) layer can also be measured and is useful.

Visual evoked potentials: Evoked potentials are electrical events that occur in the CNS in response to peripheral stimulation. Visual evoked potentials may be used in MS to detect subclinical disease and is abnormal in 50–90% of clinically definite MS. This detects abnormal myelination along the optic nerve pathway which is common in MS.

DIAGNOSIS

The diagnosis of MS is based on the concept of *dissemination in time and space*. In order to fulfill criteria for MS, both criteria must be fulfilled as described in the 2017 version of the 2010 McDonald criteria (**Table 1**).

Evidence of dissemination in space is defined as detection of lesions in more than one distinct anatomic

TABLE 1 2017 McDonald criteria.

Number of clinical attacks	Number of lesions with objective clinical evidence	Additional data needed for a diagnosis of multiple sclerosis
≥2	≥2	None
≥2	1 (as well as clear-cut historical evidence of a previous attack in a distinct anatomic location)	None
≥2	1	Dissemination in space demonstrated by an additional clinical attack indicating a different CNS site or by MRI
1	≥2	Dissemination in time demonstrated by an additional clinical attack or by MRI or demonstration of CSF-specific oligoclonal bands
1	1	Dissemination in space demonstrated by an additional clinical attack implicating a different CNS site or by MRI; *and* Dissemination in time demonstrated by an additional clinical attack or by MRI or demonstration of CSF-specific oligoclonal bands

location within the CNS. Fulfillment of dissemination in time requires confirmation of new CNS lesions over time, suggesting an ongoing disease process typical of MS rather than a monophasic disease.

PHENOTYPES OF MULTIPLE SCLEROSIS

- **Relapsing remitting MS (RRMS):** It is the most common form (about 80%), and initial presentation is considered clinically isolated syndrome (CIS).
- **Secondary progressive MS (SPMS):** Some patients will develop a progressive form of disease years after being diagnosed with RRMS.
- **Primary progressive MS (PPMS):** Up to 5–10% will present with PPMS.
- **Pediatric MS (before age 18):** Up to 3–5% present with initial symptoms at this age, takes longer to develop disability, however does so at an earlier age.

Less common variants:

- *Tumefactive MS*: It is a rapidly progressive form of MS that may render the patient stuporous, comatose, may evolve over weeks, and may be fatal. Autopsy lesions show large acute plaques of MS and may be large and confluent. The large, confluent appearance may mimic a tumor on imaging, hence the name "tumefactive" (**Fig. 5**).
- *Concentric sclerosis of Balo*: It is considered a variant due to the unusual concentric ring pattern seen on MRI and in tissue specimens that is not seen in typical MS. Sometimes named "concentric sclerosis" due to the concentric (circular) pattern of damaged myelin alternating with areas of relatively undamaged myelin. Some studies show high prevalence in southern Philippines. Patients can present with sudden acute symptoms and rapid deterioration. Axial T2 fluid attenuated inversion recovery (FLAIR) cuts on MRI and shows alternating bands of different signal intensities and resembles a "whirlpool" or "onion ring" appearance (**Fig. 6**).

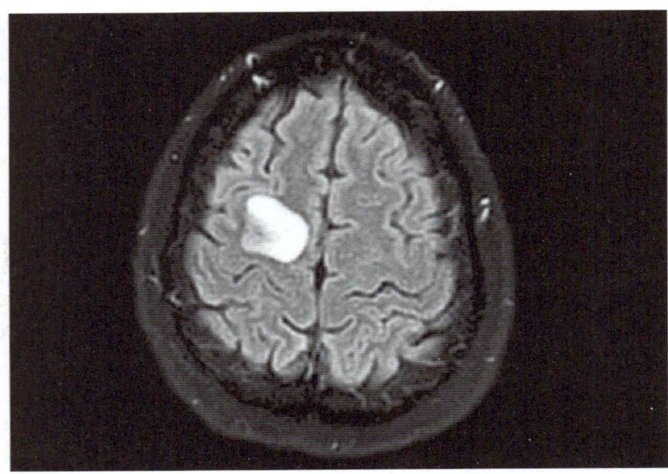

FIGURE 5: Axial T2-FLAIR (fluid-attenuated inversion recovery) image of a tumefactive multiple sclerosis (MS) lesion in the left temporal lobe.

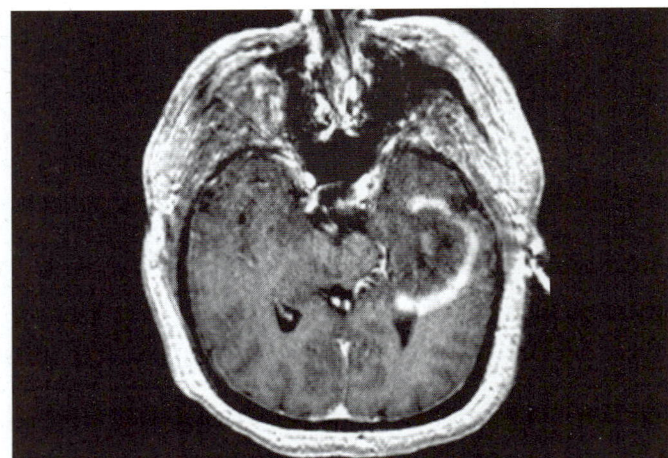

FIGURE 6: "Open ring" of contract enhancement is a common finding of acute demyelinating plaques and is less typical of tumors or abscesses.

DIFFERENTIAL DIAGNOSES

In a sense, MS is a diagnosis of exclusion and so mimics have to be ruled out. Mimics of MS may include but are not limited to:

- *Other idiopathic inflammatory demyelinating conditions of the CNS*: ADEM, and NMOSD.
- *Idiopathic nondemyelinating conditions of the CNS*: Neuro-Behcet's, systemic lupus erythematosus (SLE), Sjögren's syndrome, paraneoplastic neurologic disorders, neurosarcoidosis, and granulomatosis with polyangiitis.
- *Infectious diseases*: Lyme, human T-lymphotropic virus type-1 (HTLV-1) associated myelitis, human immunodeficiency virus (HIV) with associated CNS involvement, progressive multifocal leukoencephalopathy (PML), and neurosyphilis.
- *Metabolic disorders*: Adrenoleukodystrophy (X-linked adrenoleukodystrophy, Addison–Schilder disease), Leber's hereditary optic neuropathy (LHON), subacute combined degeneration

TREATMENT

In general, treatment can be considered in three categories: (1) Prevention of relapses and disability, (2) Treatment of acute relapses, and (3) Treatment of symptoms.

A number of immunomodulatory agents have beneficial effects for patients with RRMS, mainly a decreased relapse rate and a slower accumulation of brain lesions on magnetic resonance imaging (MRI). These disease-modifying therapies (DMTs) for MS can be grouped into: (1) infusion, (2) oral, and (3) injectable drugs (platform therapies). Injectable medications were the earliest treatments available, generally with the least efficacy (and a relatively better safety profile), and now infusions have been developed and in general have the greatest efficacy and are selected for those with more aggressive and active disease (although possibly greater risk of side effects as well). With acute relapses, treatment generally consists of a brief course of corticosteroids, often intravenous methylprednisolone, or often can also consider other oral corticosteroids such as prednisone, dexamethasone, in order to expedite recovery from the acute relapse. With severe relapses, often time plasmapheresis or intravenous immune globulin are also other considerations. *Please refer to* **Table 2** *for more information on each DMT, mechanism of action, efficacy, adverse event profiles etc.*

PROGNOSIS

Prognostication in MS is challenging and somewhat limited; however, those who are considered to have a higher risk of more active disease and risk of greater disability include:

- *Demographic*:
  - Onset of MS after age 30, even though the risk of relapse paradoxically decreases with age
  - Motor or cerebellar onset
  - Male sex
  - Nonwhite race
  - Former or current smoking
  - Comorbid cardiovascular disease
  - Obesity
  - Sedentary lifestyle
- *Clinical*:
  - Poor relapse recovery
  - Frequent early attacks
  - Presence of OCBs in the CSF
- *Radiologic*:
  - High burden of disease by T2 lesion volume on MRI
  - Ongoing disease activity by enhancing or new T2 lesions on MRI
  - Spinal cord lesion(s)
  - Presence of brain atrophy

TABLE 2 Disease modifying therapies for multiple sclerosis.

Infusion therapies	Mechanism of action	Adverse effects
Natalizumab	Monoclonal antibody against alpha-4 (α4) integrin; prevents leukocyte migration into the central nervous system (CNS)	Abdominal pain, infusion reaction, fatigue, development of neutralizing antibodies; Check JC virus antibody prior to initiation given risk of developing progressive multifocal leukoencephalopathy (PML)
Ocrelizumab	Anti-CD20	Infection [upper respiratory infection (URI)], infusion reaction
Alemtuzumab	Anti-CD52	Autoimmune thyroiditis, infections, immune thrombocytopenia (ITP), malignancies
Oral therapies		
Dimethyl fumarate	Involves nuclear factor erythroid-derived 2-related factor (Nrf2) pathways for a neuroprotective effect	Flushing, gastrointestinal disturbances
Teriflunomide	Pyrimidine synthesis inhibitor; inhibits dihydroorotate dehydrogenase	Hair thinning, hepatotoxicity, lymphocytopenia, leukopenia, gastrointestinal disturbances
Fingolimod	Sphingosine 1-phosphate (S1P) modulator	Bradycardia, bronchospasm, macular edema
Siponimod	S1P receptor modulator; binds sphingosine 1-phosphate receptors 1 and 5	Hypertension, headache, transaminitis
Ozanimod	S1P receptor agonist; sequesters lymphocytes in peripheral lymphoid organs	Upper respiratory tract infection, hypertension
Cladribine	Purine analog that is taken up by lymphocytes and interferes with DNA synthesis, thus depletes lymphocytes.	Bone marrow depression, febrile neutropenia, severe anemia, severe neutropenia, thrombocytopenia, infection
Injection therapies		
Interferon beta-1b	Enhancement of suppressor T-cell activity, reduction of proinflammatory cytokines, downregulation of antigen presentation, and reduced trafficking of lymphocytes into the central nervous system	Flu-like symptoms, nausea, transaminitis, injection site reaction
Interferon beta-1a	Enhancement of suppressor T-cell activity, reduction of proinflammatory cytokines, downregulation of antigen presentation, and reduced trafficking of lymphocytes into the central nervous system	Flu-like symptoms, nausea, transaminitis, injection site reaction
Glatiramer acetate	Copolymer of four amino acids; activates T-lymphocyte suppressor cells specific for myelin antigen	Injection site reactions and lipoatrophy
Ofatumumab	Anti-CD20	Skin rash, gastrointestinal disturbances, anemia, neutropenia, infection, fatigue

Of these, the most important factors include: Highly active disease at onset, high lesion burden, presence of infratentorial/spinal cord lesions, and/or poor relapse recovery.

NEUROMYELITIS OPTICA SPECTRUM DISORDERS

INTRODUCTION

Neuromyelitis optica spectrum disorders, previously known as *Devic's disease*, is an inflammatory CNS demyelinating disease that may mimic MS and is associated with optic neuritis, TM, and other neurologic manifestations. Aquaporin-4 (AQP4)-IgG is a serum biomarker that is found in approximately 80% of patients with this syndrome. The remaining 20% may either demonstrate anti-myelin oligodendrocyte antibody or may be seronegative.

EPIDEMIOLOGY

For AQP4-positive patients:
- Prevalence is roughly 0.5–10 per 100,000; much lesser than that of MS.
- Higher prevalence in African and Asian descents
- In regions where MS is less prevalent, NMOSD is more prevalent.
- Five to ten times more prevalent in females than males
- Can occur at any age; median age 32–41 years

PATHOLOGY

Neuromyelitis optica spectrum disorders is considered a predominantly humoral immunity-driven condition, and AQP4-IgG is considered as the pathogenic autoantibody. The site of destruction is the astrocyte, whereas with MS the site is the oligodendrocyte or its myelin extensions in MS. AQP4 levels correlate with clinical activity and may respond to immunotherapy.

Aquaporin-4-IgG causes astrocytic injury through antibody-dependent cell-mediated cytotoxicity and activation of the complement pathway. This then attracts an inflammatory cascade including T and B cells, macrophages, neutrophils, and eosinophils.

SIGNS AND SYMPTOMS

Six core clinical manifestations:
1. Optic neuritis (often severe, may be bilateral)
2. Acute myelitis
   a. Typically longitudinally extensive (three vertebral segments or more)
3. Area-postrema syndrome (episodes of intractable nausea or vomiting or hiccups)
4. Acute brainstem syndrome
5. Symptomatic narcolepsy or acute diencephalic clinical syndrome with typical diencephalic MRI lesions
6. Symptomatic cerebral syndrome with NMOSD-typical brain lesions

Other clinical features:
- Syndrome of inappropriate secretion of antidiuretic hormone (SIADH)
- Encephalopathy (ADEM or PRES-like)
- Hydrocephalus

Aquaporin-4-positive NMOSD is a highly relapsing condition, not commonly associated with a progressive course. Generally, relapses and clinical course are more disabling and severe than MS. Other autoimmune diseases commonly coexist with NMOSD, in particular SLE , Sjögren's, myasthenia gravis, and anti-phospholipid antibody syndrome.

Features of MOG-antibody-positive NMOSD (compared with AQP4):
- Optic nerve involved more commonly than the spinal cord
- More common to have simultaneous optic neuritis
- More likely to be monophasic
- Less commonly associated with other autoimmune conditions
- More infratentorial lesions and fewer supratentorial lesions
- Spinal cord lesions may be in the lower portion and may involve the conus.
- May have wider spectrum of disease and include ADEM and more common in children
- 1:1 female-to-male ratio

IMAGING

Lesions on MRI commonly include:
- *Optic nerve enhancement* may involve more than half of the length of the nerve, may be posterior and may involve the chiasm.
- Brain lesion typically surrounding regions where AQP4 expression is the highest: Adjacent to the 3rd and 4th ventricles (dorsal medulla/area postrema); often nonspecific white matter lesions (**Figs. 7 A** to **F**).
- Spinal cord lesions longitudinally extensive (3 or more vertebral segments) 85% of the time, short segment 15% of the time, on axial shows central lesion and ring or variable enhancement. T1 hypointensities and focal cord atrophy may also be seen in chronic cases (**Figs. 8 A** to **C**).

LABORATORY FINDINGS

White cell count in CSF may be elevated (up to 50 cells) and is usually of lymphocytic predominance; although in contrast with MS, neutrophils and eosinophils may also be seen. OCBs may be seen in <30% of patients.

DIAGNOSIS

The 2015 diagnostic criteria is based AQP4 status, the presence of core clinical characteristics, and MRI abnormalities.

Diagnostic criteria of patients with AQP4-IgG antibodies only require at least one core clinical characteristic. Those

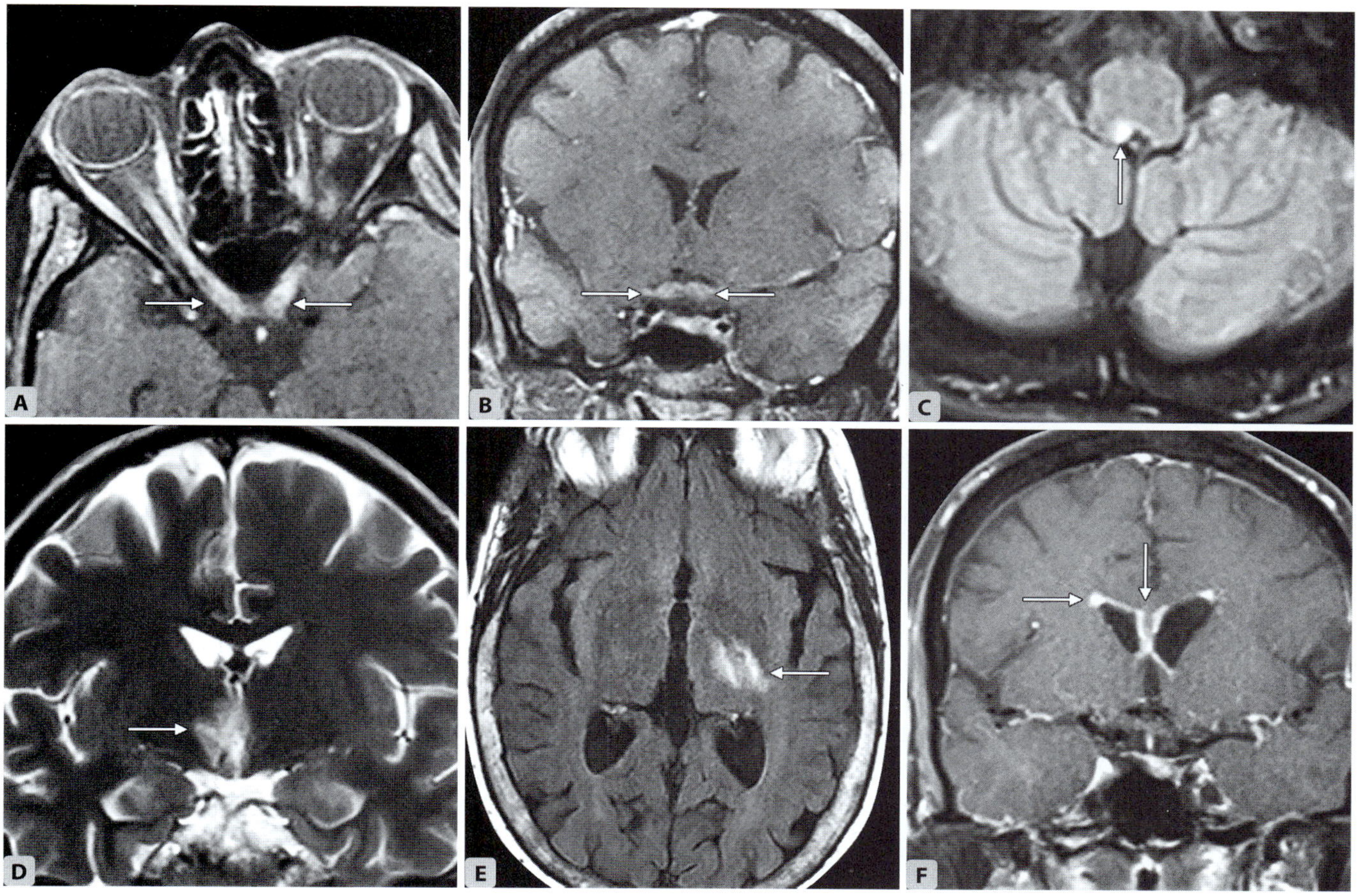

(AQP4: aquaporin-4; NMOSD: neuromyelitis optica spectrum disorders)

FIGURES 7 A to F: AQP4-positive NMOSD MRI findings: (A) and **(B)** show bilateral posterior optic nerve enhancement extending to the optic chiasm; **(C)** shows a lesion in the region of the area postrema; **(D)** shows a characteristic lesion adjacent to the third ventricle; **(E)** shows a left internal capsule NMOSD lesion; and **(F)** shows pencil-thin linear ependymal enhancement.

Source: Flanagan, E. Neuromyelitis Optica Spectrum Disorder and Other Non-Multiple Sclerosis Central Nervous System Inflammatory Diseases. Continuum Lifelong Learning in Neurology. (2019).

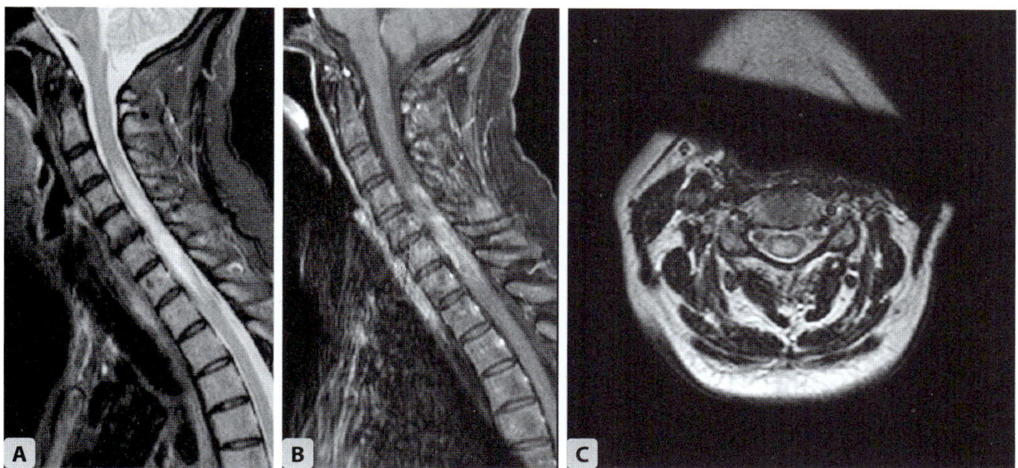

(Gd: Gadolinium)

FIGURES 8 A to C: Spinal cord MRI reveals longitudinally extensive transverse myelitis (LETM). (A) C3 to T1 lesion consistent with LETM; **(B)** Inhomogeneous patchy Gd-contrast enhancement indicating acute inflammatory changes; **(C)** central cord lesion on axial section.

without known AQP4-IgG antibodies require two or more core characteristics that must include either optic neuritis, longitudinally extensive transverse myelitis (LTEM), or area-postrema syndrome.

TREATMENT

Treatment of acute attacks and chronic treatment should be recommended in all patients given the relapsing nature of this condition.

Acute attacks: Pulse steroid therapy with or without subsequent plasma exchange is the main first-line therapy. The role of intravenous immunoglobulin (IVIG) is unclear in this setting.

Disease-modifying therapies for MS such as interferon beta, natalizumab, and fingolimod may have harmful effect on relapse rate in NMOSD and so accurate diagnosis is crucial.

For preventative treatment, there are three Food and Drug Administration (FDA)-approved treatments:

- Eculizumab (monoclonal antibody against the complement protein C5)
- Inebilizumab (anti-C19 monoclonal antibody)
- Satralizumab (anti-interleukin-6)

Other commonly used treatments include:

- Rituximab (anti CD-20 monoclonal antibody)
- Tocilizumab (anti-interleukin-6)
- Azathioprine
- Mycophenolate mofetil

PROGNOSIS

The natural history of NMOSD is that of a step-wise deterioration of visual, motor, sensory, and bladder deficits from recurrent attacks. Mortality is high with NMOSD and can be attributed to respiratory failure, which is caused by high cervical or brainstem lesions. Mortality rates among various studies range from 25 to 50%.

MYELIN OLIGODENDROCYTE GLYCOPROTEIN ANTIBODY DISORDER

Myelin oligodendrocyte glycoprotein (MOG) antibody disorder is a recently described distinct clinical syndrome characterized by the presence of autoantibodies to a glycoprotein (MOG) expressed on oligodendrocytes resulting in CNS demyelination and a NMOSD or ADEM-like clinical picture. MOG antibody disorder occurs in both children and adults, despite being more common in children. It may be monophasic or relapsing.

Common clinical presentations:

- Bilateral simultaneous or sequential optic neuritis (**Figs. 9 A** to **D**):
    - Commonly anterior involvement of the ON (contrast with AQP4 NMOSD where posterior ON and chiasmal involvement is more common)
    - Papillitis is more common when compared to ON in MS (retrobulbar involvement being common in MS).
    - Poor visual acuity at nadir with rapid and almost complete recovery
    - Commonly longitudinal lesions of the ON (common to both MOG and AQP4-NMOSD). The demographic, clinical, laboratory and radiological differential features of inflammatory demyelinating disorders MOG antibody disease, NMOSD and multiple sclerosis are given in **Table 3**.

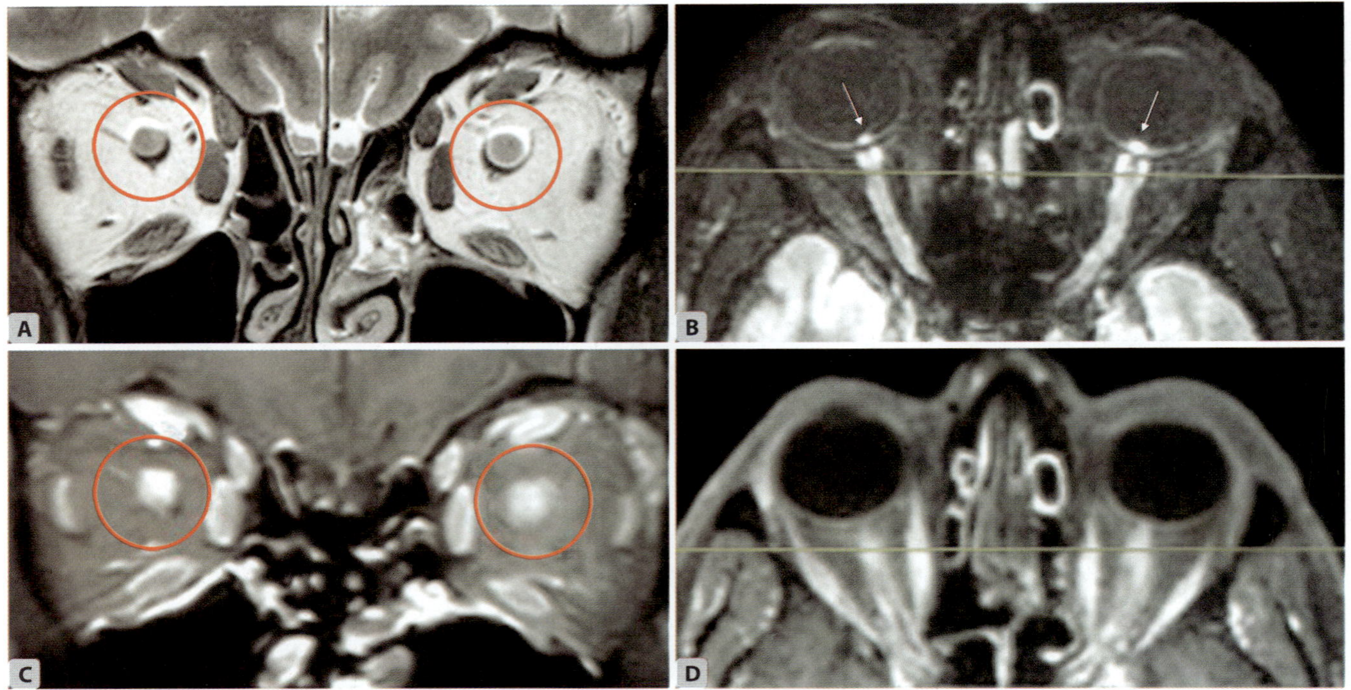

FIGURES 9 A to D: Bilateral longitudinally extensive optic neuritis in myelin-oligodendrocyte associated disorders (MOGAD).

Courtesy: Deneve M. MRI features of demyelinating disease associated with anti-MOG antibodies in adults. Journal of Neuroradiology (2019).

TABLE 3 **Demographic, clinical, laboratory and radiological differential features of inflammatory demyelinating disorders.**

	MOG antibody disease	NMOSD	Multiple sclerosis
Age of onset	Both children and adults, broad age of onset	More common in adults, mean age at onset 39 year old	Mostly young adults
Sex	No sex predominance	Predominantly females (9:1)	More common in females (3:1)
Ethnicity	No ethnic bias	Over-represented in Asian and Afro-Caribbean races	Predominantly Caucasian
Onset presentation	• 50% unilateral or bilateral ON • 20% ADEM or brainstem attacks • 20% LETM • 10% simultaneous ON and TM	• Unilateral ON • LETM • Area postrema syndrome	• Unilateral ON • Brainstem/cerebellar symptoms • Myelitis, often mild sensory
Disease course	Monophasic or relapsing, no disease progression	Relapsing, no disease progression	Relapsing and secondary progressive or primary progressive
Brain MRI	• Can have normal brain MRI (lesions were associated with ADEM or brainstem attacks) • Typical ADEM features: Poorly demarcated white and gray matter lesions often involving the thalamus and basal ganglia • Poorly demarcated brainstem lesions, often located in the pons or cerebellar peduncles, adjacent to the ventricular system • Less common selective edematous cortical lesions, typically unilateral	• Can have normal brain MRI (lesions were associated with brainstem/diencephalic/ cerebral attacks) • Brainstem and diencephalic lesions surrounding the ventricular system, including area postrema lesions • Other characteristic features include long 'pencil thin' callosal lesions, long corticospinal tract lesions	• Well-demarcated ovoid or finger-like lesions perpendicular to the lateral ventricles • Curved juxtacortical lesions • Inferior temporal lobe lesions • Small cortical lesions. • Frequent T1 lesions (black holes)
Optic nerve MRI	• Extensive (≥0.5 length) lesions involving the anterior segments • Optic chiasm usually spared • Commonly bilateral • Perioptic gadolinium enhancement	• Extensive lesions involving the posterior segments and optic chiasm • Might be bilateral	Short unilateral optic nerve lesions
New lesions on follow-up brain MRI	Rare	Rare	Accumulation of silent T2 lesions over time, new gad-enhancing lesions
Spinal cord MRI	• Usually long (at least three segments), edematous and central lesions • Short lesions in up to 25% • Conus lesions common	Usually long, edematous and central lesions, short lesions can occur	Short-segment (one or two segments), asymmetrical on axial views
CSF	• 50% elevated cells • OCB in a minority	• Elevated cells with possible neutrophils/eosinophils • OCB in a minority	• Cells typically low, unmatched • OCB present in a majority

(ADEM: acute demyelinating encephalomyelitis; AQP4: aquaporin-4; LETM: longitudinally extensive transverse myelitis; NMOSD: neuromyelitis optica spectrum disorders; OCB: oligoclonal bands)

Courtesy: Juryncztk, M, et al. Myelin oligodendrocyte glycoprotein (MOG) antibody-associated disease: practical considerations. BMJ Journals. 2019.

- Inflammatory myelopathy:
  - Commonly LETM like in AQP4-NMOSD but short segment myelitis is also reported.
  - Conus involvement and resultant sphincter dysfunction is more common on MOGAD.
  - MRI sagittal cuts show lesion extending at least three vertebral segments or more. Axial cuts show a centrally based lesion with swelling and contrast enhancement in the acute phase.

- ADEM-like presentation:
  - MOG antibodies are seen in about 50% of children with an initial ADEM-like presentation and almost in all children with multiphasic ADEM.
  - MRI shows large poorly demarcated bilateral white matter lesions, may be symmetric and unlike the classic ovoid periventricular lesions in MS.
  - A greater predilection for deep gray matter is seen.
  - Isolated brainstem attacks with fluffy T2 MRI lesions can be seen and may be indistinguishable from AQP4 NMOSD.

Clinical course: About 50% of patients relapse in the first 2–3 years and most relapses occur in the early months following the initial attack.

Diagnostic testing: The gold standard for testing is the detection of antibodies in the serum to MOG using a cell-based assay (CBA).

Management: Steroid pulse therapy followed by plasma exchange (PLEX) or IVIG are first-line therapies. A slow steroid taper is recommended after the initial pulse therapy with steroids. Long-term immunosuppression is recommended in relapsing disease. Azathioprine, mycophenolate, rituximab, and IVIG are some common steroid-sparing agents used for long-term immunosuppression.

TRANSVERSE MYELITIS

The term "myelopathy" refers to spinal cord dysfunction of any cause resulting in motor weakness, sensory changes, and autonomic (i.e., bowel and bladder) dysfunction to varying extents. TM is a subcategory of myelopathies that refers to an acquired inflammatory disorder of the spinal cord (myelitis) resulting in acute-to-subacute onset of motor, sensory, and autonomic impairment to varying extents below the affected level.

ACUTE DISSEMINATE ENCEPHALOMYELITIS (ADEM)

Acute disseminate encephalomyelitis is an inflammatory demyelinating disease of the CNS that is characterized by multifocal neurological symptoms and disturbance of cortical function (in the form of encephalopathy, seizures, or behavioral changes). This condition is strikingly more common in children and typically monophasic.

Epidemiology: The incidence worldwide is thought to be 0.07–0.64 per 100,000 in children and is much rarer in adults. A slight male preponderance is reported (M:F = 1.3:1). A majority of cases (up to 80%) occur <10 years of age. This condition is associated with a 2% mortality rate and about a third of patients are left with residual neurological deficits.

Clinical presentation: A striking feature of ADEM is an acute disturbance in cortical function which may manifest as acute alteration in the level of consciousness (mild drowsiness to a comatose state) or behavioral changes such as irritability or sometimes even frank seizures. This should be unexplained by fever, systemic illness, or postictal symptoms. The clinical course is typically rapidly progressive and hits nadir in 4–5 days. In addition to this, patients develop a polyfocal demyelination syndrome characterized by optic neuritis, other cranial nerve abnormalities, long tract signs, focal extremity weakness or sensory changes, gait and balance difficulties, incoordination, bowel and bladder dysfunction. An inflammatory myelopathy (secondary TM) can also be a part of the ADEM clinical picture (**Fig. 10**).

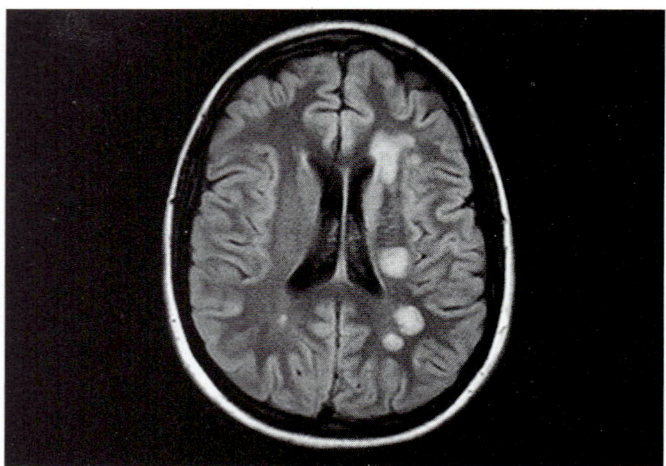

FIGURE 10: Fluffy asymmetric lesions seen in acute disseminated encephalomyelitis (ADEM) with involvement of deep gray matter.
Courtesy: Assoc Prof Frank Gaillard, Radiopaedia.org, rID: 39817.

Variants of ADEM: Acute necrotizing hemorrhagic leukoencephalitis of Weston Hurst is a hemorrhagic form of ADEM associated with a more rapidly progressive and severe clinical course than typical ADEM. Brain MRI reveals multifocal hemorrhages (typically microhemorrhages) seen on Susceptibility weighted Imaging (SWI)/Gradient Echo sequencing (GRE) and CSF may show both red and white cells. The prognosis is generally worse than typical ADEM. An association with RANBP2 mutation is reported in some acute hemorrhagic encephalomyelitis cases.

Management: In addition to obtaining MRI and CSF studies (MBP levels are elevated in most patients), a MOG antibody test is also recommended in all patients with an ADEM-like presentation and especially if there is coexisting optic neuritis, brain stem, or spinal cord lesions. Treatment consists of pulse steroid therapy during the acute phase as first-line therapy and IVIG, PLEX, cyclophosphamide, and cyclosporine as second-line therapies in refractory cases. Improvement is typically seen in hours to a few days of starting therapy.

NEUROSARCOIDOSIS

Sarcoidosis is a multisystem inflammatory disease characterized by the histological presence of inflammatory lesions called granuloma (non-caseating) on biopsy of affected tissues. Neurological complications of sarcoidosis

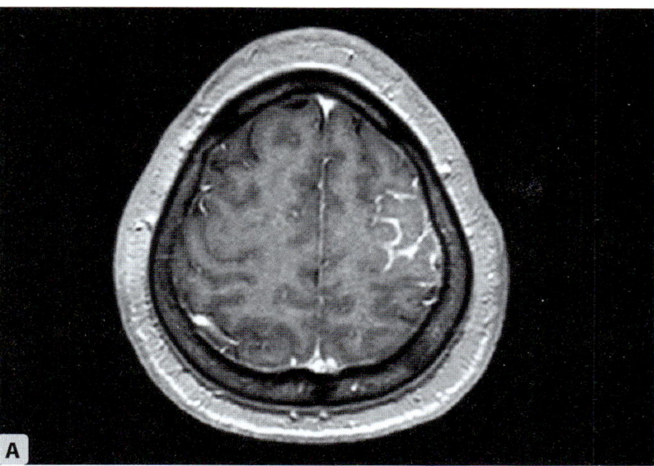

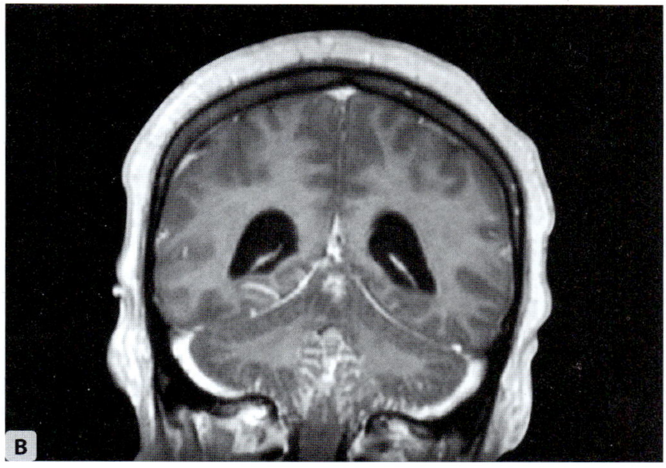

FIGURES 11 A & B: **Leptomeningeal enhancement and basal meningitis seen in neurosarcoidosis.**

(neurosarcoidosis) occur in 5–10% of all patients with this condition. About 50% of patients with neurosarcoidosis present with neurological symptoms at the time sarcoidosis is first diagnosed. Neurosarcoidosis has the potential to affect both the central and the peripheral nervous systems.

Clinical features: The condition typically presents in the age range of 30–40 years. The onset can be acute, subacute, or chronic. Clinical presentation is very heterogeneous are can be broadly classified as:

- *Constitutional symptoms*: These most commonly accompany other neurological symptoms. Headache, fatigue, and nausea are very common.
- *Cranial mononeuropathy*: Although any cranial nerve can be affected, facial nerve involvement is the most common. Both unilateral and bilateral involvements can occur. Heerfordt syndrome is a rare syndrome complex characterized by fever, uveitis, parotitis and facial nerve palsy that may occur due to sarcoid involvement of facial nerve. Other cranial nerve-related symptomatology in neurosarcoidosis are anosmia, dysgeusia, visual impairment (due to granulomatous inflammation of the optic nerves), dysarthria, dysphagia, dysphonia, vertigo and sensorineural hearing impairment, and tongue deviation/atrophy.
- *Hypothalamic and pituitary involvement*: This may lead to disturbances in thirst, sleep, appetite, temperature, and libido.
- *Brain and spinal cord involvement*: Nonspecific white matter changes, focal cerebral infarction from vasculopathy, and LTEM with a trident sign sometimes can be seen in parenchymal brain and cord involvement. Cord involvement may manifest with patchy contrast enhancement with a dural base on MRI. Chronic meningeal involvement is seen in up to 40% of patients with neurosarcoidosis and CSF may show lymphocytic pleocytosis with hypoglycorrhachia. MRI with gadolinium contrast can help demonstrate leptomeningeal or pachymeningeal involvement (**Figs. 11 A** and **B**).
- *Peripheral neuropathy*: Radiculopathy (especially cauda equine involvement), mononeuropathy, mononeuritis multiplex, sensorimotor axonal polyneuropathy, and small fiber neuropathy are common peripheral nervous system manifestations.
- *Myopathy*: Acute or chronic proximal myopathy, muscle atrophy and palpable nodules in muscles.

Diagnosis is based on Zajicek criteria. The presence of consistent neurological symptoms PLUS:

- Positive histology from the nervous system—DEFINITIVE NEUROSARCOIDOSIS
- Systemic evidence (biopsy proven from extraneural sites) or positive Kveim test or a positive PET/Gallium scan, CT chest with hilar lymphadenopathy or elevated CSF or Serum angiotensin convertase enzyme levels—PROBABLE NEUROSARCOIDOSIS
- Exclusion of other causes—POSSIBLE NEUROSARCOIDOSIS.

Workup: Besides conventional MRI imaging, PET/CT or Gallium scan may be helpful in identifying hypermetabolic sites to target biopsy. Combing fluorothymidine F-18 (FLT)-PET with fluorodeoxyglucose (FDG)-PET may increase specificity to identify hot spots of neurosarcoidosis. The most sensitive test is the Kveim test but is not performed commonly due to unavailability of the antigen.

Differentials: Tuberculosis is a very close differential and has to be ruled out prior to starting empiric immunosuppression with steroids if the diagnosis of neurosarcoidosis is not confirmed on biopsy.

Management: Spontaneous resolution may occur in some patients. Steroid therapy is the main line of therapy. Chronic steroid therapy may alone induce remission with prompt resolution of symptoms in up to 50% of cases. Mycophenolate, methotrexate, cyclosporine, thalidomide, and cyclophosphamide may be considered in steroid refractory cases. Infliximab and adalimumab are emerging as very effective options to treat neurosarcoidosis which is refractory to steroids. Cranial or spinal external beam radiotherapy (XRT) can be considered in cases refractory to first- and second-line therapies and in life-threatening circumstances.

TABLE 4 Selected inherited leukodystrophies.

Disorder	Genetics	Clinical features	Other
Alexander disease	AD; *GFAP* gene	Macrocephaly, developmental delay, seizures	MRI: Leukoencephalopathy; Pathology: Rosenthal fibers
Krabbe disease	AR; Galactocerebrosidase deficiency	Poor feeding, developmental arrest, poor head control, opisthotonic posturing, myoclonus regression, visual loss, seizures	MRI: Diffuse leukoencephalopathy
Metachromatic leukodystrophy	AR; arylsulfatase A deficiency	Weakness, hypotonia, loss of reflexes, cognitive and motor regression, optic atrophy, seizures	MRI: T2 hyperintensities in periventricular white matter sparing U fibers; Pathology: Metachromatic granules
Pelizaeus–Merzbacher disease	X-linked proteolipid protein (deficiency)	Rotary eye movements, hypotonia, involuntary movements, spasticity	MRI: Severe reduction or absence of central myelin EMG: Peripheral neuropathy
X-linked adrenoleukodystrophy	X-linked *ABCD1* gene; peroxisomal disorder	Behavioral change, neurologic dysfunction, visual loss, adrenal insufficiency, spastic paraparesis	MRI: Symmetric parieto-occipital white matter changes; may involve splenium of the corpus callosum

INHERITED DEMYELINATING SYNDROMES

Inherited disorders that affect the white matter are commonly grouped under conditions, namely leukodystrophies (**Table 4**). These are caused by diseases that affect the glial cells which results in myelin sheath and axonal damage. There are approximately 30 identified named leukodystrophies. A leukodystrophy should be suspected in a child with regression in developmental milestones and MRI is key in clarifying the diagnosis and typically show symmetric T2 hyperintensities in the white matter. Treatment is generally supportive, but treatment of seizures, spasticity, dystonia, and autonomic dysfunction is important. Genetic leukoencephalopathies are separate disorders that include metabolic disorders, primarily neuronal diseases, that affect white matter but via mechanisms other than glial pathology.

OSMOTIC DEMYELINATION SYNDROME

Osmotic demyelination syndrome (ODS) is most commonly seen to affect the central pons, and is often termed central pontine myelinolysis (CPM). CPM is a concentrated, frequently symmetric noninflammatory demyelinating condition of the central basis pontis. It is not uncommon to have concurrent demyelination outside of the pons such as in the midbrain, thalamus, basal ganglia, and cerebellum. Prolonged hyponatremia, with the vast majority having an initial serum sodium level <120 mEq/L or less, followed by rapid correction results in edema and ultimately can lead to ODS. This is not expected to occur with correction of acute hyponatremia given that there is no time for the brain to create adaptive mechanisms against brain swelling and osmotic shifts within astrocytes. It is recommended that the serum sodium should be corrected no >10 mEq/L in a 24-hour period to prevent CPM.

A patient typically presents with symptoms after 2–6 days after sodium correction and may experience dysarthria, dysphagia, paraparesis or quadriparesis, lethargy or coma, and severely affected patients may become "locked in." This means that the patient is awake, but unable to move or verbally communicate, and can usually move their eyes (primarily spared vertical eye movements) and blink but consciousness is preserved due to sparing of the reticular formation. Aggressive treatment must be pursued for minimum of 6–8 weeks given that recovery from severe deficits can occur. Deficits should not be considered irreversible before this time period.

Magnetic resonance imaging should be obtained in any case that is suspected whenever possible. However, an MRI may not show these changes for up to 4 weeks, so the possibility of CPM should not be ruled out in the acute setting (**Figs. 12 A** and **B**).

NUTRITIONAL-RELATED DEMYELINATION

Vitamin B1 insufficiency seen in Wernicke–Korsakoff syndrome complex may result in demyelination, gliosis, and relative preservation of neurons. This typically involves the mammillary bodies, the region surrounding the aqueduct and third ventricle, medial thalamus, dorsal medulla, and tectal plate. Chronic B12 deficiency can lead to demyelination of the dorsal (posterior) column and the lateral (corticospinal) columns that leads to progressive, usually symmetric sensory ataxia, paresthesias and pyramidal weakness. This syndrome is called SCD of the spinal cord. Copper deficiency can cause a syndrome similar to SCD caused by B12 deficiency. This may be caused by excessive zinc ingestion which may impair copper absorption (e.g., overuse of denture cream), gastrointestinal surgery, or other causes of acquired zinc deficiency.

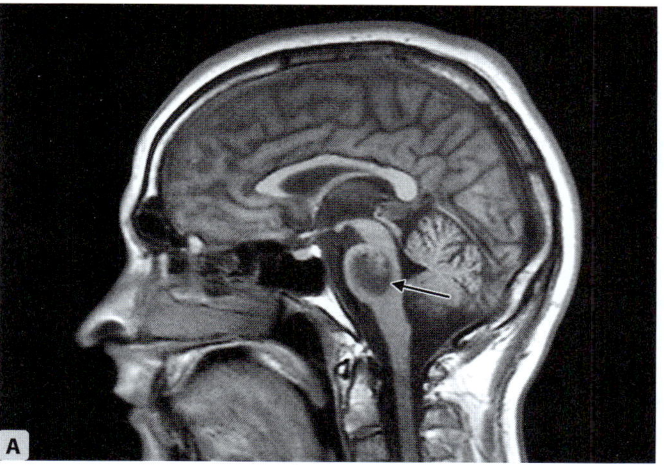

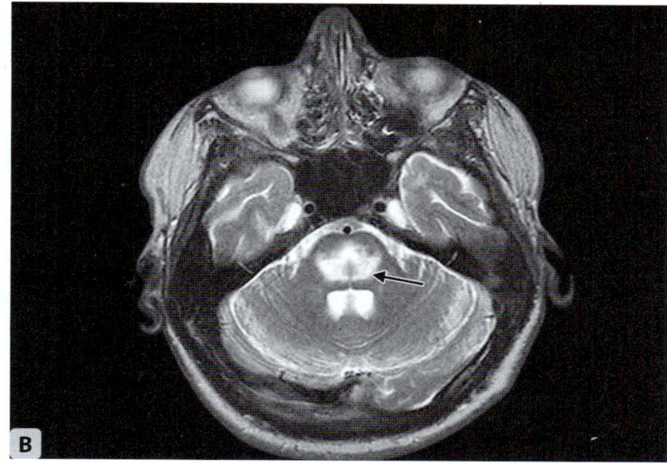

FIGURES 12 A & B: Right: Sagittal T1 hypointensity in the pons; Left: Axial T2 hyperintensity seen throughout the central pons in a **patient with ODS**.

Source: *Fleming* JD, *Babu* S. Central pontine myelinolysis. NEJM. 2008;359:e29.

OTHER UNCOMMON DISORDERS

Some other uncommon demyelinating diseases of the central nervous system are autoimmune glial fibrillary acidic protein myelopathy, chronic lymphocytic inflammation with pontine perivascular enhancement responsive to steroids (CLIPPERS), IGG4-related disease and SUSAC syndrome.

RECOMMENDED READINGS

1. Lewis SL. Multiple Sclerosis and Other CNS Inflammatory Diseases. Continuum: Lifelong Learning in Neurology. 2019;25(3):594-5.
2. Olek MJ., Narayan RN, Frohman EM, Frohman TC. (2016). Clinical features of multiple sclerosis in adults. [online] Available from http://www.uptodate.com/contents/clinical-features-of-multiple-sclerosis-in-adults?source=search_result&search=multiple+sclerosis&s electedTitle=3~150.
3. Ropper AH, Samuels MA, Klein J, Prasad S. Multiple sclerosis and other inflammatory demyelinating diseases. Adams and Victor's Principles of Neurology, 11th edition. USA: McGraw-Hill Education; 2019.
4. Yamout BI, Alroughani R. Multiple sclerosis. Seminars in Neurology. 2018;38(02):212-25.
5. Johnson RT, Griffin J, McArthur J. Neurosarcoidosis. In: Pardo-Villamizar CA (ed). Current Therapy in Neurologic Disease, 7th edition. USA: Mosby; 2006.
6. Narula S, Banwell B. Pediatric Demyelination. Continuum (Minneap Minn). 2016;22(3):897-915.
7. Cho TA, Bhattacharyya S. Approach to Myelopathy. Continuum (Minneap Minn). 2018;24(2, Spinal Cord Disorders):386-406.
8. Narayan R, Simpson A, Fritsche K, Salama S, Pardo S, Mealy M, et al. MOG antibody disease: A review of MOG antibody seropositive neuromyelitis optica spectrum disorder. Mult Scler Relat Disord. 2018;25:66-72.
9. Malli C, Pandit L, D'Cunha A, Mustafa S. Environmental factors related to multiple sclerosis in Indian population. PLoS One. 2015;10(4):e0124064.
10. Pandit L. Insights into the changing perspectives of multiple sclerosis in India. Autoimmune Dis. 2011;2011:937586.
11. Rawal S, Machnowska M, Pauranik A. Case of the week. AJNR. 2021;42(2).
12. Ömerhoca S, Akkaş SY, İçen NK. Multiple sclerosis: diagnosis and differential diagnosis. Noro Psikiyatr Ars. 2018;55(Suppl 1):S1-9.
13. Lewis SL. Neuroinfectious Disease in Isolation. Continuum: Lifelong Learning in Neurology. 2018; 24(5): 1262-3.

CHAPTER
193
Movement Disorders: The Clinical Vignette

Birinder Singh Paul, Gunchan Paul

ABSTRACT

Movement disorders are commonly encountered in the outpatient department. In this chapter, we aim to provide a practical and stepwise approach to help the residents and physicians in recognizing phenomenology of clinical syndromes. The clinical vignettes described in this chapter lead to correct classification of the movement disorders as the first step. By pattern recognition, movement disorders can be classified as akinetic-rigid syndrome or hyperkinetic (myoclonus, dystonia, chorea, and tics) disorders. Defining of the clinical syndrome in this manner results in generation of list of differential diagnosis and hence, helps to plan investigations. The diagnostic process for the most common types of movement disorders namely Parkinson's disease (PD), myoclonus, chorea, dystonia, tics, and tremors is highlighted in this chapter.

"Understanding a question is half the answer"

—Socrates

CLINICAL PRESENTATION

Clinical presentations of movement disorders are complex and have variable phenotypes with limited availability of specific biological markers that can definitely diagnose the underlying disease. Establishing the correct diagnosis in movement disorders forms the basis for subsequent diagnostic workup and management. Diagnosis of movement disorders can be greatly simplified by using a stepwise clinical approach.

First step in the diagnosis for any type of movement disorder is the recognition of the pattern of movement and establishing its clinical phenomenology. Next step involves the translation of the recognized phenomenology into specific type of movement disorder syndrome. Once this is done, generating the etiological and differential diagnosis with subsequent planning of the relevant investigations is the last step (**Fig. 1**).

RECOGNIZING THE MOVEMENT DISORDERS

There are two main categories of movement disorders, which are fairly easy to distinguish. The first phenomenology is akinetic-rigid syndromes, which correspond to slowness or poverty of movements and the second are hyperkinetic disorders (**Table 1**). The second group is heterogeneous and difficult to diagnose correctly because of overlapping characteristics. For simplification, the second group is further categorized into two main subdivisions as depicted in the **Flowchart 1**.

The next important step for diagnosis of movement disorders is recognizing the type of movement that is present in the patient. This chapter highlights the salient and individualized features of different types of hypokinetic and hyperkinetic movement disorder with which a physician must be familiar for the ease of recognition and diagnosis.

HYPOKINETIC DISORDERS (AKINETIC-RIGID DISORDERS)

The absolute criteria for diagnosing this group of movement disorder are the presence of bradykinesia or hypokinesia. The classic example is Parkinsons disease (PD), though under the umbrella of hypokinetic disorders, multiple system atrophy (MSA), progressive supranuclear palsy (PSP), dementia with Lewy body (DLB), corticobasal degeneration (CBD), and vascular parkinsonism are also included.

Bradykinesia is fundamentally progressive and fatiguing with decrement of repetitive alternative movements, in both

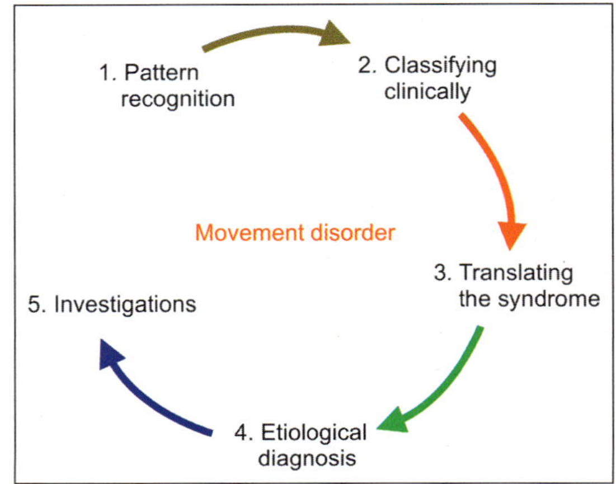

FIGURE 1: Stepwise approach to movement disorders.

TABLE 1 Types of movement disorders.

Category	Type of movement disorder	Phenomenology
Hypokinetic movements	Bradykinesia, akinesia or hypokinesia syndrome	There is progressive fatigue and decrement of repetitive alternative movements
Hyperkinetic movements		**Jerky**
	Myoclonus	Sudden brief shock like positive or negative movements
	Chorea	Randomly flowing jerky nonrhythmic movements
	Tics	Stereotype jerky movements preceded by urge which is relieved by doing movements
		Nonjerky
	Dystonia	Rapid sustained patterned twisting and repetitive movements of the limbs
	Tremors	Rhythmic oscillatory alternating movements of one or more body parts occurring at regular intervals

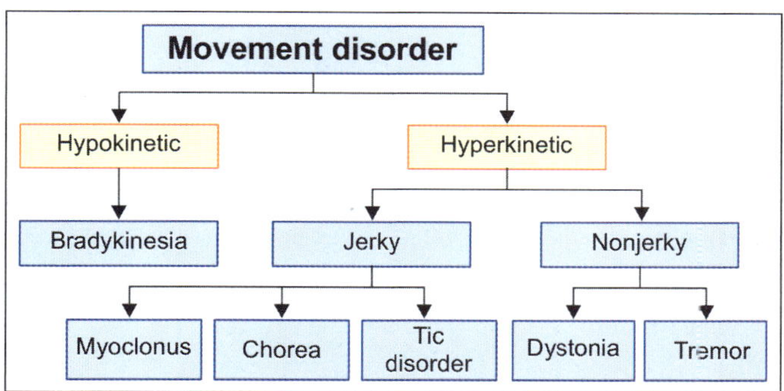

Note: Few disorder feature a combination of both categories.

FLOWCHART 1: Main categories of movement disorders.

speed and amplitude. In **Video 1**, it is noticed that when the patient is asked to make large regular repetitive alternative movements (finger and foot taps) there is reduction in amplitude and velocity on the right side as compared to left side in performing the alternative tasks. Clinician must also look for additional components of akinesia like absence or poverty of automatic movements, especially hypomania with reduced blinking or associated arm swings during walking.

Parkinson's disease being the prototype of hypokinetic-rigid disorders. Movement Disorder Society has laid down the diagnostic criteria that are widely used for the differentiating PD from secondary parkinsonism. Among the core criteria, bradykinesia is the mandatory feature for diagnosis of PD along with anyone of the following three features: (1) cogwheel rigidity, (2) rest tremors (3–5 Hz), and (3) postural instability. In addition to this, the diagnosis is reinforced by presence of one or more supportive criteria and absence of red flags and exclusions in patients having hypokinetic-rigid syndrome (**Fig. 2**).

- Lastly, clinician must know and recognize that slowness of movement without fatiguing and decrement is also seen in other disorders (**Box 1**).

HYPERKINETIC MOVEMENT DISORDERS WITH JERKY CHARACTER

Myoclonus: Myoclonus is defined as sudden, brief shock-like involuntary movements caused by muscular contraction or inhibition (negative myoclonus), seen in association with a wide variety of conditions and diseases.

The major categories of myoclonus are physiological, essential, epileptic, and symptomatic. Physiological

BOX 1 Mimics of akinetic disorders.

- Depression
- Hypothyroidism
- Spasticity
- Catatonia
- Slowing due to aging
- Frozen shoulder

Absolute exclusions

- Cerebellar signs
- Supranuclear palsy
- Cortical sensory loss
- Absence of response to levodopa
- Parkinsonism restricted to lower limbs only for >3 years
- Treatment with antidopaminergic agents

Red Flags

- Rapid deterioration of gait
- Absence of progressive motor symptoms over 5 years
- Early bulbar dysfunction
- Respiratory dysfunction
- Early autonomic failure
- Early recurrent falls
- Pyramidal tract signs
- Absence of nonmotor symptoms

Supportive criteria

- Clear and dramatic positive response to dopaminergic therapy
- Levodopa-induced dyskinesia

FIGURE 2: Movement Disorder Society clinical diagnostic criteria for Parkinson's disease.

myoclonus occurs in persons with normal neurological examination and no associated disability while essential myoclonus may be sporadic or hereditary. Epileptic myoclonus refers to presence of myoclonus in the setting of epilepsy with common example of juvenile myoclonic epilepsy. Symptomatic (secondary) myoclonus manifests in the setting of neurological or non-neurological disorders with associated abnormal cognitive functions. Symptomatic myoclonus comprise of a widely diverse group of disease processes as depicted in the **Box 2**.

Myoclonus can be classified on the basis of anatomy as cortical, brainstem, or propriospinal myoclonus syndrome. Cortical myoclonus is usually more focal action or stimulus-sensitive (touch or stretch), occurring mainly in distal muscles. In contrast, brainstem myoclonus is commonly provoked by auditory or tactile stimulus and is especially seen around the face. Propriospinal myoclonus on the other hand is generated within the spinal cord and predominantly involves trunk muscles. Hence, it is important to look for stimulus sensitivity while assessing a patient with myoclonus to establish the localization.

- Negative myoclonus (asterixis) is commonly seen in hepatic or uremic encephalopathy. Negative myoclonus can also be noted while walking producing "bouncy gait" characterized by sudden postural lapses especially noted in post anoxic myoclonus.

Chorea: Chorea is a syndrome characterized by brief, abrupt, and nonrhythmic movements resulting from a continuous flow of randomly contracting muscles. It must be remembered that all chorea has the same features regardless of the cause (**Video 2**).

- The key difference of chorea from other movement disorders is the pattern of movements that randomly changes from one body part to another conveying the impression of fidgeting. The other absolute feature that should be looked for in patients with chorea is motor impersistence as seen as milkmaid's grip (fluctuating strength of grip) or hung-up reflex (sustained contraction and choreatic movements of the leg during knee-jerk reflex (**Video 3**).

For evaluation, firstly it is important to establish the course of chorea as acute, subacute, or chronic and secondly, the body distribution pattern (focal, segmental, unilateral, or generalized).

The spectrum of acute or subacute chorea mainly includes autoimmune-mediated disorders such as anti-LGI1, anti-GAD65, anti-CASRP2, anti-GABA-A, and anti-NMDA receptor antibody-mediated encephalitis; while patients who have subacute chorea along with executive dysfunction or obsessive-compulsive complaints, diagnosis of Sydenham's chorea must also be considered. Elderly who present with chronic progressive chorea and dementia, Huntington's disease remains the most frequent cause. Pitfalls in diagnosing chorea and causes of chorea are depicted in **Boxes 3** and **4**.

- Ballismus is a violent form of chorea characterized by uncontrollable, severe, mainly proximal and large amplitude of movements. Ballismus commonly noted in clinical practice is unilateral and is known as hemiballism. It is classically noted in acute vascular insult in the contra-lateral subthalamic nucleus.

BOX 2	Clinical classification of myoclonus.
Physiologic myoclonus (healthy individual)	
• Sleep jerks (hypnic jerks)	
• Exercise induced	
• Hiccoughs	
Epileptic Myoclonus	
• Juvenile myoclonic epilepsy	
• Childhood myoclonic epilepsy	
• Myoclonic absences epilepsy	
• Photosensitive myoclonus	
• Progressive myoclonic epilepsy (Unerricht–Lundborg, Lafora body disease, Gaucher disease)	
Dementia	
• Creutzfeldt-Jakob disease	
• Dementia with Lewy bodies	
• Alzheimer disease	
Infections	
• Subacute sclerosing panencephalitis	
• AIDS (toxoplasmosis, PML, HIV encephalopathy)	
• Japanese encephalitis	
• PML	
• Syphilis	
Toxic	
• Post-hypoxia (Lance–Adam)	
• Heat stroke	
Metabolic dysfunction	
• Liver failure	
• Renal failure	
• Hyper/hypoglycemia	
• Hyper/hypocalcemia	
• Hypernatremia	
• Dialysis syndrome	
Miscellaneous	
• Mitochondrial disorders	
• Paraneoplastic syndrome	
• Opsoclonus-myoclonus syndrome	

(PML: progressive multifocal leukoencephalopathy)

Tics: Tics are semivoluntary, sudden, intermittent "stereotyped" jerky motor movements, or phonic sounds. Generally, tics are suppressible but often associated with an "inner tension" which drives further more tics. Another hallmark feature noted in tics is that they are often preceded by a premonitory sense or urge, relieved only by performing the movement.

BOX 3 Pitfalls in diagnosing chorea.

- Mild chorea can be subtle; can only be noted by carefully observing the patient with high index of suspicion
- Asking the patient to count backward with eyes closed and arm outstretched can best bring out finger chorea
- Choreatic patients themselves have few subjective complaints, especially in the early stage of the disease, hence history form partner is also important

BOX 4 Causes of chorea.

Genetic causes

- Huntington disease
- Neuroacanthocytosis
- Wilson disease
- Spinocerebellar ataxia 2, 3,17
- Ataxia-telangiectasia
- Ataxia with oculomotor apraxia
- Neuroferritinopathy
- Lesch–Nyhan disease

Immunologic

- Sydenham chorea
- Systemic lupus erythematous
- Antiphospholipid antibody syndrome
- Celiac disease
- Paraneoplastic syndromes

Drug-related

- Phenytoin
- Levodopa
- Lithium
- Ethanol

Infections

- AIDS (toxoplasmosis, PML, HIV encephalopathy)
- Japanese encephalitis
- Measles
- Neurocysticercosis
- Syphilis

Vascular

- Stroke
- Anoxia encephalopathy
- Subdural hematoma

Metabolic dysfunction

- Liver failure
- Hyper/hypoglycemia
- Hyper/hypocalcemia
- Hypernatremia

(PML: progressive multifocal leukoencephalopathy)

Simple motor tics are brief and meaningless motion, lasting <1 second, involving one group of muscles while complex motor tics are slower, longer, and more purposeful movements resembling gestures that occur in an inappropriate context. Simple phonic tics are brief and meaningless vocalization, consisting of single sound while complex phonic tics are more purposeful utterances, more intense, including words, phrases, syllables, or abnormal speech pattern (**Table 2**).

- A common diagnostic pitfall in diagnosing tics is that they are often less prominent or even absent during the clinical examination as anxiety of the patients suppresses the phenomenon.
- It may be valuable to observe the patient in the waiting room or while the patient is walking back after the visit.
- Parents can be also asked to videotape the movements of the child at home that can be later examined by the clinician.

HYPERKINETIC MOVEMENT DISORDERS WITH NONJERKY CHARACTER

Dystonia: Dystonia is a subdivision of hyperkinetic movement disorder characterized by involuntary, sustained, and repetitive movements that are directional in nature. The key feature in identifying dystonia is presence of "abnormal posture". Physiologically, these movements are a result of cocontraction of agonist and antagonist muscles.

Dystonia is clinically and etiologically a heterogeneous condition, which can be classified according to age-of-onset (early <26 years; late >26 years), distribution of movement (focal, segmental, multifocal, hemi, and generalized) or etiology (primary and secondary dystonia). Primary dystonia is characterized by presence of isolated dystonia (although tremor may be seen in some) and no other neurological deficit; while secondary dystonia has clinical features and additional neurological deficits other

TABLE 2 Type of tic disorders.

Type of tic	Examples
Simple motor	Eye blinking, facial grimacing, mouth movements, shoulder shrugging, head jerks, arm or leg jerks
Complex motor	• Echopraxia—person mimics the gesture of other • Copropraxia—production of obscene gestures • Self-injurious behaviors
Simple phonic	Throat clearing, coughing, sniffing, squeaking, hissing, grunting, braking or animal noises
Complex phonic	• Echolalia—echoing sound or words heard elsewhere • Pallialia—repetition of one's own or another person's phrases or sentences • Coprolalia—obscene words or phrases

than dystonia; hemidystonia or fixed dystonia points to secondary type of dystonia with underlying cause. There are few characteristic features that separate dystonia from other movement disorders such as:

- Abnormal posturing typically has constant directionality (torticollis with rightward head rotation will not change suddenly to a leftward torticollis and persist as rightward head movement).
- Dystonic movements are patterned and repeatedly involve the same muscle groups.
- Additional sensory tricks (geste antagoniste) are sometimes used by patients to momentarily reduce dystonia.
- Task-specific dystonia can be brought out only by action or activity of specific group of muscles and is predominantly present in specific circumstances, e.g., writer's cramp.

Tremors: Tremor is arrhythmic, sinusoidal alternating movement of one or more body parts. The key feature of tremor is presence of "rhythmicity", which means movement occurring at a regular frequency (**Video 4**). The movement does not necessarily involve a limb; tremor can affect any part of the body, including head, jaw, chin, or tongue. Like other movement disorders, tremors can be classified in various ways but an important classification system proposed by a consensus statement of the Movement Disorder Society is based on the occurrence of movement (**Table 3**).

Rest tremors are noted when the affected part is not actively moving or when the effect of gravity is removed completely; classical example is resting tremor of PD.

- It is important to differentiated postural tremor (as in essential tremor) from tremor of PD as resting tremors may mimic postural tremors when they occur in any position assumed by the affected body part that is maintained against gravity. This can be done by carefully examining how rapidly the tremor manifests after the new posture has been assumed immediately in case of essential tremors, but after a delay of several seconds in PD (termed as re-emergent tremor).
- The frequency of resetting tremor is same as that observed in the rest position.

Few disorders can have more than one type of tremors, example Holmes tremors (midbrain or rubral) have resting, postural, and intentional tremor components.

TABLE 3 Classification of tremors.

Occurrence of movement	Features	Disorder
A. At rest	Rested and supported	Parkinson's disease
B. With action		
Postural	Posture specific	Physiological enhanced tremors; essential tremors
Kinetic		
• Simple	• Present during entire movement	• Essential tremors
• Intention	• Increases toward intended movement	• Cerebellar tremors
• Task specific	• Specific activites	• Dystonic tremors
Isometric	Present during voluntary muscle contraction	Physiological
C. Combination	Various	Rubral tremor (Holmes tremor)

ASSOCIATED FEATURES

Eliciting history of certain features is important in providing important clues for establishing the diagnosing of movement disorders, such as involuntary movements induced by sudden activity (rising from chair) suggests a diagnosis of paroxysmal kinesigenic dyskinesia. Also, presence of associated non-neurological features is important, such as women who have chorea with associated migraine, recurrent spontaneous abortions, and venous thrombosis suggests a diagnosis of antiphospholipid syndrome. Similarly, family history can also be critical for diagnosing the parental consanguinity and indicates toward the genetic cause for movement disorder.

It is a must to do a detailed general physical examination in all patients with movement disorders, to look for presence of additional non-neurological signs. This includes examining the eyes for Kayser–Fleischer ring or telangiectasia in patients with dystonia or chorea, which could indicate diagnosis of ataxia telangiectasia or Wilson's disease, respectively. Similarly, presence of autonomic dysfunction (postural blood pressure changes) with features of parkinsonism raises the possibility of MSA.

DIFFERENTIAL DIAGNOSIS

The final step is generating the differential diagnosis by knitting the clinical syndrome that is determined from the phenomenology of the movements with associated features, both neurological and non-neurological. Now, the physician can proceed to a detailed diagnostic work including laboratory and radiological investigations.

- Movement disorders are learnt by continuously observing and "observing" the movement phenomenology in patients.

CONCLUSION

A systematic approach is recommended whenever clinicians approach a patient presenting with movement disorders. This chapter also has enclosed supplementary videos as examples of various movement disorders which might help in recognizing the individual movement disorder, determining the clinical syndrome and aid in learning and diagnosis.

RECOMMENDED READINGS

1. Abdo W, van de Warrenburg B, Burn D, Quinn NP, Bloem BR. The clinical approach to movement disorders. Nat Rev Neurol. 2010;6:29-37.
2. Goudreau JL. A practical approach to movement disorders: diagnosis and surgical and medical management. Neurology Aug. 2009;73:651-70.
3. Elble RJ. Tremor: Clinical features, pathophysiology and treatment. Joseph Jankovic. Neurologic Clinics-Movement disorders. Philadelphia, Pennsylvania. Saunders Elsevier, 2009;27:679-96.
4. Caviness JN. Pathophysiology and treatment of Myoclonus. Joseph Jankovic. Neurologic Clinics-Movement disorders. Philadelphia, Pennsylvania. Saunders Elsevier, 2009;27:657-77.
5. Deuschl G, Bain P, Brin M. Consensus statement of the Movement Disorder Society on Tremor. Ad Hoc Scientific Committee. Mov Disord. 1998;13:2-23.
6. Postuma RB, Berg D, Stern M, Poewe W, Olanow CW, Oertel W, et al. MDS clinical diagnostic criteria for Parkinson's disease. Mov Disord. 2001;30:1591-601.
7. B Balint , Bhatia KP . Dystonia: an update on phenomenology, classification pathogenesis and treatment. Curr Opin Neurol. 2014;27:468-76.
8. Fung VS, Jinnah HA, Bhatia K, Vidailhet M. Assessment of patients with isolated or combined dystonia: an update on dystonia syndromes. Mov Disord. 2013;28:889-98.
9. Albanese A, Asmus F, Bhatia KP, Elia AE, Elibol B, Filippini G, et al. EFNS guidelines on diagnosis and treatment of primary dystonias. Eur J Neurol. 2011;18:5-18.
10. Litvan I, Bhatia KP, Burn DJ, Goetz CG, Lang AE, McKeith I, et al. Movement Disorders Society Scientific Issues Committee report: SIC Task Force appraisal of clinical diagnostic criteria for parkinsonian disorders. Mov Disord. 2003;18:467-86.
11. Schmitz-Hübsch T, Klockgether T. An update on inherited ataxias Curr Neurol Neurosci Rep. 2008;8:310-19.
12. Norlinah IM, Bhatia KP, Ostergaard K, Howard R, Arabia G, Quinn NP. Primary lateral sclerosis mimicking atypical parkinsonism. Mov Disord. 2007;22:2057-62.
13. Cardoso F, Seppi K, Mair KJ, Wenning GK, Poewe W. Seminar on choreas. Lancet Neurol. 2006;5:589-602.
14. Gerschlager W, Münchau A, Katzenschlager R, Brown P, Rothwell JC, Quinn N, et al. Natural history and syndromic associations of orthostatic tremor: a review of 41 patients. Mov Disord. 2004;19:788-95.
15. Bhatia KP, Schneider SA. Psychogenic tremor and related disorders. J Neurol. 2007;254:569-74.
16. Nahab FB, Peckham E, Hallett M. Essential tremor, deceptively simple. Pract Neurol. 2007;7:222-33.
17. Seppi K, Schocke MF. An update on conventional and advanced magnetic resonance imaging techniques in the differential diagnosis of neurodegenerative parkinsonism. Curr Opin Neurol. 2005;18:370-75.
18. Muthugovindan D, Singer H. Motor stereotypy disorders. Curr Opin Neurol. 2009;22:131-36.
19. Saifee TA, Edwards MJ. Tardive movement disorders: a practical approach. Practical Neurology. 2011;11:341-348.
20. Mulligan C, Bronstein JM. Wilson Disease: An Overview and Approach to Management. Neurol Clin. 2020;38:417-32.

CHAPTER 194

Cerebellar Disorders

Achal K Srivastava, Divyani Garg, Mohammed Faruq

ABSTRACT

Cerebellar disorders may structurally affect the anterior cerebellum, posterior cerebellum, or both, the latter called pancerebellar disorders. A knowledge of functional anatomy aids in understanding the extent of cerebellar dysfunction, which is also relevant from the point of etiological considerations, as specific disorders may have particular structural underpinnings.

Cerebellar disorders occur due to a diverse range of etiologies. Acquired causes of cerebellar disorders include structural conditions, hypothyroidism, toxin-mediated, infectious and postinfectious conditions, and immune-mediated disorders. Acquired disorders have specific targets for therapy. Inherited cerebellar disorders are classified on the basis of the mode of inheritance into autosomal recessive cerebellar ataxia syndromes, autosomal dominant cerebellar ataxia (ADCA) syndromes, and X-linked and mitochondrial conditions. Sporadic ataxias, for example, multiple system atrophy (MSA), may also occur with no definite genetic cause.

A thorough clinical assessment, followed by meticulous diagnostic evaluation, is key to identifying the etiology. Knowledge of key clinical features coupled with genetic testing clinches the diagnosis in hereditary ataxias. Treatment is based on the underlying cause. Management of ancillary complaints, such as movement disorders, neuropathic pain, or seizures are central to improving quality of life among patients with cerebellar disorders. In this review, we highlight functional anatomy of the cerebellum, and describe acquired and inherited cerebellar disorders, along with approach to their evaluation and management.

"When suffering happens, it forces us to confront life in a different way than we normally do"

—Philip Yancey

INTRODUCTION

The word "cerebellum" in Latin stands for "little brain". Although it occupies only 10% of the brain volume, it contains over 50% of the total number of brain neurons. The normal function of the cerebellum involves coordination of the motor system, gait and balance, and also cognition. Hence, cerebellar disorders manifest with clinical features of incoordination, ataxia, dysarthria, and cognitive dysfunction. Cerebellar disorders arise from a host of diverse causes which may affect the cerebellum or its connections. In order to gain better understanding of these conditions, normal anatomy and functioning of the cerebellum must be understood. Relevant texts in neuroanatomy may be considered for detailed review of normal cerebellar anatomy. Further discussion in this chapter presumes that the reader is well-versed with the same.

CLINICAL MANIFESTATIONS

Cerebellar dysfunction leads to a wide range of clinical features, including tremor, nystagmus, dysarthria, gait ataxia, limb incoordination etc. When the disease process affects the cerebellar connections, associated symptoms and signs of brainstem dysfunction may be present.

DYSSYNERGIA

Dyssynergia is one of the main clinical manifestations of cerebellar dysfunction. Normal cerebellar function is responsible for coordination of the rate, force, and timing of the various muscle groups involved in a specific movement, to impart smoothness and harmony to the movements. As a result of cerebellar dysfunction, this flow of movements is disrupted leading to decomposition of movements, that is, the movement is fractionated into individual, uncoordinated, and bizarre components.

GAIT DISTURBANCE

Gait disturbances are the most troubling manifestation of cerebellar dysfunction. The gait becomes wide-based, with increased truncal sway, staggering walk, and impaired tandem gait. Due to instability involving the trunk, patients tend to fall in any direction. Lesions in the vermis region are usually associated with gait and truncal ataxia.

DYSMETRIA

In dysmetria, judgment errors are made regarding the direction, force, and speed of movements due to loss of coordination between agonist and antagonist muscle contraction. This may manifest as hypermetria (overshooting a target) or hypometria (undershooting a target). Lesions leading to dysmetria involve the ipsilateral cerebellar hemispheres.

AGONIST-ANTAGONIST COORDINATION

Agonist-antagonist muscles have reciprocal innervation so that contraction of the agonist is accompanied by inhibition of the antagonist to ensure uninterrupted and smooth action. In cerebellar dysfunction, the initial agonist burst may be too short or too long and may even continue into the antagonist burst. This leads to dysdiadochokinesia and rebound phenomenon. In dysdiadochokinesia, there is inability to conduct rapid alternating movement

TREMOR

The typical tremor in cerebellar dysfunction is intention tremor, which does not occur at rest but appears on movement directed towards a target. These tremors manifest as irregular movements perpendicular to the path of movement while attempting to reach a target. Cerebellar tremor may also involve proximal musculature, head, or even the entire body when severe. Lesions affecting the dentate nucleus produce intention tremor. Tremor arises because dentate nucleus lesions interrupt the connections of the cerebellum with the red nucleus and the thalamus.

DYSARTHRIA

The characteristic disorder of articulation in cerebellar disorders leads to a slow, slurred speech which may have an "explosive" character due to phonatory muscle dyssynergy. "Scanning" speech may also occur due to the same reason in which each syllable is enunciated individually with intersyllable pauses. The dysarthria may be a product of hypotonia, leading to intonation problems rather than articulatory systems. The paravermal region is associated with dysarthria.

HYPOTONIA

Loss of muscle tone or hypotonia may be seen in cerebellar dysfunction as a result of decreased tonic output of the cerebellar nuclei and subsequent facilitation of the motor cortex by the cerebellum. The deep tendon reflexes may acquire a "pendular" nature with increased to-and-fro movements of the limbs to stretch reflex. This occurs due to a combination of muscle hypotonia and loss of normal check mechanisms in cerebellar dysfunction. This is usually a feature of acute rather than chronic cerebellar lesions. The hypotonia is ipsilateral to the side of the cerebellar lesion and is more pronounced in the proximal muscles. Neocerebellar lesions are associated with hypotonia. This is because of reduced fusimotor drive, especially to the dentate nucleus, leading to reduced stretch response in myo spindle afferents.

NYSTAGMUS

The typical nystagmus seen in cerebellar disorders is a "gaze paretic" nystagmus. The patient has difficulty in maintaining eccentric gaze and repeatedly fixes gaze laterally. The nystagmus becomes more prominent on looking ipsilateral to the affected side. "Rebound" nystagmus may also be seen in which the fast component is in the direction of lateral gaze, but on returning to primary position, may overshoot to the opposite side. These are usually seen with midline lesions. Periodic alternating nystagmus occurs with uvulonodular lesions or their connections with the vestibular nuclei. Downbeat nystagmus occurs with posterior midline vestibulocerebellar lesions. Other eye signs include saccadic pursuits, opsoclonus, ocular flutter, macrosquare wave jerks, and failure to suppress the vestibulo-ocular reflex.

COGNITIVE DYSFUNCTION

Cerebellar cognitive affective syndrome (CCAS), also called Schmahmann's syndrome, features cognitive deficits in the form of executive dysfunction, language, visuospatial processing and behavioral and personality changes, and memory deficits. These are prominent with involvement of the posterior lobe of the cerebellum and vermis. This may be due to disruption of cerebellar links with various regions of the cerebral cortex including the prefrontal, parietal, temporal, and limbic regions.

ETIOLOGY

Broadly, cerebellar disorders can be classified as inherited or acquired.

ACQUIRED CEREBELLAR DISORDERS

There are diverse acquired conditions that lead to cerebellar dysfunction (**Table 1**). These range from vascular causes such as ischemic or hemorrhagic stroke, demyelination, toxin-mediated, immune-mediated, or structural compression such as due to craniovertebral junction abnormalities. Some of the common causes of acquired cerebellar dysfunction are detailed below.

Hypothyroidism: Hypothyroidism may be associated with mild incoordination and gait ataxia, in the setting of typical clinical features of hypothyroidism, and tend to affect midline cerebellum. This may be reversible on treatment with replacement thyroxine.

Toxin-mediated:

Alcohol: Alcohol is among the most frequent causes of chronic ataxia and leads to midline cerebellar dysfunction as well as degeneration. Prominently, patients develop truncal and gait ataxia. As the cerebellar hemispheres are relatively spared, involvement of the upper limbs/speech etc., are less common. Chronic alcohol abuse may lead to asymptomatic cerebellar atrophy, which may be seen on neuroimaging. Gait ataxia may be reversed to varying extents by abstinence. Thiamine must also be supplemented as thiamine depletion also contributes to gait ataxia in these patients. In Wernicke's encephalopathy, patients may develop rapidly progressive ataxia.

Antiseizure medications: Acute elevations in blood levels of antiseizure medications (ASMs), particularly phenytoin, are associated with cerebellar dysfunction. Chronic phenytoin therapy may lead to more permanent deficits due to loss of Purkinje cells. Chronic phenytoin therapy may lead to cerebellar atrophy as well, which may or may not be accompanied by clinical signs of cerebellar dysfunction. Most of the newer antiepileptic drugs, with the exception of levetiracetam and gabapentin, may increase the risk of cerebellar dysfunction to variable considerations.

Chemotherapy agents: Ataxia is a side effect of certain chemotherapy agents such as 5-fluorouracil (5-FU). High doses of 5-FU may cause cerebellar dysfunction which may be reversed with thiamine. Regular doses of 5-FU may cause cerebellar dysfunction in individuals with pyrimidine metabolism issues (dihydropyrimidine dehydrogenase deficiency). Another chemotherapy agent associated with cerebellar dysfunction in high doses is cytosine arabinoside (Ara-c).

Other toxins: Solvent abuse, such as toluene, can lead to ataxia, in combination with cognitive and pyramidal tract dysfunction. Heavy metals such as organic mercury (found in some fungicides) can lead to damage to the visual fields as well as cerebellar granule cells. This leads to ataxia and visual field constriction. Lead toxicity can also cause encephalopathy, cerebellar dysfunction, and abdominal pain, and is common in children. Bismuth toxicity leads to cognitive issues, myoclonus, and cerebellar dysfunction. Another agent that may cause cerebellar dysfunction is lithium.

Infections: Cerebellar dysfunction may be a postinfectious syndrome. In children, an acute cerebellar disorder may develop after a viral illness which may be nonspecific but may follow varicella infection also. This occurs between the age group of 5 years and 6 years. Epstein–Barr virus infection may lead to a similar syndrome among adolescents. In Bickerstaff brainstem encephalitis, a combination of ataxia, ophthalmoplegia, and lower cranial nerve palsies may occur. Another infection associated with cerebellar dysfunction is

TABLE 1 Etiological considerations in acquired cerebellar disorders.	
Etiology	**Clinical features**
Vascular	Sudden-onset cerebellar dysfunction, previous history of stroke, and neuroimaging suggesting stroke
Neoplastic	Insidious onset, progressive symptoms which may be associated with features of raised intracranial pressure
Craniovertebral junction anomalies	Associated features of lower cranial nerve palsies, pyramidal tract involvement, and short neck
Demyelinating conditions	Remitting and relapsing episodes, supportive neuroimaging, cerebrospinal fluid analysis may reveal raised protein, and presence of oligoclonal bands
Infections	
Acute cerebellitis	History of fever associated with ataxia in childhood
Postinfectious	Preceding infection/fever
Bickerstaff brainstem encephalitis	Postinfectious syndrome characterized by ataxia, areflexia, and external ophthalmoplegia
human immunodeficiency virus (HIV)	
Creutzfeldt–Jakob disease	Rapidly progressive fatal dementia associated with myoclonus
Whipple's disease	Infectious syndrome with dementia, diarrhea, ataxia, and typical oculomasticatory myorhythmia
Immune-mediated	
Paraneoplastic	Associated with malignancies. Antibodies include anti-Yo, Anti-Ri, Anti-Ta etc.
Nonparaneoplastic	Autoimmune conditions associated with antibodies, anti-glutamic acid decarboxylase (GAD) antibodies
Gluten sensitivity	Immune-mediated disease which may be related to celiac disease or nonceliac gluten sensitivity
Toxin-mediated Alcohol Antiseizure medications Chemotherapy agents Metals Solvents	Specific history of exposure to the offending agent

human immunodeficiency virus (HIV) infection. HIV may lead to cerebellar dysfunction as a result of lesions caused by lymphoma, chronic meningitis, toxoplasmosis, and progressive multifocal leukoencephalopathy. Creutzfeldt–Jakob disease (CJD) is a syndrome of rapidly progressive dementia caused by mutant prion protein (PrP). Ataxia may be a part of the illness. Whipple's disease (WD), caused by *Tropheryma whipplei*, leads to a syndrome of diarrhea, weight loss, and typically, oculomasticatory myorhythmia and oculofacial-skeletal myorhythmia. Cerebellar dysfunction is common in WD.

Autoimmune conditions:

Ataxia with gluten sensitivity: Gluten sensitivity is associated with a range of clinical manifestations. In celiac disease, antibodies occur to gliadin. It affects the small intestine and also leads to cerebellar ataxia. This may be associated with peripheral neuropathy. Diagnosis is based on the presence of antideaminated gliadin antibody, antitransglutaminase antibody, and biopsy of the small bowel. Gluten-free diet leads to remission of symptoms.

Paraneoplastic cerebellar dysfunction: Paraneoplastic cerebellar degeneration is a rapidly evolving ataxia syndrome that develops over a few months. Cerebellar dysfunction may precede the tumor diagnosis. It is a severe pancerebellar syndrome. The antibodies usually associated with this condition include anti-Hu, seen with small cell lung cancer; anti-Yo, seen with ovarian cancer; anti-Ri, seen on breast and nonsmall cell lung cancer; anti-Tr antibodies, seen in Hodgkin's lymphoma; anti-Ta, anti-Ma; and anti-CV2 antibodies.

Other immune-mediated ataxias: Antibodies to glutamic acid decarboxylase (GAD) are known to be associated with cerebellar dysfunction. Patients may also have associated peripheral neuropathy, as well as other autoimmune conditions, such as diabetes and thyroiditis. GAD is responsible for gamma-amino butyric acid synthesis and anti-GAD antibodies may bind to gamma-aminobutyric acid (GABA) receptors.

Another condition associated with cerebellar dysfunction is steroid responsive encephalopathy associated with autoimmune thyroiditis (SREAT).

INHERITED CEREBELLAR DISORDERS

Based on the pattern of inheritance, these may be classified into autosomal recessive, autosomal dominant, X-linked ataxia, and mitochondrial syndromes.

Autosomal recessive cerebellar ataxias: These conditions are summarized in **Table 2**. Further details of some individual conditions are elucidated below.

Friedreich's ataxia: Friedreich's ataxia (FA) is the most common form of inherited ataxia with usual age of onset

TABLE 2 Multisystem syndromes with prominent cerebellar dysfunction.

Disorder	Characteristic clinical findings and evaluation
Abetalipoproteinemia	Low levels of vitamin E; abnormal lipoprotein electrophoresis
Aceruloplasminemia	• Dementia, movement disorders ataxia, and retinal degeneration • Evaluation shows low serum copper with absent ceruloplasmin • Occurs due to mutations in the ceruloplasmin gene
Ataxia with CoQ10 deficiency	Abnormally low coenzyme Q levels on muscle biopsy
Ataxia telangiectasia	Elevated alpha fetoprotein and low immunoglobulin (Ig) level
Cerebrotendinous xanthomatosis	• Diarrhea, dementia, pyramidal signs, ataxia, and tendon xanthomas • Elevated serum cholestanol • Mutations in the *CYP27A1* gene
Late-onset Tay–Sachs disease	• Neuropathy, ataxia, and cognitive issues • Low hexosaminidase A; genetic mutations in hex-A gene
Niemann-Pick type C	• Vertical gaze paresis, liver, and spleen enlargement • Mutation analysis of the *NPC* gene
Refsum disease	• Hearing loss, ataxia, retinitis pigmentosa, and skin ichthyosis • Elevated phytanic acid levels; mutations in the *PHYH* and *PEX 7* genes
Wilson disease	• Cognitive issues, movement disorders, and ataxia • Presence of liver disease and Kayser–Fleischer ring • Low serum ceruloplasmin and copper levels

below 25 years. It occurs due to unstable expansion of trinucleotide repeats, GAA, in the *FRDA* gene on chromosome 9 leading to a deficiency of the protein, frataxin. Around 15% of patients may have age of onset >25 years, referred to as late-onset FA (LOFA). The typical clinical syndrome is gait ataxia, loss of proprioception in the lower limbs, and areflexia. Pathology mainly involves degeneration of dorsal root ganglion cells. Cardiac abnormalities such as hypertrophic cardiomyopathy and rhythm abnormalities may be seen in 50% of patients, as well as skeletal deformities such as scoliosis and pes cavus may be observed. The condition is progressive and patients lose ambulation over 9–15 years. A few patients develop optic atrophy and hearing impairment. Up to 10% of patients may develop diabetes. Nerve conduction studies reveal reduction of sensory potentials. Magnetic resonance imaging (MRI) brain is normal although the upper cervical cord reveals atrophy.

Ataxia with vitamin E deficiency (AVED): This is a form of young-onset ataxia due to mutations in the alpha-tocopherol transfer protein (αTTP) gene on chromosome 8 which encodes a protein required for vitamin E transport in chylomicrons. This leads to a deficiency of vitamin E, required for normal neuronal function. Ataxia with vitamin E deficiency (AVED) bears clinical similarity to FA. In addition to cerebellar dysfunction, patients develop peripheral neuropathy and retinitis pigmentosa. Titubation is a prominent clinical feature.

Abetalipoproteinemia: This occurs due to mutations in the *MTTP* gene, which codes for the microsomal triglyceride transfer protein. This leads to impaired absorption of lipid soluble vitamins, such as vitamin E and clinical manifestations resemble AVED. The patient has low levels of vitamin E and cholesterol and absent apolipoprotein B. Peripheral blood smear may reveal acanthocytes. Serum lipoprotein electrophoresis contributes to the diagnosis.

Ataxia telangiectasia: Ataxia telangiectasia (AT) is caused by mutations in the *ATM* gene on chromosome 11, which codes for a serine-threonine kinase which helps in deoxyribonucleic acid (DNA) repair. ATM presents in the first decade with progressive gait ataxia, peripheral neuropathy, and other movement disorders such as chorea. A typical finding in this condition is oculomotor apraxia, which leads to head thrust for fixation followed later by the eyes, called the eye-head lag. Telangiectasias, the pathognomonic feature, appear by 5 years of age, and have a predilection to occur on the conjunctivae, earlobes, popliteal fossa etc. Children with ATM tend to have recurrent sinopulmonary infections. They also have increased risk of hematological malignancies such as lymphoma and leukemia. Immunoglobulin A levels are decreased. Alfa fetoprotein levels are usually elevated (>10 ng/mL).

Autosomal dominant cerebellar disorders: These include spinocerebellar ataxias (SCAs) and episodic ataxias (EAs). ADCA were classified by Harding initially as follows:

- *ADCA I*: Ataxia in association with other noncerebellar signs
- *ADCA II*: Ataxia in association with visual loss
- *ADCA III*: Pure cerebellar ataxia
- Later ADCA IV was added

Spinocerebellar ataxia: Spinocerebellar ataxias (SCAs) are a large group of genetically and phenotypically heterogeneous conditions. Several SCAs occur due to unstable nucleotide repeat expansions. This leads to the phenomenon of *anticipation*, in which earlier age of onset is seen in the down generations. Various structures in the nervous system may be affected, giving rise to a host of clinical manifestations. Up to 40 genetic types have been described so far, and more continue to be described. Some of the common types are summarized in **Table 3**. SCA2 is the most common type in India. Worldwide, SCA3 is the most common type of SCA, also known as Machado-Joseph disease (MJD). Three types are described:

TABLE 3 Prominent clinical features in patients with spinocerebellar ataxia (SCA).

SCA type	Genetic abnormality/ Chromosomal region	Noncerebellar neurological features
SCA1 (ATXN1)	CAG repeats, 6p Ataxin 1	Upper motor neuron signs, saccadic slowing, sensory neuropathy, and extrapyramidal features
SCA2 (ATXN2)	CAG repeats, 12q Ataxin 2	Slow saccades prominent and peripheral neuropathy
SCA3 (Machado–Joseph disease)	CAG repeats, 14q Ataxin 3	Facial/tongue fasciculations, slow saccades, ophthalmoparesis, and extrapyramidal features
SCA5	Mutation in *SPTBN2* gene, 11p	Minor pyramidal features and prominent cerebellar presentation
SCA6	CAG repeats, 19p CACNA1A/calcium channel	Nearly purely cerebellar, minor pyramidal features, and downbeating nystagmus may be seen
SCA11	Mutation in *TTBK2* gene, 15q	Described in a small number of families; early onset
SCA12	CAG repeats, 5q *PP2R2B*	Action tremor of limbs, bradykinesia, and psychiatric features

1. *MJD-I*: The age of onset is between 10 and 30 years. Typical features include dystonia, pyramidal signs, ataxia, and ophthalmoplegia.
2. *MJD-II*: This is the most common type. Typical age of onset is between 20 and 50 years. Clinical features include ataxia and pyramidal signs.
3. *MJD-III*: This presents later than the other types, between 40 and 70 years of age, and has slowest progression. A characteristic finding is amyotrophy and peripheral neuropathy.

Among the SCAs, SCA12 is a condition which is uniquely prevalent in the northern India population and is the second most common form of SCA in India. Expansion of CAG trinucleotide repeats beyond 43 repeats in the *PPP2R2B* gene leads to cerebellar and cortical atrophy. Patients with SCA12, dominant among the Aggarwal community, present with early action tremor of the upper limbs, relatively milder gait ataxia, head tremor, and voice tremors. Age of onset is also relatively older than the other SCAs.

Episodic ataxia: These are syndromes characterized by transient episodes of ataxia, in combination with other symptoms. So far, seven subtypes (EA1 to EA7) have been delineated. Of these, EA2 is the most common subtype.

Mitochondrial diseases with cerebellar involvement: Certain mitochondrial conditions are association with ataxia such as myoclonic epilepsy with ragged red fibers (MERRF) and neuropathy, ataxia, and retinitis pigmentosa (NARP) syndromes. Other conditions include progressive external ophthalmoplegia (PEO), Kearns–Sayre syndrome (KSS), mitochondrial encephalopathy, lactic acidosis, and stroke-like episodes (MELAS).

X-linked ataxias: The most important is the fragile X-associated tremor/ataxia syndrome (FXTAS). This is an X-linked condition which leads to expansion in the *FMR1* gene. This affects the maternal grandfathers of patients with fragile X mental retardation syndrome. Typical MRI finding is T2 hyperintensity in the middle cerebellar peduncle.

Sporadic cerebellar disorders: These are progressive conditions which resemble inherited disorders, but for which no genetic correlate is known. Among adults, this is referred to as idiopathic late-onset cerebellar ataxia (iLOCA). In iLOCA, a small percentage of patients will test positive for one of the genetic mutations known to occur with cerebellar disorders, such as FA and SCA2, 3, 6, and 8.

In MSA, in addition to cerebellar dysfunction, parkinsonism and autonomic dysfunction is also seen. MSA is further subtyped as MSA-P (parkinsonism) and MSA-C (cerebellar) types. MSA-C is an important differential diagnosis for sporadic ataxias among older adults.

EVALUATION

Patients with cerebellar disorders must undergo meticulous history and examination. Helpful features to make a diagnosis include age at onset, progression, associated neurological, and nonneurological clinical features. An algorithm to aid evaluation is provided in **Flowchart 1**.

An MRI may display characteristics abnormalities such as infarction, tumors, demyelination, and meningeal infection.

In degenerative ataxia, MRI may reveal cerebellar atrophy in isolation or in combination with pontine atrophy, middle cerebellar peduncle hyperintensities etc.

Laboratory investigations include thyroid function tests, vitamin E, vitamin B1, vitamin B12, serology for syphilis, antithyroid antibodies, autoimmune antibodies including anti-GAD and anti-tissue transglutaminase (tTG) antibodies, and paraneoplastic antibodies. Cerebrospinal fluid (CSF) examination may be useful to demonstrate pleocytosis in infections and atypical cells in carcinomatous meningitis. WD may be diagnosed by CSF polymerase chain reaction (PCR).

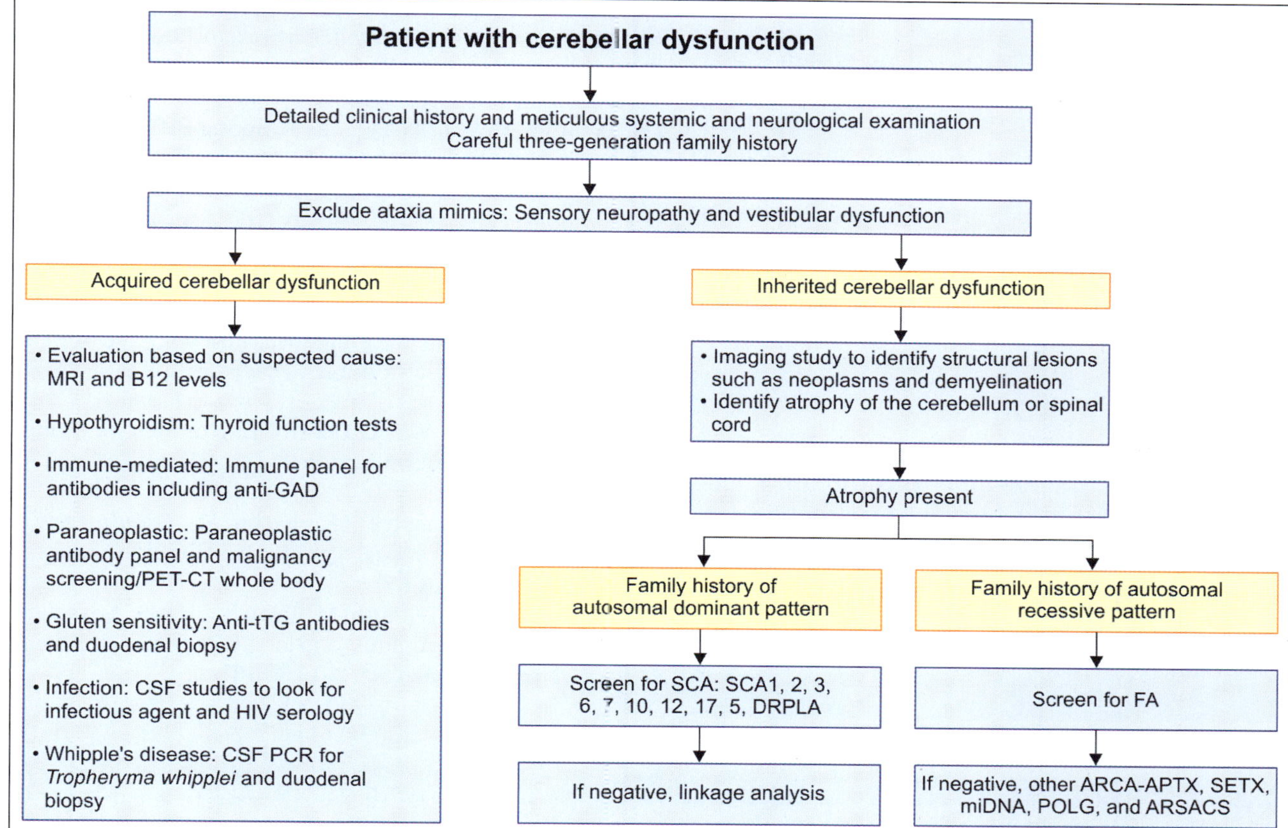

(ARCA: autosomal recessive cerebellar ataxia; ARSACS: autosomal-recessive spastic ataxia of Charlevoix-Saguenay; DRPLA: dentatorubral-pallidoluysian atrophy; FA: Friedreich's ataxia; GAD: glutamic acid decarboxylase; miDNA: mitochondrial deoxyribonucleic acid; MRI: magnetic resonance imaging; POLG: polymerase gamma; tTG: tissue transglutaminase)

FLOWCHART 1: Diagnostic evaluation of a patient with a cerebellar disorder.

Genetic testing is of utmost importance among the inherited cerebellar syndromes. DNA testing for CAG or CTG trinucleotide repeat expansions seen in SCAs may be done. For FA, GAA repeat expansions may be looked for. Mitochondrial mutations associated with MERRF, MELAS, NARP etc., may be done in suspected cases.

Clinical clues that suggest the possibility of inherited ataxias and deem genetic testing include long duration of illness and family history of a similar illness. The pattern of inheritance based on a three-generation family tree will suggest the broad genetic group to which the cerebellar disorder belongs. In a family history suggestive of autosomal dominant mode of inheritance, testing for SCAs is warranted. The initial mutation screen should assess for SCA1, 2, 3, 6, 7, and 17, as well as SCA12 in the Aggarwal clan, in which it is well described.

TREATMENT

Treatment of cerebellar disorders is specific to the etiology. Among patients with infectious causes, treatment warrants specific antimicrobial therapy. In postinfectious inflammatory syndromes such as Bickerstaff brainstem encephalitis as well as demyelinating disorders, immune therapy may be warranted. Autoimmune causes are also managed with immune therapy in the form of steroids, intravenous immunoglobulins, or plasma exchange. Paraneoplastic ataxias require treatment/removal of the underlying tumor as well as immune therapy. Toxin-mediated ataxias require removal of exposure to the offending agent. Structural causes such as a space-occupying lesion involving the cerebellum or craniovertebral junction anomalies may require surgical treatment, with or without adjunct radiation or chemotherapy in the case of tumors. Gluten sensitivity required gluten-free diet for reversal or amelioration of the cerebellar dysfunction.

Treatment of inherited cerebellar syndromes is more challenging, considering their progressive nature and lack of any definitive curative therapy. Acetazolamide is useful in the treatment of EA type 2.

Symptomatic therapy is of utmost importance to improve quality of life among these patients and involves treatment of cramps, dystonia, or other movement disorders, concomitant seizures, neuropathic pain etc., with usual management modalities.

CONCLUSION

Cerebellar disorders are a heterogeneous group which can arise from a vast array of etiologies, the identification of which is imperative to further evaluation, management, and prognosis. There are several acquired causes which lead to reversible cerebellar dysfunction with appropriate treatment. With advancements in genetic technology, more hereditary ataxias continue to be continually identified. Apart from specific therapy, symptom-based management is crucial to effectively manage these patients with cerebellar disorders.

RECOMMENDED READINGS

1. Campbell WW, DeJong RN, Haerer AF. Dejong's the Neurologic Examination: Incorporating the Fundamentals of Neuroanatomy and Neurophysiology. Philadelphia, PA: Lippincott Williams & Wilkins; 2005.
2. Daroff RB, Jankovic J, Mazziotta JC, Pomeroy S. Bradley's Neurology in Clinical Practice, 7th edition. Amsterdam, Netherlands: Elsevier; 2016.
3. Nanri K, Okuma M, Sato S, Yoneda M, Taguchi T, Mitoma H, et al. Prevalence of autoantibodies and the efficacy of immunotherapy for autoimmune cerebellar ataxia. Intern Med. 2016;55(5):449-54.
4. Beaudin M, Matilla-Dueñas A, Soong BW, Pedroso JL, Barsottini OG, Mitoma H, et al. The Classification of Autosomal Recessive Cerebellar Ataxias: a Consensus Statement from the Society for Research on the Cerebellum and Ataxias Task Force. Cerebellum. 2019;18:1098-125.
5. de Silva RN, Vallortigara J, Greenfield J, Hunt B, Giunti P, Hadjivassiliou M. Diagnosis and management of progressive ataxia in adults. Pract Neurol. 2019;19(3): 196-207.
6. Sullivan R, Yau WY, O'Connor E, Houlden H. Spinocerebellar ataxia: an update. J Clin Neurol. 2019;266: 533-44.
7. Kumar D, Srivastava AK, Faruq M, Gundluru VR. Spinocerebellar ataxia type 12: An update. Ann Mov Disord. 2019;2:48-57.
8. Agarwal A, Garg D, Faruq M, Rajan R, Goyal V, Srivastava AK. Treating hereditary ataxias—Where can we help? Ann Natl Acad Med Sci. 2019;55:182-8.

CHAPTER 195

Amyotrophic Lateral Sclerosis

Vineeth Jaison, Raviteja Kakarla, Dimple Dawar

ABSTRACT

Amyotrophic lateral sclerosis (ALS) is a progressive neurodegenerative disease affecting the motor neurons in the brain and spinal cord. The disease increases in prevalence with age and has a slight male preponderance in the younger age group. Some studies suggest an association with increased physical activity and exposure to certain toxins. Less than 10% of ALS is familial. It can affect the cranial motor neurons resulting in dysarthria and dysphagia, while cervical and thoracic segment involvement leads to weakness of the upper limbs, respiratory insufficiency, and weakness of the trunk, and lumbosacral motor neuron involvement results in weakness of the lower limbs. Cognition is also affected in a large number of patients and is the result of frontal and temporal lobe involvement.

The diagnosis requires the presence of both upper motor neuron (UMN) and lower motor neuron (LMN) signs in at least three segments and is made as a diagnosis of exclusion. Some patients worsen more rapidly than others and involvement of bulbar muscles portends a poor prognosis. The usual life expectancy of patients is 3–5 years and common cause of death is due to respiratory failure. Patients require supportive care to address the speech, swallowing, mobility, pain, and respiratory problems. Clinical trials have been unsuccessful to find a cure for this illness. Riluzole and recently edaravone are two drugs that have shown modest benefit. Several other medications are currently under study and in the last few years this field has become very fertile for research.

"Our greatest glory is not in never falling but in rising every time we fall"

—Confucius

INTRODUCTION

Amyotrophic lateral sclerosis was originally described by Jean-Martin Charcot in 1869 as a pure motor neuron disease. It is now recognized as a multisystem neurodegenerative disease, with varying clinical, genetic, and neuropathological presentations. The disease typically manifests clinically with both UMN and LMN signs involving one segment of the neuroaxis and spreading to the next, eventually resulting in death from respiratory failure. The World Federation of Neurology Research Group on Neuromuscular Diseases clubbed four sporadic diseases, namely, primary lateral sclerosis (PLS), ALS, progressive bulbar palsy, and progressive muscular atrophy (PMA) as motor neuron disease.

EPIDEMIOLOGY

The annual incidence of ALS is roughly 2 per 100,000 population with a prevalence rate of 6 per 100,000. Divided by subcontinent and economic level, the highest incidence and prevalence rate are seen in Europe [prevalence 9.62, 95% confidence interval (CI) 4.80–16.10; incidence: 2.76, 95% CI 2.00–3.64] and lowest in South Asia (prevalence 1.57, 95% CI 0.17–4.39; incidence 0.42, 95% CI 0.06–1.11).

Age is the single most important risk factor for ALS and mortality increases with age up to the eighth decade. Worldwide, the median age of onset is 55–60 years, while in India and China it has been reported to be a decade earlier. According to global burden of disease 2013, the incidence of ALS peaked between 60 and 70 years of age.

Men develop ALS more often than women in the younger age group, male:female (M:F) ratio varying between 1.11 and 2.32:1. However, there is equal distribution across the genders as age increases. Spinal onset ALS is seen in 58–82% of patients and occurs in younger individuals with a male predilection without cognitive impairment, on the other hand bulbar ALS is seen more often in elderly women. **Table 1** shows the main risk factors for ALS.

CLINICAL ANATOMY

Amyotrophic lateral sclerosis affects the motor neurons in the brain and spinal cord. **Table 2** illustrates the clinical anatomy of neuroaxis involved in ALS. ALS manifests with UMN syndrome due to the progressive destruction of the corticospinal tract (CST) and corticobulbar tract (CBT). These project to motor neurons, innervating the extremities and associated interneurons in the lateral anterior horn. Axons within these tracts provide excitatory input to alpha and gamma motor neurons, and Ia inhibitory interneurons. The LMN syndrome is due to involvement of motor neurons within the anterior horn cell which supply all the voluntary muscles of the face and trunk and extremities.

TABLE 1 Risk factors of amyotrophic lateral sclerosis.

Activity	Exercise, lower body mass index, increased muscle mass, head injury or trauma
Toxins	Smoking, heavy metals like lead and mercury, pesticides or solvents, diesel exhaust, silica, and organic dust
Occupation	Agriculture, hunting, forestry, fishing, construction work, and rural living
Environmental	Extremely low frequency magnetic fields, electric shocks

TABLE 2 Clinical anatomy of the neuroaxis involved in amyotrophic lateral sclerosis.

Neuroaxis	Tract	Origin
Brain	Corticobulbar and spinal	These tracts originate in the primary motor cortex, premotor areas, temporal cortex, and sensory cortex to converge in the internal capsule, pass through the ventral midbrain, and separate into bundles in the basis pontis
Brainstem	Corticobulbar	The corticobulbar tracts separate off and bilaterally project to the cranial motor nuclei V, VII, IX, X, and XII
	Corticospinal	In the medulla, some of the corticospinal bundles coalesce ventrally to form the pyramids with 75–90% of these fibers decussating at the pyramids to form the lateral CST. The rest travel ipsilaterally to form the ventral CST
Spinal cord	Lateral CST	These project to motor neurons, innervating the extremities and associated interneurons in the lateral anterior horn
	Ventral CST	These supply axial and postural muscles
	Anterior horn cell	Lower motor neurons are longitudinally arranged columns extending from 1 to 4 spinal segments

(CST: corticospinal tract)

CLINICAL FEATURES

TYPICAL CLINICAL FEATURES

The presence of UMN and LMN signs is characteristic of classic form of ALS which is summarized in **Table 3**.

Weakness: This is the most common presentation. It usually affects the limbs asymmetrically and spreads to neighboring myotomes in the same limb before involving the contralateral side. The dominant upper limb is more affected than the nondominant but there is no difference in the lower limbs. **Figures 1 A** and **B** show atrophied thenar eminence in a patient with ALS. An easily elicited deep tendon reflex (DTR) in a weak, atrophied, and flaccid limb should be considered a UMN sign. Fasciculations are an important sign in ALS, which are painless, involuntary, rapid twitches in muscles of the limb and trunk. These should be observed on careful examination of every patient with ALS, which is rarely noticeable to the patient. Its absence should make us rethink the diagnosis.

Bulbar involvement: Drooling or sialorrhea is a common complaint caused by decreased automatic swallowing and clearance of oral secretions, which is worsened by the coexistence of neck extensor weakness. This can lead to aspiration, which can be both silent and symptomatic and it can present as mealtime choking and coughing, nocturnal awakenings, or even fatal laryngospasm.

Respiratory involvement: Patients often complain of orthopnea, dyspnea on exertion and rest, early morning headaches, and sleep disturbances. On observation, they may use accessory muscles of respiration, have paradoxical abdominal movements, and show signs of carbon dioxide retention (bounding pulse, chemosis, papilledema, and cyanosis), weak cough, and weak sniff. Diaphragmatic and intercostal muscle involvement is very common during the course of the disease but is rare at onset. The voice may become weaker and softer at the end of long sentences and interrupted by frequent sighs.

Pain: Patient complains of pain which is secondary to immobilization leading to pericapsulitis and contractures.

Sleep: Sleep architecture is affected, leading to increased morning fatigue.

TABLE 3 Summary of UMN and LMN symptoms and signs in amyotrophic lateral sclerosis.

Area		UMN	LMN
Trunk and extremity weakness	Symptoms	Loss of dexterity, weakness, spasms, fatigue, stiffness, and slowness	More pronounced weakness, wasting of muscles, split hand, pain due to pericapsulitis, buckling of knees, and painful contractures
	Signs	Spasticity, hyperreflexia, clonus, and positive Babinski's	Decreased motor power, bulk, diminished reflexes, fasciculations, cramps, pseudoneuritic pattern (foot drop, wrist drop, and claw hand), camptocormia, and head drop
Bulbar	Symptoms	Forced speech, choking on liquids, slowed chewing, inappropriate or spontaneous crying, laughing, or yawning	Greater degrees of weakness of face, palate, and tongue
	Signs	Spastic tongue and speech, hyperactive gag, brisk cough, and jaw jerk	Asymmetrical wasting of tongue, fasciculations, hypoactive gag, weak cough, and jaw jerk

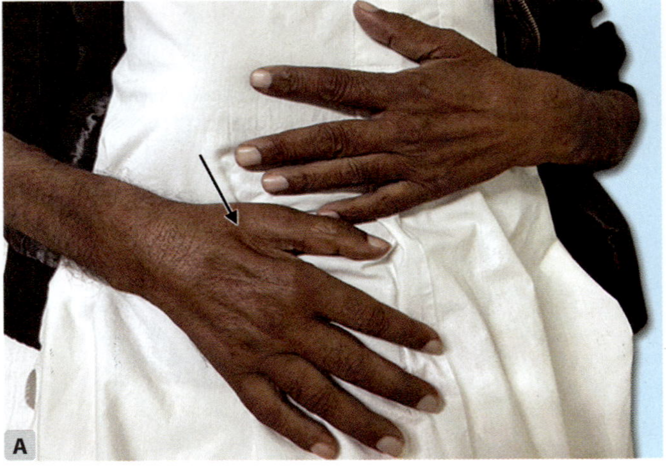

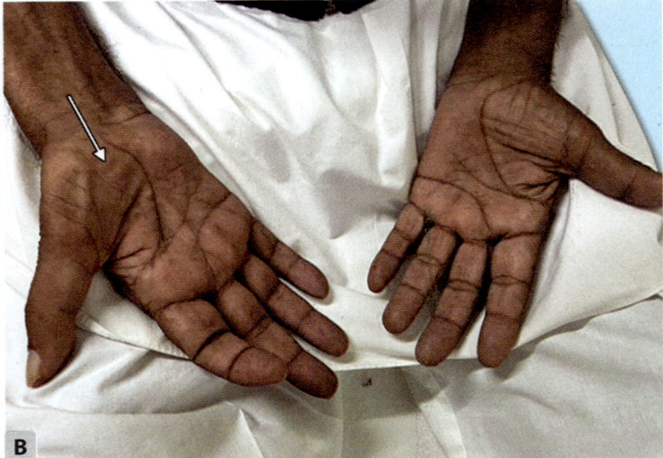

FIGURES 1 A & B: Disproportionate wasting of thenar eminence in an individual with amyotrophic lateral sclerosis (split sign). **(A)** Dorsal aspect (black arrow); **(B)** ventral aspect (white arrow).

Fatigue: Fatigue is a common complaint though its pathophysiology is unclear but it can range from disease involving the cerebral cortex down to the neuromuscular junction.

Depression: Patients often have depression, which may not be evident on initial assessment.

Weight loss: Severe weight loss disproportionate to the decrease in caloric intake can occur in patients and may represent an ALS cachexia-like state.

ATYPICAL CLINICAL FEATURES

Cognition: Around 40% of patients with ALS have cognitive impairment, while only 14% have frank frontotemporal dementia (FTD). Some patients (up to 30%) may begin with FTD onset which later evolves into ALS. The inheritance of ALS and FTD as a single trait has been seen due to the intronic expansion of GGGGCC hexanucleotide repeat within the *C9ORF72* gene.

Extraocular muscles manifestations: Extraocular muscles are relatively spared in patients with ALS. Although a study has shown visual acuity, gaze impersistence, voluntary upgaze restriction, eyelid opening apraxia, and saccadic horizontal smooth pursuits to be affected in patients with ALS as compared to similar-aged controls.

Bladder and bowel manifestations: The motor neurons of Onufrowicz that control the muscles of the pelvic floor, and the sphincter, bladder, and urethra are typically spared in ALS. Mild urgency of micturition and urinary retention may occur, while frank urge incontinence and bowel dysfunction are rare.

Sensory system manifestations: There is characteristic sparing of the sensory system, but patients may report vague sensory complaints in the distal extremities, which is not apparent on routine objective sensory testing.

Extrapyramidal manifestations: Nearly 5% of individuals with ALS may have extrapyramidal involvement which may present as impairment of retropulsion or impairment of postural reflexes.

SUBTYPES

Progressive bulbar palsy: About 19–28% of patients may present with bulbar palsy at onset. It is most commonly seen in postmenopausal women and may have worse prognosis. They usually present first with dysarthria followed by dysphagia which spreads locally and then involves the cervical, thoracic, and lumbosacral segment, respectively. Rarely, the disease may remain localized to the bulbar region (true progressive bulbar palsy).

Primary lateral sclerosis: Around 2–4% of all ALS patients present as a pure UMN syndrome called PLS that never progresses to involve the LMN. Age of onset is 50–55 years, and the rate of progression is very slow. Clinically, pure PLS can be diagnosed after 4 years of pure UMN signs with slow progression, higher level of function, and longer survival when compared to ALS.

Progressive muscular atrophy: Approximately 2% of all patients with ALS can present with a pure LMN syndrome which tends to have favorable prognosis. By definition, the condition must be pure LMN before designation as PMA for a period of time and needs reevaluation to look for the development of UMN signs.

Mills hemiplegic variant: This variant manifests with both UMN and LMN signs on one side of the body.

The flail arm and the flail leg variant: About 10% of patients with ALS can present with symmetric proximal and distal upper limb wasting with positive Babinski's sign known as "flail arm syndrome." Whereas, another 6% of patients can present with a pseudopolyneuritic variant of ALS affecting the lower limbs known as "flail leg variant." The survival in both these variants is longer than in ALS.

Familial amyotrophic lateral sclerosis: Globally, familial ALS (fALS) is observed in 5–10% of ALS patients, which may be autosomal dominant, autosomal recessive, or X-linked dominant. This number is lower in India (1–2%). fALS should be suspected when multiple generations in the same family have ALS. These usually have younger age at onset, lack male predominance, a shorter disease duration, and a predilection for the lower limbs. A mutation of large effect (presumably pathogenic) can be identified in 60–80% of fALS. The most common mutations identified are *C9orf72* (40%), SOD1 (20%), FUS (1–5%), and TARDBP (1–5%). **Table 4** illustrates the complex correlation between genes, pathology, and phenotypes. *C9orfF72* gene mutation which usually manifests as FTD-ALS is more common in the Caucasian population than among Asians. Recently, >20 genes have been reported to cause fALS.

Western pacific ALS: This unique type of ALS is found on the island of Guam in the Western Pacific. It is characterized by a combination of ALS-parkinsonism-dementia. Nearly 5% present with predominant ALS and 38% have a combination of parkinsonism and dementia. Various environmental substances including cycad seeds, aluminum, and silicon have been studied with regard to its pathogenesis. Cycad seeds have BMAA (beta-methylamino-L-alanine), which has neurotoxic effects.

CLINICAL STAGING

To monitor the progression of disease several staging systems have been described. **Table 5** demonstrates the King's staging system based on the number of affected regions of the body and the Milano-Torino (MITOS) functional staging system.

ETIOLOGY AND PATHOGENESIS

The cause of ALS remains unknown, but evidence suggests multiple molecular mechanisms that may ultimately combine to affect the loss of motor neurons

TABLE 4 Complex correlation between genes, pathology, and phenotypes.

ALS phenotypes	Predominant pathology	Associated genes
Classic ALS	TDP-43	*ALS2, SETX, TARDBP, VAPB, CHMP2b, OPTIN, PFN1, TUBA4a, UNC13a, FIG4, ELP3, NEK1, C21orf2, SIGMAR1, DCTN1, MATR3, CHCHD10, VCP, hnRNPA1, hnRNPA2b1, NIPA1, SMN1, TBK1, ATXN2, MOBP, SARM1, UBQLN2,* and *SQSTM1*
Classic ALS	SOD1	*SOD1*
Classic ALS	FUS	*FUS*
ALS with cognitive or behavioral impairment or comorbid FTD	TDP-43	*TARDBP, CHMP2b, TBK1, UBQLN2, SQSTM1, DCTN1,* and *UNC13a*
Classic ALS, ALS-FTD, FTD	TDP-43, p62, dipeptide repeats, RNA foci	*C9orf72*
Multisystem proteinopathy	TDP-43	*VCP, hnRNPA1, hnRNPA2b, SQSTM1*
Behavioral variant FTD	TDP-43	*CHMP2,* and *GRN*
Behavioral variant FTD	FUS	–
Semantic variant primary progressive aphasia	TDP-43	*GRN, C9orf72*
Semantic variant primary progressive aphasia	Tau	*MAPT*
Logopenic and nonfluent variant primary progressive aphasia	Tau	*MAPT*

(ALS: amyotrophic lateral sclerosis; FTD: frontotemporal dementia; FUS: fused in sarcoma; RNA: ribonucleic acid; SOD1: superoxide dismutase1; TDP-43: tar DNA-binding protein-43)

TABLE 5 Comparison of clinical staging in amyotrophic lateral sclerosis.

King's clinical staging	Staging	MITOS functional staging
Presymptomatic	0	Functional involvement (disease onset)
Involvement of one clinical region (disease onset)	1	Loss of independence in one functional domain
Involvement of two clinical regions	2	Loss of independence in two functional domains
Involvement of three clinical regions	3	Loss of independence in three functional domains
Substantial respiratory or nutritional failure	4	Loss of independence in four functional domains
Death	5	Death

(MITOS: Milano–Torino staging)

and their support systems which is enumerated in **Box 1**. Recent epidemiological studies have suggested a multi-hit hypothesis wherein it takes six hits for sporadic ALS to manifest. The nature of these hits may vary and in patients with genetic predisposition this number is lower. Research in fALS has informed us of many abnormalities at the molecular level.

PATHOLOGY

Gross pathology: Atrophy of the motor cortex together with grayness and atrophy of the ventral spinal roots and muscles can be seen on the specimen. The lateral columns of the spinal cord may appear gray representing sclerosis caused by gliosis.

BOX 1 Pathogenetic mechanisms in amyotrophic lateral sclerosis.

- Oxidative stress
- Glutamate excitotoxicity
- Mitochondrial dysfunction
- Neuroinflammation
- Protein aggregates
- Accumulation of neurofilaments
- Aberrant RNA metabolism

Microscopy: Lipofuscin accumulation and loss of Nissl substance are seen in the degenerating neurons. ALS is characterized by the accumulation of ubiquitinated proteins in the cytoplasm of degenerating motor neurons. TAR DNA-binding protein (TDP-43) has been seen to be a major component of neuronal inclusions.

DIAGNOSIS

CLINICAL EXAMINATION

The diagnosis of ALS is largely made on the basis of clinical examination, with ancillary testing used to confirm the clinical suspicion and to refute alternative diagnosis. World Federation of Neurology at El Escorial in Spain provided a set of clinical, electrodiagnostic, and pathological criteria for the diagnosis of ALS. This criterion divides candidates into definite, probable, possible, and suspected ALS based on the pattern of LMN and UMN involvement of bulbar, cervical, thoracic, and lumbosacral regions. The Airlie House review introduced the criterion of spread of disease from region to region and spread within a region. Other diseases that may mimic ALS need to be ruled out by radiological, pathological, and electrodiagnostic methods for this criterion to be applied. The Awaji criteria was put forward to include fasciculations as an electrodiagnostic marker for active denervation so that early cases of ALS can be identified. Recently, the Goldcoast criteria allowed the diagnosis of ALS if only one region is involved (**Table 6**).

ELECTRODIAGNOSIS

Electrodiagnosis supports the clinical examination and helps to identify the type of LMN disease (neurogenic versus myogenic) in weak muscles and pick up sensory involvement. Recently, transcranial magnetic stimulation (TMS) is being used to identify and monitor UMN disease.

- *Electromyography (EMG)*: EMG is done in all four segments (face, upper limbs, trunk, and lower limbs) especially in the weak muscles. To fulfill diagnostic criteria at least two muscles innervated by different roots and nerves need to show evidence of active denervation in the form of fibrillation, positive sharp waves, and/or fasciculations in a background of chronic denervation.
- *Nerve conduction studies (NCSs)*: Motor and sensory NCSs are usually normal in ALS. In advanced cases with severe wasting, we may see a drop in compound motor action potentials. Motor unit number estimation and motor unit number index are two methods which help us objectively to track the number of motor units over time.
- *Repeated nerve stimulation (RNS)*: RNS is usually normal in patients with ALS. Some patients may show a drop in RNS which portends a poor prognosis.
- *Single fiber EMG (SFEMG)*: This method helps identify increased jitter, which is due to unstable motor unit action potentials, a sign of ongoing denervation.
- *Transcranial magnetic stimulation*: Slowing of the central motor conduction time is seen in ALS, which is a reflection of central motor track integrity and is the difference between the latency of the response elicited by cranial versus cervical or cranial versus lumbosacral stimulation.

TABLE 6 Diagnostic criteria for amyotrophic lateral sclerosis.

Revised El Escorial diagnostic criteria for ALS (2000)	
Diagnostic certainty	**Definition**
Definite	UMN + LMN signs in three regions
Probable	UMN + LMN signs in two regions
Laboratory supported probable	UMN + LMN signs in one region/UMN signs in one or more regions with EMG evidence or acute denervation in two or more limbs
Possible	UMN + LMN signs in one region
Suspected	LMN signs only in one or more regions or UMN signs only in one or more regions
Gold coast criteria (2019)	
Progressive motor impairment documented by history or repeated clinical assessment, preceded by normal motor function	
Presence of UMN and LMN dysfunction in at least one body region (with UMN and LMN in the same body region if only one region involved) or LMN dysfunction in at least two body regions	
Investigations excluding other disease processes	

NEUROIMAGING

Imaging of the brain and spine is done to rule out other causes for the patient's symptoms. It is important to look for intrinsic/extrinsic compressive and noncompressive lesions for the UMN signs and image the roots for LMN signs.

- *Neuromuscular ultrasound*: Ultrasound can detect fasciculations better than EMG in the tongue and is less painful.
- *Magnetic resonance imaging (MRI)*: Hyperintensity of the CSTs can be prominent in patients with ALS. Voxel-based morphometry has quantified grey and white matter to detect cerebral atrophy in patients with ALS linked to cognitive impairment.

Newer modalities such as magnetic resonance spectroscopy (MRS), diffusion tensor imaging (DTI), and 5-fluorodeoxyglucose positron emission tomography (FDG-PET) also help in monitoring disease progression.

LABORATORY TESTS

Biomarkers are an important area of research to diagnose and monitor ALS with very little success. Laboratory tests are done to exclude other diseases that can present like ALS (**Box 2**).

DIFFERENTIAL DIAGNOSIS

Amyotrophic lateral sclerosis is a diagnosis of exclusion and it has both UMN and LMN features, which evolve over time. **Table 7** and **Box 3** give salient features to help differentiate ALS from other diseases.

NATURAL HISTORY AND PROGNOSIS

Predicting the course and prognosis in individual patients with ALS has been challenging despite the recent advances. Median survival remains 3 years and it is worse in patients with bulbar onset. Recent work has shown the rate of decline in function to be nonlinear with the early and late phase showing the most rapid worsening. **Table 8** lists the predictors of prognosis in ALS.

BREAKING THE NEWS

The diagnosis of ALS is devastating to any individual or family. It must be done with empathy, being careful not to take away hope and give enough time for questions. It is best to disclose the diagnosis and its implication over several meetings and guide the patient to authentic resources where they can learn at their own pace. This is also a good time to inform them of any clinical trials or ongoing research that they can participate in. If the diagnosis is in doubt, it is wise to wait till the patient fulfills the criteria and all other diseases have been ruled out.

BOX 2	Essential laboratory investigations in suspected amyotrophic lateral sclerosis.
Essential investigations:	
• Complete blood count and ESR	
• Full biochemical profile including calcium	
• CPK (>1,000 IU/L is unusual in ALS)	
• Serum protein electrophoresis	
Additional investigations in selected cases:	
• Vitamin B12 level	
• ANA by immunofluorescence, C-ANCA, P-ANCA	
• Paraneoplastic antibody screen	
• Serum leukocyte hexosaminidase levels	
• Anti-AChR, -MuSK antibodies	
• Anti-VGKC antibody	
• HIV serology	
• Lyme serology	
CSF studies	
Genetic testing:	
• *C9ORF72*	
• *SOD1*	
• *FUS*	
• *TARDP*	
Skin, nerve and/or muscle biopsy:	
• To look for ALS mimics	
CECT chest and abdomen or whole-body PET	
• To look for occult malignancy	

(AChR: acetylcholine receptor; C-ANCA: C-antineutrophil cytoplasmic antibody; MuSK: muscle-specific kinase; P-ANCA: perinuclear antineutrophil cytoplasmic antibody; VGKC: voltage-gated potassium channel)

TREATMENT

According to American Academy of Neurology guidelines the early referral of ALS patients to a multidisciplinary team improves outcomes. It often includes a dedicated neurologist, rehabilitation team, a respiratory physician, and a gastroenterologist (**Fig. 2**).

Despite an active area of research for several decades there is no cure for ALS. Till date only a few drugs have shown a modest improvement in survival.

Riluzole: It is a glutamate antagonist and given as a tablet or in liquid form dosed at 50 mg twice daily. It has shown an improvement in survival of 3 months which persists even in the final clinical stage of illness.

Edaravone: It is a free radical scavenger and administered intravenously dosed at 60 mg/day for 2 weeks every month. It has a small but significant slowing of functional decline using ALSFRS-R (ALS functional rating scale - revised) after 6 months of treatment with a recent study which showed benefits are maintained even at 1 year.

SYMPTOM MANAGEMENT

Patients with ALS suffer with various symptoms and it is necessary to identify and treat these to give them a better quality of life. **Table 9** lists some of these with the recommended pharmacological and nonpharmacological treatments.

Pain: Pain occurs late in the illness and can significantly affect the quality of life and needs to be addressed. Various treatment options are available and it is important to give active physical therapy to minimize the effect of immobilization as the disease progresses.

Dysphagia: The immediate assessment of the swallowing function is significant to plan intervention and prevent the early deterioration. Regardless of poor prognosis of ALS, adequate dysphagia management with diet and adoption of postural compensation maneuvers postpone the requirement for percutaneous endoscopic gastrostomy (PEG).

TABLE 7	Differential diagnosis of amyotrophic lateral sclerosis and appropriate investigations.	
Disorders of muscle	Inclusion body myositis	EMG, CPK, and muscle biopsy
	Polymyositis	EMG, CPK, muscle biopsy, and autoimmune screen
	Dermatomyositis	EMG, CPK, and skin and muscle biopsy
	Distal myopathies	Family history, muscle biopsy
	Myotonic dystrophy	Systemic features, genetic testing of repeat nucleotides
	Oculopharyngeal muscular dystrophy	EMG, CPK, muscle biopsy, and genetic repeat nucleotide testing

Continued...

Continued...

Disorders of neuromuscular junction	Myasthenia gravis	AChR and MuSK antibodies, RNS, and SFEMG
	Lambert–Eaton myasthenic syndrome	RNS, anti-VGKC antibodies
Disorders of motor nerves and nerve root	Multifocal motor neuropathy	NCS, EMG, and GM1 antibodies
	Chronic inflammatory demyelinating neuropathy	NCS, EMG, CSF analysis—albuminocytological dissociation
	Motor neuropathy associated with POEMS syndrome	Skeletal survey, serum protein electrophoresis
	Cramp-fasciculation syndrome	NCS, EMG
	Neuromyotonia	Anti-VGKC antibodies
	Paraneoplastic syndrome	Serum tumor markers, imaging including whole-body PET, and bone marrow biopsy
	Heavy metal poisoning	Urine or blood screens
	Mononeuritis multiplex	NCS, EMG, vasculitis screen, serology, and nerve and muscle biopsy
	Radiculoplexopathy	NCS, EMG (changes only along the root distribution) MRI
Disorders of motor neurons	Spinal muscular atrophy	*SMN* gene deletion assay
	X-linked spinobulbar muscular atrophy (Kennedy's disease)	Increased CAG repeats in DNA from blood
	Poliomyelitis or postpolio syndrome	History, NCS, and EMG
	Monomelic spinal muscular atrophy (Hirayama disease)	EMG, MRI cervical spine in flexion and extension
	Hexosaminidase A deficiency (late-onset Tay–Sachs disease)	Serum leukocyte Hex A activity and *Hex A* gene mutation analysis
CNS and spinal lesion	Syringomyelia or syringobulb a	MRI
	Tabes dorsalis	Syphilis serology
	Adrenomyeloneuropathy	Increased plasma levels of very-long-chain fatty acids
	Multiple sclerosis	MRI, oligoclonal bands, and evoked responses
	Lyme disease	Lyme serology
	Hereditary spastic paraparesis	Family history, genetic testing
	Vacuolar myelopathy	HIV testing
	Tropical spastic paraparesis	Antibodies against HTLV1 may be detected in serum and CSF, MRI
	Spinocerebellar ataxia type 3 (Machado–Joseph disease)	Genetic testing
	Adult polyglucosan disease	NCS, EMG, and biopsy
Endocrine	Thyrotoxicosis	TFT
	Hyperparathyroidism	Serum calcium, parathyroid hormone levels
	Subacute combined degeneration	Vitamin B12 concentration
	Coeliac disease	Serum testing of anti-tTg-IgA, small intestine biopsy

(AChR: acetylcholine receptor; HTLV1: human T-cell lymphotropic virus1; MuSK: muscle-specific kinase; NCS: nerve conduction study; POEMS: polyneuropathy, organomegaly, endocrinopathy, M protein, skin changes; RNS: repeated nerve stimulation; SFEMG: single fiber EMG; tTg-IgA: tissue transglutaminase-immunoglobulin A; VGKC: voltage-gated potassium channel)

BOX 3 Clues that point toward atypical motor neuron disease.

Pattern of motor involvement:
- Nonmyotomal pattern
- Nonregional spread
- Lack of concurrent UMN and LMN signs in the same spinal segments
- Insignificant wasting in a weak limb
- Extraocular weakness
- Symmetric involvement

Nonmotor involvement:
- Sensory
- Cerebellar
- Bladder or bowel involvement
- Extrapyramidal
- Cognitive or psychiatric dysfunction

Disease course:
- Absent bulbar involvement >1 year into illness
- Age of onset <35 years
- Spontaneous remissions
- Prolonged illness >5 years
- Positive family history

Associated illness:
- Malignancy
- Radiation exposure
- Electrical injury
- Poliomyelitis

TABLE 8 Prognostic indicators in amyotrophic lateral sclerosis.

	Better prognosis	Worse prognosis
Clinical features	Younger (<50 years)	Older
	Spinal onset	Bulbar onset
	Mild at diagnosis	Severe at diagnosis
	Increased time to diagnosis	Short time to diagnosis
	Slow deterioration	Rapid deterioration
	Progressive muscular atrophy	Progressive bulbar atrophy
	Primary lateral sclerosis	Some familial forms
	Flail arm or leg variant	Dyspnea onset
Examination findings	Well nourished	Malnourished
	Psychologically stable	Psychological distress
	Fasciculations mild or absent	Fasciculations widespread
Electro-physiology	Normal CMAP	Low CMAP
	No decrement on RNS	Decrement on RNS
	No jitter on SFEMG	Increased jitter on SFEMG
Laboratory investigations	Normal serum chloride	Low serum chloride
Treatment	Multidisciplinary care	No multidisciplinary care
	Riluzole, noninvasive ventilation, enteral feeding, and moderate exercise	Carbamazepine, minocycline, and diaphragmatic pacing
Genetic features	*SOD1* mutations: Glu22Gly, Gly38Arg, Asp91Ala, Gly94Cys, and Ile114Thr; reduced *EPHA4* expression	Ala5Val mutation in *SOD1*; repeat expansions in *C9orf72* or *ATXN2*; mutations in *FUS* (also associated with early onset); homozygosity for the C allele of rs12608932 in *UNC13a*

(CMAP: compound muscle action potential; RNS: repeated nerve stimulation; SFEMG: single fiber electromyography)

Nutrition management: Patients with ALS develop significant dysphagia leading to malnutrition. Identifying at risk individuals and planning for alternative methods for feeding like PEG need to be done early (**Flowchart 1**). This helps the patient to maintain body weight and improve quality of life.

Respiratory insufficiency management: The diagnosis and management of respiratory insufficiency is critical. Early discussion about all the treatment options such as noninvasive ventilation, invasive ventilation, and terminal phases should be done as soon as symptoms of respiratory problems develop. Patients and caregivers should be fully informed about the management of respiration to enable advance planning (**Flowchart 2**).

Noninvasive ventilation: It is recommended that noninvasive intermittent positive pressure ventilators (NIPPVs) or bilevel positive airway pressure can be used to provide noninvasive ventilation and they both have shown to improve quality of life and survival of the patient. This type of ventilation is recommended to the patients with daytime symptoms of nocturnal hypoventilation and mild bulbar symptoms.

Invasive ventilation: Invasive ventilation is indicated when noninvasive becomes inappropriate and no longer effective due to progression of disease. Invasive ventilation should be considered for the relevant patient with their consent. Although the use of this technique improves quality of life, but patient and caregivers should be made fully aware about the negative consequences of use of invasive ventilation, and it is essential to provide advance directions to avoid unplanned emergency intubation.

• Psychological, economical, and physical support
Caregiver, family, friends
Neurologist/ Respiratory Physician/ Gastroenterologist
• Pharmacological treatment, psychological management
• Usual care
Individual with ALS
Occupational therapist/ physiotherapist
Speech and language pathologist
• Adaptive equipment for activities of daily living (ADL)/instrumental ADL, orthosis and splinting, assistive technology
• Prevention and management of contractures, help reduce pain and spasticity, strengthening exercises
• Dysphagia and dysarthria management
• Nutritional care

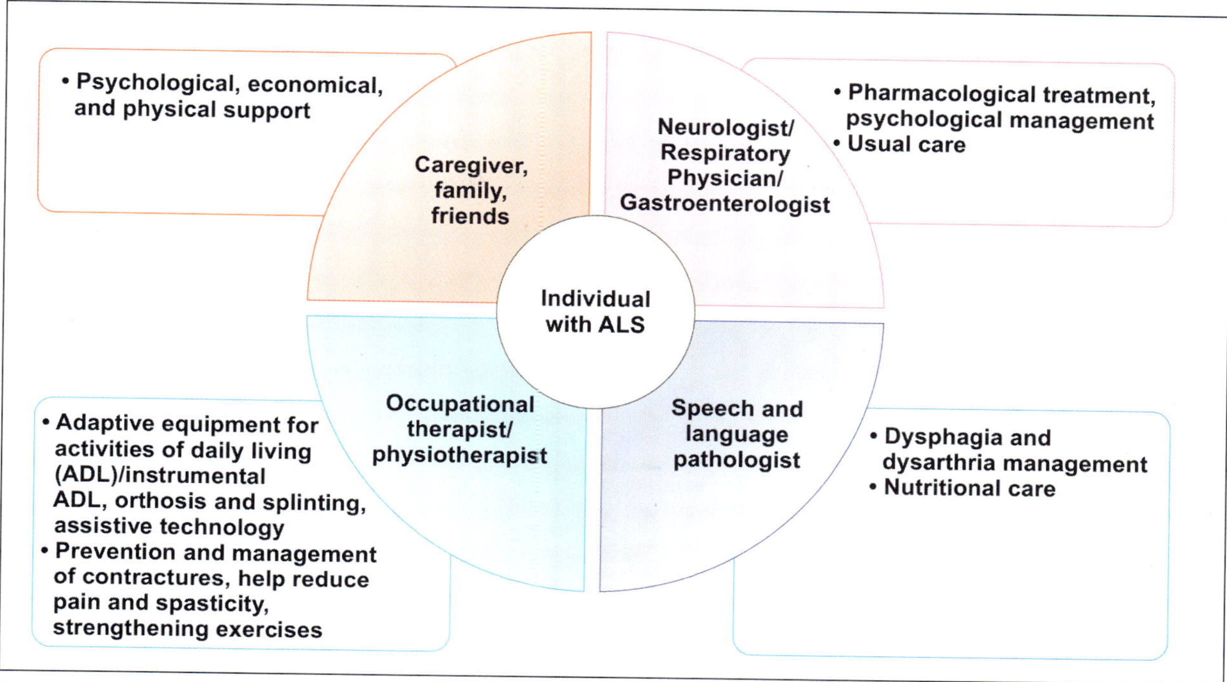

FIGURE 2: **Basic components of a multidisciplinary clinic in the care of an individual with amyotrophic lateral sclerosis (ALS).**

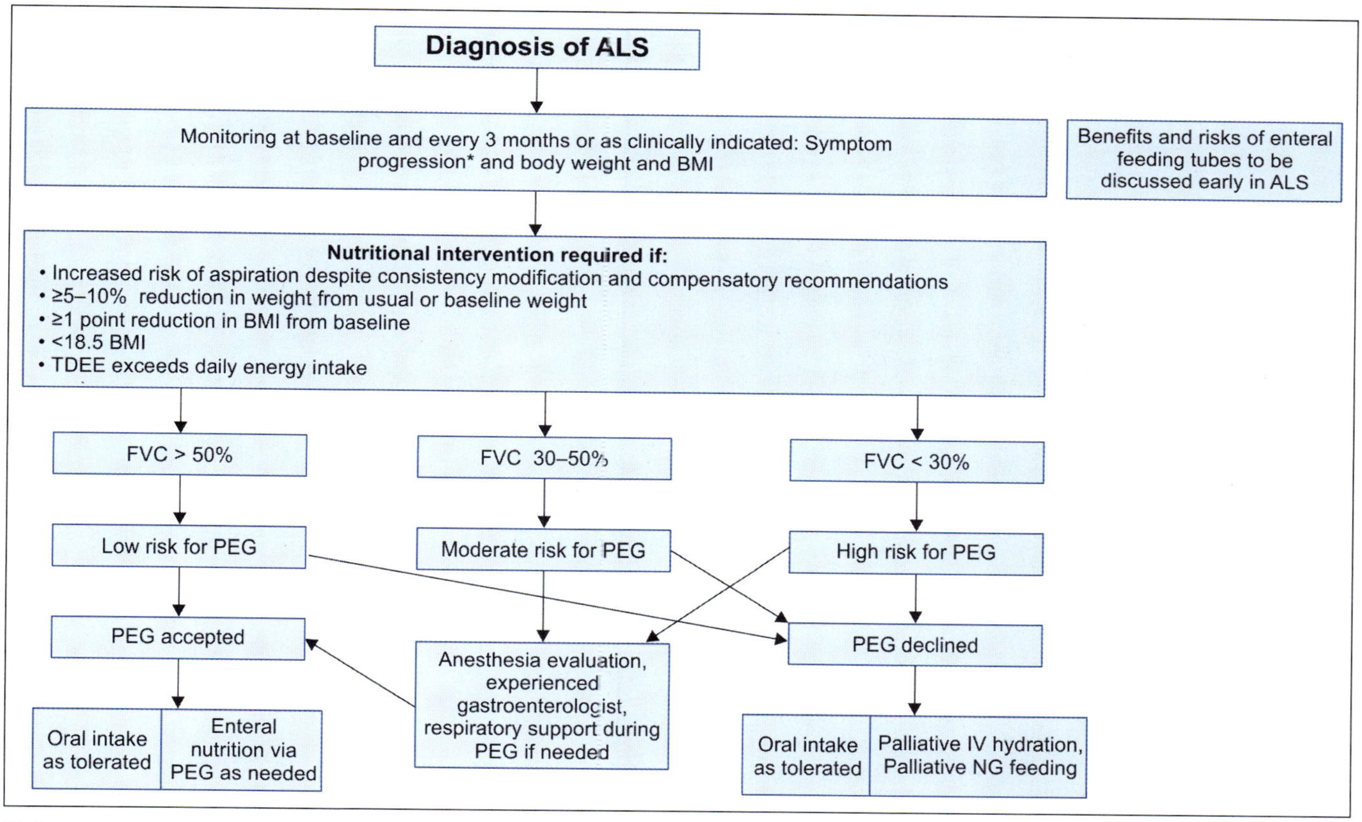

Diagnosis of ALS
Monitoring at baseline and every 3 months or as clinically indicated: Symptom progression* and body weight and BMI
Benefits and risks of enteral feeding tubes to be discussed early in ALS
Nutritional intervention required if:
• Increased risk of aspiration despite consistency modification and compensatory recommendations
• ≥5–10% reduction in weight from usual or baseline weight
• ≥1 point reduction in BMI from baseline
• <18.5 BMI
• TDEE exceeds daily energy intake
FVC > 50%
FVC 30–50%
FVC < 30%
Low risk for PEG
Moderate risk for PEG
High risk for PEG
PEG accepted
Anesthesia evaluation, experienced gastroenterologist, respiratory support during PEG if needed
PEG declined
Oral intake as tolerated
Enteral nutrition via PEG as needed
Oral intake as tolerated
Palliative IV hydration, Palliative NG feeding

*Bulbar questions in amyotrophic lateral sclerosis functional rating scale-revised.

(ALS: amyotrophic lateral sclerosis; NG: nasogastric; PEG: percutaneous endoscopic gastrostomy; TDEE: total daily energy expenditure)

FLOWCHART 1: **Algorithm for PEG insertion in patients with ALS.**

TABLE 9 Symptom management in amyotrophic lateral sclerosis.

Symptom	Pharmacological treatment	Nonpharmacological treatment
Constitutional		
Insomnia	• TCAs (i.e., amitriptyline) • Mirtazapine • Zolpidem • Benzodiazepines	• Comfort during sleep • Noninvasive ventilation
Fatigue	Modafinil	• Improve sleep • Behavioral therapy • Energy conservation techniques
Pain	• Analgesics • Acetaminophen • NSAIDs • Gabapentin • Pregabalin • Opioids	• Proper seating and positioning bracing • Physical therapy treatment like stretching and gentle exercises, TENS • Ultrasound • Ice/heat • Trigger point injections (with lidocaine and steroids)
Psychological		
Anxiety	• SSRI antidepressant (i.e., paroxetine) • Buspirone • Mirtazapine • Benzodiazepine (i.e., clonazepam)	Psychological support
Depression	• TCA • SSRI antidepressants • Mirtazapine • Venlafaxine • Bupropion	• Psychological support • Cognitive behavioral therapy
Pseudobulbar affect (emotional lability)	• Dextromethorphan/quinidine • TCA • SSRI antidepressant (i.e., sertraline)	
Otolaryngologic		
Sialorrhea	• TCA • Atropine sulfate • Glycopyrrolate • Hyoscyamine • Scopolamine transdermal patch	• Portable suction • Botulinum toxin in salivary glands • Irradiation of salivary glands
Laryngospasms	Benzodiazepines (i.e., lorazepam)	• Deep breathing • Reassurance
Gastrointestinal		
Constipation	• Docusate sodium • Senna glycoside • Bisacodyl • Lactulose • Magnesium citrate • Polyethylene glycol	• Increase hydration • Increase fiber intake • Prune or apple juice
Genitourinary		
Urinary urgency	• Oxybutynin • Tolterodine • Solifenacin • Mirabregron • Amitriptyline • Oxybutynin transdermal patch	
Erectile dysfunction	• Sildenafil citrate • Tadalafil • Vardenafil • Avanafil	
Musculoskeletal		
Spasticity	• Baclofen • Tizanidine • Dantrolene • Benzodiazepines • Cannabinoids (ITB and botulinum toxin in PLS and select cases of UMN-predominant ALS)	• Physical therapy • Stretching exercises
Cramps	• Mexiletine • Vitamin E • Phenytoin • Carbamazepine • Baclofen • Gabapentin	• Physical therapy • Massage • Hydration (tonic water)

(ALS: amyotrophic lateral sclerosis; ITB: intrathecal baclofen; PLS: primary lateral sclerosis; TCA: tricyclic antidepressant; TENS: transcutaneous electrical nerve stimulation)

TABLE 2 Certain presentations of myelopathy when pitfalls in diagnosis may occur.

Incorrect diagnosis thought of instead of myelopathy	Examples	Reasons for pitfalls in diagnosis
Motor neuron disease	Atlantoaxial dislocation, infiltrative myeloradiculopathy/myeloarachnoiditis	Combined UMN + LMN features
Stroke	Brown–Sequard syndrome/asymmetric myelitis	Unilateral motor weakness
Brachial plexopathy	Monomelic presentation of high cervical cord lesion	Unilateral upper limb weakness and pain
Lumbar canal stenosis	Conus medullaris + Cauda equina lesions	Asymmetric lower limb weakness and exercise-dependent radicular pain
Guillain–Barré syndrome	Acute myelopathy in the stage of spinal shock	Quadriplegia with generalized areflexia
Chronic neuropathy	• Myeloneuropathy • Incomplete cord involvement	Incomplete evolution of lesion or combined involvement
Peripheral vascular disorder or metabolic myopathy	Cauda conus lesions	Exercise-dependent symptoms
Hip and knee disorders	Chronic myelopathies	Spastic gait misinterpreted

TABLE 3 Differential diagnosis of myelopathies on the basis of the time course of evolution.

Hyperacute: Deficit occurs suddenly: ... seconds... minutes... hours...	• Vascular causes: Infarction, hematomyelia • Trauma
Acute (spinal cord dysfunction which lasts for at least 48 h and reaches to a maximum deficit within 3-4 weeks)	• Compressive (abscess, tumor, prolapsed disk) • Demyelination (MS/NMOSD/ADEM) • Infectious/parainfectious • Postvaccination (influenza, rabies, measles) • Systemic disease (SLE, Sjogren's syndrome, neurosarcoidosis, MCTD)
Subacute (spinal cord dysfunction occurs over weeks to months)	• Metabolic (e.g., vitamin B12 deficiency) • Compressive (tumor, tuberculosis, metastasis) • Inflammatory (systemic disorders)
Chronic (spinal cord dysfunction which is insidious in onset and gradually progressive over months to years)	• Compressive (spondylosis, tumor) • Heredodegenerative (hereditary spastic paraplegia, Friedrich's ataxia, adrenomyeloneuropathy) • Toxin (fluorosis, lathyrism) • Infections (HIV, HTLV, tabes dorsalis) • Vascular (dural AV fistula) • CNS demyelinating disease (primary progressive MS) • Craniovertebral junction anomaly/syringomyelia
Intermittent episodic symptoms	• Demyelination (MS, NMOSD, systemic inflammatory disorders) • Spinal AVM/dural AV fistula

(ADEM: acute disseminated encephalomyelitis; AVM: arteriovenous malformation; HTLV: human T-lymphotropic virus; MCTD: mixed connective tissue disorder; NMOSD: neuromyelitis optica spectrum disorder)

TABLE 4 Features of various spinal cord syndromes.

Syndrome	Common features	Certain examples
Complete transection of spinal cord	• Motor—weakness below the level of lesion • Sensory—all modalities of sensations are lost below the level of lesion • Bowel and bladder dysfunction • Initially, there is a stage of spinal shock with flaccidity, areflexia, and urine retention.	• Traumatic • Postinfectious acute transverse myelitis

Continued...

Continued...

Syndrome	Common features	Certain examples
Brown–Sequard hemicord syndrome	Ipsilateral (I/L) weakness with I/L loss of proprioception below the level of lesion; contralateral (C/L) loss of pain and temperature few segments below the level of lesion	Traumatic/demyelination/bullet injury
Central cord syndrome	Motor weakness (upper limbs > lower limbs); sensory impairment: dissociated sensory loss for pain and temperature with preserved position and vibration sense, cape-like sensory deficit may be present; bladder dysfunction (usually urinary retention)	• Syringomyelia • Ependymoma
Posterior-lateral cord syndrome	Spastic paraparesis and sensory ataxia	Subacute combined degeneration of cord (SACD): Vitamin B12 or folic acid deficiency, zinc toxicity leading to copper deficiency, HIV myelopathy, neurosyphilis
Anterior spinal cord syndrome	• Deficits below the level of lesion: • Motor—weakness • Sensory—pain and temperature loss with preserved position and vibration • Autonomic—bladder, bowel, and sexual dysfunction • Initially, there will be spinal shock with hypotonia and areflexia which is followed by gradual increase in reflexes to hyperreflexia and spasticity	Anterior spinal artery occlusion
Posterior column syndrome	• Impaired position, vibration, and light touch sensation • Sensory ataxia	• Tabes dorsalis • Posterior spinal artery syndrome
Anterior horn cells and pyramidal tract syndrome	• Asymmetric involvement of different limbs • LMN signs such as atrophy and fasciculations are seen along with UMN signs such as spasticity and hyperreflexia • Sparing of sensory and autonomic functions	Amyotrophic lateral sclerosis (*not a myelopathy*)

(LMN: lower motor neuron; UMN: upper motor neuron)

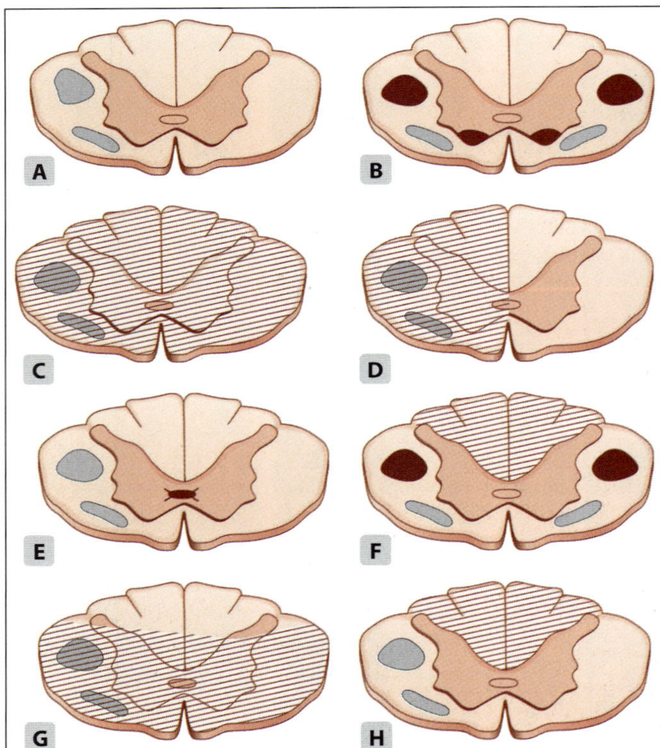

FIGURES 1 A to H: Spinal cord syndromes depending on the location of lesion in cord. (A) Normal cord; **(B)** Anterior horn cells and pyramidal tract syndrome; **(C)** Complete transection of spinal cord; **(D)** Brown–Sequard hemicord syndrome; **(E)** Central cord syndrome; **(F)** Posterior-lateral cord syndrome; **(G)** Anterior spinal artery syndrome; **(H)** Posterior column syndrome.

TABLE 5 Etiologies of compressive and noncompressive myelopathies.

Compressive	Noncompressive
• Degenerative disease (e.g., compression by osteophytes) • Traumatic (e.g., disk herniation, bone lesion) • Neoplastic (extra- or intradural tumors) • Infection (abscess) • Vascular (e.g., AV malformation, AV fistula, aneurysm) • Syringomyelia	• Infection (transverse myelitis due to viral/bacterial/fungal) • CNS demyelinating disorders (MS/NMO/ADEM) • Systemic inflammatory disease (e.g., SLE, sarcoidosis) • Spinal cord infarction • Toxic (e.g., lathyrism, nitrous oxide, radiation) • Metabolic (e.g., vitamin B12 or E deficiencies, hepatic disease) • Paraneoplastic • Degenerative (e.g., hereditary spastic paraplegia, SCA, Friedreich's ataxia)

(ADEM: acute disseminated encephalomyelitis; NMO: neuromyelitis optica;)

While the classical descriptions of myelopathies have been done in the form of compressive and noncompressive myelopathies, all etiologies of myelopathies cannot be classified as either compressive or noncompressive as some etiologies may have indeterminate or mixed etiologies. So now myelopathies have also been classified to have extrinsic lesions, intrinsic lesions, or mixed/indeterminate lesions with respect to the spinal cord involvement. The

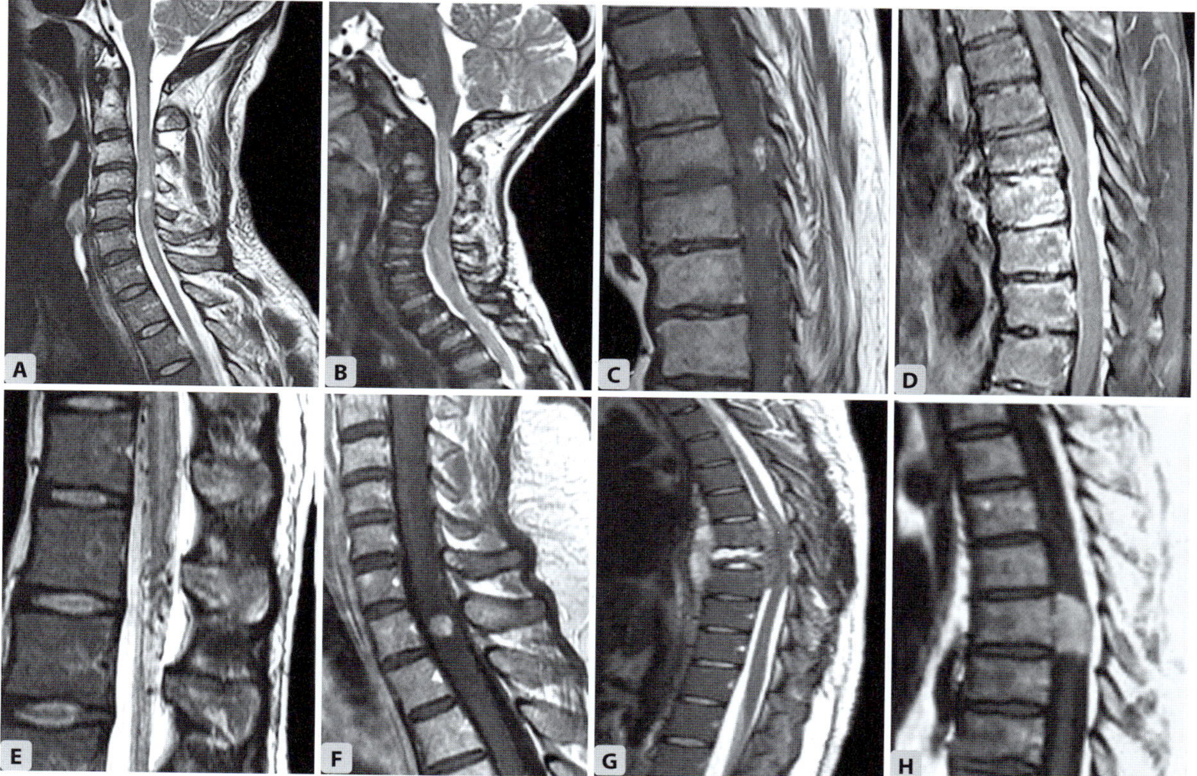

FIGURES 2 A to H: MRI patterns in different compressive myelopathy. (A) Acute post-traumatic myelopathy with a T2 hyperintense signal at C4-C5 level; **(B)** Chronic myelopathy with CV junction anomaly with T2 hyperintensity with thickening of cord; **(C and D)** T1 intensity change at endplate and postcontrast enhancement in the epidural region suggestive of epidural abscess; **(E)** T2 images showing flow voids in the dorsal cord suggestive of spinal AV malformation; **(F)** T1 contrast-enhancing intramedullary lesion: Ependymoma; **(G)** T2-enhanced spine showing osteomyelitis with discitis with cord compression secondary to TB spine; **(H)** T1 postcontrast-enhancing intraparenchymal lesion: Meningioma.

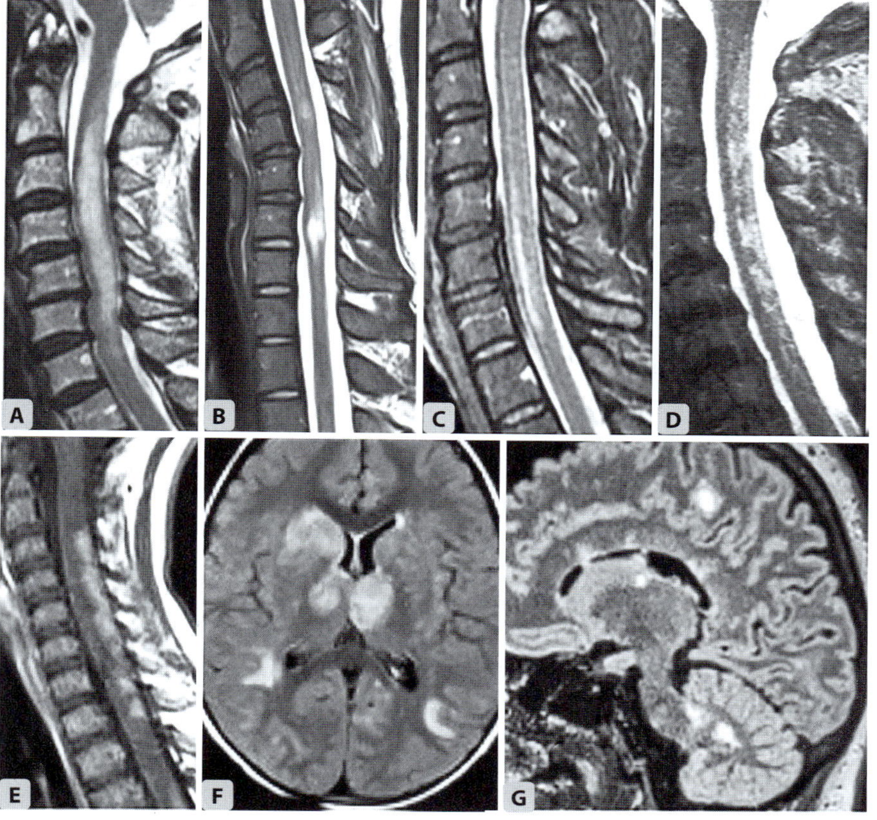

(MS: multiple sclerosis; NMOSD: neuromyelitis optica spectrum disorder; SACD: subacute combined degeneration)

FIGURES 3 A to G: MRI patterns in different noncompressive myelopathy. (A) Long-segment myelitis: In a patient with NMOSD; **(B)** Short-segment myelitis in a patient with MS; **(C)** Anterior spinal hyperintense signal in anterior spinal artery thrombosis with infarct; **(D)** Patchy posterolateral T2 hyperintense signal in SACD; **(E and F)** Patchy spinal lesions with asymmetric basal ganglia and subcortical lesion in ADEM; **(G)** MRI of brain in a patient with multiple sclerosis showing multiple juxtacortical, periventricular, and infratentorial lesions.

etiology may also be classified as congenital, genetic, traumatic, inflammatory, infective, and vascular. Such a combined approach to classify myelopathy can give further idea about the etiology of the myelopathy (**Table 7**).

TABLE 6 Some features differentiating compressive and noncompressive myelopathy.

Features	Compressive myelopathy	Noncompressive myelopathy
Radicular pain	Present	Absent
Local tenderness	Present	Absent
Onset	Gradual	Acute
Symmetry	Usually asymmetrical	Usually symmetrical

TABLE 7 Classification of myelopathies based on etiology and manner of cord involvement.

Type of lesion / Etiology	Extrinsic	Indeterminate/Mixed	Intrinsic
Genetic	Mucopolysaccharidosis		• HSP • Adrenomyeloneuropathy • SCA • Friedreich's ataxia
Congenital	Arachnoid cyst	• Syringomyelia • Craniovertebral junction anomaly • Spinal dysraphism	
Traumatic	Vertebra fracture dislocation		
Infective	• Epidural abscess • Tuberculous osteomyelitis		• Acute viral/ bacterial myelitis • Tuberculosis • Neurocysticercosis • HIV, HTLV • Syphilis
Inflammatory	• Rheumatoid arthritis • Ankylosing spondylitis		• MS • NMOSD • Postvaccinal • Idiopathic • Connective tissue disease
Vascular	Epidural hematoma	Dural AV fistula	• Infarct • Hematomyelia
Neoplastic	Metastasis		• Ependymoma • Lymphoma
Toxic	• Intrathecal methotrexate • Myodil arachnoiditis • Fluorosis	• Radiation • Electric injury • Acute myelopathy in asthma	• Lathyrism • Konzo • Nitrous oxide
Metabolic	Paget's disease		• B12 deficiency • Folic acid deficiency • Vitamin E deficiency • Copper deficiency
Degenerative	• Spondylosis • Disk prolapse		• Motor neuron disease

(HSP: hereditary spastic paraplegias; HTLV: human T-lymphotropic virus)

COMPRESSIVE VERSUS NONCOMPRESSIVE ETIOLOGIES

COMPRESSIVE MYELOPATHIES

Degenerative disease of spine: Degenerative compressive myelopathy commonly affects the cervical spine. Some degenerative and developmental causes that result in compressive cervical myelopathy are cervical spondylosis, rheumatoid arthritis, ankylosing spondylitis, basilar invagination, achondroplasia etc. Spinal canal stenosis secondary to disk herniation occurs commonly at the C6-7 level but may also occur at the C5-6 level and less frequently at the C4-5 level. The onset of symptoms in degenerative spine disease may be gradually progressive or may be sudden following carrying heavy load overhead, trauma, or fall. There is focal pain usually over the upper back region. Other features in chronic compressive cervical spine disease are weakness, gait unsteadiness, spasticity, sensory deficits, hyperreflexia of deep tendons, and Lhermitte's sign. On MRI, there is a hyperintense signal seen in cord on T2-weighted imaging (T2WI) close to the site of compression either by disk herniation or by osteophytes. There is narrowing of spinal canal with reduction in canal diameter maximally at the site of highest compression. The natural history of degenerative spondylotic disk disease is often unpredictable; while some patients develop myelomalacia with preserved activities of daily living, some patients develop progressive disability and so treatments need to be individualized according to the clinical presentation

Traumatic myelopathy: The most common cause resulting in traumatic myelopathy in India is road traffic accidents. Some other causes in decreasing frequency of occurrence are fall from height, assault, fall of object from above, and sports injury. According to one large Indian study, D12 and C5 were found to be the most common vertebral levels of injury.

Neoplastic causes of myelopathy: Tumors compressing the spinal cord can be divided into three categories: (1) Extradural, (2) intradural extramedullary, and (3) intradural intramedullary. The most common spinal tumors are extradural tumors and metastasis from other sources. Some examples of spinal tumors categorized accordingly are enlisted in **Table 8**.

MRI with gadolinium-contrast study guides the diagnosis of neoplastic causes for compressive myelopathy. While imaging of spine is essential to differentiate, there are certain clinical features that can help differentiating the site of pathology in the spinal cord (**Table 9**).

Spinal epidural abscess: Spinal epidural abscess commonly affects the lumbar spine, followed by thoracic and then cervical spine. *Staphylococcus aureus* is the most common organism with *Mycobacterium tuberculosis* being the second common organism responsible for epidural abscess. Other organisms are gram-negative bacilli, streptococci, coagulase-negative *staphylococci*, and anaerobic bacteria. The risk factors for occurrence of spinal epidural abscess are immunosuppressive states, diabetes mellitus, chronic kidney disease, alcohol abuse, chronic use of intravenous drugs, postspinal invasive procedures, local skin or soft-tissue infection, and sepsis. The common features of spinal epidural abscess are localized back pain, fever, and neurological deficit (motor weakness, sensory impairment, and/or bladder dysfunction). Spinal epidural abscess can present with neurological signs of spinal cord ischemia due to thrombosis of leptomeningeal vessels or compression of spinal arteries. MRI is the method of choice for the diagnosis. Spinal epidural abscess is a life-threatening condition which may require both medical and surgical intervention. Surgical decompression and drainage of pus are required in most patients along with intravenous antibiotics. A patient at high risk for surgery can go for antibiotic therapy with CT-guided aspiration. Empirical therapy should be started with antibiotics having methicillin-resistant *Staphylococcus aureus* (MRSA) coverage till the causative organism and antibiotic sensitivity report is available in blood culture or pus culture. Antibiotic therapy needs to be administered for 4–12 weeks and in case of associated osteomyelitis, it should be for 6–12 weeks.

Vascular malformation-associated myelopathy: Arteriovenous malformation (AVM) is commonly extramedullary,

TABLE 8 Neoplastic compressive myelopathies according to localization.

Extradural	Intradural extramedullary	Intradural intramedullary
• Lymphoma • Primary bone tumor of spine (e.g., osteoblastoma, giant cell tumor, Ewing's sarcoma) • Metastasis from other sources (e.g., carcinoma of breast, lung, prostate)	• Meningioma • Schwannomas • Malignant nerve sheath tumor • Neurofibroma • Leptomeningeal spread from other sources (e.g., leukemia, lymphoma, melanoma)	• Ependymoma • Astrocytoma • Hemangioblastoma • Cavernous angioma • Intramedullary spread from other sources (e.g., carcinoma of lung, breast, renal cell)

TABLE 9 Features differentiating intramedullary and extramedullary pathology.

Features	Intramedullary	Extramedullary
Radicular pain	Unusual	Common
Funicular pain	Common	Unusual
UMN signs	Late	Early
LMN signs	Predominant	Unusual, may occur at the segmental level
Bladder involvement	Early	Late
Trophic changes	Common	Unusual

and the most common malformation is the dural AV fistula type. Spinal AVMs can be classified into four types as enlisted in **Table 10**.

The common presentation of AVM is a gradually progressive myelopathy or sudden spinal subarachnoid hemorrhage. Usually, there is weakness of lower limbs which increases on exertion and relieves on resting. There may be pain in the back region or in lower extremities. MRI with T1 and T2WI shows posterior flow voids due to high-velocity flow with dilated perimedullary vessels causing indentation into the cord. Spinal DSA remains the diagnostic method of choice. Treatment of dural AVMs include surgical ligation or endovascular embolization.

Syringomyelia: Arnold-Chiari malformation is the congenital abnormality commonly associated with syringomyelia, while craniovertebral junction anomalies are other congenital causes. Acquired causes of syringomyelia are traumatic, chronic tubercular arachnoiditis, and intraspinal tumor. In an Indian study of 36 patients having Chiari malformation with syringomyelia, symptoms in decreasing frequency were high cervical pain, upper limb weakness, tingling and numbness, lower limb weakness and spasticity, small muscle wasting, imbalance, bladder dysfunction, and Charcot's joints. The clinical signs in the same study in a decreasing frequency were dissociated sensory loss, upper limb weakness and diminished reflexes, incoordination, wasting of small muscles of hand, lower limb weakness with Babinski sign positive, nystagmus, proprioception impairment, fasciculations, Horner's syndrome, XI cranial nerve involvement, Charcot's joints, and short neck. MRI is mainly useful for diagnosing syringomyelia. A CT scan of spine may be required for assessment of craniovertebral bone structure when the skeletal craniovertebral junction anomaly is present, to guide surgery planning. Surgical decompression is the only effective treatment for symptomatic syringomyelia.

NONCOMPRESSIVE MYELOPATHIES

In an Indian study of 80 patients having noncompressive myelopathy, 44 patients had acute myelopathy and 36 patients had chronic myelopathy. Of 44 cases with acute myelopathy, there was postinfectious myelitis in 13, neuromyelitis optica spectrum disorder (NMOSD) in 6, acute disseminated encephalomyelitis (ADEM) in 4, multiple sclerosis (MS) in 2, connective tissue disorder in 1, and idiopathic in 18. Of 36 cases with chronic myelopathy, Vitamin B12 deficiency is found in 8, MS in 2, mixed connective tissue disorder (MCTD) in 1, copper deficiency in 1, hepatic myelopathy in 1, radiation-induced myelopathy in 1, hereditary spastic paraplegia in 1, and idiopathic in 21.

Infectious/Parainfectious cause of acute transverse myelitis: Acute transverse myelitis (ATM) is defined as acute segmental spinal cord injury caused by inflammation. It can occur as a result of an infection or can occur as a parainfectious demyelination post-infection. ATM generally presents with acute onset of paraparesis/quadriparesis, sensory deficit with sensory level, and bladder dysfunction. CSF examination shows pleocytosis and increased protein than usual. MRI of spine with T2WI shows a central hyperintense signal in cord with edema. Blood tests are required for serology, culture, and detection of autoantibodies.

The diagnostic criteria for ATM are described in **Box 2**.

Acute infectious myelopathies can be caused by a plethora of varied infections including viruses, bacteria, fungi, and parasites (**Table 11**).

These patients are generally systemically ill with fever and have meningism. CSF examination would show severe pleocytosis, with raised proteins. **Box 3** delineates the

TABLE 10 Types of spinal AVMs.

Type 1	Spinal dural AV fistula
Type 2	Intramedullary glomus AVM
Type 3	Juvenile
Type 4 • Subtype 1	• Intradural perimedullary AV fistula • Single arterial supply, single small fistula, slow ascending perimedullary venous drainage
• Subtype 2	Multiple arterial supply, multiple medium fistulae, slow ascending perimedullary venous drainage
• Subtype 3	Multiple arterial supply, single giant fistula, large ectatic venous drainage

BOX 2 Diagnostic criteria for acute transverse myelitis.

- Bilateral (symmetric or asymmetric) sensory-motor and autonomic spinal cord dysfunction
- Well-defined sensory level
- Symptoms to reach up to maximum deficit between 4 hours and 21days of the onset
- Spinal cord inflammation to be demonstrated by:
  - CSF pleocytosis
  - Elevated IgG index
  - MRI showing gadolinium enhancement of spinal cord lesion
- Exclusion of causes such as vascular, neoplastic, compressive, and postradiation

(CSF: cerebrospinal fluid; IgG: immunoglobulin G)

TABLE 11 Common organisms causing acute infectious myelopathy.

Virus	Varicella zoster, herpes simplex, CMV, EBV, WNV, Zika, influenza, HIV, HTLV-1
Bacteria	TB, syphilis, Lyme disease, diphtheria, pertussis, tetanus, *Campylobacter jejuni*, mycoplasma
Fungi	Aspergillus, cryptococcus, blastomyces, coccidioides
Parasite	Cysticercosis, toxoplasmosis, schistosomiasis

(HTLV-1: human T-cell lymphotropic virus type 1; WNV: West Nile virus)

BOX 3	Clinical clues to suggest acute infectious myelopathy.
• Fever	
• Encephalopathy	
• Meningeal signs (neck rigidity/Kernig's sign)	
• Systemic infection	
• Immunocompromised state	
• Enlarged lymph nodes	
• Recurrent genital infections	
• Residence in and endemic region for parasitic infections	
• Skin rash (may give a clue to the cause to organism):	
◦ Enterovirus 71: Vesicular rash involving hands, feet, and buccal mucosa	
◦ Herpes zoster: Specific dermatomal distribution	
◦ Lyme disease: Erythema chronicum migrans	

common clinical clues which give a hint of acute infectious myelopathy.

Treatment of infection with specific antibiotics, antiviral, antifungal, or antiparasitic medication needs to be considered according to the causative organism. For reducing spinal cord inflammation, steroid therapy is usually considered in most of the cases.

Parainfectious acute myelitis differs from acute infectious myelopathy by the absence of systemic abnormalities, with patients having a history of having recovered from a recent febrile illness (usually viral) about 2–3 weeks back.

Certain patients with ATM may have no preceding illness to suggest any infectious or parainfectious etiology, and a detailed work-up for central nervous system (CNS) demyelinating diseases and systemic inflammatory disorders and infections is negative. Such patients are classified as acute idiopathic transverse myelitis.

Box 4 delineates the diagnostic criteria for acute idiopathic transverse myelitis.

BOX 4	Criteria for acute idiopathic transverse myelitis.
Inclusion criteria	
• Sensory/motor/autonomic dysfunction attributable to the spinal cord	
• Bilateral signs/symptoms (may be symmetric/asymmetric)	
• Clearly defined sensory level	
• Exclusion of extra-axial compressive etiology by neuroimaging (MRI, myelography: CT spine alone not adequate)	
• Inflammation in spinal cord demonstrated by CSF pleocytosis/elevated IgG index/gadolinium enhancement on MRI	
• If none of the inflammatory criteria is met at symptom onset, repeat MRI or CSF study between 2 and 7 days from symptom onset	
• Progression to nadir between 4 hours and 21 days following onset of symptoms (if the patient awakens with symptoms, the symptoms must become more pronounced from point of awakening)	
Exclusion criteria	
• History of radiation treatment involving spine in the last 10 years	
• Features consistent with anterior spinal artery thrombosis	
• Abnormal flow voids on cis sequence MRI of spine suggestive of AVFs	
• Brain MRI suggestive of multiple sclerosis/NMOSD	
• History of apparent optic neuritis	
• Clinical/laboratory evidence of infections such as Lyme disease, syphilis, HIV, HTLV-1, and other viruses (e.g., HSV, VZV, CMV, EBV)	
• Serologic/clinic evidence of systemic connective tissue diseases such as sarcoidosis, SLE, Sjogren's syndrome, Behcet's disease)	

(AVF: arteriovenous fistulas; HSV: herpes simplex virus; HTLV-1: human T-cell lymphotropic virus type 1; NMOSD: neuromyelitis optica spectrum disorder; VZV: varicella-zoster virus)

Central nervous system demyelinating disorders causing acute myelopathy: Multiple sclerosis, NMOSD, and ADEM are inflammatory disorders that cause CNS demyelination.

Acute disseminated encephalomyelitis: It is characterized by diffuse demyelination of cerebral white matter of spinal cord. It usually occurs post-infection or post-vaccination. It is usually a monophasic disease but may also have a recurrent form like that of MS.

Types of ADEM:

- *Monophasic ADEM*: Symptoms may evolve or fluctuate up to the period of 3 months. If symptoms re-appear during tapering or within 1 month of tapering off the steroids, then it is considered as the same episode.
- *Recurrent ADEM*: Recurrence after 3 months of symptoms that were at the time of the initial presentation. MRI findings are the same as previous though there may be an increase in the size of lesion. But there should not be any new lesion on MRI.
- *Multiphasic ADEM*: Recurrent disease that fulfills the criteria for ADEM, but there are newer symptoms that are different from the initial presentation. MRI also shows new lesions.

The common presenting features of ADEM are encephalopathy in the form of irritability or drowsiness and focal neurological deficits. In one Indian study, the common clinical features included fever at onset, decreased sensorium, cranial nerve palsy (facial, extraocular, or bulbar), motor weakness (paraparesis/quadriparesis/hemiparesis), seizures, visual problems, gait disturbance, bladder dysfunction, neck rigidity, ataxia, basal ganglia involvement (chorea/dystonia), hyperreflexia, positive Babinski sign, and autonomic involvement. In cases with a history of infection, the mean duration from the onset of prodromal symptoms to the onset of ADEM was 17 days. MRI is the investigation of choice. T2WI shows hyperintense signals bilaterally but asymmetrical typically in subcortical locations with surrounding edema. Thalami and brainstem may also be involved. T1WI with gadolinium contrast may show an open ring sign. In a small proportion of cases, the disease is more fulminant with hemorrhagic lesions which is called acute hemorrhagic leukoencephalitis. CSF examination may show CSF pleocytosis and an increased protein level in majority of cases, but the CSF picture may also be normal. Oligoclonal bands may also be present in some cases of ADEM. Steroid therapy with IV methylprednisolone administered for 3-5 days followed by oral prednisolone given for 6-8 weeks is the commonly considered therapy for ADEM. Intravenous immunoglobulin is an alternative treatment and can be considered in case of acute hemorrhagic leukoencephalitis. In case of recurrent or multiphasic ADEM, detailed evaluation of other causes such as NMOSD, sarcoidosis, lymphoma, and paraneoplastic disorders followed by treatment with cyclophosphamide, azathioprine, and rituximab would be required.

Multiple sclerosis: It is an autoimmune inflammatory demyelinating disease of the CNS. The exact cause of MS remains unknown. Higher prevalence in siblings suggests the role of genetic factors. Higher prevalence in countries with increasing latitude and among families with higher standards of living (better hygiene and sanitary facilities) suggests the role of environmental factors. Vitamin D3 deficiency is also associated with a higher risk of MS and also increases the chances of relapse. Several viruses such as Epstein–Barr virus (EBV), human herpes virus, and measles are considered as risk factors for MS.

Types of MS are as delineated in **Box 1 chapter 192** and diagnostic criteria are delineated in **Table 1 chapter 192**. The treatment of MS requires disease-modifying treatment as well as symptomatic treatment along with physiotherapy. Acute attacks are treated with intravenous steroids. Disease-modifying therapy for MS includes interferon (IFN) beta 1a, IFN beta 1b, glatiramer acetate, natalizumab, fingolimod, teriflunomide, and dimethyl fumarate. Symptomatic treatment of MS is delineated in **Table 2 chapter 192**.

Neuromyelitis optica spectrum disorders: It is a CNS demyelinating disease affecting the spinal cord and optic nerve. During an acute attack, intravenous methylprednisolone is given for 5 days followed by oral steroid therapy. In cases not responding to steroids, plasma exchange is considered. For preventing the relapses, immunosuppressive medicines such as azathioprine, mycophenolate mofetil, or rituximab need to be considered.

Myelopathy associated with systemic disease: Transverse myelitis is reported to occur with systemic inflammatory diseases such as scleroderma, systemic lupus erythematosus (SLE), Sjogren's syndrome, MCTD, antiphospholipid antibody syndrome, ankylosing spondylitis, Bechet's disease, and sarcoidosis. Myelopathy is seen most frequently with Sjogren's syndrome followed by sarcoidosis and then SLE. Investigations should include autoimmune profile, MRI, and CSF. MRI shows a hyperintense signal in cord on T2WI and variable gadolinium enhancement and CSF may show increased protein. Treatment with pulse dose of steroid is started and in case of suboptimal response, a combination of steroids with cyclophosphamide may be beneficial. A detailed general examination with assessment of classical diagnostic definition criteria of these systemic disorders is often more helpful in elucidating correct etiologic diagnosis and formulating correct management rather than ordering multiple costly investigations randomly.

Table 12 summarizes features to differentiate between MS, NMOSD, ADEM, post-vaccinal demyelination, myelitis associated with connective tissue disorders, and idiopathic ATM.

Spinal cord infarction: Spinal cord infarction is less common than cerebral infarction. The arterial supply of spinal cord is composed of single anterior spinal artery (ASA) and paired posterior spinal arteries (PSA). Spinal cord infarction is generally seen in the setting of severe atherosclerosis of spinal vessels, aortic pathology (aortic thrombosis, dissection, or aneurysm), cardioembolism, systemic hypotension, fibrocartilaginous embolism, radiation-induced vasculopathy, prothrombotic states, and during aortic surgery or percutaneous procedures such as epidural steroid injection. Spinal cord infarction can be of two types of syndromes: (1) anterior spinal artery syndrome caused by ASA occlusion and (2) posterior spinal artery syndrome caused by involvement of PSA.

Anterior spinal artery syndrome: Weakness (initially flaccid, later spastic) and loss of pain and temperature below the level of lesion, preservation of proprioception, bladder and bowel impairment, and acute back pain at the level of lesion are common features of ASA syndrome. The patient may also have autonomic dysfunction with hypotension and bradycardia.

Posterior spinal artery syndrome: It is a much rare condition than the ASA syndrome. It may occur unilaterally or bilaterally. There is loss of position and vibration below the level of lesion and total anesthesia at the level of lesion. There may be weakness which is mild and transient.

MRI shows a hyperintense lesion on T2WI and diffusion-weighted imaging (DWI) shows diffusion restriction in the ischemic area. Axial and sagittal sections are needed for better visualization of the extent of lesion. Vasculitis and thrombotic profile also need to be considered in appropriate settings.

Antiplatelet therapy with statin is initiated in patients with atherosclerotic disease. Avoiding hypotension and keeping higher mean arterial pressure (MAP) are proven to be effective. In selected patients, lumbar CSF drainage may be considered to increase spinal cord perfusion pressure. Bladder catheterization, deep venous thrombosis (DVT) prophylaxis, avoiding bedsores by regularly turning the patient side to side, and prophylactic use of proton-pump inhibitors to avoid gastrointestinal stress ulcers are the treatment to be considered to avoid complications of paraplegia/quadriplegia. Physical and occupational therapy is to be initiated at the earliest.

Metabolic and toxic myelopathies: Some common causes of metabolic and toxic myelopathies are:

TABLE 12 Summary of features to differentiate between MS, NMOSD, ADEM, postvaccinal demyelination, myelitis associated with connective tissue disorders, and idiopathic ATM.

Condition	Clinical features	MRI findings: Spine	MRI findings: Brain	CSF findings
Multiple sclerosis	• Partial myelitis, mild asymmetric involvement • Previous episodes of dysfunction with recovery	Lesion < 2 segments, peripherally located, lateral and posterior funiculi	• White matter lesions • Dawson fingers • Periventricular, juxtacortical, and infratentorial lesions with dissemination in space and time	Positive OCB, raised IgG index
NMO	Severe deficits, predominantly in women, past myelitis/optic neuritis/ area postrema syndrome, hypersomnia	Long segmental lesion > 3 segments, cord swelling, postcontrast enhancement in acute state	Hypothalamic or brainstem lesion, or subtle periventricular lesions (in about 60%)	CSF pleocytosis in acute state, no OCB in 80%, normal/mildly raised IgG index
ADEM	Acute monophasic illness in most, more in children; with encephalopathy, fever, viral prodrome preceding neurosymptoms	Variable lesion length	• Large confluent white matter lesions, • All lesions of similar duration, no old lesions	CSF pleocytosis, OCB/ IgG index may be normal or transiently raised
Postvaccinal demyelination	Monophasic illness within 3 weeks of vaccination	Variable lesion length	Variable lesion	CSF pleocytosis, OCB/ IgG index may be normal or transiently raised
Myelitis associated with connective tissue disorders	Associated connective tissue involvement: • *Sjogren syndrome*: Dry mouth, eyes, joint pain, ANA, Ro/La Ab • *Sarcoidosis*: Skin changes, hilar lymph nodes, ACE high • *Behcet's syndrome*: Oral genital ulcers, pathergy test positive	Variable	Variable	CSF pleocytosis
Idiopathic transverse myelitis	Monophasic, all exclusion criteria ruled out	Variable lesion length	Normal	CSF pleocytosis, OCB/ IgG index may be normal or transiently raised

(ADEM: acute disseminated encephalomyelitis; ATM: acute transverse myelitis; NMO: neuromyelitis optica; NMOSD: neuromyelitis optica spectrum disorder; OCB: oligoclonal band)

- Deficiency of vitamin B12, folate, vitamin E, or copper
- Exposure of toxins such as heroin, nitrous oxide, and organophosphates
- Lathyrism, Konzo
- Chronic liver disease
- Fluorosis
- Radiation therapy
- Chemotherapeutic agents such as cisplatin or intrathecal methotrexate

Manifestations of vitamin B12 deficiency: Neurological manifestations of vitamin B12 deficiency are subacute combined degeneration (SACD) and polyneuropathy. Features of SACD are paresthesia, gait difficulty, weakness in lower limbs, impaired position and vibration sense, spasticity, positive Babinski sign, abnormal tendon reflexes, positive Romberg's test, and Lhermitte's sign. MRI is needed to rule out other disorders and it can show hyperintense signals in the posterolateral cord on T2WI. Vitamin B12 levels may not correspond to the severity of disease and may be normal.

Vitamin E deficiency may cause spinocerebellar syndrome, peripheral neuropathy, and ophthalmoplegia. Copper deficiency can occur in the setting of excess zinc supplementation which can cause sensory ataxia and SCD along with optic neuropathy.

Heroin can cause transverse myelopathy, rhabdomyolysis, and stroke. Nitrous oxide inactivates vitamin B12 and causes SCD. Triorthocresyl phosphate (TOCP) is an organophosphate which causes myelopathy as a late complication. It causes spinal cord atrophy.

Consumption of lathyrus sativus as a staple diet causes neurolathyrism. It causes pain and stiffness of the lower limbs followed by weakness. It results in progressive walking difficulty. Konzo is caused by consumption of casava plant usually during draught. It causes paraparesis which is irreversible and without any sensory or bladder impairment. There is no specific treatment except for physical therapy.

Chronic liver disease rarely causes myelopathy. It presents as progressive spastic weakness of lower limbs without bladder and sensory impairment.

Fluorosis can cause compressive myelopathy due to ossification of the posterior longitudinal ligament and ligamentum flavum. Decreasing intake of fluoride-rich water and surgical treatment of compression by laminectomy relieve the symptoms of myelopathy.

Methotrexate can cause myelopathy by decreasing the folate level or by direct injury to cord causing vacuolar myelopathy.

Myodil, a contrast medium used for myelography in the past, has been described to cause myeloarachnoiditis with cauda-conus syndrome. Similar myeloarachnoiditis may also rarely develop post-spinal surgery.

Radiotherapy used for the treatment of cancers may lead to delayed-onset postradiation myelopathy after months to years.

Rarely chronic myelopathies may also occur post-exposure to *high-voltage electric current.*

Myelopathy associated with chronic infections: Human immunodeficiency virus (HIV), human T-lymphotropic virus (HTLV), and tabes dorsalis (associated with neurosyphilis) are chronic infections which can lead to chronic myelopathy.

HIV-associated myelopathy presents with a vacuolar myelopathy. It generally presents in an advanced stage of disease with low CD4 counts. It presents with chronic progressive paraparesis with tractopathy involving combined lateral and posterior column dysfunction, with bladder involvement in late stages. A normal MRI of spine, negative HTLV-1, normal vitamin B12, and no response to vitamin B12 treatment are important to consider HIV myelopathy and persons living with HIV infection. It is treated with appropriate antiretroviral drugs, and timely therapy can stabilize the course and partially reverse the signs and symptoms.

HTLV myelopathy presents with chronic spastic, predominantly motor, paraparesis, with bladder involvement and ataxia in advanced stages, with normal MRI of spine and normal CSF. It is diagnosed by HTLV antibody testing. It has an insidious progressive course, and management consists of symptomatic antispasticity treatment and rehabilitation.

Tabes dorsalis is a manifestation of chronic neurosyphilis and is now becoming very rare. It was more common in the pre-penicillin era when syphilis treatment was not available. It is important to rule out this disorder in patients with chronic myelopathy as it is treatable. It presents with predominant posterior cord syndrome with sensory ataxia, girdle pain, Lhermitte's phenomenon, with bladder involvement and impotence being seen. It is rare that patients may present with "sudden painful crisis" consisting of severe abdominal pain without any cause, which may lead to exploratory laparotomy with normal findings. One fifth of patients may have associated optic atrophy. Another classic characteristic finding (in up to 90% of patients) is the Argyll Robertson pupils (the pupils are bilaterally small and fail to constrict further in response to light, but they do respond normally to accommodation, which is a specific finding seen in neurosyphilis).

Paraneoplastic myelopathy: Paraneoplastic myelopathy is rare disorder and may occur in cancer of lungs, breast, thyroid, and Hodgkin's lymphoma. The most common antibody in paraneoplastic myelopathy is anti-Hu. Myelopathy is usually a part of encephalomyelitis. Other antibodies causing paraneoplastic myelopathy are anti-CV2/CRMP5 and antiamphiphysin. It usually involves the thoracic spinal cord. MRI shows a hyperintense signal on T2WI and also shows contrast enhancement. CSF examination shows an increased protein level. **Table 13** enlists different malignancies and antibodies associated with paraneoplastic myelopathies.

OVERALL APPROACH TO EVALUATION

Myelopathies can be suspected clinically based on specific clinical features. Specific mimics and chameleons are important to consider to avoid pitfalls in diagnosis. Once a myelopathy is suspected, its vertical level (cervical/dorsal/lumbosacral) of involvement is considered according to the clinical features of involvement. This should be followed by ascertainment of the horizontal involvement or specific patterns of involvement (e.g., hemi-cord/posterior/posterolateral etc.). Subsequently, the etiology or the cause of myelopathy should be considered based on the speed of evolution/progression of the symptoms and comorbidities.

Acute/subacute myelopathies have different causes as compared to chronic progressive myelopathies. **Flowchart 1** provides an approach to acute myelopathies and important steps in diagnosis. After the initial clinical localization and differential considerations, focused

TABLE 13 Common antibodies and malignancies causing paraneoplastic myelopathy.

Cancers associated with paraneoplastic myelopathy	Associated paraneoplastic antibody
Small cell lung cancer	• Amphiphysin • CRMP-5 • GAD • Cation channel Ab
Breast cancer	PCA2
Ovarian cancer	ANNA-2
Non-small cell lung cancer	Neuronal and muscle AChR Ab

(ANNA-2: antineuronal nuclear antibodies; CRMP-5: collapsin response-mediator protein-5; GAD: glutamic acid decarboxylase; PCA2: Purkinje cell cytoplasmic antibody type 2)

imaging of spine, with/without brain, would be required. Compressive and inflammatory/infective/vascular disorders would be subsequently considered based on imaging features. Once compressive etiologies are ruled out, a lumbar puncture for CSF study and blood markers for infections and systemic connective tissue disease as well as metabolic/toxic etiologies would be required. Chronic myelopathies generally have an insidious onset and present late into the illness, with an acute/subacute recent worsening, or they may present with some other systemic/metabolic disorder and findings of chronic myelopathy are observed. Hence, it becomes important to take detailed history and examination to diagnose such myelopathies. **Table 14** delineates important causes of chronic myelopathies and their salient features. **Table 15** enlists certain important investigations useful in patients with myelopathies and their relevance in diagnosis. After this approach, most of the patients with myelopathy would be diagnosed. About 10–20% of cases of myelopathy may present with a completely normal MRI of spine. **Table 16** discusses further points to consider in patients with myelopathy with normal MRI.

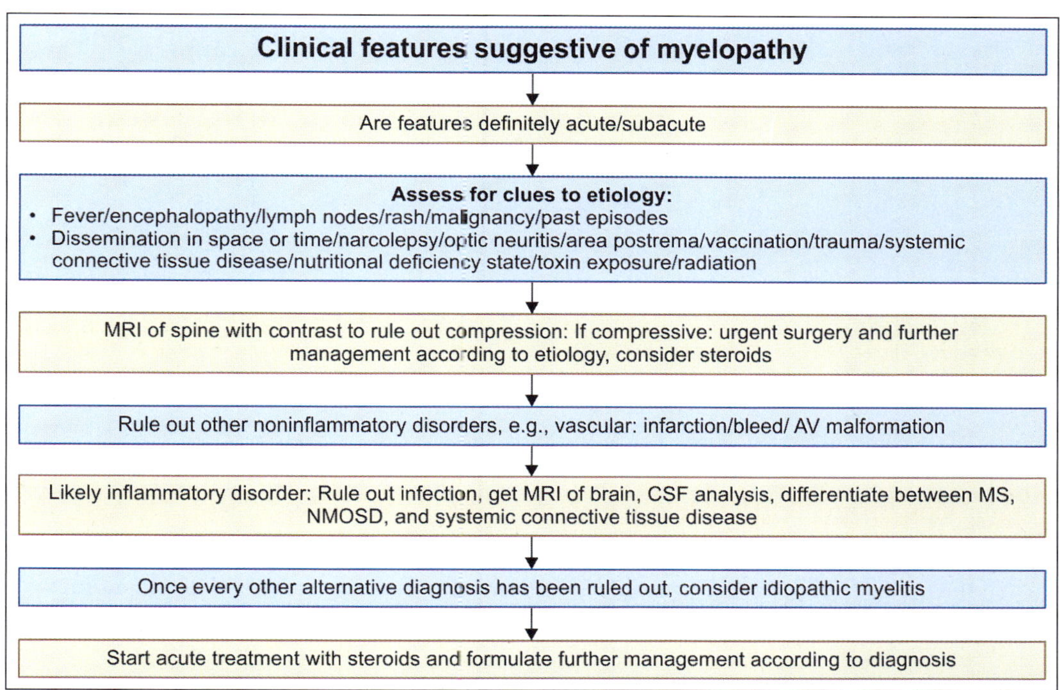

FLOWCHART 1: **Approach to acute/subacute myelopathy.**

TABLE 14 Causes of chronic myelopathies and salient features.

Etiology/Disorder	Salient features
Nutritional	• Vitamin B12/folic acid deficiency: SACD with associated polyneuropathy, macrocytic anemia, low serum levels raised homocysteine, methylmalonic acid • Copper deficiency: SACD, normal B12, folic acid, no anemia, low serum copper, high serum zinc • Vitamin E deficiency: Spinocerebellar ataxia, retinal dysfunction, low serum alphatocopherol
PPMS	Abnormal MRI of brain, short segment spine lesions, raised CSF OCB/IgG index, excluded other causes of demyelination/inflammation/infection
Spinal AV dural fistula	Elderly male with slow progressive myelopathy with T2 hyperintensity in cord with peripheral hypointensity, with perimedullary flow voids, with diagnostic spinal angiogram
Toxic myelopathy	• History of exposure: Intravenous/intrathecal methotrexate, cytarabine, cisplatin, cladribine, for chemotherapy of cancers with posterolateral cord syndrome • Konzo/lathyrism: Chronic dietary exposure to specific toxin, endemicity in the local region
Infections	• HIV vacuolar myelopathy: SACD: With normal B12, copper with positive HIV and low CD4 • Neurosyphilis: Tabes dorsalis (dorsal cord syndrome with neuropathy) with Argyll Robertson pupil and positive VDRL/TPHA/RPR • HTLV: Progressive predominant motor myelopathy with normal imaging, with abnormal HTLV Ab

Continued...

Continued...

Etiology/Disorder	Salient features
Neoplastic	• Compressive extradural lesions would present subacutely with pain (metastasis) • Extramedullary intradural: Meningioma, astrocytoma, metastasis • Intramedullary: Ependymoma • Lumbosacral filum terminale: Myxopapillary ependymoma • Recurrent progressive cord-enhancing lesions with initial response to steroids followed by no response, with negative workup for NMOSD and systemic connective tissue diseases: Primary spinal lymphoma
Delayed postradiation myelopathy	• History of >45 Gy radiation to cord, usually with combined chemotherapy, before months to years • Progressive myelopathy with sensory symptoms, T2 hyperintensity with cord swelling, variable enhancement
Genetic	• Hereditary spastic paraplegia: Positive family history, posterolateral syndrome, multiple subtypes according to features and genetic abnormality • Friedreich's ataxia/spinocerebellar ataxia: Predominant associated cerebellar dysfunction, extraocular movement abnormality, cerebellar atrophy • Adrenomyeloneuropathy: In males, predominantly motor involvement, adrenal dysfunction, typical MRI of brain and spine, low VLCFA and *ABCD1* mutation
Motor neuron disease	• Various different syndromes: Sporadic and genetic forms • Isolated UMN syndrome: Primary lateral sclerosis • Combined UMN + LMN syndromes: Amyotrophic lateral sclerosis, focal segmental amyotrophy • Isolated LMN syndromes: SMA (proximal/distal syndromes), Kennedy's disease (X-linked bulbospinal atrophy)

(HTLV: human T-cell lymphotropic virus; NMOSD: neuromyelitis optica spectrum disorder; PPMS: primary progressive MS; RPR: rapid plasma regain; SACD: subacute combined degeneration; SMA: spinal muscular atrophy; TPHA: treponema pallidum hemagglutination assay; VDRL: Venereal Disease Research Laboratory)

TABLE 15 Important investigations useful for diagnosis of myelopathies.

Investigation	Relevance
Spine MRI	• Diagnosis of compression and vascular abnormalities • Confirm parenchymal (intrinsic) cord pathologies
Brain MRI	To diagnose demyelination/leukodystrophy
Chest X-ray/CT of thorax	Diagnose tuberculosis, occult neoplasm, sarcoidosis
CSF study (cell, TC, DC, protein, glucose, OCB, IgG index)	Evidence of inflammation/infection
CSF cytology	Spinal neoplasm
Hematology, peripheral smear, B12 estimation	SACD
Panels for autoimmune disorders	For specific connective tissue disorders
Panels for infections	For diagnosing specific infection based on associated clinical features
Visual evoked potentials	For diagnosing associated optic nerve involvement
Spinal angiogram	Vascular malformations of cord
EMG NCV	For associated neuropathy/consideration of anterior horn cell disease
NMO Ab and MOG Ab	For considering NMOSD and MOG syndromes
• Paraneoplastic Ab • Whole-body PET CT scan	Paraneoplastic myelopathies
Serum copper/zinc	Copper deficiency myelopathy
VLCFA	Adrenomyeloneuropathy
Genetic testing: NGS/WES panels	Hereditary spastic paraplegia

(MOG: myelin oligodendrocyte glycoprotein; NGS: next-generation sequencing; NMOSD: neuromyelitis optica spectrum disorder; WES: whole-exome sequencing)

TABLE 16 Approach to "myelopathy" with normal imaging spine: Important considerations for review.

What else could this be?	Examples
Is the MRI quality good?	• Low Tesla scan (0.3 T/0.5 T) • Motion artifact • Gadolinium contrast not done in situations where contrast study is important • CIS sequence not taken: Posterior flow voids missed in reporting
Compressive etiology possibly missed?	• Epidural lipomatosis • Dynamic compression of cord in flexion/extension of neck
Is it a myelopathy mimic?	• Sensory ganglionopathy: Sjogren, autoimmune, toxic, paraneoplastic • Polyneuropathy: GBS/CIDP • Plexopathy: Brachial/lumbosacral • Anterior horn cell disease • Brain disorder: Parasagittal pathology, ACA disease, hydrocephalus, vascular parkinsonism
Acute presentation is on the background of subacute to chronic progressive myelopathy	• HIV, HTLV, syphilis • B12, folic acid deficiency • Nitrous oxide toxicity, lathyrism, konzo • Hereditary spastic paraplegia
Scan done too early in the disease	To repeat scan
Does the patient have a functional neurologic disorder?	Look for specific clinical features of functional symptoms

(CIDP: chronic inflammatory demyelinating polyneuropathy; HTLV: human T-lymphotropic virus)

RECOMMENDED READINGS

1. Kayal AK, Goswami M, Das M, Basumatary LJ, Bhowmick SS, Synmon B. Etiological profile of noncompressive myelopathies in a tertiary care hospital of Northeast India. Ann Indian Acad Neurol. 2017;20:41-50.
2. Hauser SL. Diseases of the spinal cord. In: Harrison's Principles of Internal Medicine, 16th ed. New York: McGraw-Hill; 2005. pp. 2438-47.
3. Doppman JL, Di Chiro G, Oldfield EH. Origin of spinal arteriovenous malformation and normal cord vasculature from a common segmental artery: angiographic and therapeutic considerations. Radiology. 1985;154(3):687-9.
4. Sivaramakrishna K, Sathyavaraprasad K. Study on syringomyelia. International J Contemp Med Res. 2017;4(10):2211-4.
5. Transverse Myelitis Consortium Working Group. Proposed diagnostic criteria and nosology of acute transverse myelitis. Neurology. 2002;59(4):499-505.
6. Polman CH, Reingold SC, Banwell B, Clanet M, Cohen JA, Filippi M, et al. Diagnostic criteria for multiple sclerosis: 2010 revisions to the McDonald criteria. Ann Neurol. 2011;69:292-302.
7. Wingerchuk DM, Banwell B, Bennett JL, Cabre P, Carroll W, Chitnis T, et al. International consensus diagnostic criteria for neuromyelitis optica spectrum disorders. Neurology. 2015;85(2):177-89.
8. Graus F, Dalmau J. Paraneoplastic neurological syndromes. Curr Opin Neurol. 2012;25(6):795-801.
9. Jacob A, Weinshenker BG. An approach to the diagnosis of acute transverse myelitis. Semin Neurol. 2008;28:105-20.
10. Marriott JJ, O'Connor PW. Differential diagnosis and diagnostic criteria for multiple sclerosis: application and pitfalls. In: Lucchinetti CF, Hohlfeld R (Eds). Blue Books of Neurology: Multiple Sclerosis 3. Philadelphia: Saunders Elsevier; 2010. pp. 19-42.

CHAPTER

197 Approach to Peripheral Neuropathy

Yogeesh PM, Vishnu VY

ABSTRACT

Peripheral neuropathies are among the most common neurological illnesses encountered by physicians in the outpatient department. Knowledge of neuroanatomy and pattern recognition are the keys to diagnose the disorders of the peripheral nerves. In this chapter, we have described the various presentations of peripheral neuropathy and its patterns. We also describe the localization of the peripheral nerve disorders based on the predominant pattern of involvement (sensory, motor, and autonomic fibers). We discuss differentials based on the duration of illness, type of fibers involved, and pattern of neuropathy. Peripheral neuropathies could be either acquired or inherited. Acquired causes account for most of the peripheral neuropathies. The chapter also describes the various classification, clinical features, and examination finding, including the peripheral neuropathies' critical differentiating components. After the clinical diagnosis, it also describes the electrophysiological approach and etiological workup for the various neuropathies.

"When you have neuropathy, Silence is NOT golden"

—The Neuropathy Association

INTRODUCTION

Peripheral neuropathies are one of the most commonly encountered neurological diseases both by physicians and neurologists in outpatient clinics. The peripheral nervous system comprises the neural elements extensions outside the brain and spinal cord. Each peripheral nerve in general consists of motor, sensory, and autonomic fibers at varying proportions. In India, epidemiological studies have shown a highly variable prevalence of peripheral neuropathies ranging from 5/10,000 to 2,400/10,000.

ANATOMY

Ventral motor (efferent) roots and dorsal (afferent) sensory roots exit the spinal cord and combine to form the mixed spinal nerve, which then comes out of the intervertebral foramen and divides into anterior and posterior rami. The posterior rami supply the muscles in the paravertebral region and the skin over it. The anterior rami supply the anterior trunk and skin over it. In the cervical and lumbosacral area, these rami form the plexus and supply the limbs' muscles and the skin overlying it. The anterior rami also communicate with the sympathetic chain in the cervicodorsal region via gray and white rami communicans. A typical mixed peripheral nerve comprises motor fibers, sensory fibers, and autonomic fibers at varied proportions. Peripheral nerves can also be purely sensory or purely motor.

Further, peripheral nerves can be divided into large myelinated fibers, thinly myelinated fibers, and small unmyelinated fibers (**Flowchart 1**).

APPROACH

A stepwise approach would be the best way to diagnose and manage peripheral neuropathy. The first step in approaching a patient with peripheral neuropathy would be to differentiate it from upper motor neuron (UMN) syndrome. Once the patient has been grouped into a lower motor neuron (LMN) syndrome, we need to differentiate whether it is neuronopathy, radiculopathy, plexopathy, peripheral neuropathy, neuromuscular disorder, and or myopathy.

There are hundreds of etiologies for peripheral neuropathies, so history, examination, and investigations should be tailored according to the clinical possibilities.

VARIOUS TYPES

Mononeuropathy: Here single nerve is involved, and the patients would present with clinical symptoms and signs in a single nerve distribution. The most common causes are entrapment neuropathies (median nerve at the carpal tunnel, the peroneal nerve at the fibular neck, the radial nerve at the spiral groove, and the lateral femoral cutaneous nerve of thigh-meralgia paresthetica). Other causes include trauma, compression, ischemia, irradiation, tumor infiltration, infection, and injury by the cold.

Mononeuropathy multiplex: Simultaneous or sequential involvement of multiple nerves are involved. It presents as asymmetrical proximal and distal onset neuropathy. Sometimes, confluent involvement of multiple nerves mimics symmetric polyneuropathy. Historically and electrophysiologically, it is essential to ascertain the pattern of involvement. Important causes are listed below (**Box 1**).

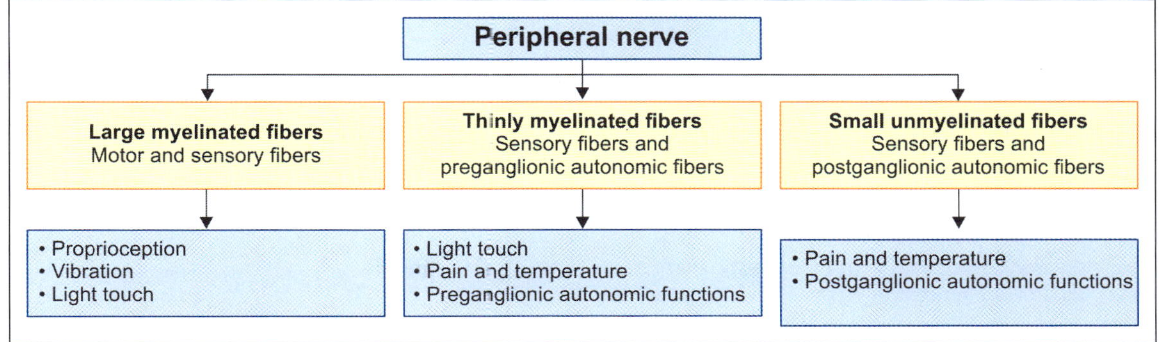

FLOWCHART 1: Classification of neuropathies based on the diameter of the impaired axon.

Polyneuropathy: Prototypical example of peripheral neuropathy is distal symmetric polyneuropathy. It is a length-dependent pattern of involvement of the sensory and motor fibers, i.e., starts at toes and progresses upward by the time symptoms reach knee, patient has symptoms in hands, and trunk is involved later. Multiple etiologies are known to cause this pattern of involvement; the most important are systemic diseases, metabolic disease, and toxins.

By the time symptoms reach the upper leg there will be involvement of the fingers in upper limbs, trunk is also involved in length dependent manner with wider involvement in lower abdomen as compared to thorax as thoracic nerves are have more longer and oblique course.

BOX 1	Causes of mononeuropathy/mononeuritis multiplex.
Diabetes mellitus	
Vasculitis	
• Primary-small (MPA, EGPA, and GPA) and medium vessel vasculitis (polyarteritis nodosa), secondary vasculitis (rheumatoid arthritis, SLE, Sjögren's and scleroderma), cryoglobulinemic vasculitis	
Sarcoidosis	
Infections	
• Leprosy (sensory predominant), HIV, Hep C, HIV, and Lyme disease	
HNPP	
• Hereditary neuropathy with liability to pressure palsies	
MMNCB	
• Pure motor	
Genetic autoinflammatory disease	
• Such as DADA-ADA2 deficiency (which mimics childhood polyarteritis nodosa)	

(ADA2: adenosine deaminase-2; DADA: deficiency of adenosine deaminase; EGPA: eosinophilic granulomatosis with polyangiitis; GPA: granulomatosis with polyangiitis; MMNCB: multifocal motor neuropathy with conduction block; MPA: microscopic polyangiitis)

Radiculopathy: Refers to the involvement of motor and sensory radicles (roots). Typically, the single root involvement presents with radicular pain. But multiple radical involvements can be seen, which can present asymmetrical onset proximal more than the distal sensory-motor LMN syndrome.

Plexopathy: They present with asymmetric onset proximal more than the distal sensory-motor pattern of involvement. Important causes include diabetes, trauma, infections, metastasis, immune-mediated, and idiopathic.

SYMPTOMS AND SIGNS

The next step in history and examination is to confirm the disease's onset, whether the disease is acute, subacute, and acute presentation of chronic neuropathy or chronic (**Boxes 2** and **3**). It helps in narrowing down the differentials (**Flowchart 2**).

Based on symptoms and signs, the particular pattern of involvement must be confirmed historically and by the clinical examination. We should assess whether the predominant involvement is motor, sensory or autonomic system (**Table 1**).

Based on the predominant type of fiber involvement (motor, sensory, and autonomic), etiological possibilities can be sorted (**Flowchart 3** and **Boxes 4** to **6**).

BOX 2	Important causes of acute neuropathy.
• Guillain–Barré syndrome (GBS)	
• Acute porphyric neuropathy	
• Toxic neuropathy	
• Critical illness neuropathy/myopathy	
• Vasculitis	
• Infectious neuropathy	
• Mimics of acute polyneuropathy	
• Botulism	
• Tick paralysis	

BOX 3	Important causes of chronic peripheral neuropathy.
•	Diabetic symmetric distal (axonal) polyneuropathy
•	Metabolic (diabetes, hypothyroid, and celiac disease)
•	Alcohol and other toxic polyneuropathy (drugs, and heavy metals)
•	Heavy metal toxicity (zinc, lead, thallium, and arsenic)
•	Immune-mediated neuropathies [chronic inflammatory demyelinating polyradiculoneuropathy (CIDP) and CIDP variants—MMN, MADSAM, and DADS—including anti-MAG neuropathy]
•	Inherited neuropathies
•	Genetic autoinflammatory disease like DADA (which mimics childhood polyarteritis nodosa)
•	Medication-induced neuropathies (nitrofurantoin, lithium, phenytoin etc.)
•	Vitamin B1, B6, B12, E, and copper deficiency
•	Vitamin B6 toxicity
•	Paraproteinemia-related neuropathies (MGUS, multiple myeloma, Waldenstrom's macroglobulinemia, and POEMS)
•	Connective tissue diseases (systemic lupus erythematosus, rheumatoid arthritis, Sjögren's syndrome, and systemic sclerosis, or scleroderma)
•	Infectious (Lyme, HIV, leprosy, and brucellosis)
•	Sarcoid neuropathy
•	Cryptogenic polyneuropathy
•	Mitochondrial (neuropathy, ataxia, retinitis pigmentosa or NARP, and myopathy and external ophthalmoplegia, neuropathy, gastrointestinal, encephalopathy or MNGIE)

(DADA: deficiency of adenosine deaminase; DADS: distal acquired demyelinating symmetric; MADSAM; multifocal acquired demyelinating sensory and motor; MAG: myelin-associated-glycoprotein; MGUS: monoclonal gammopathy of undetermined significance; MMN: multifocal motor neuropathy; POEMS: peripheral neuropathy, organomegaly, endocrinopathy, monoclonal gammopathy, and skin change)

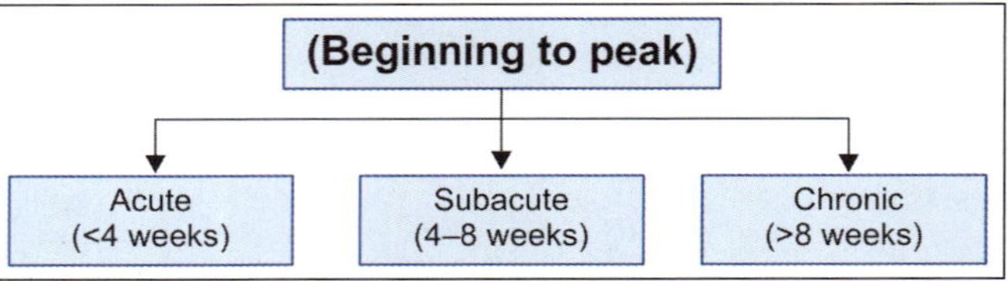

FLOWCHART 2: Classification of polyneuropathy according duration from onset to nadir of symptoms.

TABLE 1 Symptoms and signs of peripheral neuropathy.

	Positive symptoms	Negative symptoms
Motor	Cramps, twitching and myokymia (worm-like movements)	Weakness, fatigue, and wasting
Sensory	Burning, lancinating pain, tingling, pins and needles, allodynia, and hyperalgesias	Numbness, sensory ataxia, and difficulty in distinguishing hot and cold
Autonomic symptoms	Early satiety, bloating sensation, constipation, diarrhea, urinary incontinence, erectile dysfunction, abnormal sweating of skin, orthostatic hypotension, and heart rate variability	

BOX 4	Motor predominant neuropathies.
•	Porphyria
•	Lead poisoning
•	Multifocal motor neuropathy (MMN)
•	GBS (in AIDP and AMSAN)
•	CIDP (sensorimotor deficits but the presentation is usually weakness)

(AIDP: acute inflammatory demyelinating polyneuropathy; AMSAN: acute motor and sensory axonal neuropathy; CIDP: chronic inflammatory demyelinating polyradiculoneuropathy)

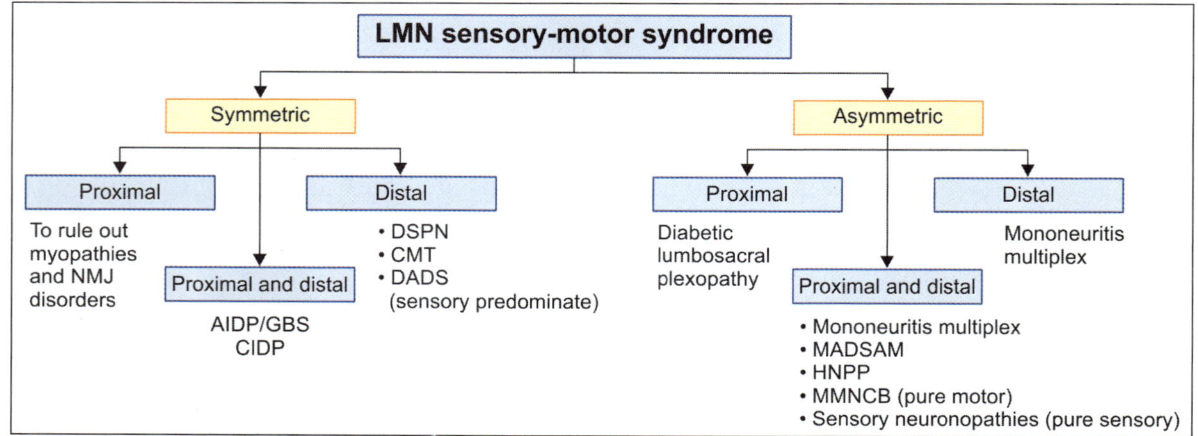

(AIDP: acute inflammatory demyelinating polyradiculoneuropathy; CIDP: chronic inflammatory demyelinating polyradiculoneuropathy; CMT: charcot marie tooth disease; DADS: distal acquired demyelinating symmetric; DSPN: distal sensory polyneuropathy; HNPP: hereditary neuropathy with liability to pressure palsies; MADSAM; multifocal acquired demyelinating sensory and motor; MMNCB: multifocal motor neuropathy with conduction block; NMJ: neuromuscular junction)

FLOWCHART 3: Patterns of involvement (LMN sensory-motor syndrome).

BOX 5	Neuropathies with predominant autonomic features.
• Diabetic autonomic neuropathy	
• Guillain–Barré syndrome	
• Toxic neuropathies (ciguatera, heavy metals, organic solvents, acrylamide, cisplatin, vincristine, paclitaxel, and amiodarone)	
• Paraneoplastic and immune-mediated neuropathies [paraneoplastic neuropathies, lupus, rheumatoid arthritis, mixed connective tissue disease (MCTD), and Sjögren's syndrome]	
• Hereditary neuropathies (porphyria, HSAN, Fabry disease, Tangier disease, allgrove syndrome, Navajo neuropathy, and multiple endocrine neoplasias)	
• Infectious diseases (HIV, botulism, Chagas disease, diphtheria, and leprosy)	
• Neuropathy related to amyloidosis	
• Vincristine neuropathy	

(HSAN: hereditary sensory and autonomic neuropathies;)

BOX 6	Sensory neuronopathies.
• Paraneoplastic syndrome	
• Immune-mediated (Sjögren's syndrome, SLE, celiac disease, and autoimmune hepatitis)	
• Chemotherapy-induced	
• Vitamin B6 toxicity	
• Friedreich's ataxia	
• Infectious (HIV, EBV, VZV, HTLV-1)	
• Miller Fisher syndrome, Bickerstaff's brainstem encephalitis	
• Cerebellar ataxia, neuronopathy, vestibular areflexia syndrome (CANVAS)	

(HTLV-1: human T-cell leukemia virus type 1; VZV: varicella zoster virus)

EXAMINATION

- General examination of the patient's vitals, blood pressure for orthostatic hypotension, and head to toe examination for any signs of systemic illness should be done. Emphasis should be given to look for signs of nutritional deficiencies, signs of connective tissue diseases, and toxicities (**Box 7**).
- Patients with inherited neuropathies [Charcot–Marie–Tooth (CMT)] presents with clumsiness in walking in childhood but usually do not complain of sensory loss, and reduced sensation to all modalities is apparent on examination. Muscle stretch reflexes are unobtainable or reduced throughout. There is often atrophy of the muscles below the knee, leading to the appearance of the so-called inverted champagne bottle legs.
- Examination for pes cavus, hammer toes, and kyphoscoliosis should be done in suspected cases of hereditary neuropathies.
- Thickening of nerves should be examined to rule out leprosy, chronic inflammatory demyelinating polyradiculoneuropathy (CIDP), neoplastic infiltration, and neurofibromatosis. Most commonly palpated nerves are the ulnar nerve at the elbow, the peroneal nerve at the fibular head, superficial radial at the dorsum of wrist and greater occipital nerve.
- Cranial nerve examination also helps in narrowing differentials like:
  - Anosmia—Refsum diseases, vitamin B12 deficiency
  - Optic atrophy in mitochondrial diseases inherited neuropathies.
  - Ophthalmoplegia in Guillain–Barré syndrome (GBS), botulism, and mitochondrial diseases.
  - Trigeminal neuropathy is associated strongly with Sjögren's disease.
  - Facial weakness is seen explicitly in many neuropathies (**Boxes 8** and **9**).
- Neuropathies associated with cancer:
  - Direct effect of the cancer by invasion or compression of the nerves.
  - Paraneoplastic
    - Sensory ganglionopathy (anti-Hu syndrome)
    - Sensorimotor neuropathy
    - Autonomic neuropathy
  - Direct toxic effect of treatment
    - Neurotoxicity secondary to chemotherapy
    - Radiation toxicity

BOX 7	Dermatological changes associated with peripheral neuropathy.
• **Amyloidosis (primary):** Purpura skin folds or flat surfaces or eyelids, papules, sometimes alopecia, rarely bullae on skin or oral mucosa	
• **Arsenic poisoning:** Dry scaly desquamation, linear hyperpigmentation of nails, and Mees lines	
• **Diabetes mellitus:** Necrobiosis lipoidica diabeticorum, and poorly healing ulcers	
• **Fabry disease:** Angiokeratoma	
• **Impaired long-chain fatty acid oxidation:** Congenital ichthyosis, and ichthyosiform erythroderma	
• **Leprosy:** Hypopigmentation and hyperpigmentation, leonine facies, erythema nodosum leprosum, Lucio phenomenon: arteritis of skin, vitiligo	
• **Lyme disease:** Target lesions	
• **Pellagra:** Erythematous photosensitive rash, erythema, vesicles, glossitis, malar and supraorbital hyperpigmentation, and rhagades	
• **Poems syndrome:** Hyperpigmentation, thickening, verrucous angiomas, and hirsutism	
• **Refsum's disease:** Ichthyosis	
• **Sarcoidosis:** Hypohidrosis, cicatricial alopecia; acute: erythema nodosum, vesicles, maculopapular rash; chronic lupus pernio, plaques, scars, and keloids	
• **Systemic lupus erythematosus:** Photosensitivity, malar rash, and discoid lupus	
• **Thallium intoxication:** Hair loss	
• **Vitamin B12 deficiency:** Black nail pigmentation (nail bed and matrix), oral aphthous ulcers	

BOX 8	Neuropathies with facial nerve involvement.
• Lyme disease, HIV	
• Sarcoidosis	
• Granulomatosis with polyangiitis	
• Sjögren's syndrome	
• Leptomeningeal carcinomatosis	
• Syphilis	
• Lymphoma, and leukemia	
• Gelsolin-related amyloidosis	
• GBS variants (pharyngo-cervico-brachial, and Miller Fisher syndrome)	

(GBS: Guillain–Barré syndrome)

BOX 9	Causes of primary demyelinating neuropathy.
• GBS	
• CIDP	
• CIDP variants [MMN, DADS, MADSAM, POEMS, MGUS, Waldenstrom's macroglobulinemia, CISP, anti-MAG neuropathy, and gait disorder, antibody, late-age onset, polyneuropathy (GALOP) syndrome]	
• Diphtheria	
• Toxic exposure (hexane, arsenic, buckthorn, and tellurium)	
• Drugs (amiodarone, gold, and taxols)	

(Anti-MAG: myelin-associated-glycoprotein; CIDP: chronic inflammatory demyelinating polyradiculoneuropathy; CISP: chronic immune sensory polyneuropathy; DADS: distal acquired demyelinating symmetric; MADSAM: multifocal acquired demyelinating sensory and motor; MGUS: monoclonal gammopathy of undetermined significance; MMN: multifocal motor neuropathy; POEMS: peripheral neuropathy, organomegaly, endocrinopathy, monoclonal gammopathy, and skin change)

- Alteration of immune status caused by immunosuppressive medications.
    - Often occur in setting of bone marrow transplantation or treatment of graft-versus-host disease (GVHD).

Motor examination: Bulk and tone would be decreased in peripheral neuropathies. The muscle weakness pattern should be confirmed, and reflexes should be examined to look for areflexia and hyporeflexia. In cases of pure small fiber, neuropathy reflexes can be preserved and can be normally absent at the ankle in the elderly population.

Sensory examination: Sensations for large (fine touch, proprioception, and vibration) and small fiber (pain, crude touch, and temperature) should be examined. The sensory examination should be done to look for dermatomal, radicular, and symmetrical length-dependent patterns and should be confirmed.

Mimics and differentiation: Pseudoneuropathy pattern of involvement in cervical myelopathy may be confused with neuropathy but can be differentiated from neuropathy by brisk reflexes and upgoing plantar.

INVESTIGATIONS

Laboratory investigations:

- *Preliminary tests*: Complete blood count, liver and renal function tests, electrolytes, fasting blood sugar (FBS), postprandial blood sugar (PPBS), vitamin B12 levels (methylmalonic acid/homocysteine levels), human immunodeficiency virus (HIV), hepatitis B surface antigen (HbsAg), anti HCV, thyroid function tests, C-reactive protein (CRP), and erythrocyte sedimentation rate (ESR)

Special investigations:

- *Connective tissue disorders*: Antinuclear antibody (ANA), antineutrophil cytoplasmic antibodies (ANCA), extractable nuclear antigens (ENA) profile, angiotensin converting enzyme (ACE) levels, rheumatoid arthritis (RA) factor, C3 levels.
- *Infections*: Venereal disease research laboratory (VDRL), HIV, HbsAg, anti HCV antibodies, and Lyme serology
- *Metabolic*: Porphobilinogen level, and glycated hemoglobin (HbA1c)
- *Paraneoplastic antibodies*: Anti-Hu specifically in smokers with suspicion of small-cell lung cancer (SCLC).
- *Paraproteinemia*: Serum and urine protein immune electrophoresis, serum protein immune fixation or serum-free light chain assay.
- *Toxins*: Heavy metal screening
- *Nutritional and malabsorption*: IgA tissue transglutaminase antibodies, endomysial antibodies, and duodenal biopsy
- *Antiganglioside antibodies*: Multifocal motor neuropathy with conduction block (MMNCB) (anti-GM1) and GBS variants (anti-GQ1b, anti-GM1, and anti-GD1a)
- *Cerebrospinal fluid (CSF) examination*: Done in cases of suspected infective, autoimmune, and malignant neuropathies. In acute inflammatory demyelinating polyneuropathy (AIDP) to look for albumin cytological dissociation after 1–2 weeks of illness.
- *Genetic analysis*: In cases of suspected hereditary neuropathies [CMTs, hereditary neuropathy with liability to pressure palsies (HNPP)], e.g., *PMP22* duplication in hereditary demyelinating neuropathy, and suspected genetic autoinflammatory disorders like deficiency of adenosine deaminase 2 (DADA2) [adenosine deaminase 2 (ADA-2 deficiency)].
- *Fat pad biopsy*: With Congo red staining to rule out amyloidosis.

Electrophysiological studies:

- *Nerve conduction studies/electromyography (NCS/EMG)*: Nerve conduction studies are done to confirm the large fiber polyneuropathy. It also helps in distinguish between axonal and demyelinating neuropathies, pattern and distribution, predominant fiber (motor, sensory or sensory-motor) involvement, superimposed compressive neuropathies, follow-up after therapeutic interventions, and also to differentiate between acquired and inherited causes (**Table 2**).

TABLE 2 Comparison between axonal and demyelinating neuropathies.

Feature	Axonal neuropathies	Demyelinating neuropathies
Motor nerve conduction studies		
Distal latency	Normal	Prolonged
CMAP amplitude	Decreased	Normal
Conduction velocity	Normal	Slow
Conduction block	Absent	Present
Temporal dispersion	Absent	Present
F wave	Normal or absent	Prolonged or absent
H reflex	Normal or absent	Prolonged or absent
Sensory nerve conduction studies		
Sensory nerve action potential (SNAP) amplitude	Decreased	Normal
Distal latency	Normal	Prolonged
Conduction velocity	Normal	Slow

(CMAP: compound muscle action potential)

Autonomic testing:
- SSR (sympathetic skin response)
- QSART (quantitative sudomotor axon reflex testing)
- TST (thermoregulatory testing)
- HRBD (heart rate variability to deep breathing)

Nerve biopsy: In today's world, with advances in serological and genetic tests, there are only a few indications for nerve biopsy. Most commonly, nerve biopsy is done to diagnose vasculitic neuropathy, in variants of CIDP when the cause remained undetermined after extensive evaluation and in cases of inconclusive hereditary neuropathy. The sural nerve, superficial peroneal, and dorsal sensory branch of the radial nerve are the most commonly selected nerves for biopsy.

Skin biopsy: It is used to diagnose small fiber neuropathy using PGP (protein gene product) 9.5 immunostaining. IENFD (intraepidermal nerve fiber density) is a reliable marker for small fiber' involvement in neuropathy. The biopsy is taken from the distal leg and thigh to differentiate between distal neuropathy and sensory neuronopathy.

Special investigations:
- *Corneal confocal microscopy*: To look for nerve fiber density, nerve fiber length and tortuosity are assessed, and its reduction corresponds to the length-dependent small fiber neuropathy and ganglionopathy.
- *Laser Doppler image flair (LDIF)*: Evaluates skin field response by vasodilation to the laser mediated heat stimulation to the skin's C fibers. The flair area depends on the receptive field of activated fibers. It helps in detecting small fiber neuropathy.
- *Meissner corpuscle density*: Here, the density of mechanoreceptors, i.e., Meissner corpuscle, is examined at the fingertip, and it has been shown to correspond to the reduction of IENFD.
- *Stimulated skin wrinkling*: This is vasoconstriction mediated by postganglionic sympathetic fibers in response to a eutectic mixture of local anesthetics by acting on calcium channels. An abnormal result predicts abnormal IEFND in sensory neuropathy.
- *Neuromuscular ultrasound*: Examination of the nerves for the thickening can also aid in the diagnosis.

CONCLUSION

Peripheral neuropathies are a heterogeneous group of disorders that require a stepwise approach for diagnosis. The most crucial step would be pattern recognition and the onset of illness. Electrophysiology helps in confirming the diagnosis, and serological tests do help in etiological diagnosis, which is essential for further management.

RECOMMENDED READINGS

1. Alport AR, Sander HW. Clinical approach to peripheral neuropathy: anatomic localization and diagnostic testing. Continuum (Minneap Minn). 2012;18(1):13-38.
2. Katona I, Weis J. Diseases of the peripheral nerves [Internet]. Handbook of Clinical Neurology, 1st edition. Netherland: Elsevier BV; 2018. pp. 453-74. [online] Available from http://dx.doi.org/10.1016/B978-0-12-802395-2.00031-6.
3. Siao P, Kaku M. A clinician's approach to peripheral neuropathy. Semin Neurol. 2019;39(5):519-30.
4. Beachy N, Satkowiak K, Gwathmey KG. Vasculitic neuropathies. Semin Neurol. 2019;39(5):608-19.
5. Kieseier BC, Mathey EK, Sommer C, Hartung HP. Immune-mediated neuropathies. Nat Rev Dis Primers. 2018;4(1):31.
6. Sommer C. Nerve and skin biopsy in neuropathies. Curr Opin Neurol. 2018;31(5):534-40.
7. London ZN. A structured approach to the diagnosis of peripheral nervous system disorders. Continuum (Minneap Minn). 2020;26(5):1130-60.
8. Vallat JM, Vital A, Magy L, Martin-Negrier ML, Vital C. An update on nerve biopsy. J Neuropathol Exp Neurol. 2009;68(8):833-44.
9. Bromberg MB. An approach to the evaluation of peripheral neuropathies. Semin Neurol. 2005;25(2): 153-9.
10. Basantsova NY, Starshinova AA, Dori A, Zinchenko YS, Yablonskiy PK, Shoenfeld Y. Small-fiber neuropathy definition, diagnosis, and treatment. Neurol Sci. 2019;40(7):1343-50.

CHAPTER

198 Guillain–Barré Syndrome

Rajinder K Bansal

ABSTRACT

Guillain–Barré syndrome (GBS) is a common cause of acute flaccid and areflexic quadriparesis, which progresses up to 4 weeks of disease onset. Although it is a disease of peripheral nerves, but cranial nerves involvement is seen in about 45–75% of patients. Facial nerve is the most common nerve involved followed by bulbar and oculomotor involvement. About 20–30% patients also have respiratory failure which requires mechanical ventilation. Autonomic involvement in the form of blood pressure and heart rate fluctuation, pupillary dysfunction, and bladder or bowel dysfunction are also seen. GBS may be triggered by many infectious and higher incidence of GBS was also seen in recent Zika virus and severe acute respiratory syndrome coronavirus 2 (SARS-CoV-2) virus pandemic. Usually there is no diagnostic difficulty in most of GBS patients, but atypical presentation with retained reflexes may pose some difficulties in diagnosis. Nerve conduction studies (NCSs) are very helpful in the second week of the disease, but some characteristic abnormalities may help during first week of the disease also.

Treatment in the form of either intravenous immunoglobulin (IVIG) or plasma exchange (PE) should be started preferably with in first 2 weeks of disease onset to prevent complications and reduce hospital stay. Absolute indication for starting treatment is if patient is unable to walk without support for 10 meters, but one should start treatment if disease is rapidly progressive or patients have bulbar dysfunction or severe dysautonomia. Steroids have not been found to useful in the treatment of GBS. About 80% of GBS patients are able to walk without support at 6 months of disease onset, but death also occur in 3–10% of patients mostly due to cardiovascular and respiratory complications. Early rehabilitation and psychological support with emphasis on preventing other complications like deep vein thrombosis (DVT) are integral part of GBS management.

"When everything else fails, there is only a single rope you can hold on to, that is hope"

—Anonymous

INTRODUCTION

Guillain-Barré syndrome is a heterogeneous group of inflammatory peripheral nerve disorders manifesting with acute onset usually with a monophasic course. It is a common cause of flaccid paralysis, which manifests as symmetrical weakness of limbs along with areflexia or hyporeflexia within 4 weeks of disease onset. Typically, the weakness starts in the legs and then progresses to arms and cranial muscles. There is respiratory involvement in about 20-30% patients. The motor weakness may be accompanied by sensory symptoms and signs in some patients. Autonomic system involvement leads to cardiac arrhythmias and blood pressure fluctuations. Even with best medical care, there is mortality of about 3-10% due to dysautonomia and other complications. After the disease progression stops, there is plateau phase for few weeks to months. About 60-80% of patients are able to walk without support after 6 months of disease onset irrespective of the treatment modality given.

The pathogenesis of GBS is not fully understood, but it is thought to be due to abnormal immune response to certain infections leading to damage to the peripheral nerves.

The diagnosis of GBS is based on good history and neurological examination. This is supported by cerebrospinal fluid (CSF) and electrophysiological examination. The electrophysiological examination helps to differentiate between different subtypes of GBS namely acute inflammatory demyelinating polyneuropathy (AIDP), acute motor axonal neuropathy (AMAN), and acute motor-sensory axonal neuropathy (AMSAN).

Guillain-Barré syndrome is not an uncommon disease and has an annual incidence of about 1-2 per 100,000 person-years and is slightly more common in men than in women (3:2). The incidence of GBS has been reported to increase during outbreaks of infectious diseases such as Zika virus epidemic and the recent coronavirus disease (COVID) pandemic.

Guillain-Barré syndrome has many atypical presentations and has many clinical variants. It is advisable to follow a stepwise pattern for diagnosis and management of GBS based on a recent publication in nature review in 2019. The various steps in management approach are discussed in this chapter.

CLINICAL FEATURES

Guillain–Barré syndrome should be suspected as a diagnosis in a patient who presents with **rapidly progressive weakness of legs and/or arms** and may be associated with distal sensory symptoms in some of the patients. Cranial nerve involvement is common and about 45–75% of patients may have cranial nerve involvement in the form of facial, bulbar, or oculomotor weakness. Most common cranial nerve involved is facial nerve followed by extraocular and bulbar muscle involvement. Deep tendon reflexes may be decreased or absent at presentation, but are usually absent in the later part of disease.

Autonomic nervous system involvement is common in the form of blood pressure and heart rate fluctuations, pupillary dysfunction, and bladder or bowel dysfunction. Some patient may feel mild-to-moderate pain which could be radicular or nonspecific muscle pain. Disease progression is usually complete by 2 weeks. If weakness progresses beyond 4 weeks, alternate diagnosis of chronic inflammatory demyelinating polyneuropathy (CIDP) should be considered.

About two-thirds of patients report preceding infection or vaccination in 6 weeks prior to onset of GBS symptoms. These preceding infections and vaccinations trigger the immune response which may causes peripheral nerve damage.

Various infections and vaccinations which have been associated with triggering of GBS pathogenesis are:
- *Campylobacter jejuni*
- Cytomegalovirus
- Hepatitis E virus
- *Mycoplasma pneumoniae*
- *Enterovirus* (EV)
- Zika virus
- SARS-CoV-2 virus
- Influenza vaccine

Atypical presentation: Atypical presentation in the form of asymmetrical onset or predominantly proximal or distal onset weakness has been reported. Sometimes cranial nerves involvement may precede the onset of the limb weakness. Some patients may have retained reflexes throughout the disease course.

GBS variants: In addition to the classical presentation of GBS described above, there are some well-known variants of GBS which one should be familiar with to avoid delay in diagnosis. These variants are:
- Pure motor variant (most common)
- Bilateral facial weakness
- Upper limb weakness (pharyngeal cervical-brachial weakness)
- Lower limb weakness (paraparetic variant)
- Miller fisher syndrome consisting of ophthalmoplegia, areflexia, and ataxia
- Pure sensory variant (rare)

Usually, these variants are not seen in the pure form but these overlap with the typical presentation of GBS.

DIAGNOSTIC CRITERIA

The diagnosis of GBS is based on history, neurological, electrophysiological, and CSF examination. The most frequently used criteria are the National Institute of Neurological Disorders and Stroke (NINDS) (1990) criteria.

These criteria were initially designed to see association between GBS and vaccinations but later on were used in clinical studies and trials.

NINDS DIAGNOSTIC CRITERIA

These diagnostic criteria for GBS were developed by the NINDS and subsequently modified in a review paper. Authors have added some features that cast doubt on the diagnosis, which were not mentioned in the original criteria and have made some adaptations to improve reliability. These criteria are not applicable for some of the variants of GBS.

Features required for diagnosis are:
- Progressive bilateral weakness of arms and legs (although only legs may be involved initially)[a]
- Absent or decreased tendon reflexes in affected limbs (at some point during clinical course)[a]

Features that strongly support diagnosis are:
- Progressive phase lasts from days to 4 weeks (usually <2 weeks)
- Relative symmetry of symptoms and signs
- Relatively mild sensory symptoms and signs (absent in pure motor variant)[a]
- Cranial nerve involvement, especially bilateral facial nerve[a]
- Autonomic dysfunction
- Radicular pain or muscular pain[b]
- Increased protein level in CSF; normal protein levels do not rule out the diagnosis[b]
- Electrodiagnostic features of motor or sensorimotor neuropathy (normal electrophysiology in the early stages does not rule out the diagnosis)[b]

Features that cast doubt on diagnosis are as follows:
- Increased numbers of mononuclear or polymorphonuclear cells in CSF (>50 × 10^6/L)
- Marked and persistent asymmetry of weakness
- Bladder or bowel dysfunction at onset or persistent during disease course[b]
- Severe respiratory dysfunction with limited limb weakness at onset[b]
- Sensory signs with limited weakness at onset[1]
- Fever at onset
- Nadir <24 hours[2]
- Sharp sensory level indicating spinal cord injury[a]
- Hyperreflexia or clonus[b]

[1] Statements in the NINDS criteria that were adapted by authors to improve readability.

[2] Additional features which were not included in the NINDS.

Note: For clarity, authors have omitted "features that rule out the diagnosis" from the original NINDS criteria for this adapted version.

- Extensor plantar responses[b]
- Abdominal pain[b]
- Slow progression with limited weakness without respiratory involvement
- Continued progression for >4 weeks after start of symptoms[b]
- Alteration of consciousness (except in Bickerstaff brainstem encephalitis)[b]

Minor adaptations were made by the authors in Nature Reviews to a simplified version of the original NINDS criteria.

INVESTIGATIONS

CEREBROSPINAL FLUID EXAMINATION

The classical CSF finding in GBS is increased CSF protein levels with normal CSF cells known as albuminocytological dissociation. But CSF protein levels may be normal in 50% patients during first week of the disease. CSF is also done to rule out presence of other abnormalities like infections or malignancy which is suggested by the presence of >50 cells/mL of CSF.

ELECTRODIAGNOSTIC STUDIES

The diagnosis of GBS may be difficult during the early phase of the disease, especially in patients with mild and atypical weakness and these patients may have retained deep tendon reflexes. Even at this early stage, NCS can help to support the diagnosis of GBS. But it is important to understand that the NCS findings may be normal during the first 3–4 days, but after 1 week most of the patients begin to show abnormal NCS findings.

- NCS abnormalities during early phase (first week of disease):
  - Prolonged F wave latencies or absent F waves suggesting involvement of proximal nerve roots.
  - *Sural sparing pattern*: A preserved sural sensory response with reduced or absent median and ulnar sensory responses is suggestive of GBS.
- *Other NCS abnormalities*: In addition to the early NCS abnormalities described above, other NCS findings in AIDP are prolonged distal motor latencies, reduced motor nerve conduction velocities, prolonged F wave latencies or absent F waves, increased temporal dispersion, and conduction blocks at noncompressible sites. These abnormalities are seen after 1 week of disease onset. NCS also help to differentiate between demyelinating and axonal variants of GBS. In axonal variant, the NCS changes are reduced compound muscle action potential (CMAP) amplitudes and reduced sensory nerve action potential (SNAP) amplitudes.

Sometimes, repeating NCS after 3–6 weeks of disease onset may help in the electrodiagnostic classification of GBS subtype into AIDP, AMAN, or AMSAN.

TREATMENT

Treatment should be started if patient is unable to walk without support for 10 meters. Treatment may also be started early if weakness is rapidly progressive and in patients with bulbar dysfunction or several dysautonomia. Treatment is effective if started within 2 weeks of disease onset with IVIG and within 4 weeks of onset with PE.

General supportive medical care is needed to prevent complications. These measures include monitoring of blood pressure, heart rate, and respiratory function and timely transfer to intensive care unit (ICU) when needed. In addition, prophylaxis for DVT, management of bladder and bowel dysfunction, early initiation of physical therapy, and psychological support are required.

INTENSIVE CARE UNIT ADMISSION

The most important reason for admission to ICU is evolving respiratory failure. Sometimes, severe dysautonomia manifesting as cardiac arrhythmias and blood pressure fluctuation is also indication for ICU admission. Another indication for ICU monitoring is swallowing dysfunction. Impending respiratory failure is defined as:

- Single breath count of <15 counts/breath
- Use of accessory respiratory muscles
- Tachypnea or tachycardia
- Vital capacity <15–20 mL/kg
- Abnormal arterial blood gas (ABG) or pulse oximetry values

Risk factors for prolonged mechanical ventilation are:

- Inability to left arms from bed after 1 week of intubation
- Axonal variant of GBS on NCS

This information can be used to consider early tracheostomy in these patients.

TREATMENT OPTIONS

Both **IVIG and PE** have been proven to be effective in treatment of GBS in many clinical trials. Early treatment is advisable to avoid irreversible nerve damage and delayed recovery. IVIG (0.4 g/kg body weight daily for 5 days or 1 g/kg daily for 2 days) and PE (200–250 mL plasma/kg body weight for five sessions) have been found to be equally effective. Whether IVIG 0.4 g/kg daily for 5 days or 1 g/kg for 2 days is better, has not been determined.

Mechanism of IVIG action is thought to be due to inhibition of Fc-mediated activation of immune cells, binding of antiganglioside antibodies to neural targets, or local complement activation. PE is considered to remove neurotoxic antibodies, complement factors, and other humoral factors responsible for inflammation. IVIG is simple to administer and has fewer treatment-related complications, so it is usually preferred over PE which requires special equipment and trained staff. It has been seen in a small trial that PE is better than IVIG in patients with AMAN. The choice of treatment may also be based on cost, patient-related factors, and availability of special equipment for PE. IVIG is more expensive, so cost may be a deciding factor in low-income countries.

Steroids: Corticosteroids in the form of intravenous (IV) methylprednisolone have not been found to useful in the treatment of GBS and oral steroids have a rather harmful effect is the outcome of GBS.

Poor response to treatment: Approximately one-third of GBS patients treated with IVIG or PE do not start improving in the first 4 weeks after treatment. Most of the times, it becomes difficult to decide whether to repeat same treatment or change to alternative treatment, because at present we do not have definite evidence for either option. In some patients, treatment with repeat dose of IVIG has been shown to be useful.

Deterioration after initial improvement: About 10% of GBS patients deteriorate again after showing initial improvement with treatment with IVIG or PE. These patients had either stabilized or improved after initial treatment. This phenomenon is known as treatment-related fluctuation (TRF). These patients may have a prolonged autoimmune response, which causes prolonged nerve damage. There is no clear evidence for retreatment with IVIG or PE, but still repeat retreatment is used because some of the patients show improvement after retreatment.

GBS with extended course: Some of GBS patients show disease progression beyond 4 weeks, which raises a question about the initial diagnosis of GBS. Actually, a diagnosis of acute-onset CIDP (A-CIDP) should be considered in these patients who have disease progression beyond 8 weeks. It is important to recognize these deteriorations because patients with TRF may improve with repeat retreatment, but those with A-CIDP will require prolonged immunomodulatory treatment.

COMPLICATIONS

The common GBS-related complications are pressure ulcers, DVT, and hospital-acquired infections such as pneumonia and urinary tract infection (UTI) which should be managed by standard preventive treatment protocols. Other common problems which GBS patients usually have are pain, anxiety, and depression. The care givers should discuss these issues with the patients and manage accordingly. So early involvement of physiotherapists, rehabilitation specialist, psychologist, and dietician are crucial for proper care of GBS patients.

PROGNOSIS

Most GBS patients including those who had required mechanical ventilation and had severe weakness will show good recovery in first year of disease onset. About 80% of GBS patients will be able to walk without support at 6 months of disease onset. Although there is good outcome in majority of patients, death occurs in 3–10% of patients mostly due to cardiovascular and respiratory complications.

Incidence of GBS in general population is 0.1%, which is much higher than the 2–5% incidence of recurrent GBS. The importance of knowing this data is to decide while giving vaccinations which have higher risk of GBS like influenza vaccine in elderly. Although prior GBS is not a contraindication for vaccination but caution may be used in people who had GBS within 1 year of planned vaccination or who developed GBS shortly after receiving same vaccination earlier.

Rehabilitation: Patients with GBS usually have long-term motor sensory deficits, fatigue, pain, and psychological distress. Before discharging these patients, these problems should be discussed with patient and family and plan to manage these problems should be discussed and explained to the family.

CONCLUSION

Guillain–Barré syndrome is about 100 years old disease and our knowledge about its pathogenesis and treatment has advanced a lot since original descriptions. Early diagnosis and starting early treatment are important because it can have varied clinical presentation. Although we have option to choose treatment between IVIG and PE, still poor response to treatment in some of the patients is an issue which has not been settled amicably. Recently observed increased incidence of GBS after viral outbreaks of Zika virus and recent SARS-CoV-2 virus outbreak raises questions about our knowledge about its pathogenesis. So continued research in developing biomarkers, prognostic models, and better therapies are needed.

RECCOMMENDED READINGS

1. Leonhard SE, Mandarakas MR, Gondim FAA, Bateman K, Ferreira MLB, Cornblath DR, et al. Diagnosis and management of Guillain–Barré syndrome in ten steps. Nat Rev Neurol. 2019;15:671-83.
2. van den Berg B, Walgaard C, Drenthen J, Fokke C, Jacobs BC, van Doorn PA. Guillain–Barré syndrome: pathogenesis, diagnosis, treatment and prognosis. Nat Rev Neurol. 2014;10(8):469-82.
3. Goodfellow JA, Willison HJ. Guillain–Barré syndrome: a century of progress. Nat Rev Neurol. 2016;12(12):723-31.
4. Walgaard C, Lingsma HF, Ruts L, van Doorn PA, Steyerberg EW, Jacobs BC. Early recognition of poor prognosis in Guillain–Barré syndrome. Neurology. 2011;76(11):968-75.
5. Kalita J, Misra UK, Das M. Neurophysiological criteria in the diagnosis of different clinical types of Guillain–Barré syndrome. J Neurol Neurosurg Psychiatry. 2008;79:289-93.
6. Willison HJ, Jacobs BC, van Doorn PA. Guillain–Barré syndrome. Lancet. 2016;388:717-27.
7. Asbury AK, Cornblath DR. Assessment of current diagnostic criteria for Guillain–Barré syndrome. Ann Neurol. 1990;27:S21-4.

CHAPTER

199 Myasthenia Gravis

S Meenakshi-Sundaram, Lakshmi Narasimhan Ranganathan, S Mahesh Kumar

ABSTRACT

Myasthenia gravis (MG) is the most common primary neurological disorder of neuromuscular transmission and is a typical example of an antibody-mediated acquired autoimmune disease. Skeletal muscle involvement with sparing of smooth muscles, selective vulnerability of some skeletal muscles than the others, diurnal fluctuations of symptoms, and pathological task-specific fatigability are its distinctive features. Ocular muscles are particularly vulnerable. Fatigable, asymmetric variable ptosis, and diplopia due to extraocular muscle weakness are the usual presenting manifestations. Bulbar, limb-girdle, and respiratory involvements are other features, the last one indicative of myasthenic crisis. Pathogenetically, there is antibody-mediated destruction of the postsynaptic neuromuscular acetylcholine receptor (AChR). Neostigmine test, neuroelectrophysiological studies [repetitive nerve stimulation (RNS) and single-fiber electromyography (SF-EMG)], and various antibody testing are employed in the diagnosis.

Acetylcholinesterase inhibitors (AChEIs) (pyridostigmine and neostigmine) are used as symptomatic medications. Immunomodulatory therapy is the key considering the autoimmune nature of the disease. Corticosteroids and steroid-sparing agents like azathioprine and mycophenolate are used on a long-term basis. Rapid immunomodulation in the form of intravenous immunoglobulin (IVIg) and plasma exchange (PLEx) is required in some situations such as myasthenic crisis. Newer therapies are rituximab, useful in antimuscle-specific kinase (MuSK) myasthenia and eculizumab, in generalized myasthenia. Thymectomy is an important option in select cases. Respiratory support may be required in myasthenic crisis.

"Take action! An inch of movement will bring you closer to your goals than a mile of intention"

—S Maraboli

INTRODUCTION

Myasthenia gravis is the most common primary neurological disorder of neuromuscular transmission. It is a typical example of an antibody-mediated, acquired autoimmune disease. The term "mys" means muscle and "asthenia" means weakness in Greek and "gravis" means serious or grave in Latin. Weakness involving the bulbar and peripheral muscles was first described by Samuel Wilks in 1877 following which the disease was recognized as a distinct clinical entity. The term "myasthenia gravis" was first used by Jolly in 1895 when he also added the term "pseudoparalytica" to denote the absence of morphological changes at autopsy. The discovery of physostigmine as the treatment for the condition was reported by Dr Mary Walker in 1934, and to date, this group of drugs continues to remain as the most important symptomatic management of the disease. Insight into the pathophysiology has resulted in a better understanding of the disease and advancements in the management have made this once-fatal disease, an essentially treatable illness.

EPIDEMIOLOGY

The exact prevalence of MG in India is not known. Worldwide the incidence rate has been reported to range from 1.7 to 21.3 cases per million and the prevalence rate from 5 to 179 cases per million. In United Kingdom, the prevalence rate is estimated to be 10 per 100,000 and in the United States, it is 14 per 100,000. Although the disease can occur at any age from childhood onward, the age distribution shows two distinct peaks. In the first, which occurs at a younger age (second and third decades) women are twice as commonly affected as men. In the second peak that occurs at a later age (seventh and eighth decades), men are more commonly affected than women. Despite being an autoimmune disease, because of an increase in life expectancy, men are now more commonly affected than women.

CLINICAL FEATURES

The onset of the disease is usually insidious and untreated the disease may progress slowly. In two-thirds of the patients maximum weakness occurs within the first year itself. The hallmarks of the disease are:

- Skeletal muscle involvement with sparing of smooth muscles
- Selective vulnerability of some skeletal muscles than the others
- Distinct fluctuation of symptoms with weakness being intermittent at least initially and showing a diurnal variation and
- Pathological fatigability

Patients with MG usually report task-specific muscle fatigue on continuous work. Those who report generalized tiredness/fatigue with demonstrable weakness are very unlikely to have MG. Provocative maneuvers demonstrate weakness of specific muscle groups in MG but not in those with generalized fatigue. **Tables 1** and **2** list the various patterns of presentation in MG and various clinical signs, respectively. **Table 3** provides the Myasthenia Gravis Foundation of America (MGFA) clinical classification that is currently used widely.

OCULAR MYASTHENIA GRAVIS

Ocular features are the presenting manifestations in half of the patients and, in nearly one-tenth, the illness remains restricted to the ocular muscles. The exact reason for this predilection of ocular muscles remains elusive and is presumed to be due to their small size. Smaller muscles have lesser "safety factor", making them vulnerable. The tendency of twitch fibers in these muscles to develop tension faster and a higher frequency of synaptic firing also renders them susceptible to fatigue. Paucity of AChR in the tonic muscle fibers responsible for sustenance of gaze is also proposed as a mechanism.

Ptosis, diplopia, and blurred vision (due to diplopia) are the usual complaints and are due to the involvement of levator palpebrae superioris and extraocular muscles. Ptosis is unilateral or bilateral and when bilateral it is often asymmetric. The degree of ptosis shows significant

TABLE 1 Clinical symptoms of myasthenia gravis.

Part of body	Symptoms
Ocular	• Double vision • Drooping of eyelids on one or both sides, usually asymmetric • Extraocular muscle weakness
Other cranial	• Difficulty in chewing—more obvious with prolonged chewing and while chewing hard food • Change in facial expression for emotions due to facial muscle weakness
Bulbar	• Difficulty in swallowing, i.e., more for liquids than solids • Difficulty in speaking • Nasal regurgitation of fluids and feeds • Constant throat clearing • Cough on feeding
Neck	Isolated neck weakness needing placement of hand for support
Respiratory	Difficulty in breathing due to respiratory muscle weakness, sometimes severe enough to cause respiratory failure
Limbs	Proximal weakness, symmetric, fluctuant, and involving upper limbs more than lower limbs. Rarely, can present as distal weakness

TABLE 2 Clinical signs of myasthenia gravis.

Ocular	• Ptosis • Extraocular muscle weakness • Strabismus • Pseudo-internuclear ophthalmoplegia (INO) • Complete pupil sparing ophthalmoparesis • Curtain sign: Ptosis of one eye, enhanced by lifting the other eyelid • Enhanced ptosis: Passively lifting a ptotic lid may cause the opposite lid to fall • Lid fatigability test: Ptosis aggravated by prolonged upgaze • Cogan's lid twitch: Patient is asked to look down for 15 s followed by a quick (saccadic) movement to the primary position—a rapid upward overshoot is seen followed by down-drift of upper lid • Lid retraction: Seen in the eye contralateral to the ptotic eye (explained by Hering's law of equal innervation) • Peek sign: When the patient is asked to keep the eyes forcefully shut, after sometime the eyelids spontaneously open as if the patient peeks through a hole, due to orbicularis oculi weakness • Quiver: On producing saccades nystagmoid jerks may be seen without any obvious weakness
Oropharyngeal	• Holds jaw with fingers to keep the mouth shut • Myasthenic sneer: When asked to smile, the patient's midlip raises but the corners of the lips do not move • Diminished gag reflex • Hypophonic voice
Neck	• Dropped head syndrome: Weakness of the neck extensors resulting in dropping of the head, seen prominently in the night
Respiratory	• Isolated respiratory muscle weakness: Severe respiratory distress requiring mechanical ventilation • Orthopnea
Limbs	• Bilateral, symmetrical, and proximal limb weakness (upper limb > lower limb) • Arm abduction test shows early fatigability • Leg abduction test shows early fatigability • Hand grip dynamometry shows abnormality

TABLE 3 Myasthenia Gravis Foundation of America-Clinical Classification.

Class	Description
I	• May involve any ocular muscle causing weakness • May have weakness of eye closure • All other muscle strength is normal
II	• Mild weakness affecting other than ocular muscles • May also have ocular muscle weakness of any variety
II-A	• Predominantly affecting limb or axial muscles or both; • May also have lesser involvement of oropharyngeal muscles
II-B	• Predominantly affecting oropharyngeal or respiratory muscles or both; • May also have lesser or equal involvement of limb or axial muscles or both
III	• Moderate weakness affecting other than ocular muscles; • May also have ocular muscle weakness of any severity
III-A	• Predominantly affecting limb or axial muscles or both; • May also have lesser involvement of oropharyngeal muscles
III-B	• Predominantly affecting oropharyngeal or respiratory muscles or both; • May also have lesser or equal involvement of limb or axial muscles or both
IV	• Severe weakness affecting other than ocular muscles; • May also have ocular muscle weakness of any severity
IV-A	• Predominantly affecting limb or axial muscles or both; • May also have lesser involvement of oropharyngeal muscles
IV-B	• Predominantly affecting oropharyngeal or respiratory muscles or both; • May also have lesser or equal involvement of limb or axial muscles or both
V	• Defined by intubation, with or without mechanical ventilation, except when employed during routine postoperative management; the use of a feeding tube without intubation places the patient in class IV-B

variability. There may be intermittent periods of blurred vision before diplopia becomes conspicuous. Asking the patient to look up for some time may be followed by progressive drooping of the eyelids. Diplopia typically worsens on prolonged gaze/on looking at a distance and is worse at night. Symptoms due to ptosis or diplopia may be interpreted by patients as visual loss. Bright sunlight often aggravates ocular signs. Asymmetric weakness of several muscles in both eyes is typical although the medial recti are most commonly affected. Symptoms may vary from time-to-time, even hour-to-hour, and are often worse in the evenings, especially following strenuous physical activity involving the affected muscle. A unique feature of MG and related neuromuscular diseases are the fatigability of affected muscles on repeated action, often to the point of total paralysis, yet with complete recovery with rest. Caution must be exercised while attributing a subtle, albeit perceptible difference in palpebral fissure width between the two sides to MG, while it is actually physiological (seen in one-third of normal persons). Apparent appearance of ptosis during fatigue, which also tends to recover with rest, may also simulate MG. Under such circumstances presence of orbicularis oculi weakness, innervated by the facial nerve, provides a clue, checked by asking the patient to keep his eyes tightly closed. Fatigue causes the patient to open his eyes partially (peek sign). Cold often improves the ocular signs; the basis of ice pack test, done for diagnosing the disease. Another distinctive feature of myasthenia is ophthalmoplegia with pupillary sparing since pupils are comprised of smooth muscles.

BULBAR INVOLVEMENT

Bulbar involvement is characterized by dysphagia, typically more severe for liquids than solids. Patients also report nasal regurgitation of fluids and feeds due to palatal weakness. They may have dysarthria and dysphonia. Talking for prolonged-periods or counting numbers may cause progressive hypophonia and, at times, development of a hoarse voice with nasal quality. It may even proceed to anarthria. Weakness of the soft palate causes nasal speech (rhinolalia) due to the inability to seal off the nasal cavity from the oral cavity. Voice sounds may have an abnormal resonance. On pronouncing, the patient may experience special difficulty with the velar sounds. Labials and linguals are also affected since much of the air needed for their production escapes through the nose. The speech resembles that of a patient with a cleft palate. Characteristically, the sound of "b" becomes "m", "d" becomes "n", and "k" becomes "ng". Asking the patient to count from 1 to 100 may be a clue to identify bulbar weakness. The intensity of the sound when the patient pronounces one may be loud and this may progressively decline. Jaw muscle weakness may result in the patient keeping his or her mouth open. A typical patient may be seen holding the jaw to prevent it from dropping. Patients also report chewing difficulty. Patients may be able to eat freely as they begin the act of eating but would not be able to complete it easily. Neck muscle weakness can result in a typical neck drop. MG is one of the causes of floppy head syndrome.

LIMB-GIRDLE PRESENTATION

Limb-girdle involvement as an initial manifestation is seen in only 5–10%. Typically patients have proximal weakness, more pronounced in the arms than in the legs. Rare patients have distal weakness. Asking the patient to keep the arm abducted, called the arm abduction time, is a useful bedside test for identifying shoulder girdle muscle weakness. Asking the patient to repeatedly stand up from a squatting position (called situps) may be a test for lower limb muscle involvement.

RESPIRATORY MUSCLE INVOLVEMENT

Respiratory involvement is usually a heralding manifestation of myasthenic crisis. Myasthenic crisis is characterized by respiratory distress. While dyspnea, tachypnea, and use of accessory muscles of respiration are features of respiratory distress, it should be remembered that as myasthenic crisis worsens the accessory muscles also become involved and are fatigued. When this happens, despite dangerous respiratory impairment, patients may have no signs of distress. Myasthenic crisis may occur spontaneously or is precipitated by infections, surgery, or medications.

Clinical clues for the diagnosis of MG in a patient who has equivocal clinical features include the total absence of sensory involvement, normal pupils despite ocular motor paresis, and preserved reflexes. Fatigability and diurnal fluctuations are important historical clues. In some patients with long-standing MG, weakness may remain permanent, referred to as myasthenic myopathy (**Box 1**).

PATHOGENESIS

The site of abnormality in MG is the postsynaptic neuromuscular receptor. Antibodies directed against these receptors result in destruction of the same. T-cell-dependent antibody-mediated attack on postsynaptic membrane damages the postsynaptic muscle membrane leading to reduction of the density of AChR. A schematic diagram of the pathogenesis of MG is depicted in **Flowchart 1**.

BOX 1 Bedside tests for fatigability in patients with myasthenia gravis.

- Patient is instructed **to look up** for sustained upgaze for >60 s and observed for ptosis
- **Peek sign:** Sustained eye closure brings out fatigue of orbicularis oculi and results in involuntary opening of the eyes
- Patient is asked to drink 100 mL of water (1/2 cup) and observed for coughing, throat clearing, nasal regurgitation, and difficulty in swallowing
- **Speech:** Patient is asked to count aloud starting from 1 to 50 and observed for dysphonia and dysarthria. More severe the disease, earlier the abnormality in these parameters manifests before completing counting till 50
- Patient is instructed to **lift the head to 45°** in supine position and sustain for 100 s and observed for fatigue
- **Arm abduction test:** Patient is instructed to outstretch (abduct) the arm in 90° position while sitting and keep it sustained for 4 min and observed for fatigability
- **Hand dynamometry:** The intactness of hand grip is assessed using hand dynamometry
- **Leg abduction test:** Patient is instructed to outstretch the leg and keep it sustained for 100 s and observed for fatigability

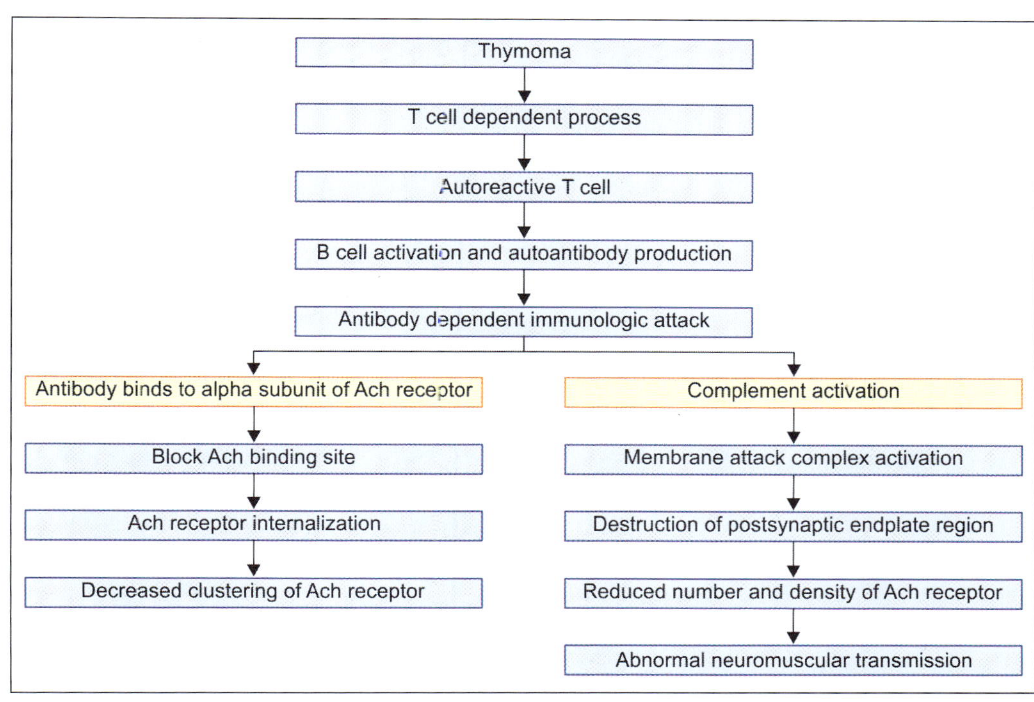

(Ach: acetylcholine)

FLOWCHART 1: Schematic diagram depicting the pathogenesis of myasthenia gravis.

DIAGNOSIS

The diagnosis of MG must be suspected in any patient who presents with fluctuating weakness, diplopia, bulbar symptoms, and fatigue. The various investigations that are pursued in patients suspected with MG are discussed below.

ICE-PACK TEST

This is based on the fact that cold improves neuromuscular transmission. A disposable glove-filled with ice is applied over the ptotic eye for 2–5 minutes. The interpalpebral fissure distance is estimated before and after the application of the ice pack (**Fig. 1**). Improvement in ptosis by at least 2 mm suggests MG. This test has a sensitivity of about 80% in ocular myasthenics.

NEOSTIGMINE TEST

Neostigmine is an inhibitor of acetylcholinesterase and response to this agent is the basis of this test, done after written consent. Special precautions are to be taken in patients with cardiac disease and chronic obstructive pulmonary disease. Atropine sulfate (0.8 mg), preadministered serves two purposes. It counters the muscarinic side effects of neostigmine, especially cardiac arrhythmias, and helps to identify placebo responders.

Neostigmine is administered (0.03 mg/kg or 1.5 mg intramuscularly) and the patient is assessed every 10 or 15 minutes for 2–3 hours, objectively. Palpebral fissure measurement, range of eye movements, single breath count, and situps are documented. False-positive responses are seen in disorders other than MG affecting the neuromuscular junction, like congenital myasthenic syndrome, Lambert–Eaton syndrome, and also ocular myopathy and intracranial aneurysms.

NEUROELECTROPHYSIOLOGICAL EVALUATION

Repetitive nerve stimulation test: A supramaximal stimulus of 0.1 ms duration is given at a rate of 3–5 Hz. A train of ten impulses is given. The first and the fourth or fifth compound muscle action potentials (CMAP) evoked in response are compared. Decrement >10% is abnormal. It is important to visualize the profile of the response. The decrement occurs between the first and second response, then the second and third, and so on, till the fifth. The changes are neither sudden nor irregular. Beyond the fifth, the CMAP amplitude rises again. This results in an envelope-shaped response that characterizes MG. Following forceful brief muscle contraction for 10 seconds, there may be temporary repair of the decrement. However, after a minute or two after a sustained forceful contraction for 60 seconds, there is a decrease in presynaptic calcium concentration and metabolic exhaustion. The first CMAP of the RNS response is now smaller than the pre-exercise amplitude and the decrement becomes more pronounced. RNS should be tested over weak muscles.

Testing several muscles maximizes the yield. Facial muscles, biceps (musculocutaneous), deltoid (axillary), trapezius (spinal accessory), hypothenar (ulnar), thenar (median), extensor digitorum brevis (fibular), and tibialis anterior (fibular) are some of the muscles that can be sampled. An air-conditioned electrophysiology laboratory may mask decremental response since cooling facilitates neuromuscular transmission. Prior warming of the muscles mitigates this problem. Proximal and facial muscles are generally not affected by cooling.

False-positive decremental responses are known in conditions like amyotrophic lateral sclerosis (ALS) and organophosphorus poisoning. Sensitivity of RNS test ranges from 53 to 100% in generalized and 10–48% in ocular MG. Normal and abnormal responses are provided in **Figure 2**.

Single-fiber electromyography: Single-fiber electromyography (SF-EMG) is the technique of selectively recording the action potentials of a single muscle fiber that is voluntarily contracting. The subject is asked to gently contract a muscle. The timing of activation of one muscle fiber in a motor unit is compared to another. Interpotential interval (IPI) is the time difference between the activation of the two fibers. This time interval between the two

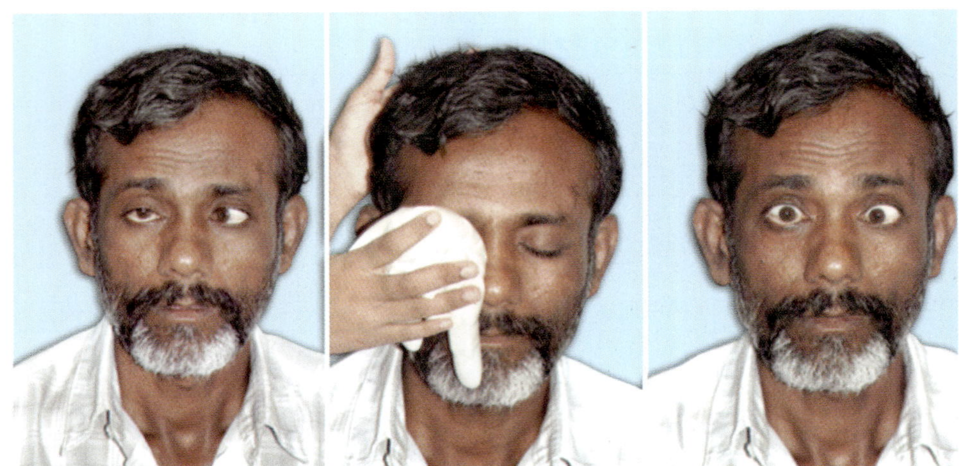

FIGURE 1: Ice pack test showing improvement in right-sided ptosis in a patient with myasthenia gravis.

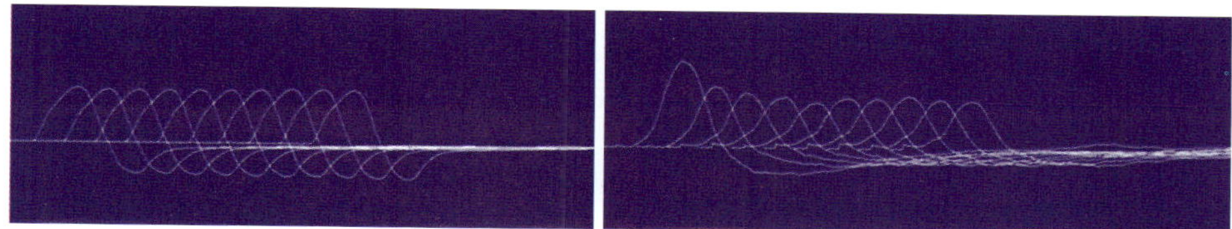

FIGURE 2: Repetitive nerve stimulation test showing normal response (left) and abnormal response (right). The abnormal response typically shows an envelope pattern.

muscle fibers is evaluated over a series of nerve action potentials. This is known as jitter. Increased variability is seen in MG referred to as abnormally increased jitter. Jitter is quantified as the mean consecutive difference (MCD). MCD is the mean difference between consecutive intervals and is a measure of the IPI between the two muscle fibers. An increased MCD compared to controls suggests neuromuscular transmission defect as in MG. When the variability is more pronounced there is an occasional failure of transmission referred to as neuromuscular "blocking". Clinical weakness is myasthenia correlates with this blocking rather than increased jitter. SF-EMG is complementary to the RNS test and is useful in situations when RNS is negative as in some patients with ocular MG. Normal jitter in a weak muscle excludes MG.

SEROLOGICAL TESTING

Acetylcholine receptor antibodies: There are three such antibodies namely binding, blocking, and modulating antibodies. Binding antibodies, the most commonly tested type are highly specific for MG. They may also be seen in low titers in conditions like Lambert Eaton syndrome, motor neuron disease, and polymyositis. When a false-positive result is suspected, demonstration of blocking antibodies helps to clarify the nature of the disease. Levels of AChR-antibodies (AChR-Ab) do not correlate with the severity of the illness and hence are not useful as markers for improvement.

Anti-muscle-specific kinase antibodies: These are seen in one-half-of patients with generalized MG who are AChR-Ab negative. MuSK-MG is a distinct clinical syndrome with oculobulbar manifestations, characteristics of which are provided in **Box 2**.

Anti-low density lipoprotein receptor-related protein 4 antibodies: These are seen in 1% of patients with generalized MG. Similar to MuSK-MG, such patients have no association with thymic involvement. They are younger and have milder course.

Seronegative myasthenia gravis: At least one of the antibodies listed above is seen in 94% of patients with generalized MG, seronegative patients are those who do not have any of these and have better outcomes since their presentation is often purely ocular.

Thymoma and antibodies: Markers for the thymoma in patients with MG include antistriated muscle antibodies and antititin antibodies.

BOX 2 **Characteristics of muscle-specific kinase (MuSK)-associated myasthenia gravis.**

- Oculobulbar and facial involvement at presentation rather than purely ocular form
- Female predominance
- Onset at any age but more common in elderly people
- Neck extensors more involved than neck flexors
- Muscle atrophy, involving tongue, face, sometimes limb, and shoulder girdle muscles and paraspinal muscles
- Less common involvement of limbs
- Paradoxical worsening with acetylcholinesterase inhibitors in some
- Less frequent thymic involvement and poor response to thymectomy
- More responsive to rituximab

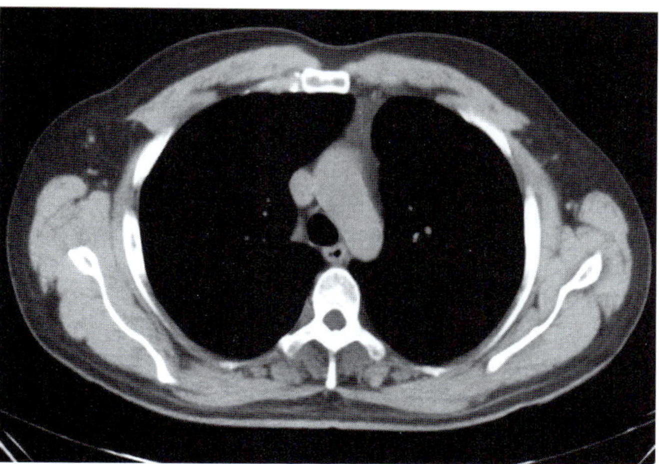

FIGURE 3: Axial image of CT scan of the chest showing diffuse enlargement of the thymus suggestive of thymic hyperplasia.

IMAGING

All patients with MG require computed tomography (CT) scan of the chest to evaluate for thymic hyperplasia (**Fig. 3**) or mass (**Fig. 4**). The sensitivity of this test is 91.7%. Cranial MRI is required in some where the diagnosis is not straightforward.

OTHER TESTS

The frequency of a second autoimmune disorder in MG is 13–22%, highest for females and early onset MG. Patients with respiratory disturbances are monitored with pulmonary

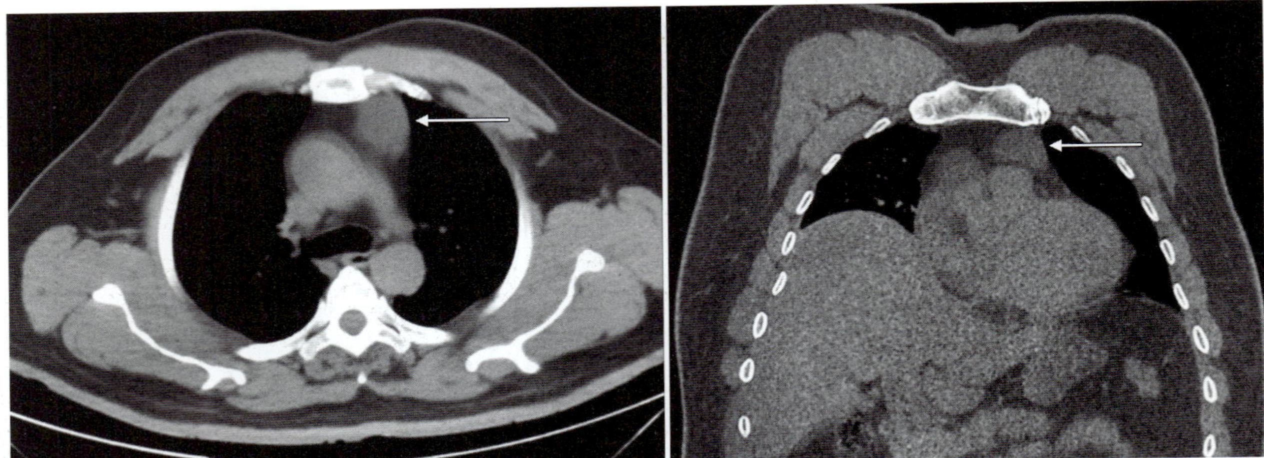

FIGURE 4: Axial (left) and coronal (right) images of CT scan of the chest showing well-defined lobulated soft tissue mass lesion in the anterior mediastinum (white arrow) which is not invading the ascending aorta or main pulmonary artery.

TABLE 4 Other tests to be done in patient with myasthenia gravis.

Test	Autoimmune disease
Antinuclear antibodies	Systemic lupus erythematosus and autoimmune hepatitis
Extractable nuclear antigen profile (ENA)	Rheumatoid arthritis and Sjögren syndrome
Antithyroid antibodies	Autoimmune thyroiditis (Hashimoto's disease)
Thyroid function tests	Autoimmune thyroiditis

function tests to detect impending myasthenic crisis (**Table 4**).

TREATMENT

The cornerstones of management of MG are:

- Symptomatic treatment
- Immunomodulatory therapy
  - Long-term immunomodulation
    - Corticosteroid therapy
    - Steroid-sparing agents: Immunosuppressants
  - Rapid immunotherapy
    - IVIg
    - PLEx
    - Pulse methylprednisolone
- Surgical management
- Management of myasthenic crisis

SYMPTOMATIC TREATMENT

Pyridostigmine and neostigmine are AChEIs useful as symptomatic medications. The former is more commonly used given its longer duration of action. A typical starting dose is 30 mg thrice daily, uptitrated based on the clinical response. The dosage is highly individualized, some requiring higher and some lower dosages. The interval between the dosages is also variable, and is modified according to the requirements. For instance, the drug is usually administered along with food to minimize the gastrointestinal adverse effects, but a patient who is particularly troubled by dysphagia will benefit by taking the medication 30–45 minutes before the anticipated food intake. Many patients do not need medications at bedtime. However, when symptoms are troublesome in the night or patients are weak in the morning upon getting up, AChEIs are administered in the night as well. The timed-release preparation (180 mg sustained-release form), may be useful in this situation. However, the benefits of such sustained-release agents are variable, owing to their erratic absorption. Hence some patients may be woken up in the night time at the anticipated hours of worsening and extra doses of the regular form are administered. The variability of the response makes the timed-release form unsuitable for regular daytime use.

Dosages needed to elicit response may vary between the various muscles of the same individual. For instance, the ocular muscles may not respond well and patients may report the persistence of diplopia despite high doses. Further hiking of the doses may invite undesirable adverse effects. It is prudent to inform the patient beforehand of this possibility. Such patients may be advised about nonpharmacologic measures to overcome this problem, for instance, the use of crutch glasses for ptosis. The dosage may vary from 60 mg thrice daily to even 120 mg every 4 hourly or sometimes even higher, but generally, it must not exceed 960 mg/day. Oral neostigmine has a shorter duration of action and the equivalent doses compared to pyridostigmine is about 25%, i.e., 60 mg of pyridostigmine roughly corresponds to 15 mg of neostigmine. Neostigmine is more useful in patients who are admitted to the intensive care area with myasthenic crisis since it can be administered parenterally. A peculiar situation to remember is MuSK-myasthenia where patients may not respond well to the usual doses and may require higher doses or sometimes paradoxically worsen with these agents.

Cholinergic side-effects (**Box 3**) are well-known following initiation of therapy with AChEIs, resulting from an accumulation of acetylcholine at the muscarinic receptors of the smooth muscles and autonomic glands. Glycopyrrolate (1 mg thrice daily, titrated to 8 mg/day) is a useful adjunct to mitigate these adverse effects. Loperamide can be used to counteract the gastrointestinal adverse effects of these agents.

BOX 3	Cholinergic side effects of acetylcholinesterase inhibitors.
• Pin point pupis	
• Lacrimation	
• Urination	
• Sweating	
• Bronchospasm	
• Loose stool	
• Emesis	
• Bradycardia	

IMMUNOMODULATORY THERAPY

Long-term immunomodulation:

Corticosteroid therapy: Steroid is the key immunomodulatory agent used. An algorithm for corticosteroid use in MG is provided in **Flowchart 2**. Gastric ulcer prophylaxis, calcium, and vitamin D supplementation, and monitoring and treating any complications well-known with long-term steroid therapy are quintessential in the management.

Steroid-sparing agents: Immunosuppressants

First-line agents: Azathioprine and mycophenolate mofetil

Second-line agents: Cyclosporine, tacrolimus, and methotrexate

These medications are often started immediately after starting the steroid or more typically once the maintenance dose of steroid is reached. Standard precautions, as for any immunosuppressive medications, are to be followed during their use. Patients typically require immunosuppression for several years.

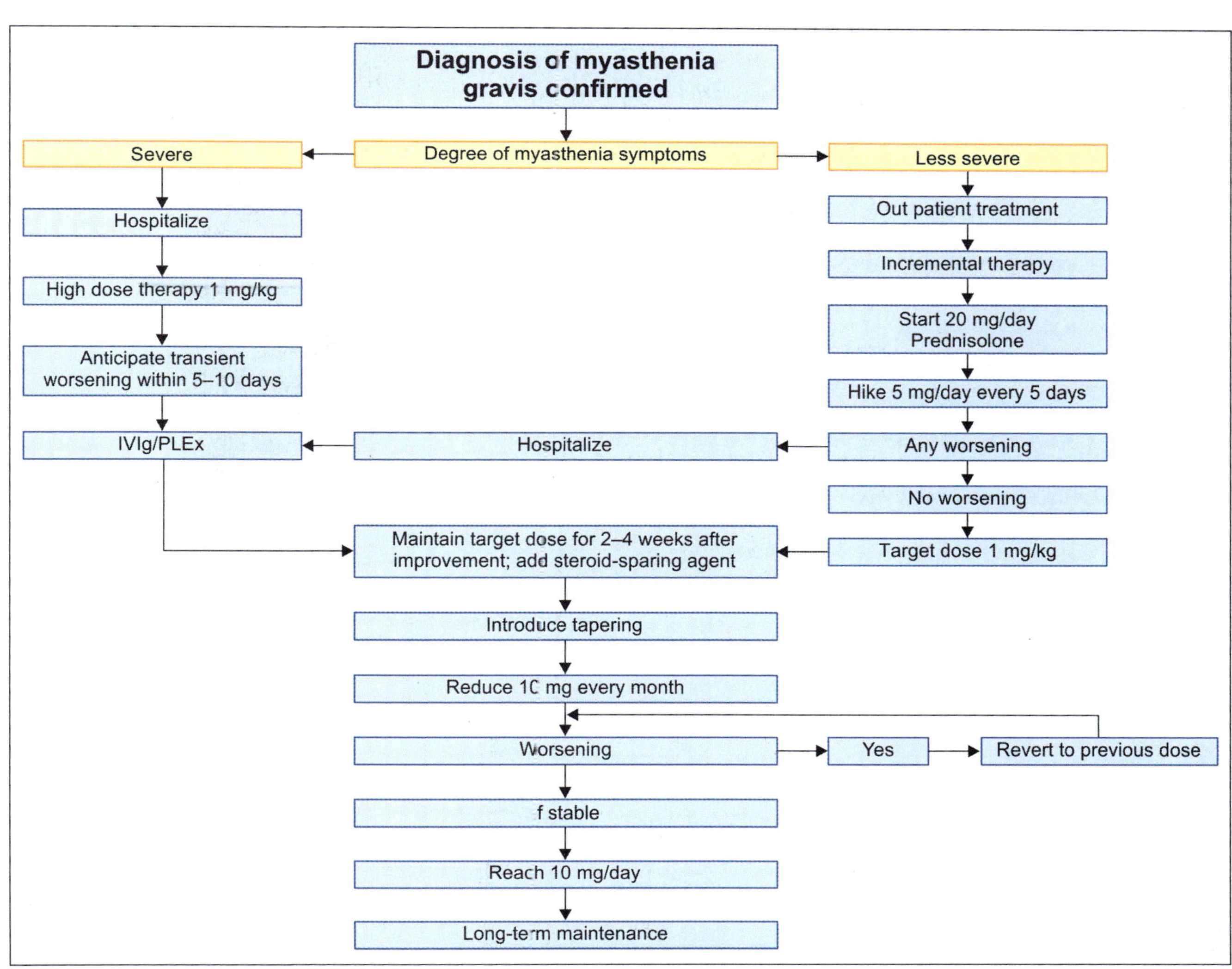

(IVIG: intravenous immunoglobulin; PLEx: plasma exchange)

FLOWCHART 2: Algorithm for prednisolone dosage in myasthenia gravis.

Rapid immunotherapy:

Plasma exchange and intravenous immunoglobulin: These are indicated in myasthenic crises (MG grade 5, on mechanical ventilation), impending crisis in severe MG (grade 4/4B) with dysphagia, respiratory dysfunction, or generalized weakness, and when a patient with mild (2/2B) or moderate (3/3B) MG is worsening or not responding to other immunosuppressant therapies, and as a prethymectomy procedure in symptomatic patients to treat respiratory and bulbar weakness before surgery. PLEx therapy usually consists of five exchanges done on alternate days (3–5 L of plasma per exchange). IVIG is administered at a dose of 400 mg/kg daily for 5 days. Response to treatment generally occurs after 2 days with PLEx and after 4–5 days with IVIg and the effects can last for several weeks. In patients with highly refractory MG, chronic PLEX may be useful for long-term disease control.

Pulse methylprednisolone: Pulse methylprednisolone 2G/day for 1–2 days has been used in patients with exacerbations but carries a risk of precipitating respiratory involvement. It is generally avoided in patients with myasthenic crisis needing IVIg or PLEx since it carries the risk of precipitating critical illness myopathy.

Newer advances: In clinical trials, rituximab appeared to be more favorable in new-onset generalized MG, fared better than conventional immunosuppressant therapy, and showed relatively greater benefit when used earlier in the disease course. Rituximab is particularly useful in MuSK-associated MG. Eculizumab, a monoclonal antibody that inhibits the complement component C5 and prevents activation of the membrane attack complex (MAC), is approved for the treatment of generalized, AChR-positive MG.

SURGICAL MANAGEMENT: THYMECTOMY

An algorithmic approach to thymectomy in MG is provided in **Flowchart 3**.

MANAGEMENT OF MYASTHENIC CRISIS

Patients with crisis or impending crisis are admitted to the intensive care area and closely monitored with frequent clinical assessments (keeping in mind the pitfall mentioned in section "Respiratory Muscle Involvement") and laboratory parameters (**Table 5**). Forced vital capacity, peak inspiratory pressure, tidal volume, and acid-base gas analysis (ABG) are useful tools. Upper airway weakness can lead to respiratory failure by oropharyngeal collapse or tongue obstruction and by increasing the work of already fatigued respiratory muscles against a closed airway. Signs of bulbar weakness include nasal regurgitation, dysphagia, rhinolalia quality to speech, jaw weakness (jaw closure weaker than jaw opening), bifacial paresis, and tongue weakness. The parameters to be monitored during mechanical ventilation of myasthenic patients are provided in **Box 4**.

DRUGS TO BE AVOIDED IN MYASTHENICS

It is essential to provide myasthenics with such when they are being treated for minor ailments by their family physicians, since they worsen neuromuscular transmission (**Box 5**).

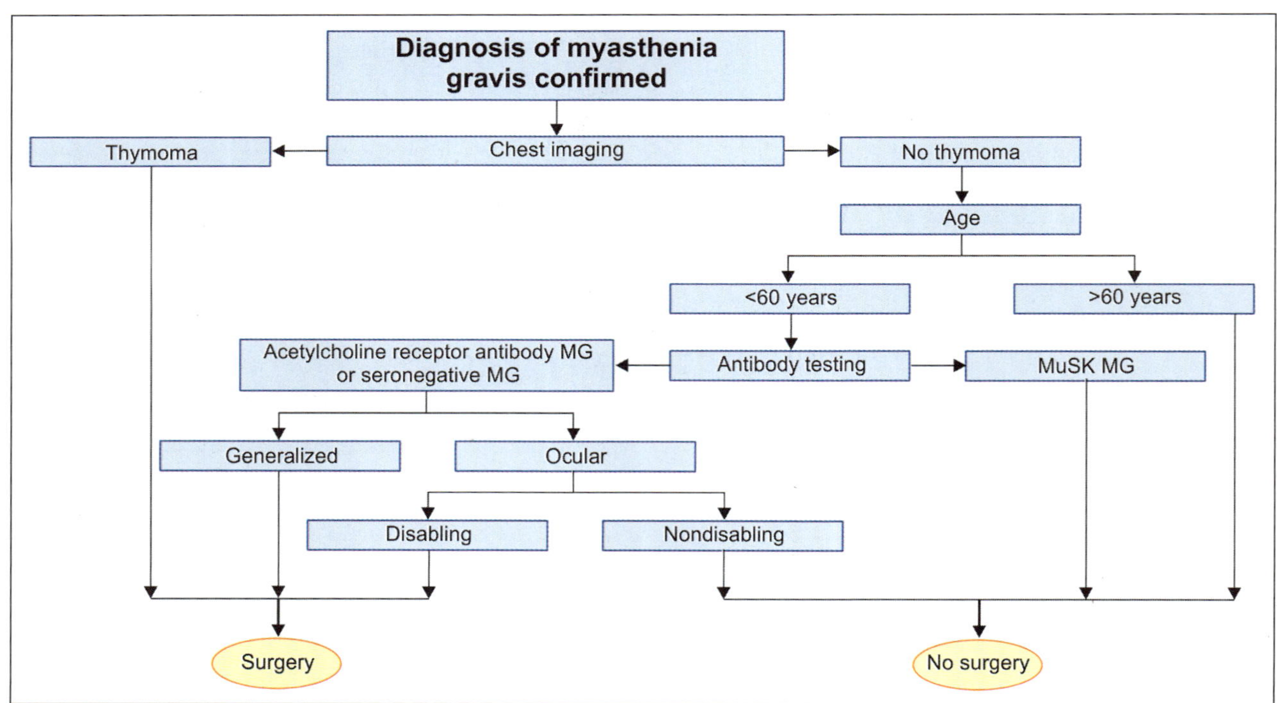

FLOWCHART 3: Algorithm for thymectomy in myasthenia gravis.

TABLE 5	Parameters to be monitored in myasthenic crisis.
Parameters monitored	**Findings in myasthenic crisis**
Vital capacity (VC)	VC <1 L (or <20–25 mL/kg)
Negative inspiratory force (NIF)	NIF <20 cm H_2O
Positive expiratory force (PEF)	PEF <40 cm H_2O
Single breath count	Difficulty counting to 20 in a single breath

BOX 4 Mechanical ventilation in myasthenia gravis.

- Patients should be placed on an assisted ventilator setting with tidal volumes of 8–10 cc/kg ideal body weight and pressure support of 8–15 cm H_2O to prevent atelectasis and to minimize the work of breathing
- Use of depolarizing agents (succinylcholine) should be cautious as they are less potent in myasthenics because very few functional postsynaptic AchR are available
- Nondepolarizing agents (e.g., vecuronium) have high potency and reduced doses are required for paralysis
- Weaning from the ventilator should be initiated after the patient demonstrates clinical improvement, typically at a vital capacity of >15 mL/kg
- Independent risk factors for prolonged intubation (>14 days) are age >50 years, peak vital capacity <25 mL/kg on post-intubation days 1 to 6, and a serum bicarbonate >30 mmol/L

BOX 5 List of drugs to be avoided in patients with myasthenia gravis (Mnemonic: ABCD is the IQ of MP).

- Aminoglycosides
- Beta blockers
- Chloroquine
- Depolarizing neuromuscular blockers like succinylcholine and D-tubocurarine
- Iodinated contrast agents
- Quinine and quinolones
- Magnesium and macrolides
- Penicillamine

VACCINATIONS

Patients with MG require annual pneumococcal and flu vaccinations since they have the risk of contracting these infections due to immunosuppressant treatment. Also, these infections can trigger or aggravate myasthenia, a risk that outweighs the risk of the potential for worsening of the myasthenia as a complication of vaccination.

PROGNOSIS

The prognosis is generally good in treated patients. Nearly 33% of people relapse over a duration of 10 years. The term gravis, used before the advancements in therapy, indicated the severity of the disease but mortality has now decreased with the advancements in modern medicine. The mortality rate in the MG population was 5.88% at a 10-year follow-up. The majority of deaths occurred at 5–10 years after the onset of the disease, and rarely within 5 years.

ACKNOWLEDGMENT

We are thankful to Dr K Ravi Kumar and Dr Abhilash Somasundaram, residents, Institute of Neurology, Madras Medical College, Chennai for helping us prepare this chapter.

RECOMMENDED READINGS

1. McCarter SJ, Burkholder DB, Klaas JP, Martinez-Thompson JM, Boes CJ. The Mary Walker effect: Mary Broadfoot Walker. J R Coll Physicians Edinb. 2019;49(3):255-9.
2. Carr AS, Cardwell CR, McCarron PO, McConville J. A systematic review of population based epidemiological studies in Myasthenia Gravis. BMC Neurol. 2010;10:46.
3. Aragonès JM, Roura-Poch P, Hernández-Ocampo EM, Alonso F, Pont-Lluelles M, Xandri I, et al. Myasthenia gravis: A disease of the very old. J Am Geriatr Soc. 2014;62(1):196-7.
4. Singhal BS, Bhatia NS, Umesh T, Menon S. Myasthenia gravis: a study from India. Neurol India. 2008;56(3):352-5.
5. Jaretzki A 3rd, Barohn RJ, Ernstoff RM, Kaminski HJ, Keesey JC, Penn AS, et al. Myasthenia gravis: Recommendations for clinical research standards. Task Force of the Medical Scientific Advisory Board of the Myasthenia Gravis Foundation of America. Neurology. 2000;55(1):16-23.
6. Nair AG, Patil-Chhablani P, Venkatramani DV, Gandhi RA. Ocular myasthenia gravis: A review. Indian J Ophthalmol. 2014;62(10):985-91.
7. Rodolico C, Toscano A, Autunno M, Messina S, Nicolosi C, Aguennouz M, et al. Limb-girdle myasthenia: clinical, electrophysiological and morphological features in familial and autoimmune cases. Neuromuscul Disord. 2002;12(10):964-9.
8. Wendell LC, Levine JM. Myasthenic crisis. Neurohospitalist. 2011;1(1):16-22.
9. Meriggioli MN, Sanders DB. Myasthenia gravis: diagnosis. Semin Neurol. 2004;24(1):31-9.
10. Fakiri MO, Tavy DLJ, Hama-Amin AD, Wirtz PW. Accuracy of the ice test in the diagnosis of myasthenia gravis in patients with ptosis. Muscle Nerve. 2013;48(6):902-4.
11. Luo H, Xie S, Ma C, Zhang W, Tschöpe C, Fa X, et al. Correlation Between Thymus Radiology and Myasthenia Gravis in Clinical Practice. Front Neurol. 2019;9:1173.
12. Narayanaswami P, Sanders DB, Wolfe G, Benatar M, Cea G, Evoli A, et al. International consensus guidance

for management of myasthenia gravis: 2020 update. Neurology. 2021;96(3):114-22.
13. Sanders DB, Wolfe GI, Benatar M, Evoli A, Gilhus NE, Illa I, et al. International consensus guidance for management of myasthenia gravis: Executive summary. Neurology. 2016;87(4):419-25.
14. Mehndiratta MM, Pandey S, Kuntzer T. Acetylcholinesterase inhibitor treatment for myasthenia gravis. Cochrane Database Syst Rev. 2014;2014(10):CD006986.
15. Brauner S, Eriksson-Dufva A, Hietala MA, Frisell T, Press R, Piehl F. Comparison Between Rituximab Treatment for New-Onset Generalized Myasthenia Gravis and Refractory Generalized Myasthenia Gravis. JAMA Neurol. 2020;77(8):974-81.
16. Albazli K, Kaminski HJ, Howard JF Jr. Complement Inhibitor Therapy for Myasthenia Gravis. Front. Immunol. 2020;11:917.
17. Liu C, Wang Q, Qiu Z, Lin J, Chen B, Li Y, et al. Analysis of mortality and related factors in 2195 adult myasthenia gravis patients in a 10-year follow-up study. Neurol India. 2017;65(3):518-24.
18. Gupta A, Goyal V, Srivastava AK, Shukla G, Behari M. Remission and relapse of myasthenia gravis on long-term azathioprine: An ambispective study. Muscle Nerve. 2016;54(3):405-12.
19. Sanghani N, Hanumanthu R, Shah S, Souayah N. Myasthenia Gravis after Vaccination in Adults the United States: A Report from the CDC/FDA Vaccine Adverse Event Reporting System (1990–2017). Neurology. 2018;(Suppl):437.
20. Seok HY, Shin HY, Kim JK, Kim BJ, Oh J, Suh BC, et al. The impacts of influenza infection and vaccination on exacerbation of myasthenia gravis. J Clin Neurol. 2017;13(4):325-30.

CHAPTER 200

Disorders of Muscle

Rakesh K Singh, Vikram Aglave, Satish V Khadilkar

ABSTRACT

Evaluation of flaccid weakness can be a challenge. Reaching a clinical diagnosis of myopathy needs a proper approach. Various myopathies present a diagnostic conundrum. Understanding the nuances of various common myopathic symptoms and signs, help to navigate through this complex landscape. While muscle weakness is universal in myopathies, further characterization depends on identifying typical features.

Confirmation of myopathy is not difficult with easy availability of tests and electrophysiology laboratories. Muscle magnetic resonance imaging (MRI) is a relatively new diagnostic tool. Access to advanced genetic tests, though costly, has further refined our diagnosis. Family history needs special emphasis. It not only aids the diagnosis of genetic myopathies, but also helps in family counseling. Ours being an inbred community, consanguinity is more common.

Spectrum of myopathies in India is quite diverse, with muscular dystrophies and inflammatory myopathies, being commoner. Duchenne and limb-girdle muscular dystrophies (LGMDs) are very well described in our population. Natural history of these common myopathies is better known today. Reversible myopathies, such as toxic and metabolic myopathies are increasingly recognized. Neurorehabilitation care has vastly improved.

Skeletal muscle weakness or myopathies result from myriad of causes. Broadly, they are either due to abnormal genetic mutations or acquired causes. Muscular dystrophy is defined as progressive degeneration of muscle fibers, due to abnormal genetic mutations.

"Being challenged in life is inevitable, being defeated is optional"

—Roger Crawford

APPROACH

Symmetrical, hip-girdle or proximal weakness has differentials. After ruling out spasticity, key to lower motor neuron and finally muscle localization is a meticulous examination. Nerve (or root) diseases with proximal weakness, are often with sensory dysfunction, hence can be easily identified. Myopathies are pure motor, as are anterior horn cell (AHC) disorders (**Flowchart 1**). The differentiation can be difficult at times. Neuromuscular disorders, like myasthenia, have recognizable presentation

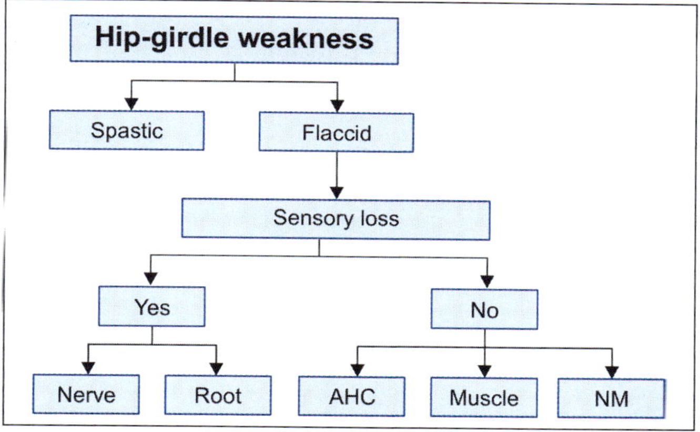

(AHC: anterior horn cell; NM: neuromuscular)

FLOWCHART 1: An approach: Hip-girdle or proximal weakness.

TABLE 1 Difference between disorders of anterior horn cell and muscle.

	Anterior horn cell	Muscle
Atrophy	Significant wasting is more than weakness	Weakness is more than wasting
Symmetry	Asymmetrical	Symmetrical
Distribution	Proximal + distal	Proximal
Reflexes	Early reflex change	Hyporeflexia as per weakness
Fasciculations	Prominent	Absent

with fluctuating muscle weakness, affecting ocular, bulbar, and limb muscles (**Table 1**).

In general, most myopathies will typically present with the following features:

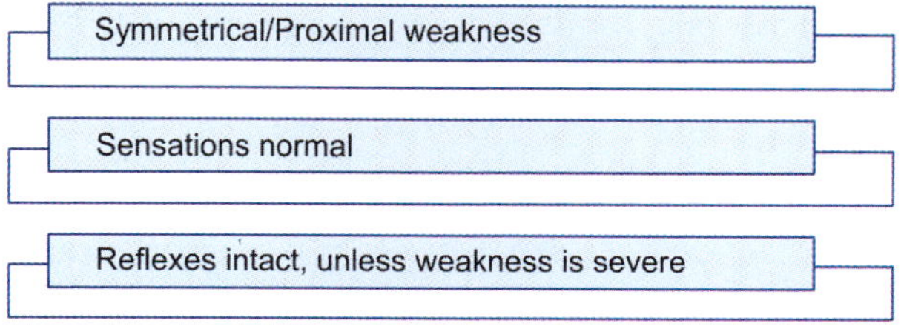

HISTORY

AGE OF ONSET

Early to teen age onset of weakness signals muscular dystrophy. Adulthood and late onset cases are usually acquired myopathies. Inflammatory myopathies, which are treatable, can present at all age groups.

DURATION

Chronic weakness (Years)	
Progressive	Muscular dystrophy
Nonprogressive	Congenital myopathies
Acute (Days) to Subacute (Months)	Acquired myopathies

FAMILY HISTORY

- Affected family member confirms the muscular dystrophy.
- Specifically ask about any family member using walking aids or has calf enlargement.
- Horizontal transmission and consanguinity implies autosomal recessive (AR) myopathy.
- Vertical transmission (especially father to son) favors autosomal dominant (AD) myopathy.
- Maternal inheritance (mother to daughter), hints at mitochondrial myopathy.
- Be aware of pseudodominance of autosomal recessive conditions.
- Unlike western free societies, we tend to marry within our own community, thus increasing the prevalence of AR disorders, which can then appear in all generations, mimicking AD.
- *Extramuscular attributes*: Apart from muscle weakness, genetic myopathies or muscular dystrophies can have varying extramuscular manifestations, among the family members. These are often considered as isolated diseases, but are part of the same disease, as in the index case.

DM/BMD—cardiomyopathy/myalgias
Myotonic dystrophy—cataracts
FSHD—scapular winging, and facial weakness
Mitochondrial—diabetes, and short stature

(DM/BMD: Duchenne muscular/Becker muscular dystrophy; FSHD: facioscapulohumeral muscular dystrophy)

"NEGATIVE" AND "POSITIVE" SYMPTOMS

Myopathies present with various negative and positive symptoms. Direct questioning of them, helps in proper evaluation.

- Negative symptoms
  - Weakness
  - Exercise intolerance
  - Muscle atrophy
  - Fatigue
- Positive symptoms
  - Myalgias/Cramps
  - Contractures
  - Muscle stiffness
  - Myoglobinuria

Most common symptom of myopathy is muscle weakness: Inquiry about "weakness" may sound easy but can be tricky. This is due to varying interpretations of the term "weakness" by patients. Sensory complaints such as numbness or nonspecific aches and pains can be mistaken for weakness and vice versa.

Fatigue, complained by patients, can be difficult to decipher. Exertional fatigue can have cardiopulmonary reasons, but do consider myasthenia gravis, before labeling as nonspecific.

Also, be clear whether the weakness is *persistent* or *episodic* weakness. While persistent or constant weakness is a regular feature of myopathies, episodic weakness is classically due to myasthenia gravis, periodic paralysis, and metabolic myopathies.

While inquiring about the muscle weakness, *it is important to ask specific questions regarding the actual functional impairments* that is "what you cannot do". This depends upon the weakened muscle groups. While the hip-girdle muscles are most frequently affected, leading to up squat difficulty, and climbing stairs, weakness of various other muscle groups cause distinctive difficulties (**Table 2**).

This approach highlights two important aspects of muscular dystrophies (not seen in acquired myopathies).

1. *Distinct patterns of weakness*: Muscular dystrophies are numerous and phenotypically diverse. They are characterized by various identifiable patterns of weakness. Each pattern and distribution of weakness has certain specific causes. Weakness of certain muscle groups point toward specific causes of myopathy.

- Proximal weakness
- Distal weakness
- Scapuloperoneal weakness
- Facial weakness
- Neck muscle weakness
- Ptosis/Ophthalmoplegia

2. *Differential weakness*: A unique feature of muscular dystrophies, whereby certain muscle groups are preferentially weak, while others nearly spared. This selectivity of weakness can be seen even within the same muscle causing a part of it to atrophy and other hypertrophy ("Lump and Bump" appearance).

Acquired myopathies, in contrast, commonly presents with proximal weakness with diffuse and nearly equal weakness of all muscle groups.

Following is the MRC (Medical Research Council) grading of muscle power (**Table 3**).

TABLE 2 Functional impairment and muscle weakness.

Functional impairment	Muscle weakness
Ptosis/Diplopia	• Extraocular muscles • Levator palpebrae
Eye closure weakness	Orbicularis oculi
Inability to drink through straw	Lower facial muscles
Inability to raise head from supine position	Neck flexor
Inability to raise head from prone position	Neck extensor
Inability to get up from bed/turn side to side	Truncal muscles
Inability to raise arms above head	Proximal arm muscles
Inability to do buttoning/unbuttoning	Distal hand muscles
Inability to open jars, doorknobs	Forearm muscles
Inability to descend stairs, buckling of knees	Quadriceps femoris
Waddling gait	Hip abductors
Inability to get up from floor or low chair	Hip and knee extensors
Inability to walk on toes	Calf muscles
Scraping of toes while walking/high steppage gait	Tibialis anterior

TABLE 3 The Medical Research Council grading of muscle power.

Score	Description
0	No contraction
1	Trace or just a flicker of contraction
2	Active movement, with gravity eliminated
3	Active movement, against gravity
4	Active movement, against gravity and resistance
5	Normal power

PHYSICAL SIGNS

DIFFERENT PATTERNS OF WEAKNESS

Proximal lower limb weakness: Hip-girdle weakness, or the so-called limb-girdle pattern, despite being the most common, is least specific for etiology, and is seen in both muscular dystrophies and acquired causes of myopathies. Presence of differential weakness, would however, point to the former.

Patients complain of difficulty in up squat from floor or low chair, and climbing stairs. Due to Indian culture of defecation in squatting posture, up squat difficulty comes to medical attention early in the disease course.

Following postural changes are also worth identifying, as they point to specific muscle weakness.

- *Lordosis*: An inward curve of spine, occurs due to hip extensor weakness. Lordosis and toe walking are common in Duchenne muscular dystrophy (DMD).
- *Gower's maneuver*: The typical maneuver results due to profound weakness of hip extensors and quadriceps muscles in DMD.

  Here, the child in supine position, when asked to get up, first rolls into a prone position. Then, with the extended arms, pushes the "butt up" and forms a triangle. This is followed by the classic climb upon himself, using the extended arms to raise the trunk straight.
- *Waddling*: Occurs due to bilateral hip abductor (Gluteus medius) weakness. While most myopathies waddle, LGMDs do not waddle due to intact hip abductor power.

- *Genu recurvatum*: Is hyperextension of knee, with backward bending. This suggests quadriceps weakness.
- *Hip abduction sign*: When asked to up squat, hips splay out, at times making an angle of 90% between them. This is due to preferential hip adductor weakness, (and intact hip abductors), common in LGMD.

Proximal upper limb weakness: Shoulder girdle muscle weakness commonly occurs along with hip-girdle weakness, in both genetic and acquired myopathies. Patients complain of inability to do overhead activity.

Predominant or isolated shoulder girdle weakness (pure motor) has distinct differentials as shown in the **Table 4**.

"Man in barrel syndrome" is characterized by bilateral proximal upper limb weakness (brachial diplegia), with intact power of facial, neck, and lower limb muscles. With no arm movements, patients appear to be trapped in a "barrel". This is classically due to bilateral watershed infarcts [anterior and middle cerebral arteries].

Distal weakness: Generally, myopathies are proximal and remain so, during the course of the disease. However, distal myopathies are not uncommon.

They present with early and predominant weakness of distal muscles like:

Weak muscle	Example
• Tibialis anterior (foot drop) • Inability to stand on toes	*GNE* myopathy
• Gastrocnemius • Inability to stand on heels	Miyoshi myopathy

Extensor digitorum brevis (EDB) a small distal muscle, located on the side of foot, which helps differentiate the causes of foot drop. It remains strong in myopathic but wasted in neuropathic causes.

Scapuloperoneal or proximal arm/distal leg weakness: This is unique and diagnostic pattern, with scapular muscle weakness (causing winging of scapula) and foot drop.

Examples with additional classical features.

FSHD: Facial weakness
Emery–Dreifuss: Contractures/cardiac conduction defects
Calpainopathy: Hip abduction sign/abdominal hernia
Pompe's disease: Diaphragmatic palsy

(FSHD: facioscapulohumeral muscular dystrophy)

TABLE 4	Distinct differentials of predominant or isolated shoulder girdle weakness.
Symmetrical	• Inflammatory myopathy • Myasthenia
Asymmetrical	• Anterior horn cell disease • FSHD

(FSHD: facioscapulohumeral muscular dystrophy)

Facial weakness: Bifacial weakness is an important diagnostic clue. Patients cannot bury eye lashes tightly and they remain open in sleep. Drinking through a straw or blowing up a balloon is difficult.

Early and prominent bifacial weakness is classical of facioscapulohumeral muscular dystrophy (FSHD) and myotonic dystrophy. Congenital myopathies, such as nemaline, also have facial weakness with long and thin facies.

Common examples of diseases with prominent bifacial weakness.

Muscle	NM junction	Nerve	AHC
Myotonic dystrophy	Myasthenia	Polyneuritis cranialis	Fazio-Londe
FSHD	Botulism	GBS	Brown–Vialetto–Van Laere syndrome
Nemaline/ Central core myopathy	OP poisoning	Sarcoid/ Lyme's	

(AHC: anterior horn cell; FSHD: facioscapulohumeral muscular dystrophy; GBS: Guillain-Barré syndrome; NM: neuromuscular; OP: organophosphate

Ptosis with or without ophthalmoparesis: Ptosis can be easily detected by the patient or their relatives.

Asymmetrical, painless, and fluctuating ptosis is classical of myasthenia gravis.

Ptosis with eye closure weakness (or facial muscle weakness) implies either myasthenia gravis or myopathy. Further grouping of ptosis can be done with or without ophthalmoparesis (**Table 5**).

Ptosis with chronic and progressive ophthalmoparesis is unique to only few myopathies, the classical being mitochondrial myopathies. Due to chronicity and symmetry, diplopia does not occur.

Oculopharyngeal muscular dystrophy (OPMD), an autosomal dominant myopathy, seen in elderly, presents with asymmetrical ptosis, followed by ophthalmoparesis and prominent dysphagia.

Neck muscle weakness: Weakness of neck flexors manifest in inability to lift the neck from pillow.

Weakness of neck extensors manifest in "Dropped head syndrome".

TABLE 5	Ptosis with or without ophthalmoparesis.
Ptosis without ophthalmoparesis	• Myasthenia • FSHD/Myotonic dystrophy • Mitochondrial myopathies
Ptosis with ophthalmoparesis	• Myasthenia • Mitochondrial myopathies • OPMD • Congenital myopathies

(FSHD: facioscapulohumeral muscular dystrophy; OPMD: oculopharyngeal muscular dystrophy)

Neck flexor weakness: Inflammatory myopathies/ Myasthenia gravis
Neck extensor weakness: ALS/Polymyositis/Myasthenia gravis

(ALS: amyotrophic lateral sclerosis)

MUSCLE HYPERTROPHY

Enlargement of muscle bulk is characteristic of inherited myopathies.

It is of two types: Pseudo and True.

1. *"Pseudo" hypertrophy* occurs due to fatty and connective tissue replacement of muscle fibers, most seen in calf muscles, but also in EDB, deltoid and triceps.
2. *"True" hypertrophy* is a feature of myotonia congenita and neuromyotonia (Isaacs syndrome) where the fibers enlarge due to continuous muscle fiber activity, leading to herculean appearance.

Calf pseudohypertrophy is sine qua non of muscular dystrophy: Occurs in almost 90% of patients of DMD. The muscle feels doughy and is weak. Also, develops quite early in DMD, and is often noted by it parents. Other causes of enlarged calves are sarcoglycanopathy and spinal muscular atrophy (SMA).

Hypothyroidism is a treatable cause of muscle enlargement (Hoffman syndrome).

MUSCLE ATROPHY OR WASTING

Prominent atrophy of muscles is a classic feature of AHC diseases, where atrophy is more than weakness. Reverse is true for myopathies.

However, significant muscle atrophy can be a characteristic feature of certain dystrophies, as shown in the **Table 6**.

Combination of hypertrophy and atrophy: Results in special signs, and diagnostic of various muscular dystrophies.

Poly hill sign	FSHD	Multiple mounds of muscle noted in arm abduction
Lump and bump	Dysferlin	Biceps show selective wasting
Valley sign	DMD	Valley between deltoid and infraspinatus

(DMD: Duchenne muscular dystrophy; FSHD: facioscapulohumeral muscular dystrophy)

TABLE 6 Characteristic feature of certain dystrophies.

Muscular dystrophy	Wasted muscles
Myotonic dystrophy 1	Face, jaw, neck, and leg muscles
FSHD	Shoulder and periscapular muscles/ asymmetric wasting
LGMD	Hip adductor muscle wasting and weakness
Dysferlinopathy	Calf wasting

(FSHD: facioscapulohumeral muscular dystrophy; LGMD: limb-girdle muscular dystrophy)

CONTRACTURES

Persistent shortening of muscles causes joint contractures.

Early contractures are of diagnostic value.

EDMD: Extensive and early contractures in neck, spine, and elbow, even before muscle weakness develops.
Collagenopathies • Bethlem: Finger joint contractures/Keloid • Ullrich: Contractures with distal joint laxity
DMD: Early toe walking due to ankle contractures.

(DMD: Duchenne muscular dystrophy; EDMD: Emery-Dreifuss muscular dystrophy)

Painful, transient, and exercise induced contractures are distinctive of McArdle's disease.

MYOTONIA

Percussion myotonia is diagnostic of myotonic muscle diseases, which are either dystrophic or nondystrophic.

Myotonia is defined as slow muscle relaxation, after contraction.

It is checked by tapping the thenar eminence with hammer, and observing the slow relaxation of the abducted thumb. Also, ask the patient to forcefully clench the fist and then release it.

Myotonia improves with repeated exercises (warm up phenomenon).

Paradoxical myotonia or paramyotonia, worsens with exercises and cold.

It is best seen by asking the patient to repeatedly shut the eyelids tightly.

Myotonic dystrophy (DM1) is the most common myopathy worldwide. It is a multisystem disease.

Nondystrophic myotonias are chloride channelopathies, and not dystrophies. They lead to Herculean muscles, a true muscle hypertrophy.

CARDIO-RESPIRATORY INVOLVEMENT

Respiratory muscles are commonly affected in myasthenia and motor neuron disease. Among myopathies, early and prominent respiratory insufficiency is a classic manifestation of acid maltase deficiency (or Pompe's disease), even before significant muscle weakness ensues.

Pompe's disease is treatable by enzyme replacement therapy.

Vital capacity can be checked clinically by asking the patient to take a deep breath and count.

Single breath count <20 indicates reduced vital capacity.

Myopathies with early respiratory failure
• Acid maltase deficiency • Myotonic dystrophy • Nemaline

Cardiac functions are significantly affected in many myopathies, and should be detected early, as they are amenable to treatment (**Table 7**).

TABLE 7	Cardiac dysfunction (congestive heart failure and arrhythmias).
Congestive heart failure	**Arrhythmias**
• Acid maltase deficiency	• Andersen–Tawil syndrome
• DMD/BMD	• EDMD
• EDMD	• Myotonic dystrophy
• LGMD 1A/1B	• Mitochondrial myopathy

(DMD/BMD: Duchenne muscular dystrophy/Becker muscular dystrophy; EDMD: Emery–Dreifuss muscular dystrophy; LGMD: limb-girdle muscular dystrophy)

Following positive symptoms are quite specific for diagnosis.

MYALGIAS

Generalized aches and pains are some of the most nonspecific symptoms and are often due to nonmuscular reasons.

In general, myopathies are painless. However, following can have significant pains.

Infectious myositis	Trichinosis/Pyomyositis
Statin	Improves with withdrawal
Hypothyroid	Improves with thyroxine replacement
Osteomalacic	Improves with vitamin D supplementation

Polymyalgia rheumatica, occurs in elderly with diffuse myalgias and is often associated with temporal arteritis. If untreated, it can lead to sudden blindness.

CRAMPS/STIFFNESS

Cramps are defined as painful, transient, and involuntary muscle contraction.

Physiological cramps: Nocturnal calf cramps and pregnancy induced.

Pathological cramps: *Cramps, during exercise*, are classical of McArdle disease. First few minutes into exercise, muscle cramps and pain occur, followed by painful contracture, (if exercise is continued), often associated with red colored urine, due to myoglobinuria. Patients are taught about "second wind phenomenon", where they need to slow down or stop the exercise for few moments, following which they can continue exercising without developing further pain.

Cramps, at rest, can be a feature of neuromyotonia (Isaacs syndrome). This is associated with myokymia. a slow arrhythmic, visible skin undulations. These are treatable autoimmune diseases.

Cramps at rest and triggered by activity and noise, especially in low back muscles, occurs in stiff person syndrome. Glutamic acid decarboxylase (GAD) antibodies are positive in half of cases.

Hypothyroid myopathy is a treatable cause of cramps/myalgias.

MYOGLOBINURIA

Acute muscle damage or rhabdomyolysis occurs due to multiple causes. This releases myoglobin in urine, turning it dark reddish brown. Rarely, it can lead to acute renal failure.

Direct inquiry about passage of red urine, especially in patients with exercise induced muscle pains, is of great diagnostic value. It clearly suggests metabolic myopathies such as McArdle's disease or carnitine palmitoyltransferase (CPT) deficiency (**Table 8**).

Myopathy is a general term referring to an abnormality of the muscle.

Myopathies can be broadly categorized into genetic or hereditary and acquired (**Table 9**).

INDIVIDUAL MYOPATHIES

HEREDITARY/GENETIC MYOPATHIES

Among hereditary myopathies:

Disorders of the structural proteins and enzymes: Muscular dystrophies
Disorders of the ion channels or channelopathies: Non-dystrophic myotonias and periodic paralyses
Disorders of the glycogen and lipid metabolism: Metabolic myopathies

Most common hereditary myopathies are muscular dystrophies.

Muscular dystrophies are gradually progressive disorders that occur at all ages with varying degrees of severity. The important features include selective involvement, significant wasting and weakness, and sometimes hypertrophy of selective muscles. Traditionally classified on clinical grounds, currently they are classified based on the distinct molecular component involved and the inheritance pattern.

Some common muscular dystrophies and their subgroup diseases are shown in **Table 10**. The phenotypic features of some common muscular dystrophies are given in **Fig. 1**.

TABLE 8	Metabolic myopathies: McArdle's disease and carnitine palmitoyltransferase deficiency.
McArdle's disease	**Carnitine palmitoyltransferase deficiency**
Disorder of glycogen metabolism	Disorder of fatty acid metabolism
Pain occurs after <2 min of high intensity exercise	Pain occurs after >30 min of low intensity exercise
Second wind phenomenon helps	Continuous glucose intake helps

TABLE 9 Categorization of myopathy.

Myopathy	
Hereditary or Genetic	**Acquired**
Muscular dystrophies • Dystrophinopathies • Limb-girdle dystrophies • Congenital muscular dystrophies • Distal myopathies • Hereditary inclusion body myopathies • Other dystrophies **Metabolic myopathies** • Disorders of carbohydrate metabolism • Disorders of lipid metabolism **Mitochondrial myopathies** **Congenital myopathies** **Ion channelopathies** • Sodium channel disorders (hyperkalemic PP, PMC, PAM) • Calcium channel disorders (hypokalemic PP) • Chloride channelopathies (myotonia congenita) • Potassium channelopathies (ATS)	**Idiopathic inflammatory myopathies** • Polymyositis • Dermatomyositis • Inclusion body myositis • Necrotizing autoimmune myopathy **Inflammatory myopathies associated with CTDs:** SLE, MCTD, RA, and systemic sclerosis **Endocrine myopathies** • Hyper/Hypoparathyroidism • Hyper/Hypothyroidism • Diabetes • Steroid myopathy **Toxic myopathy** • Drugs: Statins, other lipid lowering drugs, chloroquine, zidovudine, colchicine, amiodarone • Snake bite and insect bite **Others** • Infections: Parasitic/Viral/ Bacterial • Critical illness myopathy • Osteomalacic myopathy

(ATS: Andersen–Tawil syndrome; CTDs: connective tissue diseases; MCTD: mixed connective tissue disease; PAM: potassium-aggravated myotonia; PMC: paramyotonia congenita; PP: periodic paralysis; RA: rheumatoid arthritis; SLE: systemic lupus erythematosus)

X-LINKED DYSTROPHIES

DUCHENNE MUSCULAR DYSTROPHY

Duchenne muscular dystrophy is the *most common and rapidly progressive childhood onset muscular dystrophy*, with an incidence of 1 in 3,500 live births. It is due to absent dystrophin protein which is a subsarcolemmal protein that provides mechanical stability to the sarcolemma. It is encoded by the large 79 exon dystrophin gene on chromosome Xp21, and DMD most frequently involves gene deletion in around 60–70%, duplication in 5–10%, and point mutations in rest, resulting in absent dystrophin protein.

Affected boys are normal at birth or may have delayed motor milestones. Around 2–3 years of age, weakness is noticed in the form of frequent falls, toe walking, and characteristic use of hands to climb up themselves when rising from the ground (*Gower's sign*). Running, jumping, and hopping are invariably affected. Calf enlargement is present in the majority, while *Valley sign* is also a helpful sign, due to selective loss of muscles forming the posterior axillary fold with hypertrophied deltoids and infraspinatus. *Contractures of heel cords* and iliotibial bands become apparent around 5–6 years of age. Proximal girdle muscles are more affected, and lower limbs are more severely affected than upper limbs. Around 8–10 years, the patients require assistance for walking and rising, and eventually become wheelchair bound by around 12 years of age. Progressive fixed contractures and scoliosis lead to pulmonary functional impairment, eventually leading to fatal chest infections and death. *Cardiomyopathy* is present in all, but rarely symptomatic. *Intellectual impairment* with lower IQ, which is usually nonprogressive and affects verbal abilities more, is common (**Fig. 2**).

TABLE 10 Classification of muscular dystrophies.

Disease	Inheritance	Affected protein
X-linked dystrophies		
Duchenne/Becker	XR	Dystrophin
Emery–Dreifuss	XR	Emerin
Scapuloperoneal	XR	*FHL1* protein
Limb-girdle muscular dystrophies (LGMDs)		
LGMD1A	AD	Myotilin
LGMD1B	AD	Lamin A and C
LGMD1C	AD	Caveolin-3
LGMD1D	AD	*DNAJB6*
LGMD1E	AD	Desmin
LGMD1F	AD	Transportin-3
Congenital muscular dystrophies (MDC)		
Walker–Warburg Syndrome	AR	*POMT1*
Muscle-eye-brain disease	AR	*POMGnT1*
Rigid spine syndrome	AR	Selenoprotein N1

Continued...

Continued...

Disease	Inheritance	Affected protein
Distal myopathies		
Welander	AD	TIA1
Udd	AD	Titin
Markesbery–Griggs	AD	*ZASP*
Nonaka	AR	*GNE*
Other dystrophies		
Myotonic dystrophy 1	AD	*DMPK*
Myotonic dystrophy 2	AD	*ZNF9*
Myofibrillar myopathy	AD	Myotilin/ZASP/Filamin-c/BAG-3
Hereditary inclusion body myositis		
hIBM with FTD and Paget disease	AD	*VCP*

(FSHD: facioscapulohumeral muscular dystrophy; FTD: frontotemporal dementia; HIBM: hereditary inclusion body myopathy; IBM: inclusion body myopathy; PABP2: polyadenylate-binding protein 2; POMT2: protein O-mannosyl-transferase 2)

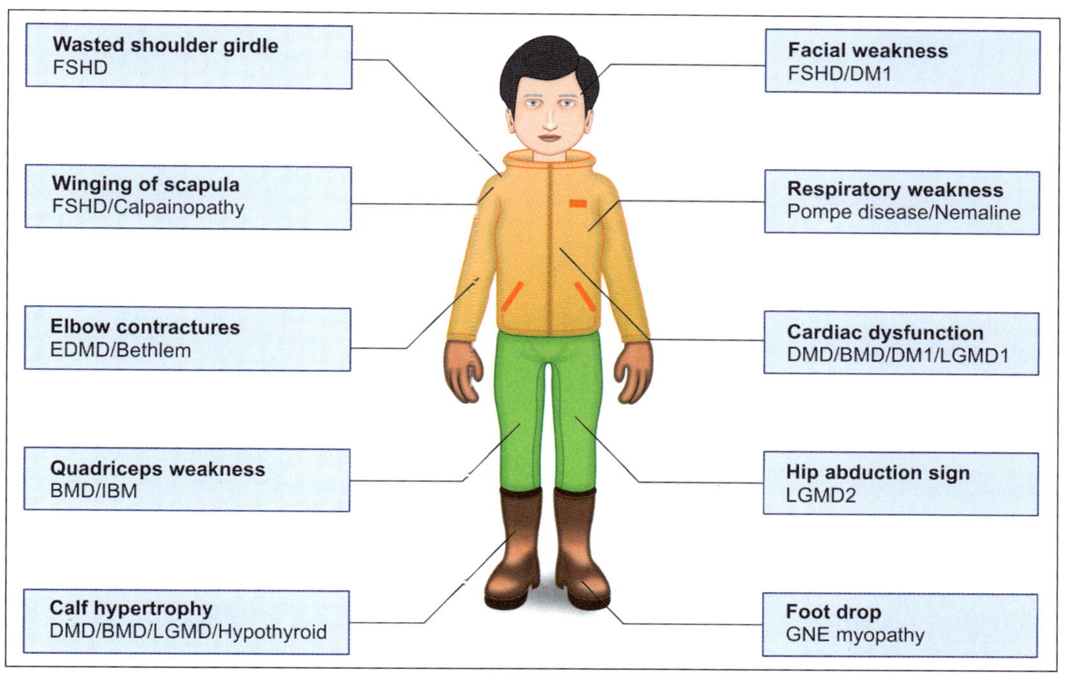

(BMD: Becker muscular dystrophy; DM1: myotonic dystrophy 1; DMD: Duchenne muscular dystrophy; EDMD: Emery–Dreifuss muscular dystrophy; FSHD: facioscapulohumeral muscular dystrophy; GNE: glucosamine-2-epimerase/N-acetylmannosamine kinase; IBM: inclusion body myositis; LGMD: limb-girdle muscular dystrophies)

FIGURE 1: The classical phenotypic features of common muscular dystrophies.

Salient features of Duchenne muscular dystrophy:

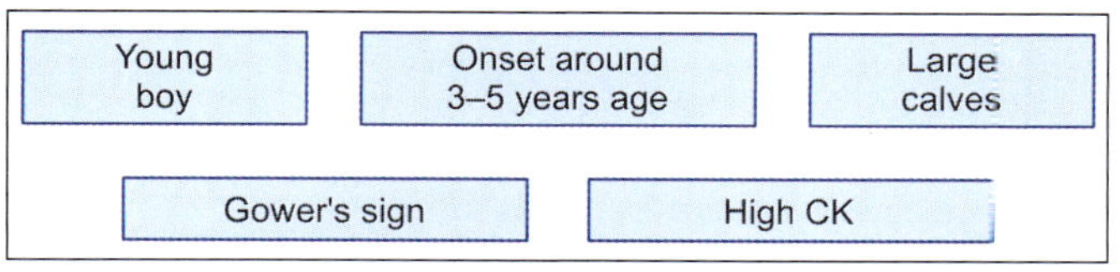

Creatine kinase (CK) levels are high at birth, progressively increase to 20–100 times upper normal limit by 3 years of age.

Definite diagnosis requires molecular diagnosis with:

- Multiplex polymerase chain reaction (PCR) which screens deletions in 19–32 exons (70% sensitivity).
- Multiplex ligation-dependent probe amplification (MLPA) which screens deletions, duplications as well as point mutations.

Treatment: Prednisolone 0.75 mg/kg in various regimens, started around the time of increased falls (8 years) has been shown to slow down the progression to wheelchair confinement by up to 3 years, however the therapy is poorly tolerated by some.

Eteplirsen, an exon 51 skipping antisense oligonucleotide, can be used in 14% patients with specific deletions by converting out of frame mutations to in-frame mutations resulting in production of protein with some dystrophin activity.

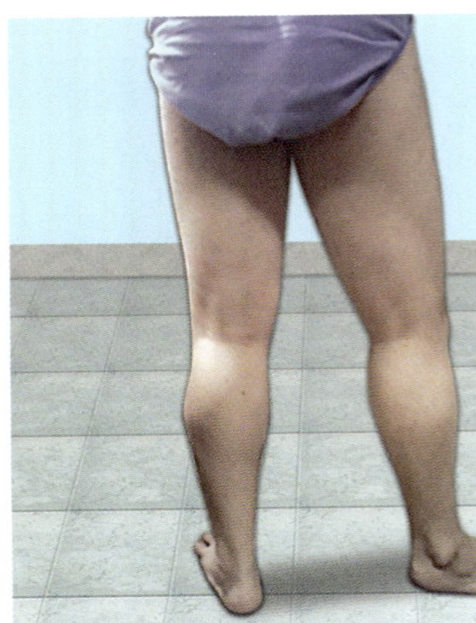

FIGURE 2: Calf pseudohypertrophy.

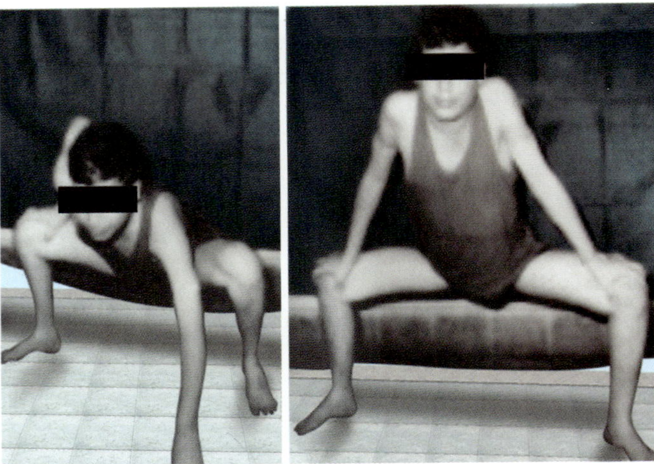

FIGURE 3: Hip abduction sign: Splaying of thighs while upsquatting.

BECKER MUSCULAR DYSTROPHY

Although clinically and genetically like DMD, the cause is usually an in-frame mutation resulting in production of some dystrophin protein. It has a later age of onset from second to fourth decade and a more slowly progressive course. Unlike DMD, patients are still ambulatory beyond 12 years of age. Cardiomyopathy is quite common. Steroids have not been shown to be beneficial.

LIMB-GIRDLE MUSCULAR DYSTROPHY

Limb-girdle muscular dystrophies are distinct group, with chronic progressive hip and shoulder-girdle weakness. As per mode of inheritance, it is classified into, autosomal dominant LGMD1 and recessive LGMD2. Following are some of the commonly seen LGMDs, in India, with their typical weakness patterns.

Calpainopathy: Scapular winging/Shoulder girdle weakness/Hip abduction sign/Ankle contractures/ Abdominal hernia (**Fig. 3**)
Dysferlinopathy: Prominent distal muscle weakness/ Diamond sign on quadriceps/Biceps lump
Sarcoglycanopathy: Calf hypertrophy. Can mimic DMD (**Fig. 4**)

(DMD: Duchenne muscular dystrophy)

Next generation sequencing with Sanger sequencing is the mainstay of genetic diagnosis of various LGMDs.

EMERY–DREIFUSS MUSCULAR DYSTROPHY

It is a rare, early onset X-linked recessive muscular dystrophy due to mutations in *Emerin* gene (Xp28). Weakness and wasting typically involves scapuloperoneal and tibial muscles first and then limb-girdle muscles and the most affected muscle is the biceps brachii.

Following are the two hallmarks of Emery–Dreifuss muscular dystrophy (EDMD).

1. Contractures
   - Contractures affecting the elbows, ankles, neck, and spine causing more disability than weakness, usually symptomatic in second or third decade.

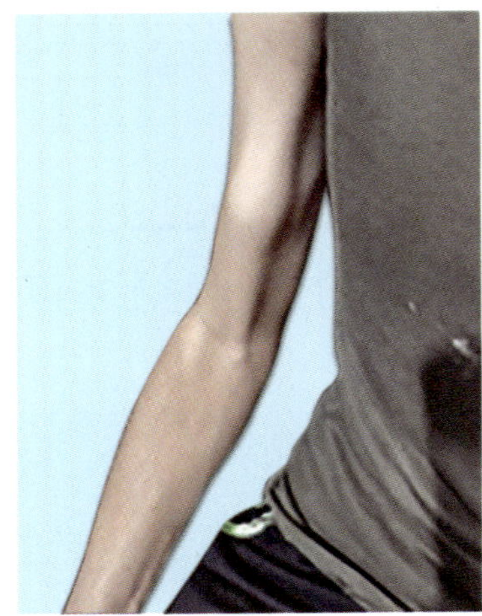

FIGURE 4: Biceps lump: Selective atrophy of distal half of biceps muscle.

2. Cardiomyopathy
   - Resulting in atrioventricular conduction disturbances and sudden death is common, and results in death usually in the fourth decade.

Management of cardiomyopathy and arrhythmias with implantable defibrillators or pacemakers may be lifesaving.

FACIOSCAPULOHUMERAL DYSTROPHY

Facioscapulohumeral dystrophy is a gradually progressive autosomal dominant disease with markedly variable clinical expression.

Onset is usually during teenage years, ranging from early childhood to adulthood.

Three classical features are as follows:

- Facial weakness
- Asymmetrical shoulder weakness
- Beevor's sign

Facial muscle weakness with inability to smile, whistle or close eyes is the initial manifestation, but patients are usually brought to medical attention with onset of asymmetric shoulder girdle weakness. Biceps, triceps, trapezius, and proximal one-fourth of deltoid are selectively affected with relative sparing or mild hypertrophy of infraspinatus, distal three-fourths deltoid, brachioradialis and extensor digitorum communis (EDC), resulting in the classic "poly-hill sign", "chicken wing scapular winging", and "Popeye sign". Beevor's sign can be positive due to selective lower abdominal muscle weakness (**Figs. 5** to **7**).

Creatine kinase is mild to moderately elevated. Treatment is supportive.

MYOTONIC DYSTROPHY

Two types are known. Common, Type 1 and a rarer, Type 2 [proximal myotonic myopathy (PROMM)].

Type 1 is a multisystem disorder, affecting both skeletal and smooth muscles, along with eye, heart, and central nervous system.

It occurs due to abnormal trinucleotide expansion CTG, in noncoding region of *DMPK* gene.

Type 1 is characterized by:
Autosomal dominant inheritance
Typical face: Hatchet like face with frontal balding and swan neck
Wasted muscles: Facial/Sternocleidomastoid/Anterior tibial
Cataracts
Clinical myotonia

Case vignette: 40-year-old female presented with progressive difficulty getting up from sitting and climbing stairs, for 4 months followed by difficulty raising arms for 2 months. On examination, diffuse hip-girdle weakness more than shoulder muscles weakness. No differential weakness noted, (that is all muscles of hip are equally weak). CK values are elevated (**Fig. 8**).

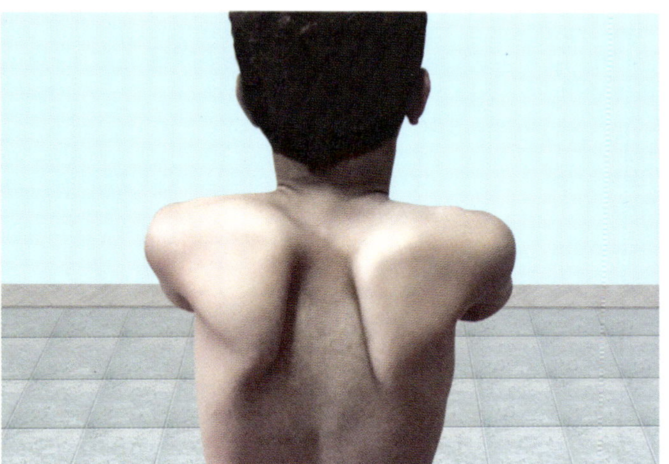

FIGURE 5: Winging scapula: Prominent winging, due to serratus anterior weakness.

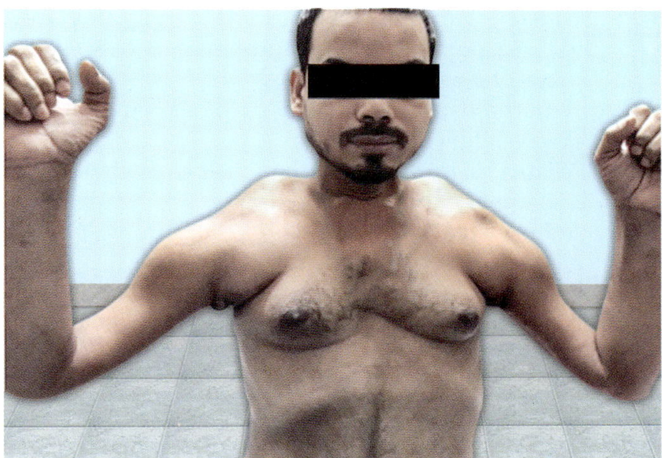

FIGURE 7: Chicken wing: Note the scapula rising from behind, toward neck, giving a wing appearance and Popeye sign: Wasted arm compared to forearm.

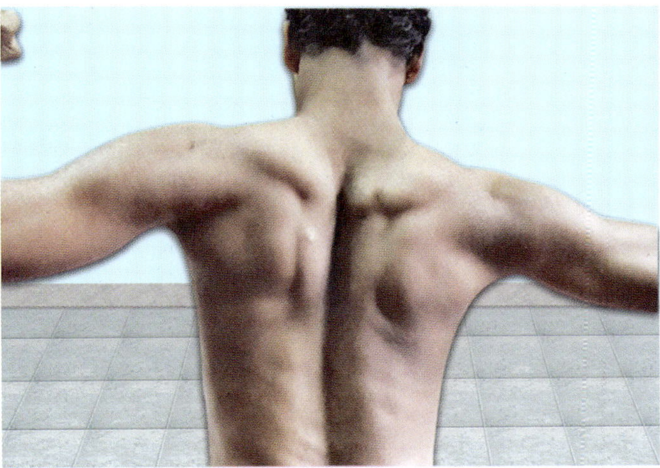

FIGURE 6: *Poly hill sign*: Multiple bony and muscle mounds.

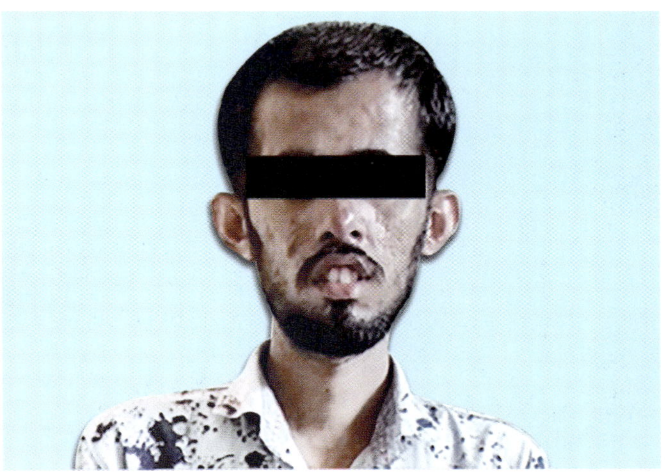

FIGURE 8: Myotonic dystrophy face: Note the frontal balding, wasted temporalis and masseter, wasted sternocleidomastoid (swan neck).

Is this hereditary or acquired myopathy?

This is an acquired myopathy, due to the following features.

Short duration/no selective weakness/rapid involvement of shoulder girdles after hip-girdle weakness.

She has rash on eyelids and back, suggestive of dermatomyositis.

IDIOPATHIC INFLAMMATORY MYOPATHIES

These are a diverse group of disorders with several common features:

Acute to subacute onset and progression, proximal muscle weakness (without differential weakness) with elevated CK, electromyography (EMG) showing active myopathic changes, and muscle biopsy showing inflammation and muscle necrosis.

They include:

- *Polymyositis*: Proximal weakness with truncal and neck muscle involvement.
- *Dermatomyositis*: Proximal weakness with following typical skin changes:
  - *Gottron papules*: Erythematous papules over metacarpophalangeal/interphalangeal (MCP/IP) joints of dorsal hand (**Fig. 9**).
  - *Heliotrope rash*: Reddish/Purple rash on or around the eyelids (**Fig. 10**).
  - *"Shawl" sign*: Erythematous rash over chest, neck and upper back.
  - *Subcutaneous calcification*: Lumps of painful calcium deposits below skin.
- *Inclusion body myositis*: Asymmetrical, selective muscle weakness with early long finger flexors, and quadriceps involvement.
- *Necrotizing myopathy*: Severe course with poor prognosis.

Definitive diagnosis requires myositis-specific auto antibody testing and muscle biopsy, showing characteristic features in each type.

Polymyositis: Endomysial inflammatory cell infiltrating non-necrotic myofibers
Dermatomyositis: Perifascicular atrophy
Inclusion body myositis: Rimmed vacuoles with endomysial inflammatory cells
Necrotizing myopathy: Widespread myonecrosis without inflammation

Treatment requires aggressive acute and chronic immunosuppression.

Overlap syndrome: It is inflammatory myopathy associated with connective tissue diseases.

Antisynthetase syndrome: An inflammatory myopathy associated with mechanic hands, Raynaud's phenomenon, arthritis, and interstitial lung disease (ILD).

POMPE'S DISEASE

A treatable metabolic myopathy, resulting due to deficiency of lysosomal enzyme, acid-alpha glucosidase (GAA), and manifests with progressive hip and truncal muscle weakness. Early respiratory failure, due to diaphragmatic and accessory muscle weakness, causes serious morbidity.

Three classical forms are known as:

Infantile onset	Fulminant cardiomyopathy and poor survival
Juvenile onset	Less severe cardiomyopathy
Adult onset	Predominantly skeletal and respiratory muscle weakness

Diagnosis is done by measuring the GAA activity in dried blood sample. Muscle biopsy shows periodic acid-Schiff (PAS) positive glycogen deposits.

Enzyme replacement therapy, Lumizyme, significantly improves the outcome.

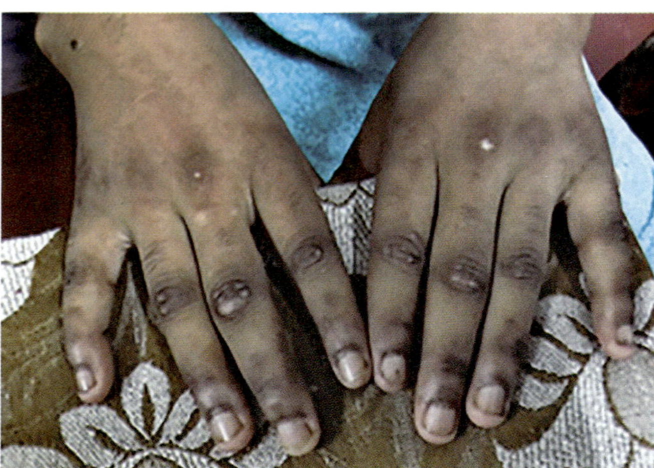

FIGURE 9: Gottron's papules.

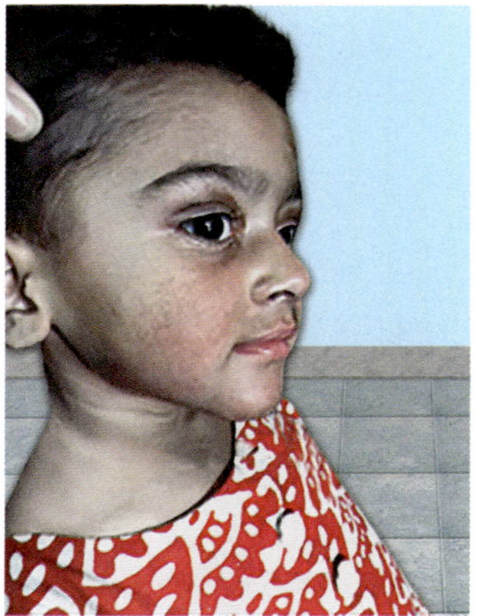

FIGURE 10: Heliotrope and malar rash.

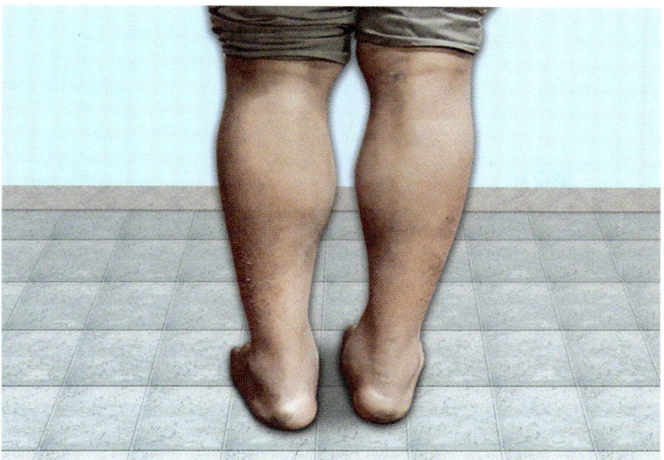

FIGURE 11: ***Hoffman syndrome*: Calf hypertrophy: Before treatment.**

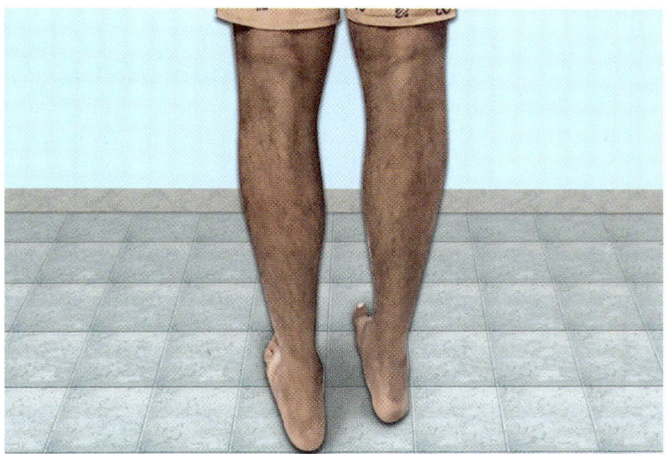

FIGURE 12: ***Hoffman syndrome*: Regression of calf hypertrophy: Post-treatment.**

HYPOTHYROID MYOPATHY

Myalgias and hip-girdle weakness, is a common feature of both congenital and acquired hypothyroidism, especially long standing and untreated. Rarely, weakness can develop in subclinical cases.

Two forms are common depending on age of the patient.

Kocher-Debre-Semelaigne syndrome occurs in children, characterized by generalized muscular hypertrophy, cretinism, and myxedema.

Hoffman syndrome develops in adults, with pseudohypertrophy of muscles, especially calves and muscle stiffness (**Figs. 11** and **12**).

Myoedema is a typical feature of hypothyroid myopathy. It is demonstrated by tapping the muscle with hammer, which forms a transient "mound" at the site of stimulus.

Hypothyroid myopathy reverses with early and prompt treatment of hypothyroidism.

STERIOD MYOPATHY

Exogenous glucocorticoid induced myopathy is common (2–20%), more with fluorinated compounds such as, dexamethasone, betamethasone, and triamcinolone. Fast twitch glycolytic fibers (type 2) are mainly affected. Occurs in two forms:

1. *Acute*: Usually in intensive care unit (ICU) settings, with rapid development of flaccid paralysis. Patients are on ventilator and exposed to high doses of steroids along with sepsis and neuromuscular blockade.
2. *Chronic*: Often occurs after > 4 weeks of exposure. Pelvic girdle is weaker than arms. Cranial muscles are spared.

   Creatine kinase values and EMG studies are normal.

   Reducing the dose, alternate day regimen and switching to nonfluorinated compounds, reverses the weakness.

STATIN MYOPATHY

Use of statin is ever increasing.

Two types of myopathies occur with statins:

1. *Toxic myopathy*: Commonly causes myalgia pains with mild weakness, which sometimes worsens into severe myopathy and rhabdomyolysis. Usually, it is self-limiting, and subsides with prompt withdrawal of the statin. Following approach can be used:

If CK is <5 times the upper limit/No weakness: Observe or lower the dose of statin
If CK is >5 times the upper limit/With weakness: Stop the statin
Once CK normalizes, restart with low dose of rosuvastatin

   All statins can cause myopathy. Worse being cerivastatin (now banned). Safest is rosuvastatin, followed by atorvastatin.

2. *Necrotizing myopathy*: Rarely, statins can trigger an autoimmune myopathy, which worsens despite statin withdrawal. CK values are remarkably high. This needs aggressive immunotherapy for recovery.

GNE MYOPATHY

A unique distal myopathy, seen in third decade of life, begins with foot drop (due to tibialis anterior weakness), and gradually progresses to involve the posterior thigh muscles. There is striking sparing of quadriceps muscle, even late in the disease, hence sometimes called, "quadriceps sparing myopathy". Distal hand muscles are often involved during illness. Beevor's sign (upward movement of umbilicus, with neck flexion) is frequently noted in the Indian patients.

Muscle biopsy classically shows rimmed vacuoles.

The myopathy is the result of mutation in *GNE* gene, which codes for an enzyme, N-acetylglucosamine epimerase/N-acetylmannosamine kinase (*GNE*), which is needed to produce sialic acid. The mutation leads to deficient sialic acids in muscles, supplementation of which is being tried for treatment (**Figs. 13** and **14**).

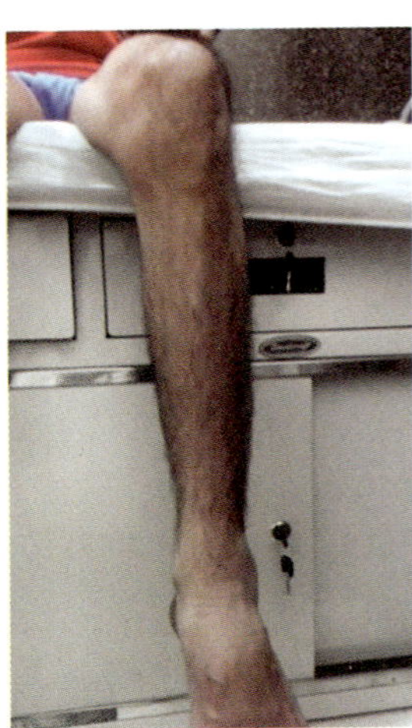

FIGURE 13: ***GNE myopathy*: Foot drop.**

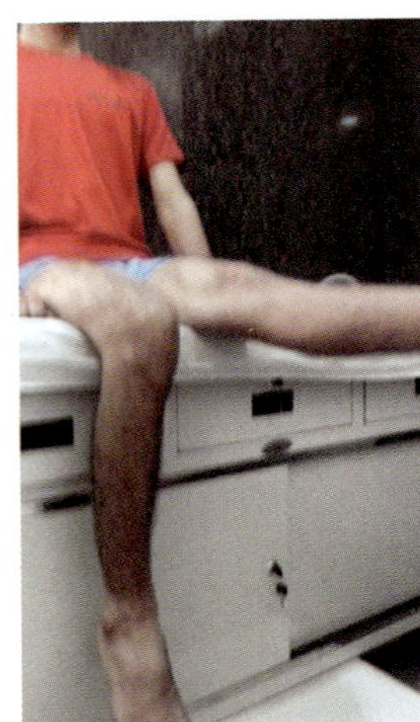

FIGURE 14: ***GNE myopathy*: Normal quadriceps strength.**

CONCLUSIONS

- Clinical diagnosis of myopathy depends upon meticulous history and examination.
- Muscle hypertrophy and differential weakness of muscles are the two cardinal signs of muscular dystrophy.
- Family history and consanguinity should be asked in detail.
- Treatable causes of myopathies should always be sought after.
- Judicious use of genetic tests is advisable.

RECOMMENDED READINGS

1. Ropper A, Robert BH. Principals of Neurology: Adams and Victor, 8th edition. USA: McGraw-Hill Professional; 2005.
2. Khadilkar SV, Shetty K. Clinical approach to muscle disease. In: Singh G, Prabhakar S (Eds). Differential Diagnosis in Neurology. New Delhi: Jaypee Brothers Medical Publishers Pvt. Ltd.; 2016.
3. Hauser SL, Harrison TR, Josephson SA (Eds). Harrison's Neurology in Clinical Medicine. McGraw-Hill Medical Pub. Division; 2006.

CHAPTER

201

COVID Neurology

Vibhor Pardasani

ABSTRACT

Although primarily a respiratory virus, severe acute respiratory syndrome coronavirus-2 (SARS-CoV-2) is known to have several neurological associations. Some of these are protean, nonspecific and mild including headache and dizziness while others are strongly suggestive though not diagnostic such as hyposmia and hypogeusia. Rarely, infected patients can have serious and at times life-threatening neurological complications involving the central as well as peripheral nervous system (PNS). While definitive causal association with SARS-CoV-2 can also be established by presence of virus in the appropriate neural tissue, presence of temporal relation and exclusion of other infectious and neurologic causes can establish this virus as the etiologic factor with reasonable confidence. Early in the pandemic, it was postulated that stroke in Coronavirus disease (COVID) patients primarily affects younger populations and is attributable to large artery disease. However, as more evidence emerged it became known that association of stroke is with severe COVID illness with deranged systemic parameters.

The management of acute respiratory distress syndrome (ARDS) in COVID is similar to its management in non-COVID patients and the use of steroids was considered even before data from clinical trials emerged. Similarly, even though there may never be good randomized trials for management of neurological complications of COVID, therapy would be guided by clinical experience with similar complications occurring in absence of COVID. While the world still waits for the wonder antiviral against SARS-Cov-2, neurological management would be supportive with judicious use of immunomodulatory agents when required.

"The only true wisdom is in knowing that you know nothing"

—Socrates

INTRODUCTION

A novel coronavirus, SARS-CoV-2, first reported from Wuhan, China, in December 2019, resulted in a severe outbreak of worldwide pandemic. The COVID-19 presents with a variety of symptoms chiefly fever, cough, breathlessness, and fatigue. As the pandemic spread and more people got involved, it became apparent that neurologic involvement in COVID-19 may be important in some patients. Some patients of COVID-19 present with neurologic symptoms such as headache, dizziness, or a cerebrovascular event. A subset of patients also reports isolated, sudden onset of anosmia and ageusia as early indicators of SARS-CoV-2 infection. However, a few patients also manifest long-term neurologic complications from COVID-19 infection.

NEUROLOGIC MANIFESTATIONS

Much before the pandemic caused by SARS-CoV-2, six coronaviruses were already known to infect humans. The epidemic of SARS in 2002–2003 was caused by SARS-CoV and Middle East respiratory syndrome (MERS) in 2012 was caused by MERS-CoV. Both these and the other more innocuous coronaviruses have had involvement of the central nervous system (CNS) and PNS, albeit at the rate of <1%. This included encephalitis including brainstem encephalitis, acute disseminated encephalomyelitis (ADEM), cerebrovascular disease, neuropathy, and myopathy.

ANOSMIA AND AGEUSIA

Loss of smell (anosmia) and taste (ageusia) have been reported commonly as symptoms of COVID-19, at times even in isolation, without systemic or respiratory symptoms. Although olfactory dysfunction can commonly occur with any viral illness with mucosal inflammation, and development of anosmia and hyposmia in the absence of nasal obstruction or rhinorrhea represents possible involvement of the olfactory system. The human olfactory epithelium expresses two key genes involved in SARS-CoV-2 infection—angiotensin-converting enzyme 2 (ACE2) and transmembrane protease, serine 2 (TMPRSS2). Some reports isolated the expression of ACE2 to the non-neuronal support cells of the olfactory epithelium rather than neurons of the olfactory bulb. A few clinical reports describe fluid-attenuated inversion recovery (FLAIR) hyperintensities of bilateral olfactory bulbs and right gyrus rectus in magnetic resonance imaging (MRI) in patients with acute anosmia with signal resolution and slight reduction in olfactory bulb thickness on follow-up imaging. Direct viral involvement in olfactory areas of the brain remains a possibility in the pathogenesis of anosmia.

ENCEPHALITIS

Encephalitis manifesting as alteration in consciousness, seizures, fever, headache, vomiting, and focal neurological deficits requires diagnostic features of imaging changes, cerebrospinal fluid (CSF) pleiocytosis, or focal abnormalities on electroencephalogram (EEG). Encephalitis can manifest right from the time of onset of respiratory symptoms to a few weeks later. It usually affects individuals with severe respiratory symptoms more than those with milder course. For a definitive diagnosis, reverse transcription-polymerase chain reaction (RT-PCR) for SARS-CoV-2 should be positive in the CSF. However, in absence of such direct microbiological evidence, the diagnosis can be made if other causes of encephalitis have been excluded in a patient with RT-PCR positive in respiratory secretions.

There are no characteristic clinical features, CSF findings, and patterns of cerebral involvement on MRI or EEG findings that would point specifically toward COVID encephalitis. There is no specific treatment for SARS-CoV-2 encephalitis. Whether viral infection associated with axonal damage or inflammatory response thereof or both contribute to the pathology are not definitively known. Whether any specific agents in the form of antivirals or anti-inflammatories including steroids have any role in the management of COVID encephalitis are also poorly understood.

ENCEPHALOPATHY

Symptoms of altered behavior, cognition, or consciousness when brain inflammation has not been proven is termed as encephalopathy. In relation to COVID, the causes include hypoxia, drugs, toxins, and other metabolic derangements including hyponatremia or hypernatremia, hypocalcemia or hypercalcemia, renal dysfunction, liver dysfunction, and hypoglycemia or hyperglycemia. The inflammatory and cytokine storm, notoriously talked of in severe infection, and also contribute to encephalopathy with inflammatory markers such as interleukin (IL-6), IL-8, IL-10, and tumor necrosis factor-α being directly implicated in states of confusion.

The approach to encephalopathic state in a SARS-CoV-2 positive patient remains the same as that in any general patient. If hypoxia and CO_2 retention have been excluded, one needs to look at any acute change in metabolic parameters including electrolytes and do neuroimaging.

ACUTE NECROTIZING ENCEPHALOPATHY

Another pattern of CNS involvement by SARS-CoV-2 is rapidly developing confusional state with characteristic MRI features of hemorrhagic rim enhancing lesions within the thalami, medial temporal lobes, and subinsular regions, termed as acute necrotizing encephalopathy (ANE). ANE is a known complication of viral illnesses in children and was also reported in adults during the novel influenza A H1N1 pandemic. It is hypothesized to be immune mediated, with most cases preceded by fever and upper respiratory infection and characterized by elevated CSF and serum cytokines.

ACUTE DISSEMINATED ENCEPHALOMYELITIS

Acute disseminated encephalomyelitis is a postinfectious syndrome of multifocal demyelination involving the brain with/without the spinal cord that usually follows a systemic infection. It has been found to occur following COVID, though not at any unusually high rate. It is treated with corticosteroids or other immunotherapies such as intravenous immunoglobulins and plasma exchange. If the time interval between the systemic infection and ADEM is short or if the virus is detected in the CSF, one needs to be judicious with the use of immunotherapies so as to avoid flaring up of the infection itself.

STROKE

Early in the COVID-19 pandemic, the number of patients hospitalized worldwide for stroke showed an unexplained fall. Later, as lockdowns in various parts of the world were eased, the reported incidence of both ischemic strokes (ISs) as well as intracerebral hemorrhage (ICH) went up to the baseline levels at roughly the same proportions. Both IS and ICH are known to occur in patients with COVID-19 disease and are associated with a more severe course of the disease.

A confirmed or presumed infection with SARS-CoV-2 in patients with acute stroke should not lead to different treatment than for other stroke patients. The management protocols including the ones with intravenous thrombolysis and mechanical thrombectomy remain the same provided that appropriate hygiene measures are observed.

Early in the COVID-19 pandemic, an *unusually higher number of strokes* were reported in younger patients and were large vessel IS in some case series. However, as the infection spread around the world, association with cerebrovascular disease was found mostly in critically ill patients with a proinflammatory and coagulopathic state. Pulmonary thrombosis and embolism were also found in moderate to severely ill patients infected with SARS-CoV-2. A prophylactic approach using anticoagulation with low-molecular-weight heparin in patients with elevated D-dimer levels was recommended and used to reduce the risk of thrombotic disease.

In severe or fatal COVID-19 cases, *coagulopathy, including elevated D-dimer levels,* prolonged prothrombin time, and reduced platelet counts have been consistently found. In one study, hyperfibrinolysis, as reflected by elevated serum D-dimer, was present in 97% of COVID-19 nonsurvivors at admission and 71.4% of nonsurvivors met the criteria for disseminated intravascular coagulation. In other words, severely affected patients, who are also more likely to have baseline stroke risk factors as comorbidities, are more susceptible to cerebrovascular disease.

In addition, patients with preexisting cerebrovascular conditions are more likely to have worse clinical outcomes after SARS-CoV-2 infection. This might possibly be due to plasmin, which is a significant factor in fibrinolysis, contributing to enhanced virulence, and pathogenicity of SARS-CoV-2.

A study conducted across seven centers in India for 6 months found that stroke associated with COVID-19 is associated with higher severity, morbidity, and mortality in short as well as long-term. Presence of COVID-19 was found to be an independent risk factor for stroke mortality.

GUILLAIN–BARRÉ SYNDROME

Guillain–Barré syndrome (GBS) and its variants have been frequently reported in close temporal association with SARS-CoV-2 infections worldwide. Since it is a postinfectious illness, there is a possibility of a causal association. However, the incidence of reported GBS cases over the initial 10–12 months of the pandemic has not been particularly higher than expected in the general population over that period of time. No specific clinical pattern of involvement or course has been found to be associated with post-COVID GBS. The association between COVID-19 and GBS warrants further data to support a causal relationship between them. However, unpublished epidemiologic data on incidence of GBS for the last 6 months of 2020 in Europe and the US, when the number of COVID cases shot up dramatically, remained entirely flat thereby excluding any significant causal link. An analysis of the genetic and protein structure of SARS-CoV-2 to check whether the virus had any obvious propensity to trigger an immune response causing GBS was unyielding too. The management of GBS in the presence of COVID-19 remains unchanged with intravenous immunoglobulins or plasmapheresis being the primary modalities. There is no evidence that GBS is more or less severe or response to treatment is altered in the context of the viral epidemic.

INTENSIVE CARE UNIT-ACQUIRED WEAKNESS

Certain COVID-19 patients requiring intensive care with invasive ventilation may develop ICUAW ("intensive care unit-acquired weakness"). This might be either CIP ("critical illness polyneuropathy") or CIM ("critical illness myopathy") or a combination of the two. The incidence of ICUAW, in general as also with COVID association, increases with the severity and duration of the intensive care treatment and may be compounded by sepsis, multiorgan failure, hyperglycemia, parenteral nutrition, and certain medications (sedatives, antibiotics, corticosteroids, and muscle relaxants). This clinical picture is characterized by weakness and atrophy of the entire musculature, including the respiratory muscles with or without sensory disturbances. In general, the prognosis of CIM is better than CIP. Supportive therapy and physiotherapy with early mobilization are the key factors that determine the prognosis and duration of this neurological weakness.

MULTIPLE SCLEROSIS AND COVID-19

Since it is the immune system provides vital defense against viral infections, there was the understandable concern for people taking immunosuppressive agents, as immune compromised people are particularly vulnerable to infections and complications thereof. Multiple sclerosis (MS) is a major neurological disease that causes disability and is largely managed with immunomodulatory drugs, also termed as disease modifying therapies (DMT). There had been a *concern that patients with MS who are receiving DMT may be at higher risk of COVID-19 infection, especially severe infectious complications.* The big question during the pandemic was whether to discontinue DMT for patients already taking these drugs and delay those who were newly diagnosed. Therefore, to understand the risks posed to people with MS using DMT, it is crucial to understand the mechanisms of action, the impact of the treatments on infection-risk, vaccination responses, and the mechanisms of pathology and immunity to SARS-CoV-2. Being a novel disease condition, there are several gaps in our knowledge. However, understanding can be gained from the study of SARS-CoV infection, as well as other coronaviruses, and lower respiratory tract infections.

It is well known that although CD4, T-helper 17 (TH17) T cells are the central mediators of MS, all active DMT inhibit memory B cell activity in a hierarchical (low to high degree of inhibition) fashion that reflects their therapeutic activity. SARS-CoV-2 elimination is largely mediated by CD8 T cells and the innate immune responses. Targeting memory B cell subsets or TH17 cells with DMT is not likely to prevent this viral elimination process. In response to viral infections, antibody secreting cells can be generated by germinal center cells independent of the CD27+, and memory B cell pathway. Even vaccine responses are generated from the immature/naive B cell compartments that regenerate most rapidly following B cell depleting therapies. Once formed, antiviral responses reside within the long-lived plasma cell pool with lymphoid tissue and bone marrow. Plasma cells being relatively quiescent avoid the action of agents targeting proliferating cells. Once formed, plasma cells may not be particularly well targeted by the current DMT, except hematopoietic stem cell therapy (HSCT) that purges the lymphoid tissues. Most DMTs have no major long-term impact on CD8 T cells to limit protection against COVID-19. There is little impact on the formation of immature B cells within lymphoid tissue that will provide antibody-mediated protection from infection/reinfection or mounting response to vaccination.

MECHANISMS OF NEUROLOGICAL DISEASE

Autopsy studies in COVID-19 patients with severe CNS manifestations detected virus in frontal lobe neurons by electron microscopy despite negative CSF PCR testing. Viral particles were also identified in brain capillary endothelial cell indicating a potential direct hematogenous route for CNS spread. Besides this, CNS invasion could be achieved by several routes, including trans-synaptic transfer across infected neurons, entry via the olfactory nerve or leukocyte migration across the blood-brain barrier.

Viral invasion into the brain through the olfactory bulb—the only part of the CNS not protected by dura—is one important plausible route for SARS-CoV-2, especially since anosmia is one of the common characteristic feature of COVID-19. This entry route is also thought to be used by the herpes simplex virus, the most common cause of sporadic viral encephalitis. The ACE2 receptor, to which SARS-CoV-2 binds for entry into cells, is found in brain vascular endothelium as well as smooth muscle.

Damage within the central or the PNS might be caused directly by the virus or by *immune responses activate by the infection.* SARS-CoV-2 or related coronaviruses are not known to be highly neurovirulent, unlike herpes simplex virus, some enteroviruses, and some arboviruses, which can cause uncontrolled neuronal destruction.

The association of cerebrovascular disease in COVID-19 is probably due to a *coagulopathy-like state.* SARS-CoV-2 is known to cause endothelial damage, activating inflammatory, and thrombotic pathways. Thrombocytopenia with elevated D-dimer and C-reactive protein in severe COVID-19 and stroke are consistent with a virus-associated microangiopathic process. A vasculitis process in which the virus replicates in the arterial wall triggering local inflammation, similar to the one reported with Varicella Zoster virus is also possible though as yet unproven mechanism of stroke causation.

DRUGS USED IN COVID-19

Chloroquine and hydroxychloroquine (HCQ), initially developed as antimalarial drugs, were postulated to work in COVID-19 by preventing viral entry via ACE2 binding although human in vivo studies are lacking. There is limited evidence of benefit in the clinical setting. Neurologic adverse effects include irritability, psychosis, peripheral neuropathy, and neuromyopathy. *HCQ is well known to exacerbate weakness in myasthenia gravis* and is contraindicated for patients with this disease. There are reports of myasthenia aggravation when HCQ was used as antiviral in COVID-19. It also lowers the seizure threshold and interacts with several antiepileptic drugs, including lacosamide and lamotrigine. Tocilizumab is a monoclonal antibody to the IL-6 receptor that may attenuate cytokine release in patients with severe inflammatory disease. Neurologic adverse effects include headache and dizziness.

COVID VACCINES

In this pandemic and with ongoing worldwide mass vaccination campaign, it is important for clinicians to recognize and manage neurological complications or other side-effects, if any, associated with COVID-19 vaccination. There are a *few isolated cases of GBS, transverse myelitis, and facial palsy* reported following vaccine administration when used in clinical trials. However, due to absence of significant numbers and no apparent causal link, the trials were not halted and even when mass vaccination drives were initiated there were no reports of any associated neurologic side-effects. There have been worldwide reports of *systemic thrombosis* following the administration of the COVID vaccines especially Astra-Zeneca vaccine. These include coronary as well as cerebral thrombotic events. However, since the incidence has been low and the potential benefit is immense, vaccination is strongly recommended in patients with stroke as well as those with stroke risk factors, just like the general population. Hence, the risk of neurological complications associated with COVID-19 vaccination is low and the benefits of the vaccination, especially against severe COVID, outweigh any potential risks or side-effects.

RECOMMENDED READINGS

1. Ahmad I, Rathore FA. Neurological manifestations and complications of COVID-19: a literature review. J Clin Neurosci. 2020;77:8-12.
2. Ellul MA, Benjamin L, Singh B, Lant S, Michael BD, Easton A, et al. Neurological associations of COVID-19. Lancet Neurol. 2020;19(9):767-83.
3. Sharifian-Dorche M, Huot P, Osherov M, Wen D, Saveriano A, Giacomini PS, et al. Neurological complications of coronavirus infection; a comparative review and lessons learned during the COVID-19 pandemic. J Neurol Sci. 2020;417:117085.
4. Chen X, Laurent S, Onur OA, Kleineberg NN, Fink GR, Schweitzer F, et al. A systematic review of neurological symptoms and complications of COVID-19. J Neurol. 2021;268(2):392-402.
5. Niazkar HR, Zibaee B, Nasimi A, Bahri N. The neurological manifestations of COVID-19: a review article. Neurol Sci. 2020;41(7):1667-71.
6. Paterson RW, Brown RL, Benjamin L, Nortley R, Wiethoff S, Bharucha T, et al. The emerging spectrum of COVID-19 neurology: clinical, radiological and laboratory findings. Brain. 2020;143(10):3104-20.
7. Fotuhi M, Mian A, Meysami S, Raji CA. Neurobiology of COVID-19. J Alzheimers Dis. 2020;76(1):3-19.
8. Ahmed MU, Hanif M, Ali MJ, Haider MA, Kherani D, Memon GM, et al. Neurological Manifestations of COVID-19 (SARS-CoV-2): A Review. Front Neurol. 2020;11:518.
9. Needham EJ, Chou SH, Coles AJ, Menon DK. Neurological Implications of COVID-19 Infections. Neurocrit Care. 2020;32(3):667-71.
10. Baker D, Amor S, Kang AS, Schmierer K, Giovannoni G. The underpinning biology relating to multiple sclerosis disease modifying treatments during the COVID-19 pandemic. Mult Scler Relat Disord. 2020;43:102174.
11. Berlit P, Bösel J, Gahn G, Isenmann S, Meuth SG, Nolte CH, et al. "Neurological manifestations of COVID-19" - guideline of the German society of neurology. Neurol Res Pract. 2020;2:51.

MULTIPLE CHOICE QUESTIONS

To access the multiple choice questions of this Section online, kindly scan the QR code.

CHAPTER 202

Clinical Approach to Respiratory Problems

Surinder K Jindal, Aditya Jindal

ABSTRACT

Over one-third of outpatients seen in clinical practice suffer from one or the other respiratory symptom. A systematic clinical approach is essential to make a meaningful, comprehensive diagnosis—the key to an effective management. Good history-taking is the most essential component of respiratory diagnosis. Physical examination provides limited information but essential to assess the overall assessment and functional status. Plain chest skiagram and routine laboratory investigations are essential for almost all new patients seen in the clinic. Chest X-ray is one of the most useful investigations which lead the clinician how to proceed further. Special investigations such as the lung function tests and the chest computed tomography scan, as well as the disease-specific immunological, microbiological or biochemical tests are undertaken as per needs in an individual case. Invasive and semi-invasive procedures such as fiberoptic bronchoscopy, pleurocentesis, and thoracoscopy are necessary to obtain biopsy specimens for cytological or histopathological examinations.

A good diagnosis is not only required to initiate treatment but also to anticipate treatment outcome and disease prognosis. But for an occasional case, an accurate diagnosis is often possible with the availability of modern techniques. The need to start empirical treatment without a confirmed diagnosis is rather rare if a logical approach is followed. This is also essential to avoid unnecessary costs, delay, and discomfort to the patient.

"A wise man proportions his belief to the evidence"

—David Hume

INTRODUCTION

Over one-third of patients seen in routine clinical practice are reported to complain of one or the other respiratory symptom. A patient with respiratory disease may often present with symptoms of cough and phlegm or expectoration which point to the underlying disease. It is not uncommon that a patient may complain of nonspecific symptoms such as fever, malaise, fatigue, anorexia, and weight loss. Even breathlessness and chest pain may not always mean the presence of a lung disease.

Respiratory problems can be broadly classified to involve the various components of the respiratory system as follows:

- Diseases of the lung parenchyma and airways
- Diseases of pleura, chest wall and mediastinum
- Diseases of the respiratory control

More than one component is involved in most diseases. Moreover, a disease may frequently involve other organ systems besides the lungs. It is important to systematically proceed to arrive at the diagnosis for appropriate management. Typically, the approach starts with a good history-taking and physical examination followed by laboratory investigations, radiology and endoscopy etc. as per needs in an individual patient.

HISTORY-TAKING

A good history-taking may in fact point to the broad underlying diagnosis in almost half the patients. One must follow the principles of history-taking listed in manuals of clinical examination. Inquiry into the details of both general and respiratory symptoms is critical to make a good diagnosis. History of past and concurrent illnesses or comorbidities is an important component. It is significantly helpful to lead to the diagnosis. The golden rule is—"Listen to the patient patiently." Following points should be specifically considered:

- Current symptoms—presence, severity, and duration of different symptoms. There are multiple causes of different symptoms—the most common (cough, expectoration, hemoptysis, chest pain, and breathlessness) of them are listed in this chapter (**Table 1**).
- Presence of general and/or other organ-specific symptoms may frequently lead to the diagnosis of a systemic illness.
- Previous history of a respiratory disease, diabetes, cardiovascular, gastrointestinal, or other chronic illnesses is important.
- Inquiry into personal and occupational exposures is of great significance in respiratory medicine. Tobacco-smoking, biomass domestic fuel combustion, and

TABLE 1 Causes of five common respiratory symptoms.

Cough	Hemoptysis	Wheezing	Chest pain	Breathlessness
• Upper airway cough syndrome—allergic; infections • Pneumonia • Tuberculosis • Asthma and COPD • Bronchitis and bronchiectasis • Lung tumors • Other lung parenchymal diseases: ILDs • Cardiac causes: ◦ Congestive heart failure ◦ Pulmonary embolism • Drugs: ACE inhibitors • Psychogenic/habit cough • Unexplained	• Infections: TB ◦ Bronchitis ◦ Bronchiectasis ◦ Lung abscess ◦ Pneumonia ◦ Aspergillosis ◦ Other infections • Tumors: ◦ Carcinoid ◦ Malignant • Cardiovascular: ◦ Mitral stenosis ◦ Thromboembolism ◦ Aortic aneurysm • Systemic: ◦ Vasculitides ◦ Goodpasture syndrome ◦ Idiopathic pulmonary hemosiderosis ◦ Hematologic ◦ Trauma • Miscellaneous: ◦ Broncholithiasis ◦ Cryptogenic ◦ Foreign body aspiration	• Bronchial asthma • COPD • Bronchitis • Bronchiectasis • Upper airway cough syndrome—allergic; infections	• Pleural diseases: Effusion, tumors pneumothorax • Gastroesophageal reflux disease • Pneumonia • Lung tumors • Pulmonary thromboembolism • Angina and myocardial infarction	• All pulmonary and cardiac conditions listed as causes for cough and wheezing • Lack of exercise/obesity • Anemia • Neuromuscular diseases • Renal: Renal failure, metabolic acidosis • Pregnancy • Psychiatric: ◦ Anxiety ◦ Depression ◦ Hyperventilation syndrome

(ACE: acetyl converting enzyme; ILD: interstitial lung disease)

exposures to occupational dusts (both organic and inorganic in nature) are important risk factors for various lung diseases and are therefore important in their diagnosis, management, and prevention strategies.
- History of past as well as current medication for different diseases. Particular attention should be paid to the concurrent drug therapy.

PHYSICAL EXAMINATION

GENERAL PHYSICAL EXAMINATION

It is quite important for an astute physician to get at the diagnosis. Typically, one needs to look at the general build and nutrition of the patient, status of consciousness, vital signs (Respiratory Rate, Pulse, and Blood Pressure), presence of any respiratory distress, cyanosis, jaundice, or any kind of pigmentation. Body weight, height, and BMI should be noted as possible in an individual case. General muscle mass and presence of edema over the ankles and/or elsewhere on the body should be carefully looked for.

Presence of some common physical signs may point to the presence of an underlying disease or complication (**Table 2**). Absence of a finding does not imply that the disease or the complication is absent. In today's medical practice, it is relatively uncommon to find many of these physical findings since the diagnoses are made relatively earlier than in the past. Face and neck examination may reveal the presence of abnormal venous engorgement, jugular venous pulse, facial edema or enlargement of lymph node, parotid, and salivary glands. Other sites of possible lymph node enlargement such as the axillae and groins should be carefully palpated. Presence of clubbing of the nails over the finger tips is a significant pointer to the presence of a chronic or subacute lung disease although the same may be present in some cardiac, gastrointestinal, or liver diseases. Koilonychia and other types of nail dystrophies and pigmentation may point to the presence of anemia or other nutritional deficiencies or diseases.

It is also important to carefully take a look at the key findings on examination of other organ systems which are relevant in a patient with a potential respiratory disease. Some of the important sites include skin, eyes, mouth, and joints which should be carefully looked at. Abdominal examination should be done for engorged veins, ascetic fluid, enlargement of liver and spleen, or presence of any other abdominal mass. Cardiac examination should be done for any abnormal pulsation, cardiac enlargement, and murmurs. Examination of the neuromuscular system and spine should be done for any neurological deficit or muscular dystrophies which are frequently relevant in respiratory diseases.

TABLE 2 Important signs as pointers to different diseases.

Physical sign	Disease and/or disease-complication
• General appearances and nutrition: Anemia, wasting	Chronic systemic disease, malignancy
• Cyanosis	Hypoxemia—pulmonary or cardiac, right to left shunts
• Bluish pigmentation of lips/finger tips	Cold exposure; methemoglobinemia or sulphemoglobinemia
• Abnormal venous engorgement, jugular venous pulse, facial edema and chemosis	• Superior vena cava obstruction • COPD with pulmonary hypertension (chronic cor pulmonale)
• Enlargement of lymph nodes	Tuberculosis, metastases, lymphomas
• Parotid and salivary glands	Sarcoidosis, other immune diseases, drugs
• Nasal lesion	Granulomatosis with poly-angiitis (Wegener's granulomatoisis)
• Clubbing of the nails over the finger tips	• Bronchiectasis, lung abscess, lung cancer, idiopathic pulmonary fibrosis. • Infective endocarditis; congenital heart disease • Ulcerative colitis, cirrhosis, Celiac disease • Tuberculosis, sarcoidosis, drugs, idiopathic
• Koilonychia, nail dystrophies and pigmentation	Anemia or other nutritional deficiencies or diseases
• Skin and/or eye lesions: ○ Erythema nodosum ○ Malar rash over face ○ Subcutaneous nodules	• Systemic lupus erythematosus, dermatomyositis • Metastases • Tuberculosis
• Eye lesions—phlyctenular conjunctivitis Iridocyclitis	Tuberculosis, sarcoidosis
• Horner Syndrome	Recurrent laryngeal nerve palsy—lung cancer
• Flapping tremors of hands	Chronic respiratory failure

CHEST EXAMINATION

The standard clinical method of chest examination includes the steps of inspection, palpation, percussion, and auscultation. For a medical student, it is important to undertake the detailed stepwise examination as described in books on clinical methods. It is however time-consuming and physicians frequently do an abbreviated shortcut in a busy outpatient clinic. Both *inspection* and *palpation* can help to identify any asymmetry and mediastinal shift to suggest the presence of lung collapse, fibrosis, or pleural disease. Similarly, *percussion* can help to identify the presence of pleural effusion, pneumothorax, and a mass lesion. *Auscultation* will identify the intensity of breath sounds and presence (or absence) of air entry, presence of abnormal chest sounds, crackles, or wheezes. Some of these signs may prove to be diagnostic of an underlying disease.

One can make a fairly accurate clinical diagnosis with good history-taking and physical examination. Chest roentgenogram (CXR) and other relevant laboratory tests are however generally necessary to make a confirmed, final diagnosis and start treatment. This is particularly so in patients with early disease before the development of clinically identifiable signs. In today's medical practice, at least some of the tests are a part and parcel of clinical examination. For example, CXR, routine hematological and biochemical investigations are essentially required for all the patients.

INVESTIGATIONS

CHEST ROENTGENOGRAPHY

A plain CXR: [Posteroanterior (PA) view] is almost an essential component of a clinical diagnosis before starting treatment for a new patient. It is a simple and cheap investigation which is highly sensitive and specific than simple physical examination. Each type of abnormal shadow has distinct characteristics which are fairly suggestive. Further investigations may be required whenever the doubt arises. Following important information can be obtained from a plain film:

Abnormal lung parenchymal opacities: CXR can detect the presence of lung infiltrates, consolidation, collapse, cysts, bullae, nodules, or masses. Parenchymal opacities are typically defined as alveolar or interstitial based on the following characteristics:

- Alveolar opacities—usually localized to a lobe or a segment, fluffy and homogenous, presence of air bronchogram
- Interstitial—distinct reticular, nodular or reticulo-nodular, liner or irregular, more diffuse (often bilateral), fuzzy borders of surrounding structures such as the heart, diaphragms, or pleurae
- Pleural diseases—presence of effusion, pleural thickening, or pneumothorax
- Mediastinal lesions—widening, lymph node enlargement, or presence of other abnormal masses
- Chest wall lesions—deformity, bony rib lesions, and spine abnormalities/erosions
- Heart and great vessels—CXR may provide fairly useful information about the heart size and enlargement of its chamber, aorta, and pulmonary arteries.

Further radiological imaging is required whenever there is an abnormality and diagnosis is not clear. Computed tomography (CT) scan helps to differentially resolve the lesions more clearly as well as to identify small lesions which might not have been visible on plain films. High-resolution CT (HRCT) scanning should be undertaken for interstitial diseases while contrast-enhanced scanning is more useful for localized lung opacities as well as for mediastinal and pleural lesions. CT scanning is also helpful to undertake image-guided procedures for lung lesions.

Chest ultrasound is helpful to identify and guide aspiration for pleural and mediastinal lesions. Magnetic resonance imaging is usually not required for lung diseases except in certain specific conditions such as mediastinal vascular lesions. Positron emission tomography (PET) is of great help to identify malignant lesions and their metastatic sites. PET-FDG (fluorodeoxyglucose) scanning is finding increasing utility for the diagnosis of immune diseases such as sarcoidosis and vasculitides. Pulmonary angiography or CT-pulmonary angiography is needed for diagnosis of pulmonary thromboembolism.

Radiology of bones and joints, cardiovascular, gastrointestinal, or other organ systems is required whenever there is such suspicion.

ROUTINE LABORATORY INVESTIGATIONS

Laboratory investigations are necessary to know about organ system involvement and complications. A routine **hemogram** includes the assessment of hemoglobin, total leukocyte count (TLC), differential leukocyte count (DLC), and blood film examination. Erythrocyte sedimentation rate (ESR) is useful only if done from a fasting blood sample. These routine tests can provide useful leads to the presence of conditions which are either important as risk factors for or indicate the presence of a complication of a lung disease. Some of the important clues to different lung diseases are listed as under:

- *Hemoglobin:*
  - Anemia—nutritional, chronic infections, or other chronic diseases; hematological or other malignancies
  - Polycythemia—chronic lung disease, long-standing hypoxia
- *TLC:*
  - Leukocytosis—acute ongoing infection, active inflammatory disease
  - Leukopenia—some viral infection, drugs
- *Platelet count:* Reduced in some viral infections, e.g., dengue; platelet-lowering drugs; hematological malignancies
- *Blood film examination:* Presence of immature cells points to the presence of a hematological malignancy.

Routine **biochemical investigations** include the estimation of blood sugar, serum bilirubin and liver enzymes, blood urea, and serum creatinine levels. Raised levels indicating abnormality provide clue to the presence of diabetes, liver, or renal dysfunction or failure. Other tests may be needed to confirm diagnosis or for other purposes. Similarly, involvement of other organ systems is assessed with appropriate laboratory tests whenever there is a clinical suspicion.

MICROBIOLOGICAL INVESTIGATIONS

Respiratory system is a common site for both community and hospital-acquired infections by different microorganisms including bacteria, viruses, and fungi. Tuberculosis (TB) is one of the most important respiratory infections. For several decades, any lung disease was almost always identified as TB. Even now, any new patient reporting with cough and/or other respiratory symptoms in India is required to be tested for TB. Therefore, sputum smear should always be examined for acid-fast bacilli (AFB). Role of other microbiological tests such as the tuberculin hypersensitivity test, gamma interferon release assay, molecular tests such as Gene X-pert MTB and others is discussed in the TB chapter.

Sputum and other respiratory specimens should also be examined with smear and culture tests for other microorganisms. Serological tests are also needed in suspected cases of different infections. TB serology however is not helpful and is always avoided. Fungal and viral serology is helpful in differential diagnosis of an infective disease.

SPECIAL LABORATORY INVESTIGATIONS

Some patients require special laboratory tests which are not routinely required in every patient. Some such tests are listed below:

- **Immunological tests** for interstitial lung disease (ILD) due to suspected connective tissue disease—rheumatoid factor, antinuclear factor (ANF) and antineutrophilic cytoplasmic autoantibodies (ANCA), and other autoantibodies
- Vasculitides—ANCA and other auto-antibodies
- Viral pneumonia such as due to SARS-CoV-2 infection—lactate dehydrogenase (LDH), D-dimer, and C-reactive protein
- Sarcoidosis—acetyl converting enzyme (ACE) and other autoantibodies
- **Pleural fluid**—routine biochemistry, cytology, and ADA (adenosine deaminase activity)
- Pulmonary thromboembolism—serum D-dimer assay and tests for hemoglobinopathies
- **Lung cancer markers**

The list of special and specific investigations is however keeps expanding with addition of newer knowledge and technology. But one must be cautious in clinical practice to apply the same before the results are validated and recommended as per standard guidelines and principles.

PULMONARY FUNCTION TESTS

Pulmonary function test (PFT) is not specific for a particular disease-diagnosis but tells about the broad categorization, severity, and therapeutic response. It helps to characterize a disease as obstructive or restrictive in nature. One should always be careful to interpret a PFT pattern as diagnostic of a clinical disease. Routinely, PFT includes the measurements of lung volumes, capacities, and flows with the help of spirometry.

The common spirometric parameters are: Vital and forced vital capacity (FVC), forced expiratory volume (FEV1), forced expiratory flows (FEF200–1200 and FEF25–75%), and FEV1/FVC ratio. Spirometry does not measure residual volume, functional residual capacity, and total lung capacity. Peak expiratory flow (PEF) is a useful personal measure of airways obstruction but relatively insensitive for clinical practice. Spirometry following bronchodilator inhalation is required to look for bronchoreversibility. But for infections, spirometry is required in almost all patients with a lung disease. The following list provides some of the important diseases with spirometric abnormalities:

- **Obstructive**—bronchial asthma, chronic obstructive pulmonary disease (COPD), and bronchiectasis
- **Restrictive**—ILDs, pleural diseases, chest wall abnormalities, myopathy, and diseases of central nervous system affecting the central regulatory control
- **Mixed pattern**—COPD, bronchiectasis, and hypersensitivity pneumonias

Other PFTs include measurements of diffusion capacity for carbon monoxide (DLCO), total lung volume, airways resistance, and body plethysmography. 6-minute walk or exercise test is done to check for endurance and tolerance in response to treatments in different categories of patients. Measurements of oxygen saturation and partial pressures of blood gases (oxygen and carbon dioxide) are routinely required in all patients in intensive care units (ICU) and suffering from severe illnesses.

INVASIVE AND SEMI-INVASIVE INVESTIGATIONS

Fiberoptic bronchoendoscopy (FOB): FOB is the most important investigation which has revolutionized the pulmonary practice. FOB done with the help of flexible, fiberoptic bronchoscope is routinely done under local anesthesia as an outdoor procedure. It is useful for following purposes:

- Inspection of bronchial tree for obstruction, tumors, ulcers, secretions, or other changes
- Biopsy of an endobronchial abnormality—plaques, ulcers, and masses
- Biopsy of lung parenchyma with transbronchial techniques; transbronchial cryobiopsy is preferred as it provides a larger sample size.
- Endobronchial ultrasound (EBUS)—guided needle aspiration for masses, enlarged lymph nodes
- Bronchoalveolar lavage (BAL) for alveolar exudates
- Radial EBUS-guided needle aspiration for peripherally situated masses (**Box 1**)

BOX 1 Indications and uses of fiberoptic bronchoscope.

It is useful for following purposes:

- Inspection of bronchial tree for obstruction, tumors, ulcers, secretions, or other changes
- Biopsy of an endobronchial abnormality—plaques, ulcers, and masses
- Biopsy of lung parenchyma with transbronchial techniques; transbronchial cryobiopsy is preferred as it provides a arger sample size
- Endobronchial ultrasound (EBUS)-guided needle aspiration for masses, enlarged lymph nodes
- Bronchoalveolar lavage (BAL) for alveolar exudates
- Radial EBUS-guided needle aspiration for peripherally situated masses

Therapeutic indications: Removal of bronchial secretions or plugs; foreign bodies; control of hemoptysis with thermocautery or electrocoagulation; laser ablation; and others. Therapeutic FOB is better performed under general anesthesia often with the help of rigid bronchoscopy. It can also be used for placement of tracheal and bronchial stents for bronchial strictures and malignancies causing narrowing of lumen.

Pleurocentesis, pleurodesis, and thoracoscopy: Pleurocentesis is frequently required for cases with pleural effusion and empyema for both diagnosis and treatment. Pleural fluid is examined for the underlying cause of effusion such as TB, bacterial or fungal infection, malignancy, or an immune disorder. Therapeutically, it is required for relief of respiratory distress due to breathlessness. Intercostal tube or pigtail-catheter placement for drainage is required in patients with large or recurrent effusions, empyema, hemothorax, chylothorax, and pneumothorax. Pleurodesis is done in cases of recurrent effusion, pneumothorax, and malignancies.

Thoracoscopy is a useful addition in the armamentarium of pulmonary physicians. It is used for inspection of both parietal and parenchymal pleural surfaces and biopsy of nodules or masses. Sometimes, it can also be used for biopsy of the peripheral lung nodules or mediastinal masses. Thoracoscopy is frequently employed for pleurodesis. To avoid complications which can be sometimes serious, medical thoracoscopy should be done only in expert hands by experienced physicians and mostly for diagnostic indications only.

Mediastinoscopy: Endoscopic mediastinoscopy can also be done for inspection of the mediastinum and biopsy of enlarged lymph nodes or mediastinal masses. It is better done by a trained thoracic surgeon in view of the potential surgical complications. Factually, the diagnostic mediastinoscopy is rarely needed these days since EBUS and/or esophagoscopic ultrasound (EUS)-guided procedures will provide the diagnosis in most patients with mediastinal diseases.

Percutaneous needle aspiration or biopsy: Tissue specimens for cytohistopathological examination of peripherally situated nodules or masses can be obtained through percutaneous approach by fine needle aspiration or trucut needle biopsy. Image (ultrasound or CT scan) guidance is helpful to exactly localize the lesion for biopsy.

Surgical biopsy: Open surgical biopsy is rarely required for diffuse ILD when adequate tissue is not obtained on endoscopic cryobiopsy or thoracoscopy. It may also be needed sometimes for an obscure mass which cannot be when other endoscopic and percutaneous approaches have failed.

All attempts should be made to reach a final, confirmed diagnosis for effective management. A good diagnosis is also important to anticipate outcomes of treatment, progress, and prognosis of the underlying disease. But for an occasional case, a comprehensive diagnosis is possible with the availability of modern techniques. A logical approach is however essential to avoid unnecessary costs, delay, and discomfort.

RECOMMENDED READINGS

1. Jindal SK. Anatomy and Architecture: A Clinical Perspective. In: Jindal SK (Ed). Textbook of Pulmonary & Critical Care Medicine, Vol 2. New Delhi: Jaypee Brothers Medical Publishers; 2017. pp. 12-9.
2. Gupta PR. History and Physical Examination. In: Jindal SK (Ed). Textbook of Pulmonary & Critical Care Medicine, Vol 2. New Delhi: Jaypee Brothers Medical Publishers; 2017. pp. 217-25.
3. Jindal SK. Approach to Systemic Manifestations of Pulmonary Disease. World Clinics Pulm Crit Care Med. 2013;2(2):227-37.
4. Verghese A, Brady E, Kapur CC, Horwitz RI. The bedside evaluation: ritual and reason. Ann Intern Med. 2011;155(8):550-3.
5. Moore-Gillon J. The respiratory system. In: Michael Swash (Eds.) Hutchison's Clinical Methods, 21st Edition. Philadelphia: Saunders; 2002. pp. 60-78.
6. Morice AH, Fontana GA, Belvisi MG, Birring SS, Chung KF, Dicpinigaitis PV, et al. ERS guidelines on the assessment of cough. Eur Respir J. 2007;29(6): 1256-76.
7. Diederich S. Radiological diagnosis of pulmonary metastases: Imaging findings and diagnostic accuracy. Radiology. 2004;44(7):663-70.
8. Kritek P, Choi A. Approach to the Patient with Disease of the Respiratory System. Harrison' Principles of Internal Medicine, 20th edition. New York: McGraw-Hill Professional; 2018.
9. Irwin RS. Symptoms of respiratory disease. In: ACCP Pulmonary Medicine Board Review, 25th edition. Northbrook, IL: American College of Chest Physicians; 2009. pp. 415-56.
10. Smyrnios NA, Irwin, RS. Wheeze. In: Irwin RS, Curley FJ, Grossman RF (Eds). Diagnosis and Treatment of Symptoms of the Respiratory Tract. Armonk, New York: Futura Publishing Company, Inc; 1997. pp. 117-53.
11. Prasad R, Garg R, Singhal S, Srivastava P. Lessons from patients with hemoptysis attending a chest clinic in India. Ann Thorac Med. 2009;4(1):10-2.

CHAPTER 203

Air Pollution: Health Effects in Current Scenario and Way Forward

Randeep Guleria, Vartika Mathur, Pawan Tiwari

ABSTRACT

Air pollution is known to be detrimental to health and environment since ancient times. However, there was a surge of pollutants in the atmosphere due to a rapid increase in urbanization and industrialization in the last century. Rapid and unplanned industrialization, especially in developing countries, has altered our environment in a negative manner. This has led to significant increase in premature deaths and air pollution-associated disability-adjusted life years (DALYs), especially in developing countries such as China and India.

Air pollution is now also being linked to many noncommunicable diseases and infectious diseases. Moreover, the coronavirus disease 2019 (COVID-19) pandemic data has suggested an increase in mortality due to COVID in areas where pollution levels were high. Thus air pollution mitigation and control is the need of the hour. Efforts are essential from all levels, be it legislative, administrative, community, or individual.

This chapter elaborates on the burden of air pollution-related diseases, vulnerable population, methods of measuring air pollution exposure and health risks associated with pollutants released from various anthropogenic sources with an emphasis on Indian scenario. We have also described the current status and strategies employed by government and public for reducing air pollution in India and suggest the way forward in mitigating air pollution.

"Man is the only animal that fouls his owns nest"

—Anonymous

INTRODUCTION

Air pollution has been recognized as a health hazard since ancient times. According to *Charaka Samhita*, "The polluted air is mixed with bad elements. The air which is against the virtues of season, full of moisture, speedy, hard, icy cool, hot dry, terribly roaring, colliding from two or three sides, bad smelling, oily, full of dirt, smoke, sand, and steam creates diseases in body and is polluted." Studies on Greenland ice cores demonstrate rise in greenhouse emissions from 100 BC to AD 1800 attributable to ancient Roman, Indian, and Chinese civilizations. Ancient Romans termed their city's cloud of smoke as infamis aer ("infamous air"). Roman Emperor Justinian labeled clean air as the basic right.

London suffered from sea coal burning in the 13th century, leading to multiple royal attempts at banning the practice. However, the great surge in air pollution had come with rapid industrialization and urbanization in 20th century. This led to multiple attempts at workable solutions at air pollution mitigation in Europe and North American cities. However, it took two large-scale disasters, namely the Donora Smog (Donora, Pennsylvania, 1948) and the London Smog (London, 1952) with >4,000 casualties for public opinion and administration to take concrete galvanized steps to curb air pollution. United States Congress passed Clean Air Act in 1963 and strengthened it in 1970. Moreover, in 1960s, it was found that acid rains that caused destruction of forests and aquatic ecosystems in northern hemisphere were a result of air pollutants emitted thousands of miles away. This led to 32 countries of the European Union signing the *Convention on Long-Range Transboundary Air Pollution (abbreviated as Air Convention or CLRTAP)* in 1979 that came into force in 1983. Despite these, with rapid industrialization and increased use of fossil fuels, the scourge of air pollution engulfed the developing world as well. China, India, and other developing nations reported gradually worsening ambient air quality.

BURDEN OF AIR POLLUTION IN INDIA

According to the *Global burden of disease (GBD) study* (2016), air pollution accounted for 6.4 million (5.7–7.3 million) deaths in 2015. Household air pollution (HAP) from solid fuel use was responsible for 2.8 million [95% uncertainty interval (UI) 2.2–3.6 million] deaths and 85.6 million (66.7–106.1 million) DALYs. In India alone, it was estimated that >1.09 million premature deaths, could be attributed to ambient air pollution (AAP). While in India, data shows that the numbers have risen by 24% over the past decade; in China, deaths have stabilized with a 3% drop. The annual deaths attributed to air pollution in India in 2015 alone were >4 times as compared to the European Union. It is estimated that global deaths due to AAP could double by 2050.

There has been an increase in ambient PM2.5 exposure (by 10%) and ozone (by 14–25%) in India since 1990. The estimated population-weighted mean concentrations in India was 74.3 $\mu g/m^3$ for 2015, which increased to 89.9 $\mu g/m^3$ (95% UI 67.0–112.0) in 2017. Up to 76.8% of Indian population had PM2.5 exposure >40 $\mu g/m^3$, which is higher than the recommendations of the Indian national ambient air quality standard (NAAQS). Highest exposures (>125 $\mu g/m^3$) were in Delhi, Uttar Pradesh, and Haryana. Average household level PM2.5 exposures were estimated to be 337 $\mu g/m^3$, 204 $\mu g/m^3$, and 285 $\mu g/m^3$ for women, men, and children, respectively in a recent study, as opposed to the World Health Organization air quality interim target (WHO-AQG IT-1) of 35 $\mu g/m^3$. In India (2017), of the 1.24 million (1·09–1·39) deaths, i.e., 12.5% of total deaths, were attributable to air pollution. Of these, 0.48 million (0.39–0.58) were attributable to HAP. Notably, 51.4% deaths were amongst people aged <70 years.

India contributed 26.2% of the global air pollution DALYs in 2017. AAP-attributable DALYs were highest in the states of Uttar Pradesh, Delhi, Punjab, Haryana, and Rajasthan whereas those related to HAP were highest in Chhattisgarh, Rajasthan, Madhya Pradesh, and Assam. Improvement is air pollution is estimated to improve life expectancy in 2017 by 1.7 years (1.6–1.9); and >2 years in Rajasthan, UP, and Haryana. These were greater than the Global burden of disease (2010) estimates, in which, 627,000 premature deaths and 17.8 million DALYs were attributable to AAP. **Figure 1** gives a comparative perspective of air pollution-attributable morbidity and mortality in India.

VARIOUS AIR POLLUTANTS

Air pollutants can be classified on the basis of their sources of emission, size criteria, and production or their states of matter (**Table 1**).

Though air pollution affects people across all age groups and is associated with increased risk of diseases of multiple organ systems, some population groups are deemed to be at increased risk. These are outlined in **Table 2**.

METHODS TO MEASURE EXPOSURE

Atmospheric air pollutants enter human body primarily through inhalation. Factors that affect their penetration and retention in respiratory tract include physical properties such as size, solubility of the pollutant, concentration in inspired air, amount inhaled per unit time (including the respiratory rate and tidal volume) as well as the duration of exposure. Adverse effects also depend upon the potency or reactivity of the pollutant. For example, highly water-soluble gases (SO_2) and large particles (PM10) remain in the upper airways and tracheobronchial tree, whereas the others, such as *ozone, ammonia, and fine particles (PM2.5) reach the alveoli.*

Fine and ultrafine particulate matter deposit on the alveolar surface, and gases such as carbon monoxide

Number	Factor
1	Top environmental cause of disease and death
	One million deaths in 2017
	One in 10 deaths in India is attributable to air pollution
2	Of 10 Indians breathe clean air (mean annual exposure)
	Times exposure to air pollutants for average Indian vs. world average
	Years increase in life expectancy with improvement in air quality
3	Time exposure to air pollutants in Delhi, Haryana, and UP
	Years added to life in Delhi, Haryana, and UP if air pollution controlled
4	Lakh deaths due to household air pollution in 2017 in India
	Out of 10 air pollution-related deaths are in persons <70 years of age

FIGURE 1: Important facts and comparative figures for air pollution-attributable morbidity and mortality in India.

TABLE 1 Overview of classification of various air pollutants.

Classification	Description	Comments
On the basis of sources		
Natural	Due to various natural processes	• Volcanic eruptions, dust storms • Wild fires • Various organic and inorganic decays
Anthropogenic (man-made)	Human activity generated	• Industrial activities • Fossil fuel burning
On the basis of size		
Particulate matter <10 µm (PM10)	Coarse particles of size <10 µm	Composition and biologic effects of PM depends on its source
PM2.5	Fine particles <2.5 µm	
PM0.1	Ultrafine particles <0.1 µm	
On the basis of production		
Primary	Directly emitted from sources	Sulfur and nitrogen dioxides, carbon monoxide, others
Secondary	Formed by interactions between primary pollutants	Ozone, nitric acid, carbonic acid
On the basis of states of matter		
Gaseous	Present in gaseous state at usual temperature and pressure	Sulfur and nitric oxides, carbon monoxide
Particulate	Present as particles at usual temperature and pressure	Particulate matter of various sizes, pollens

readily permeate the alveolar capillary membrane and bind to hemoglobin. Mechanisms for pollutant removal via mucociliary clearance are effective only in upper airways and tracheobronchial tree. The ultrafine particles are removed primarily via the macrophages, which is a slower and less effective mechanism. Ultrafine particles are said to permeate and circulate to various organ systems and capillary beds. Exercise greatly increases minute ventilation and total exposure to pollutants per unit time.

Other than inhalation, direct deposition on skin, mucus membranes of exposed surfaces, and conjunctiva may result in exposure to air pollutants which can cause local as well as systemic adverse effects.

Following terms are commonly used to measure air pollutant exposure in scientific studies:

- *Concentration*: Amount of pollutant present in air
- *Exposure*: Duration of contact of pollutant with the body, i.e., concentration of pollutant multiplied by time duration for which subject is exposed to the pollutant
- *Dose*: Amount of pollutant that enters the body
- *Biologically effective dose*: Amount of pollutant reaching the target organs, which can then cause adverse health effects
- *Total personal exposure*: Time-weighted mean concentration of pollutant in the ambient environment of the exposed person

TABLE 2 Vulnerable population and risks of diseases.

Population segments	Risks of various diseases attributable to air pollution
Pediatric age group	• Low birth weight • Antecedent asthma • Decreased lung growth • Increased risk of allergies and atopy • Learning disabilities
Elderly	• Lower respiratory tract infection • Macro- and microvascular events such as myocardial infarction or stroke • Exacerbation of preexisting respiratory diseases
Preexisting cardiovascular disorders	Increased risk of myocardial ischemia
Preexisting chronic respiratory disorders	• Acute exacerbation of asthma or chronic obstructive pulmonary disease • Acute myocardial infarction or stroke
Women of childbearing age group	Increased risk of lower respiratory tract infections, tuberculosis, and lung cancer (especially with indoor air pollution)

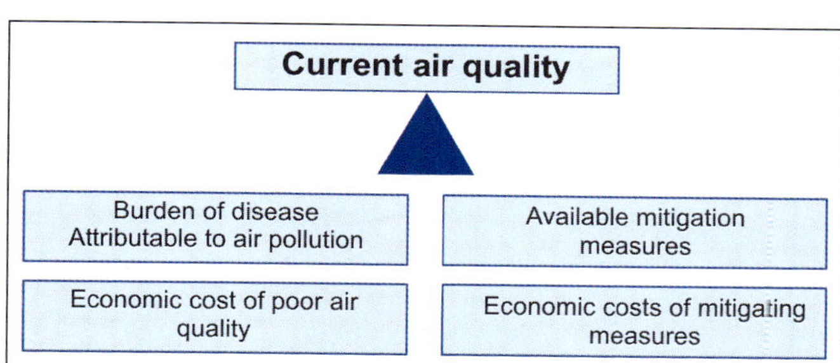

FIGURE 2: Factors considered during derivation of air quality standards.

Air quality standards have been developed and implemented worldwide for measurement of levels of various air pollutants. This is based on various factors including burden of air pollution-attributable diseases, socioeconomic factors, and feasibility of implementation (**Fig. 2**). Air quality standards of various countries and that of the WHO are shown in **Table 3**.

PATHOPHYSIOLOGICAL MECHANISMS

Air pollutants exert their harmful health effects via a variety of pathophysiological mechanisms. Among them, notable mechanisms are:

- Direct irritation of the mucus membranes, e.g., nitric dioxide, ammonia
- Inflammation of respiratory epithelium via production of toxic oxygen species and inflammatory mediators, e.g., nitrogen dioxide, ozone, particulate matter
- Endothelial activation and inflammation, e.g., fine and ultrafine particulate matter
- Induction or promotion of carcinogenesis, e.g., diesel fumes, polycyclic aromatic hydrocarbons
- Promotion or activation of platelet activation and coagulation, e.g., fine particulate matter
- Increasing airway reactivity, e.g., enhanced allergic response to pollens after high exposure to fine particulate matter or gaseous pollutants

ADVERSE HEALTH EFFECTS

Major causes of death due to air pollution are ischemic heart disease, cerebrovascular diseases, chronic obstructive pulmonary disease (COPD), lower respiratory tract infections, and lung cancer (**Table 4**). Moreover, various studies have associated air pollution with increase in noncommunicable and infectious diseases. A recent evidence of this was given through several studies that suggested an increase in mortality due to COVID-19 in areas with high pollution levels.

Respiratory diseases (combined) are known to contribute to nearly 43% of all mortality and about 50% of DALYs due to AAP. Studies from various areas of India have reported positive correlations between higher levels of AAP and premature mortality, along with increased morbidity and mortality due to respiratory diseases.

Adverse respiratory effects of AAP range from decline in lung function, increased respiratory symptoms, asthma/COPD exacerbations and lung cancer. Short-term exposures also increase cardiorespiratory mortality. Pande et al. (2002) demonstrated increased emergency visits for asthma (21.3%), COPD (24.9%), and acute coronary events (24.3%) with increased AAP exposure. A more recent study from AIIMS has also shown an increase in emergency visits in children and adults following increased levels of AAP for up to 6 days. In addition, HAP is known to cause acute lower respiratory tract infections in children and adults and increased risk of tuberculosis (TB). In a recent meta-analysis, pooled odds ratios were 2.37 [95% confidence interval (CI) 1.59, 3.54] for chronic bronchitis and 2.33 (1.65, 3.28) for TB. About 2.4 (95% CI 1.4–3.1) of 5.6 million cases of chronic bronchitis and 0.3 (95%CI 0.2–0.4) of 0.76 million cases of TB could be attributed to HAP due to biomass cooking fuel. Although there are a few ongoing cohort studies, only limited data is available to date to ascertain chronic health effects of air pollution in India.

CURRENT ACTIONS AND WAY FORWARD

All ancient civilizations evolved methods of coexisting with the environment. India, known as a country with eco-friendly civilization, has always been in sync with the environment through its cultural and religious beliefs. Modern India needs to go back to the roots of this harmony between man and nature. In the current scenario, a campaign to improve the quality of air while continuing development is the need of the hour. We need to strike a sustainable balance between economy and ecology, which requires legislative, administrative, community, and individual efforts.

TABLE 3 Comparison of air quality standards across the world.

Ambient pollutant	Common sources	Averaging time	Indian National Standard (2009)	WHO guidelines	Chinese guidelines	European guidelines	United States guidelines
PM10 (μg/m³)	Fossil fuel combustion, industry, surface dust	Annual	60	20	40–70	40	-
		24 hours	100	50	50–150	50	150
PM2.5 (μg/m³)	Fossil fuel and wood or residue crop burning, industry	Annual	40	10	15–35	25	12–15
		24 hours	60	25	35–75	-	35
SO_2 (μg/m³)	Fossil fuel combustion, industry, manufacturing	Annual	50	-	20–60	-	-
		24 hours	80	20	50–150	125	-
NO_2 (μg/m³)	Vehicular pollution, fossil fuel burning, industrial	Annual	40	40	40	40	99.6
		24 hours	80	-	80		-
		1 hour		200	200	200	188
CO (mg/m³)	Vehicular pollution	8 hours	2.0	10	-	10	~10.3
		1 hour			10		
Ozone (μg/m³)	Secondary pollutant, derived from reactions between nitric oxides and hydrocarbons	8 hourly	100	100–160	100–160	120	140
Lead (μg/m³)	Petroleum, dust-containing lead	Annual	0.5	0.5–1.0	0.5	0.5	0.15 quarterly average
Ammonia (μg/m³)	Industries, fossil fuel burning, agriculture slurry and fertilizers	24 hours	400	-	-	-	-
		Annual	100	-	-	-	
Benzene (μg/m³)	Vehicular exhaust, industrial emissions, indoor fossil fuel burning and tobacco smoking	Annual	5	-		5	-
Benzopyrene (ng/m³)	Tobacco, wood and coal tar smoke, forest fires, volcano eruptions	Annual	1	-	1	1	-
Arsenic (ng/m³)	Mining, coal and wood burning, industrial waste disposal, tobacco smoke, forest fires, and volcanic eruptions	Annual	6	-	6	6	-
Nickel (ng/m³)	Fuel oil burning, mining, municipal waste burning	Annual	20	-	-	20	-

TABLE 4 Health effects due to common air pollutants/contaminants and their sources.

	Sources	Persons at risk	Associated diseases
Carbon monoxide	• Incomplete burning of coal and petroleum, vehicular exhaust • Indoor fossil fuel burning	• Smokers • Preexisting cardiovascular disease or chronic lung disease	• Acute myocardial ischemia • Cardiac arrhythmias • Lower respiratory tract infections
Nitrogen oxides	• Fossil fuel burning • Industrial emission	• Ambient exposure • Occupational	• Incident asthma and COPD or exacerbation
Sulfur oxides	• Fossil fuel burning • Industrial emission	• Ambient exposure • Miners	• Incident asthma and COPD or exacerbation
Ozone	• Secondary pollutant from action of sunlight on hydrocarbons and nitrogen oxides • Vehicle exhaust • O_3, a secondary pollutant	• Preexisting cardiovascular or cerebrovascular disease • Preexisting asthma or COPD	• Incident asthma and COPD or exacerbation
Fine particulate matter	• Vehicular pollution • Burning of fossil fuels, wood, coal, crop residues	• Children, pregnant females • Preexisting cardiovascular or cerebrovascular disease • Preexisting asthma or COPD	• Low birth weight • Developmental delay • Learning disability • Incident asthma • Exacerbation of asthma or obstructive airway diseases • Acute cardiovascular or cerebrovascular disease • Lung cancer • Alzheimer's disease • Increased risk of influenza or lower respiratory tract infections
Formaldehyde		• Asthmatics • Obstructive airway disease	• Occupational asthma • Lung cancer
Fungal spores	• Old buildings	• Persons with preexisting allergic or obstructive airway diseases	• Allergic disorders • Hypersensitivity pneumonitis
Pollens	• Pollinating flora	• Atopic individuals • Preexisting allergics or asthmatics	• Exacerbation of allergic diseases and asthma
Radon	• Soil, rocks, underground sources • Granite • May accumulate indoors from underground sources	• Residents of exposed buildings • Uranium miners • Underground workers	• Lung cancer
Asbestos	• Construction material (mixed cement or rooftop sheets) • Demolition or dismantling of old buildings • Scrapping industry • Ship dismantling • Mining	• Miners • Construction and shipyard workers • Residents of buildings where asbestos used	• Asbestosis • Mesothelioma • Lung cancer
Volatile organic compounds	• Solvents • Paints or binders • Alcohol based propellants • Drycleaning liquids, waxes and polishing compounds	• Occupational and indoor exposure	• Malignancies including lung cancer

VARIOUS EFFORTS AND LEGISLATIONS IN INDIA

Various efforts and legislations in this direction in India are outlined below:

- The Factories Act, 1948: This focused indirectly on air quality for workforce in factories.
- Air (Prevention and Control of Pollution) Act, 1981: This was the first act aimed at controlling air pollution in India. It paved the way for establishment of pollution control organizations at central and state levels.
- National Air Quality Monitoring Programme, 1981: Led to monitoring of air quality nationwide
- The Environment (Protection) Act, 1986: This was enacted in aftermath of the Bhopal Gas tragedy. It strengthened the 1981 Air Pollution Act.
- Motor Vehicle Act, 1988: Established emission norms and limits for motor vehicles
- Taj Trapezium Case, Agra, 1996: This was related to air pollution around the Taj Mahal in Agra. This led to relocation of the implicated industries in the area.
- Delhi Air Pollution Case, 1998: This led to Supreme Court Verdict for compressed natural gas (CNG) adoption by public transport buses in Delhi NCR, and resulted in short-term improvement in air quality in the area.
- Bharat stage emission standards (BSES), 2000: These were adopted from the European emission standards. Stage III norms were enforced in 2010, and stage VI norms have been implemented since 2020.
- The Ozone-Depleting Substances (Regulation and Control) Rules, 2000: This act deals with prohibition on investments on ozone-depleting substances.
- Revised National Air Quality Standards, 2009: Revised emission standards for 12 air pollutants including SO_2, NO_2, PM10, PM2.5, Ozone, Lead, Arsenic, Nickel, CO, NH3, Benzene, and Benzo[a]pyrene (particulate phase). These were broadly based on the first interim targets given by the WHO.
- Air Quality Index (AQI), 2015: Implemented real-time monitoring and reporting of AOI across major cities
- India became signatory to the Paris Accord, 2017: This led to self-committed targets for reducing emissions and reduce air pollution.
- Ujjwala Yojana, 2016: This has led to clean fuel delivery to crores of poor households, leading to improved indoor air quality.
- Graded Response Action Plan in Delhi National Capital Region, 2017: AQI-based graded response to mitigate air pollution in Delhi NCR
- National Action Plan, 2016: Comprehensive plan to reduce air pollution

Sustainable development goals have set air pollution-related indicators for monitoring the progress. For addressing AAP, "avoid-shift-improve" framework has been proposed. The "Avoid" refers to changes in town or land use planning, financial disincentives (higher taxes on fuels, congestion pricing, increasing parking fees), limiting vehicle use, or declaring highly congested areas vehicle free. "Shift" refers to shifting to alternative cleaner modes of transport. These include electric powered metros, buses, cars, and two wheelers. Promoting nonmotorized vehicles such as bicycles will have positive health impact along with reducing air pollution. "Improve" refers to tighter emission and fuel standards. Compliance to current emission standards requires strict implementation and monitoring at all levels. Adopting more stringent norms for PM2.5 may save even more lives.

Shift from coal toward renewable energy: For example hydroelectricity, wind, and solar power for electricity production is equally important. Tight standards for particulate matter should be enforced for power plants. Industry and power plants should be relocated away from densely populated areas. Periodic compliance monitoring and imposition of penalties for aberrations and noncompliance are also required. Dust from roads can be controlled through proper street design, green cover, adopting newer methods for cleaning roads to avoid resuspension of road dust in air. Enforcement of good construction practices and safe disposal and recycling of construction and demolition waste is required to reduce construction-related dust production. Other measures include penalties and moratorium on construction activities ignoring dust production or waste disposal standards. Large sources such as industries and power plants need to adopt clean technologies to reduce emissions.

Local industries and brick kilns utilizing coal or agricultural residue contribute to poor urban air quality. Phasing out old technology, implementing emission standards, and promoting alternative building material may limit AAP from this source. Similarly, crop residue disposal practices need to be improved, by promoting eco-friendly disposal methods, crop cycling, and financial incentives.

Graded public response systems based on daily AQI are the need of the hour for all major cities, including warnings for at-risk population groups, school holidays, limitation of usage of personal automobiles (using odd-even schemes or other methods), increasing frequency of public transport, and provision of free or subsidized public transport during days of poor AQI. Public warning systems should explicitly inform people regarding general health risks as well as risks to vulnerable groups, and type of remedial measures to be taken. Daily reporting of cardiovascular and respiratory casualty visits or admissions during periods of high pollution should also be done; this will create necessary public awareness and improve understanding of short-term effects of air pollution.

Household air pollution mitigation requires a community-level approach. Ensuring access to clean fuels such as liquid petroleum gas (LPG), electric and biogas will require continuous fiscal support and robust distribution systems. Biomass stoves emission standards should be as per the WHO emission rate targets. Awareness initiatives should concentrate on changing attitudes and practices of people, ensuring uptake, and utilization of clean cooking practices.

Healthcare providers need to be trained to educate their patients on harm-reduction strategies from air pollution. Robust large epidemiologic and clinical research on adverse effects of air pollution is also needed.

CONCLUSION

The menace of air pollution continues to cause environmental, economic, and health-related adverse effects, and is one of the most important health emergencies faced by the world and, more so by developing countries including India. Air pollution, both indoor and outdoor, lead to both acute and chronic diseases across spectrum of ages either directly or through environmental degradation. This was evident from the increased COVID-19-related mortality in areas with increased air pollution. Various legislative, administrative, community-based, and personal interventions are needed for improving air quality in our country. Clinicians should be aware of the diseases that can be caused or aggravated by air pollution.

RECOMMENDED READINGS

1. Balakrishnan K, Dey S, Gupta T, Dhaliwal RS, Brauer M, Cohen AJ, et al. The impact of air pollution on deaths, disease burden, and life expectancy across the states of India: the Global Burden of Disease Study 2017. Lancet Planet Health. 2019;3(1):e26-39.
2. Cohen AJ, Brauer M, Burnett R, Anderson HR, Frostad J, Estep K, et al. Estimates and 25-year trends of the global burden of disease attributable to ambient air pollution: an analysis of data from the Global Burden of Diseases Study 2015. Lancet. 2017;389(10082):1907-18.
3. Guleria R, Mathur V, Dhanuka A. Health effects of changing environment. Natural resource management: Ecological perspectives. Cham: Springer; 2019. pp. 95-107.
4. Guleria R, Tiwari P. Air Pollution: Health Hazards and Prevention. J Cardiac Crit Care TSS. 2019;3(01):01-4.
5. Health Effects Institute. State of Global Air 2020. Special Report. Boston, MA: Health Effects Institute; 2020.
6. Khilnani GC, Tiwari P. Air pollution in India and related adverse respiratory health effects: past, present, and future directions. Curr Opin Pulm Med. 2018;24(2):108-16.
7. Pande JN, Bhatta N, Biswas D, Pandey RM, Ahluwalia G, Siddaramaiah NH, et al. Outdoor air pollution and emergency room visits at a hospital in Delhi. Indian J Chest Dis Allied Sci. 2002;44(1):13-9.
8. Pandey A, Brauer M, Cropper ML, Balakrishnan K, Mathur P, Dey S, et al. Health and economic impact of air pollution in the states of India: the Global Burden of Disease Study 2019. Lancet Planet Health. 2020;5(1):e25-38.

CHAPTER 204

Bronchial Asthma

SK Chhabra, Mansi Gupta

ABSTRACT

Bronchial asthma is a chronic respiratory disease that occurs all over the globe, affecting millions of people irrespective of age and gender. The earlier belief that it was uncommon in the developing and poor countries is no longer valid, and millions continue to suffer from it, including in India. It causes substantial morbidity, and notwithstanding continued efforts to develop standardized approach to management and availability of effective drugs, remains significant cause of mortality. Mainly an airways disease, the pathophysiological hallmarks include airway inflammation, airflow limitation, and bronchial hyperresponsiveness. Allergies, viral infections of the upper respiratory tract, exercise, exposure to nonspecific irritants including air pollution and occupational environment are often identified as triggers that precipitate symptoms of asthma. The main symptoms include breathlessness with wheezing, often with cough and nasal symptoms. The characteristic pattern of symptoms that occur with intermittency and variability is virtually diagnostic and confirmed further by demonstration of airway obstruction and bronchodilator responsiveness.

A stepwise approach is advocated for management with inhaled corticosteroids (ICS) being the drugs of choice and other drugs including long-acting beta-2 agonists (LABA), long-acting muscarinic antagonist (LAMAs), tiotropium, theophyllines, as add-ons to achieve the desired goals of treatment. Inhalational route is preferred for administration of drugs because of rapid onset of action, lower doses, and fewer adverse effects. Less than 5% asthmatics are severe cases where usual pharmacological treatment fails to provide adequate control. Adjuvant treatment in selected cases includes specific allergen immunotherapy and bronchial thermoplasty. Recent strides in personalized therapy through introduction of biological agents that specifically target IgE, IL-5, or their receptors have opened new vistas in therapeutic options.

"Student: Dr Einstein, Aren't these the same questions as last year's final exam?
Dr-Einstein: Yes; But this year the answers are different"

—Albert Einstein

DEFINITION

Scadding defined asthma as an abnormality of function, *"a disease characterized by wide variations over short periods of time in resistance to flow in intrapulmonary airways."* While this definition captured the clinical concept of asthma, it did not incorporate the essential features of its pathophysiology. The Global Initiative for Asthma (GINA) 2020 update describes asthma as *"A heterogeneous disease, usually characterized by chronic airway inflammation; defined by respiratory symptoms such as wheeze, shortness of breath, chest tightness, and cough that are variable over time and in intensity, along with a variable expiratory flow limitation."* This definition epitomizes our current understanding of this disease. Although it is typically associated with variable airflow limitation, it may become persistent in some patients with long-standing disease. Moreover, patients experience episodic flare-ups in their symptoms known as exacerbations, which are a major cause of morbidity and can be potentially life-threatening.

EPIDEMIOLOGY

Asthma affects an estimated 300 million individuals worldwide. Annually, the World Health Organization (WHO) has estimated that 15 million disability-adjusted life-years are lost and 250,000 asthma deaths are reported worldwide. The prevalence of asthma has been found to be vary between 1% and 20% or even more in numerous studies carried out in several countries, including India. Studies on children have consistently showed 2–3 times higher prevalence. While geographical, environmental, and ethnic factors may contribute to this wide range, methodological differences including definition, sampling, and tools for diagnosis also contribute to this variation. Nevertheless, the total disease burden for highly populated countries such as India is huge. Due to large number of asthmatics, the economic burden imposed on direct costs of outpatient management and hospitalizations and indirect costs due to socioeconomic consequences is substantial.

Majority of patients have their onset in childhood and young adulthood. While asthma can set in at any age, new-onset asthma in later life is less common and is sometimes considered a distinct phenotype. Asthma is more common in boys in childhood, with a male-to-female ratio of 2:1 until puberty, but later in middle and adulthood, the prevalence has no gender bias. Interestingly, some studies have found asthma to be more severe in females. Approximately 15–20% of adults with recently diagnosed asthma experience disease remission within 5 years.

Genetic factors play a major role in the predisposition to asthma. A family history of asthma or other atopic disorders is common, especially in early-onset asthma. Environmental factors play a greater role in the precipitation of asthma. Factors that have been implicated include urbanization, air pollution, passive smoking, and change in exposure to environmental allergens. It is also estimated that 5–20% of new cases of adult-onset asthma can be attributed to occupational exposures.

PATHOPHYSIOLOGY AND PATHOLOGY

The pathophysiology of asthma involves the following components:

- Airway inflammation
- Bronchial hyperresponsiveness
- Airways obstruction

AIRWAY INFLAMMATION

Asthma is a chronic inflammatory disease involving large and small airways. There is also evidence for considerable variability in the pattern of airway inflammation, thus indicating phenotypic differences that may influence treatment responses. Several different cells have been identified such as mast cells, eosinophils, epithelial cells, macrophages, and activated T lymphocytes. T lymphocytes play an important role in the regulation of airway inflammation through the release of numerous cytokines.

Airway inflammation in asthma may represent a loss of normal balance between "opposing" populations of two types of Th (T helper) lymphocytes: (1) Th1 and (2) Th2. Nearly three fourths of asthmatics have eosinophil-dominated (Th2) inflammation. Th2 generates a family of cytokines (IL-4, IL-5, and IL-13) that can mediate eosinophilic inflammation, characteristic of allergic/atopic asthma. IL-5 leads to stimulate production, recruitment, activation, and survival of eosinophils, while IL-4 leads to IgE production from B lymphocytes and subsequent binding to mast cells. IL-13 increases goblet cell differentiation, activation of fibroblasts, elevation of bronchial hyperresponsiveness, and switching of B-cell antibody production from IgM to IgE.

A wide range of stored toxic substances, free oxygen radicals, and newly formed mediators including cytokines released from eosinophils and mast cells perpetuate and maintain airway inflammation. The various constituent airway cells, such as fibroblasts, endothelial cells, and epithelial cells, contribute to the chronicity of the disease. Other factors such as adhesion molecules (e.g., selectins, integrins) are critical in directing the inflammatory changes. Finally, cell-derived mediators influence smooth muscle tone and produce structural changes and airway remodeling. The airway inflammatory response comprising varying degrees of cellular infiltration, airway edema, and mucus secretion, also contributes to airflow obstruction and bronchial hyperresponsiveness. Persistent or inadequately controlled inflammation contributes to desquamation of epithelium, smooth muscle hyperplasia, and airway remodeling leading to persistent airflow limitation in severe/long-standing cases.

BRONCHIAL HYPERRESPONSIVENESS

Bronchial hyperresponsiveness is an exaggerated response to numerous exogenous and endogenous stimuli. The mechanisms involved include direct stimulation of airway smooth muscle and indirect stimulation by pharmacologically active substances from mediator-secreting cells such as mast cells or nonmyelinated sensory neurons. The degree of hyperresponsiveness generally correlates with clinical severity of asthma. Although an intrinsic characteristic of asthma, it can be modulated by airways inflammation and thus varies over time in intensity.

AIRWAYS OBSTRUCTION

Airflow obstruction occurs due to a variety of phenomena including acute bronchoconstriction, airway edema, chronic mucous plug formation, and airway remodeling. It causes increased airway resistance and decreases expiratory flow rates resulting in hyperinflation. The resulting overdistention alters pulmonary mechanics and increases the work of breathing. These physiological changes are responsible for breathlessness and may be completely reversible with bronchodilators and sometimes even without treatment once the exposure to the causative trigger ceases.

CLINICAL FEATURES

The cardinal symptom of asthma is breathlessness, usually associated with wheezing. Cough is often present with small quantity of sputum that may be difficult to expectorate. Unless complicated by other conditions such as pneumonia, tuberculosis, allergic bronchopulmonary aspergillosis (ABPA), and bronchiectasis etc., patients do not report fever, chest pain, purulent sputum, or hemoptysis. The pattern of symptoms gives vital clue for diagnosis. The intermittency and variability in symptoms are characteristic, and a good history is often sufficient to make diagnosis. Patients typically experience episodic occurrence of symptoms (usually more than one) with periods of relative or complete remission; symptoms are worse at night or early morning, vary over time and in severity, occur typically with change of seasons, often triggered by factors such as change in weather, allergen, or irritant exposure (dust, smoke, fumes, and odors), exercise, laughter, emotional stress, viral respiratory infections etc., and respond well to bronchodilators. Atypical presentations include isolated cough, especially in children occurring with the same characteristic intermittency and variability (labeled as cough variant asthma), exertional dyspnea with little wheeze (labeled as late-onset asthma) and chest heaviness. Sneezing, rhinorrhea, and nasal congestion with irritation are symptoms suggestive of allergic rhinitis that often coexist in majority of allergic asthmatics.

Based on the recognizable clusters of clinical, demographic, and/or pathophysiological characteristics, various phenotypes have been identified which do not necessarily correlate with specific pathological process and/or response to treatment.

The most common phenotypes are:

- *Allergic asthma*: Early onset (mostly in childhood); easily recognized; associated with past and/or family history of allergic disease manifestations, such as allergic rhinitis, eczema, and food allergy, respond well to ICS treatment
- *Nonallergic asthma*: Noneosinophilic/neutrophilic/paucigranulocytic inflammation, poor/short-lived response to ICS
- *Adult-onset asthma*: Late-onset, mainly women, nonatopic/allergic variant, require high doses of steroids or are steroid refractory.
- *Asthma with obesity*: Usually late-onset disease with little eosinophilic inflammation, chronic persistent respiratory symptoms.
- *Asthma with persistent airflow limitation*: Long-standing disease with/without adherence to medications, airflow limitation is persistent or partially reversible, associated with airway remodeling, frequent exacerbations common; poor response to steroids

INVESTIGATIONS

The diagnosis of asthma is largely based on the characteristic history. However, documentation of variability of airflow limitation confirms the diagnosis. In most patients with asthma, only the following investigations are required:

Chest radiograph: May be normal or show signs of hyperinflation (**Fig. 1**). Presence of parenchymal shadows suggest

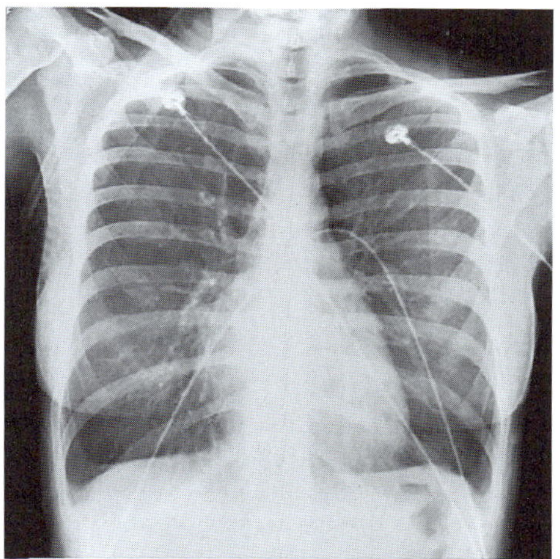

FIGURE 1: Hyperinflation on chest radiograph in a young girl with symptoms suggestive of acute severe asthma.

comorbidities and complications including pneumonia, tuberculosis, ABPA, or bronchiectasis.

Blood counts: May show variable degree of eosinophilia. Documentation of eosinophil count has recently become an important criterion for phenotyping for targeted therapy.

Spirometry: Spirometry is required to confirm airways obstruction and its variability. The expiratory flow limitation/airways obstruction is detected by reduced forced expiratory volume in 1 second (FEV1) with a reduced ratio of FEV1/FVC (forced vital capacity) below lower limit of normal using an ethnically appropriate equation. An increase in FEV1 of >12% and 200 mL from baseline (after 10–15 min of giving 200–400 µg of salbutamol) is consistent with diagnosis of asthma. In asthma, lung function may vary between completely normal and severely obstructed in the same patient at different times (**Fig. 2**).

- *Peak expiratory flow rates (PEFR)*: This is a mechanical hand-held device to measure PEFR that can be used for home monitoring. Documenting daily diurnal PEFR variability (calculated from twice daily PEFR measured through same meter averaged over 2 weeks) of >10% in adults supports the diagnosis of asthma.
- *Fraction of exhaled nitric oxide (FENO)*: It is a surrogate for eosinophilic inflammation. It has emerged as a useful tool for phenotyping and monitoring response to treatment. Values <20 ppb indicate a controlled level of inflammation and those >50 ppb are distinctly abnormal with doubtful range in-between. Serial estimations are more useful than one-off estimations.

Other investigations:

- *Other lung function tests*:
  - Diffusion capacity for carbon monoxide is normal in asthma. It is useful in differentiating asthma from chronic obstructive pulmonary disease (COPD) where it is reduced.
  - Impulse oscillometry is not used in a clinical setting.
- *Computed tomogram (CT) of the chest*: It is not indicated in uncomplicated asthma but may be required to confirm ABPA (central bronchiectasis and hyperattenuated mucus) or emphysema or for other differential diagnosis.
- *Immunological workup*:
  - A total IgE assay is useful for phenotyping as well as to suspect and monitor ABPA.
  - Skin tests for allergen hypersensitivity: These tests are performed for type 1 hypersensitivity response to aeroallergens. These are performed when strong allergy is suspected, pharmacological treatment and allergen avoidance are not yielding acceptable control, and immunotherapy is planned.
  - Estimation of IgE and IgG antibodies to *Aspergillus* species is required as part of the diagnostic criteria for ABPA.
- *Bronchial challenge tests*: Several types of bronchial challenge tests may have clinical or research applications. These tests performed in laboratory settings with emergency management facilities as these may cause a severe reaction.
  - *Exercise*: Running or jogging in cold dry air or on a cycle ergometer for 6–8 minutes may cause a 10% decline in FEV1 [exercise-induced asthma (EIA)] shortly after exercise is stopped.
  - *Histamine/methacholine inhalation*: Gradually increasing doses of aerosolized histamine or methacholine are given by aerosolization to produce controlled bronchospasm and quantify bronchial hyperresponsiveness.

		Measured	LL	Pred	% Pred	Post	% Chg
FEV1	[L]	1.32	2.50	3.11	42	2.82	115
FVC	[L]	2.81	2.82	3.50	80	3.30	17
FEV1 (%) FVC	[%]	47	78	89	52	86	83
FET 100	[sec]	14.1				3.5	–75

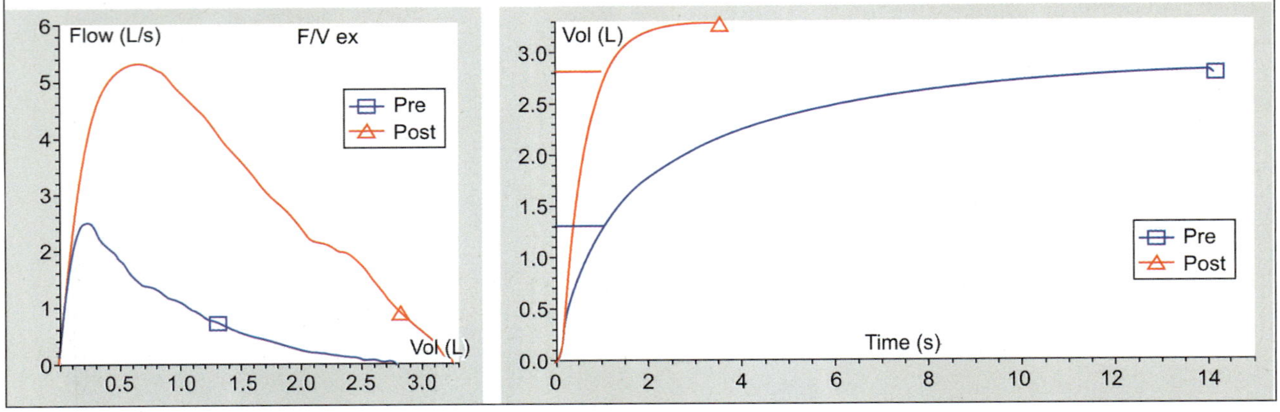

(FET: forced expiratory time; % Chg: percentage change; FEV1: forced expiratory volume in 1 second; FVC: forced vital capacity; LL: lower limit; % Pred: percentage predicted)

FIGURE 2: Spirometry with bronchodilator responsiveness testing in a young girl with symptoms suggestive of bronchial asthma.

- *Allergen challenge*: Controlled inhalation of a suspected allergen or an occupational sensitizing agent can be used to confirm causative agents.

DIFFERENTIAL DIAGNOSES

While a classical presentation with typical features discussed above is diagnostic in most cases, it is pertinent to point out that *"All that wheezes is not asthma."* A review of diagnosis is required when an apparent asthmatic is not responding to treatment or has additional clinical features on presentation and diagnostic workup. Some of the common conditions that closely mimic asthma have been tabulated in **Table 1**. The other differentials include hypersensitivity pneumonitis (acute/subacute), eosinophilic lung diseases (e.g., tropical pulmonary eosinophilia), aspirin or nonsteroidal drug-exacerbated respiratory disease (AERD or Samter's triad), angiotensin-converting enzyme (ACE) inhibitor-related chronic cough, sarcoidosis, malignancies with central airway obstruction etc. Rarely, asthma-like symptoms have also been reported in pulmonary hypertension, pulmonary embolism, eosinophilic granulomatosis with polyangiitis (EGPA), lymphangioleiomyomatosis (LAM) etc. However, any of these above-mentioned alternative diagnoses may coexist with asthma and should be searched for in all cases of difficult-to-treat asthma.

MANAGEMENT OF CHRONIC ASTHMA

The management is aimed at achieving following long-term goals through a multimodality approach consisting of patient education, pharmacotherapy, nonpharmacological therapies, and adjunctive therapies:

- To achieve good symptom control and maintain normal activities of daily living
- To minimize the risk of asthma-related deaths, exacerbations, persistent airflow limitation, and side effects due to medications

In control-based management cycle, pharmacotherapy and nonpharmacological treatments are adjusted in a continuous cycle (see **Flowchart 1**). Some alternative

TABLE 1 Differential diagnoses of asthma.

Conditions mimicking asthma	Diagnostic clues
Chronic rhinosinusitis (CRS), chronic upper airway cough syndrome (CUACS)	• Seen in both adults and children, subacute/chronic onset • Sneezing, itching, nasal blockage, throat irritation, postnasal drip, nasal polyposis etc. • Seasonal variations may be present
Gastroesophageal reflux disease (GERD)	• Seen more commonly in adults, adolescent children, obese; subacute/chronic onset • Heart burn, symptoms after meals/lying down, epigastric discomfort, nausea, vomiting
Inducible laryngeal obstruction	• Seen in adolescents and young adults commonly • Sudden-onset symptoms: Wheeze/stridor, shortness of breath, cough • Reversible narrowing of the laryngeal opening seen on laryngoscopy • Due to external triggers such as exercise, irritants, and emotional stress • Classically described as paradoxical vocal cord motion (PVCM), aka vocal cord dysfunction
Inhaled foreign body	• Seen in children <12 years, elderly with predisposing risk factors • Sudden/subacute-onset symptoms: Shortness of breath, cough, unilateral wheeze
Hyperventilation, dysfunctional breathing	• Seen in adolescents and young adults commonly • Sudden onset, associated with triggers • Dizziness, paresthesia, sighing etc.
Chronic obstructive pulmonary disease (COPD)	• Seen in adults >40 years, smoking/occupational noxious exposures/young onset (apha-1 AT deficiency) • Shortness of breath (exertional), cough, typically lack seasonal variability/remission periods in symptoms
Bronchiectasis	• Seen in both adults and children, subacute/chronic onset • Chronic productive cough, excessive sputum production, repeated infections • Seen with sinusitis (primary ciliary dyskinesia), gastrointestinal symptoms (cystic fibrosis)
Congestive heart failure (CHF)	• Seen in adults/elderly, subacute/chronic onset • Risk factors: CAD, valvular heart disease etc.; children (congenital heart diseases) • Nocturnal symptoms, orthopnea, paroxysmal nocturnal dyspnea, pedal edema etc. • Associated with additional auscultatory findings—fine crepitations, murmurs etc.
Infections: • *Bacterial (e.g., tuberculosis)* • *Viral* • *Fungal*	• Seen in both adults and children, acute or subacute onset • Associated with fever, productive cough, constitutional symptoms ± hemoptysis • Radiological evidence of parenchymal involvement with microbiological confirmation

(AT: antitrypsin; CAD: coronary artery disease)

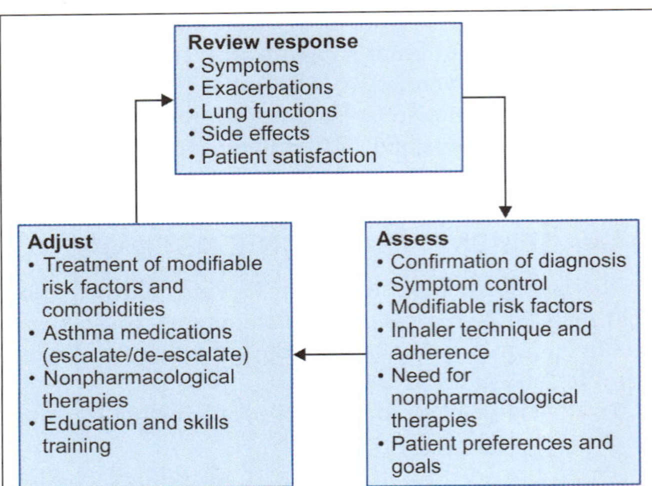

(GINA: Global Initiative for Asthma)

FLOWCHART 1: Personalized asthma management cycle for control-based asthma care (Adapted from GINA guidelines, 2021).

strategies used for adjusting asthma treatment include treatment guided by sputum or blood eosinophilia, and treatment guided by fractional concentration of exhaled nitric oxide (FENO). However, these strategies are not currently recommended as per the standard guidelines.

PATIENT EDUCATION

Patients should be provided with education material about the disease, information about the available treatments, training in essential skills such as inhaler technique, and advised on the warning signs of worsening asthma control. The need for avoidance of risk factors, ensuring adherence to controller medications, training in asthma self-assessment and management plan should be emphasized on a regular basis.

PHARMACOTHERAPY

The choice of medications, devices, and doses is based on individual patient needs, assessment of symptom control, risk factors, patient preferences, and practical issues such as cost, availability, and ability to use and adhere. The medications for long-term treatment fall into three categories: (1) *controller medications,* (2) *reliever (rescue) medications,* and (3) *add-on therapies.* It is essential to record the level of symptom control, lung functions, and potential risk factors for exacerbations, existing comorbidities, and other factors that may impact adherence (**Table 2**) before treatment and at regular intervals thereafter. The various inhaled drugs available for asthma are listed in **Table 3** along with their range of doses and adverse effects.

Inhaled corticosteroids: Given the dominant role of airway inflammation in asthma, ICS are the agents of choice for all patients irrespective of age, gender, and clinical severity. All adults and adolescents with asthma should receive ICS-containing controller treatment to control symptoms and reduce their risk of acute exacerbations. Even, apparently mild asthmatics are at risk of serious adverse events. Almost 30–37% of adults with acute asthma, 16% of patients with near-fatal asthma, and 15–20% of adults dying of asthma had reported symptoms less than weekly in previous 3 months. The ICS-containing controllers are given daily on regular basis, or in very mild asthma, combined with LABA combination for symptomatic relief on an as-needed basis. Low-dose ICS provides most of the clinical benefit for most asthmatics; however, due to variable ICS responsiveness, few patients may need medium- or high-dose ICS despite good adherence and technique. Long-term use of high-dose ICS is discouraged due to increased risk of local and systemic side-effects.

Long-acting beta-2 agonists have proved to be drugs of great utility when combined with ICS. They have additional anti-inflammatory actions and in patients not responding adequately to low-dose ICS, adding a LABA has been a more effective strategy than doubling the dose of latter. LABAs are not given as monotherapy. It is no longer recommended to treat asthma with short-acting b2-agonists (SABAs) alone, because their regular or frequent use is associated with adverse effects such as β2-receptor downregulation, decreased bronchoprotection, and rebound hyperresponsiveness. Overuse of SABAs is also associated with adverse clinical outcomes such as increased risk of emergency department presentations, exacerbations, and mortality. With the advent of Single Maintenance and Reliever Therapy (SMART), where single inhaler serves as both controller and reliever, the GINA 2020 guidelines introduced a paradigm shift in strategy advocating a preference for the combination of budesonide and formoterol as a reliever.

The treatment plan for chronic stable asthma has been advised in a *"Stepwise" approach* (**Flowchart 2**). While the treatment can be scaled up by adding more controller drugs to achieve the goals, this approach also allows a step-down once the control is achieved, thus giving minimum therapy to maintain adequate control. The initial controller therapy step may be decided based on the presenting symptoms and asthma control, as given below:

- **Step 1:** Symptoms less than twice a month
- **Step 2:** Symptoms twice a month or more, but less than daily
- **Step 3:** Symptoms on most days and/or waking with asthma once a week or more
- **Step 4/5:** Symptoms on most days and/or waking with asthma once a week or more with low lung functions (includes patients with frequent exacerbations requiring oral corticosteroids)

Asthma is a variable condition, and periodic treatment adjustments are needed for day-to-day adjustments in reliever medications, short-term step-up (for 1–2 weeks) of controller medications or a sustained step-up (for at least 2–3 months) of treatment. It is also recommended to review the patients every 1–3 months initially for their symptoms, risk factors, exacerbations etc., and 3–12 months thereafter. The treatment should be reviewed at every visit and

TABLE 2 Assessment of asthma patients before and during treatment (at regular intervals).

Symptom control	Modifiable risk factors	Comorbidities
In past 4 weeks, has the patient had: 1. Daytime asthma symptoms >2/week? 2. Any night-time waking due to asthma? 3. SABA reliever for symptoms >2/week? 4. Any activity limitation due to asthma? • *Well-controlled asthma:* None of the above present • *Partly controlled asthma:* 1–2 of the above present • *Uncontrolled asthma:* 3–4 of the above present	• ≥1 severe exacerbation and/or emergency department visit for asthma in last 1 year • Low baseline FEV1 (<60% predicted) • Smoking/exposure to tobacco smoke • Obesity • Allergen exposure if sensitized • Confirmed food allergy • Sputum eosinophilia • Major psychological problems • Major socioeconomic problems	• Obesity • Gastroesophageal reflux • Anxiety and depression • Food allergy and anaphylaxis • Rhinitis and /or sinusitis • Nasal polyps

(FEV1: forced expiratory volume in 1 second; SABAs: short-acting beta-2-agonists)

TABLE 3 Inhaled drugs used in management of asthma in adults.

Drug	Recommended doses	Common side-effects
Inhaled corticosteroids		
• Beclometasone dipropionate (pMDI-HFA) • Budesonide (DPI) • Fluticasone propionate (DPI) • Fluticasone furoate (DPI) • Ciclesonide (pMDI-HFA) • Mometasone furoate (pMDI-HFA)	200–400 µg/ day 200–800 µg/day 250–500 µg/day 50–100 µg/day 80–320 µg/day 200–400 µg/day	Hoarseness, cough, sore throat, dryness of mouth, oral thrush, dysphonia, dysphagia, minor nasal bleeds
Inhaled beta-2 agonists		
• **Short-acting beta-2 agonists:** ◦ Salbutamol (albuterol) pMDI-HFA Via nebulizer ◦ Levosalbutamol (levalbuterol) pMDI-HFA Via nebulizer • **Long-acting beta-2 agonists:** ◦ Formoterol (DPI) ◦ Salmeterol (DPI)	3–4 times/day (maximum 4–6 hourly) 100 µg/actuation 2.5 mg/respule 50 µg/actuation 0.31/0.63 mg/respule 12–48 µg/day 50–100 µg/day	Tachycardia, palpitations, musculoskeletal tremors, visual blurring, nervousness, headache, sore throat, nasal symptoms, hypokalemia, increase in blood glucose levels
Inhaled antimuscarinic agents		
• **Ipratropium bromide (short-acting)** ◦ pMDI-HFA ◦ Via nebulizer • **Tiotropium (long-acting)** ◦ pMDI ◦ Soft mist inhaler	3–4 times/day (maximum 4–6 hourly) 17 µg/actuation 500 µg/respule 9–18 µg/day 2.5–5 µg/day	Visual disorders, dry mouth, constipation, micturition difficulties and tachycardia

(DPI: dry-powder inhaler; HFA: hydrofluoroalkane; pMDI: pressurized metered-dose inhalers)

de-escalated to achieve minimum effective drug doses based on the achievement and maintenance of good symptom control over past 3–6 months to minimize the potential side effects.

NONPHARMACOLOGICAL INTERVENTIONS

- Cessation of smoking
- Avoidance of exposure to environmental tobacco smoke and suspected aeroallergens
- Regular physical activity and healthy diet
- Weight optimization
- Breathing and calming exercises
- Maintaining good mental health and dealing with emotional stress
- Avoidance of drugs, medication, foods, food-chemicals causing worsening of asthma
- Avoidance of occupational exposures

ADJUNCTIVE THERAPIES

- **Allergen-specific immunotherapy** (subcutaneous immunotherapy (SCIT) and sublingual immunotherapy (SLIT) have been tried in carefully selected patients with

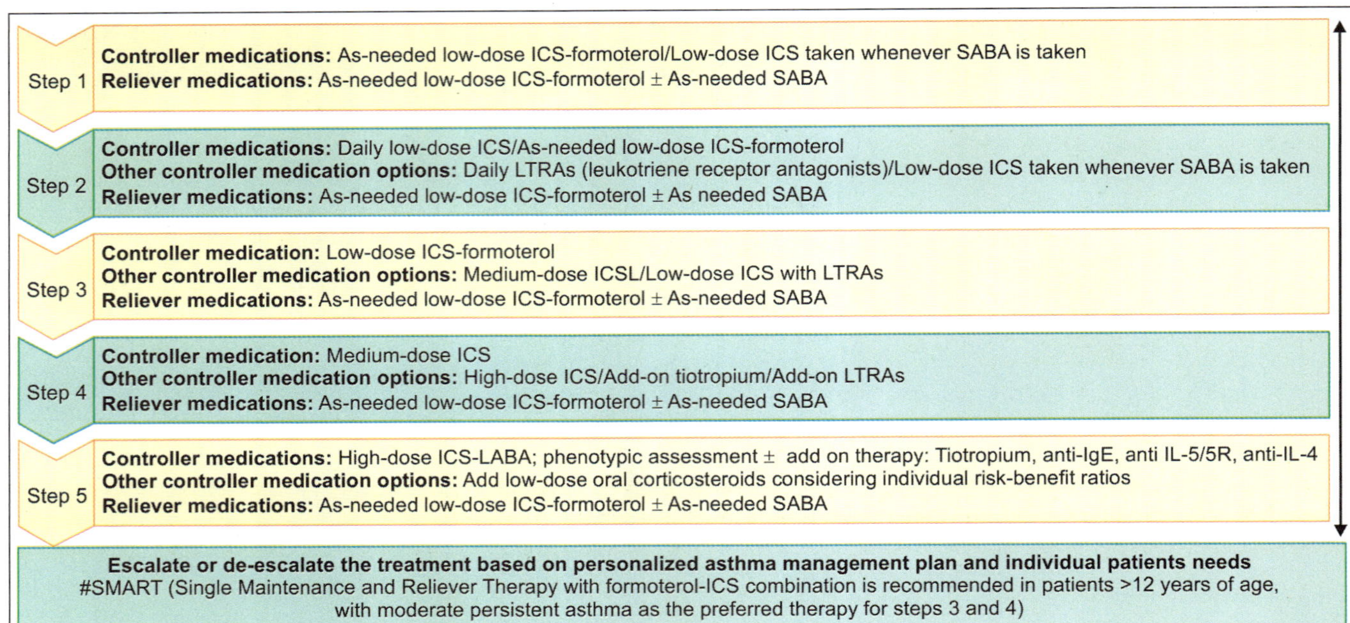

(GINA: Global Initiative for Asthma; ICS: inhaled corticosteroids; SABA: short-acting beta-2-agonist; LABA: long-acting beta-2-agonist)

FLOWCHART 2: Stepwise approach to asthma management (Adapted from GINA guidelines, 2021).

persistent allergic asthma and/or rhinoconjunctivitis. It is reserved for patients with strongly suspected allergy to one or two agents, where avoidance of allergen and regular pharmacotherapy fails to achieve adequate control. Use of standardized extracts for testing of hypersensitivity and for treatment is of critical importance.

- **Targeted biological therapy** such as anti-IgE, anti-ILR, and anti-IL-5/5R may be considered as adjunctive therapy in severe refractory allergic asthma with features of Th2 inflammation (sputum/blood eosinophilia, raised FENO). Agents such as omalizumab, mepolizumab, and benralizumab have been documented to reduce the frequency of exacerbations and use of oral corticosteroids in such patients. At present, these drugs are limited in wider applicability due to the need for parenteral administration and high costs.
- **Bronchial thermoplasty** might be considered in patients with persistent asthma who place low value on harms (short-term worsening symptoms and unknown long-term adverse effects) and high value on potential benefits (improvement in quality of life, small reduction in exacerbations). It involves controlled delivery of therapeutic radiofrequency energy to airway wall using specialized equipment bronchoscopically and reducing the smooth muscle layer mass in airways. High costs and requirement of expertise are limitations to its wider use.

MANAGEMENT OF ACUTE SEVERE ASTHMA

Acute severe asthma or "exacerbation" is acute worsening of symptoms and lung functions as compared to the patient's baseline status. It may present as a complication in patients with prior diagnosis of asthma (even in mild, well-controlled patients) or may even be the first clinical presentation. It usually results from external triggers or poor adherence to controller medications. Delay in recognition of worsening symptoms and action-taking by the patient are major reasons for an acute exacerbation becoming severe enough to require hospitalization and even intensive care management. Some patients have a propensity for severe exacerbations developing out of the blue (*brittle asthma*). The importance of an acute exacerbation lies in the risk of death that it carries lending an urgency in its management.

While acute worsening in symptoms is more sensitive measure of onset of an exacerbation, acute decline in lung functions (FEV1, PEFR etc.) are more reliable indicators of its severity. The severity ranges from mild-to-life-threatening exacerbations requiring hospitalizations and ICU care. The decision for hospitalizations is based on patient's clinical status, lung functions, response to treatment, recent and past history of hospitalizations and exacerbations, and ability to manage a patient at home. It is important to identify the possible risk factors in patients susceptible for asthma-related deaths (**Box 1**).

A schema for management of an acute exacerbation according to severity and response is shown in **Flowchart 3**. The *treatment in emergency department* involves rapid clinical assessment, aiming for rapid achievement of clinical stability (relieving airflow limitation, reducing tachypnea and respiratory distress, address hypoxemia, prevention of respiratory muscle fatigue), while addressing factors responsible for delayed response to treatment and life-threatening complications. Objective assessments of certain parameters such as measurement of FEV1, PEFR, and oxygen saturation (spO_2) by pulse oximetry are necessary as history and physical examination may not indicate the severity. Lung function testing may not be possible during an acute episode as these tests require patient cooperation. Respiratory distress and reduced or falling spO_2 are key pointers to the development of a life-threatening acute exacerbation.

BOX 1	Risk factors for increased asthma-related deaths (Adapted from the GINA guidelines, 2021).
•	History of near-fatal asthma requiring intubation or mechanical ventilation
•	Hospitalization or emergency department visits for asthma during last 1 year
•	Not on regular ICS-based long-term controller medications
•	Currently using or recently stopped oral corticosteroid therapy for asthma control
•	Overuse of SABAs (more than one canister of salbutamol per month)
•	Poor adherence to medications or the written asthma-action plan
•	History of psychiatric disease or psychosocial problems
•	Food allergy in patients with asthma

(ICS: inhaled corticosteroids; GINA: Global Initiative for Asthma; SABAs: short-acting beta-2-agonists)

The initial treatment includes repetitive administration of short-acting inhaled bronchodilators (usually salbutamol and ipratropium bromide), use of systemic steroids, and controlled flow oxygen supplementation. SABAs should be administered every 20 minutes in first 1 hour for rapid reversal of airflow limitation, via pressurized metered-dose inhalers (pMDIs)/spacer or as dry-powder inhalers (DPIs) or via a nebulizer. The requirement is titrated with clinical response and if possible, objective improvement in PEFR (>60–80% for 3–4 hours). The oxygen saturation should be maintained between 93% and 95% with controlled oxygen therapy for best clinicophysiological outcomes. *The need for ICU admission* should be assessed accurately, and invasive mechanical ventilation (IMV) should not be delayed in patients showing poor initial response or rapid clinical deterioration. The role of noninvasive ventilation (NIV) in acute severe asthma remains controversial due to weak evidence in its support. However, it may be tried in selected patients by an experienced intensivist under close supervision.

Patients should be *discharged after attaining clinical stability for 2–4 hours in the emergency department* and/or showing an objective improvement with a post-treatment PEFR > 60%. They should also receive optimum doses of

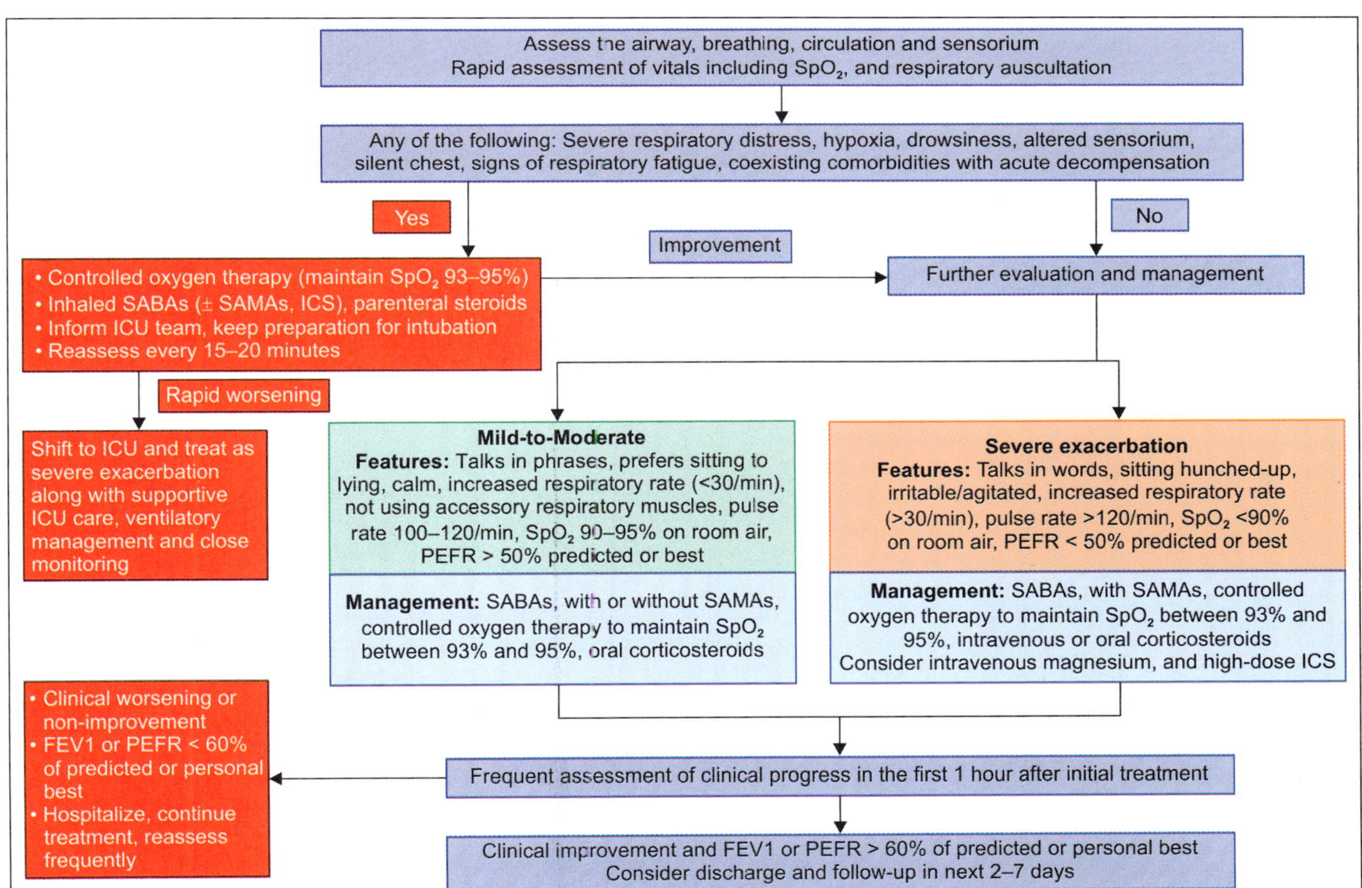

(FEV1: forced expiratory volume in 1 second; ICS: inhaled corticosteroids; PEFR: peak expiratory flow rates; SABA: short-acting beta-2 -agonist; SAMA: short-acting muscarinic antagonists)

FLOWCHART 3: Management of acute severe asthma in emergency department.

ICS-LABA, with or without add-on therapies along with short course of oral corticosteroids for 5–7 days. In addition, for patients who require hospitalization, the risk factors for repeated exacerbations should be explored and addressed prior to discharge. The patients should be advised to follow-up within 2–7 days of their exacerbation and follow their personalized written asthma self-management plan stringently.

SUMMARY

Bronchial asthma is a common chronic respiratory disease with airway inflammation and bronchial hyperresponsiveness characterized by variable airflow limitation. The intermittent and variable symptoms of breathlessness, wheeze, cough, and nasal symptoms have a characteristic pattern that strongly suggest the diagnosis which can be confirmed by spirometry to document airflow limitation and response to bronchodilators. Inhaled corticosteroids are the first-line therapy and other drugs such as LABAs, LAMAs, and theophylline are added or withdrawn in a stepwise manner to achieve best control of symptoms with minimum drug doses. Personalized therapy based on phenotyping of patients and targeting of specific molecular pathways including IgE and IL-5 is a newer modality for severe asthma.

RECOMMENDED READINGS

1. Mims JW. Asthma: definitions and pathophysiology. Int Forum Allergy Rhinol. 2015;5(Suppl 1):S2-6.
2. Padem N, Saltoun C. Classification of asthma. Allergy Asthma Proc. 2019;40(6):385-8.
3. Tilles SA. Differential diagnosis of adult asthma. Med Clin North Am. 2006;90(1):61-76.
4. Mauer Y, Taliercio RM. Managing adult asthma: The 2019 GINA guidelines. Cleve Clin J Med. 2020;87(9): 569-75.
5. Agnihotri NT, Saltoun C. Acute severe asthma (status asthmaticus). Allergy Asthma Proc. 2019;40(6):406-9.
6. Cloutier MM, Dixon AE, Krishnan JA, Lemanske RF Jr, Pace W, Schatz M. Managing asthma in adolescents and adults: 2020 Asthma Guideline Update from the National Asthma Education and Prevention Program. JAMA. 2020;324(22):2301-17.
7. Global Initiative for Asthma. Global strategy for the diagnosis and prevention. Global Initiative for Asthma (updated 2021) [https://ginasthma.org › gina-reports].

CHAPTER

205 Chronic Obstructive Pulmonary Disease

Raja Dhar, Shyam Krishnan, Tarang Kulkarni

ABSTRACT

Chronic obstructive pulmonary disease (COPD) is a major healthcare burden globally with a prevalence of 10.1% and a mortality rate of over 3 million deaths worldwide. The term COPD encompasses various clinical entities with multiple causes resulting in airflow limitation that is not fully reversible. It occurs because of a complex inflammatory cascade triggered by exposure of the lungs to various noxious stimuli (tobacco use, biomass fuel, and environmental pollution etc.). Spirometry forms the backbone in the diagnosis of COPD.

Early detection and prompt treatment with bronchodilators/anti-inflammatory agents, smoking cessation, increasing physical activity, vaccination, and treatment of comorbidities are key measures to reduce the burden of the disease. With a better understanding of the disease, different COPD phenotypes have been identified allowing for precision medicine to be in-vogue in the management of COPD. In this chapter we elaborate on different aspects of COPD including pathophysiology, diagnosis and management of COPD, and its different phenotypes.

"A wise man proportions his belief to the evidence"

—David Hume

INTRODUCTION

Chronic obstructive pulmonary disease is a common respiratory disorder which poses a major healthcare burden both, in our country as well as globally. It is also one of the leading causes of mortality worldwide accounting for around 3 million deaths. COPD is a heterogenous disease with pulmonary and extrapulmonary components. It is still being debated whether COPD is a "single disease" or a "syndrome". In this chapter, we treat it as a clinical syndrome which encompasses chronic respiratory symptoms (cough, breathlessness etc.), structural lung abnormalities, impaired lung function, or a combination of these findings often accompanied by multiple comorbid disorders.

The acronym COPD, though sounding general, describes two very complex pathological processes (chronic bronchitis and emphysema) related to inhalation of noxious fumes, as a single entity. Although believed to affect older individuals there is now increasing evidence to suggest that exposure to risk factors early in life contributes to the development of COPD. More recently it was observed that a certain cohort of individuals with smaller lungs at birth, eventually have a decline in lung function in relation to pollution and poverty which results in COPD. The introduction of the spirometer measuring the forced expiratory volume in 1 second (FEV1) and forced vital capacity (FVC) has been fundamental to diagnose, classify, and measure the progression of COPD. Further advances in imaging, laboratory techniques have helped us to identify different phenotypes of COPD patients thus helping in curating patient specific management plans.

HISTORICAL PERSPECTIVE

Bonet (1679) and Morgagni (1769) made some of the earliest references to emphysema. Morgagni described 19 cases where the lungs were "turgid" particularly from air. The description of chronic bronchitis and bronchiolitis was given by Badhlam in 1814 where he used the word "catarrh" to describe the cardinal symptoms of chronic cough and mucous hypersecretion. Laënnec (1821) in his treatise of diseases of the chest described explicitly the emphysema component and elaborated that emphysematous lungs were hyperinflated and did not empty well. The spirometer invented by John Hutchinson in 1846 became key in the diagnosis and management of COPD after it evolved to measure FEV1 and FEV1/FVC% based on Tiffneau's and Gaensler's work.

Some of the early concepts in pathogenesis of COPD were illustrated by *the Dutch* and *the British hypothesis*. The Dutch hypothesis first put forward the concept that both genetic and environmental factors can determine whether one would have obstructive airway disease. The British hypothesis proposed that hypersecretion in the respiratory tract caused by an infection causes chronic respiratory tract stenosis.

DEFINITION

It was at the ninth Aspen Emphysema Conference where William Briscoe is believed to have first used the term COPD, and later the CIBA Guest Symposium 1959 and the ATS committee on diagnostic standards 1962 laid foundations for the current definition.

The Global Initiative for Chronic Obstructive Lung Disease (GOLD) 2021 document defines COPD as *"A common, preventable, and treatable disease that is characterized by persistent respiratory symptoms and airflow limitation that is due to airway and/or alveolar abnormalities usually caused by significant exposure to noxious particles of gases and influenced by host factors including abnormal lung development."*

EPIDEMIOLOGY

Chronic obstructive pulmonary disease is still underdiagnosed in many parts of the world including India. Despite the complexities in conducting prevalence studies, reliable data is emerging which provide close to actual numbers. According to the *Global Burden of Disease study 2017*, the global prevalence of COPD stands at 10.1%, affecting many people in low-income, middle-income, and wealthy countries. The years of life lost prematurely increased 13.2% between 2007 and 2017. COPD led to 3.2 million deaths in 2017 and by 2040 a figure of 4.4 million yearly deaths is expected. India has 18% of the global population and an increasing burden of chronic respiratory diseases. According to the same study, the number of cases of COPD in India increased from 28.1 million (27.0–29.2) in 1990 to 55.3 million (53.1–57.6) in 2016, an increase in prevalence from 3.3% (3.1–3.4) to 4.2% (4.0–4.4). COPD contributed to 75.6% of the total disability adjusted life-years (DALYs) due to chronic respiratory diseases in 2016 (**Fig. 1**). Globally, COPD is the third leading cause of mortality. In India after ischemic heart disease, COPD was the second leading cause of disease burden, contributing 8.7% (7.8–9.5) of the total deaths and 4.8% (4.3–5.3) of the total DALYs.

PATHOPHYSIOLOGY

Presence of *persistent and fixed airflow obstruction* is central to the pathophysiology of COPD. This persistent airflow limitation usually results after exposure to noxious stimuli such as cigarette smoking, biomass fuel exposure, and several genetic factors. The inflammatory cascade leading to fibrotic changes and later emphysema is depicted in the **Flowchart 1**. These effects eventually result in hyperinflation and progressive air trapping which contributes to dyspnea and worsening quality of life (QoL).

Chronic obstructive pulmonary disease has also been associated with *systemic manifestations* such as cor pulmonale, muscular weakness, ischemic heart disease, depression, osteoporosis, pulmonary hypertension etc., (**Box 1**). These extrapulmonary manifestations not only complicate COPD management, but also lead to an increased healthcare costs, hospital admissions, and ultimately mortality. It has been hypothesized that these extrathoracic manifestations result from "spill-over" of inflammatory cytokines from the lungs to other parts of the body. This has been supported by various studies reporting a raised blood of CRP, tumor necrosis factor-alpha (TNF-α), and other cytokines in COPD patients.

Note: On exposure to noxious stimuli, an inflammatory cascade mediated by cytokines and chemokines such

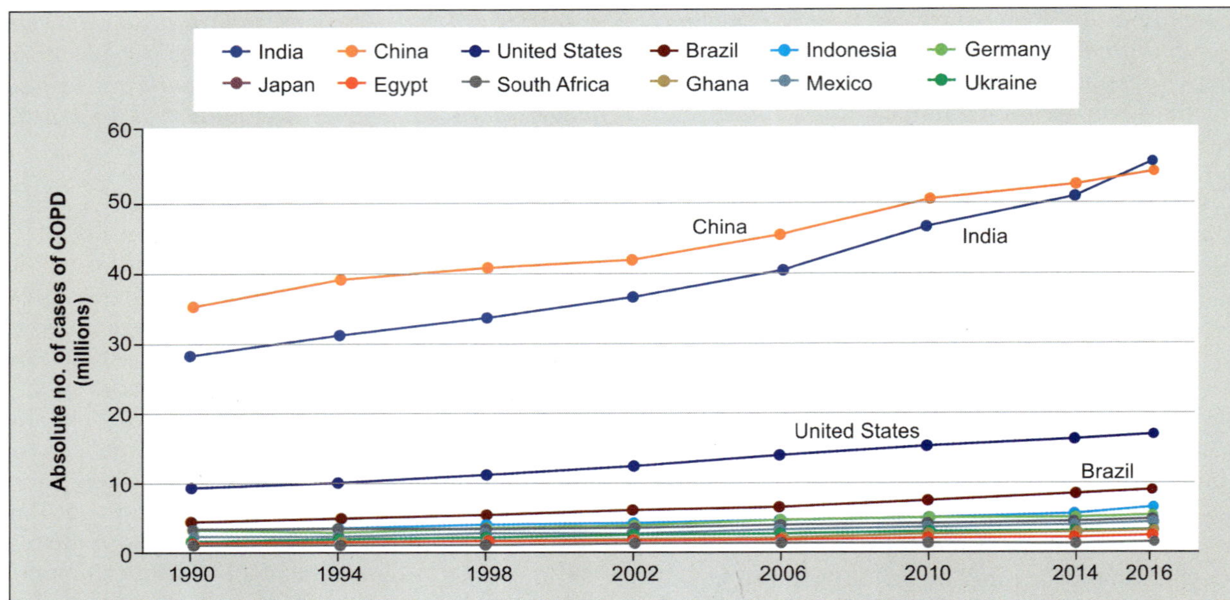

FIGURE 1: Prevalence of chronic obstructive pulmonary disease (COPD) in selected ountries, 1990–2016.

Source: Data are from the Global Burden of Disease (www.healthdata.org/gbd).

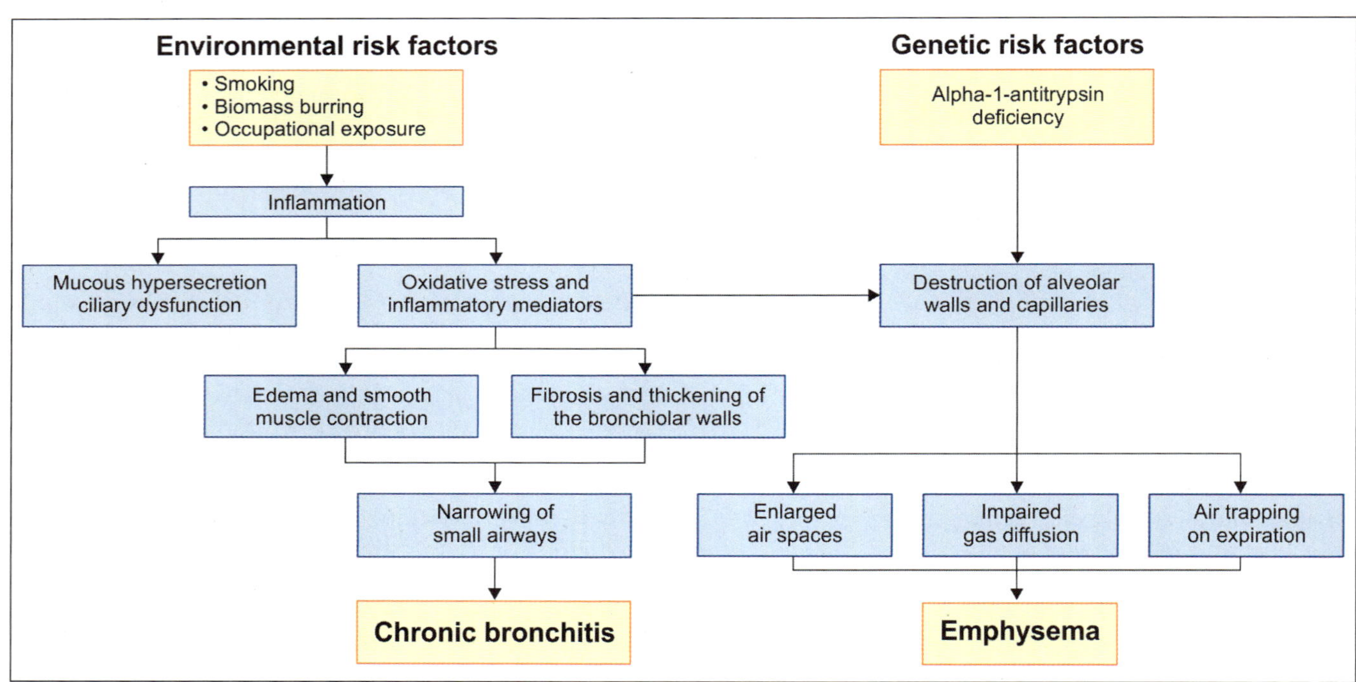

FLOWCHART 1: Flowchart depicting the pathophysiology of chronic obstructive pulmonary disease.

as IL-8, IL-6, IL-10, TNF-α, LTB-4, and several oxygen reactive species is initiated. There is also a release of various proteolytic enzymes such as elastase, matrix metalloproteinases (MMP), cathepsin-G etc., which lead to damage to the elastic lung tissue. Elastic proteolysis leads to a development of reduced recoil pressures and thereby promoting significant airway narrowing. This leads to air trapping and later fibrotic remodeling and fixed airflow obstruction.

RISK FACTORS

The definition of COPD emphasized the importance of exposure to noxious particles and gases. Along with cigarette smoking, biomass fuel exposure has also been recognized to be the most important causative factor for COPD.

Cigarette smoking: Cigarette smoking/biomass exposure when coupled with genetic predisposition is likely to result in further decline of FEV1 over an individual's lifetime.

BOX 1	Extrapulmonary manifestations and associations of chronic obstructive pulmonary disease.
• Pulmonary hypertension	
• Ischemic heart disease	
• Diabetes mellitus	
• Metabolic syndrome	
• Osteoporosis	
• Anemia	
• Skeletal muscle wasting	
• Obstructive sleep apnea	
• Depression	

Exposure to biomass fuel: In the Indian scenario, exposure to biomass fuel remains an important risk factor for COPD, especially in the rural population. In a prevalence study from rural India, it was found that up to 85% of COPD patients had never smoked in their lives. Biomass fuel exposure COPD is associated with more small airways obstruction, lesser degree of emphysema, and a predominantly eosinophilic inflammation. In an Indian study comparing Indian nonsmoking COPD (NS-COPD) and smoking COPD (S-COPD) patients, it was observed that NS-COPD is generally seen in younger patient with an equal male to female predominance. These patients had a preserved lung function and had a slower decline in FEV1 when compared to their S-COPD counterparts. Air pollution has also been recognized as an important risk factor for COPD in recent times. Long-term exposure of NO_2, $PM_{2.5}$, PM_{10}, and residence near a road has been associated with development of COPD and worsening lung function. Similarly, certain occupations have also been linked with increased risk of development of COPD. Exposure to vapors, gas, dust, or fumes in occupations such as heavy equipment operators and construction workers have been implicated in increasing risk.

Presence of **alpha-1 antitrypsin (AAT) deficiency** has also been associated with development of COPD, especially in young individuals. About 1–5% patients with COPD are estimated to have AAT. The gene encoding AAT deficiency (*SERPINA-1*) is located on the long arm of chromosome 14 and is generally inherited by autosomal dominant transmission. It is associated with emphysema and bronchiectasis along with extrapulmonary features such as liver cirrhosis, panniculitis, inflammatory bowel disease etc. Emphysema in a young individual with basal predominance should with/without family history of lung disease raise suspicion of AAT deficiency.

CLINICAL FEATURES

Dyspnea, cough, and sputum production are generally described as the three cardinal symptoms of COPD. Wheezing and chest tightness are also sometimes encountered. While shortness of breath is usually the first encountered symptom, the order of the symptoms in COPD is variable.

Flowchart 2 mentioned below depicts the pathophysiology of COPD in the chronic bronchitis and emphysema phenotype.

COPD PHENOTYPES

Wilhelm Johannsen, in 1909, first used the terms "genotype" and "phenotype". The term "phenotype" refers to the observable physical properties of an organism; these include the organisms appearance, development, and behavior. Based on the clinical, radiological, and pathological features, two main phenotypes were described: Emphysema or the "pink puffer" and chronic bronchitis or the "blue bloater type". As the knowledge of COPD evolved it was proposed that phenotyping COPD patients will allow for classification of patients into distinct prognostic and therapeutic subgroups for both clinical and research purposes. In the tables given below we have outlined the current accepted COPD phenotypes with their definition and the emerging phenotypes (**Tables 1** and **2**).

MANAGEMENT

The *goals for treatment* of stable COPD broadly includes two areas:

1. Reduction of symptoms
2. Risk reduction

The classes of medication used to treat COPD, however, do not show a long-term improvement of lung function, in fact modification of decline of lung function is also not proven conclusively in clinical trials.

Treatment can be divided in the following broad sections.

BRONCHODILATORS

Bronchodilators are drugs which improve lung function by increasing FEV1 with also a change in other spirometric variables. They form the backbone in the management of COPD.

Beta agonists:

- The principle action of beta agonist is relaxation of the airway smooth muscles. They stimulate the beta-2 adrenergic receptors which increases cyclic AMP levels thus preventing bronchoconstriction. For a single as needed dose in COPD there seems to be no advantage of routinely using short-acting beta agonist (SABA) over conventional long acting beta-2 agonist. The long-acting bronchodilators which act for 12 hours or more have a greater benefit as compared to the short-acting bronchodilators.
- The various categories of long-acting beta-2 agonist (LABA) bronchodilators are:
  - *LABA*: Formoterol and Salmeterol are used twice daily, and in various trials they have shown some improvement in FEV1 and dyspnea scores. They also seem to reduce exacerbations and hospitalizations without effective mortality to any great extent.
  - *Ultra LABAs*: The newer ultra LABAs like indacaterol also seem to have similar effect in FEV1, dyspnea

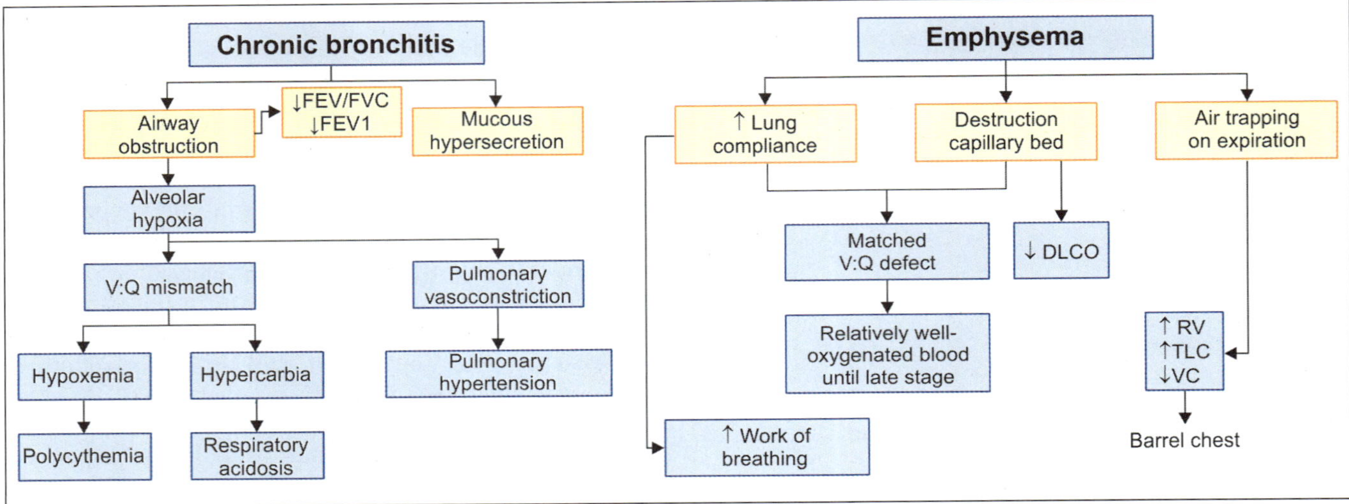

(DLCO: diffusing capacity of the lung for carbon monoxide; FEV1: forced expiratory volume in 1 second; FVC: forced vital capacity; RV: residual volume; TLC: total lung capacity; VC: vital capacity)

FLOWCHART 2: Flowchart depicting the pathophysiology of COPD in the chronic bronchitis and the emphysema phenotype.

TABLE 1 Table listing the accepted COPD phenotypes.

COPD phenotype	Definition
Chronic bronchitis	The presence of productive cough >3 months per year in 2 or more consecutive years
Emphysema	Presence of emphysema confirmed on imaging
Asthma-COPD-overlap	Persistent airflow limitation with several features usually associated with asthma and several features usually associated with COPD (typically is asthmatic smoker)
Frequent exacerbator	Presence of frequent exacerbations (2 or more per year)
No or one non severe exacerbation in a calendar year	Presence of rare exacerbations (no or just one exacerbation)

Source (for Table 2 also): Corlateanu A. Chronic obstructive pulmonary disease and phenotypes: a state-of-the-art. Pulmonology. 2020;26(2):95-100.

TABLE 2 Table listing the emerging COPD phenotypes.

COPD phenotype	Definition
Pulmonary cachexia phenotype	Body mass index lower than 21 kg/m^2
Overlap COPD and bronchiectasis	HRCT confirmation of bronchiectasis and definite COPD diagnosis
Upper lobe-predominant emphysema phenotype	CT findings consistent of predominant upper lobe emphysema
The fast decliner phenotype	Rapid decline of lung function
The comorbidities or systemic phenotype	High comorbidities burden, predominantly cardiovascular, and metabolic
α1-antitrypsin deficiency	Genetic condition caused by deficiency of α1-antitrypsin
Non smoking COPD	Induced by biomass exposure

scores, QoL, and reducing exacerbation rates. Indacaterol causes a cough in a minority of patients after inhalation. Newer drugs which are yet to come to the market such as vilanterol and olodaterol are taken once daily. These newer ultra LABAs also have demonstrated an improvement in lung function and symptoms.

Adverse effects:

- *Resting sinus tachycardia*: This is probably the most common side effect. They tend to worsen cardiac rhythm disturbances in susceptible individuals.
- *Increase in tremors*: This effect is noticed when high doses are prescribed.
- *Hypokalemia*: It is seldom seen when used alone. Usually seen when combined with other hypokalemia inducing agents like thiazide diuretics etc.
- A fall in PaO_2 can be seen transiently in patients prescribed SABA and LABA. The cause is uncertain.

Antimuscarinic agents: They block the bronchoconstrictor effect of acetylcholine M3 muscarinic receptors expressed in airway smooth muscles. Here too there are short-acting antimuscarinic bronchodilators (SAMA) like ipratropium and oxytropium, and long-acting antimuscarinic bronchodilators (LAMA) such as tiotropium, glycopyrronium, aclidinium, and umeclidinium. They have a prolonged binding effect on the M3 muscarinic receptors with a faster dissociation from M2 receptors. This helps in having a more duration of action with bronchodilatation. Ipratropium in randomized controlled trials (RCT) and systematic reviews shows a small benefit in improved bronchodilatation over SABA. Health-related QoL and requirement of oral steroids are less compared with SAMA over SABA.

LAMA treatment with tiotropium also causes an improvement in QoL. Most importantly tiotropium seems to improve effect of pulmonary rehabilitation. LAMA is more effective compared to LABA in reducing exacerbations and hospitalizations. Hence, if we have to choose a long-acting bronchodilator, we choose a LAMA over LABA for monotherapy in COPD patients.

Adverse effects: A LAMA is poorly absorbed and hence the troublesome systemic effects seen with atropine is generally not seen with LAMAs.

- One of the common side effects which the patients complain is dryness of mouth.
- Rarely patients complain of urinary symptoms (retention) and an increase in cardiovascular events in patients prescribed LAMA (both with tiotropium and glycopyrronium).

Methylxanthines: Their position in management of COPD is controversial. In India, the use of methylxanthines with theophylline as a prototype methylxanthine is common. It is metabolized by cytochrome P450 enzyme cascade. The clearance of methylxanthines decreases with age which translates into greater toxic side effects. There is a little bit of evidence that they have a small advantage over placebo in patients with COPD. Hence, theophylline can be added to traditional bronchodilators described above in alleviating breathlessness and improving QoL in a small section of COPD patients. Their role in reducing exacerbations is not well established.

Adverse effects:

- The toxicity is dose related and mainly cardiac in nature, arrhythmias being one of the common side effects.
- Gastrointestinal (GI) side effects (nausea and vomiting) are also encountered in a small population of patients. Cautious use of theophylline hence is advocated.

Combination bronchodilators: It has been observed that combining bronchodilators with different mechanisms and separate durations of actions enhance the effect and do not worsen the side effect profile of the components either.

Hence, treatment with formoterol and tiotropium seems to have a bigger impact on FEV1 than either component prescribed alone. This is not a molecule effect but more a class effect and happens across the board in which ever LABA or LAMA we choose to use. Studies have shown that there is a reduction of exacerbations as well as improvement of QoL when a LABA-LAMA is used in combination. Moreover, when a LABA-LAMA combination is used a lower dose of either component can be used which translates into a lesser side effect profile for these drugs.

ANTI-INFLAMMATORY TREATMENT

Use of inhaled corticosteroids: Inhaled corticosteroids (ICS) do not have an effect in improving FEV1 or reducing mortality. In fact in the TORCH (TOwards a Revolution in COPD Health) study, the use of fluticasone propionate by itself or in combination increased mortality when compared with placebo or with salmeterol/fluticasone combo. However, other studies have not indicated an increase in mortality with inhaled steroids.

Some recent studies in moderate COPD have shown that fluticasone furoate with vilanterol is associated with delayed decline of FEV1 as compared with placebo or vilanterol alone by an average of 9 mL/year. However, in most cases the use of ICS by itself (without bronchodilators) is not recommended by current guidelines.

Inhaled corticosteroids with long-acting bronchodilators: Most of the studies in patients with moderate-to-severe COPD show that patients respond better to an ICS with LABA combination as compared to either of the mono components. This increased effect happens as far as lung function, health status, and reducing exacerbations is concerned. An RCT which was conducted in the primary healthcare settings in UK compared LABA-ICS with usual care. It showed an 8.4% reduction in moderate-to-severe exacerbations and improvement of COPD assessment test (CAT) scores with no difference in healthcare contact or pneumonias.

Blood eosinophils: Recent studies have shown that blood eosinophil count can be a good surrogate marker to predict effect of ICS in preventing future exacerbations. The effect of ICS is better if the blood eosinophil count >300 cell/μL. The higher the eosinophil count, the better the effect of ICS in reducing exacerbations. On the other side if blood eosinophils are <100 cells/μL, these patients seldom respond to ICS as far as reduction of exacerbations is concerned. Between eosinophil count of 100 and 300 cells/μL, an individual call needs to be taken according to symptom burden and risk of exacerbations. When we talk about predicting ICS response based on exacerbations, the response is higher with patients with a higher exacerbation rate or >1 hospitalization rate in the previous year. Smoking status, ethnicity, and geographical location are all factors which influences ICS effect.

Adverse effects: There is high-quality evidence that shows ICS increase the incidence of pneumonia. There are also other side effects which have been reported which include oral candidiasis, hoarseness of voice, skin bruising, osteoporosis, poor diabetes control, and cataracts. Data on the last few side effects are not robust. Incidence of pneumonia is higher in smokers, patients with low BMI, elderly (over 55 years), poor dyspnea scores, and severe airflow limitation. As mentioned before patients with eosinophil counts <100 or 2% is at a greater risk of developing pneumonia. The risk of nontuberculous mycobacteria (NTM) or tuberculosis has also been reported in meta-analysis and RCTs.

Withdrawal of inhaled corticosteroids: There are a couple of trials which have looked at gradual step down of dose of ICS. They have looked into its effect on lung function, symptoms, and exacerbation rates. The most robust study the WISDOM (Withdrawal of Inhaled Steroids During Optimized bronchodilator Management) trial showed that gradual withdrawal of ICS did not increase exacerbation rates but showed a modest decline in lung function. Subgroup analysis has also shown that the risk of exacerbations is greater if the blood eosinophil count is >300 cells/μL. Hence, withdrawal of ICS in patients with high eosinophil count should be done with caution.

Triple inhaler therapy: Inhaled corticosteroids (LAMA/LABA/ICS) combination can improve lung function, QoL, and reduce incidence of exacerbations. Adding a LAMA to existing ICS/LABA combination improves lung function and reduces exacerbation risk. However, unfortunately mortality benefit seems to be elusive in the prescription of inhaled respiratory medications in patients with COPD. Large RCTs have not shown survival benefit with salmeterol/fluticasone or vilanterol/fluticasone combination. With triple therapy there seems to be a somewhat statistically better mortality rate. De-escalation of ICS on triple therapy should be done with caution, as they can deteriorate unless all parameters are considered before de-escalating.

Oral corticosteroids: Oral steroids have numerous side effects including increased risk of infections, muscle weakness (myopathy), osteoporosis, decreased functionality, and respiratory failure in patients with severe COPD. Hence, OCS will only play a role during management of acute exacerbations. Only a very small percentage of patients will benefit with long-term OCS, hence the guidelines will try and tell you to not keep your patients on maintenance long-term steroids therapy.

Phosphodiesterase-4 inhibitors: The principle action is to reduce inflammation. Roflumilast is a drug which is prescribed once daily and has no bronchodilator effect. It reduces exacerbations and is beneficial in the chronic bronchitis phenotype of patients. These patients will have spirometrically graded severe to very severe COPD (GOLD D) with history of multiple exacerbations.

They should be used as only add on drugs, added to bronchodilators. Benefits is more with patients with previous hospitalization.

Adverse effects: These drugs have more adverse effects than inhaled medications. They have more GI symptoms (nausea, decreased appetite, and diarrhea) and cause sleep disturbances, depression, and headache. Hence, they should be avoided in patients with depression.

Other anti-inflammatory drugs: Certain other drugs such as vitamin D, anti-TNF-α antibody, leukotriene modifiers etc., have not been adequately tested and hence not recommended in patients with stable COPD.

ANTIBIOTICS

Older studies showed that use of prophylactic long-term antibiotics have no effect in reducing exacerbations in patients with COPD. However, later studies demonstrated the use of low dose macrolides (azithromycin 250 mg/day or 500 mg three times per week or erythromycin 500 mg two times per day) and their anti-inflammatory effect can be tried in patients with GOLD D COPD. These two drugs can be used for a duration of 6 months to 1 year for their exacerbation reducing property. There is a risk of antimicrobial resistance, prolonged QTc, impaired hearing etc., by use of long-term low dose macrolides. These need to be addressed with the patient before prescribing these drugs.

MUCOLYTICS

Use of mucolytics with N-acetyl cysteine/carbocysteine can reduce exacerbations and improve health status. This effect is greater in the frequently exacerbating and the chronic bronchitis phenotype of patients. Their benefit is that they are comparatively safe as compared to the other medications mentioned above.

NONPHARMACOLOGICAL TREATMENTS

Pulmonary rehabilitation: It is defined as "a comprehensive intervention based on through patient assessment followed by patient-tailored therapies that include, but not limited to, exercise training, education, self-management intervention aiming at behavior change, designed to improve the physical and psychological condition of people with chronic respiratory disease, and to promote the long-term adherence to health-enhancing behaviors."

It has significant benefits in COPD and is thought to be an intervention which improves shortness of breath, health status, and exercise tolerance more than the drugs itself.

Oxygen therapy and ventilatory support: Long-term administration of oxygen in COPD patients (>15 hours/day) with chronic respiratory failure severe resting hypoxia is shown to improve mortality and resting hypoxia. Breathlessness in COPD patients can be relieved by oxygen administration even in the absence of hypoxia, but such an intervention has not shown to improve mortality. Administration of oxygen should be done cautiously as there is a risk of worsening hypercapnia with over oxygenating COPD patients.

Ventilatory support: During exacerbations of COPD, in patients who have type II respiratory failure (uncompensated), noninvasive ventilation (NIV) is the standard of care and this reduces morbidity and mortality. In patients who are chronically hypercapnic and experience frequent exacerbations, using NIV at home can help to reduce hospital admissions and future exacerbations. However, home NIV is difficult to manage and is of benefit only if significantly large pressures are used in these patients.

Surgical intervention: Lung volume reduction surgery (LVRS) is a surgical procedure where portions of lungs are resected to reduce hyperinflation and make the respiratory muscles more effective pressure generators. LVRS increases the elastic recoil of lung thus improves expiratory flow rates and reduce exacerbations.

Lung transplantation: Lung transplantation in a select group of COPD patients is shown to improve health status and functional capacity but does not prolong survival. Most transplants which happen in COPD are double lung transplants. Bilateral lung transplant is shown to have longer survival than single lung transplantation. The median survival for COPD who have had a double lung transplant is 7 years while it is 5 years for those who have had a single lung transplant.

Bronchoscopic interventions: Due to the morbidity and mortality associated with LVRS newer bronchoscopic interventions have been introduced to reduce hyperinflation. This includes endobronchial valve placement, targeted thermal vapor ablation, use of nitinol coils etc. These technologies are not yet licensed for use in India. Further trials are needed for them to be used in COPD patients.

Vaccination: Chronic obstructive pulmonary disease patients need to follow the vaccination schedule according to the Indian vaccination guidelines. Vaccination is important for the elderly and patients with comorbidities.

MANAGEMENT ACCORDING TO GOLD GRADES OF COPD

GOLD A: It is best managed with short-acting bronchodilators. It could be a SABA or a SAMA or both. Use of a single long acting bronchodilator, the preferred option being a LAMA, could be useful in certain patients with GOLD A COPD. The evidence is evolving in a way that early use of long-acting bronchodilators is preferred over short-acting bronchodilators in patients with COPD.

GOLD B: Therapy here should start with a long-acting bronchodilator. Evidence is more robust with early initiation of LAMA. Adding LABA to LAMA helps in maximizing bronchodilator effect and reduces exacerbations as compared to monotherapy with individual agents.

GOLD C: Initial therapy should consist of a single long-acting bronchodilator (in this case a LAMA). We would add in a LABA or in certain cases an ICS depending on the phenotype of patients. Doing an eosinophil count in the stable state in these patients will help in phenotyping these patients.

GOLD D: For patients with very severe symptoms (CAT > 20), increased dyspnea, a LAMA + LABA should be chosen as initial treatment. An advantage of using a LABA over a LAMA has not been consistently demonstrated. In certain patients with blood eosinophils >300/mL, adding an ICS might be a first choice when we combine with a LABA. It would also be the first choice in patients with asthma-COPD overlap or a history of asthma. The worry about ICS is the incidence of pneumonia, hence the risks should be weighed in before prescribing ICS.

FOLLOW-UP TREATMENT

Follow-up pharmacological treatment should be based on the principle of review, assess, and adjust as needed. During each review, patient should be examined for the grade of breathlessness and evaluated for risk of exacerbations. Assessment for inhaler technique and adherence should be done. The need for nonpharmacological interventions such as smoking cessation, pulmonary rehabilitation, oxygen therapy etc., should be assessed at each visit. The requirement for escalation and de-escalation of pharmacological treatment, changing of devices as required, and subsequent review of clinical response should be done on a regular basis.

Palliative end of life and hospice care: It encompasses two different approaches. One is symptom control and the second is management of patients who are "end of life" from COPD. The aim is to relieve suffering and to support the families to the best possible extent, regardless of the stage of the disease and requirement of other therapies. This is for patients who continue to experience symptoms despite having optimal treatment in the way of cough, fatigue, poor QoL, depression, anxiety, and other psychosocial factors.

COPD EXACERBATIONS

Acute exacerbation of COPD represents an important event in the patient's disease course. According to the GOLD-2020 guidelines, acute exacerbation of COPD is defined as an acute worsening of symptoms that results in additional therapy. These exacerbations are important since they significantly impact the disease progression, health status, and rates of hospitalization and readmission. Due to this significant negative impact of exacerbations on patients health, several investigators have suggested alternate terminologies like COPD attacks, COPD flare ups, lung attacks etc. Using these terms not only attempt to increase awareness but also to capture the immense burden of this disease on patients health.

Classification of acute exacerbations of chronic obstructive pulmonary disorder (AE-COPD) was updated in the recent GOLD-2020 guidelines. This classification was based upon the level of healthcare management needed to treat the exacerbation. Exacerbations termed as "mild" are those treated with (SABAs) only, whereas exacerbations termed as "moderate" are those treated by SABA with antibiotics and/or oral corticosteroids. Severe exacerbations are classified as exacerbations associated with respiratory failure, requiring mechanical ventilation.

Respiratory infections have been identified to be most common triggers for exacerbations. It has been estimated that almost 70% of exacerbations have been triggered by respiratory viral infections. While viral and bacterial infections seem to be more commonly seen triggers several atypical bacteria have also been identified. Various risk factors have been identified which predict an increased risk of future exacerbations. Advanced age, COPD disease duration, history of COPD related hospitalization, peripheral blood eosinophilia, and presence of multiple comorbidities have been associated with an increased COPD exacerbation risk. In the ECLIPSE (Evaluation of COPD Longitudinally to Identify Predictive Surrogate Endpoints) study, the single most important predictor of increased exacerbation risk was history of previous exacerbations. FEV1 level was previously thought to be a predictor of increased exacerbation risk; however, this hypothesis has been challenged in recent times. This phenomenon led to a paradigm shift to GOLD guidelines in 2017 in the COPD refined ABCD assessment tool.

MANAGEMENT OF ACUTE EXACERBATIONS

The initial evaluation of an exacerbation of COPD is aimed at confirming the diagnosis of an exacerbation, assessing the severity, and etiology. It is also important to rule out the comorbidities (if any) as the contributing factors during an exacerbation and to decide if the patient needs outpatient management or hospitalization.

Global Initiative for Chronic Obstructive Lung Disease recommends certain factors to be taken into consideration when deciding between outpatient management and hospitalization for the treatment of COPD exacerbations. The following factors should be considered when evaluating the patient for hospitalization (**Box 2**).

Home management is generally recommended in mild exacerbations. Treating of these mild exacerbations includes intensification of bronchodilators and a course of glucocorticoids and oral antibiotics on a case to case basis. Bronchodilators in this case can either be administered through a metered dose inhaler (MDI) with a spacer or via a nebulizer, although, most studies do not show an advantage of drug delivery via nebulizer over MDI with spacer. The GOLD guidelines recommend oral antibiotics for moderately or severely ill patients with COPD exacerbations who have increased cough and sputum purulence.

The mainstay of hospital management includes airflow limitation reversal with inhaled short-acting bronchodilators, systemic glucocorticoids, and treating infection while also ensuring proper oxygenation and avoiding the need for invasive mechanical ventilation. Adequate oxygenation by using supplemental oxygen should be closely monitored to avoid hypercapnia in COPD patients. Continuous monitoring of pulse oxygen saturation by maintaining target SpO_2 between 88 and 92% and titrating supplemental oxygen can avert hypercapnia and lower the mortality.

When combined with bronchodilator therapy, systemic corticosteroids have been shown to improve symptoms, lung function, relapse rate at one month, and decrease the length of hospital stay. The GOLD guidelines recommend using the equivalent of prednisone 40 mg once daily for 5 days for the management of most COPD exacerbations.

In some exacerbations of COPD, especially if severe, with features such as severe dyspnea with impending respiratory muscle fatigue, tachypnea with excessive accessory muscle use, and respiratory acidosis. NIV is the preferred mode of ventilation, wherever required, in patients with COPD exacerbation. NIV has been shown to improve many clinical outcomes related to an exacerbation of COPD and can be administered through various interfaces including full face masks, nasal prongs, or nasal masks (**Box 3**). Patients not responding/worsening on NIV should be considered as candidates for invasive mechanical ventilation.

PREVENTION OF EXACERBATION

Each COPD exacerbation is a risk factor for further exacerbations. Also, each exacerbation leads to drop in lung function and the lung function never returns to baseline even after treatment of exacerbation. Attempts should be made to prescribe strategies that would prevent further exacerbations, even in stable COPD and in patients with no history of exacerbations (**Table 3**).

BOX 3 Indications of IMV in AE-COPD.

- Failed response to NIV
- Worsening respiratory acidosis on NIV
- Intolerance to NIV
- Contraindications for use of NIV (e.g., facial deformities, poor mentation, and worsening GCS)

(AE-COPD: acute exacerbations of chronic obstructive pulmonary disorder)

BOX 2 Indications of hospitalization in AE-COPD.

- Significant worsening of symptoms from the baseline status, such as resting breathlessness, high respiratory rate, tachypnea and accessory muscle use, confusion, and drowsiness
- Appearance of new signs such as cyanosis, worsening confusion/new onset confusion, and edema of the peripheries
- Failure to respond to initial management
- Acute respiratory failure
- Inadequate home support and other local factors also need consideration

(AE-COPD: acute exacerbations of chronic obstructive pulmonary disorder)

TABLE 3 Preventive strategies for COPD exacerbation.

Nonpharmacologic therapy	Pharmacologic therapy
• Smoking cessation • Pulmonary rehabilitation • Vaccination (influenza and pneumococcal) • Action plan/self management plan	• Long-acting inhaled bronchodilators (LAMAs and LABAs), with or without inhaled corticosteroids • Roflumilast • N-acetylcysteine(NAC) • Low dose macrolides

(LABA: long-acting beta-2 agonist; LAMA: long-acting muscarinic antagonist)

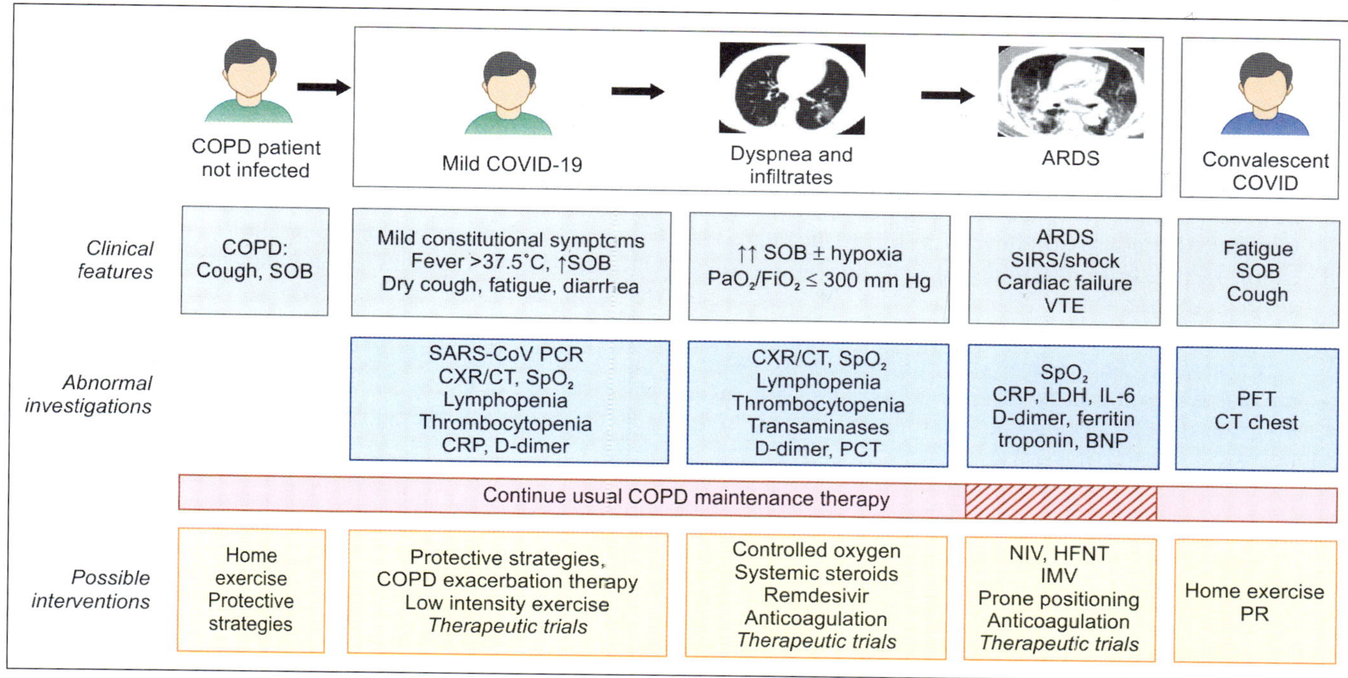

(HFNT: high flow nasal therapy; IL-6: interleukin 6; IMV: invasive mechanical ventilation; PCT: procalcitonin; PR: pulmonary rehabilitation; SOB: shortness of breath)

FIGURE 2: Image showing the severity of coronavirus disease 2019 (COVID-19) in chronic obstructive pulmonary disease (COPD) patients and the possible interventions at each stage.

Source: Halpin et al. 2020 Global Initiative for the Diagnosis, Management, and Prevention of Chronic Obstructive Lung Disease. The 2020 GOLD Science Committee Report on COVID-19 and Chronic Obstructive Pulmonary Disease.

COVID-19 AND COPD

The coronavirus disease 2019 (COVID-19) pandemic has affected over 100 million people globally since its onset. During these extraordinary times, caring for patients with COVID-19 and underlying COPD poses particular challenges. Certain treatments relevant to treating patients with COPD, such as nebulized bronchodilators and NIV, are thought to carry an increased risk of viral spread via aerosols. Though there is no data to suggest that COPD patients are at an increased risk of contracting COVID-19 infection but treating COPD patients effectively in the context of COVID-19 is important since patients with COPD are at an increased risk of poor outcomes (**Fig. 2**). The GOLD 2021 document has lucidly put forward an algorithm to help identify and treat patients with COPD and severe acute respiratory syndrome coronavirus 2 (SARS-COV-2) infection.

CONCLUSION

Chronic obstructive pulmonary disease is a chronic disease which is emerging as an important cause of morbidity and mortality globally. In India, given the combined risk factors of smoking, biomass exposure, and air pollution, COPD poses a huge burden to our healthcare infrastructure. Long-term good quality pharmacological and nonpharmacological treatment is essential in maintaining control and to ameliorate symptoms of this disease process. The respiratory community should endeavor to improve the QoL in individuals who are suffering from this disease process. We hope that this chapter will help to understand the intricacies in the management of COPD.

RECOMMENDED READINGS

1. Global Initiative for Chronic Obstructive Lung Disease (GOLD). (2019). Global Strategy for the Diagnosis, Management and Prevention of Chronic Obstructive Pulmonary Disease: 2019 Report. [online] Available from http://www.goldcopd.org .
2. Alqahtani JS, Oyelade T, Aldhahir AM, Alghamdi SM, Almehmadi M, Alqahtani AS, et al. Prevalence, severity and mortality associated with COPD and smoking in patients with COVID-19: A rapid systematic review and meta-analysis. PLoS One. 2020;15(5):e0233147.
3. Barnes PJ, Celli BR. Systemic manifestations and comorbidities of COPD. Eur Respir J. 2009;33(5): 1165-85.
4. Salvi SS, Barnes PJ. Chronic obstructive pulmonary disease in non-smokers. The Lancet. 2009;374(9691): 733-43.
5. Siddiqui SH, Pavord ID, Barnes NC, Guasconi A, Lettis S, Pascoe S, et al. Blood eosinophils: A biomarker of COPD exacerbation reduction with inhaled corticosteroids. Int J Chron Obstruct Pulmon Dis. 2018;13:3669-76.

6. Crim C, Calverley PMA, Anderson JA, Celli B, Ferguson GT, Jenkins C, et al. Pneumonia risk in COPD patients receiving inhaled corticosteroids alone or in combination: TORCH study results. Eur Respir J. 2009;34(3):641-7.
7. Chong J, Leung B, Poole P. Phosphodiesterase 4 inhibitors for chronic obstructive pulmonary disease. Cochrane Database Syst Rev. 2017;9(9):CD002309.
8. Spruit MA. Pulmonary rehabilitation. Eur Respir Rev. 2014;23(131):55-63.
9. McCarthy B, Casey D, Devane D, Murphy K, Murphy E, Lacasse Y. Pulmonary rehabilitation for chronic obstructive pulmonary disease. Cochrane Database Syst Rev. 2015 ;2:CD003793.
10. Cranston JM, Crockett AJ, Moss JR, Alpers JH. Domiciliary oxygen for chronic obstructive pulmonary disease. Cochrane Database Syst Rev. 2005;(4):CD001744.
11. Elliott MW. Noninvasive ventilation in acute exacerbations of COPD. Eur Resp Rev. 2005;14(94):39-42.
12. Dhar R, Ghoshal AG, Guleria R, Sharma S, Kulkarni T, Swarnakar R, et al. Clinical practice guidelines 2019: Indian consensus-based recommendations on pneumococcal vaccination for adults. Lung India. 2020;37(7):19-29.
13. Kim J, Lee CH, Lee MG, Shin KC, Yoo KH, Lim SY, et al. ; KOLD, KOCOSS investigators. Acute Exacerbation According to GOLD 2017 Categories in Patients with Chronic Obstructive Pulmonary Disease. Arch Bronconeumol (Engl Ed). 2019;55:414-20.

CHAPTER

206

Occupational Lung Diseases

Surinder K Jindal, Trinath Dash

ABSTRACT

Occupational lung diseases include a wide spectrum of health problems varying from nonspecific symptoms to serious diseases. Occupational lung diseases vary with the type, severity, and duration of exposure. Occupational asthma, hypersensitivity pneumonitis, and pneumoconioses constitute the three main groups which are often identified. Both occupational asthma and hypersensitivity pneumonitis commonly occur as immunological disorders due to organic, antigenic exposures. On the other hand, pneumoconioses occur due to deposition of inorganic dusts in the lung parenchyma. While clinical manifestations are not always distinct, the relationship of exposure with onset of symptoms is important for diagnosis. Chest radiology and exposure history are often adequate to make the diagnosis. Lung biopsy is rarely required. Treatment essentially consists of removal of the offending agent even though this may not be possible in most cases who are managed with symptomatic treatment. Chronic, persistent exposure can frequently result in diffuse fibrosis, permanent lung damage, and chronic respiratory failure. Besides the adoption of personal, environmental, and engineering measures, surveillance and screening strategies are important for disease prevention.

"If you don't think it's safe, it probably isn't"

—Jerry Smithr

INTRODUCTION

A large number of occupations are associated with generation of dusts and fine particles which remain suspended in the environmental air. Respiratory system is constantly exposed to the environment more than any other organ. Lungs are therefore most prone to suffer from adverse effects and diseases due to the presence of occupational emissions and pollutants in the working environment (**Box 1**). Many of these workplace exposures are specific to the occupation and the type of work being done. These are generally confined to the select population of workers engaged in these occupations. On the other hand, there are several other pollutant-related diseases which can affect any individual. The occupation-related lung diseases can be broadly categorized into the following main groups:

- Nonspecific health and respiratory effects
- Occupational asthma
- Hypersensitivity pneumonias (HPs)
- Pneumoconioses or inorganic dust deposition diseases
- Toxic gases and fumes inhalation.

BOX 1 **Adverse effects and respiratory diseases attributed to different occupational exposures.**

- **General health effects:**
  - Systemic symptoms: Malaise, fatigue, and body aches
  - Respiratory symptoms–cough, phlegm
  - Lung function deterioration
  - Infections—upper respiratory tract, pneumonias, and tuberculosis
- **Organic dust exposure:**
  - Occupational asthma
  - Hypersensitivity pneumonias: Agricultural exposures, drug and chemical industry
  - Miscellaneous interstitial lung diseases
- **Inorganic dust deposition diseases:**
  - Silicosis
  - Coal workers pneumoconiosis
  - Asbestosis
  - Others: Metal-induced lung disease
- **Toxic gases and fumes:**
  - Asphyxiation–CO_2, nitrogen, and methane
  - Irritation: NH_3, chlorine, SO_2, O_3, and phosgene
- **Carcinogenesis:**
  - Lung cancer

NONSPECIFIC HEALTH EFFECTS

Work in mills, foundries, manufacturing industry, shipping, mines, and other places which involve the blue-collar jobs is frequently associated with environmental dusts. Inhalation of these dusts is often responsible for following nonspecific adverse health and respiratory effects.

- General aches and pains, malaise, fatigue, and insomnia
- Nonspecific cough and phlegm production
- Long-term exposure results in impairment of respiratory function and symptoms of breathlessness.
- Upper respiratory infections and chronic bronchitis as well as pneumonias, tuberculosis, and exacerbations of asthma or chronic obstructive pulmonary disease (COPD) may occur with an increased frequency.

Indoor air pollution is an important aspect of several different kinds of occupations. Domestic cooking is an important occupation in which a majority of women are engaged in both rural and urban areas. They are constantly exposed to smoke generated by combustion of biomass fuels such as the dried cattle dung, wood, and forest residue. This indoor household air pollution (HAP) is responsible for adverse health effects, COPD, and other systemic diseases (cataracts, hypertension, cardiovascular, and cerebrovascular disease). Other fossil fuels such as the gas, kerosene, and liquid petroleum gas (LPG) have been similarly shown to relate to the presence of respiratory symptoms, lower respiratory tract infections (LRTIs), asthma, and COPD.

Respiratory infections are particularly common in children living in polluted dwellings. Tuberculosis is also more likely to spread among close inmates living together in closed dwellings. The incidence is further enhanced due to the significant presence of other risk factors such as tobacco smoking, malnutrition, poor living conditions, and HAP among these populations.

Long-term indoor work in the offices, workshops, and laboratories also expose even white-collared workers to chemical and physical pollutants including volatile organic compounds (VOC) such as formaldehyde (which originate from building materials, furnishings, resins, cosmetics, paper products, and other sources) may be responsible for sick building syndrome—mucosal irritation and neurobehavioral impairment. Indoor presence of radon daughter and asbestos fibers is another important carcinogenic health hazard. Low relative humidity of the air causes dryness of the eyes and the respiratory tract. Excessive electromagnetic hyper-sensitivity or the "dirty electricity" in indoor environment is shown to cause deleterious effects in patients with asthma, diabetes, multiple sclerosis, chronic fatigue, fibromyalgia, and others.

OCCUPATIONAL ASTHMA

Occupational asthma is defined as the occurrence of symptoms of asthma following an exposure to a known or an unidentified triggering agent at a workplace. Characteristically, the symptoms consist of chest tightness, cough, wheezing, and/or breathlessness. A patient with previously known asthma can also develop exaggerated symptoms following work. Characteristically, there is a lag period required after an exposure for sensitization to the causative agent. Typically, the agent can either be a protein, a chemical, or some other allergen. Allergic response is demonstrated typically by antigen-specific immunoglobulin E (IgE). A large number of both chemical and biological immunological agents are listed among causes of occupational asthma (**Table 1**).

Agents: Occupational exposures can incite airway reactions either as specific or as nonspecific stimuli. Chemical agents like SO_2 and chlorine, other agents like flour may induce asthma as nonspecific stimuli. Some important chemical agents are diisocyanates (e.g., toluene, diphenylmethane, naphthalene, and hexamethylene used in polyurethane foam manufacture, printing on flexible packaging, spray paints), acid anhydride (used as adhesives, surface coating), polyamines (as plastic coatings), and complex platinum salts. There are several biological agents which can induce asthma, e.g., small mammal's (rats, mice, rabbits, and guinea pigs) urine proteins, locusts, grain flour, and contaminants like mite and mold. Most of these agents are recognized in Western countries for statutory compensation. From India, there

TABLE 1 Some important allergens identified as causes of occupational asthma.

Agents causing asthma	Occupation/Industry
• **High-molecular-weight compounds:**	
◦ Bovine proteins	• Dairy work
◦ Egg white/yolk	• Egg processing
◦ Birds	• Bird breeding, poultries
◦ Sea animals: Fish, prawns	• Food processing, fish farming
◦ Cereals, legumes, and seeds	• Food processing, farming, granary storing and milling, baking
◦ Insects and worms	• Food processing, farming, granary storing and milling, sericulture, and laboratories
◦ Enzymes	• Detergent, drug and medical industry, baking, and food processing
◦ Miscellaneous	• Confectioneries, pharmaceutical industry, printing, farming, and food industry
• **Low-molecular-weight compounds:**	
◦ Wood dusts	• Timber industry, sawing
◦ Antibiotics	• Pharmaceutical industry
◦ Metal salts	• Metal work—plating, welding
◦ Chemicals, dyes, insecticides	• Chemical, dyeing, plastic and resin industries, laboratories, and foundries
◦ Miscellaneous	• Pharmaceutical industry, fumigation, and electronics

are only occasional and sporadic published reports on occupational asthma. This however does not imply that the disease is rare. It is perhaps not recognized in routine clinical practice.

Diagnosis of occupational asthma is suspected from the history of a temporal relationship between symptoms and occupational exposure. As the condition progresses over several months, symptoms tend to become more severe, to start earlier and last longer, to have nocturnal symptoms, and to persist on the weekends. The physical examination may be nonspecific but tends to be insensitive. It is important to establish objectively a relationship between work and asthma symptoms. This can be demonstrated by allergen-specific challenge tests or occupational exposure tests.

Pulmonary function testing is usually required in order to make the diagnosis of occupational asthma. It is however important to do the tests both at and away from work. Skin testing with common allergens, such as the house dust, danders, and grass and tree pollens may be useful in determining the atopic status of an individual. Presence of specific IgE antibodies to occupational allergens is helpful to make a diagnosis. Serologic testing is highly specific but less sensitive indicator of sensitization than skin testing. Specific inhalation challenge test is the gold standard in the confirmation of the diagnosis.

General management of occupational asthma consists of inhaled corticosteroid and bronchodilator therapy as for any other type of asthma. It is important to remove the causative exposure for an effective management plan. Frequently, it may require a change in the job which may not be possible all the time. Patient must be educated about the importance of this measure. All other personal, professional, and engineering measures should be adopted and implemented to minimize the exposure.

HYPERSENSITIVITY PNEUMONIAS

Pulmonary diseases caused by exposure to organic dusts. In this category of occupational hazards, the offending agents are organic in nature such as the biological products, dusts of sugar cane, moldy hay, enzyme detergents, pigeon excreta, or microorganisms. Patients exposed to these organic dusts may develop allergic rhinitis, asthma, chronic bronchitis or HP and interstitial fibrosis. Allergic rhinitis is usually mild and may be accompanied by redness of eyes. Pulmonary symptoms and signs are more outstanding and patients may complain of cough, expectoration, wheezing, chest pain, chills, and shortness of breath. HP is a delayed type of hypersensitivity reaction which develops after repeated work exposure to an occupational agent with formation of antigen and antibody complexes which cause cellular and vascular injury in the lung parenchyma. Some of the important HPs and the causative exposures are listed in **Table 2**.

COMMON HPs: *Byssinosis* is a specific type of hypersensitivity reaction to inhalation of cotton fibers. It has been extensively described in industrial workers of cotton and textile mills mostly from the Western India. *Farmer's lung, psittacosis or Bird fancier lung and bagassosis* are also common in India. HPs may present with features of bronchoconstriction. There is a delayed hypersensitivity reaction 4–8 hours following antigenic exposure. In byssinosis, known as Monday morning fever, the patient develops cough, chest tightness, bronchoconstriction, and constitutional symptoms on getting exposed to the antigen after a restful weekend. Symptoms are generally reversible and regress on removal from the dusty surroundings. Interstitial lung disease (ILD) and pulmonary fibrosis occurs in chronic HP due to persistent exposure. These patients will complain of progressive cough and breathlessness, ultimately developing respiratory insufficiency. Chronic

TABLE 2 Important hypersensitivity pneumonias and the causative occupational exposures.

Type of hypersensitivity pneumonitis	Occupational exposure/antigen
Farmer's lung	Moldy hay–thermophilic actinomycetes
Bagassosis	Moldy bagasse (sugar cane)—thermophilic actinomycetes
Mushroom worker's disease	Moldy compost and mushroom—thermophilic actinomycetes
Malt worker's lung	Contaminated barley—*Aspergillus clavatus*
Compost lung	Compost—*Aspergillus*
Ventilator lung	Contaminated humidifiers, air conditioners, heating systems—thermophilic actinomycetes
Bird fancier's lung	Domestic birds—bird proteins
Psittacosis	Pigeons/Parakeets—droppings, feathers, proteins
Budgerigar fancier's lung	Wood cutting
Woodman's disease	Contaminated basement—fungi
Basement lung	Contaminated hot tub water—*Mycobacterium avium* complex
Hot-tub lung	

HP-ILD may be difficult to differentiate from other forms of pulmonary fibrosis. Advanced disease with extensive fibrosis will present with hypoxia and chronic respiratory failure.

Diagnosis of HP is made from exposure-symptom relationship. It is typically a delayed, Arthus-type of hypersensitivity and symptoms usually occur after 4–6 hours of exposure. General systemic symptoms of fever, malaise, fatigue, and body aches are common. Respiratory symptoms such as cough, chest tightness, breathlessness, and wheezing may not be as prominent as in occupational asthma. Chest X-ray and CT scan may show fine miliary or granular shadows, predominantly involving the upper lobes. Patients with chronic HP typically complain of progressive cough and breathlessness like any other ILD. Radiology may also be indistinguishable. Demonstration of specific IgE antibodies to the causative allergen is helpful for diagnosis. Lung biopsy may be required in some cases to distinguish from other causes of ILD.

Treatment of organic dust-induced lung disease includes both general and specific measures. Removal of the affected person from the source of antigen exposure is the most important step. Symptomatic treatment of HP consists of anti-inflammatory drugs, inhaled corticosteroids, and bronchodilators. Chronic HP is treated as any other type of pulmonary fibrosis. There is some evidence to suggest the role of antifibrotic drugs in addition to the use of immunosuppressants. Patients with extensive fibrosis will require oxygen support and other management strategies for chronic respiratory failure.

PNEUMOCONIOSES

Due to the deposition of inorganic dusts inhaled by workers: Pneumoconioses result due to the deposition of inorganic dusts inhaled by workers engaged in dusty occupations such as mines, factories, and foundries. Generally, up to a kilogram of dust may enter the respiratory tract in a working life span of 30 years. It is more in people living in dusty and smoky environments. The health hazards depend upon the fibrogenic reaction induced by the inhaled dust based on the presence of silica. The other important factors are:

- Particle size of the inhaled dust; generally, particles above 80 μ are filtered out by the nose while those between 1 and 80 μ can cause pulmonary damage.
- Duration of exposure
- Host's defense system

A sizable load of dust is cleared by the mucociliary system of the tracheobronchial tree. Smaller particles are engulfed by the macrophages and removed via the lymphatics. Dust deposition disease is likely to result if these defense systems are defective or choked. Clinical picture of pneumoconiosis is highly variable. Dust deposition in the lung parenchyma remains asymptomatic for long periods of time. Symptoms appear only after a significant progression of disease has taken place. Earlier diagnosis is based on routine radiographic screening of workers involved in occupations risked with high exposure levels to different mineral dusts. Mineral dust fibrosis is progressive and to a large extent irreversible unless the exposure is discontinued. Various types of pneumoconioses are described below:

Types of pneumoconioses:

- *Silicosis*: Silicosis is an enormous problem reported from several parts of India among workers of silica, copper, mica, lead and zinc mines, slate pencil and other stone cutting units, quartz grinding and agate industries, iron and steel foundries, pottery, ceramic, glass manufacturing and in people working with metal casting, scaling, grinding, polishing and manufacturing of paints and rubber. Commonly it causes progressive interstitial pulmonary fibrosis. Pleural involvement is also common. Cough in simple silicosis is usually dry but mucoid expectoration is also reported. Clinical picture may be complicated by tobacco smoking, and/or concomitant infections, especially tuberculosis (e.g., silicotuberculosis). Such patients may present with expectoration, hemoptysis, and general constitutional symptoms. Occasionally, pneumothorax may also occur. Disease progression in these patients is faster. Acute silicosis may develop within a period of months following massive exposure. Chronic cor pulmonale generally develops in a matter of a few years after the onset of breathlessness. Hypoxemia and respiratory failure develop more prominently and earlier in patients with severe degree of pulmonary fibrosis.

Diagnosis is based on chest roentgenography in the presence of following findings:
- Diffuse involvement, predominantly of upper and mid zones
- Dense, nodular, or reticulonodular shadows of varying sizes
- Calcification may occur occasionally. Eggshell calcification of hilar lymph nodes is quite characteristic.
- Pleural plaques and calcification may also occur.
- Large opacities due to agglomeration of nodules are seen in progressive massive fibrosis (PMF). These masses of dense fibrosis are often surrounded by bullae.
- Cavitation may indicate the evidence of silico-tuberculosis.

Computed tomographic scanning of the lungs is not considered essential for the diagnosis but may help to define the lung involvement in the presence of ILD.

- *Coal Workers' Pneumoconiosis (CWP)*: CWP is reported in about 3% in miners, while PMF is rare. Lung damage is usually attributable to the presence of silica dust. Coal dust consists of carbon (60–80%), apart from 50 different elements and oxides—including silica—higher the quality of coal, higher the silica content in the dust.
- *Asbestosis*: Commercial use of asbestos has been banned in several countries. High environmental levels of air-borne asbestos fibers are reported in different chrysotile asbestos mills. Following health hazards have been reported due to asbestos exposure:
  - Asbestosis in people working in the asbestos mines. The prevalence in workers of asbestos cement factories and textile industry is variably described from 3% to 9%. Sporadic cases are seen in people who accidentally inhale asbestos fibers from unconventional sources such as the ragged bags and sheets containing asbestos fibers.
  - Interstitial lung disease: Asbestos is a fibrogenic dust. It is an important cause of progressive fibrosing ILD.
  - Pleural plaques and mesotheliomas
  - Malignancies: Respiratory cancers have been described several years after exposure. Lung cancer risk gets multiplied among smokers exposed to asbestos.

Miscellaneous pneumoconiosis: Some of the other metals which have been implicated include beryllium, metals, and alloys such as cobalt, zinc, cadmium, manganese, chromium, nickel, and others. Most of them are inert dusts and do not cause fibrosis. They do not produce symptoms and are incidentally diagnosed on chest radiography in exposed workers.

TOXIC GASES AND FUMES INHALATION

Inhalation of toxic gases can cause both direct and indirect pulmonary damage. The Bhopal tragedy of 1984 which resulted in over 2,000 deaths due to the leakage of poisonous methyl diisocyanate gas from a Union Carbide fertilizer plant is the classical example of acute accidental exposure. Asphyxiation caused by massive inhalation is usually the immediate deaths. Pulmonary edema and acute respiratory distress syndrome can result due to the direct damage caused to the alveolo-capillary membrane. Other manifestations of exposure to gases and fumes may vary from simple, irritative cough, irritation of eyes, and nose to severe pneumonias, neurological damage, convulsions, and coma. Damage may also occur to the liver, heart, brain, and kidneys.

Direct mucosal and alveolar damage: Toxic gases may injure the respiratory tract depending upon the physical and chemical properties and duration and concentration of the exposure. Highly soluble gases like ammonia and sulfur dioxide cause maximal injury to the proximal and large airways causing bronchitis, bronchiolitis, atelectasis, and pneumonia. The less soluble gases (chlorine, oxides of nitrogen) may produce distal injury at alveolar level causing pneumonia, pulmonary edema, and severe respiratory distress.

Systemic toxicity: Inhalation of fumes of metal oxides (e.g., zinc, copper, magnesium, cadmium, nickel, tin, iron, selenium, antimony, and manganese) may cause systemic reaction like fever and other constitutional symptoms besides respiratory symptoms. This is called "metal fume fever". This occurs, for example, during welding of galvanized iron or during cleaning of zinc-coated water tanks. "Polymer fume fever" can occur due to inhalation of fumes of degradation products of poly tetrafluoroethylene (Fluon, Teflon) when it is heated to high temperature.

CONCLUSION

In summary, occupational diseases are far more prevalent than reported. In the past, this was attributed to the lack of an organized occupational healthcare service structure. Screening facilities for health hazards were relatively sparse. Moreover, the need for industrialization required for an expanding economy had outweighed most other considerations. The sparse practice of medical reporting amongst Indian physicians had also been responsible for a relative underassessment of the problem. But the problems are rather enormous. Concerted efforts are required to manage and prevent the problem.

RECOMMENDED READINGS

1. Jindal SK, Aggarwal AN, Jindal A. Household air pollution in India and respiratory diseases: Current status and future directions. Curr Opin Pulm Med. 2020;26(2):128-34.
2. Mortimer K, Gordon SB, Jindal SK, Accinelli RA, Balmes J, Martin WJ II. Household air pollution as a major avoidable risk factor for cardiorespiratory disease. Chest. 2012;142(5):1308-15.
3. Jindal SK, Jindal A. COPD in Biomass exposed nonsmokers: a different phenotype. Expert Rev Respir Med. 2020;16:1-8.
4. Tarlo SM, Lemiere C. Occupational asthma. N Engl J Med. 2014;370(7):640-9.
5. Patel S, Ram U, Ram F, Patel SK. Socioeconomic and demographic predictors of high blood pressure, diabetes, asthma and heart disease among adults engaged in various occupations: evidence from India. J Biosoc Sci. 2020;52(5):629-49.
6. Cullinan P, Munoz X, Suojalehto H, Agius R, Jindal S, Sigsgaard T, et al. Occupational lung diseases: from old and novel exposures to effective preventive strategies. Lancet Respir Med. 2017;5(5):445-55.
7. Quirce S, Vandenplas O, Campo P, Cruz MJ, de Blay F, Koschel D, et al. Occupational hypersensitivity pneumonitis: an EAACI position paper. Allergy. 2016;71(6):765-79.
8. Singh S, Collins BF, Sharma BB, Joshi JM, Talwar D, Katiyar S, et al. Hypersensitivity pneumonitis: Clinical manifestations - Prospective data from the interstitial lung disease-India registry. Lung India. 2019;36(6): 476-82.
9. Jindal SK. Silicosis in India: Past and present. Curr Opin Pulm Med. 2013;19:163-8.
10. Jindal SK, Aggarwal AN, Gupta D. Dust-induced interstitial lung disease in the tropics. Curr Opin Pulm Med. 2001;7(5):272-7.

CHAPTER 207 Pneumonia and Other Respiratory Infections

DJ Christopher, Barney J Isaac

ABSTRACT

Pneumonia is not an uncommon infectious disease. It is an acute infection of the lung parenchyma and thus presents with respiratory symptoms and signs. It can be either community or hospital acquired. Community-acquired pneumonia (CAP) is a significant cause of morbidity and mortality worldwide. It is commonly caused by bacteria and viruses. Severity assessment scores help in deciding the need for hospital admission as well as the need for critical care. It is an important cause of sepsis which increases its mortality. Prompt diagnosis and treatment of sepsis are required for best outcomes. Antibiotics are the cornerstone of treatment. Vaccination is advocated in the high-risk group to prevent pneumonia. Hospital-acquired pneumonia (HAP) is a significant cause of increased length of hospital stay and mortality. It is called ventilator-associated pneumonia (VAP), when it occurs in the setting of invasive ventilation. Risk factors for multidrug resistance pathogens are important to identify, to start appropriate empirical antibiotic treatment. Culture and drug susceptibility testing of appropriate samples may help in the choice of antibiotics.

"Never forget it is not pneumonia, but a pneumonic man who is your patient"

—William W Gull

PNEUMONIA

INTRODUCTION

Pneumonia is a common infectious disease that presents with respiratory symptoms and signs. It is caused by a wide range of microorganisms, particularly bacteria. If promptly diagnosed and appropriately treated, the morbidity and mortality can be reduced significantly. There are known factors which predispose to pneumonia. In this chapter, we will delve into details of pneumonia and touch upon other respiratory infections.

DEFINITION

Pneumonia is an acute infection of the lung parenchyma. It can either be caused by organisms acquired from the community, when it is called *community-acquired pneumonia*, or it could be acquired from the hospital and termed *hospital-acquired pneumonia (HAP)*, which is also called nosocomial pneumonia. HAP is defined as pneumonia that develops ≥48 hours after admission to a hospital. At times, CAP may also develop in the hospital, if infection with community-acquired organism was in incubation period at the time of admission, then it is likely to manifest within 48 hours. VAP is a subtype of HAP which occurs 48 hours after endotracheal intubation or tracheostomy. *Healthcare-associated pneumonia (HCAP)* was a term used till recently, which was referring to pneumonia that develops after visiting a healthcare facility like outpatient visits, nursing homes, daycare dialysis units, hospitalization within the previous 3 months etc. In such situations, resistant pathogens are more likely to be encountered. However, this terminology has been withdrawn owing to rampant use of inappropriate broad spectrum antibiotics on account of this categorization.

EPIDEMIOLOGY

Community-acquired pneumonia is a significant cause of morbidity and mortality worldwide; however, there is significant variation due to geographic distribution, host factors, and age. In the US, the incidence of CAP is 16–23 per 1,000 individuals per year; 30% of these require admission resulting in it being the second most common cause for hospitalization. In India, only sparse data is available mostly from cross-sectional studies, from tertiary care institutes. These studies have reported a mortality rate of 5–30% for CAP. Lower respiratory tract infections account for 20% of all deaths due to infectious diseases in India. HAP is the second most common nosocomial infection and it prolongs the hospital stay and the cost of treatment significantly. HAP is diagnosed in 5–10 per 1,000 hospital admissions and the risk increases by 6- to 20-fold in those who are mechanically ventilated, when it is termed VAP. The mortality is significantly higher (37% and 47%) in the two Indian studies that have reported mortality from VAP.

ETIOLOGY

Bacteria and viruses are the etiological agents that cause CAP. Studies show that microbiological identification is not possible in up to 40–70% of samples. The most common etiological agent is *Streptococcus pneumoniae*, accounting for around 30% of all CAPs. These rates vary based on the prevalence of pneumococcal vaccination in the population; in US, it contributes only to 10–15% of all CAPs whereas in India it contributes to 35% of CAPs. The other common bacteria causing CAP are *Klebsiella pneumoniae*, *Staphylococcus aureus*, and *Haemophilus influenzae*. *Mycoplasma pneumoniae* and *Legionella pneumophila* are common causes of atypical CAP. Atypical CAP is characterized by less severe symptoms, patchy interstitial infiltrates, resistance of the causative organisms to β-lactams and their inability to show up on gram stain and traditional cultures. Studies which have looked at viruses as etiological agents have identified them in up to 36% samples of CAP. Influenza A and B viruses and, more recently, the severe acute respiratory syndrome coronavirus 2 (SARS-CoV-2) are common viruses causing CAP. **Table 1** lists the bacteria and viruses that cause CAP.

The common etiology of HAP is bacteria and is listed in **Table 2**. In India, gram-negative bacilli are the most common cause with *Pseudomonas* and *Acinetobacter* being the leading causes, whereas in the west, methicillin-resistant *S. aureus* (MRSA) is emerging as the leading cause. Of late, there is an increased recognition of viruses in the etiology of HAP. Etiology of HAP is dependent on the presence of risk factors for infections with multidrug resistant (MDR) bacteria. These have been listed in **Table 3**. Prolonged hospital stay and prior intravenous antibiotic therapy are

TABLE 1 List of organisms causing community-acquired pneumonia.

Category	Organism
Typical bacteria	• *Streptococcus pneumoniae (most common cause)* • *Haemophilus influenzae* • *Klebsiella pneumoniae* • *Staphylococcus aureus* • *Moraxella catarrhalis* • Group A streptococci • *Escherichia coli* • Microaerophilic bacteria and anaerobes (associated with aspiration)
Atypical bacteria	• *Legionella pneumophila* • *Mycoplasma pneumoniae* • *Chlamydia pneumoniae* • *Chlamydia psittaci* • *Coxiella burnetii*
Viruses	• Influenza A and B viruses • Severe acute respiratory syndrome coronavirus 2 (SARS-CoV-2) • Other coronaviruses • Rhinoviruses • Parainfluenza viruses • Adenoviruses • Respiratory syncytial virus • Human metapneumovirus • Human bocaviruses

TABLE 2 List of organisms causing hospital-acquired pneumonia.

Gram-negative bacilli	• *Pseudomonas aeruginosa* • *Acinetobacter* species • *Klebsiella pneumoniae* • *Escherichia coli* • *Enterobacter* species
Gram-positive cocci	• *Staphylococcus aureus*, including methicillin-resistant *S. aureus* (MRSA) • *Streptococcus* species

TABLE 3 Risk factors for MDR pathogens.

Category	Risk factors
MDR VAP	• Septic shock at time of VAP • ARDS preceding VAP • 5 or more days of hospitalization prior to the occurrence of VAP • Acute renal replacement therapy prior to VAP onset
MDR HAP	Prior intravenous antibiotic use within 90 days
MRSA VAP/HAP	
MDR *Pseudomonas* VAP/HAP	

(HAP: hospital-acquired pneumonia; MDR: multidrug resistant; VAP: ventilator-associated pneumonia)

the two most important risk factors for being infected by an MDR pathogen. The other factor which may influence the type of pathogens is whether the HAP developed while on the ventilator (VAP) as opposed to non-VAP HAP. However, there is inadequate data on this difference.

RISK FACTORS

The risk factors which increase the risk of developing pneumonia are different for community-acquired and hospital-acquired pathogens except for few factors like age and chronic lung diseases. These have been given in **Table 4**.

PATHOGENESIS

Conventionally, it has been thought that infective organisms are transmitted from person to person either as droplets or aerosols. These deposit in the nasopharynx and get microaspirated into the pulmonary alveoli. If the inoculum is sufficient and/or if the host immune mechanisms are overwhelmed, there is replication of the pathogen. A combination of virulence factors of the organism and the host immune response results in damage to the lung parenchyma resulting in the pathological features of pneumonia. The concept and discovery of the lung microbiome have provided alternate hypothesis that the altered alveolar microbiome could be a predisposing factor to the development of pneumonia. The pathology of pneumonia has four stages, namely (1) consolidation, (2) red hepatization, (3) gray hepatization, and (4) resolution.

CLINICAL FEATURES

The common symptoms of pneumonia are fever, productive cough, shortness of breath, and pleuritic chest pain. Elderly patients and immunocompromised individuals may not present with fever. Pleuritic chest pain occurs when the parietal pleura is involved either by a peripheral consolidation causing a pleural inflammation or a parapneumonic effusion. Bronchial breathing and crackles are the most common physical findings. However, increased vocal fremitus, increased vocal resonance,

TABLE 4 Risk factors of CAP and HAP.

Community-acquired pneumonia	Hospital-acquired pneumonia
Demographics	**Demographics**
Age >65 years	Older age
Comorbidities	**Comorbidities**
• Chronic lung diseases • Chronic heart disease, particularly CHF • Stroke • Diabetes mellitus • Malnutrition • Immunocompromising conditions • Viral respiratory tract infection • Impaired airway protection	• Chronic lung disease • Depressed consciousness • Aspiration • Chest or upper abdominal surgery • Malnutrition • Chronic renal failure • Anemia • Multiple trauma
Treatment related	**Previous hospitalization**
High-dose inhaled corticosteroids	
Habits	**Treatment related**
• Alcohol overuse (>80 g/day) • Smoking	• Previous antibiotic exposure, especially broad spectrum • Agents that increase gastric pH [H2 blockers, antacids, and proton pump inhibitors (PPIs)]
Environmental factors	**ICU and ventilation related**
• Crowded living conditions (e.g., prisons and homeless shelters) • Residence in low-income settings • Exposure to environmental toxins (e.g., solvents, paints, or gasoline)	• Reintubation or prolonged intubation • Mechanical ventilation for acute respiratory distress syndrome • Frequent ventilator circuit changes • Presence of an intracranial pressure monitor • Number of central venous catheter placements and surgeries • Use of muscle relaxants or glucocorticoids • Paralysis • Total opioid exposure

(CAP: community-acquired pneumonia; HAP: hospital-acquired pneumonia)

bronchophony, and egophony can be elicited in a lobar consolidation.

DIAGNOSIS

When CAP is clinically suspected, a chest radiograph is obtained to confirm the diagnosis. It may reveal a lobar consolidation with air bronchogram (**Fig. 1 A**) or patchy interstitial infiltrates. Leukocytosis and an elevated C-reactive protein (CRP) (>20 mg/L) are laboratory parameters which support the diagnosis. However, in the outpatient setting, an appropriate clinical picture with radiograph is enough to clinch the diagnosis and initiate

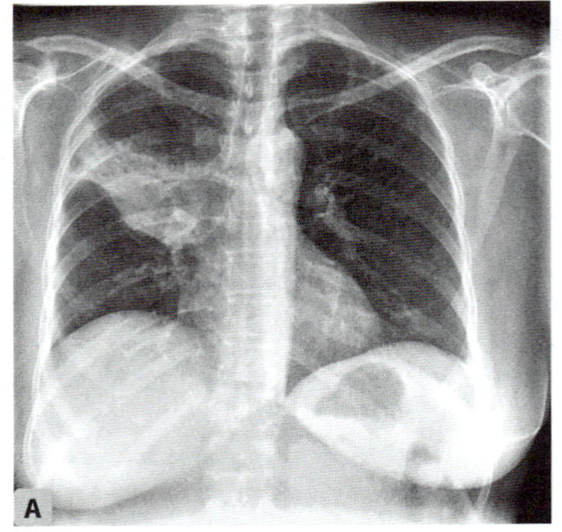

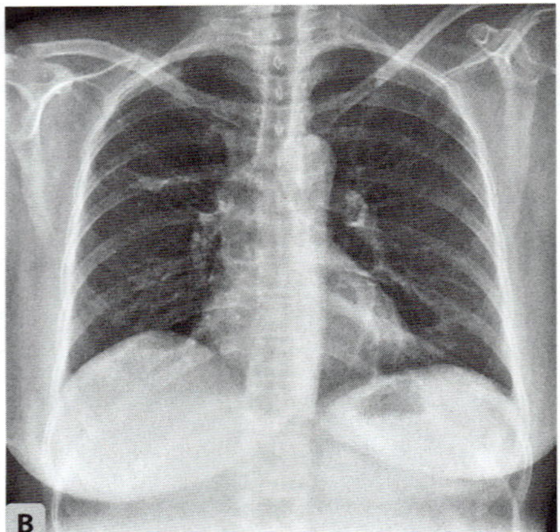

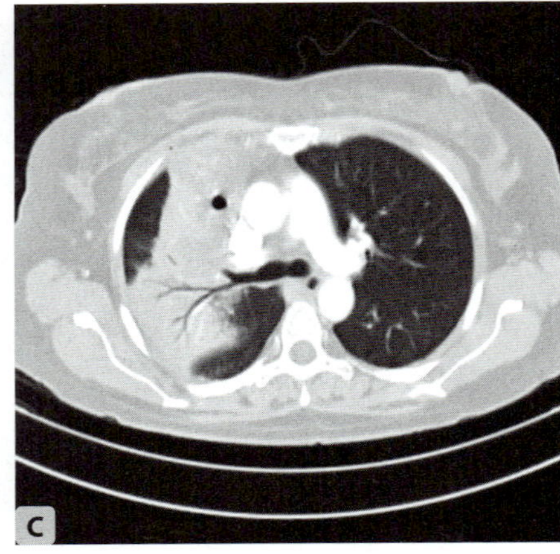

(HRCT: high-resolution computed tomography)

FIGURES 1 A to C: Chest radiograph of a 39-year-old lady with productive cough and fever for a week; **(A)** at presentation, showing right upper lobe consolidation with air bronchogram; **(B)** after 1 month, following treatment with antibiotics; and **(C)** HRCT of the same patient showing right upper lobe consolidation with air bronchogram.

treatment. This should be followed by careful reassessment. A sputum test for bacterial culture is advocated only if there is a need for admission. Its yield varies from 35 to 65% and could direct antibiotic therapy, especially when clinical response is inadequate. Blood cultures are recommended for patients who are admitted with severe CAP. Urinary antigen tests are point-of-care tests in detecting *Pneumococcus* and *Legionella* with good sensitivity but low specificity and hence their routine use is not recommended. Computed tomography (CT) scan of the thorax (**Fig. 1 C**) is needed only if alternate diagnoses like malignancy are suspected or if there is inadequate clinical response.

For the diagnosis of HAP/VAP, the Centers for Disease Control and Prevention (CDC) criterion is widely used and is presented in **Box 1**. In all those clinically diagnosed using this criterion, sputum culture should be sent in non-VAP HAP and endotracheal aspirates should be sent for VAP or in those who get subsequently intubated.

BOX 1 Modified CDC criteria for diagnosis of HAP/VAP.
Chest radiographic opacities (new, progressive, or persistent infiltrate or cavitation) and at least two of the following:
1. Fever > 38°C or >100.4°F
2. Leukopenia (<4,000 WBC/μL) or leukocytosis (≥12,000 WBC/μL)
3. Altered mental status with no other recognized cause in the elderly
4. New onset of purulent sputum, or change in character of sputum, or increased respiratory secretions, or increased suctioning requirements
5. Worsening gas exchange (e.g., desaturations, increased oxygen requirements, or increased ventilator demand)
6. New onset or worsening cough, dyspnea, or tachypnea
7. Rales or bronchial breath sounds

(CDC: Centers for Disease Control and Prevention; HAP: hospital-acquired pneumonia; VAP: ventilator-associated pneumonia)

DIFFERENTIAL DIAGNOSIS

Pneumonia is a clinicoradiological diagnosis and non-infectious causes of pulmonary infiltrates would form the bulk of the differential diagnoses, while chronic infections like tuberculosis would also be among the differentials. These have been given in **Table 5** with the features that could differentiate them from pneumonia.

MANAGEMENT

Treatment of CAP involves assessment of severity to decide on the appropriate site of care and identifying risk factors of MDR pathogens to choose the appropriate antibiotics. The CURB-65 (confusion, urea, respiratory rate, blood pressure, age > 65), CRB-65 (confusion, respiratory rate, blood pressure, age > 65), PSI (Pneumonia Severity Index), and ATS/IDSA (American Thoracic Society/ Infectious Disease Society of America) criteria are the most widely used for deciding on the severity of CAP. The CURB-65 and CRB-65 are provided in **Table 6** and are easy to apply and useful in determining the location of care, particularly in the decision of hospitalization versus providing outpatient treatment. The CRB-65 is entirely clinical and has hence gained more acceptability in comparison with CURB-65 in the prediction of mortality. A CRB-65 score of 2 and above warrants admission. Oxygen saturation below 92% requires in-patient management and is an important parameter which is not part of these screening scores. The PSI is a score obtained from 20 parameters which include demographics, place of residence, comorbidities, physical examination findings, and laboratory and radiographic findings. It categorizes patients into classes I to V. It has been extensively validated in predicting mortality as opposed to the CURB-65 and

TABLE 5 Differential diagnosis of CAP.

Differential diagnosis	Features that can help differentiate
Acute pulmonary embolism	Predisposing factors of pulmonary embolism, presence of deep vein thrombosis, and hypoxia out of proportion to the pulmonary infiltrates
Acute pulmonary edema	Underlying cause for pulmonary edema like congestive cardiac failure; resolution of pulmonary infiltrates in a day or two with diuretic therapy
Alveolar hemorrhage	Fleeting opacities, quick resolution, underlying conditions which can cause alveolar hemorrhage
Atelectasis	Volume loss, resolution with chest physiotherapy
Pulmonary vasculitis	Constitutional symptoms, multiple opacities, other organ involvement
Lung cancer	Risk factors for lung cancer, hemoptysis
Allergic broncho-pulmonary aspergillosis (ABPA)	History of asthma, fleeting opacities, elevated immunoglobulin E
Chemical pneumonitis	History of aspiration
Connective tissue diseases	Underlying rheumatoid arthritis (can present with nodules), SLE (pneumonitis)
Interstitial lung diseases	Features of sarcoidosis, organizing pneumonia, hypersensitivity pneumonitis
Tuberculosis	Constitutional symptoms, prolonged history, hemoptysis, upper lobe infiltrates
Hydatid cyst	Rounded opacity, persistent shadows noted on review of previous radiographs
Exacerbation of bronchiectasis	Mucous plugging can mimic pneumonia

(CAP: community-acquired pneumonia)

CRB-65 scores, but is time consuming and unwieldy to use. The ATS/IDSA criteria were laid out in 2007 and are presented in **Table 7**. They are useful in identifying severe CAP among hospitalized patients and help in deciding the need for critical care. These criteria can also be used to determine need for critical care for non-VAP HAP that develops in the in-patient wards. An algorithm depicting this approach is shown in **Flowchart 1**.

TABLE 6 CURB-65 and CRB-65 scoring.

Parameter	Description	Score
Confusion	Present	1
	Absent	0
Urea (only for CURB-65)	≥7 mmol/L or ≥42.8 mg/dL	1
	<7 mmol/L or <42.8 mg/dL	0
Respiratory rate	≥30/min	1
	<30/min	0
Blood pressure	Systolic ≤ 90 mm Hg or diastolic ≤ 60 mm Hg	1
	Systolic > 90 mm Hg and diastolic > 60 mm Hg	0
Age	Age ≥ 65 years	1
	Age < 65 years	0
Maximum	**CURB-65**	**5**
	CRB-65	**4**

(CURB-65: confusion, urea, respiratory rate, blood pressure, age > 65; CRB-65: confusion, respiratory rate, blood pressure, age > 65)

TABLE 7 ATS/IDSA severity criteria.

Major criteria	Minor criteria
One major or three minor criteria qualify as severe CAP	
• Septic shock with need for vasopressors • Respiratory failure requiring mechanical ventilation	• Respiratory rate ≥ 30 breaths/min • PaO_2/FIO_2 ratio ≤ 250 • Multilobar infiltrates • Confusion/disorientation • Uremia (blood urea nitrogen level ≥ 20 mg/dL)* • Leukopenia (white blood cell count < 4,000 cells/mL) • Thrombocytopenia (platelet count < 100,000/mL) • Hypothermia (core temperature < 36°C) • Hypotension requiring aggressive fluid resuscitation

* BUN of 20 mg/dL = 42.8 mg/dL of urea (also see Table 6).

(ATS: American Thoracic Society; CAP: community-acquired pneumonia; FiO_2: fraction of inspired oxygen; IDSA: Infectious Disease Society of America)

ANTIBIOTICS

The empirical choice of antibiotic for CAP is directed against the common pathogen *S. pneumoniae*. It is also based on the site of care (outpatient vs. in-patient), the presence of comorbidities and the severity of CAP based on the ATS/IDSA criteria in **Table 7**. Patients can be divided into four categories based on these, as shown in **Table 8**, and appropriate empirical antibiotics should be initiated. The timing of antibiotic is crucial, and it should be administered as early as possible. The doses of the commonly used antibiotics are given in **Table 9**. Fluoroquinolones should not be used as empirical therapy, particularly in high tuberculous burden countries like India, where it is known to increase the risk and prevalence of drug-resistant tuberculosis. However, in an exceptional situation of confirmed hypersensitivity to β-lactams, levofloxacin 750 mg once a day can be used if tuberculosis is not under consideration.

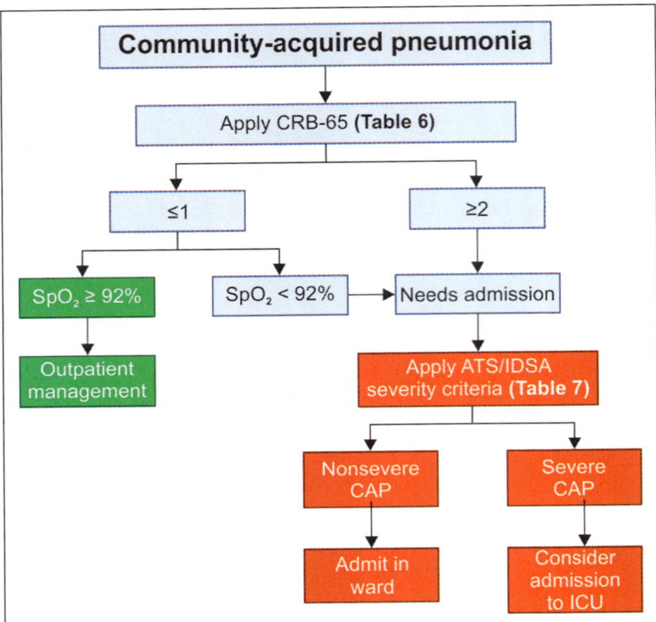

(ATS: American Thoracic Society; CAP: community-acquired pneumonia; IDSA: Infectious Disease Society of America; CRB-65: confusion, respiratory rate, blood pressure, age > 65)

FLOWCHART 1: Algorithm for the management of CAP.

TABLE 8 Empirical antibiotic choice in CAP in the absence of risk factors for *Pseudomonas* or MRSA.

Category	Empirical choice of antibiotic	Route	Duration
Outpatient without comorbidities*	β-lactams or macrolides	Oral	3–5 days
Outpatient with comorbidities*	β-lactams + macrolides	Oral	5 days
Inpatient nonsevere (refer **Table 7**)	β-lactams + macrolides	IV and switch to oral once tolerating orally	5–7 days
Inpatient severe (refer **Table 7**)	β-lactams + macrolides	IV	7 days

*Chronic heart disease, chronic respiratory disease, chronic liver disease, chronic renal disease, diabetes mellitus, alcohol overuse (>80 g/day), malignancies, use of antimicrobials in the previous 3 months.

(CAP: community-acquired pneumonia; MRSA: methicillin-resistant *S. aureus*)

Prior isolation of MRSA or *Pseudomonas* in respiratory samples or admission requiring parenteral antibiotics in the previous 90 days warrants antibiotics cover with antipseudomonal antibiotics (piperacillin-tazobactam, cefepime, cefoperazone, cefoperazone-sulbactam, ceftazidime, meropenem, and imipenem) and anti-MRSA antibiotics (vancomycin and linezolid). Other recognized risk factors for *Pseudomonas* are tracheostomy, bronchiectasis, need for invasive ventilation or vasopressors, and very severe COPD. When these antibiotics are initiated, results from sputum or endotracheal aspirates and blood culture will help to de-escalate or modify the empirical therapy.

TABLE 9 Doses of common antibiotics used to treat pneumonia.

Antibiotic	Dose
Amoxicillin	0.5–1 g thrice daily (PO or IV)
Coamoxiclav	625 mg thrice a day to 1 g twice daily (PO)/1.2 g thrice daily (IV)
Azithromycin	500 mg daily (PO or IV)
Ceftriaxone	1–2 g twice daily (IV)
Cefotaxime	1 g thrice daily (IV)
Cefepime	1–2 g 2–3 times a day (IV)
Ceftazidime	2 g thrice daily (IV)
Piperacillin–tazobactam	4.5 g four times a day (IV)
Imipenem	0.5–1 g 3–4 times a day (IV)
Meropenem	1 g thrice daily (IV)

Empirical antibiotic choice for HAP should be based on updated local antibiogram data and risk factors of MDR pathogens (**Table 3**). Antipseudomonal and anti-staphylococcal covers are mandatory. If there are no risk factors for MDR pathogens, then a single antipseudomonal agent and MSSA cover are sufficient. If MRSA risk factors are present, then vancomycin or linezolid should be initiated. Dual antipseudomonal cover should be initiated if there are risk factors for MDR *Pseudomonas*. The recommended duration of antibiotics is 7 days, unless clinically warranted to continue for longer.

In both CAP and HAP, after initiation of empirical antimicrobial therapy, once specific microbes have been identified, de-escalation should always be planned based on the sensitivity pattern. In other situations, when there is lack of clinical improvement, the culture reports could enable appropriate antibiotics escalation.

RESPIRATORY SUPPORT

Oxygen should be administered through nasal prongs or a venturi mask to maintain saturation ≥ 92%. In patients with severe COPD or those known to have type 2 respiratory failure, the target oxygen saturation should be 89–92% to prevent suppression of hypoxemic drive and resultant worsening of type 2 respiratory failure. If the clinical condition worsens to fulfill indications for invasive mechanical ventilation, then it should be instituted. Acute respiratory distress syndrome (ARDS) is managed using standard ventilatory protocols recommended by the ARDS network group. Noninvasive ventilation is indicated when there is an exacerbation of underlying obstructive airway disease, resulting in an acute on chronic type 2 respiratory failure. Apart from this, the role of noninvasive ventilation is controversial in pneumonia.

OTHER TREATMENT

Pneumonia increases the risk of thromboembolism several folds and hence prophylactic anticoagulation should be commenced for all hospitalized patients, unless contraindicated. There is no role for corticosteroids except in refractory septic shock.

ASSESSING RESPONSE TO TREATMENT

The most important aspect of assessing response to treatment in pneumonia is clinical. One needs to look for defervescence and improvement in symptoms of cough and breathlessness along with objective evidence of improvement in vital signs, particularly respiratory rate, blood pressure and oxygen requirement/saturation or arterial partial pressure of oxygen/fraction of inspired oxygen (PaO_2/FiO_2) ratio. There is no role for the routine monitoring of CRP, white blood counts, or procalcitonin in assessing response to treatment. A chest radiograph is also not needed if there is clinical response. However, if there is a clinical worsening, these and other appropriate tests are required, to ascertain the cause of worsening which could be progression of pneumonia, development of pleural effusion/empyema, sepsis, or an alternate or additional diagnosis. A repeat chest X-ray to ensure resolution of consolidation (**Fig. 1 B**) is required after about 6 weeks for those who have persistent symptoms or sign or who are at a higher risk of malignancy, particularly smokers and those above 50 years of age.

PREVENTION

The two key factors in the prevention of pneumonia are smoking cessation and vaccination. All current smokers should be advised to quit, with appropriate counseling and necessary pharmacological treatment. Vaccination is available against *Pneumococcus* and influenza infections. The two pneumococcal vaccines available are PPSV23 (23-valent pneumococcal polysaccharide vaccine) and PCV13 (13-valent pneumococcal conjugate vaccine). These are recommended for high-risk individuals and based on age. The influenza vaccine is recommended as a yearly vaccine for the high-risk group, as the strains keep changing every year. The schedule for these vaccines is available in the specific guidelines which are updated from time to time.

COMPLICATIONS

EMPYEMA

Empyema is a common complication of pneumonia. It results from the spread of infection to the adjacent pleural space and results in formation of pus in the pleural cavity. A complicated parapneumonic effusion, characterized by abnormal pleural fluid biochemical tests (pH < 7.2, glucose < 40 mg/dL or < 2.2 mmol/L, LDH > 1,000 IU/L) or microbiological features (Gram stain positive or bacterial culture positive) also indicates spread of infection to the pleural space. The pleural fluid culture serves as an important source to ascertain the etiological agent causing the pneumonia. In addition to giving appropriate antibiotics preferably through a parenteral route, the management will involve drainage of pus/pleural fluid in these situations.

SEPSIS

Pneumonia is the most common cause of sepsis. It occurs secondary to bacteremia, resulting in a systemic inflammatory response syndrome, which could progress to septic shock. It significantly increases the duration of hospital stay and the risk of mortality. Appropriate intravenous antibiotics, adequate fluid resuscitation, timely initiation of inotropes, and ventilatory management when needed are the key management principles. These should be administered in line with the surviving sepsis guidelines to decrease the morbidity and mortality to the maximum.

LUNG ABSCESS

Lung abscess is a pus-filled cavity of >2 cm diameter in the lung parenchyma which is caused due to liquefaction necrosis of lung tissue. It usually occurs when the infection is due to oropharyngeal or gastric aspiration. It can also happen postobstruction or by hematogenous spread. Due to the thick wall around it causing difficult penetration of antibiotics, prolonged duration of antibiotics up to 6 weeks is usually required. When large in size and if there is inadequate response to antibiotic treatment, either a percutaneous drainage or surgical excision needs to be considered based on the size of the abscess and general condition of the patient.

SPECIAL SITUATIONS

ASPIRATION PNEUMONIA

There are several predisposing factors for aspirating orogastric contents into the lung. It could either cause a chemical pneumonitis or a bacterial pneumonia. The latter can present as a CAP or as HAP when it occurs during hospitalization. These infections are predominantly anaerobic and are at increased risk of developing lung abscess and empyema. Antibiotic therapy should be directed with adequate anaerobic coverage. The underlying predisposing factor that led to the aspiration should be found and addressed appropriately.

POST-OBSTRUCTIVE PNEUMONIA

An endobronchial obstruction of a lobar or segmental or main bronchus, usually secondary to malignancy, can result in pooling of secretions distally and development of pneumonia. This can present in someone with a known endobronchial lesion or can present de novo as a CAP. In the latter, it can result in delayed resolution/improvement or inadequate improvement. Presentation with hemoptysis either during or preceding the current illness can provide a clue. When suspected, a CT scan followed by bronchoscopy will be needed. Bronchoscopy may be planned once the patient stabilizes from the acute infection. Sometimes, endobronchial debulking may be required to augment drainage and resolution of the pneumonia.

PNEUMONIA IN IMMUNOCOMPROMISED

The respiratory infections that occur in immunocompromised individuals are different and require special mention. The immunocompromising conditions include neutropenia (due to immunosuppression or underlying disease), long-term steroid use, use of biological agents, drug-induced T-cell suppression and lymphocyte depletion, certain autoimmune conditions and hematological malignancies, infection with human immunodeficiency virus, and solid organ transplantation. Bacteria (particularly caused by *S. pneumoniae*) are still the most common cause of pneumonia in this group. Viruses including cytomegalovirus, fungi including *Aspergillus* and *Pneumocystis jirovecii* and *Nocardia* are the other notable causative agents of pneumonia which usually do not cause infection in an immunocompetent host. The evaluation and treatment of pneumonia in this population need to take into consideration all these etiologies, and is based on the type of immunosuppression.

OTHER RESPIRATORY INFECTIONS

ACUTE BRONCHITIS

Acute bronchitis is a self-limiting condition which is caused by inflammation of the larger airways presenting with acute cough in the absence of pneumonia or an alternate diagnosis to explain the cough, preferably in the absence of a chronic lung disease. It is usual caused by viral infections, the most common being influenza A and B viruses. It usually resolves in 2–3 weeks; it does not warrant initiating antibiotics.

ACUTE UPPER RESPIRATORY INFECTIONS

These include acute pharyngitis, acute laryngitis, and acute epiglottitis. These are usually of viral etiology but could also be bacterial. Pharyngitis presents with throat pain, whereas laryngitis presents with change in voice. Acute epiglottitis, also called croup, is a disease which usually affects children.

SUMMARY

Pneumonia is a fairly common acute infection of the lung parenchyma causing significant morbidity and mortality. It can be either community acquired or hospital acquired. It is predominantly caused by bacteria. Based on severity scores, a decision on need for admission to ward or the ICU is made. Prompt initiation of antibiotics and other supportive treatment results in good outcomes. Vaccinating high-risk groups may reduce its incidence.

RECOMMENDED READINGS

1. Kalil AC, Metersky ML, Klompas M, Muscedere J, Sweeney DA, Palmer LB, et al. Management of Adults With Hospital-acquired and Ventilator-associated Pneumonia: 2016 Clinical Practice Guidelines by the Infectious Diseases Society of America and the American Thoracic Society. Clin Infect Dis. 2016;63(5):e61-111.
2. Metlay JP, Waterer GW, Long AC, Anzueto A, Brozek J, Crothers K, et al. Diagnosis and Treatment of Adults with Community-acquired Pneumonia. An Official Clinical Practice Guideline of the American Thoracic Society and Infectious Diseases Society of America. Am J Respir Crit Care Med. 2019;200(7):e45-67.
3. Gupta D, Agarwal R, Aggarwal AN, Singh N, Mishra N, Khilnani GC, et al. Guidelines for diagnosis and management of community-and hospital-acquired pneumonia in adults: Joint ICS/NCCP(I) recommendations. Lung India. 2012;29(Suppl 2):S27-62.
4. Lim WS, Baudouin SV, George RC, Hill AT, Jamieson C, Le Jeune I, et al. BTS guidelines for the management of community acquired pneumonia in adults: update 2009. Thorax. 2009;64(Suppl 3):iii1-55.

CHAPTER

208

Tuberculosis: Epidemiology, Pathology, and Diagnosis

D Behera, Ranjan Kumar Behera

ABSTRACT

Tuberculosis is an ancient disease and is one of the common infectious diseases causing significant mortality in the world. Despite continuous measures to curtail the disease, nearly 10 million new cases were reported in the world in 2019. India still continues to be harboring the largest number of TB cases of the world. Although there is an increased trend in notifying the disease in recent years, such new case registration was reduced by 40% in 2020 due to COVID-19 pandemic in India.

M. tuberculosis is carried in droplet nuclei of 1–5 microns in diameter. Infectious droplet nuclei are generated when persons who have pulmonary or laryngeal TB disease cough, sneeze, shout, or sing. Depending on the environment, these tiny particles can remain suspended in the air for several hours. *M. tuberculosis* is transmitted through the air, not by surface contact. Transmission occurs when a person inhales droplet nuclei containing *M. tuberculosis*, and the droplet nuclei traverse the mouth or nasal passages, upper respiratory tract, and bronchi to reach the alveoli of the lungs. This necessitates airborne infection control measures.

Although sputum microscopy was the hallmark of diagnostic method of tuberculosis at the initial method, current availability of rapid molecular tests like Cartridge Based Nucleic Acid Amplification test (CBAAT) using either the Gene Xpert or TrueNat is the first diagnostic approach. This not only gives the species identification, but also gives information about the status of the rifampicin sensitivity or resistance helping the approach of universal drug sensitivity testing. Further, liquid culture methods using MGIT platform has eased the diagnostic approach shortening the duration of mycobacterial growth so that one gets the result early.

"Knowing is not enough; we must apply. Willing is not enough; we must do"

—Johann Wolfgang von Goethe

INTRODUCTION

Tuberculosis (TB) is an ancient infectious disease known to mankind for many centuries. It is caused by the bacillus *Mycobacterium tuberculosis*, discovered by Robert Koch in 1882. This communicable disease is a major cause of ill health with significant socioeconomic impact for the patient, family, the nation, and above all the world, and is one of the top 10 causes of death worldwide. It is the leading cause of death from a single infectious agent and ranks above human immunodeficiency virus/acquired immunodeficiency syndrome (HIV/AIDS). The disease is spread when people who are sick with TB expel bacteria into the air; for example, by coughing or sneezing. The disease typically affects the lungs (pulmonary TB) but can also affect other sites (extrapulmonary TB). About a quarter of the world's population is infected with *M. tuberculosis*.

Tuberculosis can affect anyone anywhere, but most people who develop the disease are adults, there are more cases among men than women, and 30 high TB burden countries account for almost 90% of those who fall sick with TB each year. TB is a disease of poverty, and economic distress, vulnerability, marginalization, stigma, and discrimination are often faced by the people affected by TB. TB is curable and preventable.

EPIDEMIOLOGY

GLOBAL SCENE

As per the global TB report 2020, an estimated 10.0 million (range, 8.9–11.0 million) people suffered from TB in 2019 in the world. This number is declining very slowly in recent years. An estimated, 1.2 million (range, 1.1–1.3 million) people died due to TB (among HIV-negative people) in 2019 which is a reduction from 1.7 million in 2000. An additional 208,000 deaths (range, 177,000–242,000) occurred among HIV-positive people (a reduction from 678,000 in 2000). The disease commonly affected men (aged ≥ 15 years) who accounted for 56% of the all cases in 2019 while women accounted for 32% and children (aged < 15 years) for 12%. Among all those affected, 8.2% were people living with HIV. The underdeveloped regions of the World Health Organization (WHO) had the highest burden of TB in 2019:

- Southeast Asia (44%)
- Africa (25%)
- Western Pacific (18%)
- Eastern Mediterranean (8.2%)
- Americas (2.9%)
- Europe (2.5%)

Two-thirds of the total global number of TB cases were reported from eight countries: (1) India (26%), (2) Indonesia (8.5%), (3) China (8.4%), (4) Philippines (6.0%), (5) Pakistan (5.7%), (6) Nigeria (4.4%), (7) Bangladesh (3.6%), and (8) South Africa (3.6%). The remaining 22 high-burden countries as listed by the WHO accounted for 21% of the global total. The distribution is shown in **Figure 1**.

The TB incidence rate (new cases in a year) at national level varies widely in the world. It is from less than five to more than 500 cases (new and relapse) per 100,000 populations per year. In 2019, low incidence of TB (<10 cases per 100,000 populations per year) was reported from 54 countries in 2019 and most of these countries were in the WHO Region of the Americas and European Region, with a few countries in the Eastern Mediterranean and Western Pacific regions.

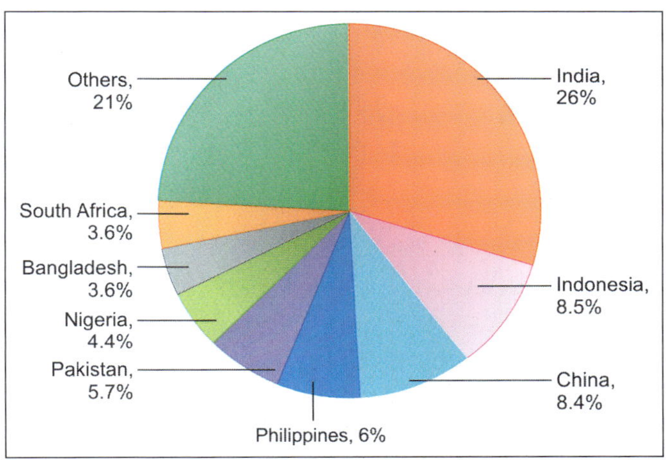

FIGURE 1: Distribution of tuberculosis (TB) in the 30 high-burden countries of the world in 2019.

In 2019, about a half-a-million people developed rifampicin-resistant TB (RR-TB) world over in 2019 out of which 78% had multidrug-resistant TB [MDR-TB, resistance to both rifampicin and isoniazid (INH)]. India (27%), China (14%), and the Russian Federation (8%) contributed the largest numbers to this pool. Nearly 3.3% of new TB cases and 17.7% of previously treated cases had MDR/RR-TB globally in 2019. The highest proportions (>50% in previously treated cases) were in countries of the former Soviet Union. Around 123 countries of the world have reported the presence of XDR-TB (extensive drug-resistant TB) in their population. The proportion of XDR-TB among MDR-TB patients is 6.2% worldwide

INDIAN SCENARIO

India has the highest number of TB cases in the world. It was estimated that the incidence of TB in India was 26.9 lakh cases in 2019 (WHO). A record high notification of 24 lakh cases was made in 2019; an increase of over 12% as compared to 2018. Of the 24 lakh TB cases, 90% (*N* = 21.6 lakhs) were incident TB cases (new and relapse/recurrent). This translates to an incident notification rate of approximately 159 cases/lakh against the estimated incidence rate of 199 cases/lakh population; thus, closing the gap between the estimated and notified incident cases to just 40 cases per lakh population, or an approximate of 5.4 lakh missing cases across India. The estimated and case notification over the past three years is depicted in **Figure 2**.

Case notification in India in the year 2020 was reduced by 40% due to coronavirus disease-2019 (COVID-19) pandemic. Overall, the age distribution of TB diagnosed incident cases shows a predominance in the adolescent and young adult age groups between 15 and 30, indicating ongoing disease transmission. However, there is a wide variation in the age distribution patterns among the states. In southern states of Kerala, Karnataka, Tamil Nadu, Andhra Pradesh along with the UTs of Puducherry, Lakshadweep, and Andaman and Nicobar, there is a general elderly prevalence of TB toward the age 50-year ranges. However, in most of the other states, the incidence is similar to that of the country with predominance in the 15–30-year groups. This indicates the need to further optimize program performance and the need to push novel interventions to accelerate progress toward TB elimination in those states.

India and WHO carried out the first National Anti-TB Drug Resistance Survey (NDRS) during 2014–1916. The survey carried out drug susceptibility testing (DST) for 13 anti-TB drugs using the automated liquid culture system (the mycobacteria growth indicator tube, MGIT 960). The main findings were—MDR-TB in 6.19% of cases (2.84% among new and 11.60% among previously treated TB patients). Additional resistance to any fluoroquinolones was observed in 21.82%, and 3.58% of cases to any second-line injectable drugs amongst all MDR-TB cases. XDR-TB was present in 1.3% of cases. During 2007–2018, India tested 2,798,599 patients using cartridge-based nucleic amplification test (CBNAAT) and line probe assays (LPAs). These tests detected 236,725 drug-resistant TB patients. In 2019, the program notified a total of 66,359 MDR/RR-TB cases and 56,500 (85%) of them put on treatment, which is an improvement of 7.6% over last year as reported by the India TB Report, 2020.

The TB estimated in India in the year 2019 is shown in **Table 1**.

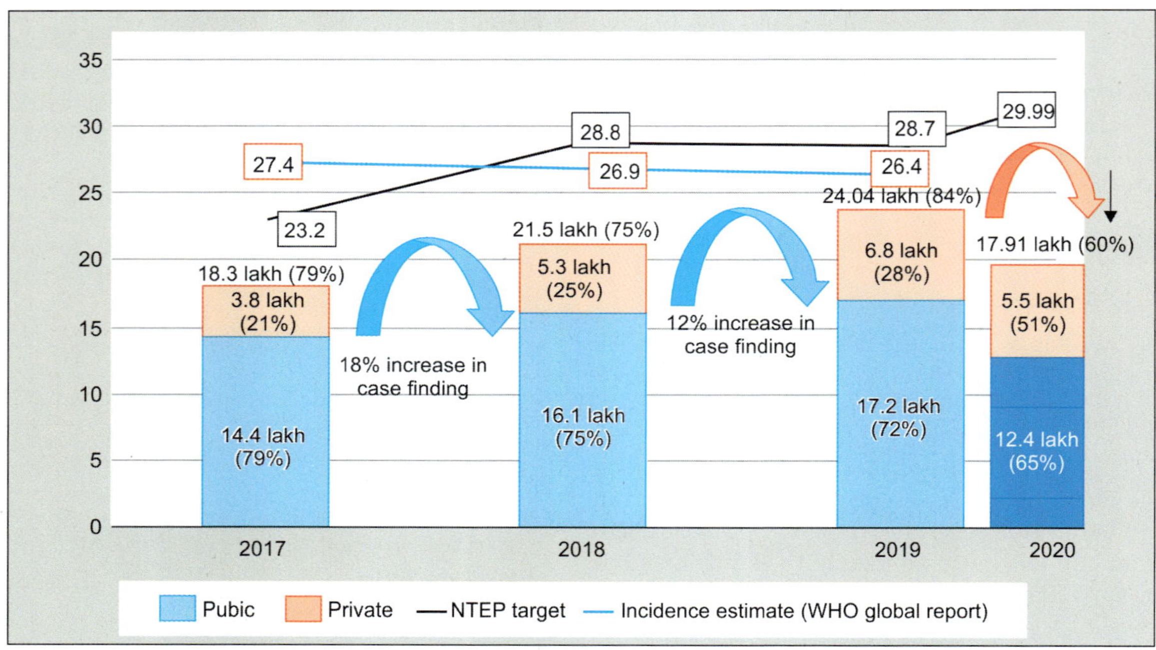

FIGURE 2: Tuberculosis (TB) estimates, total TB cases notification (from public and private sectors) from 2017 to 2020 by the NTEP (National TB Elimination Program).

Source: India TB report and global TB report 2018, 2019, 2020. Values in lakhs.

TABLE 1 TB estimates in India in 2019.

Estimates of TB burden (2019)	Rate	Numbers	Global position (rates)	% Global burden
Incidence of TB	193/lakh population	26.4 Lakh	39th	27%
Mortality of TB (including TB-HIV)	33/lakh population	4.45 lakh	35th	32%
Multidrug-resistant TB	9.1/lakh population	1.24 lakh	35th	27%
Incidence of TB-HIV	5.2/lakh population	71,000	59th	9%

PATHOPHYSIOLOGY

Mycobacterium tuberculosis is carried in airborne particles, called droplet nuclei of 1–5 microns in diameter. Infectious droplet nuclei are generated when persons who have pulmonary or laryngeal TB disease cough, sneeze, shout, or sing. Depending on the environment, these tiny particles can remain suspended in the air for several hours. *M. tuberculosis* is transmitted through the air, *not* by surface contact.

TRANSMISSION

Transmission occurs when a person inhales droplet nuclei containing *M. tuberculosis*, and the droplet nuclei traverse the mouth or nasal passages, upper respiratory tract, and bronchi to reach the alveoli of the lungs. The infectious dose of *M. tuberculosis* is very low, usually 1–5 tubercle bacilli. After inhalation of a droplet nucleus, it passes down the bronchial tree without settling on the respiratory epithelium and implants in a respiratory bronchiole or alveolus beyond the mucociliary system. Here the bacilli may multiply with no initial resistance from the host.

The first implant can occur anywhere in the lungs. However, the cavitary lesion characteristic of the tuberculous disease is often located in the apical regions in the lung. Even, if the primary implant can occur anywhere in the lungs, for the progression from infection to disease, the tubercle bacilli must gain access to the vulnerable regions in the apex of the lungs. Specific immunity is usually adequate to limit further multiplication of the bacilli. The host remains symptomatic, and the lesions heal. Overall, in approximately 5% of all infected persons, control of the dividing organisms is inadequate, and disease occurs within 1 year of infection. In another 5%, containment of the organism fails at a time much more after the acquisition of infection, and disease results. Thus, overall, 10% of persons infected with *M. tuberculosis* will develop clinical TB sometimes during their lives. This figure of course will vary in different countries.

A possible timetable of development of TB in various organs after the first infections is shown in **Table 2**.

TABLE 2 Timetable of tuberculosis after primary infection.

Type of tuberculosis	Time after infection	Comments
Miliary tuberculosis and tuberculous meningitis	Within 6 months	• Common in children under the age of 5 years • Meningitis may be a terminal event in the cryptic miliary disease in elderly
Pleural effusion	6–12 months	Common in young adults
Progressive primary or postprimary disease	1–2 years	• Common at puberty • The primary disease can progress with increasing infiltration and cavitation
Skeletal tuberculosis	1–5 years	Common in spines
Genitourinary and cutaneous tuberculosis	5–15 years	

PRIMARY INFECTION

When infection with *M. tuberculosis* occurs in a person who has had no previous exposure to tubercle bacillus, it is referred to as a "primary infection "or primary disease. The usual route of invasion is by the lungs. The bacilli will be deposited in the alveoli and a small patch of caseous bronchopneumonia develops. This encapsulates later. This is the *"primary focus" or "Ghon focus."* The regional lymph node is soon involved and together they are called the *"primary complex" (parenchymal lesion + lymph node)*. The bacilli reach the lymph node within less than one hour of reaching the lung and often the blood. Attraction of neutrophils and macrophages to the site of infection leads on to the cascade of events. The primary infection can develop at any lung zone, but is common in the lower part of the upper lobe or in the upper part of the lower lobe, chiefly in the right upper lobe. It is seldom found in the apex. The lesion is usually situated nearer to the pleura. The lymph glands beyond the regional nodes first affected, may become involved by lymphatic spread both upward toward the neck and downward to the abdomen. It is hypothesized that the first implant can occur anywhere in the lung, and the cavitary lesion is often located in the apical region of the lungs.

The primary foci may follow one of the following consequences—(1) most primary foci become quiescent and calcify; (2) some of the calcified foci, especially those in the lymph nodes may recrudesce at a later age and become the source of progressive pulmonary/extrapulmonary TB; and (3) a primary lesion may also, soon after formation, becomes the center of progressive disease either by liquefaction and subsequent eruption into the (1) bronchi, (2) vessels, or (3) by transmission of bacilli to the hilar nodes and then to the blood stream.

The fate of a primary focus can thus be summarized as—the early development of primary focus starts with the multiplication of bacilli during the first few days and some migration of leukocytes occurs to the alveoli. Epithelioid cell formation appears as the first recognizable, characteristic *tubercular lesion called "tubercle" 6–8 days after inhalation.* The epithelioid cells are macrophages, which develop pale foamy cytoplasms rich in lipid and crowd together. Some mononuclear cells fuse to form the multinucleated or Langhans giant cells. The center of the lesion liquefies causing caseation necrosis, the characteristic of a tubercular granuloma. The small foci enlarge and undergo caseation necrosis. This becomes arrested soon and a capsule is formed in the collapsed tissue around the focus, which mainly consists of fibrous tissue. 3–6 weeks after inhalation, the primary focus is fully developed and sometimes calcified in the center. After lymphocytic demarcation of the central caseous area, recrudescence may cause further fresh caseation outside the ring of lymphocytes. The calcified lesions may contain acid-fast bacilli (AFB) on histological section.

REACTIVATED OR POSTPRIMARY TUBERCULOSIS

The primary infection is usually contained. But potential for reactivation of infection, however, is always present. The primary lesion sometimes progresses and the pathological changes will then be similar to those seen in reactivation TB. The main difference between the primary infection and reactivation is that, while in the former involvement of the regional lymph node is an essential component of the pathology, in the later regional lymph node is not necessarily involved. Due to an early bacteremia following the formation of a primary lesion in the hilar glands, the bacilli are carried by the lymphatics to the right heart and thence again into the lungs. *These foci are called "Simon foci." Thus these are essentially postprimary lesions* commonly seen both radiologically and at necropsy in chronic disseminated and extrapulmonary TB. They also occur in a large number of primarily infected individuals as accidental findings. In case of primary intestinal TB, small calcified nodules may sometimes be seen in liver, which originates in a direct hematogenous transmission of the bacilli to the liver from the intestine via the portal vein.

Reactivated pulmonary TB is most often seen in the upper lung zones and is limited in extent most frequently to the posterior segment of the upper lobe or apex of the lower lobe. The high alveolar PO_2 in the upper zones relative to the other lung zones due to high ventilation-perfusion ratios is believed to predispose to reactivation at these sites. Softening and liquefaction of the caseous material, which may discharge, into a bronchus with resultant cavity formation, follow proliferation of tubercle bacilli in the caseous center. Hemorrhages may result from extension of the caseous process into vessels within the cavity walls. Spread of caseous and liquefied material through the bronchial tree may disseminate the infection to other lung zones with or without the development of a vigorous inflammatory exudates or tuberculous pneumonia. Sometimes this type of reaction is due to a hypersensitivity reaction to tubercular protein released by the dead bacilli, and is called "epituberculosis."

Rupture of a caseous pulmonary focus into a blood vessel may result in miliary TB with the formation of multiple 0.5–2 mm tuberculous foci in the lung and in other organs of the body. Encroachment on bronchi of pulmonary or lymph node caseous material may give rise to tuberculous bronchitis. Rupture of caseous glands into trachea or major bronchi causes collapse of lung or even sudden death by suffocation particularly in young children. Vasculitis secondary to TB affecting the affected vessels like pulmonary or cerebral is not an uncommon finding. *On the basis of a large autopsy study of cases of pulmonary TB, the lesions are divided into four main types:*

1. *Nodular type*—small and large
2. *Fibrocaseous type*:
   i. With cavity
   ii. Without cavity
3. *Miliary lesions*
4. *Mixed nodular and fibrocaseous*

DIAGNOSIS

Diagnosis of TB is a constellation of clinical features, radiological changes, and laboratory tests. The definite diagnostic test for TB is the demonstration of *M. tuberculosis*. However, isolation of mycobacteria is possible only in about 60–70% of cases. Although smear positivity is quite specific (see below), such positivity is only seen in up to 50% of cases. Therefore, a number of tests have been used in the diagnosis of TB (**Flowcharts 1** and **2**).

Various diagnostic tests used for diagnosing TB can be classified as:

- Tests used for diagnosing latent TB infection (LTBI)
- Tests used to diagnose active TB disease (drug sensitive/resistant strains)

Various tests used to diagnose LTBI include:

- Tuberculin skin test (TST)
- Interferon-γ release assays (IGRAs)

LATENT TB INFECTION

Tuberculin skin test: The standard 5 tuberculin unit (5TU) dose of purified protein derivative standard (PPD-S) is defined as the delayed skin test activity contained in a 0.1 mg/0.1 mL (1 in 10,000 dilutions) dose of PPD-S. The standard test dose of a commercial PPD preparation is defined as the dose of the product that is biologically equivalent to that contained in 5TU of PPD-S (i.e. it elicits reactions of equivalent size ± 20%). Products labeled 1TU and 250TU do not necessarily contain one-fifth and 50 times the biologic activity of 5TU PPD-S. Instead, these preparations contain one-fifth and 50 times the concentration of antigen determined to be bioequivalent to 5TU PPD-S. Evaluation

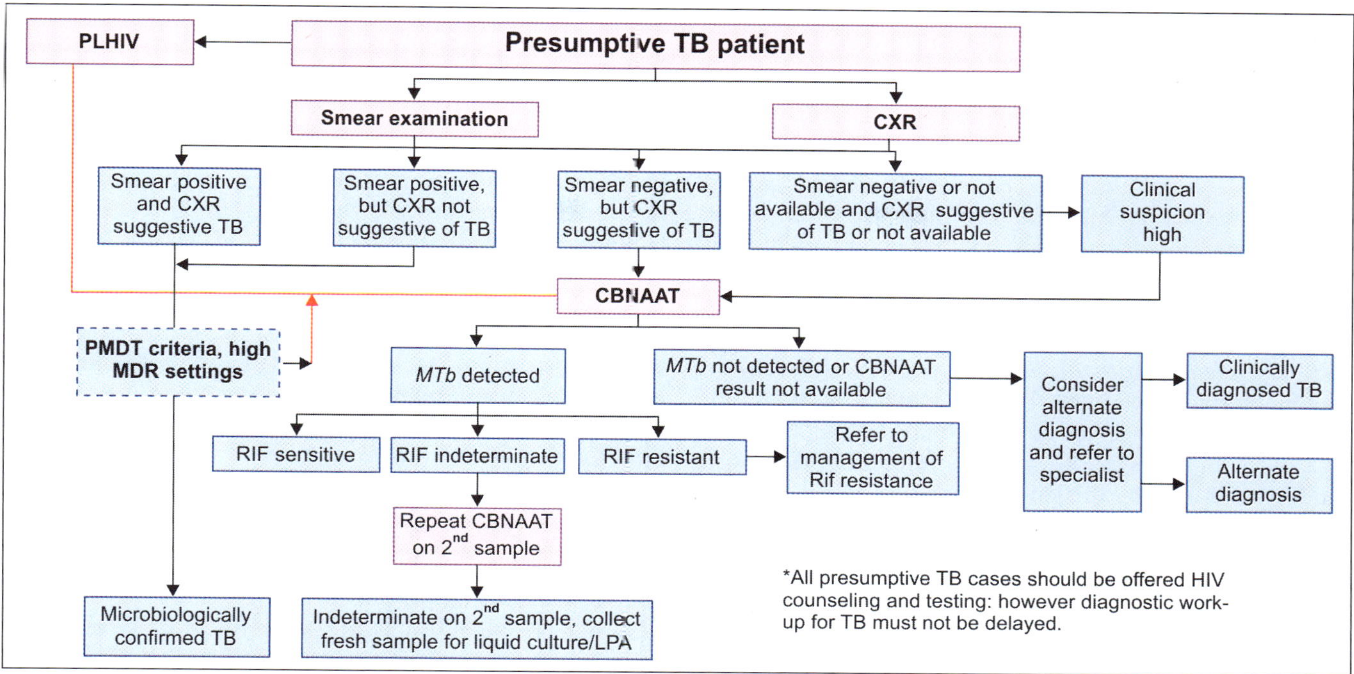

(CBNAAT: cartridge-based nucleic amplification test; CXR: chest X-ray; LPA: line probe assay; *MTb*: *Mycobacterium tuberculosis*; MDR: multidrug-resistant; PLHIV: people living with HIV)

FLOWCHART 1: Diagnostic algorithm for pulmonary tuberculosis.

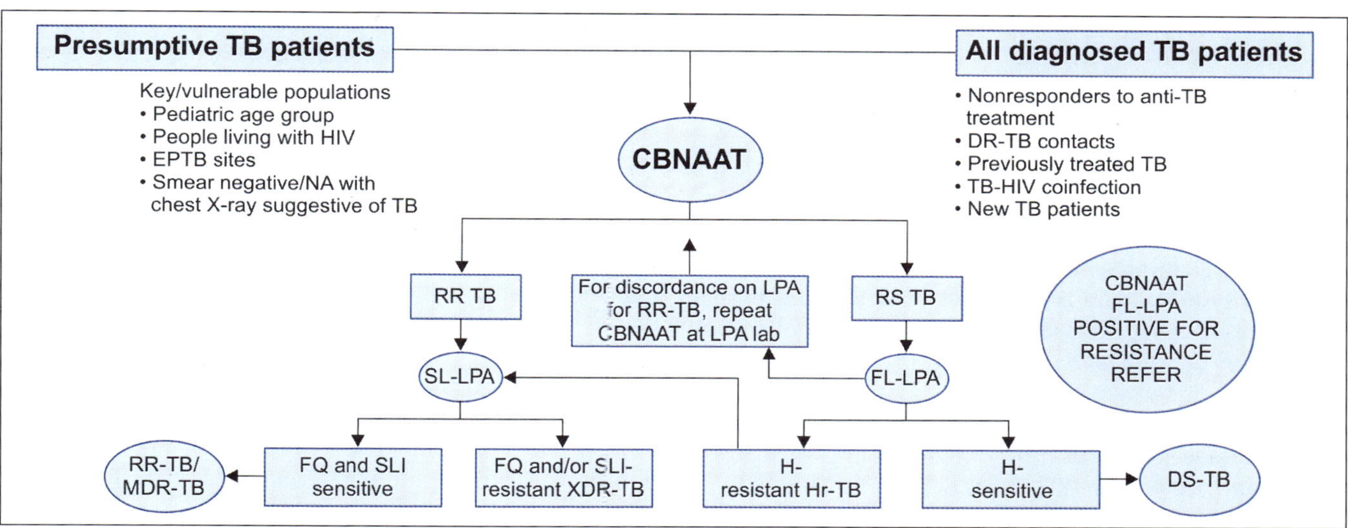

(CBNAAT: cartridge-based nucleic amplification test; DR: drug resistant; FQ: fluoroquinolone; MDR: multidrug-resistant; RR: rifampicin-resistant; SL-LPA: second line–line probe assay; SLI: second-line injectable; TB: tuberculosis; XDR: extensive drug-resistant)

FLOWCHART 2: DR-TB diagnostic algorithm.

of the biologic activity of 1TU and 250TU products has not been required. The 250TU products are sometimes useful in assessing the immunologic status of patients. Both the 1TU and 250TU products have limited usefulness in the diagnosis of TB infection.

Reactions to tuberculin begin at 5–6 hours, are maximal at 48–72 hours, and subside over a period of days. In a few persons (those who are elderly or those who are being tested for the first time), reactions may develop slowly and may not peak until after 72 hours. Immediate hypersensitivity reactions to tuberculin or constituents of the diluents can also occur. These reactions begin shortly after injection, disappear by 24 hours, and are not likely to be confused with delayed hypersensitivity reactions.

The interpretation should be done as follows depending on the diameter of the induration:

Negative	Positive	Strongly positive
0–5 mm	6–14 mm	+15 mm

Interferon-gamma release assays (IGRA): Diagnoses of both TB infection and disease still remain problematic, especially among children and the immunocompromised. Immunologic tests have contributed remarkably in the diagnosis of many viral infections, even when there is difficulty in isolating the causative organism. For TB, the situation is much more complex. The human body relies mainly on cellular immune response to defend against the tubercle bacillus/humoral responses are variable and inconsistent, and no serologic test has been conclusively found to be useful for the diagnosis of either TB infection or disease. The TST has been the golden test for diagnosis of LTBI for many years. However, as TST is cross-reactive to *BCG (Bacille Calmette-Guérin)* and nontuberculous mycobacteria, a relatively high specificity is attainable often at the expense of sensitivity, which is also suboptimal regardless of the cut-off value among infants, young children, the elderly, the severely malnourished, and the immunocompromised.

Principles of IGRAs rely on the understanding of advances in immunology and genomics and *M. tuberculosis* genome. A number of relatively specific antigens have been discovered in the pathogenic *M. tuberculosis* complex:

- The early secretory antigen target 6 (ESAT-6)
- Culture filtrate protein 10 (CFP-10)
- TB7.7

These are encoded by genes located in the region of difference (RD-1) of the bacillary genome. They are absent in all BCG strains and most environmental mycobacteria (with the exception of *M. szulgai, M. marinum, M. flavescens,* and *M. kansasii*).

These IGRA are *in vitro* T-cell-based assay tests for diagnosis of LTBI:

- QuantiFERON-TB Gold (QFT-G)
- QuantiFERON-TB Gold in-Tube (QFT-G-IT) (Cellestis Limited, Carnegie, Victoria, Australia)
- T-SPOT.TB test (Oxford Immunotec, Oxford, UK)

QuantiFERON-Gold is new class of *in vitro* assay that measures interferon release by sensitized T-cells after stimulation by *M. tuberculosis* antigens. It measures the immune reactivity to the organism.

QuantiFERON-TB Gold-in-tube assay is a whole blood enzyme-linked immunosorbent assay (ELISA) measuring interferon-γ production (ESAT-6, CFP-10, and TB7.7).

The T-SPOT.TB test is an enzyme-linked immunospot (ELISPOT) assay of peripheral blood mononuclear cells (PBMC) to detect the number of interferon-γ-producing T-cells (ESAT-6 and CFP-10). IGRAs include both internal positive and negative controls. It is presumed that these tests are more sensitive in HIV cases and more specific than tuberculin test and in infections with NTM. However, there is limited data on these two IGRAs in high-burden settings in children, in HIV-positive persons to differentiate between infection and disease.

WHO guidelines: The 2018 WHO guidelines recommend that either a TST or IGRA can be used to test for LTBI. There is no strong evidence that one test should be preferred over the other to predict progression to active TB disease. The choice will depend on test availability, cost and the health infrastructure. However, neither the TST nor IGRA can be used to diagnose active TB disease nor for the diagnostic workup of adults suspected of having active TB. LTBI testing by TST or IGRA is not a requirement for initiating preventive treatment in people living with HIV or children aged < 5 years who are household contacts with a pulmonary TB patient. The evidence reviewed and the recommendations in the 2018 consolidated guidelines apply to the use of QuantiFERON®-TB Gold In-Tube and T-SPOT®.TB only. Any new or generic test should be subjected to proper validation according to WHO guidelines. It is further emphasized that either TST or IGRAs can be used to identify candidates to LTBI treatment in high- and upper-middle-income countries with estimated TB incidence less than 100 per 100,000. IGRAs should not replace TST in low and other middle-income countries.

ACTIVE TB DISEASE

Diagnosis of TB of can be divided into *direct methods* and *indirect methods*. Direct methods include the detection of either the bacilli or their DNA and indirect methods include tests like demonstration of antigens, antibodies, or other biological products in various specimens.

Histologic examination of diseased tissue like biopsy or fine needle aspiration cytology biopsy specimens like lymph node, pleura, transbronchial biopsy specimen of lung tissue etc., which reveal characteristic granulomatous lesions with necrosis are fairly specific of TB even if the bacilli are not demonstrated in the specimen.

Direct sputum smear microscopy is the easiest and cheapest method of diagnosing pulmonary TB. Because the identification of organism is critical to get a confirmed diagnosis of TB, it is important that careful attention be given to the collection and handling of specimens. Success in isolating mycobacteria from clinical materials depends on the manner in which specimens are handled after their collection.

A series of at least two to three single specimens on different days should be collected from sputum-producing patients [the recent Revised National Tuberculosis Control Program (RNTCP) guidelines require two samples]. The Ziehl–Neelsen method is usually used to detect AFB in the smear (**Fig. 3**).

With the adaptability of universal DST approach of the national program, the sputum smear is no more the preferred test (it is CBNAAT now). The smear is used only for following up the TB cases.

Fluorescent light-emitting diode microscopy: Light-emitting diodes (LED) have been developed to offer the benefits of fluorescence microscopy without the associated costs. The accuracy of LED microscopy is equivalent to that of international reference standards, it is also more sensitive than conventional Ziehl–Neelsen microscopy and it had qualitative, operational, and cost advantages over both conventional fluorescence and Ziehl–Neelsen microscopy. LED microscopy was statistically significantly more sensitive by 6% (95% CI 0.1–13%), with no appreciable

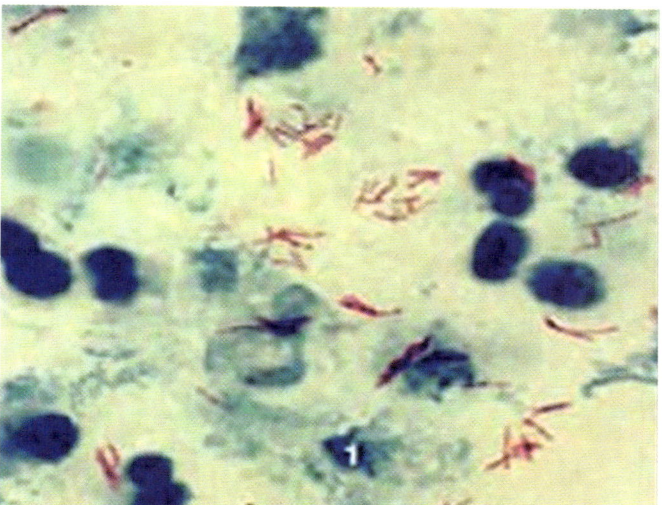

FIGURE 3: **Ziehl–Neelsen staining method showing AFB.**

loss in specificity, when compared with direct Ziehl-Neelsen microscopy.

Culture of mycobacteria: The culture is much more sensitive than microscopy, being able to detect as few as 10 bacteria/mL of digested, concentrated material. Moreover, culture provides precise species identification. Sensitivity of sputum culture is approximately 81% in pulmonary TB, with a higher sensitivity of 96% in cavitary form of the disease. False-positive cultures are mainly because of laboratory contaminations; nevertheless, the specificity of culture positivity is as high as 98.5%.

Numerous culture media are available. However, most of them fall under two general categories:

1. Egg-potato-based media
2. Agar-based media

The most popular egg-based media are the Lowenstein-Jensen (LJ) buffered egg-potato medium and American Trudeau Society egg yolk-potato flour medium. Among the *agar-based media*, Middlebrook 7H10, Middlebrook 7H11, and Dubos oleic-albumin agar are important. Incubation of inoculated media in an atmosphere of 5–10% carbon dioxide enhances both the number of positive isolations and the actual number of cultivable colonies.

The culture media can also be divided into solid and liquid media. Various solid media are LJ medium, LJ with Na pyruvate, LJ without asparagine, Synthetic Middlebrook 7H10, 7H11 oleic acid albumin agar, selective 7H10 medium, Tarshi's fresh blood agar medium, and Ogawa medium. Liquid media are usually used in the cultivation of mycobacteria when the specimens contain very small number of bacilli since positive cultures could be more often obtained in these media with a larger inoculum. These liquid media include Kirchner-Herman medium, Dubos medium, Sula's medium, Youman and Karlson's medium, Proskauer and Beck medium, and 7H9 synthetic medium.

Although a number of molecular diagnostic methods have been shown to have the potential to provide direct detection of *M. tuberculosis* complex from clinical specimens within a few hours, culture still represents the cornerstone on which a definitive diagnosis of TB and other mycobacterioses relies in addition to have information on drug susceptibility. In recent years, rapid, reliable methods for culture detection of AFB have been developed that are regarded as of absolute priority. Currently, mycobacterial culture can be performed with conventional solid media and by one of the available broth-based methods. Of these, the radiometric semiautomated BACTEC 460TB system (Becton Dickinson, Sparks, Md.) was the first system to permit the significantly earlier detection of mycobacteria that was once considered as the "gold standard." However, as it had several drawbacks, like the use of radioactive material, and reading of cultures was labor-intensive and is associated with a potential risk of cross-contamination. Furthermore, the use of needles for inoculation of the vial involves the risk of stick injury.

In recent years, several new *nonradiometric technologies for growth and detection of AFB* have been introduced; among these, the fluorimetric MGIT (Becton Dickinson) and the MB-Redox system (Biotest, Dreieich, Germany) are manual, while the ESP Culture System II (AccuMed, Chicago, Ill.), the MB/BacT system (Organon Teknica, Turnhout, Belgium), the BACTEC 9000 MB system (Becton Dickinson), as well as the BACTEC MGIT 960 system (Becton Dickinson) are fully automated, continuously monitoring, walk-away systems.

The BACTEC MGIT 960 system is a noninvasive, nonradiometric system that uses the same technology used by manual MGIT and the BACTEC 9000 MB system and uses a liquid media. A ruthenium pentahydrate oxygen sensor embedded in silicon at the bottom of a tube containing 8 mL of modified Middlebrook 7H9 broth fluoresces following the oxygen reduction induced by aerobically metabolizing bacteria within the medium. A compact instrument incubates and tests, according to on-board algorithms, up to 960 culture tubes.

This is more useful in detecting the drug-resistant cases particularly MDR- and XDR-TB.

While culture on the egg-based solid media, known as LJ medium, may take as long as 4–6 weeks, *liquid culture systems [BACTEC and MGIT (Becton Dickinson)]* offer a more sensitive and rapid alternative to conventional solid culture and may detect growth in 1–3 weeks. The mycobacterial growth indicator tube or MGIT contains a fluorescent compound at the bottom of the tube which is quenched by oxygen. As *Mycobacterium tuberculosis (MTB)* grows, the oxygen in the tube is used and the fluorescent compound is detected. Potentially, the MGIT technology can yield results in <8 days. Automated MGIT allows for drug susceptibility through the addition of critical concentrations of streptomycin, INH, rifampin, and ethambutol.

Rapid methods of detection: As many national programs have adopted the UDST (Universal DST) approach, *CBNAATs* are the first-line tests instead of smear microscopy. *GeneXpert and TrueNat* are the currently available tests those confirm the presence of *M. tuberculosis* and inform about the rifampicin-sensitivity pattern. Various other molecular tests are depicted in **Table 3**.

TABLE 3 WHO-endorsed molecular tests for pulmonary TB detection and drug susceptibility testing.

Technology	Method/ Principle	Usefulness	Sensitivity (%)	Specificity (%)	Turnaround time (hours)	Amenable to rapid test-and-treat?
Xpert MTB/RIF	qPCR	• MTB diagnosis and • RIF resistance detection	85 (pooled), 96 (RIF resistance)	• 99 (MTB detection) • 98 (RIF resistance)	<2	Yes, especially on Omni platform
Xpert MTB/RIF ultra	qPCR/melting temperature analysis (RIF resistance)	MTB diagnosis and RIF resistance detection	90 (pooled), 94 (RIF resistance)	• 96 (MTB detection) • 98 (RIF resistance)	<2	Yes, especially on Omni platform
First-line probe assays (e.g., GenoType MTBDRplus and NIPRO	PCR, hybridization	Diagnosis of RIF and INH resistance	• 98 (RIF resistance) • 84 (INH resistance)	• 99 (RIF resistance) • >99 (INH resistance)	<5	No
Second-line probe assays (e.g., GenoType MTBDRsl)	PCR, hybridization	Diagnosis of FLQ and SLID resistance	• 86 (FLQ resistance) • 87 (SLID resistance)	• 99 (FLQ resistance) • 99 (SLID resistance)	<5	
Loopamp MTBC assay	Loop-mediated isothermal amplification	MTB diagnosis	78 (pooled)	98 (MTB detection)	<2	No
Truenat MTB plus	Micro RT-PCR	MTB diagnosis	80 (pooled)	96 (MTB detection)	<2	Yes, on Truelab platform
Truenat MTB-RIF Dx	Micro RT-PCR	Diagnosis of RIF resistance	84 (RIF resistance)	97 (RIF resistance)	<2	Yes, on Truelab platform

(FLQ: fluoroquinolone; SLID: second-line injectable drugs; SSM+/C–: sputum smear microscopy positive/culture negative)

RECOMMENDED READINGS

1. WHO. (2020). Global Tuberculosis Report 2020. [online] Available from who.int/teams/global-tuberculosis-programme/tb-reports/global-tuberculosis-report-2020.
2. Central TB Division Ministry of Health and Family Welfare, Nirman Bhawan, New Delhi. (2020). India TB Report 2020, National Tuberculosis Elimination Program, Annual Report. [online] Available from www.tbcindia.gov.in
3. MacLean E, Kohli M, Weber SF, Suresh A, Schumacher SG, Denkinger CM, et al. Advances in molecular diagnosis of tuberculosis. J Clin Microbiol. 2020;58:e01582-19.
4. Hunter RL. The pathogenesis of tuberculosis: The early infiltrate of post-primary (adult pulmonary) tuberculosis: A distinct disease entity. Front Immunol. 2018;9:2108.
5. Behera D. Chapter 11: Tuberculosis. Text Book of Pulmonary Medicine, Vol I, Second Edition. New Delhi: Jaypee Brothers Medical Publishers; 2010. pp. 455-787.

CHAPTER
209
Management of Pulmonary Tuberculosis

Deepak Aggarwal

ABSTRACT

Management of pulmonary tuberculosis (PTB) has seen major changes in terms of diagnostics and treatment in the last five decades. Introduction of rapid molecular assays like line probe assay (LPA) and nucleic acid amplification test (NAAT) has not only enhanced the sensitivity of microbiological diagnosis but also improved the treatment protocols by facilitating use of drug susceptibility test-guided treatment in place of old conventional regimens. The treatment of drug-sensitive tuberculosis (DS-TB) has remained unchanged over the last 35 years with a 6-month short course therapy containing four first-line anti-TB drugs. However, evidence-based use of new drugs bedaquiline (Bdq) and delamanid in recently approved all oral regimens as well as introduction of shorter multidrug-resistant (MDR) TB regimen has been a paradigm shift in the drug-resistant TB (DR-TB) management. These developments will take a couple of years before their impact on TB control/elimination becomes evident.

"The easiest way to do anything is properly"

—KJ Parker

INTRODUCTION

Tuberculosis is one of the oldest infectious diseases known to mankind. It is caused by the bacillus *Mycobacterium tuberculosis* (MTB) that usually spreads by airborne route. Lungs are the most common site of disease, though the infection can virtually involve any part of the human body. TB is ranked among the top 10 causes of death worldwide and is the leading cause of mortality from a single infectious agent. As per the Global TB report 2020, an estimated 10.0 million (range, 8.9–11.0 million) people got TB and half-a-million developed rifampicin-resistant (RR) TB in 2019. Currently, India accounts for 26% of the global burden of TB and has estimated total TB incidence of 193/100,000 population.

Management of pulmonary tuberculosis (PTB) has seen sea changes over the last half-a-century. Important changes include institution of short course chemotherapy, domiciliary treatment, intermittent therapy before the year 2000 to introduction of molecular diagnostic tests, daily DOTS, newer anti-TB drugs, and all oral regimens for DR-TB after 2000. With these new advances, the focus of program managers has also changed from TB control to TB elimination. Under National TB Elimination Program (previously Revised National Tuberculosis Control Program), Government of India has committed to end TB by 2025, 5 years ahead of the global target under Sustainable Development Goals (SDG). To achieve the targets, the Government has rolled out National Strategic Plan (NSP) 2017–2025 that has set out the strategic directions and key initiatives for all stakeholders driven by "DETECT–TREAT–PREVENT–BUILD" approach. The present chapter describes the current approach to management of PTB based on the World Health Organization (WHO) recommendations and National Tuberculosis Elimination Program (NTEP) guidelines.

DIAGNOSIS

Timely and accurate diagnosis is the cornerstone to successful management of PTB. Pulmonary TB usually presents with subacute to chronic onset of cough, fever, and weight loss. Early identification of people with suggestive clinical features (presumptive TB) is the most important and, often the time-limiting step in TB diagnosis. Under NTEP, presumptive pulmonary TB is defined by presence of any of the symptoms and signs suggestive of TB including cough > 2 weeks, fever > 2 weeks, significant weight loss, hemoptysis, any abnormality on chest X-ray. The suspicion for TB should be high in patients with immunocompromised status like diabetes, HIV, cancer, and patients on immunosuppressants or steroids who may present with minimal or atypical symptoms.

DIAGNOSTIC TOOLS

All patients with TB suspicion are subjected to microbiological tests and imaging for the confirmation of the diagnosis. **Table 1** enlists important microbiological tests and their roles in the management of PTB. Demonstration of the acid-fast bacilli (AFB) or its nucleic acid in sputum has remained the standard method for TB diagnosis. Apart from sputum, lower respiratory samples like bronchoalveolar lavage can also be used for evaluation, particularly in patients with negative sputum result but high index of suspicion.

Smear microscopy: Since the last century, demonstration of bacteria on sputum microscopy has remained the most

TABLE 1 Different microbiological tests for the diagnosis of pulmonary tuberculosis.

Investigation	Types	Recommended roles
1. Smear microscopy	• Ziehl-Neelsen staining • Fluorescence staining	Diagnosis and monitoring, defining cure
2. Culture	• Solid (Lowenstein-Jensen) media • Automated liquid culture systems, e.g., MGIT 960	Diagnosis, monitoring, DST, and defining cure
3. Rapid molecular diagnostic testing	• Line probe assay for MTB complex and detection of RIF and INH resistance • Nucleic acid amplification test (NAAT)	Diagnosis and DST

(DST: drug-susceptibility testing; MTB: *Mycobacterium tuberculosis*)

TABLE 2 Features of line probe assay and nucleic acid amplification test.

Parameter	Line probe assay (LPA)	Nucleic acid amplification test (NAAT)
1. Principle	Involves reverse hybridization of PCR-amplified DNA products on nitrocellulose strips containing probes specific for detection of MTB and mutations	Involves isolation of DNA by sonication and subsequent amplification by PCR. Clinically relevant, rifampicin resistance inducing mutations in the RNA polymerase beta (rpoB) gene is detected in the MTB genome in a real-time format using fluorescent probes called molecular beacons
2. Samples that can be tested	Sputum and positive culture isolates	Pulmonary and extrapulmonary samples and tissue
3. Turnaround time	72 hours	2 hours
4. Detects MTB DNA sequence	Yes	Yes
5. Resistance coding genes that are detected currently	• Rifampicin (rpoB) • Isoniazid (katG, inhA), • Fluoroquinolone class resistance (gyrA, gyrB) • Second-line injectable class resistance (rrs, eis)	• Rifampicin (rpoB)

(DNA: deoxyribonucleic acid; MTB: *Mycobacterium tuberculosis;* RNA: ribonucleic acid)

widely used and acceptable testing tool for PTB diagnosis. Besides diagnosis, it can be used for monitoring and defining cure in PTB patients (**Table 1**). Being a simple and inexpensive test with high reliability and specificity, it is suitable for use in peripheral health institutions under programmatic conditions. However, visualizing bacteria in smears requires the presence of 5–10 thousand AFB per mL of the sputum. Hence, it can miss patients in the initial phase of disease when the bacillary load is low as well as certain patient populations like children and patients living with human immunodeficiency virus (HIV) (PLHIV).

Culture: Culture of biological specimen is considered the gold standard test for the diagnosis of TB. It has high sensitivity and can grow AFB from the sputum sample containing as low as 100 bacilli/mL. In addition, it also permits identification of mycobacterial species as well as performing drug-susceptibility testing (DST) on culture isolate (phenotypic DST). However, due to long turnaround time, it is not suitable for routine use in high-burden countries like India. The most common culture method endorsed by WHO and adopted by NTEP is liquid culture (LC) using Middlebrook 7H9 broth—the Mycobacterial Growth Indicator Tube (MGIT). It gives faster results than on solid media with a turnaround time of 42 days.

Rapid molecular assays: Rapid molecular assays are polymerase chain reaction (PCR)-based technologies with various modifications that detect not only DNA sequences specific for MTB complex but also presence of putative resistance genes to different anti-tubercular drugs (genotypic DST). Line probe assay (LPA) and nucleic acid amplification test (NAAT) are the two rapid molecular assays recommended for use under the program. **Table 2** enlists salient differentiating features of LPA and NAAT.

DIAGNOSTIC ALGORITHM

Diagnosis of PTB involves two steps: (1) confirmation of the diagnosis, and (2) evaluation for drug resistance. Those patients who are smear negative are subjected to NAAT. Flowchart 1 in Chapter 208 (taken from NTEP training module) shows sequential steps required for the confirmation of PTB. Accordingly, two types of TB cases are identified.

1. **Microbiologically confirmed TB:** Presumptive TB patient with biological specimen positive for AFB (smear or culture) or positive for TB through quality assured rapid diagnostic molecular test.
2. **Clinically diagnosed TB:** A presumptive TB patient who is not microbiologically confirmed, but diagnosed

with active TB on the basis of X-ray, histopathology, or clinical signs with a decision to treat the patient with a full course of anti-TB treatment (ATT).

TREATMENT

Domiciliary administration of a DST-/non-DST-guided multiple-drug regimen under direct observation is the basic principle behind PTB treatment. The goals of treatment include achieving relapse-free cure, breaking the chain of transmission of disease by rendering patient noninfectious and minimizing and preventing drug resistance.

PRINCIPLE OF CHEMOTHERAPY

- **Bacteriological basis:** In an untreated smear-positive pulmonary TB lesion, there are naturally occurring DR mutants to different antitubercular drugs at different frequencies. Roughly, the frequency of occurrence of DR mutants is ~1 in 10^6 to isoniazid (H), ~1 in 10^6 to streptomycin (S), and ~1 in 10^8 to rifampicin (R). Based on these frequencies, the chances of naturally occurring organisms that is resistant to both H and R would be roughly ~1 in 10^{14}. Hence, administering multiple drugs during the intensive phase (IP) would achieve rapid killing of actively multiplying bacteria including the resistant mutants and decrease their chances of selection and further multiplication. Thereafter, lesser number of drugs given over longer time in continuation phase (CP) will eliminate persisters (extracellular intermittently multiplying and intra-/extracellular acidic environmental slowly multiplying mycobacteria) which are responsible for relapses (**Table 3**).
- **Pharmacological basis:** While giving chemotherapy, it is important to achieve peak serum level of all drugs simultaneously so as to have maximum bactericidal effect. Hence, it is recommended to administer all the drugs at the same time.

DRUG-SENSITIVE TUBERCULOSIS

Drug-sensitive TB (DS-TB) is defined when the resistance to both H and R is not detected in the biological specimen. Previously, the regimens for the DS-TB were classified as category I and II based on previous history of TB treatment. But now with the initiation of universal DST to rifampicin, these treatment categories have been abandoned. *Currently, the ATT for DS-TB comprises four drugs (HRZE) given daily for initial 2 months (IP) followed by three drugs (HRE) for next 4 months (CP).* In slight deviation to this protocol, American Thoracic Society (ATS)/Centers for Disease Control and Prevention (CDC) guidelines on DS-TB recommend that three drugs (R, H, and Z) regimen can be given without ethambutol in the IP if baseline patient's isolate is susceptible to both H and R. CP may be extended by 12–24 weeks in certain forms of TB like central nervous system (CNS) TB, skeletal TB, and disseminated TB, based on clinical decision on a case-to-case basis. Under NTEP, anti-tubercular drugs are given as fixed-dose combination (FDC) based on fixed weight bands and on daily basis. Apart from ATT, steroids are added as adjunctive therapy in patients with TB pericarditis, meningeal TB, and miliary TB that can be tapered over 6–8 weeks, depending on clinical improvement. Management of comorbidities, nutritional supplementation, and abstinence from smoking and alcohol are other measures that have shown to improve treatment outcome in TB.

It is important to check compliance to anti-TB drugs and the same should be reiterated to the patient at each visit. Treatment response is evaluated clinically (resolution of fever, weight gain etc.) along with serial sputum smear examinations and X-rays done at regular intervals. Cure is defined when a microbiologically confirmed TB patient becomes sputum smear or culture negative at the end of the complete treatment. However, a patient is said to have failed ATT, if his biological specimen is positive by smear or culture at the end of treatment. Any follow-up positive sputum should be subjected to NAAT and further decision regarding ATT is to be taken on the basis of DST results.

DRUG-RESISTANT TUBERCULOSIS

Resistance to first-line and second-line anti-TB drugs has been a major roadblock in the elimination of TB from India. As per WHO Global TB report, India contributed highest number of MDR-TB cases in the world with an incidence rate of 9.1/100,000 population in 2019. The treatment success rate has been dismal with less than half (49%) of all notified MDR-TB patients achieving treatment success. In order to improve the dismal picture, major changes have been incorporated in the management of

TABLE 3 Grading of different types of activities of first-line anti-TB drugs.

Drugs	Adult dosage (per day)	Early bactericidal	Sterilizing activity	Prevention of emergence of drug resistance
Isoniazid (H)	5 mg/kg (4–6 mg/kg)	++++	++	++++
Rifampicin (R)	10 mg/kg (8–12 mg/kg)	+++	++++	+++
Pyrazinamide (Z)	25 mg/kg (20–30 mg/kg)	++	+++	+
Ethambutol (E)	15 mg/kg (12–18 mg/kg)	+	–	++

DR-TB under the TB elimination program. These include universal DST, intensifying baseline DST to first-line and second-line drugs and redesigning DR-TB regimens based on WHO guidelines, 2019.

Types of drug resistance:

- *Mono-resistant (MR) TB*: Disease in which biological specimen is resistant to one first-line anti-TB drug only.
- *Poly-drug-resistant (PDR) TB*: Disease in which biological specimen is resistant to more than one first-line anti-TB drug, other than both isoniazid and rifampicin.
- *Multidrug-resistant TB:* Disease in which biological specimen is resistant to both isoniazid and rifampicin with or without resistance to other first-line drugs, based on the results from a quality-assured laboratory.
- *Rifampicin-resistant TB*: Disease in which resistance to rifampicin is detected using phenotypic or genotypic methods, with or without resistance to other anti-TB drugs excluding H. Patients, who have any rifampicin resistance, should also be managed as if they are MDR-TB case.
- *Extensively drug-resistant (XDR) TB*: A MDR-TB case whose biological specimen is additionally resistant to a fluoroquinolone (ofloxacin, levofloxacin, or moxifloxacin) and a second-line injectable anti-TB drug (kanamycin, amikacin, or capreomycin) from a quality-assured laboratory.

Classes of anti-TB drugs for DR-TB: Currently, the drugs recommended for treatment of DR-TB are divided into three groups based on their relative benefits and harms. WHO Guideline Development Group (GDG) analyzed the data on relative efficacy and safety of individual drugs from the meta-analysis of individual patient data (IPD-MA), 2018 and Phase III Trial 213 of delamanid and classified the drugs into three groups (**Table 4**). These drugs include the two new drugs Bdq and delamanid that have recently been added to the TB drugs armamentarium. Bdq is a diarylquinoline that specifically targets mycobacterial ATP synthase, an enzyme essential for the supply of energy to MTB. Its unique feature is its extended half-life as a result it is present in plasma up to 5.5 months post-stopping Bdq. Its strong bactericidal and sterilizing properties make it an ideal agent for use in TB treatment. Delamanid is another bactericidal agent with 38 hours of half-life. Previously called as OPC-67683, it is a dihydro-nitroimidazooxazole derivative which acts by inhibiting the synthesis of mycobacterial cell wall components.

Integrated DR-TB algorithm: Evaluation of baseline drug resistance to rifampicin by rapid DST (NAAT) is an important step in the management of all notified, bacteriologically confirmed and clinically diagnosed TB patients and is termed as universal DST. This integration of DST with the TB diagnosis has been the most important change in the DR-TB management that detects rifampicin resistance at baseline in all diagnosed TB patients. **Flowchart 1** illustrates the management strategies for DR-TB right from the time the result of NAAT is available. Patients with rifampicin resistance "not detected" are evaluated for mono-resistance to isoniazid. If H is found to be resistant, patient is started on H mono/poly DR-Tb regimen while awaiting the results of second-line-LPA (for checking fluoroquinolone status). The patients with rifampicin resistance are considered for shorter MDR-TB regimen after ruling out the DST and non-DST-based exclusion criteria mentioned in the **Table 5**. The patients who are not eligible for shorter MDR-TB regimen are initiated on all oral longer MDR-TB regimen. In case of additional resistance on LC-DST, the all oral longer MDR-TB regimen is appropriately modified.

TABLE 4 Groups of anti-TB drugs recommended for drug-resistant tuberculosis.

Groups and steps	Drugs	
Group A: Include all three medicines	Levofloxacin OR	Lfx
	Moxifloxacin	Mfx
	Bedaquiline	Bdq
	Linezolid	Lzd
Group B: Add one or both medicines	Clofazimine	Cfz
	Cycloserine OR	Cs
	Terizidone	Trd
Group C: Add to complete the regimen and when medicines from group A and B cannot be used	Ethambutol	E
	Delamanid	Dlm
	Pyrazinamide	Z
	Imipenem-cilastatin OR	Ipm-Cln
	Meropenem	Mpm
	Amikacin OR	Am
	Streptomycin	(S)
	Ethionamide OR	Eto
	Prothionamide	Pto
	p-aminosalicylic acid	PAS

Treatment regimens for DR-TB: As previously mentioned, three standards DR-TB regimens have been approved for three different sets of drug resistance/criteria. **Table 6** mentions the drug composition of all the three regimens. The number in parenthesis refers to the duration of therapy in months. As shown in the **Table 6**, duration of shorter MDR-TB regimen is 9–11 months with 4–6 months of IP containing injectables and 5 months of CP. The all oral H mono/poly DR-TB regimen and all oral MDR-TB regimens do not have separate IP/CP.

As per WHO consolidated guidelines on DR-TB treatment 2019, all oral regimens should include all three group A agents and at least one group B agent (**Table 4**) so that treatment consists of four drugs that are likely to be effective and at least three drugs are continued for the remaining duration of treatment after Bdq is stopped. In view of high probability of discontinuation of linezolid due to toxicity, fifth drug cycloserine has been included in the all oral longer MDR-TB regimen for India. This regimen will also be used for treatment of XDR-TB patients with 20 months duration. Further monitoring and evaluation for treatment outcome is done using clinical, microbiological, and radiological parameters.

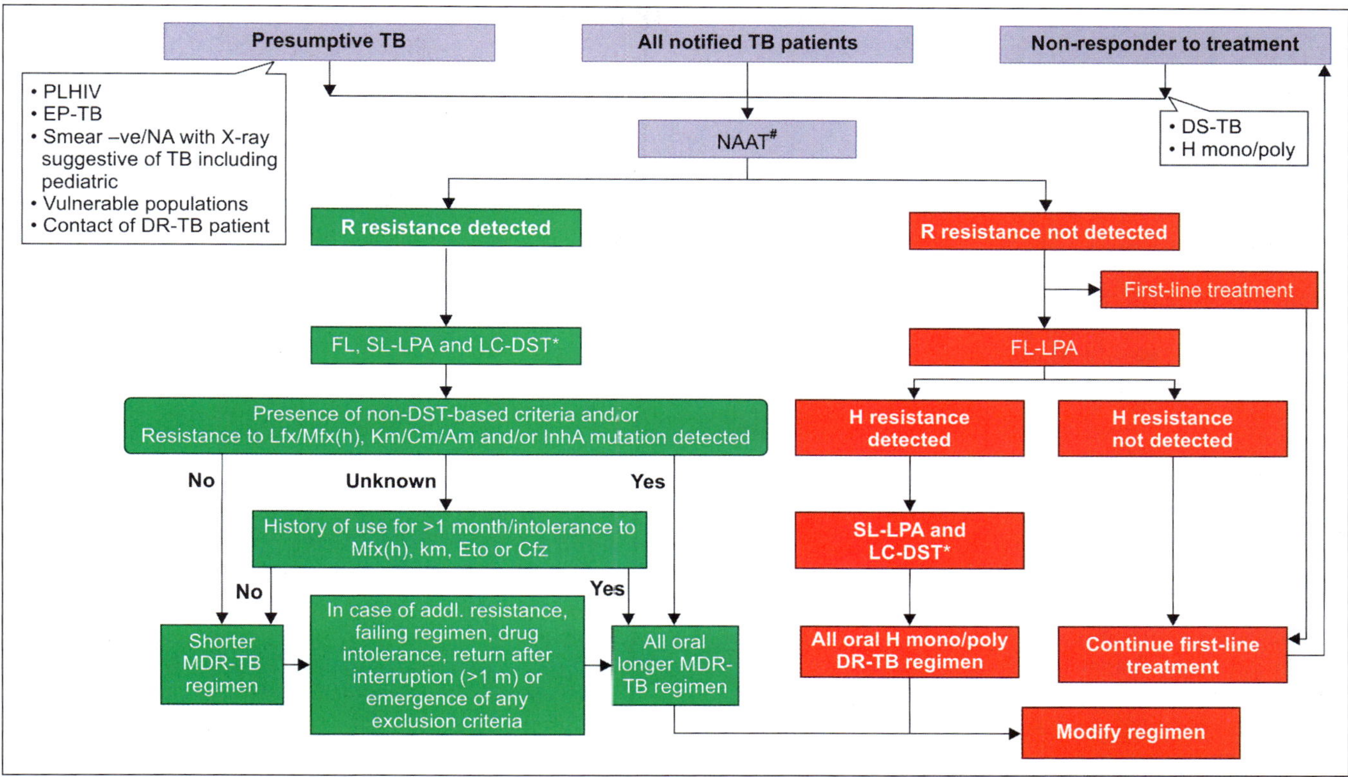

NAAT include CBNAAT and TruNAAT; * LC-DST will be done as per the diagnostic algorithm; ** Refer table of exclusion criteria for shorter MDR-TB regimen.

(CBNAAT: cartridge-based nucleic acid amplification test; DST: drug sensitivity testing; DR: drug-resistant; EPTB: extrapulmonary tuberculosis; FL: first-line; LC: liquid culture; LPA: line probe assay; MDR: multidrug-resistant; PLHIV: patients living with human immunodeficiency virus; SL: second-line)

FLOWCHART 1: Integrated drug-resistant TB algorithm.

Source: Central TB Division. Guidelines on programmatic management of drug-resistant tuberculosis in India. New Delhi: Central TB Division, MoHFW, Government of India; 2019.

TABLE 5 Criteria for patients to receive standard DR-TB regimen.

Standard DR-TB regimen	Inclusion criteria	Exclusion criteria
All oral H mono/poly regimen	Isoniazid-resistant TB with confirmed result for rifampicin-resistance not detected (RS)	No specific criteria except drug interaction/intolerability with any other drug used concomitantly
Shorter MDR-TB regimen	Patient with rifampicin-resistant pulmonary or extrapulmonary TB	DST-based criteria: • If DST/DRT result for FQ or SLI is resistant or • Presence of InhA mutation (for Eto) or • Resistance to Z (whenever available) • History of use for > 1 month/intolerance to Mfx(h), Km, Eto, or Cfz Non-DST based criteria: • Pregnancy • Any extrapulmonary disease in PLHIV • Disseminated, meningeal, or central nervous system TB • Intolerance to any drug in the shorter MDR-TB regimen or risk of toxicity from a drug in the shorter regimen (e.g., drug–drug interactions)
All oral longer regimen for MDR/RR-TB	Patients in whom shorter MDR-TB regimen cannot be considered due to any reason	None

(DR: drug-resistance; DRT: drug-resistance testing; DST: drug-susceptibility testing; FQ: fluoroquinolone; PLHIV: patients living with human immunodeficiency virus; SLI: second-line injectable drug)

TABLE 6 Standard regimen for initiating treatment of MDR/RR-TB or H mono-poly DR-TB.

Type of drug resistance and drug regimen	Intensive phase	Continuation phase
1. H mono/poly DR-TB regimen (R resistance not detected and H resistance)	(6) Lfx R E Z	
2. MDR/RR-TB		
Shorter MDR-TB regimen	(4–6) Mfx^h Km/Am Eto Cfz Z H^h E	(5) Mfx^h Cfz Z E
All oral longer MDR-TB regimen	(18-20) Bdq(6) Lfx Lzd Cfz Cs	

(DR: drug-resistance; MDR: multidrug resistant; RR: rifampicin-resistant; TB: tuberculosis)

FUTURE OPTIONS

Current treatment guidelines for TB being practiced worldwide are the outcome of 65 years of clinical trials, observational studies, and expert consensus statements. In the last few years, the number of ongoing clinical trials has increased tremendously, as a result, next 5 years should likely bring major changes in TB treatment. The main targets of these trials are to shorten the treatment duration and/or design more effective regimens using new drugs in different combinations.

Shortening the duration is being tried by incorporating fluoroquinolone (e.g., TBTC study), increasing the dose of rifampin (RIFASHORT trial), or selecting patients with less severe disease (Predict TB trial). TRUNCATE-TB is a multiarm, multistage trial that incorporates high dose of rifamycins and various combinations of linezolid, clofazimine levofloxacin, and Bdq into four 2-month treatment regimens for DS-TB. Similar to DS-TB, trials in DR-TB have also aimed to shorten the duration of therapy. It is best exemplified by the famous "Bangladesh regimen" that was proved to be noninferior to 20-month standard of care in STREAM (Standard Treatment Regimen of Anti-tuberculosis Drugs for Patients with MDR-TB) trial. It is now recommended by WHO guidelines 2019 and adopted by NTEP for treatment of MDR-TB.

CONCLUSION

Systematic use of rapid molecular assays for TB diagnosis and DST has revolutionized the management of PTB. Besides shortening the time to diagnosis, it helps in designing DST-guided effective anti-TB regimens thus ensuring high treatment success rates. There is urgent need to upscale the quality assured laboratory network with facilities for rapid molecular assays and LC. Together, institution of highly effective regimens containing new anti-TB drugs backed by evidence for its efficiency and safety is another step toward TB elimination. We need to wait for couple of years before the treatment outcomes from these regimens start pouring in. Nevertheless, there is need for large scale, well-designed randomized control trials evaluating new drugs and regimens so as to make TB treatment shorter, safer, and more effective.

RECOMMENDED READINGS

1. Ministry of Health and Family Welfare, Government of India, National TB Elimination Programme. (2020). Training modules (1-4) for programme managers and medical officers.[online] Available from www.tbcindia.gov.in
2. Revised National Tuberculosis Control Programme. Guidelines on programmatic management of drug resistant Tuberculosis in India. New Delhi: Central TB Division, MoHFW, Government of India; 2019. pp. 195.
3. Behera D. Management of Tuberculosis. In: Jindal SK (Ed). Text Book of Pulmonary and Critical Care Medicine, 2nd edition. New Delhi: Jaypee brothers Medical Publishers; 2017. pp. 492-500.
4. World Health Organization. (2020). Global Tuberculosis report 2020. [online] Available from https://www.who.int/publications/i/item/9789240013131
5. World Health Organization. (2019). WHO consolidated guidelines on drug-resistant tuberculosis treatment. [online] Available from https://www.who.int/tb/publications/2019/consolidated-guidelines-drug-resistant-TB-treatment/en/
6. Nahid P, Dorman SE, Alipanah N, Barry PM, Brozek JL, Cattamanchi A, et al. Official American Thoracic Society/Centers for Disease Control and Prevention/Infectious Diseases Society of America Clinical Practice Guidelines: Treatment of Drug-Susceptible Tuberculosis. Clin Infect Dis. 2016;63(7):e147-95.
7. World Health Organization. (2017). Guidelines for treatment of drug-susceptible tuberculosis and patient care (2017 update). [online] Available from https://www.who.int/tb/publications/2017/dstb_guidance_2017/en/
8. Ministry of Health and Family Welfare, Government of India, Revised National Tuberculosis Control Programme. (2016). Technical and Operational Guidelines for TB Control in India. [online] Available from https://tbcindia.gov.in/index1.php?lang=1&level=2&sublinkid=4573&lid=3177
9. Lee A, Xie YL, Barry CE, Chen RY. Current and future treatments for tuberculosis. BMJ. 2020;368:m216.

CHAPTER
210 Extrapulmonary Tuberculosis

Uma Devaraj, Priya Ramachandran

ABSTRACT

In the year 2019, the incidence of tuberculosis (TB) in India was estimated to be 26.9 lakh cases contributing to 26% of the global burden of TB. In approximately 80% of the population, infection with *Mycobacterium tuberculosis* (*M. tb*) causes pulmonary TB. However, the percentage of extrapulmonary tuberculosis (EPTB) is 15–20% in immunocompetent population and rises to 45–50% in HIV-infected population. A high proportion of the EPTB is seen between 30 years and 50 years. Any organ can be invaded by *M. tb* and the myriad symptoms and signs of EPTB depend on the specific organ, site involved and severity. The clinical manifestations are nonspecific and can mimic other noninfectious conditions.

Extrapulmonary tuberculosis results in sequelae such as gibbus, hydrocephalus, or sinus tracts. A high degree of clinical suspicion and diligent work-up is necessary to establish a diagnosis of EPTB. All patients with EPTB should be evaluated for presence of pulmonary TB and also tested for HIV infection as per national guidelines.

Treatment principles for EPTB are very similar to that of PTB with standard 6 months of antituberculous therapy (ATT). A 2-month intensive phase with four drugs [isoniazid (INH), rifampicin, pyrazinamide, and ethambutol] followed by a 4-month continuation phase with INH, rifampicin, and ethambutol is recommended. In some conditions like central nervous system (CNS) and skeletal TB, the duration of therapy is increased from 6 to 12 months. Adjunctive corticosteroid therapy limits the inflammatory process and reduces residual scaring in conditions like CNS, pericardial, and ocular TB.

"The cure for bad politics is the same as the cure for tuberculosis. It is living in the open"

—Woodrow Wilson

INTRODUCTION

Tuberculosis spreads by airborne transmission through droplet nuclei. Not all persons exposed to the bacilli develop active TB. In many individuals, the inhalation of droplet nuclei does not lead to infection because either they do not reach the alveoli or are cleared by the innate immune system, mainly the macrophages. EPTB results when *M. tb* evades the macrophages and spreads to distant organs by lymphohematogenous route (**Fig. 1**).

Establishing the diagnosis is a challenge in EPTB as it is a paucibacillary disease (**Flowchart 1**). Imaging techniques such as computed tomography/magnetic resonance imaging (CT/MRI)/ultrasound help the diagnostic approach and in obtaining samples of tissue or fluid for microbiological and histopathological studies. Isotopic techniques such as positron emission tomography-CT (PET-CT) may detect inflammatory activity early but findings may be nonspecific.

Mantoux test, gamma interferon release assay (IGRA), immunoglobulin G (IgG), and/or IgM estimation cannot be used for diagnosis of disease as they neither differentiate infection from active disease nor help monitor the response to treatment.

Definitive diagnosis of EPTB, however, requires the detection of *M. tb*. A variable percentage (30–50%) of EPTB may be smear-negative. Microbiological culture, the gold standard test, takes a few days (liquid culture) to few weeks (solid culture media) to detect *M. tb*.

Molecular methods like cartridge-based nucleic acid amplification technique (CB-NAAT), which is based on the amplification of *M. tb*-specific genetic fragments facilitate rapid diagnosis and detect gene mutations responsible for antimicrobial resistance. The determination of the enzyme adenosine deaminase (ADA) in body fluids is useful, though cutoff for the positivity is not clear in all fluids.

An attempt to establish a microbiological diagnosis must be made in all cases of EPTB. This is helpful to differentiate whether the cause of lack of response to treatment is due to worsening from drug resistance or immune reconstitution inflammatory syndrome (IRIS).

The various manifestations of EPTB based on the site/organs involved will be discussed in the following paragraphs.

LYMPH NODE TUBERCULOSIS

Tubercular lymphadenitis, also called scrofula, is the most common presentation of EPTB contributing 40–58.7% of all EPTB. Though described across all age groups, the median age affected with lymph node (LN)-TB is 40 years. Any group of LNs can be involved, with the cervical LNs being most frequently involved, followed by mediastinal, axillary, mesenteric, hepatic, portal, perihepatic, and inguinal LNs.

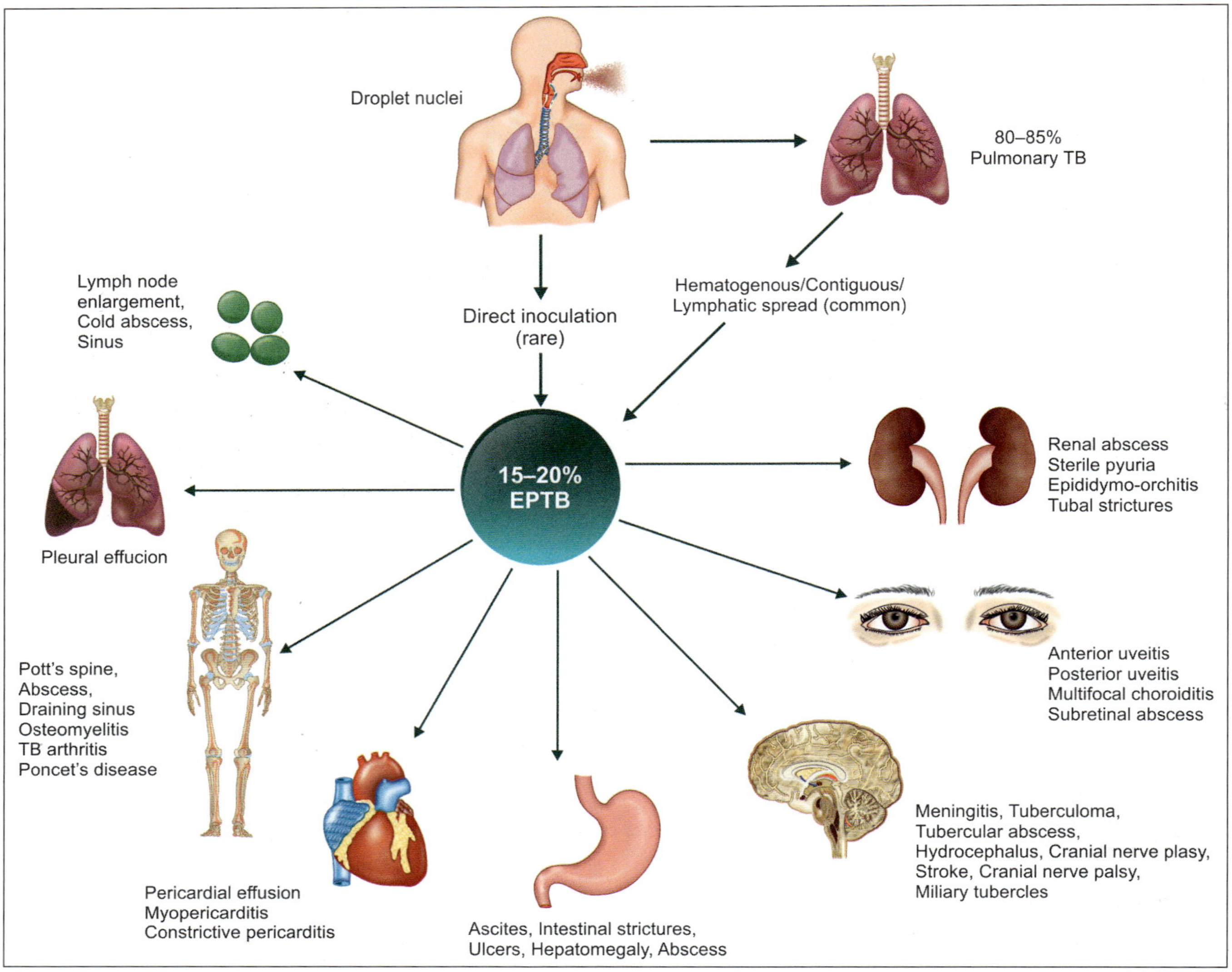

FIGURE 1: Spread of *Mycobacterium tuberculosis* and manifestations of extrapulmonary tuberculosis.

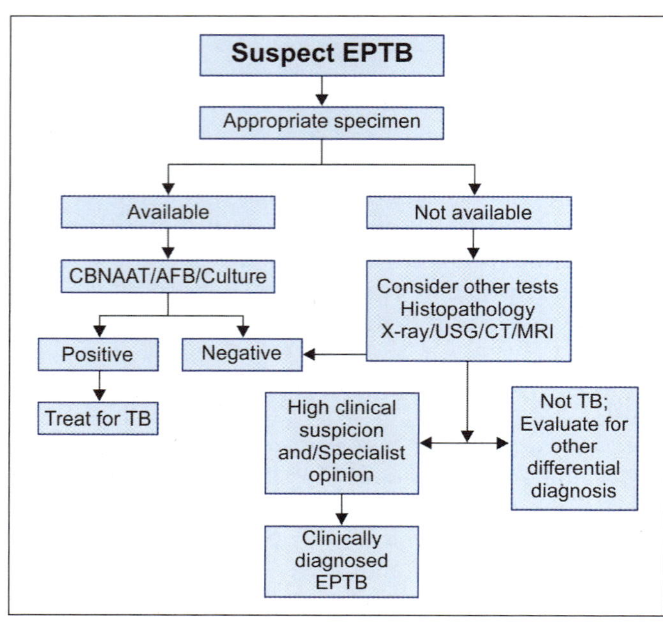

(EPTB: extrapulmonary tuberculosis; CB-NAAT: cartridge-based nucleic acid amplification technique)

FLOWCHART 1: Diagnostic algorithm for EPTB.

CLINICAL PRESENTATION

The presentation LN-TB varies depending on the anatomical location of LN and the immune status of the patient. It ranges from chronic painless neck swelling, abdominal pain with or without constitutional symptoms of fever and weight loss, or chronic cough with systemic symptoms depending on the LN site involved.

The LNs are usually described as either single or multiple, firm, nontender, mobile, and matted with overlying skin showing no erythema. Associated fever is uncommon, seen in 20–50% of the cases in immunocompetent patients and 60–80% in HIV-infected patients. Sometimes the nodal enlargement leads to development of a cold abscess, which can breakdown and form a draining sinus.

Compression of the larger airways leading to bronchial or tracheal stenosis can be secondary to mediastinal LN-TB (**Fig. 2**).

DIAGNOSIS

Radiological investigations such as chest X-ray (CXR), ultrasound examination, or CT scan are useful to demonstrate presence of enlarged LNs. Diagnosis is confirmed by fine

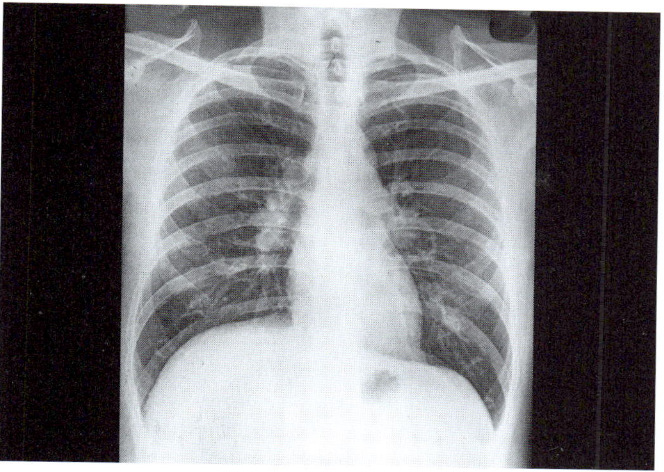

FIGURE 2: Bilateral hilar lymph node enlargement—mediastinal node TB.

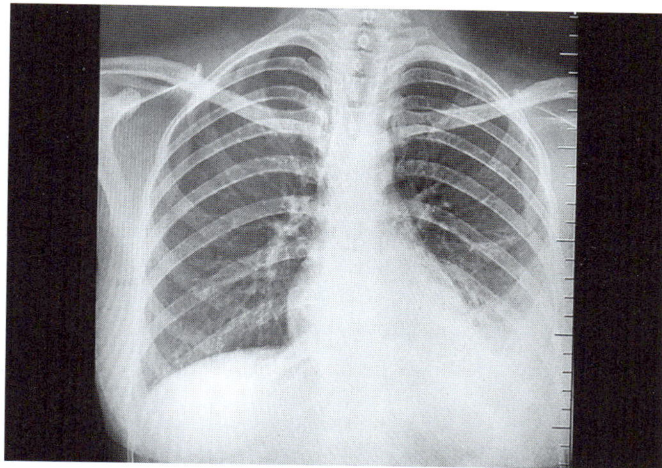

FIGURE 3: Tubercular pleural effusion.

needle aspiration cytology (FNAC) demonstrating caseating granulomatous inflammation and/or acid-fast bacilli (AFB). CB-NAAT has a sensitivity of 83.1% and specificity of 93.6% to diagnose TB. It is adjunctive to culture of the aspirate and cytology in FNAC specimens.

TREATMENT

Treatment of LN-TB is similar to that of pulmonary TB. Paradoxical reaction with increase in size of the nodes on treatment is seen in 3.8–10% of nonhuman immunodeficiency virus (HIV) coinfected patients and up to 50% in HIV-TB coinfected patients. There are no specific criteria to define improvement or cure. However, complete resolution of nodes or persisting lymphadenopathy less than 15 mm can be taken as a sign of cure.

PLEURAL TUBERCULOSIS

Pleural TB, the second most common type of EPTB, constitutes 28–39.43% of EPTB. Pleural TB usually represents type IV hypersensitivity response to the presence of mycobacterial antigens released into pleural space due to rupture of a subpleural caseous focus in the lung. Although the effusion is known to resolve spontaneously, treatment of TB effusion is essential, as untreated patients are at risk of developing active TB infection later. TB effusion is usually seen in younger age group, mean age being 31–50 years.

CLINICAL PRESENTATION

Usually, the effusion presents as an acute febrile illness, associated with dry cough, pleuritic chest pain, and sometimes with dyspnea and weight loss. In 75–90% of patients, the tubercular effusion is a unilateral moderate effusion.

DIAGNOSIS

Clinical examination added to a unilateral homogenous opacity in chest radiograph helps in identifying the presence of effusion (**Fig. 3**). Diffuse thickening of visceral and parietal pleura separated by fluid ("split pleura" sign) is evident on chest CT scan. Ultrasound is the best modality to confirm and aid in real-time image guidance for pleurocentesis. Pleural fluid is straw colored, often lymphocyte predominant exudate, with ADA levels above 40 IU/L. The initial fluid analysis can show polymorphonuclear-rich exudate in 11% of patients. An ADA level of >70 IU/L suggests that the effusion is highly likely to be pleural TB. The IGRA tests such as the QuantiFERON-TB Gold or Elispot test demonstrate poor sensitivity and specificity in pleural fluid.

Although Ziehl–Neelsen stain of pleural fluid yields positive results in less the 10% of patients, culture yields positive results in up to 70% of cases, using newer liquid culture media. CB-NAAT has higher sensitivity (90%) and specificity (100%) in pleural biopsy specimens than in pleural fluid (50% and 99%, respectively). Induced sputum culture yields *M. tb* in up to 55% even with no obvious parenchymal infiltrates on CXR. Demonstration of caseating granulomas or AFB by microscopy or CBNAAT in pleural tissue obtained by blind or thoracoscopic pleural biopsy substantiates diagnosis of TB effusion.

TREATMENT

With ATT, symptom resolution may take from 2 weeks to 8 weeks duration and often up to 12 weeks for radiological resolution of effusion. In presence of a large effusion, therapeutic drainage relieves breathlessness and reduces risk of residual pleural thickening. Corticosteroids do not reduce the incidence of pleural fibrosis or adhesions and hence are not indicated in treatment of TB effusion.

ABDOMINAL TUBERCULOSIS

Abdominal TB constitutes 11% of EPTB and can affect gastrointestinal tract, LNs, peritoneum, or any solid viscera in the abdominal cavity. *M. tb* reaches the abdomen either by swallowing of infected sputum or milk or by lymphohematogenous route in patients with active pulmonary TB or contiguous spread from adjacent organs.

CLINICAL PRESENTATION

It varies depending on the site involved. Abdominal pain, distension, fever, and loss of appetite and weight are common symptoms. Sometimes chronic diarrhea can occur. The ileocecal region is the most common site of involvement in gastrointestinal TB, where the lesions can be ulcerative or hypertrophic or form a stricture. Intestinal obstruction and vomiting may also be the presenting feature of gastrointestinal TB.

A doughy feel on abdominal palpation, hepatomegaly, ascites, and rarely a palpable mass in the abdomen are some of the clinical signs seen in abdominal TB. Hematochezia and constipation are present when the rectum is affected. A persistent discharging perianal sinus or fistula should also raise a suspicion of tuberculous etiology.

DIAGNOSIS

Evaluation by ultrasound demonstrates loculated or free ascites, thickened bowel wall, splenic microabscesses, enlarged mesenteric, retroperitoneal LNs, and/or peritoneal and omental thickening. A contrast enhanced CT scan of the abdomen also clearly delineates circumferential wall thickening of the small intestine along with lymphadenopathy. Other modalities of investigation such as esophagogastroduodenoscopy, capsule endoscopy, colonoscopy, and laparoscopy are helpful in noting characteristic findings and obtaining tissue samples. The LNs/other viscera can also be subjected to FNAC/biopsy to confirm the diagnosis. In the presence of ascites, fluid analysis shows a lymphocytic exudate with ADA levels above 30 IU/L. Hepatic involvement causes abnormalities in liver function tests with elevated alkaline phosphatase and gamma-glutamyl transferase levels. Treatment is with the standard 6-month regimen of ATT.

TUBERCULOSIS OF THE CARDIOVASCULAR SYSTEM

Tuberculosis of the heart has high morbidity and mortality, second only to CNS-TB. It can manifest as pericarditis, myocardial TB with or without aneurysm formation, and TB aortitis. *In India, 60–70% of the pericardial effusions are due to TB.* The pathogenesis of TB pericarditis, akin to pleural effusion, is secondary to hypersensitivity reaction to *M. tb.*

CLINICAL PRESENTATION

The pericardial involvement can present as either acute pericarditis, effusive pericarditis, myopericarditis, or constrictive pericarditis. Effusive pericarditis is the most common presentation. The presentation depends on the volume and rapidity of fluid accumulation, impediment to cardiac function due to fluid accumulation or loss of visceral pericardial compliance, and the severity of inflammation.

In the acute pericarditis phase, patients present with chest pain, pericardial friction rub, and widespread ST elevation without effusion. Later the presentation changes to features of heart failure and/or cardiac tamponade due to accumulation of moderate to large pericardial effusion (**Figs. 4 A and B**). Patients present with sinus tachycardia, pulsus paradoxus, raised central venous pressure, peripheral edema, increased cardiac dullness, muffled heart sounds, hepatomegaly, and ascites.

DIAGNOSIS

Pericardial fluid is predominantly a lymphocytic exudate. The ADA cutoff of 35 IU/L is suggestive of tubercular etiology. Demonstration of tubercle bacilli in the pericardial fluid or tissue by either direct examination, CB-NAAT, or culture is the definitive diagnostic modality for tuberculous pericarditis. QuantiFERON TB gold is an additional test that aids in diagnosis.

TREATMENT

Standard 6-month ATT is recommended. Adjuvant steroids are recommended, regardless of HIV status. Prednisolone, 1 mg/kg/day is given for 4–6 weeks in tapering doses. Alleviation of cardiac tamponade can be achieved by echocardiographic-guided pericardiocentesis and drainage of fluid. Reduced incidence of constrictive pericarditis has been reported when patients are treated with pericardial fluid drainage. Surgical pericardiectomy remains the only definitive treatment for tuberculous constrictive pericarditis. Recovery rate of up to 60% and 18% mortality has been so far reported.

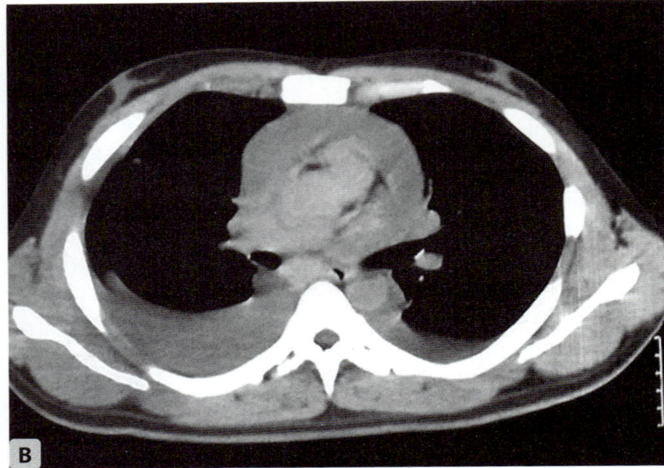

FIGURES 4 A & B: Tuberculous pericardial effusion with bilateral pleural effusion in a 27-year-old male.

OCULAR TUBERCULOSIS

Prevalence of tubercular uveitis is 5.6–10.5% in India. TB can affect any part of the eye with most common manifestation being posterior uveitis. Other rare presentations are endophthalmitis, panophthalmitis, and optic neuropathy. Obtaining a tissue sample is difficult and hence in many situations, ancillary and laboratory investigations in the background of a clinical setting support a TB diagnosis.

CLINICAL PRESENTATION

Patients with anterior, intermediate, posterior or panuveitis present with complaints of blurred vision, redness of eye, eye pain, photophobia, floaters, and flashing lights in the eye. Granulomatous anterior uveitis or posterior uveitis, including choroidal/disk granuloma, multifocal choroiditis, and subretinal abscess are manifestations of ocular TB.

Eales' disease is tubercular retinal vasculitis, an occlusive disease with or without active retinal periphlebitis, peripheral neovascularization with recurrent vitreous hemorrhages.

DIAGNOSIS

Exclusion of other causes of uveitis in the presence of characteristic clinical features, corroborative infiltrates in CXR or CT scan, positive Mantoux or IGRA test helps to confirm the diagnosis. Rarely, invasive tests such as intraocular sampling with molecular tests are considered. Characteristic features of posterior segment disease may be detected by investigations such as fundus autofluorescence, fluorescein angiography, indocyanine green angiography, and optical coherence tomography.

TREATMENT

Adjunctive corticosteroids are indicated to manage the type IV hypersensitivity reaction to tubercular proteins in ocular TB. Steroids also reduce the macular edema secondary to the inflammation. Steroids are started with ATT, with a dose of 1 mg/kg/day, tapered over 6–12 months.

TUBERCULOSIS OF CENTRAL NERVOUS SYSTEM

Tuberculosis of the nervous system (CNS-TB) is seen in 1–5% of all patients with TB and is more common in those with HIV (10%). Children <5 years of age, immunocompromised individuals [HIV, treatment with steroids, and tumor necrosis factor-α (TNFα) inhibitors] are at greater risk of CNS-TB.

Studies published by Rich and McCordock in 1933 have helped us understand the pathogenesis of CNS-TB. Hematogenous spread of infection to the brain results in the formation of a caseating vascular focus, the "Rich focus," which is the key pathway for the tubercle bacilli to enter the subarachnoid space. *M. tb* multiplies in the microglial cells, the resident macrophages in the CNS. A dense exudate is formed after release of the bacilli into the subarachnoid space, more in interpeduncular fossa and suprasellar region anteriorly, prepontine cistern, and around the spinal cord. Hydrocephalus ensues due to the blockage of flow of cerebrospinal fluid (CSF) because of encapsulation of the arteries and nerves by the exudate. Tubercles that enlarge without rupturing result in tuberculoma and abscess formation.

Subjects with TB meningitis (TBM) present with symptoms of classic meningitis like fever, headache, meningismus, focal neurological deficits, behavioral changes, and altered sensorium. Up to 50% of adults will have evidence of active TB on chest imaging.

DIAGNOSIS

Radiological imaging plays an important part in diagnosis of CNS-TB. Leptomeningeal uptake both in CT and MRI and basal exudates are suggestive of TBM (**Fig. 5**). CSF analysis shows a lymphocytic fluid with elevated protein levels, and low glucose. Standardized cutoff values for ADA for the diagnosis of TBM have not been established. CSF smears are positive in 20% of subjects. Hence, CSF for CB-NAAT is the first-line test over conventional microscopy in patients with suspected TBM (**Table 1**).

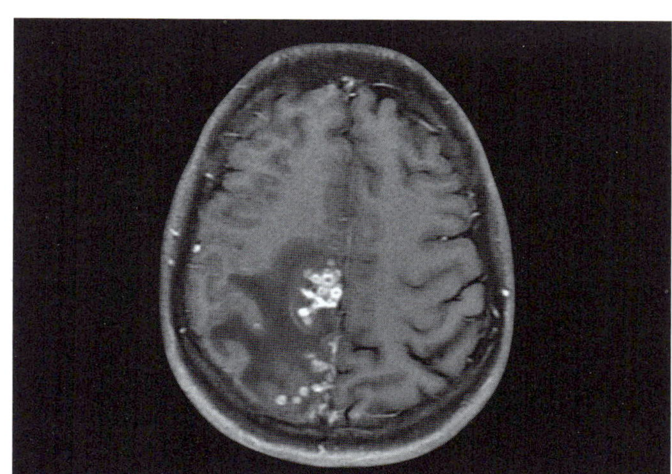

FIGURE 5: Tuberculoma with meningeal enhancement.

TABLE 1 Radiological and clinical features of CNS–TB.

Form of CNS-TB	Clinical presentation	Imaging features
Meningitis	Subacute presentation Symptoms—neck stiffness, photophobia, vomiting, and altered sensorium *Neurological deficits*: Hemiparesis, cranial nerve palsies	*CT and MRI*: Basal meningeal enhancement MR-DWI (MR-diffuse weighted imaging)–symmetrical restricted diffusion of cortical and adjacent subcortical structures

Continued...

Continued...

Form of CNS-TB	Clinical presentation	Imaging features
Miliary TB	Acute presentation *Symptoms*: Fever, headache, altered sensorium, and seizures	Pulmonary miliary shadows *MRI*: Small focal lesions *T2-weighted imaging*: Isointense with hypointense center *T1-weighted imaging*: Postcontrast rim enhancement
Tuberculoma/ Abscess	Subacute presentation *Symptoms*: Fever, headache, seizures, focal deficits, and rupture into subarachnoid space—Meningitis	*CT:* Postcontrast—ring enhancing lesions (caseating) Central calcification (target sign) *MRI:* Hypointense on T1 WI, *MR spectroscopy*: Lipid peaks suggestive of mycobacteria in abscess
Tubercular spondylosis (extradural) **Spinal tuberculosis (intradural)**	Subacute presentation *Symptoms*: Back pain, radicular, cauda equina or sensory disturbances, bladder and bowel dysfunction, and paraparesis/paralysis	*MRI*: Paraspinal abnormal signal with a thin and smooth abscess wall Subligamentous spread with preservation of the intervertebral space. Meningeal and radicular enhancement Intramedullary spinal tuberculoma Syringomyelia

TREATMENT

While INH and pyrazinamide cross the blood-brain barrier, rifampicin and ethambutol have significantly less penetration. Treatment duration is for 6–12 months with adjuvant steroids.

COMPLICATIONS

Central nervous system-TB is fatal in 20% of subjects. Mental retardation, seizures, persistent neurological deficits, and hydrocephalus are dreaded complications seen in up to 30%.

SKELETAL TUBERCULOSIS

During the process of dissemination, *M. tb* can get lodged in any bone and causes inflammatory (Poncet's disease) or infective process.

Spinal TB is the most common form of osteoarticular TB. Infection begins with inflammation of the anterior aspect of vertebral bodies and then spreads. Eventually, the infection extends to adjacent soft tissues with the formation of paravertebral abscesses. The posterior aspect of vertebral bodies is involved increasing the risk of spinal cord compression. The paravertebral abscess can rupture resulting in a draining sinus. Pott's disease most commonly affects the lower thoracic region or upper lumbar region. The most common symptom is local pain, swelling, and deformities (gibbus) with constitutional symptoms like fever and weight loss. Diagnosis of spinal TB in the early (inflammatory) stage is essential to prevent the development of spinal deformity and neurological deficit.

Skeletal TB diagnosis is established through a combination of clinical evaluation, imaging features, AFB smear, mycobacterial culture, histologic and/or cytologic evaluation, and molecular methods.

Computed tomography scan delineates bone destruction better than radiography and is useful for percutaneous biopsy of infected bone and/or soft tissue (**Figs. 6 A to G**). MRI

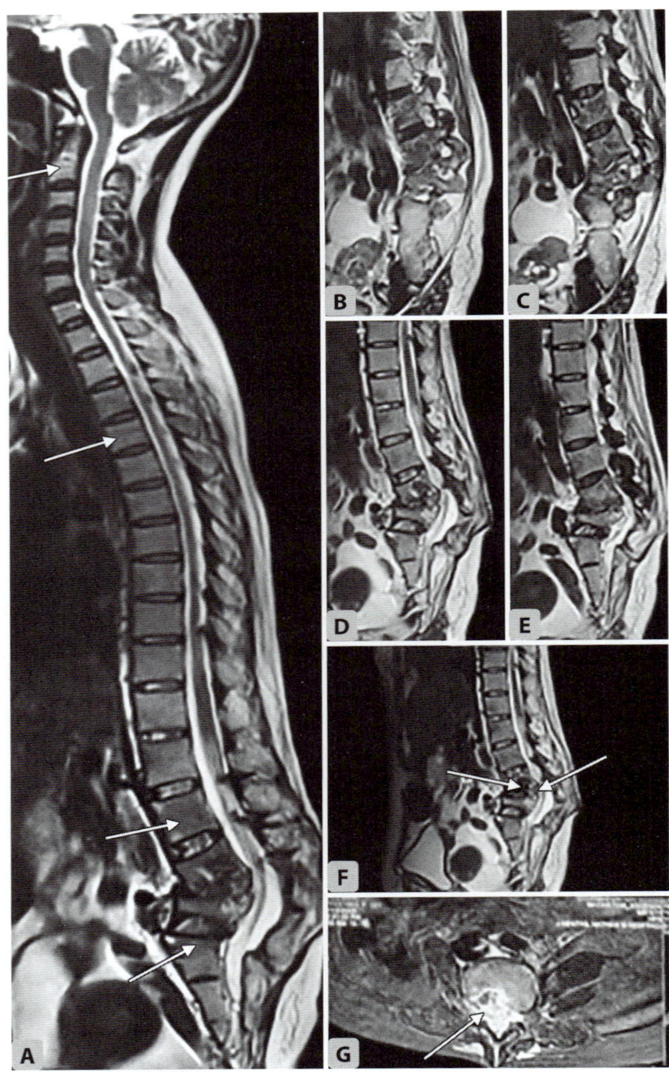

FIGURES 6 A to G: Compression fracture L2, L3 vertebrae, and gibbus formation—spinal TB.

TABLE 2 Clinical characteristics, evaluation, and treatment of EPTB.

Site	Prevalence	Symptoms and signs	Investigations	Treatment
Lymph node TB	40–58%	Enlarged LN, draining sinus	Lymph node aspiration/biopsy	ATT—6 months
Pleural TB	28–39%	Fever, cough, and pleuritic chest pain; effusion signs	CXR, ultrasound, pleurocentesis, and pleural biopsy	ATT—6 months
Abdomen	11%	Distended, subacute intestinal obstruction Doughy abdomen	Aspiration of ascitic fluid; biopsy of lesion	6 months ATT ± surgery
CNS-TB	5–10%	Headache, altered sensorium, and seizures	CSF analysis; *Imaging*: Tuberculoma, basal meningitis, and ring enhancing lesions	ATT for 6–12 months + steroids ± surgery
Eye	5.6–10.5%	Eye pain, redness, blurred vision, and floaters; uveitis	Ophthalmic examination; Mantoux/IGRA; and CXR	ATT, local/systemic steroids
Bone and joints	1–2%	Swelling, pain, and draining sinus	*Imaging*: Contiguous lesions of vertebral bodies, osteomyelitis. Aspiration of joint fluid/pus/tissue biopsy	ATT: 6–12 months, ± surgery
Pericardial effusion	1–2%	Chest pain, breathlessness, hypotension, and cardiac failure	Aspiration of pericardial fluid	6 months ATT + steroids; ± surgery
Genitourinary	4%	Sterile pyuria, Infertility	Urine analysis; biopsy of involved area	ATT: 6 months; ± surgery
Adrenal	Rare	Nausea, vomiting, weight loss, and hypotension	CT abdomen-bilateral enlarged adrenals/ calcification	ATT + steroids

(CB-NAAT: cartridge-based nucleic acid amplification technique; HPE: histopathological examination; IGRA: gamma interferon release assay)

findings include contiguous vertebral body involvement with preservation of disk spaces, marrow edema, prevertebral, and paravertebral septate loculated collections.

The indications for surgery and type of surgery performed (decompression, instrumented stabilization, or deformity correction) are case-specific decisions.

Duration of treatment is 6–12 months of standard ATT regimen. Steroids are indicated if there is spinal cord compression.

GENITOURINARY TUBERCULOSIS

This rare form of TB contributes to 4% of all EPTB. Patients present with increased frequency, urgency of urination and nocturia associated with dysuria and/or hematuria. Systemic symptoms of fever, weight loss, and night sweats are seen in few patients. Infertility, menstrual problems, pelvic mass, or unexplained abdominal pain in premenopausal woman or vaginal bleeding in postmenopausal woman should make one suspect genitourinary TB (GU-TB). In males, GU-TB presents as scrotal pain or swelling for 2 weeks or more, or with discharging sinuses in the scrotum. Presence of sterile pyuria should raise the possibility of GU-TB.

Urine examination, tissue specimens by FNAC or biopsy aid in diagnosis. Ultrasound, CT, and MRI scans are ancillary investigations to establish diagnosis.

ADRENAL TUBERCULOSIS

It manifests commonly with weakness, fatigue, anorexia, nausea, vomiting, weight loss, hypotension, and skin hyperpigmentation. *M. tb* spreads to the adrenal glands hematogenously. More than 90% of the gland must be destroyed before insufficiency and clinical manifestations appear. CT scan shows bilateral adrenal enlargement in active disease, while atrophy and calcification are apparent with inactive disease.

Adrenal biopsy is not required for primary adrenal insufficiency with bilateral adrenal enlargement in a patient with proven extra-adrenal TB. Treatment is with standard ATT and replacement doses of steroids.

CUTANEOUS TUBERCULOSIS

It can manifest as tuberculous chancre, acute miliary TB, orificial TB, scrofuloderma, and metastatic abscess (tuberculous gumma) which are multibacillary. Paucibacillary forms—lupus vulgaris and TB verrucosa cutis are less common. Hypersensitivity reactions to *M. tb* antigens can present as erythema nodosum, papulonecrotic tuberculid, and lichen scrofulosorum.

KEY MESSAGES

- 15–20% of TB infection manifests as EPTB, higher percentage in HIV-TB coinfection.
- HIV testing is mandatory in patients with EPTB.
- Look for signs of dissemination and pulmonary involvement in all subjects (**Table 2**).
- Though empirical ATT can be started in certain conditions, such as ocular or pericardial TB, tissue samples from the involved sites from presumptive EPTB patients for smear microscopy/CB-NAAT/culture for

M. tb/histopathological examination, helps to confirm the diagnosis.

- Treatment with four-drug standard ATT for 6 months is indicated for all EPTB. Duration of therapy is extended to 12 months for CNS and skeletal TB.
- Adjunctive therapy with systemic corticosteroids is indicated in ocular, cardiac, and CNS tuberculosis.

RECOMMENDED READINGS

1. WHO. (2020). Global Tuberculosis Report 2020. [online] Available from https://www.who.int/publications/i/item/9789240013131.
2. Prakasha SR, Suresh G, D'Sa IP, Shetty SS, Kumar SG. Mapping the pattern and trends of extrapulmonary tuberculosis. J Glob Infect Dis. 2013;5:54-9.
3. Department of Medicine, All India Institute of Medical Sciences, New Delhi WHO Collaborating Centre (WHO-CC) for Training and Research in Tuberculosis Centre of Excellence for Extra-Pulmonary Tuberculosis, Ministry of Health and Family Welfare Government of India. Index-TB Guidelines . Delhi: Ministry of Health and Family Welfare; 2016.
4. Velingker A, Lawande D, Dcosta L. (2018). Clinico-Epidemiological Profile of Extra Pulmonary Tuberculosis in Western India. [online] Available from https://www.ijcmr.com/uploads/7/7/4/6/77464738/ijcmr_1878_v2.pdf.
5. Gandhare A, Mahashur A. The extrapulmonary disease: Tuberculosis of the lymph nodes: Many facets, many hues. Astrocyte. 2017;4:80-6.
6. Debi U, Ravisankar V, Prasad KK, Sinha SK, Sharma AK. Abdominal tuberculosis of the gastrointestinal tract: Revisited. World J Gastroenterol. 2014;20:14831-40.
7. Light RW. Update on tuberculous pleural effusion. Respirology. 2010;15:451-8.
8. Sarker ZM, Mahmud AK, Chowdhury AJ, Hasnat MA, Alam MR, Paul HK et al. Tuberculous pleural effusion. Mymensingh Med J. 2011;20:66-70.
9. Porcel JM. Biomarkers in the diagnosis of pleural diseases: A 2018 update. Ther Adv Respir Dis. 2018;12:1-11.
10. Cherian A, Thomas SV. Central nervous system tuberculosis. Afr Health Sci. 2011;11:116-27.

CHAPTER 211 Nontuberculous Mycobacterial Pulmonary Disease

Vishwanath Upadhyay, Surendra K Sharma

ABSTRACT

Nontuberculous mycobacteria (NTM) are ubiquitously present in the environment. These organisms are generally considered to be less virulent than *Mycobacterium tuberculosis (M. tb)*, and can cause diseases in both immunocompromised and immunocompetent hosts. As compared to *M. tb*, person-to-person transmission does not occur except with *Mycobacterium abscessus* NTM species among cystic fibrosis (CF) patients. Lung is most commonly involved, and NTM-pulmonary disease (NTM-PD) occurs frequently in patients with prior lung disease.

Rapid molecular tests are now available for confirmation of NTM diagnosis at species and subspecies level. Drug susceptibility testing (DST) is not routinely done except in nonresponsive disease due to slowly growing mycobacteria (SGM) or infection due to rapidly growing mycobacteria (RGM) especially *M. abscessus*.

While decision to treat patients with NTM-PD is made carefully, the treatment is given for 12 months after sputum culture conversion except in *Mycobacterium kansasii* for a total duration of 12 months. Pulmonary disease due to *M. kansasii* is similar to pulmonary tuberculosis and responds well to first-line antituberculosis (TB) drugs. Additional therapeutic measures include pulmonary rehabilitation and correction of malnutrition. Treatment response in NTM-PD is variable and depends on isolated NTM species and severity of underlying pulmonary disease. Surgery is reserved for patients with localized disease with good pulmonary functions. Future studies should focus on development and validation of nonculture-based rapid diagnostic tests for early diagnosis, and discovery of newer drugs with greater efficacy and lesser toxicity than the currently available.

"It is through science that we prove, but through intuition that we discover"

—**Henri Poincare**

INTRODUCTION

Nontuberculous mycobacteria are known by several names environmental mycobacteria, atypical mycobacteria or anonymous mycobacteria, mycobacteria other than *M. tb* (MOTT) and its close relatives, *M. africanum, M. bovis, M. canetti, M. caprae and M. pinnipedii*, and *M. leprae*. NTM are ubiquitously distributed in our environment and have been isolated from air, soil, dust, plants, natural, and drinking water sources including biofilms, wild animals, milk, and food products. NTM are characterized by a thin peptidoglycan layer surrounded by a thick outer lipid-rich coating that enables their attachment to rough surfaces, survival in adverse conditions and by offering resistance to antibiotics and disinfectants, helping NTM survival in low oxygen and carbon concentrations.

Based on their growth characteristics from the subculture, NTM are divided into RGM (<7 days) and SGM (≥7 days) (**Box 1**). At present, there is no evidence for latency of NTM. Taxonomy of the genus mycobacteria includes nearly 200 species and 13 subspecies. With the availability of molecular diagnostic tools such as deoxyribonucleic acid (DNA) sequencing, many new NTM species have been identified in recent years although some of these may not be clinically relevant. Because of a heavy reliance on smear microscopy in high TB burden countries for TB diagnosis, the NTM diagnosis is frequently missed due to lack of awareness among healthcare workers and poor access to laboratory resources.

EPIDEMIOLOGY

DISEASE BURDEN

Table 1 describes distribution of various NTM species in our environment. **Table 2** details major differences between NTM and *M. tb*. Recent reports suggest of *M. abscessus* transmission and *M. massiliense* among CF patients. The NTM diagnosis is not notifiable to public health authorities in many countries. NTM lung infection rates, defined as individuals with NTM-positive cultures and those with defined NTM-PD, increase with age and differ considerably among various countries. Many studies have suggested increases in prevalence rates over the last four decades. USA data suggest that the current prevalence of NTM-positive culture ranges between 1.4 per 100,000 and 6.6 per 100,000,

BOX 1 Common NTM species causing NTM-PD.

Slowly growing non tuberculous mycobacteria (>7 days):

- *M. avium* complex (MAC)
- *M. kansasii*
- *M. xenopi*
- *M. simiae*
- *M. szulgai*
- *M. malmoense*

Rapidly growing nontuberculous mycobacteria (<7 days):

- *M. abscessus*
- *M. fortuitum*
- *M. chelonae*

(NTM-PD: nontuberculous mycobacteria-pulmonary disease)

MAC incudes *M. intracellulare*, *M. avium* and *M. chimaera* species.

M. abscessus include *M. abscessus subspecies abscessus, M. abscessus subspecies bolletii, M. abscessus subspecies massiliense.*

Source (for Boxes 1, 2, 3, 4, 5, 8 and Tables 1 and 2, and Flowchart 1 also): Corlateanu A. Chronic obstructive pulmonary disease and phenotypes: a state-of-the-art. Pulmonology. 2020;26(2):95-100. Sharma SK, Upadhyay V. Epidemiology, diagnosis and treatment of nontuberculous mycobacterial diseases. Indian J Med Res. 2020;152:185-226.

TABLE 1 Environmental niches of NTM.

Types of sources	Sources	Commonly isolated NTM
Natural water sources	Streams, rivers, lakes, ponds, and seawater	*M. avium* complex (MAC), *M. fortuitum, M. chelonae, M. kansasii, M. gordonae, M. xenopi, and M. marinum*
Man-made water sources	Drinking water supply pipelines Cold and hot water tanks Hot-tubs, indoor and outdoor pools Household plumbing, showerheads, and faucets Hospital plumbing and water supply Ice machines and commercial ice Bottled drinking water	MAC, *M. kansasii, M. gordonae, M. xenopi, M. abscessus, M. fortuitum, M. chelonae, M. scrofulaceum*, and *M. szulgai*
Aerosols	Showers, hot-tubs, humidifiers, indoor swimming pools, and heater-cooler units in hospitals	MAC, *M. kansasii, M. gordonae*, and *M. abscessus*
Other sources*	Natural soil dust, potting soil, peat moss, and domestic dust	MAC, *M. fortuitum, M. chelonae, and M. kansasii*

M. avium complex: *M. intracellulare, M. avium*, and *M. chimaera*

M. abscessus subspecies: *M. abscessus* subspecies *abscessus*, *M. abscessus* subspecies *massiliense*, and *M. abscessus* subspecies *bolletii*

*Contaminated tattoo inks: *M. haemophilum* skin disease; contaminated metal working fluids: *M. immunogenum* skin disease.

TABLE 2 Differences between nontuberculous mycobacteria and *Mycobacterium tuberculosis.*

Characteristics	Nontuberculous mycobacteria (NTM)	*Mycobacterium tuberculosis (M. tb)*
Nomenclature	*Preferred name*: Nontuberculous mycobacteria (NTM). Other names include mycobacteria other than tuberculosis (MOTT), atypical mycobacteria, anonymous mycobacteria, and environmental mycobacteria	• *Mycobacterium tuberculosis* (*M. tb*): Member of *Mycobacterium tuberculosis* complex (MTBC) • Other species in MTBC: *M. africanum*, *M. bovis*, *M. canetti*, *M. caprae*, and *M. pinnipedii*
NTM species distribution	Nearly 200 species. Regional variation of NTM species due to climatic and geographical factors	*M. tb strains*: Beijing (most pathogenic), Cameroon, CAS, EAI, Haarlem, LAM, and Manu (Indian)
Microscopic morphology	Absence of characteristics serpentine cords in acid-fast smears	Characteristic serpentine cording seen as rope-like aggregates
Growth in cultures	• Rapidly growing mycobacteria (<7 days) • Slowly growing mycobacteria (≥7 days)	Slowly growing mycobacteria (≥14 days)
Transmission	Person-to-person transmission does not occur except *M. abscessus* among cystic fibrosis patients	*M. tb* is highly transmissible in cavitary PTB with and high bacillary loads
Route of entry	*Sources*: Inhalation, ingestion, or direct inoculation. Route for NTM-PD inhalation is airborne	Smaller cough droplet nuclei (<1–10 μM) carrying *M. tb* reach terminal bronchioles and alveoli and establish infection
Pathogenicity	Opportunistic organisms	Highly pathogenic and obligate parasites
Virulence	Generally, NTM have low virulence *M. kansasii* is more virulent among NTM	Highly virulent
Latent infection	No evidence of latency	*Latent TB infection*: Important source of future cases
Case notification	NTM disease notification is practiced only in a few countries	Systematic TB notification is encouraged WHO annually publishes Global TB Report
Risk factors	• Preexisting lung disease • Impaired mucociliary function or in individuals with heterozygous for CFTR mutations • GERD	• TB can involve both healthy and destroyed lungs • *Risk factors*: Malnutrition, tobacco smoking, chronic alcohol intake, diabetes mellitus, overcrowding, HIV/AIDS, head or neck cancer, leukemia, or Hodgkin's disease, drugs including corticosteroids, TNF-α inhibitors, or receptor blocker
Radiographic patterns in pulmonary disease	• Cavitary in elderly smokers with COPD patients • Nodular/bronchiectatic (NB) • Hypersensitivity pneumonitis-like pulmonary disease due to MAC	• Primary complex (usually in children) • Progressive pulmonary disease • Miliary PTB • *Postprimary PTB*: Cavitary, atelectasis, and consolidation • Sequelae such as fibrotic and calcified lesions
Drug susceptibility testing (DST)	Phenotypic and genotypic DST for selected drugs *MAC*: macrolides (clarithromycin) and amikacin *M. kansasii*: rifampicin and clarithromycin *RGM species*: Macrolides, amikacin, sulfamethoxazole, doxycycline, minocycline, tigecycline, and cefoxitin linezolid. Status of *erm* (41) gene in *M. abscessus* should be known	Universal DST should be performed As per sensitivity profile of *M. tb*, disease should be categorized into DS-TB, Hr-TB, MDR/RR-TB, and XDR-TB
Treatment	Following treatment guidelines on NTM diseases: • American Thoracic Society (ATS), 2007 • British Thoracic Society (BTS), 2017 • ATS/ERS/ESMID/IDSA, 2020	National guidelines should be followed for treatment of drug sensitive and DR-TB
Treatment outcomes	Treatment outcomes differ among NTM species and subspecies	Treatment outcome in drug-sensitive TB is good Treatment of DR-TB is challenging and global success rate is 56%
Prevention	Exposure to NTM from environmental sources *especially* household water systems, hospital settings, and soil should be avoided	Exposure to smear positive PTB should be avoided to prevent *M. tb* transmission

(CAS: Central Asian strain; CFTR: cystic fibrosis transmembrane regulator gene; DS-TB: drug sensitive-TB; EAI: East African Indian strain; *erm:* erythromycin ribosome methylation; ERS: European Respiratory Society; ESMID: European Society of Clinical Microbiology and Infectious Diseases; Hr-TB: isoniazid resistant-TB; IDSA: Infectious Disease Society of America; LAM: Latin American-Mediterranean strain; MDR/RR-TB: multidrug resistant/rifampicin resistant-TB; SGM; slowly growing mycobacteria; RGM: rapidly growing mycobacteria; TNF-α: tumor necrosis factor-α; XDR-TB: extensively drug-resistant TB)

Note: Underlying esophageal disease must be ruled out in NTM-PD due to RGM especially *M. fortuitum*.

BOX 2	Factors contributing to increased NTM burden.
• Genetic evolution in NTM due to mutations leading to increased virulence	
• Environmental and climatic changes due to increased human-manufactured infrastructure	
• Changes in host immunity due to increased life expectancy and immunocompromised population	
• Increased incidence of chronic lung diseases	
• Decreasing "herd immunity" due to declining TB burden especially in high-income countries	
• Widespread availability of computed tomography (CT) scanning and laboratory infrastructure for NTM diagnosis	
• Increasing awareness among medical personnel about NTM disease	
• Sharp rise in NTM publications by laboratories and practicing physicians	

while UK data suggest that NTM-positive culture incidence increased from 4 per 100,000 to 6.1 per 100,000 between 2007 and 2012. Similarly, a study from Canada reported significant increases in prevalence of NTM-PD from 29.3 cases/100,000 in 1998–2002 to 41.3/100,000 in 2006–2010. Various factors that are responsible for these increases in incidence and prevalence are listed in **Box 2**.

RISK FACTORS

Various risk factors for NTM-PD are described in **Box 3**. Preexistent lung disease is mostly present in these patients. In the absence of obvious structural lung disease, patients may have quantitatively impaired ciliary function or may be heterozygous for CF transmembrane regulator (CFTR) gene mutations. Certain environmental factors such as water sources and reservoirs have also been reported as risk factors (**Box 4**).

PATTERNS

Chronic pulmonary disease is the most common form of NTM disease. *Three patterns of pulmonary involvement have been described*—(1) fibrocavitary (FC) type, which usually occurs in the upper lobe with history of smoking in an older male patient with prior lung disease such as chronic obstructive pulmonary disease (COPD), bronchiectasis, and CF; (2) nodular/bronchiectatic type of pattern occurring in postmenopausal, non-smoking females, and predominantly having right middle lobe and left lingular bronchiectasis with a few lung nodules. These patients may have other features such as mitral valve prolapse, silicosis, and pectus excavatum, high prevalence of gastroesophageal reflux disease (26–44%), increased adiponectin, decreased leptin and estrogen levels and abnormalities in fibrillin gene; (3) hypersensitivity pneumonitis-like NTM-PD or "hot tub lung" occurring due to exposure to aerosols from indoor hot tub.

BOX 3	Host-related risk factors for NTM-pulmonary disease.
• Destroyed lungs due to TB or other diseases like pneumoconioses	
• Bronchiectasis (especially middle lobe and lingula) due to any cause	
• Chronic obstructive pulmonary disease	
• Lung cancer	
• Thoracic skeletal abnormalities (kyphoscoliosis)	
• Pulmonary alveolar proteinosis	
• Rheumatoid arthritis with lung involvement	
• Primary ciliary dyskinesia	
• Gastroesophageal reflux disease*	
• Lady Windermere syndrome†	
• Cystic fibrosisCFTR gene polymorphism‡	
• Alpha 1 antitrypsin deficiency‡	

(CFTR: cystic fibrosis transmembrane regulator gene)

* In gastroesophageal reflux disorders, RGM are commonly involved in the disease *especially* as *M. fortuitum*.

† NTM disease especially nodular-bronchiectatic type in nonsmoking postmenopausal white women who are taller and lean with scoliosis, pectus excavatum, and mitral valve prolapse syndrome than their peers.

‡ Rare genetic abnormalities.

BOX 4	Environmental risk factors for NTM-pulmonary disease.
• Soil exposure	
• Showers and hot tubs	
• Municipal water supply	
• Kitchen sink biofilms, ice machines, refrigerator taps	
• Indoor swimming pool use in past 4 months	
• Outdoor swimming pool use for at least once a month	
• Infection from spa, Jacuzzi, whirlpool footbath, saunas, and pedicure procedures	

SPECIES AND PULMONARY DISEASE

Because of variable virulence of NTM species, it is important to identify NTM species and subspecies in the case of *M. abscessus* for management of NTM-PD. It has been reported that only 25–60% patients with positive respiratory specimens fulfill clinical, radiographic, and microbiologic criteria of NTM-PD. Patients in whom *M. kansasii* and *M. malmoense* are isolated from respiratory specimens frequently meet clinical disease criteria, as these NTM isolates are clinically highly relevant, whereas 40–60% with *Mycobacterium avium* complex (MAC), *M. abscessus*, and *M. xenopi* and <20% patients with *M. chelonae* and *M. fortuitum* meet clinical disease criteria.

The potential to produce specific clinical type of lung disease also varies among NTM species. While *M. kansasii*, *M. xenopi*, and *M. malmoense* commonly cause FC disease but rarely cause nodular-bronchiectatic disease, MAC and *M. abscessus* cause both types of NTM-PDs and MAC and *M. immunogenum* cause hypersensitivity pneumonitis-like NTM-PD.

Mycobacterium avium complex is the most common NTM isolated from respiratory secretions in almost all international studies in patients with NTM-PD. While single strain of MAC species is repeatedly isolated in the cavitary type, several strains of MAC species may occur simultaneously, or the strain may change sequentially in nodular-bronchiectatic type. Relapse versus new reinfection of MAC infection after treatment completion can be differentiated by MAC genotyping.

While tap water was the source of *M. avium* infection and soil was the source of *M. intracellulare* infection in one study from North America. Studies have also suggested that patients with *M. intracellulare* lung disease tend to present at an advance stage with adverse prognosis than patients with *M. avium* lung disease. *M. chimaera* has low virulence than *M. avium* and *M. intracellulare*. Significant geographic variation exists in the distribution of NTM species in the United States. Whereas MAC was the most common species isolated in the South, *M. abscessus*/*M. chelonae* was proportionately higher in the West in one study. MAC species has regional variation: while *M. avium* is dominantly found in South America and Europe and *M. intracellulare* in South Africa and Australia. Recurrence rates also differ among MAC species.

The second common NTM species also has geographical variation: while *M. abscessus* is the second most common cause of NTM-PD in USA, *M. kansasii* in some European countries including UK, *M. xenopi* in some parts of Europe and Canada and *M. malmoense* in northern Europe are the second most common causes of NTM-PD. *M. kansasii*, one of the slowly growing NTM, is most virulent. About 80% of NTM-PD due to RGM results from *M. abscessus*. There are three subspecies of *M. abscessus*—(1) *M. abscessus* subspecies *abscessus* is the most common pathogen (45–65%); followed by (2) *M. abscessus* subspecies *massiliense* (20–55%) and (3) *M. abscessus* subspecies *bolletii* (1–18%). Patients with gastroesophageal disease may have NTM-PD due to RGM such as *M. fortuitum*.

CLINICAL FEATURES

Respiratory symptoms and signs in NTM-PD vary depending on the clinical type. Patients with cavitary type have constitutional symptoms such as fever, anorexia, progressive fatigue, malaise, and weight loss. Additional features may include shortness of breath, cough with expectoration, and hemoptysis due to prior underlying lung disease. Patients with nodular bronchiectasis usually have milder respiratory symptoms and nagging cough may be prominent. Clinical and radiographic presentation in *M. kansasii* pulmonary disease is similar to *M. tb.* Patients with hypersensitivity pneumonitis-like NTM-PD have subacute onset of respiratory symptoms involving young subjects without preexisting lung disease and the prognosis is good.

DIAGNOSIS

CRITERIA FOR DIAGNOSIS

Healthcare provider should carefully assess causality association of the isolated NTM species with patient's symptoms and signs. Approximately, one-third of NTM species are potentially pathogenic for humans. It is possible that an individual with a particular NTM isolate may not have an active disease or it may not be clinically relevant. American Thoracic Society (ATS) and Infectious Disease Society of America (IDSA) (2007) and British Thoracic Society (BTS) (2017), ATS/ERS/ESMID/IDSA (ATS/European Respiratory Society/European Society of Clinical Microbiology and Infectious Diseases/IDSA), 2020 have published guidelines to standardize the diagnosis of NTM disease. Clinical and microbiological criteria for diagnosis of NTM pulmonary disease are detailed in **Table 3**.

DIFFERENTIAL DIAGNOSIS

Because of similar clinical features and radiographic appearances, diseases such as tuberculosis, recurrent pulmonary aspirations, pneumonitis, bronchiectasis, histoplasmosis, aspergillosis, and lung cancer should be considered in the differential diagnosis and should be appropriately ruled out. In the laboratory, the presence of *Pseudomonas aeruginosa*, *Staphylococcus aureus*, *Nocardia*, and *Aspergillus* in the specimens must be carefully tested.

INVESTIGATIONS

SPECIMEN COLLECTION AND PROCESSING

A proper sample collection is imperative to establish a correct laboratory diagnosis of NTM disease. In case of NTM-PD patients, utmost care should be given to avoid contamination while collecting sputum specimens. **Box 5** details precautions for samples collection, transportation, and laboratory processing.

LABORATORY TECHNIQUES

Besides traditional staining and culture-based techniques, newer techniques have been used to identify NTM at species and subspecies levels. High-pressure liquid chromatography (HPLC), matrix-assisted laser desorption/ionization time-of-flight (MALDI-TOF), line probe assay, and gene sequencing (*rpoB*, *hsp65*, 16S rRNA, 16S-23S rRNA ITS sequence and *erm* genes) and whole genome sequencing are modern techniques used for NTM species and subspecies identification. MALDI-TOF-MS is the most rapid technique which identifies around 160 NTM species. At present, gene sequencing is considered as gold standard to identify NTM species and subspecies. The diagnostic algorithm for NTM isolation is described in **Flowchart 1**.

TABLE 3 Clinical and microbiologic criteria for diagnosis of nontuberculous mycobacterial pulmonary disease.*

Clinical	Pulmonary or systemic symptoms	Both clinical and radiologic criteria required
Radiologic	Nodular or cavitary opacities on chest radiograph, or a high-resolution computed tomography scan that shows bronchiectasis with multiple small nodules	
Microbiologic†	Appropriate exclusion of other diagnoses • Positive culture results from at least two separate expectorated sputum samples. If the results are nondiagnostic, consider repeat sputum AFB smears and cultures *or* • Positive culture results from at least one bronchial wash or lavage *or* • Transbronchial or other lung biopsy with mycobacterial histologic features (granulomatous inflammation or AFB) and positive culture for NTM or biopsy showing mycobacterial histologic features (granulomatous inflammation or AFB) and one or more sputum or bronchial washings that are culture positive for NTM	

(AFB: acid-fast bacilli; NTM: nontuberculous mycobacteria)

* Expert consultation should be obtained when NTM are recovered that are either infrequently encountered or that usually represent environmental contamination. Patients who are suspected of having NTM pulmonary disease but do not meet the diagnostic criteria should be followed until the diagnosis is firmly established or excluded. Making the diagnosis of NTM, pulmonary disease does not *per se*, necessitate the institution of therapy, which is a decision based on the potential risks and benefits of therapy for individual patients.

† When two positive cultures are obtained, the isolates should be the same NTM species (or subspecies in the case of *M. abscessus*) in order to meet disease criteria.

Source (for Tables 4, 5, 6, 7, 8 also): Reproduced with permission of the © ERS 2020: Daley CL, Iaccarino JM, Lange C, Cambau E, Wallace RJ, Andrejak C, et al. Treatment of nontuberculous mycobacterial pulmonary disease: An official ATS/ ERS/ESCMID/IDSA clinical practice guideline. Clin Infect Dis. 2020;71:905-13.

BOX 5 Precautions for specimen collection and laboratories diagnosis of NTM.

- Individuals should not rinse their mouths with tap water or other fluids before submitting the respiratory specimens
- Use a sterile, leak proof, and disposable plastic container is recommended
- Specimen should be kept at 2–8°C, if transport is delayed >1 hour and should not be kept >1 week
- Use of tap water or stored distilled water should be avoided in laboratory procedures
- Use of 70% alcohol and 5% phenol as disinfectant is recommended for bench surface cleaning and biosafety filters
- Plastic ware and glassware used in laboratory should be autoclaved at 131°C under 15 psi pressure
- Incubation temperature for every species may vary between 27°C and 45°C and requires constant monitoring

Techniques such as HPLC, MALDI-TOF, and LPA have limitations because limited number of NTM species is detected. Also, these techniques have low discriminatory power to identify genetically closely related NTM species. LPA is the most widely used technique in National TB Elimination Program (NTEP) laboratories in India for NTM species identification.

DRUG SUSCEPTIBILITY TESTING

Drug susceptibility testing for NTM is controversial because of discrepancy between *in vitro* susceptibility results and the treatment response. DST should follow Clinical and Laboratory Standards Institute (CLSI) guidelines. Both phenotypic and genotypic DST for MAC and *M. kansasii* are performed for initial and recurrent isolates. RGM species (and subspecies) show different drug resistance patterns and DST should be selectively done for following antibiotics: Macrolides, amikacin, tobramycin, imipenem, trimethoprim-sulfamethoxazole, doxycycline, minocycline, tigecycline, cefoxitin, and linezolid. Information on an active *erm* (41) gene is important in RGM (*especially* in *M. abscessus* subspecies) because of presence of inducible resistance to macrolides. Constitutive resistance to macrolides can occur due to mutation in 23S rRNA gene. **Table 4** describes the recommendations on DST for important NTM species.

TREATMENT

Various scientific bodies have published guidelines for the management of NTM diseases. While ATS/IDSA guidelines (2007) deal with both pulmonary and extrapulmonary NTM diseases. BTS guidelines (2017) and ATS/ERS/ESCMID/IDSA guideline (2020) deal specifically with NTM-PD.

Treating physician should be well versed with the knowledge of various NTM species in his geographical area. Despite repeated isolation of NTM, laboratory contamination and colonization in the host must be ruled out. Subsequently, underlying predisposing structural lung disease should be identified and its severity evaluated. NTM-PD should be stratified into mild-moderate (nonsevere) and severe NTM-PD (**Box 6**) on the basis of patient's systemic signs and symptoms, chest radiographic appearances, and microbiologic features (acid-fast smear status, bacillary load, mycobacterial culture, NTM species, and subspecies characterization). The conventional microbiological outcomes include smear status, culture conversion, and relapse (**Box 7**). Recent ATS/ERS/ESCMID/

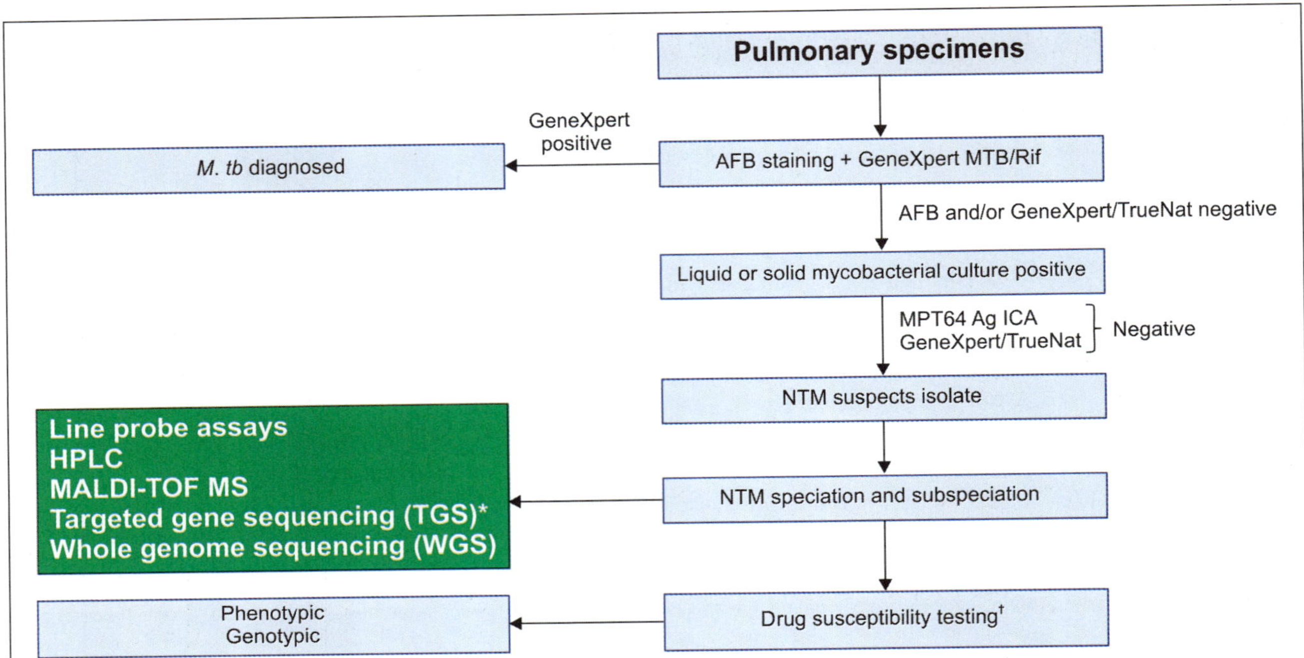

(*M. tb*: *Mycobacterium tuberculosis*; MPT64Ag ICA: *M. tb* MPT64 antigen immunochromatographic assay; MALDI-TOF MS: matrix-assisted laser desorption-ionization time-of-flight mass spectrometry)

* For NTM species and subspecies (for MAC and *M. abscessus*) identification sequencing of target genes such as: *rpo*B, *hsp*65, 16S rRNA, 16S-23S rRNA ITS region, *erm* gene, *dnaJ*, *sec* A1, and *rec* A has been reported in literature. A multilocus target gene sequencing approach is recommended for NTM speciation and subspeciation.

† DST in generally done in nonresponsive patients with MAC and *M. kansasii* disease. Phenotypic (on 3–5 and 14 days) and genotypic [for *erm* (41) gene] DST in *M. abscessus* disease.

FLOWCHART 1: Laboratory diagnosis of NTM pulmonary disease.

TABLE 4 Recommended phenotypic and genotypic DST in important NTM species.

NTM species	Name of drug	Phenotypic DST	Genotypic DST	
		MIC cutoff	*Genes associated with mutations*	*Type of resistance*
***M. avium* complex**	Clarithromycin*	>32 µg/mL	23S rRNA (*rrl*) gene	Acquired resistance
	Amikacin: • Parenteral • Liposomal	 >64 µg/mL >128 µg/mL	16S rRNA (*rrs*) gene	Acquired resistance
M. kansasii	Rifampicin Clarithromycin*	>2 µg/mL ≥32 µg/mL	*rpoB* gene Not recommended	Acquired resistance Acquired resistance
M. abscessus	Clarithromycin*	≥8 µg/mL	Dysfunctional *erm* (41) gene (if susceptibility observed at day 3–5 and 14) †Functional *erm* (41) gene (if resistance observed at day 14) 23S rRNA gene (if resistance observed at day 3–5 and 14)	Macrolide susceptible (in subspecies *M. abscessus. massiliense*) Inducible resistance (in subspecies *M. abscessus—abscessus* and *M. abscessus—bolletii*) Constitutive resistance(it can occur in any *M. abscessus* subspecies)
	Amikacin	>64 µg/mL	16S RNA (*rrs*) gene	Acquired resistance

(DST: drug susceptibility testing; MIC: minimum inhibitory concentration)

* Clarithromycin is used as a class agent for macrolides.

† Presence of T instead of C at 28th nucleotide position in *erm* (41) gene confers *M. abscessus* resistance against clarithromycin.

BOX 6	Definitions of mild-moderate and severe NTM-PD.

- **Mild-moderate (nonsevere disease):**
  - Mild-moderate symptoms
  - No signs of systemic illness
  - Absence of lung cavitation and extensive lung disease
  - AFB smear-negative in the pulmonary specimens
- **Severe disease:**
  - Presence of severe symptoms and signs of systemic illness
  - Presence of lung cavitation and extensive lung involvement
  - Pulmonary specimens positive for AFB smear

(AFB: acid-fast bacilli; NTM-PD: nontuberculous mycobacteria-pulmonary disease)

Source (for Box 7 also): Adapted from Haworth CS, Banks J, Capstick T, Fisher AJ, Gorsuch T, Laurenson IF, et al. British Thoracic Society Guideline for the management of non-tuberculous mycobacterial pulmonary disease (NTM-PD) BMJ Open Respir Res. 2017;4(1):e000242.

BOX 7	Definitions for microbiological outcomes NTM-PD.

Culture conversion:

Three consecutive negative mycobacterial sputum cultures collected over a minimum of 3 months, with the time of conversion being the date of the first of the three negative mycobacterial cultures. In patients unable to expectorate sputum, a single negative mycobacterial culture of a CT-directed bronchial wash is indicative of culture conversion.

Recurrence:

Two positive mycobacterial cultures following culture conversion. Genotyping may help to distinguish relapse from reinfection

Refractory disease:

Failure to culture-convert after 6 months of nontuberculous mycobacterial treatment.

IDSA guidelines (2020) suggest treatment initiation rather than watchful waiting, especially in the context of positive acid-fast bacilli (AFB) sputum smears and/or cavitary lung disease. Whereas, a watchful waiting is preferred in patients with mild disease because of the following: higher chances of drug intolerance and adverse drug reactions and poor response to treatment in some NTM species (e g., *M. abscessus*). In such cases before initiating the treatment, the patient should be counseled about potential adverse effects of drugs, the uncertainties of benefits of antimicrobial therapy, and the possibility for recurrence including reinfection (specifically in nodular-bronchiectatic disease setting). It is suggested that treatment regimens should be designed by experts in the management of complicated NTM infections.

DRUG REGIMENS

Nontuberculous mycobacteria-PD due to MAC is generally treated with a drug regimen, consisting of three to four antibiotics, administered either daily or thrice weekly depending upon the severity of disease, patient's tolerance of drugs, and occurrence of side effects and the therapy is continued for at least 12 months following sputum culture conversion. *M. kansasii*-related NTM-PD is treated with ant-TB drugs consisting of rifamycin, isoniazid, and ethambutol. Pyrazinamide is not recommended for *M. kansasii* pulmonary disease as the organism is naturally resistant to pyrazinamide (a prodrug) due to reduced pyrazinamidase activity preventing conversion of the drug into pyrazinoic acid which is an active bactericidal compound. A significant proportion of patients with NTM-PD discontinues the prescribed treatment because of lengthy duration and occurrence of side effects. The treatment regimens vary depending on the isolation of NTM species, clinical phenotypes and drug susceptibility profiles leading to varying therapeutic response. The variable treatment response is related to several factors such as NTM species (*M. avium vs. M. abscessus*) and subspecies (*M. abscessus* subspecies *massiliense vs. M. abscessus* subspecies *abscessus*), disease phenotype (FC vs. nodular bronchiectatic), and the treatment regimen (drug treatment regimen with macrolide vs. without macrolide).

Mycobacterium avium complex-related NTM-PD is treated with a drug regimen comprising rifampicin (or rifabutin in HIV-positive individuals to avoid drug-drug interactions), ethambutol, and macrolide (azithromycin or clarithromycin; some patients tolerate azithromycin better). There is *in vitro* synergy of antimycobacterial action between rifampicin and ethambutol as the latter destabilizes mycobacterial cell wall and facilitates rifampicin entry into the mycobacteria to its target site, the RNA polymerase. These two drugs also prevent development of macrolide resistance. Neither isoniazid nor moxifloxacin is very much active against MAC, clofazimine and amikacin are good alternatives. BTS guidelines (2017) recommend intermittent three-times-weekly treatment for noncavitary (nonsevere) MAC-PD due to potential benefits, better treatment adherence and comparable efficacy. As per guidelines, intravenous or nebulized amikacin can be added as fourth drug for the initial 3 months in patients with severe or macrolide-resistant MAC-PD (**Table 5**). The pooled treatment success rates in MAC-PD in the five systematic reviews ranged from 32 to 65% and 12 to 16% of the enrolled patients had not completed treatment.

Patients with clarithromycin-resistant MAC-PD should be treated with rifampicin, ethambutol and isoniazid or a quinolone and intravenous amikacin, or nebulized amikacin (if intravenous amikacin is not tolerated or impractical to administer or is contraindicated) for initial 3 months. The treatment of macrolide-resistant (MR)-MAC-PD is challenging because of poor sputum culture conversion rates (15–36%) and high mortality rates at 2-year (9–15%) and 5-year (47%). A recent systematic review and meta-analysis of nine studies reported poor treatment

TABLE 5 Recommended treatment regimens for *M. avium* complex, *M. kansasii*, and *M. xenopi* pulmonary disease.

Organism	Number of drugs	Preferred drug regimen	Dosing frequency
***M. avium* complex**			
Nodular-bronchiectatic	3	• Rifampicin (rifabutin) • Ethambutol • Azithromycin (clarithromycin)	Three times weekly
Cavitary	≥3	• Rifampicin (rifabutin) • Ethambutol • Azithromycin (clarithromycin) • Amikacin IV (streptomycin)*	Daily (three times weekly may be used with aminoglycosides)
Refractory†	≥4	• Rifampicin (rifabutin) • Ethambutol • Amikacin liposome inhalation suspension or amikacin IV (streptomycin)* • Azithromycin (clarithromycin)	Daily (three times weekly may be used with aminoglycosides)
M. kansasii			
	3	• Rifampicin (rifabutin) • Ethambutol • Azithromycin (clarithromycin)	Daily
	3	• Azithromycin (clarithromycin) • Rifampicin (rifabutin) • Ethambutol	Three times weekly
	3	• Rifampicin (rifabutin) • Ethambutol • Isoniazid	Daily
M. xenopi			
	≥3	• Rifampicin (rifabutin) • Ethambutol • Azithromycin (clarithromycin) and/or moxifloxacin • Amikacin*	Daily (three times weekly may be used with aminoglycosides)

Alternative drugs for patients who are intolerant of or whose isolate is resistant to first-line drugs include clofazimine, moxifloxacin, and linezolid. Some experts would consider bedaquiline or tedizolid

* Consider for cavitary, extensive nodular/bronchiectatic disease or macrolide-resistant MAC. Amikacin or streptomycin may be given three times a week.

† *Refractory disease*: Sputum culture positive after 6 months of guideline-based therapy. Amikacin liposome inhalation suspension (ALIS) has been shown to improve culture conversion when added to guideline-based therapy in treatment refractory patients with MAC pulmonary disease.

outcomes in MR-MAC-PD with overall 21% sputum culture conversion rate and 10% one-year all-cause mortality with no difference between nodular bronchiectatic (NB) and FC type of MR-MAC-PD. Despite the combination of multiple antibiotics including amikacin liposomal inhalation solution (ALIS) and surgical resection, the treatment outcomes of MR-MAC-PD were poor.

Table 5 describes treatment regimens for *M. kansasii* pulmonary disease. One-time isolation of *M. kansasii* from sputum sample is considered pathogenic and should be treated immediately. *M. kansasii*-pulmonary disease is treated with a treatment regimen similar to pulmonary TB. Although, MICs of isoniazid for *M. kansasii* are higher as compared to *M. tb*, therefore, macrolide (clarithromycin or azithromycin) is preferred over isoniazid for the treatment of *M. kansasii*.

Treatment regimen for *M. xenopi* pulmonary disease has been detailed in **Table 5**. While four-drug regimen (rifampicin, ethambutol, macrolide, and moxifloxacin) is used to treat nonsevere disease, intravenous amikacin or nebulized amikacin is added to the regimen as a fifth drug for severe disease. Treatment response of macrolide containing response in patients with *M. malmoense* NTM-PD is better than MAC or *M. xenopi*. Treatment for other slowly growing can be extrapolated from common NTM species. Isolation of *M. simiae* is rarely associated with true infection. Limited success is seen in *M. simiae* infection with rifampicin and ethambutol-based drug regimen and a combination of amikacin and clofazimine may be used to construct a drug regimen to treat the infection.

The treatment details of pulmonary disease due to *M. abscessus* are provided in **Table 6** and antibiotic

TABLE 6 Treatment regimens for *M. abscessus* by macrolide susceptibility (mutational and inducible resistance).

Macrolide susceptibility pattern		*Number of drugs‡*	*Preferred drugs*	*Frequency of dosing*
Mutational*	**Inducible†**			
Susceptible	**Susceptible**	Initial phase ≥3	• *Parenteral (choose 1–2)*: ◦ Amikacin ◦ Imipenem (or Cefoxitin) ◦ Tigecycline • *Oral (choose 2)*: ◦ Azithromycin (clarithromycin)§ ◦ Clofazimine ◦ Linezolid	Daily (three times weekly may be used for aminoglycosides)
		Continuation phase ≥2	• *Oral/inhaled (choose 2–3)*: ◦ Azithromycin (clarithromycin)§ ◦ Clofazimine ◦ Linezolid ◦ Inhaled amikacin	
Susceptible	**Resistant**	Initial phase ≥4	• *Parenteral (choose 2–3)*: ◦ Amikacin ◦ Imipenem (or cefoxitin) ◦ Tigecycline • *Oral (choose 2–3)*: ◦ Azithromycin (clarithromycin) ◦ Clofazimine ◦ Linezolid	Daily (three times weekly may be used for aminoglycosides)
		Continuation phase ≥ 2	*Oral/inhaled (choose 2–3)*: • Azithromycin (clarithromycin) • Clofazimine • Linezolid • Inhaled amikacin	
Resistant	**Susceptible or resistant**	Initial phase ≥4	• *Parenteral (choose 2–3)*: ◦ Amikacin ◦ Imipenem (or Cefoxitin) ◦ Tigecycline • *Oral (choose 2–3)*: ◦ Azithromycin (clarithromycin) ◦ Clofazimine ◦ Linezolid	Daily (three times weekly may be used for aminoglycosides)
		Continuation phase ≥2	*Oral/inhaled (choose 2–3)*: • Azithromycin (clarithromycin) • Clofazimine • Linezolid • Inhaled amikacin	

* Mutational resistance: none present: isolate determined to be phenotypically susceptible at 3–5 days of incubation in culture. Present: isolate determined to be phenotypically resistant at 3–5 days of incubation or sequencing identifies *rrl* mutation know to confer resistance.

† Inducible resistance: Functional *erm* (41) gene: Isolate determined to be resistant after 14 days of incubation or sequencing identifies functional gene sequence. Nonfunctional *erm* (41) gene: Isolate determined to be susceptible after 14 days of incubation or sequencing identifies truncated sequence or C28 mutation (in subspecies *abscessus*).

‡ Initial phase refers to the time that the parenteral agents are being given. Continuation phase refers to the subsequent phase of therapy that typically includes oral antimicrobial agents sometimes paired with inhaled agents.

§ Azithromycin (clarithromycin) is active in this setting and should be used whenever possible.

Azithromycin (clarithromycin) activity is unlikely but can be added for its immunomodulatory effects but should not be counted as active against *M. abscessus* with a functional *erm* (41) gene. In this setting, frequent sputum cultures should be obtained to detect potentially new organisms like *M. avium* complex.

combination is administered according to the DST profile. A precise identification of subspecies along with information on *erm* (41) gene is important in *M. abscessus* infection because of a variable treatment response. The treatment outcomes among three subspecies of *M. abscessus* differ due to *erm* (41) gene and inducible and constitutive resistance to macrolides (**Table 4**). Presence of T instead of C at 28th nucleotide position in *erm* (41) gene confers *M. abscessus* resistance against clarithromycin. In patients with lung infection due to *M. fortuitum,* underlying gastroesophageal reflux disease should be carefully evaluated and treated.

INHALED ANTIBIOTICS

Similar to TB treatment, drug treatment regimens comprising three to four drugs are used for treating NTM-PD for longer periods with high discontinuation rates (9–39%) due to significant side effects. Use of inhaled drugs in bronchial asthma, COPD and *P. aeruginosa* infections in CF patients has demonstrated successful treatment outcomes while achieving higher drug concentrations at the disease site without simultaneous development of significant systemic side effects. Similar approach can be followed in NTM-PD to achieve higher drug concentrations at infected pulmonary sites with minimal extrapulmonary exposure to avoid side effects. Inhaled amikacin along with other oral drugs is already used in patients with severe NTM-PD. Development of inhaled clofazimine suspension for administration via nebulizer device in NTM-PD treatment is in progress. In addition, studies using inhaled recombinant granulocyte-macrophage colony-stimulating factor and exogenous nitric oxide gas are in progress to evaluate their antibacterial effect on *M. abscessus.* Dosing guidelines for drugs used in the management of NTM-PD are provided in **Table 7**.

Monitoring of drug toxicities: Drugs required for treatment NTM-PD have many potential adverse events (**Table 8**). During follow-up period, side effects of treatment should be checked by regular clinical as well as laboratory monitoring of these systems and if required, necessary modification in the treatment can be done.

TABLE 7 Dosing guidelines for drugs used in the management of nontuberculous mycobacterial pulmonary disease.

Drug	Daily dosing	Thrice weekly dosing	Hepatic impairment	Renal impairment
Oral				
Azithromycin	250–500 mg/ day	500 mg/day	N/A	N/A
Ciprofloxacin	500–750 mg twice/day	N/A	N/A	250–500 mg dosed at intervals according to CrCl
Clarithromycin	500 mg twice/day	500 mg twice/day	N/A	Reduce dose by 50% if CrCl < 30 mL/min
Clofazimine*	100–200 mg/day	N/A	Caution in severe hepatic impairment	N/A
Doxycycline	100 mg once to twice a day	N/A	N/A	N/A
Ethambutol	15 mg/kg/day	25 mg/kg/day	N/A	Increase dosing interval (e.g., 15–25 mg/kg, three times/week)
Isoniazid	5 mg·kg^{-1} up to 300 mg/day	N/A	Caution	N/A
Linezolid	600 mg once or twice/day†	N/A	N/A	N/A
Moxifloxacin	400 mg per day	N/A	N/A	N/A
Rifabutin	150–300 mg/day (150 mg per day with clarithromycin)	300 mg/day	Caution	Reduce dose by 50% if CrCl < 30 mL/min
Rifampicin (rifampin)	10 mg/kg (450 mg or 600 mg)/day	600 mg/day	Caution	N/A
Trimethoprim/ Sulfamethoxazole	800 mg/160 mg tab twice daily	N/A	Caution	Reduce dose by 50% if CrCl 15–30 mL·min^{-1}
Parenteral				
Amikacin (IV)	10–15 mg/kg/day‡, adjusted according to drug level monitoring§	15–25 mg/kg/day‡, adjusted according to drug level monitoring§	N/A	Reduce dose or increase dosing interval (e.g., 15 mg/kg, two to three times per week)
Cefoxitin (IV)	2–4 g two to three times daily (maximum daily dose is 12 g/day)	N/AC	N/A	Reduce dose or increase dosing interval

Continued...

Continued...

Drug	Daily dosing	Thrice weekly dosing	Hepatic impairment	Renal impairment
Imipenem (IV)	500–1000 mg, two to three times/day	N/A	N/A	Reduce dose or increase dosing interval
Streptomycin (IV or IM)	10–15 mg/kg/day, adjusted according to drug level monitoring	15–25 mg/kg/day, adjusted according to drug level monitoring	N/A	Reduce dose or increase dosing interval (e.g., 15 mg/kg, two to three times/week)
Tigecycline (IV)	25–50 mg once or twice/day†	N/A	25 mg once or twice daily in severe hepatic impairment	N/A
Inhalation				
Amikacin liposome inhalation suspension	590 mg/day	N/A	N/A	N/A
Amikacin, parenteral formulation	250–500 mg/ day	N/A	N/A	N/A

* Clofazimine availability varies by country. In the United States, an investigational new drug application is required.

† Most experts recommend once daily dosing of linezolid and tigecycline due to the high rate of drug-related adverse reactions associated with twice daily dosing.

‡ The use of the described regimens for 15 weeks was associated with permanent ototoxicity in approximately one-third of patients, and the risk was associated with age and cumulative dose. Given the high rates of ototoxicity, risks and benefits should be carefully considered in light of the goals of therapy. Clinicians should consider lower dose ranges and probably rely on intermittent dosing when more prolonged therapy is employed.

§ *Drug level monitoring*: Trough <5 mg/L; peak with daily dosing 35–45 µg/mL; peak with intermittent dosing 65–80 µg/mL.

TABLE 8 Common adverse drug reactions and monitoring recommendations.*

Drug	Adverse reactions	Monitoring
Azithromycin	Gastrointestinal, tinnitus/hearing loss hepatotoxicity, prolonged QTc	Audiogram, LFT, and ECG (QTc)
Clarithromycin	Gastrointestinal, tinnitus/hearing loss Hepatotoxicity, prolonged QTc	Audiogram, LFT, and ECG (QTc)
Ethambutol	Ocular toxicity and neuropathy	Visual acuity and color discrimination
Rifampicin (rifampin)	Hepatotoxicity, cytopenias Hypersensitivity, orange discoloration of secretions	LFT and CBC
Rifabutin	Hepatotoxicity, cytopenias Uveitis, hypersensitivity, orange discoloration of secretions	LFT, CBC, and visual acuity
Isoniazid	Hepatitis, peripheral neuropathy	LFT
Linezolid	Peripheral neuropathy, optic neuritis Cytopenias	Visual acuity and color discrimination, CBC
Moxifloxacin	Prolonged QTc, hepatotoxicity, tendinopathy	ECG (QTc) and LFT
Clofazimine	Tanning of skin and dryness, hepatotoxicity, prolonged QTc	LFT and ECG (QTc)
Doxycycline	GI upset, photosensitivity, and tinnitus/vertigo	Clinical monitoring
Trimethoprim/Sulfamethoxazole	GI upset, cytopenias, hypersensitivity, and photosensitivity	CBC

Continued...

Continued...

Drug	Adverse reactions	Monitoring
Amikacin (intravenous)	Vestibular toxicity, ototoxicity Nephrotoxicity, electrolyte disturbances	Audiograms BUN, creatinine Ca^{2+}, Mg^{2+}, K^{+}
Amikacin liposome inhalation suspension	Dysphonia, vestibular toxicity, ototoxicity, nephrotoxicity, cough, and dyspnea	Audiograms, BUN, and creatinine
Cefoxitin	Cytopenias, hypersensitivity	CBC
Imipenem	Rashes, cytopenias, and nephrotoxicity	CBC, BUN/Creatinine
Tigecycline	Nausea/vomiting and hepatitis/pancreatitis	LFT, amylase/lipase

(QTc: corrected QT; Ca^{2+}: calcium; Mg^{2+}: magnesium, K^{+}: potassium)

Note: Monitoring frequency should be individualized based on treatment regimen, age, comorbidities, concurrent drugs, overlapping drug toxicities, and resources.

* The expert panel recommends that patients have a complete blood count, liver function tests, and metabolic panel every 1–3 months in patients on oral therapy and weekly when on intravenous therapy.

SURGICAL INTERVENTION

Surgery may be considered in carefully selected individuals with NTM-PD who have localized structural lung disease and good pulmonary functions without having impaired gas exchange. Role of a team comprising pulmonary and/or infectious disease specialist, respiratory therapist, and nutrition expert is crucial for a successful surgical outcome. Patients should be advised to pay special attention to maintain adequate calorie intake and body mass index especially if surgical intervention is considered. Monitoring of prealbumin level can serve as a useful marker of nutrition. In some individuals along with antibiotic regimen, probiotic therapy can be helpful.

NONPHARMACOLOGIC TREATMENT

In addition to pharmacological therapy, other nonpharmacological measures can be tried for treating the prior lung disease. These include techniques for mucus clearance such as nebulization using hypertonic saline, aerobic exercises, chest physiotherapy, postural drainage, use of oscillating positive expiratory pressure devices, and high-frequency chest wall oscillation.

BOX 8	Measures for preventing NTM-PD.

Measures to reduce health care-and hygiene-associated NTM disease:

Avoid the following:

- Cleaning of endoscopes with tap water
- Contamination of clinical specimens with tap water and ice
- Use of benzalkonium chloride as a skin disinfectant prior to local injections

Household and personal measures:

- Avoid using saunas, hot tubs or any water with an aerator. Hot water usage should be done in proper ventilation
- Replacement of shower heads at regular intervals; maintain water heater temperature ≥ 54.4°C
- Use sterilized water in humidifiers; avoid ultrasonic humidifiers
- Take steps to reduce gastroesophageal reflux disease (GERD); avoid foods that may trigger it and avoid vulnerable body positions that may cause aspiration

NTM-associated hypersensitivity lung disease: Ensure regular cleaning of indoor pools, hot tubs and hot water pipes.

(NTM: nontuberculous mycobacteria)

PREVENTION

Box 8 details various preventive measures to reduce NTM disease in various settings, especially those due to contamination of disinfectants, ice, wounds, injection sites, catheters, endoscopes etc. can be prevented by proper sterilization.

FUTURE PROSPECTS

Future studies should try to explore the role of risk factors for developing NTM-PD so that the benefit of screening can be offered to high-risk individuals for early diagnosis and treatment. Recent studies have established a role of human-to-human transmission of *M. abscessus* among CF patients; further research should focus on studying mechanisms contributing to patient-to-patient transmission of other NTM species to prevent further spread. Newer nonculture-based methods should be developed for early identification and speciation of NTM from respiratory specimens as present methods rely heavily on mycobacterial culture for identification and further characterization of NTM species causing significant delay in treatment. Future research should focus on understanding the role of DST in predicting treatment outcomes in NTM-PD. Efforts should be directed toward drug discovery and to constitute more effective and less toxic drug regimen for shorter periods for treatment of NTM-PD especially due to *M. abscessus* as this NTM species responds poorly to treatment with frequent relapses occurring after stopping the treatment.

RECOMMENDED READINGS

1. Griffith DE, Aksamit T, Brown-Elliott BA, Catanzaro A, Daley C, Gordin F, et al. An official ATS/IDSA statement: Diagnosis, treatment, and prevention of nontuberculous mycobacterial diseases. Am J Respir Crit Care Med. 2007;175:367-416.
2. Haworth CS, Banks J, Capstick T, Fisher AJ, Gorsuch T, Laurenson IF, et al. British Thoracic Society Guideline for the management of non-tuberculous mycobacterial pulmonary disease (NTM-PD). BMJ Open Respir Res. 2017;4:e000242.
3. Daley CL, Iaccarino JM, Lange C, Cambau E, Wallace RJ, Andrejak C, et al. Treatment of nontuberculous mycobacterial pulmonary disease: An official ATS/ERS/ESCMID/IDSA clinical practice guideline. Clin Infect Dis. 2020;71:905-13.
4. Clinical and Laboratory Standards Institute. Susceptibility testing of mycobacteria, Nocardiae, and other aerobic actinomycetes, 3rd ed. Wayne, PA: CLSI; 2018.
5. Sharma SK, Upadhyay V. Epidemiology, diagnosis and treatment of non-tuberculous mycobacterial diseases. Indian J Med Res. 2020;152:185-226.
6. Sharma SK, Sharma R, Singh BK, Upadhyay V, Mani I, Tripathi M, *et al.* A prospective study of non-tuberculous mycobacterial disease among tuberculosis suspects at a tertiary care centre in north India. *Indian J Med Res.* 2019;*150*:458-67.
7. Parte AC. LPSN—List of Prokaryotic names with standing in nomenclature (bacterio.net), 20 years on. *Int J Syst Evol Microbiol.* 2018;*68*:1825-9.

CHAPTER

212 Interstitial Lung Diseases

Vijay Hadda, Irfan Shekh, Irshad Ahmad Banday

ABSTRACT

The interstitial lung diseases (ILDs) are a heterogeneous group of acute and chronic diffuse lung diseases that are characterized by varying degrees of inflammation and fibrosis. Occurrence of ILDs may be related to known underlying disease, environmental exposure, or without any known etiological context and pose a diagnostic and therapeutic challenges to the clinicians. There is no single diagnostic test for a specific ILD; a confident diagnosis requires careful multidisciplinary discussion incorporating all clinical and radiological features, with or without bronchoalveolar lavage (BAL) fluid cytology or lung histopathology.

The spectrum of various ILDs varies from center to center. In practice, idiopathic pulmonary fibrosis (IPF), chronic hypersensitivity pneumonitis (HP), connective tissue disease (CTD)-associated ILDs, and sarcoidosis are commonly encountered ILDs. The drugs used for treatment of ILDs include corticosteroids, immunosuppressive agents, and antifibrotics. The choice of therapy depends on the underlying ILD. Despite treatment, many patients would develop respiratory failure requiring oxygen therapy or ventilatory support. For such patients, lung transplant is the only life-saving option.

"Diagnosis is not the end, but the beginning of practice"

—Martin H Fischer

INTRODUCTION

The ILDs are a heterogeneous group of acute and chronic diffuse lung diseases that are characterized by varying degrees of inflammation and fibrosis. ILDs may be related to known underlying disease, environmental exposure, or without any known etiological context and pose a diagnostic and therapeutic challenges to the clinicians. Majority of these disorders are characterized by progressively increasing fibrosis and are associated with significant morbidity and mortality, despite use of currently available treatment options.

There is a significant advancement in the understanding of the clinical, radiological, and pathological features of these disorders. Also, with discovery of antifibrotic drugs (pirfenidone and nintedanib) the management of some of the ILDs, especially IPF and systemic sclerosis (SSc) associated ILD has changed significantly. Therefore, it is essential to differentiate various subtypes of ILDs from each other as there are significant differences amongst them in the risk factors, pathogenesis, treatment, and outcomes. This chapter aims to provide insights of recent advances in classification, diagnosis, and management of various types of ILD.

SPECTRUM

For many years, ILDs were being diagnosed and classified without any universally accepted criteria. In an effort to minimize variable and confusing diagnostic criteria for ILDs, the American Thoracic Society (ATS)/ European Respiratory Society (ERS) proposed consensus criteria for classification of ILDs in 2002 and subsequently updated in 2013. These guidelines emphasize the need for multidisciplinary discussion (MDD) among expert pulmonologists, radiologists, rheumatologists, and pathologists familiar with ILD to facilitate accurate diagnosis of ILD. Based on the MDD, ILDs were broadly classified into four categories: (1) ILDs with known causes (drugs, connective diseases, occupational exposure, hypersensitivity pneumonitis (HP), infections etc.), (2) granulomatous diseases (sarcoidosis), (3) idiopathic interstitial pneumonia (IIPs), and (4) other forms of ILDs (pulmonary Langerhans cell histiocytosis, lymphangiomyomatosis etc.). All IIPs can be further divided in to various clinicopathological entities (**Table 1**).

There is lack of data on incidence and prevalence of various ILDs based on benchmark classification proposed by ATS/ERS consensus statements on IIPs. The annual incidence of ILDs, diagnosed with variable criteria, has been reported between 1 and 31.5 per 100,000.

Globally, commonly reported ILDs include - IPF (19.9–43.4%), non-IPF (6.1–27.3%), sarcoidosis (7.8–44.7%), CTD-ILDs (2% to 34.8%), HP (0 to 47.3%), occupational lung disease (2% to 13.9%), drug/radiation (1.1–5%) and unclassifiable (0.2–30.9%).

Data regarding spectrum of ILDs from India is limited to few studies. A multicenter registry reported HP 47.3% (513 out of 1,084 patients) as the most prevalent ILD, contrary to the data from a tertiary care center in north India which reported sarcoidosis (42.2% out of 803 patients) as the most common ILD. At our center, IPF and CTD-ILDs form the bulk of ILDs. The spectrum of ILDs among Indians is shown in **Table 2**.

MULTIDISCIPLINARY TEAM

Diagnosis of ILD is suspected in a patient who presents with unexplained dyspnea and/or cough that is usually of chronic or subacute onset and chest radiograph or computer tomographic (CT) scan of the thorax shows bilateral parenchymal densities (nodules, airspace densities, or fibrosis). Once suspected, the diagnosis of specific ILD usually requires a multidisciplinary discussion (MDD). The MDD is a dynamic communication between pulmonologist, radiologist, and pathologist, if a cytopathological (bronchoalveolar fluid) or histopathological (lung biopsy) sample is obtained. Addition of the rheumatologist in the MDD may help in reducing the number of cases which remain in the unclassifiable group. The focus of the MDD remains the

TABLE 1 The ATS/ERS classification of idiopathic interstitial pneumonias.

2002 classification	2013 classification
• Idiopathic pulmonary fibrosis (IPF) • Nonspecific interstitial pneumonia (NSIP) • Desquamative interstitial pneumonia (DIP) • Acute interstitial pneumonia (AIP) • Respiratory bronchiolitis-interstitial lung disease (RB-ILD) • Cryptogenic organizing pneumonia (COP) • Lymphocytic interstitial pneumonia (LIP)	• Major idiopathic interstitial pneumonias: ◦ Idiopathic pulmonary fibrosis ◦ Idiopathic nonspecific interstitial pneumonia ◦ Respiratory bronchiolitis-interstitial lung disease ◦ Desquamative interstitial pneumonia ◦ Cryptogenic organizing pneumonia ◦ Acute interstitial pneumonia • Rare idiopathic interstitial pneumonias: ◦ Idiopathic lymphoid interstitial pneumonia ◦ Idiopathic pleuroparenchymal fibroelastosis • Unclassifiable idiopathic interstitial pneumonias

(ATS: American Thoracic Society; ERS: European Respiratory Society)

TABLE 2 Spectrum of various ILDs among Indians.

Types of ILD	Singh et al. (N-1,084)	Dhooria et al. (N-803)	Kumar et al. (N-289)	AIIMS, New Delhi* (N- 1,039)
IPF	148 (13.7%)	170 (21.2%)	80 (27.68%)	231 (22.31%)
Non-IPF	136 (12.5%)	74 (9.2%)	81(28.02%)	281 (27.04%)
Sarcoidosis	85 (7.8%)	339 (42.2%)	108 (37.37%)	145 (13.9%)
Hypersensitivity pneumonitis	513 (47.3%)	86 (10.7%)	7 (2.42%)	96 (9.2%)
CTD-ILD	151 (13.9%)	102 (12.7%)	13 (4.49%)	227 (21.8%)
Drug induced	3 (0.3%)	6 (0.7%)	-	-
Occupational	33 (3.0%)	7 (0.9%)	-	2 (0.2%)

* Unpublished data from authors' own institute.

(ILD: interstitial lung disease; IPF: idiopathic pulmonary fibrosis) integration of the detailed clinical data [onset, progression, smoking, history of exposure, drugs, any feature of CTD, pulmonary function test (PFT) etc.], pattern of the ILD on the CT scan or histopathology.

CLINICAL DATA

The clinical data including presentation *(acute, subacute, or chronic), progression and clinical course*, specific history assessment (with regard to smoking or occupational exposure), exposure to drugs, and any signs or symptoms of CTD (e.g., SSc, rheumatoid arthritis, or myositis) are important for making diagnosis of a specific ILDs. Smoking is commonly associated with IPF, desquamative interstitial pneumonia (DIP), respiratory bronchiolitis-interstitial lung disease (RB-ILD), and pulmonary LCH. Most of the ILDs present as chronic illness; however, acute onset is common for acute HP, acute interstitial pneumonia, diffuse alveolar hemorrhage, cryptogenic organizing pneumonia, acute eosinophilic pneumonia, and acute exacerbation of ILDs. Number of drugs including antibiotics (cephalosporins, nitrofurantoin, and minocycline), antiarrhythmics (amiodarone and tocainide), chemotherapeutic agents (all trans-retinoic acid, alpha-interferon, bleomycin, busulfan, carmustine, cyclophosphamide, gefitinib, mitomycin-C, vinorelbine), antipsychotics, and others are associated with pulmonary toxicity. Hence, a detailed history of drug exposure is paramount during evaluation of patient with ILD. The detailed list of drugs that are associated with lung infiltrates may be found at the website PNEUMOTOX online.

Connective tissue diseases are commonly associated with ILDs and the features can be subtle. Hence, a careful assessment for the presence of the indicators of CTDs are required. History of joint pain or swelling, digital ulcer, mechanic's hands, Gottron's papules, dry eyes or mouth, skin rash, oral ulcers, Reynaud's phenomenon, gastroesophageal reflux, myalgia or muscle weakness, and parotid enlargement may point toward underlying CTD. Examination of skin (for any rash), finger tips, joints (synovitis), eyes, lymph nodes, and muscle weakness is crucial during assessment. Some of the features of CTD are shown in **Figure 1**.

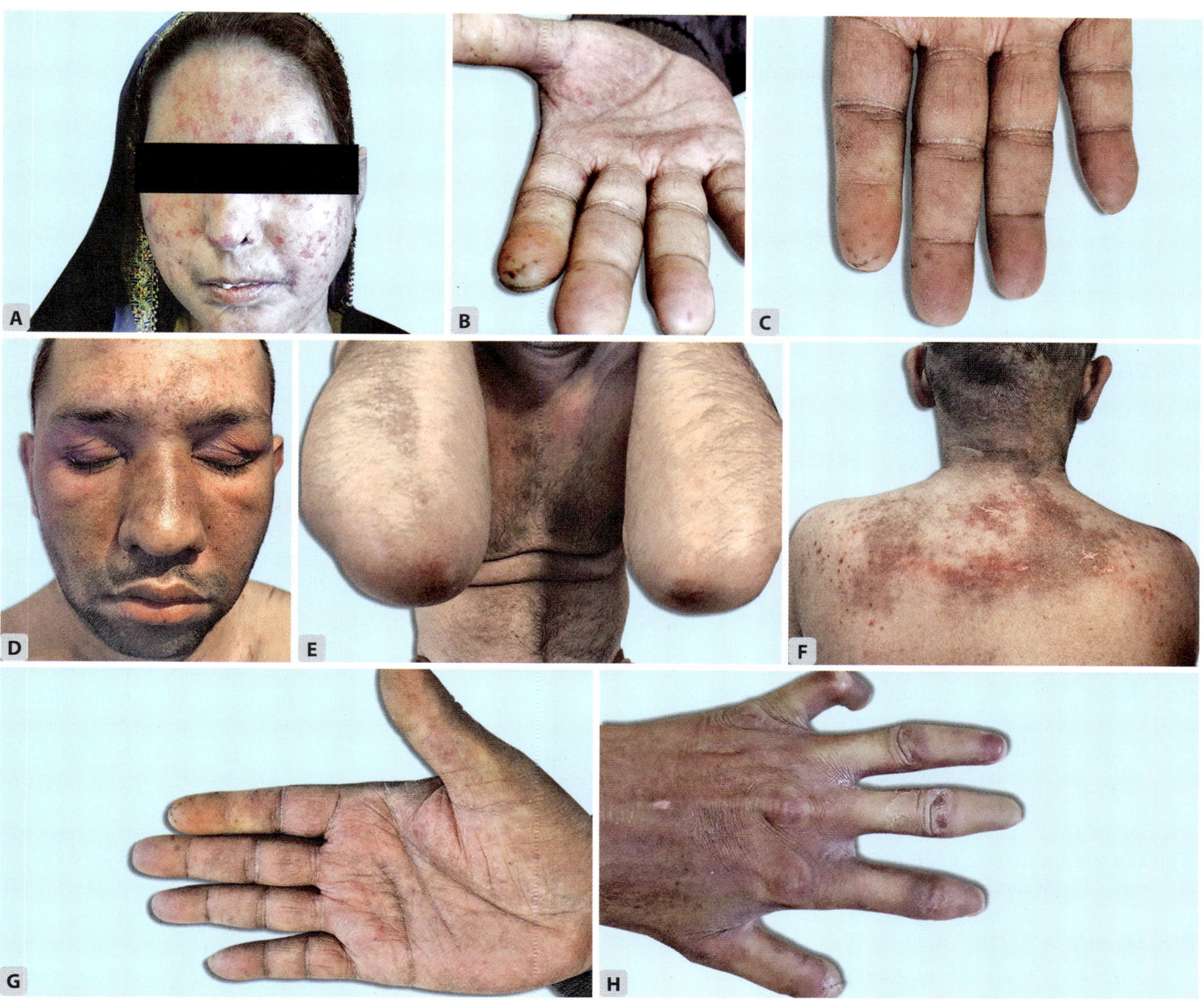

FIGURES 1 A to J: *Continued...*

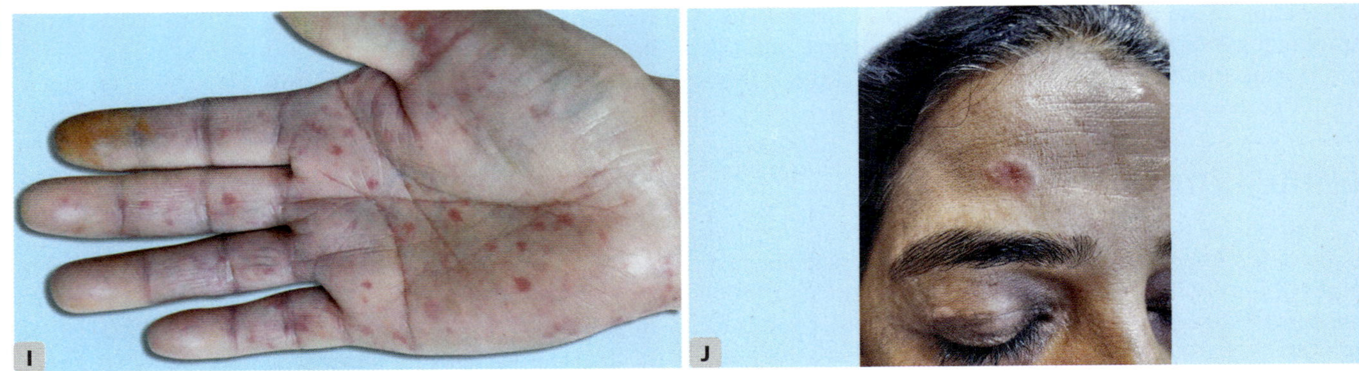

FIGURES 1 A to J: Various signs suggestive of underlying CTDs. (A) Cutaneous rash of SLE; **(B and C)** Healed distal digital ulcers due small/ medium vessel vasculitis; cutaneous signs of dermatomyositis—**(D)** heliotrope rash; **(E)** Gottron's papule; **(F)** shawl sign; and **(G)** mechanic hand; **(H)** sclerodactyly and resorption of digit in scleroderma; **(I)** skin rash of vasculitis; **(J)** papular lesion of sarcoidosis.

TABLE 3 Common serological tests and their association with various CTDs.

Serological tests	Associated CTD
ANA	Scleroderma, SLE, MCTD
Anti-Ro (SSA)	Sjögren's syndrome, polymyositis
Anti-La (SSB)	Sjögren's syndrome
Jo-1, CK, aldolase, myositis-associated antibodies	Polymyositis, dermatomyositis
Jo-1, myositis-associated antibodies	Anti-synthetase syndrome
Scl-70, anticentromere antibody	Scleroderma
RF, CCP	Rheumatoid arthritis
RNP, antihistone antibody	Mix connective tissue disease
p-ANCA, c-ANCA	ANCA-associated vasculitis

(CCP: cyclic citrullinated peptide; c-ANCA: cytoplasmic ANCA; p-ANCA: perinuclear ANCA)

INVESTIGATIONS

Serological analysis is indispensable both for the screening for subclinical and confirmation of clinical diagnosis of CTD. Various serological tests available and their association are shown in the **Table 3**. It is suggested that antinuclear antibody (ANA), rheumatoid factor (RF), and anti-cyclic citrullinated peptide (CCP) should be done in all IIPs.

SEROLOGICAL TESTS

Serological tests assessing the precipitin levels against some fungi (*Alternaria alternata, Cladosporium herbarum, Penicillium chrysogenum,* and *Aspergillus fumigatus*) and pigeon proteins (droppings and feathers) are commercially available. A raised level of precipitins against these antigens may indicate the exposure; however in absence of clinical setting, the utility of these tests is questionable. Also, there is lack of standardization of these tests, hence routine use of these tests is not recommended.

PULMONARY FUNCTION TESTS

Spirometry, body plethysmography, diffusion capacity of lungs (DLco) and 6-minute walk tests are commonly used tests for objective assessment of functional impairment during rest or on activity. Irrespective of type, all ILDs are characterized by a restrictive pattern with reduced lung volumes on spirometry and body plethysmography and impaired DLco. Hence, these tests are used for severity assessment, follow-up, and for prognosis rather than for diagnosis of specific ILD. It is recommended that all patients with ILDs should be evaluated with spirometry and DLco at baseline and subsequently, once in 3–6 months during follow-up.

RADIOLOGY

Chest radiograph is the first imaging modality that is usually performed for assessment of respiratory symptoms. The chest radiograph finding only can be suggestive of ILDs; however, it has limited role in recognition of the pattern, severity, and extent or making specific diagnosis of ILDs. The distribution of the lung infiltrates may help in differential diagnoses of ILDs. Sarcoidosis, HP, occupational lung diseases, chronic eosinophilic pneumonia, and Berylliosis are upper-lobe dominant disease; whereas IPF, nonspecific interstitial pneumonia (NSIP), CTD-ILD, asbestosis, and DIP predominantly affect lower lobes.

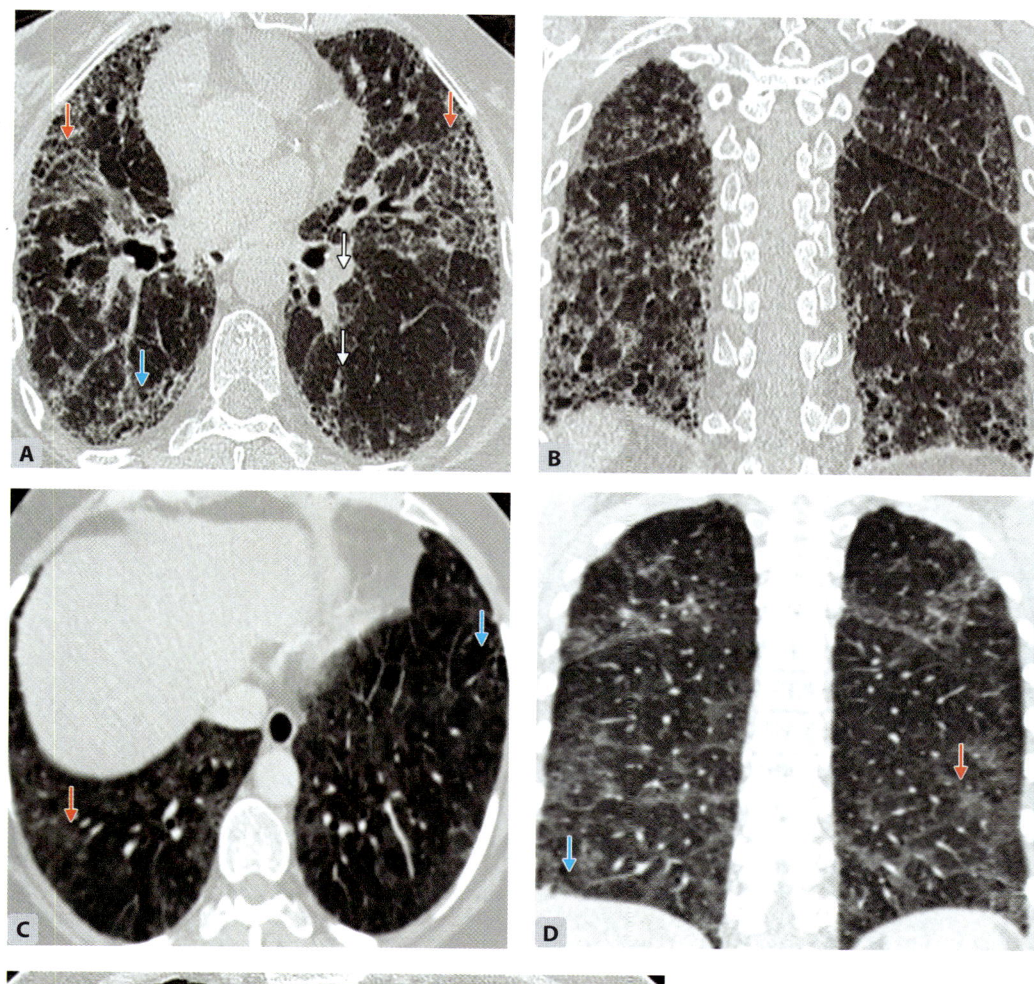

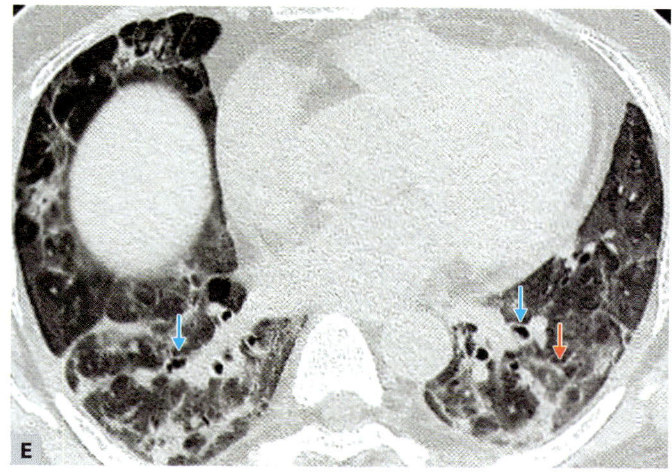

(GGO: ground-glass opacity; HRCT: high-resolution computed tomography; NSIP: nonspecific interstitial pneumonia; UIP: usual interstitial pneumonia)

FIGURES 2 A to E: The radiological features of various IIPs: (A) UIP—axial lung window of HRCT shows sub-pleural honeycombing (red arrows) without dominant GGO or air-trapping. Tractional bronchiolectasis (blue arrow) and reticulations (white arrows) are also seen. **(B)** The coronal lung window shows lower and basal predominance; **(C)** NSIP—axial and **(D)** coronal lung window shows ground-glass predominant opacities (red arrows) with apicobasal gradient visible on coronal image. Basal and sub-pleural reticulations (blue arrow) are seen without honeycombing. *Organizing pneumonia (OP) in a COVID-RTPCR positive patient.* **(E)** Axial lung window shows background ground glass with patchy consolidations due to OP predominantly in subpleural (red arrow) and peribronchial distribution (blue arrows).

High-resolution computed tomography (HRCT) is the essential tool for recognition of the pattern, severity, and extent of the ILD. A good-quality HRCT obtained following recommended protocols is required for evaluation of ILDs. In some cases, HRCT scan can be diagnostic for specific diagnosis without further need of lung biopsy. HRCT (in particular, the fibrosis score) can also help determine the prognosis in ILDs, and quantitative computed tomography (CT) over time interval may be used for evaluating disease progression. **Figures 2** and **3** show HRCT scan patterns of various IIPs and few common ILDs, respectively.

LUNG BIOPSY

Lung biopsy is not mandatory for making a confident diagnosis of specific ILDs. During MDD, ILD diagnoses should be categorized as confident, provisional, or unclassifiable depending on the level of diagnostic confidence based on clinical context, serological tests and HRCT findings. Lung biopsy and bronchoscopy should be reserved for the minority of cases where a careful MDD failed to achieve a confident diagnosis. The risk of complications (including acute exacerbations of underlying disease) and mortality

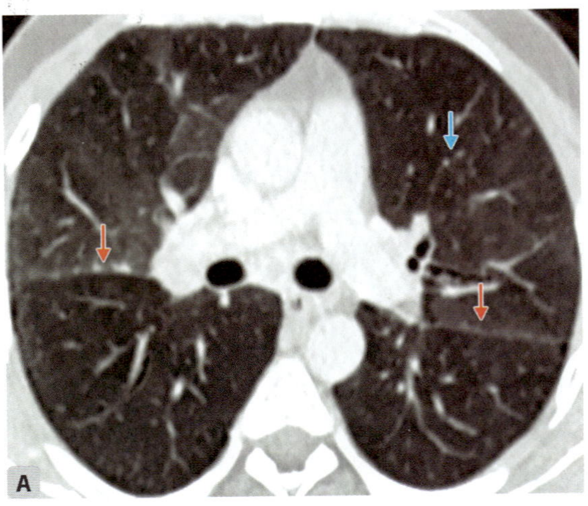

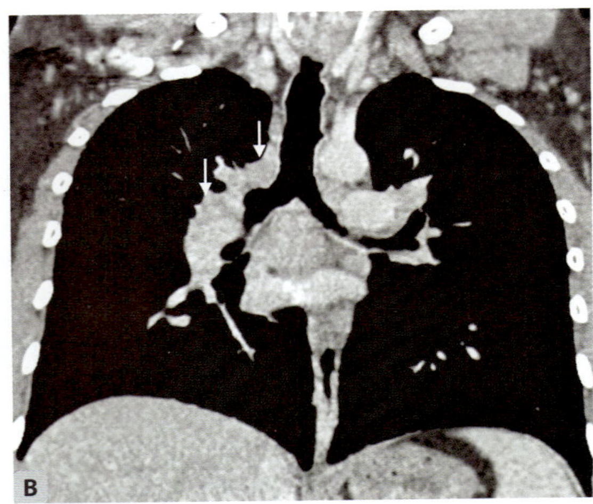

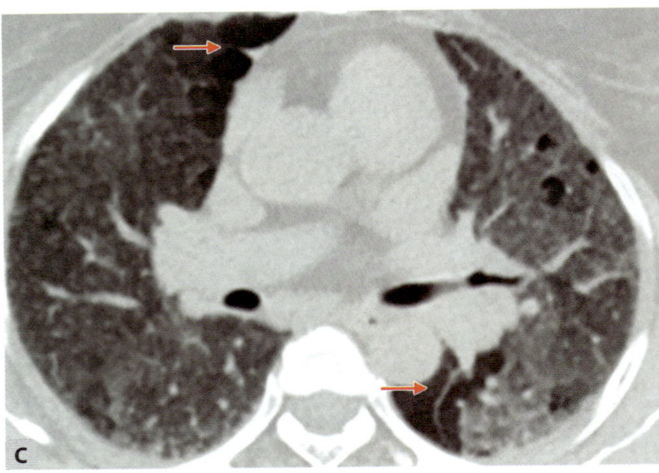

(GGO: ground-glass opacity)

FIGURES 3 A to C: HRCT features of few other commonly encountered ILDs: (A) *Sarcoidosis*—An axial lung window shows fissural (red arrows) and peribronchovascular nodules (blue arrow). **(B)** Coronal mediastinal window shows mediastinal and hilar nodes (white arrows); **(C)** *Hypersensitivity pneumonitis*—axial lung window image shows GGO and centrilobular nodules with areas of mosaic attenuation (red arrow).

must be considered before a biopsy is undertaken. When indicated, lung biopsy can be obtained by surgeons [thoracotomy or video-assisted thoracic surgery (VATS)] or by interventional pulmonologist [transbronchial lung biopsy (TBLB) or transbronchial cryobiopsy]. BAL has a limited role in the diagnosis of IIPs; however, it can be used to rule out infection, hemorrhage, malignancy etc.

Transbronchial lung biopsy: Transbronchial lung biopsy is mostly performed using the flexible bronchoscope, with or without fluoroscopic guidance, under conscious sedation. Although it is relatively easy to obtain TBLB, the small size (median size 5 mm) and associated crush-artifacts limit the role of TBLB in the workup of several ILDs. The overall diagnostic yield of TBLB is around 25–75% but it varies largely depending on the underlying ILD. It can be as low as 20–30% for IPF (as it is lower lobe predominant and subpleural pathology) and as high as 80–90% for nonfibrotic ILDs. TBLB may be diagnostic for ILDs with peribronchovascular and centrilobular involvement such as sarcoidosis, diffuse alveolar hemorrhage (DAH), pulmonary alveolar proteinosis, lymphangitic carcinomatosis, and in some cases of HP. The complications of TBLB include bleeding (1–4%), pneumothorax (1–6%), and death (<0.05%).

Transbronchial cryobiopsy: Transbronchial cryobiopsy is relatively a newer technique used by interventional pulmonologists. This technique involves a cryoprobe that is placed under bronchoscopy guidance in one of the distal segments of the lung, the activation of the probe, and shearing out the lung tissue frozen and adhered at the tip. With this technique, we get a larger specimen as compared to TBLB with a diagnostic yield ranges from 51 to 98% [pooled estimate 83%; 95% confidence interval (CI) 73–94%]. Complications include moderate-to-severe bleeding and pneumothorax.

Surgical lung biopsy: Currently, surgical lung biopsy (VATS) is the gold standard as far as tissue samples are concerned. It plays an important role in providing pathologic results, thus complementing the diagnostic rationale for suspected ILD. The biopsy site should be guided by HRCT manifestations. Biopsy should be taken from at least two affected lobes, and care should be taken to avoid biopsy from most advanced area. The median diagnostic yield of surgical lung biopsy is 95% (range, 42–100%). The mortality after surgical lung biopsy is reported to be 3.6% (95% CI 2.1–5.5%).

MAJOR INTERSTITIAL LUNG DISEASES

IDIOPATHIC PULMONARY FIBROSIS (IPF)

Idiopathic pulmonary fibrosis is a *prototype of ILD* characterized by chronic progressive fibrosing interstitial pneumonia of unknown etiology, and is associated with

BOX 1 Diagnostic criteria for idiopathic pulmonary fibrosis.

In the presence of UIP on HRCT

- Exclusion of known causes of ILD (Exposure, drugs, and CTD)
- UIP pattern on HRCT
- Abnormal pulmonary function tests (showing restrictive pattern, reduced TLC or VC with normal or increased FEV_1/FVC ratio and/or impaired DLco)

In absence of surgical lung biopsy

Major criteria:

- Exclusion of known causes of ILD (Exposure, drugs, and CTD)
- Radiological (HRCT) suggestive of definite UIP pattern
- Abnormal pulmonary function tests (showing restrictive pattern, Reduced TLC or VC with normal or increased FEV1/ FVC ratio and/or impaired gas exchange)
- BAL or TBLB showing no features of alternate diagnosis

Minor criteria:

- Age > 50 years
- >3 months of illness
- Unexplained dyspnea on exertion
- On clinical examination: Typical end inspiratory crepitations (Velcro type) predominantly heard in basal area
- On clinical examination: Typical end inspiratory crepitations (Velcro type) predominantly heard in basal area

(BAL: bronchoalveolar lavage; DLco: diffusion capacity of lungs; FEV_1/ FVC: forced expiratory volume in 1 second/ forced vital capacity; TBLB: transbronchial lung biopsy; TLC: total lung capacity; UIP: usual interstitial pneumonia)

usual interstitial pneumonia (UIP) pattern on HRCT and /or histopathology. UIP pattern includes subpleural and basal predominance; the distribution is often heterogeneous. Abnormalities include honeycombing with or without traction bronchiectasis/bronchiolectasis. GGOs are not a dominant feature (**Figs. 2 A** and **B**). Fibrosis, architectural distortion, honeycombing, scattered fibroblastic foci, patchy distribution, and involvement of the periphery of the acinus or lobule are characteristic findings on lung biopsy. It has heterogeneous appearance at low magnification with alternating areas of normal lung, inflammation, fibrosis, and honeycombing. The diagnosis of IPF can be made in absence in of the lung biopsy also when HRCT shows a UIP pattern. The diagnostic criteria of IPF are summarized in the **Box 1**.

Idiopathic pulmonary fibrosis is usually seen in smokers in their 50s (male > females) and presents with dyspnea on exertion with or without chronic nonproductive cough, often refractory to antitussive agents. Constitutional symptoms are uncommon. Examination shows a typical fine end inspiratory crackles (Velcro) heard over basal area. Clubbing is seen in 25–50% of patients. Features of cor pulmonale are seen in late stages of IPF. Pulmonary function testing shows a restrictive pattern with reduced total lung capacity (TLC) or vital capacity (VC) with normal or increased FEV_1/FVC (forced expiratory volume in 1 second/forced vital capacity) ratio and/or impaired gas exchange (DLco).

Idiopathic pulmonary fibrosis is usually a progressive disease with a *median survival ranging from 2.5 to 3.5 years* from the time of diagnosis. Occasionally, periods of rapid decline are seen which may represent accelerated disease, secondary bacterial/viral infection, exacerbation of ILD, and improvement in lung function test/radiologic abnormalities are rare.

NONSPECIFIC INTERSTITIAL PNEUMONIA (NSIP)

Idiopathic nonspecific interstitial pneumonia is a *diagnosis of exclusion* that requires an in-depth evaluation for the presence of associated clinical or subclinical CTDs, drugs, infections, exposure etc. NSIP may account for about 25 % of all IIPs.

The characteristic radiological findings of NSIP include peripheral, basal, symmetric, predominantly lower lobe reticular and ground-glass opacities (GGOs) with traction bronchiectasis, consolidation and subpleural sparing, honeycombing is generally absent (**Figs. 2 C** and **D**). Presence of spatial and temporal homogeneity and subpleural sparing distinguishes NSIP from IPF. Histology of NSIP involves uniform alveolar and interstitial mononuclear cell inflammation with preserved lung architecture that is almost always accompanied by fibrosis.

The clinical features are poorly understood. This disease entity neither has a predilection for any gender nor for the smokers. However, the disease affects patients with almost a decade younger (40–50 years of age) than IPF and can affect children also. Clinical presentation is usually with gradual-onset dyspnea, cough, fatigue, and weight loss. Few patients can present with subacute onset of symptoms. Finger clubbing is less common and can be observed in 10–35% of patients. Chest examination reveals basal crackles; there may be inspiratory squeak in some patients. PFTs are characterized by a restrictive ventilatory defect and a low DLco. Course of NSIP is highly variable, some patient may remain stable or improve with treatment but others progress to end-stage fibrosis. The prognosis of NSIP is influenced by the underlying conditions, lung functions, and histopathology (cellular vs. fibrotic) at the time of diagnosis, and use of immunosuppressive therapy; CTD-associated NSIP has a better prognosis that idiopathic NSIP. Overall, NSIP has a better survival than IPF with a reported 5-year survival of 82% whereas IPF has median survival of 5 years.

Cryptogenic organizing pneumonia: This clinical entity was described by Davison and colleagues in 1983 as cryptogenic organizing pneumonia (COP) and by Epler in 1985 as bronchiolitis obliterans organizing pneumonia (BOOP). The term COP is preferred because it conveys the essential features and avoids confusion with airway disease as constrictive bronchiolitis that can be confused with BOOP. Organizing pneumonia pattern may be associated with various autoimmune disorders, infections, malignancy, drugs/fumes/toxins, eosinophilic pneumonia etc.

Clinical features include variable degrees of cough and dyspnea of relatively short duration (median <3 months) affecting patients in their 50s. Constitutional symptoms such as weight loss, intermittent fever, sweating, and myalgia are common. Both genders are affected equally, though nonsmokers outnumber smokers. Usually the features are confused with lower respiratory tract infections and patients end up taking multiple courses of antibiotics before the diagnosis. Widespread crackles are usual and typical signs of consolidation as well as clubbing are usually absent. Raised erythrocyte sedimentation rate (ESR), C- reactive protein (CRP), and blood neutrophil counts are common. Radiologically, COP is characterized by presence of bilateral or unilateral patchy consolidation involving subpleural region (**Fig. 2 E**). Lower lobes are more frequently involved. COP can be present in variable ways; however, if suspected, the diagnosis can be made easily by TBLB.

Cryptogenic organizing pneumonia responds well to corticosteroids leading to remission in majority of the patients but relapses are common. Relapse usually occurs on reduction (<15 mg/day) or discontinuation of corticosteroids. Thereby, these patients should be treated for a longer course of corticosteroids (minimum 6 months).

RESPIRATORY BRONCHIOLITIS ILD

It is an entity characterized by symptomatic ILD associated with pathologic lesions of respiratory bronchiolitis. HRCT features of RB-ILD include upper-lobe predominant centrilobular GGOs, thickening of central and peripheral airways with associated centrilobular emphysema, and air trapping. On histopathological evaluation, bronchiolocentric accumulation of pigmented alveolar macrophages with mild bronchiolar fibrosis and chronic inflammation is seen.

DESQUAMATIVE INTERSTITIAL PNEUMONIA (DIP)

It is a form of IIP associated with smoking. Both RB-ILD and DIP affect cigarette smokers of 30–40 years of age with a male-to-female ratio of 2:1. It is characterized by the presence of increased numbers of pigmented macrophages evenly dispersed within alveolar spaces. HRCT findings include lower lung-predominant GGO with peripheral and patchy or diffuse distribution and uniform distribution with occasional interlobular septal thickening. PFTs demonstrate a restrictive abnormality and decreased DLco. Significant overlap between RB-ILD and DIP is seen in clinical, radiological, and pathological findings, and they are considered to reflect different degrees of severity of the small airways and parenchymal reaction to cigarette smoking, with DIP being the end spectrum of RB-ILD.

ACUTE INTERSTITIAL PNEUMONITIS

Acute interstitial pneumonitis (AIP) is a form of IIP that presents acutely with severe dyspnea of short duration of few days. Patients usually give a history of upper respiratory viral-like illness—fever, myalgia, arthralgia, and chill preceding the respiratory illness. It is characterized by widespread signs of consolidations. HRCT of thorax will show GGOs, bronchial dilatation, and architectural distortion. Histopathology will show acute and/or organizing phases of diffuse alveolar damage. Most of the patients require mechanical ventilation. AIP closely mimics ARDS—acute onset, low PaO_2/FiO_2, bilateral infiltrates without evidence of left heart failure. It is associated with high mortality rates.

LYMPHOID INTERSTITIAL PNEUMONIA

Lymphoid interstitial pneumonia (LIP) is a histological variant of diffuse pulmonary lymphoid hyperplasia with ILD being a predominant feature. Overall, the incidence of LIP is low; and clinical features are poorly described. The presentation is similar to other chronic ILDs with slow and gradually increasing cough and dyspnea. In some cases, there may be lymph node enlargement, especially in the presence of Sjögren's syndrome. Because of rarity of idiopathic LIP, all patients with LIP need extensive evaluation for underlying CTD and immune deficiency.

IDIOPATHIC PLEUROPARENCHYMAL FIBROELASTOSIS

Pleuroparenchymal fibroelastosis (PPFE) is a rare form of ILDs that has been described both in children and elderly; however, most common age is between 40 and 70 years. PPFE is characterized by chronic interstitial and pleural fibrosis in the upper lobe. Approximately, 50% of patients have history of recurrent infections and pneumothorax is common. In majority (60%) of the patients, this is a progressive disease.

UNCLASSIFIABLE INTERSTITIAL PNEUMONIA

It is reported that approximately 12% of all IIPs are unclassifiable. Most of the IIPs may remain unclassifiable due to inadequate, nonspecific, or conflicting clinical, radiological, or histopathological findings, or because of lack of surgical lung biopsy. Unclassifiable IIP was first defined in the international guidelines in 2013, meaning the disease has been largely unrecognized and further investigation is needed for improved understanding. The risk factors for the prognosis of unclassifiable IIP are not very clear.

Clinical features include exertional dyspnea, dry cough, and crackles on examination with no evidence of known causes of ILDs. HRCT findings may vary markedly, with mixed patterns. The prognosis for unclassifiable IIPs may be slightly better than that of IPF but the mortality rate is still high (estimated to be 31% at 5 years). A low DLco, UIP-like fibrotic pattern on HRCT (a high fibrosis score, the presence of honeycombing, or the presence of UIP, or a possible UIP pattern) may have a poor prognosis similar to patients with IPF. The extent of fibrosis, which can be measured by quantitative CT analysis, may help to predict outcomes in patients with unclassifiable IIP.

PULMONARY LANGERHANS' CELL HISTIOCYTOSIS

It is an uncommon idiopathic ILD, histologically characterized by the destruction of distal airways by bronchocentric granulomas containing Langerhans cells. Pulmonary Langerhans' cell histiocytosis (LCH) is commonly grouped with bronchiolitis-associated interstitial lung disease (RB-ILD), and DIP as smoking-related ILDs. Clinically, pulmonary LCH equally affects men and women, and is associated with smoking history, typically affects young adults. HRCT findings include a combination of cysts and nodules with centrilobular distribution and upper and middle lung predominance sparing the costophrenic angle. The cyst walls are usually round (sometimes can be confluent and bizarre) and thin but can be as thick as several millimeters and usually <1 cm in size; however, the cysts can be larger (≥2–3 cm). Combinations of small nodules of varying sizes (1–5 mm, 5–10 mm, or larger) are seen, with indistinct margins. Cavitation of the nodule is often seen and is associated with a relatively thick wall. Lung volumes are normal or increased in most patients. Prognosis varies from complete remission after smoking cessation to development of cystic lung disease.

CONNECTIVE TISSUE DISEASE ILD

Connective tissue diseases, also known as collagen vascular diseases, encompass a spectrum of systemic immune diseases in which T- and B-cells produce circulating autoantibodies leading to inflammation and organ damage including involvement of lungs. While the causes of these diseases are unknown, both genetic and environmental factors appear to contribute. ILDs occur in approximately 15% of all patients with CTDs, with higher rates reported in conditions such as SSc and rheumatoid arthritis (RA), with varying rates of mortality. CTD-ILDs remain among the most common diagnoses at many centers. The risk of CTD-ILDs appears to be higher in women and in patients <50 years of age. On HRCT, NSIP is the most common pattern. CTD-ILD may present with UIP pattern, in that case it is important to differentiate the disease from IPF. The prevalence, main features, and ILD patterns of various CTD-ILDs are shown in **Table 4**.

HYPERSENSITIVITY PNEUMONITIS

Hypersensitivity pneumonitis, also known as extrinsic alveolar alveolitis, is a complex, diffuse ILD caused by repeated exposure and sensitization to a myriad of inhaled antigens, most commonly avian, microbial (especially molds), or chemical. This is among the most prevalent ILD along with IPF- and CTD-ILDs worldwide. The principal forms of HP are acute, subacute, and chronic. Acute/subacute HP is predominantly characterized by influenza-like symptoms (e.g., fever, cough, and dyspnea) usually 2–9 hours after exposure to an antigen, and may last or increase over a period of hours or days. Patients with chronic HP have progressive course with predominant symptoms being dyspnea on exertion, cough, fatigue, and weight loss. The chronic form of HP arises from repetitive, low-level exposure over a long period of time but in half of the patients the causative antigen may remain unknown. More recently,

TABLE 4 Summary of the prevalence, features, and HRCT patterns of various CTD-ILDs.

Disease and prevalence of ILD	Clinical features	ILD pattern
Systemic sclerosis: ILD detectable: Up to 75%, clinically significant: 25–45%	Raynaud's phenomenon, sclerodactyly, digital ulcers/pits, telangiectasia, skin thickening, GI involvement	• **Most common:** NSIP • **Other:** UIP, OP • PAH • Pulmonary lymphoma, aspiration pneumonia
Rheumatoid arthritis: ILD detectable: 30–60% Clinically evident: 10–30%	Polyarthritis, rheumatoid skin nodules	• **Most common:** UIP • **Other:** NSIP, OP bronchiectasis, bronchiolitis, nodules, pleural disease ± effusion
Idiopathic inflammatory myopathy (IIM): ILD seen in 30–50%, up to 80% in anti-synthetase syndrome	Proximal symmetrical muscle weakness Gottron's papules, Heliotrope rash, Shawl sign, Mechanic's hands	• **Most common:** NSIP • **Other:** OP, UIP, AIP/DAD • Respiratory muscle weakness
Systemic lupus erythematosus: • ILDs detectable: Up to 30% • Clinically evident: 3–11%	Photosensitive and/or malar rash, oral ulcers, alopecia, serositis	• **Most common:** NSIP • **Other:** LIP, OP, UIP, FB, AIP/DAD, DAH, pleuritis • Shrinking lung syndrome
Mixed connective tissue disease: ILDs can be seen in 20–85%	Swollen hands, synovitis, myositis, acrosclerosis, Raynaud's phenomenon	• **Most common:** NSIP • **Other:** UIP, OP • Pleuritis, DAH, respiratory muscle weakness, aspiration pneumonia
Sjögren's syndrome: ILD can be seen in 10–30%	• Sicca symptoms • Enlarged parotid glands	• **Most common:** NSIP • **Other:** OP, LIP, UIP, FB • MALT lymphoma, amyloidosis, bronchiectasis

(AIP: acute interstitial pneumonia; DAD: diffuse alveolar damage; DAH: diffuse alveolar hemorrhage; FB: follicular bronchiolitis; LIP: lymphoid interstitial pneumonia; MALT: mucosa-associated lymphoid tissue; NSIP: nonspecific interstitial pneumonia; OP: organizing pneumonia; UIP: usual interstitial pneumonia) the ATS/JRS/ALAT (American Thoracic Society/Japanese Respiratory Society/Asociación Latinoamericana del Tórax) suggested to classify HP into fibrotic and nonfibrotic forms. The search for a cause of chronic HP may include the detailed history of exposure and consideration of specific circulating immunoglobulin G antibodies.

Chronic fibrotic HP frequently present with UIP pattern closely resembling to IPF, hence can be difficult to diagnose. Potential radiological features that distinguish chronic HP from IPF/UIP include upper-lobe predominance, presence of GGOs, centrilobular nodules, mosaic attenuation, and air trapping. The diagnosis can be supported by lymphocyte predominance on BAL although the absence of BAL finding should not exclude the diagnosis of fibrosing HP. The histological findings of HP include fibrosis in bronchiolocentric pattern, infrequent or inconsistently distributed fibroblast foci, poorly formed granulomas, giant cells, inflammation, organizing pneumonia, or chronic bronchiolitis.

An international group of experts suggested following diagnostic criteria for chronic HP: (1) identification of a causative antigen, (2) temporal relation between exposure and disease, (3) mosaic attenuation on chest imaging, and (4) poorly formed nonnecrotizing granulomas on pathology.

The natural history of fibrosing HP with a UIP pattern is similar to IPF; progression occurs despite the treatment with an appropriate agent. However, some patients with chronic fibrosing HP may stabilize over time in response to therapy. The median survival from the time of diagnosis chronic HP is approximately 5 years. The extent of fibrosis on HRCT in these patients with chronic HP is predictive of mortality. Potential fatal acute exacerbations of HP have also been reported.

SARCOIDOSIS

Sarcoidosis is a rare multisystemic, inflammatory disease of unknown etiology. Nearly 90% of patients with sarcoidosis have some form of pulmonary involvement. Signs and symptoms of pulmonary sarcoidosis include dry cough, chronic dyspnea on exertion, chest tightness, and wheezing.

Approximately 20% of patients with pulmonary sarcoidosis may develop pulmonary fibrosis (stage IV sarcoidosis), which is associated with significant morbidity and mortality in these patients. Pulmonary fibrosis predominantly affects the upper lobes (posterior segments), airway-centered without air trapping and it follows the bronchovascular bundles. Imaging tends to reveal faint reticulations to dense linear bands, cystic lung disease, traction bronchiectasis, and airway distortion. A UIP pattern of lung injury is uncommon, although honeycombing may be seen in the upper zones of the lungs.

The natural history of lung function decline in patients with sarcoidosis is not well established. A 10-year mortality rate of 16% has been reported in patients with stage 4 sarcoidosis. Acute exacerbations are not reported in stage 4 pulmonary sarcoidosis.

ILD RELATED TO OCCUPATIONAL EXPOSURE

Inhalation of various dusts related to occupational exposure may lead to the development of pulmonary fibrosis and ILDs. The most known diseases caused by occupational exposure include asbestosis (caused by asbestosis fibers) and silicosis (free crystalline silicon dioxide or silica). Also, the exposure to farming, livestock, metal dust, coal, sand and dust arising from the preparation of dental prosthetics have been linked to the development of ILDs. ILDs related to other occupational exposures are mainly diagnosed from history of exposure to offending agent and typical HRCT patterns.

DIAGNOSIS

The final diagnosis of the specific ILDs requires a multidisciplinary approach (MDD) that integrate all clinical, radiological, and other tests (e.g., peripheral blood tests, PFT) carefully thought and reviewed to determine whether or not additional procedures are needed and whether such procedures are likely to be helpful in reaching confident diagnosis. MDD also assess the need of more invasive testing such as bronchoscopy with BAL and/or TBLB or lung biopsy. Finally, all information is integrated to reach a final diagnosis with level of confidence. Various patterns on HRCT and/or the lung biopsy help in differential diagnoses. **Flowchart 1** has shown a simplified approach for the diagnosis of ILDs. The differential diagnosis of various patterns are shown in **Table 5**.

MANAGEMENT

Once confident diagnosis is established, then next step is to plan treatment and monitoring of the disease activity. The important management issues while managing ILDs

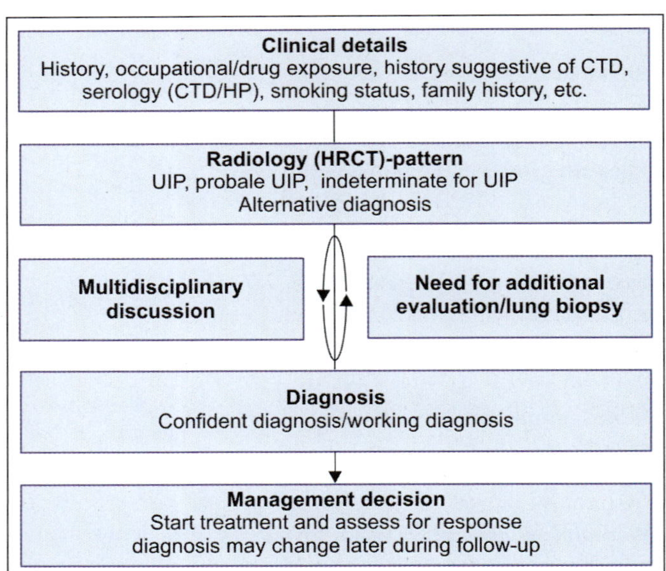

(ILDs: interstitial lung diseases; UIP: usual interstitial pneumonia)

FLOWCHART 1: A simplified approach for the diagnosis of ILDs.

TABLE 5 Differential diagnoses of various patterns of ILDs.

HRCT/Biopsy pattern	Differential diagnosis
UIP	IPF, asbestosis, HP, CTD-ILD, drug toxicity, familial IPF, Hermansky–Pudlak syndrome
NSIP	Idiopathic NSIP, CTD-ILD, HP, drug-induced, infection, immune deficiency
OP	Idiopathic, infections, distal obstruction, aspiration pneumonia, drugs, fumes and toxic exposure, CTDs, HP, eosinophilic lung disease, reparative process—abscess, vasculitis, neoplasm etc.
AIP	Conditions associated diffuse alveolar damage—infection, CTDs, drugs, inhalation, sepsis, transfusion associated lung injury etc.
RB-ILD	DIP, bronchiolitis, NSIP
DIP	UIP, RB-ILD, NSIP, eosinophilic pneumonia, hemosiderosis, venoocclusive disease
LIP	Idiopathic, infection (*Pneumocystis jirovecii*, hepatitis B, EBV), CTD (Sjögren's syndrome, rheumatoid arthritis, SLE), immune deficiency (HIV, SCID), drugs/toxin exposure

(AIP: acute interstitial pneumonia; CTD-ILD: connective tissue disease-interstitial lung disease; DIP: Desquamative interstitial pneumonia; HP: hypersensitivity pneumonitis; IPF: idiopathic pulmonary fibrosis; LIP: lymphoid interstitial pneumonia; NSIP: nonspecific interstitial pneumonia; OP: organizing pneumonia; RB-ILD: respiratory bronchiolitis-interstitial lung disease; SCID: severe combined immunodeficiency; UIP: usual interstitial pneumonia)

include whether disease is stable or progressive, whether to administer pharmacological agent, or whether disease is already end stage of fibrosis that is unlikely to respond to therapy in that case supportive, palliative care, and workup for lung transplant is the best approach. Basic principles of ILDs include avoidance of exposure, pharmacotherapy (immunosuppressive therapy and antifibrotics), supportive care, and management of comorbidities. The treatment of ILDs has been summarized in **Table 6**.

AVOIDANCE OF EXPOSURE

If any causative exposure such as drugs, toxins, or exposure is identified that should be eliminated. Avoidance from environmental exposures may require more extensive remediation, for example, in addition to removal of birds from the home, extensive cleaning of upholstery, window coverings, and ventilation systems may be required. Despite all these measures, the complete removal of all residual antigen may not be achieved, and removal of the patient from the location may be required. Presence of extensive water damage and mold growth, significant demolition, and reconstruction may be necessary. If exposure is occupational, alteration in the job, changing the substances used, or use of protective respiratory equipment may be effective; for few patients, complete removal from the suspected exposure may be the only option.

IMMUNOSUPPRESSIVE THERAPY

Certain forms of ILD, including COP, CTD-ILD, and sarcoidosis may demonstrate a favorable response to corticosteroids and other immunosuppressive agents. However, an assessment should be made regarding the likelihood of response (end stage fibrotic lesion may not respond) as well as the relative risks and benefits of the therapy.

In disorders such as CTD-ILD, when a more prolonged course of therapy is anticipated, the early addition of steroid-sparing medications, such as azathioprine or mycophenolate mofetil, should be used. Severe cases of CTD-ILD may require drugs such as cyclophosphamide and rituximab, which carry increased risk for severe side effects. If no clinical improvement is seen after 3–6 months of therapy, discontinuation of immunosuppressive therapy should be strongly considered.

ANTIFIBROTIC THERAPY

For progressive fibrotic lung diseases, particularly IPF, antifibrotic agents, pirfenidone and nintedanib, have been approved by FDA and are in usage for last few years. The exact mechanism of antifibrotic action of pirfenidone is not known; however, it has anti-inflammatory, antioxidative, and antiproliferatory properties. Nintedanib is a tyrosine kinase inhibitor and exhibits its antifibrotic action via inhibition of receptors for platelet-derived growth factor, fibroblast growth factor, and vascular endothelial growth factor (VEGF) and of nonreceptor tyrosine kinases of the Src family. Trials showed that both pirfenidone and nintedanib decreased the rate of decline in FVC, acute exacerbations, all-cause mortality, and respiratory-related mortality in patients with IPF; both drugs have been evaluated and used for other fibrotic ILDs.

SUPPORTIVE CARE

Supportive therapy that may improve quality of life and decrease respiratory symptoms include oxygen supplementation and pulmonary rehabilitation. Patients with ILD are encouraged to maintain saturations >90% both at rest and with exercise. Pulmonary rehabilitation may lead to increased muscle strength and improved endurance. Other benefits include ongoing education regarding oxygen use, breathing and pacing techniques, and social support. Also, these patients frequently suffer from anxiety and depression; pulmonary rehabilitation may benefit patients by identifying these issues leading to appropriate specialist referrals to psychiatrist.

ADDRESS THE COMORBIDITIES

Common comorbidities observed among patients with ILD include gastroesophageal reflux (GERD), coronary artery disease, obstructive sleep apnea (OSA), pulmonary hypertension, and osteoporosis (related to corticosteroids use and less sun exposure due to reduced outdoor activity). Every attempt should be made to identify and provide management of these comorbidities.

TABLE 6 Treatment summary of various ILDs.

ILD	Main therapy	Other therapy
IPF	Antifibrotic drugs: • Nintedanib - Dose : 150 mg BD • Pirfenidone - Dose: 40 mg/Kg (maximum of 2,403 mg in three divided doses)	• Combination of N-acetyl cysteine, Corticosteroids and azathioprine combination (PANTHER trial) should NOT be used • Lung transplantation in progressive disease
NSIP	• Avoiding of inciting agent (drug/inhalational exposure) • Corticosteroids: Optimal dose and duration not known (usually 0.5–1 mg/kg to a max of 60 kg, tapered based on clinical response) • Other immunosuppressive: ◦ Azathioprine: 25–50 mg/day to max of 200 mg/day ◦ Mycophenolate mofetil: Target dose of 1.5–3 g daily in two divided doses	• In refractory disease: ◦ Cyclophosphamide ◦ Rituximab ◦ Calcineurin inhibitors—cyclosporine and tacrolimus (limited data) • Methotrexate not chosen in idiopathic NSIP because of potential pulmonary toxicity
COP	• Corticosteroids: Optimal dose and duration not known usually 0.5–1 mg/kg to a maximum of 60 kg, taper based on clinical response • Other immunosuppressive: ◦ Azathioprine: 25–50 mg/day to maximum of 200 mg/day	• Cyclophosphamide (in refractory disease). • Macrolide antibiotics (case reports)
AIP	• General supportive critical care • High-dose systemic steroids (case series)	• Other immunosuppressive therapy (vincristine, cyclophosphamide, cyclosporine and azathioprine) • Lung transplantation
Hypersensitivity pneumonitis	• Avoidance of exposure • Corticosteroids (dose and duration depends upon clinical response) • Other immune suppressants (who have not responded to steroids): ◦ Azathioprine: 25–50 mg/day to maximum of 200 mg/day ◦ Mycophenolate mofetil: Target dose of 1.5–3 g daily in two divided doses	• Rituximab (in case of refractory disease) • Antifibrotics: Nintedanib and pirfenidone (for fibrotic HP) • Lung transplantation
Sarcoidosis	• Observation • Corticosteroids (dose equivalent of 10 mg prednisolone for at least 3 months) • Steroid-sparing agents: Methotrexate (5–7.5 mg/week, maximum of 10–15 mg/week)	• Azathioprine, leflunomide (10-20mg/day), mycophenolate mofetil • In refractory disease: ◦ TNF-α antagonists : Infliximab and adalimumab
CTD-ILD	• Corticosteroids • Mycophenolate mofetil • Antifibrotic: Nintedanib and pirfenidone • DMARDS	• Cyclophosphamide pulses (for refractory disease) • Rituximab (for refractory disease) • Other immunosuppressive: azathioprine

(AIP: acute interstitial pneumonia; COP: cryptogenic organizing pneumonia; DMARDs: disease-modifying antirheumatic drugs; HP: hypersensitivity pneumonitis; IPF: idiopathic pulmonary fibrosis; NSIP: nonspecific interstitial pneumonia)

PALLIATIVE CARE

Symptom control is particularly important for patients with all stages of ILD. Pulmonary rehabilitation should be encouraged in all patients to improve dyspnea. The breathlessness due to advanced ILD can be treated with oxygen supplementation, low-dose opiates, and anxiolytics. Cough can be quite problematic and difficult to control in these patients; low-dose opiates and low-dose corticosteroids are occasionally used to treat cough. Understanding their long-term risk and evaluation for acid and nonacid reflux should be considered whenever intractable cough persists.

LUNG TRANSPLANTATION

Although lung transplantation has been significantly associated with morbidity and mortality. However, for many patients with advanced ILDs with respiratory failure, lung transplant is the only potentially life-extending alternative. The timing of listing for lung transplant is complicated in ILD because of difficulties in prediction of progression and exacerbation that can change the entire course of illness. Lung transplant is most frequently done for IPF and for those with advanced disease, survival after lung transplantation is superior to the natural history of their disease. However, this intervention requires a strong social support system as well as the emotional and physical ability to tolerate a complex medical regimen of immunosuppressive therapy.

RECOMMENDED READINGS

1. Raghu G, Mehta S. Interstitial lung disease (ILD) in India: Insights and lessons from the prospective, landmark ILD-India registry. Lung India. 2016;33(6):589-91.
2. American Thoracic Society/European Respiratory Society. International Multidisciplinary Consensus Classification of the Idiopathic Interstitial Pneumonias. This joint statement of the American Thoracic Society (ATS), and the European Respiratory Society (ERS) was adopted by the ATS board of directors, June 2001 and by the ERS Executive Committee, June 2001. Am J Respir Crit Care Med. 2002;165(2):277-304.
3. Travis WD, Costabel U, Hansell DM, King TE, Jr, Lynch DA, Nicholson AG, et al. An official American Thoracic Society/European Respiratory Society statement: Update of the international multidisciplinary classification of the idiopathic interstitial pneumonias. Am J Respir Crit Care Med. 2013;188(6):733-48.
4. Coultas DB, Zumwalt RE, Black WC, Sobonya RE. The epidemiology of interstitial lung diseases. American journal of respiratory and critical care medicine. 1994;150(4):967-72.
5. Thomeer M, Demedts M, Vandeurzen K. Registration of interstitial lung diseases by 20 centres of respiratory medicine in Flanders. Acta Clin Belg. 2001;56(3):163-72.
6. López-Campos JL, Rodríguez-Becerra E. Incidence of interstitial lung diseases in the south of Spain 1998-2000: the RENIA study. Eur J Epidemiol. 2004;19(2):155-61.
7. Singh S, Collins BF, Sharma BB, Joshi JM, Talwar D, Katiyar S, et al. Interstitial Lung Disease in India. Results of a Prospective Registry. Am J Respir Crit Care Med. 2017;195(6):801-13.
8. Dhooria S, Agarwal R, Sehgal IS, Prasad KT, Garg M, Bal A, et al. Spectrum of interstitial lung diseases at a tertiary center in a developing country: A study of 803 subjects. PLoS One. 2018;13(2):e0191938.
9. Kumar R, Gupta N, Goel N. Spectrum of interstitial lung disease at a tertiary care centre in India. Pneumonol Alergol Pol. 2014;82(3):218-26.
10. Singh S, Sharma BB, Bairwa M, Gothi D, Desai U, Joshi JM, et al. Management of interstitial lung diseases: A consensus statement of the Indian Chest Society (ICS) and National College of Chest Physicians (NCCP). Lung India. 2020;37(4):359-78.
11. Mathai SC, Danoff SK. Management of interstitial lung disease associated with connective tissue disease. BMJ. 2016;352:h6819.
12. Sheth JS, Belperio JA, Fishbein MC, Kazerooni EA, Lagstein A, Murray S, et al. Utility of Transbronchial vs Surgical Lung Biopsy in the Diagnosis of Suspected Fibrotic Interstitial Lung Disease. Chest. 2017;151(2):389-99.
13. Dhooria S, Agarwal R, Sehgal IS, Aggarwal AN, Goyal R, Guleria R, et al. Bronchoscopic lung cryobiopsy: An Indian association for bronchology position statement. Lung India. 2019;36(1):48-59.
14. Raghu G, Collard HR, Egan JJ, Martinez FJ, Behr J, Brown KK, et al. An official ATS/ERS/JRS/ALAT statement: idiopathic pulmonary fibrosis: evidence-based guidelines for diagnosis and management. Am J Respir Crit Care Med. 2011;183(6):788-824.

CHAPTER 213

Bullous Lung Disease

Anant Mohan, Tejas M Suri

ABSTRACT

Bullous lung diseases are characterized by presence of pulmonary bullae. A bulla is defined as an airspace with a diameter > 1 cm with a wall < 1 mm in thickness. Often bullae may expand to occupy more than one-third of a hemithorax and are then referred to as giant bullae. Primary bullous lung disease may occur in young male smokers with underlying normal lung parenchyma. Bullae may also occur secondary to pulmonary and systemic diseases, especially chronic obstructive pulmonary disease (COPD). In the latter situation, underlying lung is emphysematous, and the condition is known as bullous emphysema. The diagnosis is radiological and usually requires a high-resolution computed tomography (HRCT) of chest. Bullous lung disease may be complicated by secondary spontaneous pneumothorax, fluid collection within bulla, infection, or superimposed lung cancer.

Medical management of bullous lung disease includes symptomatic treatment with inhaled bronchodilators and glucocorticoids, vaccination, pulmonary rehabilitation, and supportive care according to COPD guidelines. Symptomatic patients with progressive bullous enlargement and relatively normal surrounding lung parenchyma are ideal candidates for surgical bullectomy. Newer approaches including bronchoscopic interventions and lung transplantation are being explored for management of advanced bullous lung disease.

"Your breath is your anchor"

—Anonymous

INTRODUCTION

Bullous lung diseases are a heterogenous group of conditions which are characterized by the presence of bullae in the lung. A bulla is an air-filled structure with a diameter of at least 1 cm (often up to several centimeters) and a wall thickness of < 1 mm. Bullae are detected on chest imaging [chest radiograph or computed tomography (CT)] as sharply demarcated radiolucent structures. They may be surrounded by emphysematous lung, or less commonly normal lung parenchyma. It is essential to differentiate bullae from other radiolucent structures such as blebs, cavities, emphysema, and pneumatoceles (**Table 1**).

In this chapter, we will review the etiopathogenesis, clinical and imaging features, and medical and surgical management of pulmonary bullae.

ETIOLOGY

Based on etiology, bullae may occur as a primary abnormality or secondary to various pulmonary and systemic causes (**Box 1**). It is essential to differentiate primary bullous lung disease from secondary causes of pulmonary bullae because this has important implications for management and prognosis.

Primary bullous lung disease is characterized by the presence of bullae with surrounding normal lung parenchyma. These persons may have no underlying pulmonary or systemic disease. Most patients are young male smokers in third or fourth decade of life. Certain agents such as tobacco smoking, cannabis (marijuana), and e-cigarette smoking have been causally implicated. Patients with primary bullous lung disease may have presence of "giant bullae", i.e., bullae which occupy more than one-third of a hemithorax. Furthermore, in

BOX 1 Etiology of bullous lung disease.

Primary:

- Primary bullous lung disease
- Idiopathic giant bullous emphysema/vanishing lung disease

Secondary:

- *Bullous emphysema:*
  - Chronic obstructive pulmonary disease (COPD)
  - Alpha-1 antitrypsin deficiency
  - HIV-related emphysema
- *Fibrotic lung disease:*
  - Sarcoidosis
  - Idiopathic pulmonary fibrosis
  - Pneumoconiosis (e.g., silicosis, progressive massive fibrosis)
  - Post-tuberculosis sequelae
  - Post-COVID-19 fibrosis
- *Systemic disorder:*
  - Marfan syndrome
  - Ehlers–Danlos syndrome
  - Neurofibromatosis type-1
  - Fabry disease
  - Salla disease
  - Cutis laxa
- *Intravenous drug use:*
  - Heroin
  - Cocaine
  - Crushed oral tablets of methadone

TABLE 1 Characteristics of radiolucent lung lesions.

	Characteristics	Borders	Clinical associations
Bulla	Air-filled space > 1 cm (often enlarged to more than one-third or half of hemithorax)	Thin, sharp wall < 1 mm made of connective tissue from pleura or alveolar septa	Primary bullous lung disease, bullous emphysema
Bleb	Air-filled space usually <1 cm	Surrounded by elastic layers of visceral pleura	Primary spontaneous pneumothorax
Cyst	Rounded air-filled space in lung parenchyma	Thin epithelial or fibrous wall (<2 mm)	Langerhans cell histiocytosis, lymphangioleiomyomatosis, Birt–Hogg–Dubé syndrome
Cavity	An air-filled space created within a mass, nodule, or consolidation due to drainage on contents	Wall thickness is variable (usually >2 mm); thinner wall in benign lesions and thicker in malignant lesions	Infections, malignancies, and vasulitides
Pneumatocele	Gas-filled space in lung formed by parenchymal necrosis and air trapping by check-valve mechanism	Usually thin walled	Post-traumatic, postinfectious; often transient
Emphysema	Destruction of alveolar walls distal to terminal bronchiole; can be centrilobular, paraseptal, or panlobular	No discernible walls	Smoking, alpha-1 antitrypsin deficiency

a subset of patients, these bullae may enlarge rapidly to replace majority of the normal lung parenchyma, which is progressive compressed, leading to a situation termed as the "vanishing lung syndrome."

The presence of bullae *secondary to existing pulmonary or systemic diseases* is more common than primary bullous lung disease. Most commonly, bullae are surrounded by centriacinar or paraseptal emphysema. This condition is termed as "bullous emphysema" and the epidemiology resembles that of COPD. Bullous emphysema predominantly affects the lung apices. In addition to cigarette and *bidi* smoking, biomass fuel exposure is an important risk factor in the Indian subcontinent. Bullous emphysema which is diffuse or basal predominant may occur in patients with alpha-1 antitrypsin deficiency. These patients tend to develop bullous lung disease at relatively younger age with lesser smoke exposure. Similarly, subjects with human immunodeficiency virus (HIV) infection tend to have more rapid development of bullous emphysema at a younger age and with lower tobacco smoke exposure compared to those without HIV.

Bullae may also appear in advanced lung fibrosis due to various causes including sarcoidosis and pneumoconiosis. Systemic connective tissue disease such as Marfan syndrome and Ehlers–Danlos syndrome are uncommon causes of pulmonary bullae. Intravenous (IV) use of illicit drugs (heroin or crushed oral tablets of methylphenidate) has also been linked to pulmonary bullae.

PATHOGENESIS

Our understanding of the pathogenic mechanisms of bulla formation is incomplete. The traditional theory suggested that bullae are formed due to air trapping by a check valve obstructive mechanism in the small airways. This would lead to development of a positive pressure within the bulla. However, studies have revealed the presence of a negative pressure within the bulla, which approximates the pleural pressure. This has led to the contemporary theory that the bulla is formed because of increased compliance compared to the adjacent lung parenchyma which leads to its selective inflation. Further, most bullous disorders have apical predominant bullae as the pleural pressures are more negative near lung apices. Consequently, the bullae are subjected to greater distending pressures near lung apices. Gravitational factors may also be preventive against bulla formation near lung bases.

The increased compliance leading to bulla formation may be a consequence of alveolar wall destruction due to emphysema. This often results in diffuse bullous emphysema with multiple and bilateral bullae. The connective tissue from the alveolar septa is incorporated into the bullous wall. Patients with HIV are believed to have accelerated emphysematous changes due to upregulation of matrix metalloproteinases, which participate in alveolar wall breakdown. In contrast, patients with primary bullous lung disease are assumed to have focal defects leading to increased compliance of the bulla in comparison to the surrounding lung.

It has been found that marijuana smokers take deeper inhalations and hold breath for longer than tobacco smokers. Whether the Valsalva maneuvers performed during smoking cigarettes or marijuana contribute to barotrauma, irritant deposition and consequent bulla formation in susceptible individuals are unclear. Interestingly, IV drug users tend to have bullae involving the bases of the lung. In IV drug users, the cutting agents, or inert fillers such as talc, cellulose, or corn starch are incriminated as they are believed to distribute preferentially to the well perfused lung bases, where they may lead to local injury.

CLINICAL FEATURES

Patients with bullous lung disease may have a varied presentation depending on the size of the bullae and the extent of emphysema in the surrounding lung parenchyma.

Many young patients with primary bullous disease with normal lung parenchyma may be asymptomatic, with the bullae being an incidental finding on chest radiography. These patients may become symptomatic with dyspnea or cough as the bullae enlarge and compress adjacent lung parenchyma, thereby compromising ventilation. The natural history of pulmonary bullae is that of progressive enlargement, albeit at a highly variable rate. Progressive dyspnea and respiratory failure may ensue, particularly among patients with giant bullae and vanishing lung syndrome. Such giant bullae lead to hyperinflation of the chest with downward displacement of the diaphragm, which leads to mechanical disadvantage to diaphragm function. Physical examination may reveal reduced breath sounds and hyperresonance over the affected hemithorax.

On the contrary, patients with bullous emphysema have more prominent symptoms earlier in the disease course. The clinical features resemble those of COPD and include cough, sputum production, dyspnea, and wheeze. Progressive disease may result in hypercapnic respiratory failure and pulmonary hypertension.

Sometimes, the first presentation of bullous lung disease involves acute breathlessness or chest pain due to occurrence of complications such as pneumothorax or infection. Rarely, hemoptysis may occur and may indicate superimposed infection or malignancy.

INVESTIGATIONS

IMAGING

The diagnosis of bullous lung disease is typically made on chest imaging, including *radiography and CT of the thorax*. On chest radiographs, bullae appear as areas of radiolucency with curvilinear demarcation (**Fig. 1**). However, radiographs have a low sensitivity and may miss about half of the cases of bullous lung disease. Hence, HRCT of the chest is the preferred modality.

The Fleischner Society has defined bulla as an airspace > 1 cm in diameter, with a thin wall which is <1 mm in thickness. The bullae may enlarge to several centimeters in size; a bulla occupying more than one-third of the hemithorax is described as a "giant bulla." The wall of a bulla

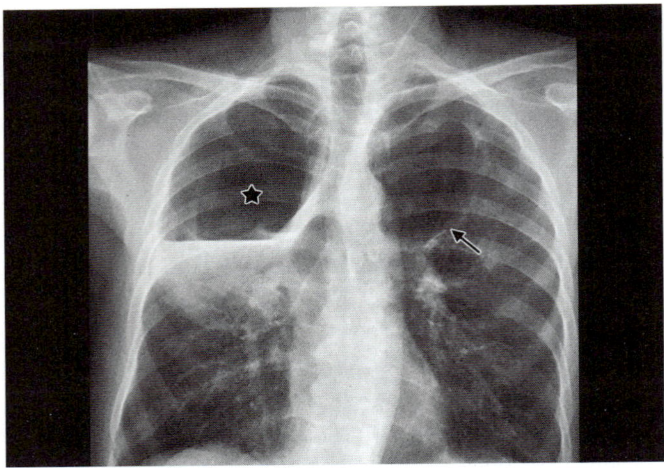

FIGURE 1: Chest radiograph shows presence of bilateral bullous lung disease complicated with air fluid level in the right lung *(star)*. Note the sharply demarcated thin arcuate margin of the bulla in the left lung *(arrow)*.

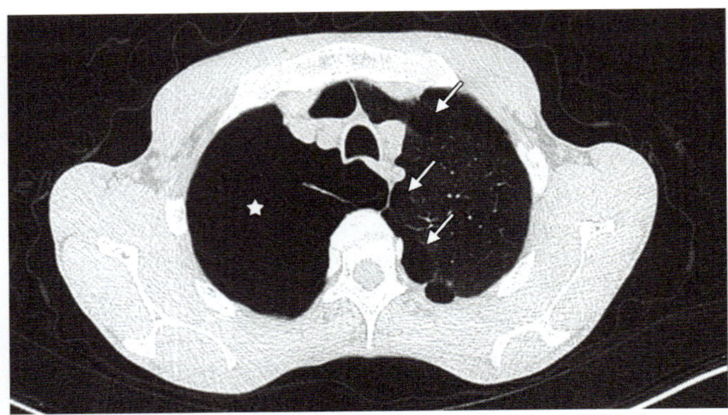

FIGURE 2: High-resolution computed tomography of chest shows presence of bilateral primary bullous lung disease in a young male patient. There is appearance of "hairline shadows" which are thin arcuate demarcations of the bulla with the remaining lung parenchyma (*arrows* in left lung). There is pneumothorax *(star)* in right lung (better appreciated in **Fig. 3**).

TABLE 2 Favorable and unfavorable factors for surgical candidacy of patients with bullous lung disease.

Favorable factors	Unfavorable factors

• Primary bullous lung disease with normal surrounding lung parenchyma
• Crowding of bronchovascular structures in adjacent lung parenchyma
• Giant bulla (occupying greater than one-third of hemithorax)
• Higher bullous volume (difference of TLC using body plethysmography and helium dilution/nitrogen washout)
• Perfusion scan showing well-matched localized defect with bulla
	• Underlying COPD with diffuse bullous emphysema
	• Multiple bullae without a dominant giant bulla
	• *Impaired lung function*:
	  ◦ FEV_1 < 40% predicted
	  ◦ DLCO < 40% predicted
	• *Respiratory failure*:
	  ◦ $PaCO_2$ > 45 mm Hg
	• *Comorbidities*:
	  ◦ Pulmonary hypertension
	  ◦ Cardiovascular disease

(DLCO: diffusing capacity of the lung for carbon monoxide; FEV_1: forced expiratory volume in the first second)

appears as a thin "hairline shadow" (**Fig. 2**). Additionally, CT scans are useful to assess the remaining lung parenchyma, which may be often crowded or atelectatic. The remainder of the lung may appear normal in primary bullous disorders or emphysematous in case of bullous emphysema. CT scan is also useful to assess for presence of complications including pneumothorax, air-fluid level, or superimposed lung cancer (see below).

Radionuclide imaging can be used to assess the functional status of the lungs prior to surgery. Perfusion scans are useful to demonstrate the lack of contribution of the bullous segment to gas exchange; this may predict an improvement in respiration following bullectomy (**Table 2**).

PULMONARY FUNCTION TESTS

Pulmonary function tests (PFTs) include spirometry, lung diffusion study, and lung volume assessment. **Spirometric parameters**, including forced expiratory volume in the first second (FEV_1) and the forced vital capacity (FVC) are usually normal in patients with primary bullous lung disease with surrounding normal lung parenchyma. However, patients with bullous emphysema have reduced FEV_1/FVC ratio and FEV_1 suggestive of obstructive lung disease akin to COPD.

The lung diffusion study is performed using diffusing capacity of the lung for carbon monoxide (DLCO). This may be normal in patients with pulmonary bullae and surrounding normal lung parenchyma. However, the DLCO is reduced in patients with emphysema.

The lung volumes including the total lung capacity (TLC) at maximal inspiration and residual volume (RV) after maximal expiration can be assessed using either of two methods. The first method is body plethysmography and measures the volume of the entire lung including the bullous regions. The second method uses helium gas dilution or nitrogen washout and does not assess the volume of poorly ventilated regions such as bullae. Hence, the difference of the TLC assessed using the two methods can help in approximating the volume of the bullae. Since patients with bullous lung disease have air trapping and hyperinflation of the lungs, body plethysmography usually reveals elevated TLC and RV.

There is an important role for PFTs in assessing patients with bullous lung disease for suitability for undergoing bullectomy. Although, there is insufficient prospective trial data to define specific cut-offs based on PFTs for contraindicating surgery, observational data suggests that surgical fitness can be assessed using spirometry and lung diffusion testing (**Table 2**). In studies of patients with FEV_1 values between 30 and 60% of predicted who underwent bullectomy, those with more severe obstructive lung disease and diffuse emphysema had poorer postoperative outcomes and increased risk of mortality. Hence, reduced values of FEV_1 and DLCO (<40% of predicted) may be contraindications for bullectomy.

LABORATORY TESTING

A complete blood count is useful to detect the presence of anemia (which may contribute to dyspnea) and secondary polycythemia (which may indicate chronic hypoxemia). An arterial blood gas evaluation is also helpful in patients who are in respiratory failure or are being considered for surgery. Elevated arterial partial pressure for carbon dioxide ($PaCO_2$ > 45 mm Hg) is associated with worse postoperative outcomes and is a contraindication for bullectomy.

There is limited role for blood tests in the etiologic evaluation of bullous lung disease. In selected patients with basal-predominant bullous disease, alpha-1-antitrypsin levels may be obtained. Further, HIV testing should be considered in all patients.

COMPLICATIONS

As previously mentioned, complications of bullous lung disease may be an initial manifestation or an exacerbating feature in existing bullous lung disease. The important complications of bullous lung disease are discussed in this section.

PNEUMOTHORAX

Patients with bullous lung disease are at an increased risk for **spontaneous pneumothorax**. The patients present with acute onset of dyspnea and chest pain. As the underlying lung is diseased, this is referred to as secondary spontaneous pneumothorax. Such patients may develop prolonged air leak, tension pneumothorax, or respiratory failure at a higher risk than primary spontaneous pneumothorax. Hence, all bullous lung disease patients with pneumothorax should be admitted and treated with drainage of the pleural air. As there is a high risk of recurrence, an attempt should be made to prevent the same. In patients with primary bullous lung disease with a giant bulla, a bullectomy along with pleurodesis may be performed by a video-assisted thoracoscopic surgery (VATS) approach. However, in patients with diffuse emphysema, pleurodesis is done without bullectomy.

It is important to note that the radiolucent appearances of pneumothorax and bullous lung disease may be confused for each other. In this regard, the configuration of the margin is helpful. In case of bullae, the thin wall is usually concave (forms an obtuse angle) in relation to the

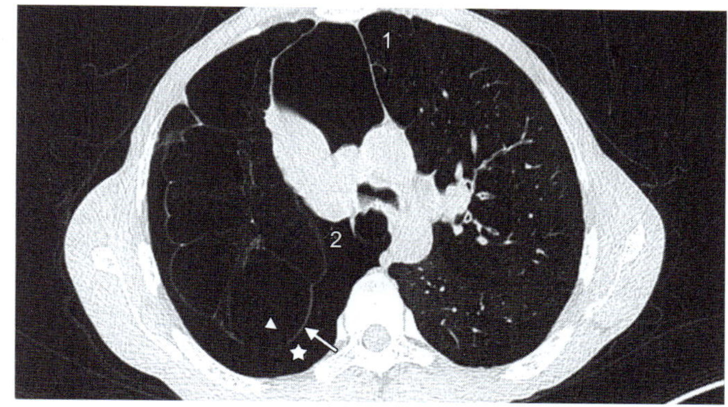

FIGURE 3: A lower section of the high-resolution computed tomography of chest of the same patient as **Figure 2**. The bilateral bullous lung disease is complicated by right-sided pneumothorax. Note the obtuse angle which the bulla forms with the chest wall in the left lung *(angle 1)* versus the acute angle which the pneumothorax forms with mediastinal wall in the right lung *(angle 2)*. **The double wall sign (arrow)** is seen separating the air in the bulla *(triangle)* from the air in the pleural cavity *(star)*.

chest wall. In contrast, the pleural line in pneumothorax is convex (forms an acute angle) in relation to the chest wall (**Fig. 3**). Further confusion may arise when a patient with underlying bullous lung disease has superimposed pneumothorax. A useful radiological sign observed in this situation is the "double wall sign," wherein air is seen on both sides of the margin: pneumothorax on one side, and bulla on the other (**Fig. 3**). Furthermore, the margin is usually convex toward the chest wall in keeping with the orientation of the pleural line in pneumothorax. The radiological discrimination of pneumothorax and bulla using HRCT of chest is imperative as inappropriate placement of chest drain in a bulla may lead to prolonged air leak and need for subsequent lobectomy.

AIR-FLUID LEVEL

Chest radiography is unable to distinguish whether an air fluid level is within a bulla or an infected or malignant cavity (**Fig. 1**). Hence, an HRCT of chest is useful in this situation to determine the wall thickness and reach the diagnosis of bullous lung disease. The occurrence of a new air-fluid level in a patient of known bullous lung disease may also clinch this diagnosis. An air-fluid level within a bulla can occur in numerous contexts: (1) benign, sterile fluid collections, (2) infected bullae, and (3) malignancy. In a series (Chandra et al.) of 52 patients with fluid containing bullae, over one-third were asymptomatic and only 10% had severe lung infection.

Benign fluid collections may be reactionary to adjacent pneumonia (analogous to parapneumonic pleural effusions) or incidental. Patients usually require treatment only if they have clinical, radiological, or microbiological diagnosis of pneumonia. Treatment need not continue till resolution of the air-fluid level as this may take several months after clinical improvement.

Infected bullae on the other hand occur due to primary infection within a bulla. Common etiological agents are methicillin-resistant *Staphylococcus aureus* (MRSA),

Bacteroides, and *Pseudomonas aeruginosa*. The patients usually present with fever, cough, sputum production, and chest pain. Microbiological testing of blood, sputum, or bronchoscopic specimens has low yield. Antibiotic selection should be similar to that for pneumonia in COPD patients and therapy is usually required for at least 6 weeks. In patients with persistent systemic features of infection, percutaneous image-guided drainage using a thin-bore catheter may be needed for source control and microbiological culture. Such drainage may be complicated by pneumothorax or empyema.

CARCINOMA LUNG

Patients with bullous lung disease are at *increased risk for the development of carcinoma lung*. The carcinoma may develop from the wall of the bulla and may appear radiologically as a nodule projecting outward or inward from the bullous wall or as a thickening of the wall. On occasion, it may present as a new air-fluid level, hemorrhage, or pneumothorax. Uptake on positron emission tomography (PET) may provide a clue to the diagnosis. Obtaining tissue for diagnosis of carcinoma arising from bullous wall is challenging. Bronchoscopy may be used for preoperative airway assessment but has low yield for pathological diagnosis. Suspicion of malignancy may guide decision of bullectomy or lobectomy. However, consideration must be given to the extent of emphysema and PFTs while assessing fitness for surgery.

MANAGEMENT

The management of bullous lung disease depends on the following factors: presence of symptoms, radiological extent of bullae, and status of surrounding lung parenchyma. Accordingly, patients may be candidates for medical, surgical, or novel approaches.

MEDICAL MANAGEMENT

Asymptomatic patients with primary bullous lung disease and normal surrounding lung parenchyma may be observed without any active management. Smoking cessation must be emphasized, and necessary aid provided. Clinical, radiological, and PFT follow-up may detect progression of bullous lung disease and need for intervention.

In symptomatic patients with bullous lung disease and bullous emphysema, medical management is along the lines of COPD management. Bronchodilators, inhaled glucocorticoids, vaccinations for influenza and pneumococcus, and pulmonary rehabilitation are advised as per COPD guidelines. Patients with respiratory failure may require long-term oxygen therapy (LTOT) or home noninvasive ventilation.

SURGICAL MANAGEMENT

Surgical management is advisable for symptomatic patients with pulmonary bullae. In the absence of prospective trials, there are no guidelines for selecting patients for bullectomy. The favorable features for surgery include presence of giant bulla with compression of adjacent lung parenchyma and absence of underlying emphysema (**Table 2**). Unfavorable features associated with postoperative morbidity include diffuse emphysema, severe obstruction, or impaired DLCO. Comorbidities like uncontrolled cardiovascular disease or pulmonary hypertension also portend an unfavorable outcome of surgery.

Bullectomy is usually performed by open or VATS-guided approaches. Open thoracotomy may employ a posterolateral incision. Presence of bilateral bullae may necessitate a median sternotomy. In appropriately selected patients, bullectomy may result in improvement of symptoms, lung function, exercise capacity, and blood gases. Prospective studies have demonstrated that benefits may persist for >5 years following surgery without recurrence of bullae. However, in a series (Palla et al.) of 41 consecutive patients who underwent bullectomy, 1-year and 5-year mortality rates were 7.3% and 12.2%, respectively. The mortality occurred exclusively in the subgroup of patients with underlying diffuse emphysema. An Indian series (Lone et al.) of 54 patients has also confirmed improvement in subjective dyspnea, FEV_1, and FVC postoperatively. In this series, patients with diffuse underlying emphysema had lesser improvements and increased risk of mortality.

Patients with predominantly bilateral apical bullous emphysema may also be candidates for *lung volume reduction surgery (LVRS)* as per existing recommendations for COPD. Finally, patients with severe obstruction (e.g., FEV_1 < 25% of predicted value), respiratory failure, pulmonary hypertension, or frequent exacerbations may be candidates for lung transplantation.

NEW APPROACHES

Patients with symptomatic bullous emphysema who are unfavorable surgical candidates may be considered for bronchoscopic management. A case report (Lee et al.) has described the use of bronchoscopic lung volume reduction (BLVR) using one-way endobronchial valve for successful management of a giant emphysematous bulla. Absence of collateral ventilation should be confirmed prior to BLVR. Further prospective studies are required to assess the feasibility of bronchoscopic approaches to management of bullous lung disease.

CONCLUSION

In conclusion, bullous lung diseases are relatively uncommon pulmonary ailments but carry considerable morbidity. They may be primary or secondary to preexisting lung disease; both types differ in risk factors, patient profile, and treatment modalities. Medical options are limited, while surgical treatment using bullectomy may be beneficial in selected patients but may be associated with increased postoperative morbidity or mortality. Alternative approaches including LVRS, BLVR, and lung transplantation can be considered, however, evidence for their efficacy is sparse.

RECOMMENDED READINGS

1. Agarwal R, Aggarwal AN. Bullous lung disease or bullous emphysema? Respir Care. 2006;51(5):532-4.
2. Mishra R, Patel R, Khaja M. Cannabis-induced bullous lung disease leading to pneumothorax. Medicine (Baltimore). 2017;96(19):e6917.
3. Chandra D, Rose SR, Carter RB, Musher DM, Hamill RJ. Fluid-containing emphysematous bullae: a spectrum of illness. Eur Respir J. 2008;32(2):303-6.
4. Lone YA, Dar AM, Sharma ML, Robbani I, Sarmast AH, Mushtaq E, et al. Outcome of the surgical treatment of bullous lung disease: a prospective study. Tanaffos. 2012;11(2):27-33.
5. van Berkel V, Kuo E, Meyers BF. Pneumothorax, bullous disease, and emphysema. Surg Clin North Am. 2010;90(5):935-53.
6. Sharma N, Justaniah AM, Kanne JP, Gurney JW, Mohammed TL. Vanishing lung syndrome (giant bullous emphysema): CT findings in 7 patients and a literature review. J Thorac Imaging. 2009;24(3):227-30.
7. Palla A, Desideri M, Rossi G, Bardi G, Mazzantini D, Mussi A, et al. Elective surgery for giant bullous emphysema: a 5-year clinical and functional follow-up. Chest. 2005;128(4):2043-50.
8. Lee EG, Rhee CK. Bronchoscopic lung volume reduction using an endobronchial valve to treat a huge emphysematous bullae: a case report. BMC Pulm Med. 2019;19(1):92.
9. Waitches GM, Stern EJ, Dubinsky TJ. Usefulness of the Double-wall sign in detecting pneumothorax in patients with giant bullous emphysema. Am J Roentgenol. 2000;174(6):1765-8.

CHAPTER 214

Sarcoidosis

Karan Madan

ABSTRACT

Sarcoidosis is a granulomatous disease that can affect virtually any organ, of which pulmonary involvement is the most common. The condition is characterized by the demonstration of noncaseating granulomas in tissue biopsy. The epidemiological profile and clinical presentation are variable. The diagnosis may be incidental in many patients. Differentiating sarcoidosis from mediastinal tuberculosis (TB) is also challenging in high TB prevalence settings.

Radiologically, a presentation with mediastinal lymphadenopathy and lung nodules is the most common. Bronchoscopic and endosonographic modalities are the cornerstones to diagnosis in a majority, as pulmonary involvement is present in more than 90% of the patients. Many patients are asymptomatic, and the disease course is variable. The clinical course may range from spontaneous remission, treatment-induced remission, relapses, or persistent disease activity.

Many patients with minimal or no symptoms and no evidence of threatening organ involvement may be observed, and disease may spontaneously remit. Corticosteroids are the mainstay of pharmacotherapy. The usual course of treatment, once initiated, is 6–12 months. The dose of steroids is gradually tapered. Other drugs like antimetabolites, cytotoxic drugs, and anti-tumor necrosis factor (TNF) agents like infliximab may be used in some patients with relapsed and refractory disease. Reliable indices of disease activity assessment are lacking, and usually, a combination of clinical, radiological, and lung function is used to follow-up treatment response in pulmonary sarcoidosis.

"I learned very early the difference between knowing the name of something and knowing something"

—Richard Feynman

INTRODUCTION

Sarcoidosis is a multisystem granulomatous disease with uncertain etiology. The condition affects all age groups and races and is characterized by nonnecrotizing granulomas in tissue biopsy specimens. Uncommonly, necrotizing granulomatous inflammation may also be evident. The clinical course ranges from spontaneous remission, relapses, or persistent disease activity. The diagnosis requires the exclusion of other possible causes of granulomatous inflammation.

There is a geographical variability in disease presentation, outcomes, and the frequency and type of organ involvement also differ across various ethnic backgrounds. The etiology is unclear. The pathogenic mechanism is hypothesized as an abnormal inflammatory response to an unidentified antigenic trigger leading to granulomatous organ system involvement. Intrathoracic involvement is the most common, and lungs and lymph nodes are most commonly involved. A myriad of extrapulmonary manifestations may occur. The other organs that may be affected include the eye, skin, kidney, heart, central nervous system (CNS), joints, bones, liver, spleen, and others. The respiratory system's involvement is usually the most common reason patients seek clinical evaluation and is the most common reason for the associated morbidity and healthcare utilization due to the disease.

EPIDEMIOLOGY

Sarcoidosis was initially thought to be uncommon in tropical and high TB endemic settings like India. However, sarcoidosis is a frequent indication for pulmonary physicians' referral to evaluate undiagnosed mediastinal lymphadenopathy in India. The exact prevalence of sarcoidosis in India is difficult to estimate as systematic population-based prevalence data are lacking. However, several studies highlighting the clinical profile of sarcoidosis in India have been published.

Globally a higher prevalence of sarcoidosis is found in *Scandinavian countries*. The demographic profile is also different. Data from the west indicate a younger age of onset and most patients are younger than 40 years. However, *data from India* suggest that the age of onset may be older (usually in the fourth or fifth decade). A female predominance of the disease in western literature is also not corroborated by the studies from India. Studies from India indicate that the gender distribution may be equal or a slight male predominance.

The phenotypic differences in disease presentation are also present. Acute presentation of the disease like Lofgren's syndrome and Heerfordt syndrome is uncommon in India. A familial clustering may be evident in some patients highlighting the possibility of genetic susceptibility.

CLINICAL PRESENTATION

The clinical presentation of sarcoidosis is variable and depends on the type of organ involvement. Pulmonary/intrathoracic involvement is the most common and occurs in more than 90% of patients. Constitutional symptoms are common, and fatigue may be a significant symptom. The most typical symptoms include cough, shortness of breath, fatigue, weight loss, and fever. Many patients may report dull aching chest pain. Hemoptysis is rare and pleural involvement is also uncommon. Patients may also report symptoms of airway obstruction like wheezing. The prevalence of obstructive defect on spirometry is variable, and its prevalence in India patients has been likely overestimated in many studies.

Eye involvement may be present in the form of conjunctival nodules and uveitis. Uveitis is the most common ocular manifestation, and acute presentation is typical. Some patients may present with chronic recurrent uveitis. Other ocular manifestations may include keratoconjunctivitis sicca, lacrimal gland enlargement, or retinal vasculitis. Skin involvement may occur and may consist of plaque-like lesions, maculopapular involvement, erythema nodosum etc. Lupus pernio is rarely described in Indian patients. Peripheral lymphadenopathy may also occur, and joint symptoms are frequently reported. Mostly the signs are arthralgias, and some patients may complain about obvious joint swellings.

Cardiac involvement is a potentially life-threatening manifestation. The presentation of cardiac sarcoidosis ranges from ventricular arrhythmias, cardiomyopathy, heart block, and sudden cardiac death. In many patients with cardiac sarcoidosis, mediastinal lymphadenopathy or pulmonary parenchymal involvement may be apparent. In these patients, a diagnosis may be made on a noncardiac tissue biopsy.

Neurosarcoidosis may have protean manifestations depending on the site of involvement. Hypercalcemia and hypercalciuria may occur and may rarely lead to acute renal failure. Rarely glomerulonephritis may lead to renal dysfunction. However, most patients do not have organ-threatening or life-threatening manifestations and respond well to treatment.

DIAGNOSIS

The diagnosis of sarcoidosis is confidently established with integration of clinical, radiological, and pathological findings.

IMAGING

An abnormal **chest radiograph** is a common finding in a majority of patients at presentation. The abnormality is usually a prominence of bilateral hila or the right paratracheal stripe (**Fig. 1**). The staging of pulmonary sarcoidosis on chest radiographs (**Scadding's classification**) is as follows: Stage 0, normal; stage 1, bilateral hilar enlargement; stage 2, bilateral

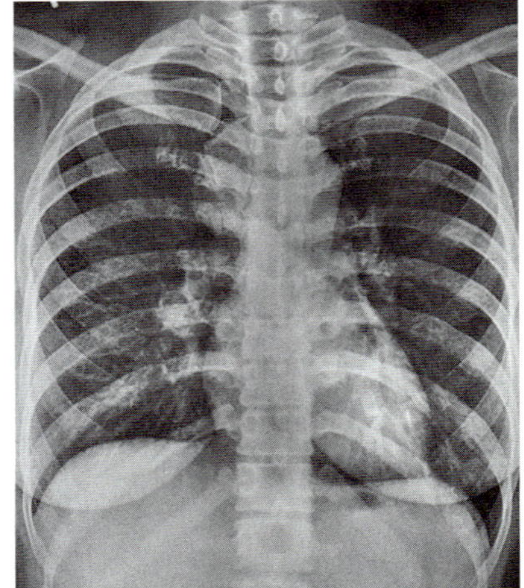

FIGURE 1: Chest radiograph showing widening of right paratracheal stripe suggesting the presence of paratracheal lymphadenopathy.

hilar enlargement with lung parenchymal infiltrates; and stage 3, lung infiltrates without hilar enlargement. The relevance of the Scadding's classification is now often debated following the widespread utilization of computed tomography (CT) scans.

A CT scan of the thorax: A CT scan of the thorax is one of the most useful imaging modalities in the diagnostic and management algorithm of patients with sarcoidosis. On CT, the nodal involvement is excellently discernible, and the character of the involved lymph nodes is also assessed (**Fig. 2**). The presence of homogenous and multistation lymph node involvement characterizes sarcoidosis. When present, pulmonary parenchymal involvement is characterized by the presence of perilymphatic nodules (peribronchovascular, fissural, subpleural, and interlobular septal involvement) (**Fig. 3**). Some authors have highlighted that a typical radiological pattern combined with the clinical findings may be diagnostic of sarcoidosis. However, a tissue diagnosis is preferable, and this is especially important in TB endemic stings. CT scan is also useful for response monitoring. CT scans also allow the assessment of pulmonary fibrosis and the presence of pulmonary artery hypertension (indicated by the presence of an enlarged pulmonary artery). The role of magnetic resonance imaging (MRI) in the diagnostic and monitoring algorithm of pulmonary sarcoidosis is not yet clearly established (**Fig. 4**).

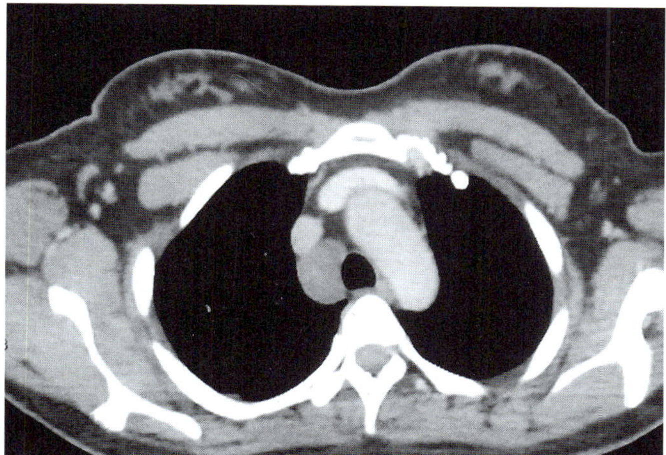

FIGURE 2: CT thorax mediastinal window section showing the presence of a homogenous, nonnecrotic lower paratracheal lymph node.

Recently, there are reports of the utilization of *positron emission tomography (PET)* scanning in sarcoidosis. Fluorodeoxyglucose (FDG)-PET scans combined with CT imaging (FDG-PET-CT) may help to assess the extent of disease involvement and response to treatment.

BRONCHOSCOPIC MODALITIES

As intrathoracic involvement is common, bronchoscopic approaches are the cornerstone for diagnosis of sarcoidosis in most patients. In case, another easily accessible peripheral site for tissue biopsy is available; the same may lead to the diagnosis. These include biopsy from the skin, peripheral lymph node, or the conjunctiva. Recent guidelines suggest that lymph node biopsy may be avoided in patients with a typical presentation of sarcoidosis. However, evidence to support the same is weak, and in case a biopsy is not performed, patients must be kept under close clinical observation and follow-up.

The bronchoscopic modalities are used for sampling of mediastinal lymph nodes or the lung parenchyma. The modalities can be conventional bronchoscopy centered or endosonographic modalities. The various bronchoscopic modalities for diagnosis of sarcoidosis include:

- *Lymph node aspiration modalities*:
  - Transbronchial needle aspiration (TBNA)
  - Endobronchial ultrasound-guided TBNA (EBUS-TBNA)

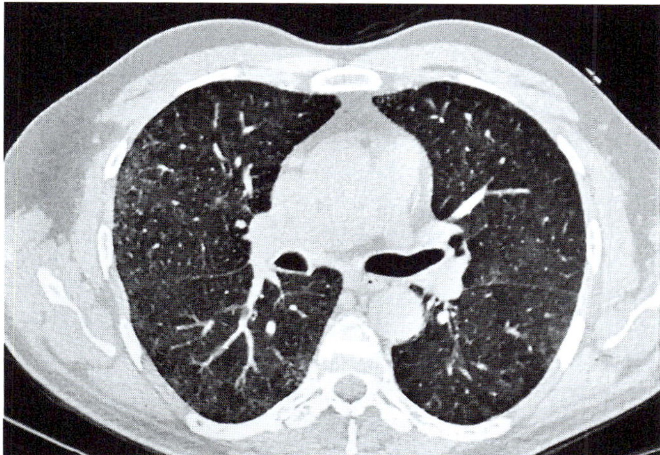

FIGURE 3: CT thorax lung window section showing multiple nodules with ground-glass opacity and fissural and pleural nodularity.

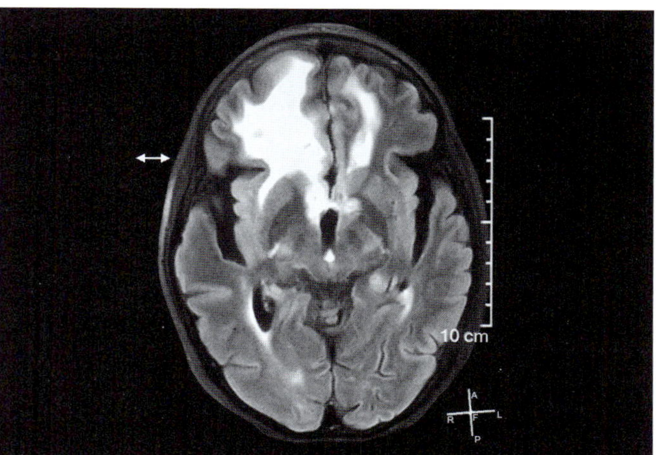

FIGURE 4: Magnetic resonance imaging (MRI) of brain showing extensive frontal lobe hyperintensities in a patient with neurosarcoidosis.

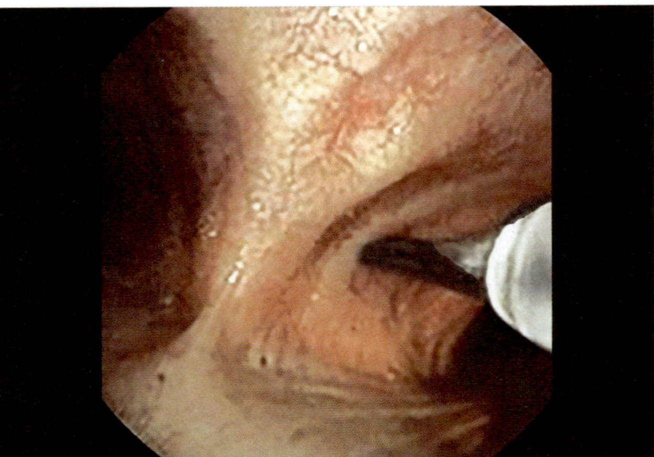

FIGURE 5: Bronchoscopic image showing transbronchial needle aspiration (TBNA) being performed from the subcarinal lymph node station.

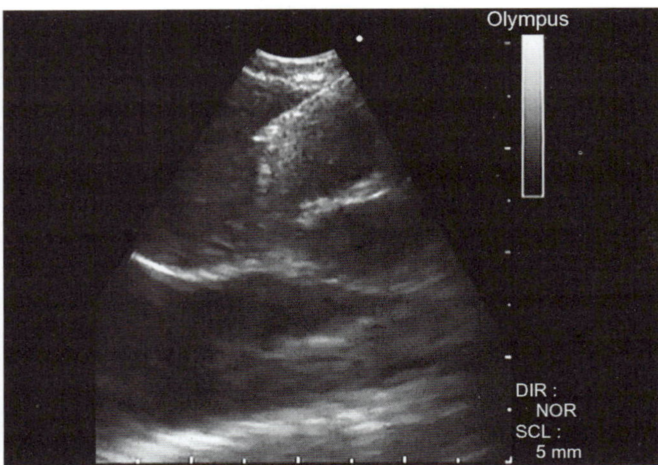

FIGURE 6: Sonographic image showing the endobronchial ultrasound-guided (EBUS) needle inside the lower paratracheal lymph node.

- Endoscopic ultrasound with bronchoscope-guided fine needle aspiration (EUS-B-FNA)
- Endoscopic ultrasound-guided FNA (EUS-FNA)
- *Lung biopsy modalities*:
  - Endobronchial biopsy (EBB)
  - Transbronchial lung biopsy (TBLB)
  - Transbronchial lung cryobiopsy (TBLC)
- Bronchoalveolar lavage (BAL)

LYMPH NODE ASPIRATION

Transbronchial needle aspiration is performed using a standard adult flexible bronchoscope (**Fig. 5**). The procedure involves introducing a flexible needle catheter (usually 21G or 19G) through the bronchoscope's working channel, followed by needle puncture of the bronchial wall. The procedure is performed by the bronchoscopist based on the knowledge of the anatomical landmarks. The yield of conventional TBNA as a standalone procedure is moderate and is safe and efficacious, especially for lymphadenopathy, at the lower right paratracheal and subcarinal lymph node stations.

ENDOSONOGRAPHIC MODALITIES

The evaluation of mediastinal lymphadenopathy has been revolutionized since the advent of various endosonographic procedures. Endosonographic modalities are based on dedicated bronchoscopes or endoscopes with an integrated ultrasound transducer at the distal end. These modalities allow real-time ultrasonographic visualization of the mediastinal lymph nodes and aspiration using dedicated needle assemblies. During **EBUS-TBNA**, a dedicated ultrasound bronchoscope is used, and real-time aspiration may be performed from lymph nodes near the tracheobronchial tree (**Fig. 6**). As a standalone modality, EBUS-TBNA has the widest mediastinal reach among the available endosonographic modalities. The EBUS bronchoscope may also be introduced through the esophagus to aspirate lymph nodes near the esophagus, a procedure described as EUS-B-FNA. The advantage of this approach is less cough due to the avoidance of tracheal introduction of the bronchoscope. It provides good access to the left-sided paratracheal, subcarinal, paraesophageal, and pulmonary ligament lymph nodes.

Gastroenterologists perform EUS-FNA, and there is a dedicated ultrasound endoscope for this indication. The EUS scope's size is larger than the EBUS bronchoscope, and the access is limited to the esophageal accessible lymph node stations. EBUS centered approaches are recommended as the preferred diagnostic modalities for the evaluation of sarcoidosis. The yield of TBNA is lower than EBUS-TBNA as a standalone procedure. TBNA-based approach in combination with EBB and TBLB may be used when EBUS-TBNA is not available.

LUNG AND BRONCHIAL BIOPSY

Before the advent of endosonography, bronchoscopic diagnosis of sarcoidosis was predominantly centered on the conventional bronchoscopic biopsy modalities. EBB involves a pinch biopsy of the bronchial mucosa using a small biopsy forceps (usually 2.0–2.8 mm) during diagnostic bronchoscopy. In many patients with pulmonary sarcoidosis, an endobronchial granularity is apparent. During TBLB, similar biopsy forceps are used to obtain multiple biopsies from the distal lung parenchyma. Even with normal radiological imaging, lung biopsy may show granulomas. TBLB carries a risk of pneumothorax and bleeding. Fluoroscopic guidance may be used to minimize the risk of pneumothorax by maintaining a distance from a pleural surface during the biopsy.

The yield of needle aspiration modalities in isolation may be suboptimal. Recent evidence supports the combination of lymph node aspiration combined with EBB and TBLB to optimize diagnostic yield to detect granulomas. In case ROSE (rapid on-site evaluation) of aspirates can be performed, EBB and TBLB may be avoidable in many patients.

Because of the small size of biopsy specimens obtained with small bronchoscopic biopsy forceps, another recently described modality is TBLC. In contrast to small biopsy forceps, TBLC utilizes a flexible thin cryoprobe (usually 1.9–2.4 mm), which may be introduced through a flexible bronchoscope channel. The cryoprobe freezes a spherical part of the lung tissue and allows lung biopsies that are considerably larger than the conventional TBLB. The role of TBLC in the diagnostic algorithm of sarcoidosis remains investigational.

BRONCHOALVEOLAR LAVAGE

An elevated CD4:CD8 T lymphocyte ratio in the BAL may support a diagnosis but is seldom performed, and its utility in TB endemic settings has not been studied in detail.

Although surgical approaches like mediastinoscopy have a higher diagnostic yield for detecting granulomas than EBUS, a surgical procedure may be associated with significant morbidity and are not preferred.

TREATMENT

A diagnosis of sarcoidosis is not by itself an indication of initiation of pharmacotherapy. The disease course is highly variable, and a standardized management protocol is difficult to formulate. Many patients are asymptomatic, and the disease may undergo spontaneous remission in a large proportion of patients. Asymptomatic patients without any evidence of significant functional or organ system impairment may be observed, and the disease may improve spontaneously in many.

Treatment in pulmonary sarcoidosis aims to reduce the burden of granulomatous inflammation and improve organ function if any impairment is present. Treatment aims to prevent irreversible organ damage and improve the quality of life. *Corticosteroids are the mainstay of pharmacotherapy*. Most recommendations on the dosage and duration of treatment are based on expert opinion. Randomized controlled trials to provide high-quality evidence for treatment recommendations are lacking. Once corticosteroid treatment is initiated, it is usually continued for 6–12 months. Another challenge during the treatment and follow-up of these patients is a lack of standardized and reliable measures to assess disease activity. The follow-up and assessment of response to treatment are performed based on clinical, radiological, and lung function testing parameters. Lung disease is one of the major indications of long-term pharmacotherapy.

The second-line drugs may be required in patients who either fail to respond to corticosteroids, relapse, or develop side effects of corticosteroid treatment. The second-line agents for sarcoidosis treatment include methotrexate, azathioprine, mycophenolate mofetil, leflunomide, and infliximab. The anti-TNF monoclonal antibody infliximab is usually reserved for persistent disease refractory to treatment with corticosteroids and another immunomodulatory agent. As the second-line agents, both methotrexate and azathioprine are efficacious. However, the risk of increased infections (with azathioprine) and hepatic toxicity (with methotrexate) need to be carefully monitored.

CONCLUSION

Sarcoidosis is a common cause of mediastinal lymphadenopathy. The clinical presentation is varied, and many patients are asymptomatic. Diagnosis requires careful integration and interpretation of clinical, radiological, and tissue biopsy findings. Mediastinal TB is a close differential diagnosis in TB prevalent populations. Many patients do not require pharmacotherapy and improve spontaneously. A close clinical follow-up is required during clinical management.

RECOMMENDED READINGS

1. Spagnolo P, Rossi G, Trisolini R, Sverzellati N, Baughman RP, Wells AU. Pulmonary sarcoidosis. Lancet Respir Med. 2018;6(5):389-402.
2. Madan K, Dhungana A, Mohan A, Hadda V, Jain D, Arava S, et al. Conventional Transbronchial Needle Aspiration Versus Endobronchial Ultrasound-guided Transbronchial Needle Aspiration, With or Without Rapid On-Site Evaluation, for the Diagnosis of Sarcoidosis: A Randomized Controlled Trial. J Bronchology Interv Pulmonol. 2017;24(1):48-58.
3. Sharma SK, Mohan A. Sarcoidosis: global scenario & Indian perspective. Indian J Med Res. 2002;116: 221-47.
4. Singha A, Liao SY, Herman DD, Crouser ED, Maier LA, Baughman RP, et al. Summary for Clinicians: Clinical Practice Guideline for the Diagnosis and Detection of Sarcoidosis. Ann Am Thorac Soc. 2020;17(12):1510-15.
5. Guleria R, Jyothidasan A, Madan K, Mohan A, Kumar R, Bhalla AS, et al. Utility of FDG-PET-CT scanning in assessing the extent of disease activity and response to treatment in Sarcoidosis. Lung India. 2014;31(4):323-30.
6. Sharma SK, Soneja M, Sharma A, Sharma MC, Hari S. Rare manifestations of Sarcoidosis in modern era of new diagnostic tools. Indian J Med Res. 2012;135(5):621-9.

CHAPTER

215 Pulmonary Eosinophilic Disorders

Aditya Jindal

ABSTRACT

Pulmonary eosinophilic disorders are defined as the syndromic conditions characterized with peripheral and/or pulmonary eosinophilia. Some of the important primary lung conditions involving the lungs include acute and chronic eosinophilic pneumonias while secondary pulmonary eosinophilia may be seen in parasitic infestations and infections with other microorganisms (bacteria, fungi, and tuberculosis). Various systemic eosinophilic diseases with lung involvement may characteristically include eosinophilic granulomatosis with polyangiitis (EGPA) [Churg–Strauss syndrome (CSS)] and idiopathic hypereosinophilic syndrome (HES). Some other syndromes which are also characterized with eosinophilia include tropical pulmonary eosinophilia (TPE) (usually secondary to microfilarial infection of the lungs), allergic bronchopulmonary aspergillosis, and hypersensitivity pneumonias. Eosinophilia can also occur following administration of certain drugs, toxins, and following radiation. Although not diagnostic, variable degrees of raised eosinophil counts may also be seen in other different conditions such as interstitial lung diseases, sarcoidosis, idiopathic pulmonary fibrosis and organizing pneumonia, Langerhans cell histiocytosis (LCH), and connective tissue diseases. Eosinophilia is also an important feature of allergic phenotypes of bronchial asthma.

Diagnosis of pulmonary eosinophilic disorders is made in the presence of respiratory symptoms, radiological presence of infiltrates, and raised eosinophil count in the peripheral blood. Peripheral blood eosinophilia may, however, be absent. Pulmonary eosinophilia in such a situation can be demonstrated on induced sputum or bronchoalveolar lavage fluid examination. Transbronchial lung biopsy may be required in such cases when the underlying diagnosis is not clear. Treatment of pulmonary eosinophilia essentially depends upon the primary cause of eosinophilia.

Eosinophils are important cells in the etiopathogenesis of several systemic and pulmonary diseases. Eosinophilic lung diseases include conditions associated with peripheral and/or pulmonary eosinophilia. As a part of the human leukocyte system, eosinophils have a variety of functions to perform. They are especially important in the defense against helminthic infestations—eosinophilic products are lethal to the larval stages of these parasites. They also exert an important role in allergic disorders, parasitic, and neoplastic diseases.

"Health is not valued till sickness comes"

—Thomas Fuller

MATURATION OF EOSINOPHILS

Eosinophils share a common immediate precursor with basophils which under the influence of cytokines, such as interlukin-5 (IL-5), GM-CSF and IL-3 differentiate toward the eosinophilic lineage. IL-5 produced by T cells and endothelial cells in the bone marrow, promotes the release of eosinophils into the bloodstream.

The mature eosinophil varies from 12–17 μm in diameter and has a bilobed nucleus in an eosinophilic cytoplasm. It is characterized by the presence of various granules in the cytoplasm, which are clearly visible on electron microscopy. *There are two types of granules:* (1) primary and (2) secondary. Primary granules are rounded, membrane-limited structures and contain Charcot–Leyden crystal protein. The secondary granules are somewhat oval and consist of a dense core clearly visible in a less dense matric. The core of these granules is formed by major basic protein (MBP) while the matrix contains various other enzymes such as eosinophil-derived neurotoxin (EDN), eosinophil cationic protein (ECT), and eosinophil peroxidase. Additionally, dense lipid bodies that are not membrane bound and contain enzymes for metabolizing arachidonic acid, are present. These serve as sites of eicosanoid synthesis.

After a brief intravascular stay of 3–8 hours following its release, the *mature eosinophil enters various tissues*—predominantly those having an epithelial-environment interface such as the respiratory, gastrointestinal, and genitourinary tracts. Once in tissues, survival depends upon the local production of cytokines regulating eosinophil apoptosis. It is eventually phagocytosed by tissue macrophages after a few days. Eosinophils have a diurnal variation in response to the level of endogenous steroids with higher levels in the morning. There is an increase in the total eosinophil count in the blood following parasitic infestations, allergic reactions, and after administration of certain drugs. On the other hand, eosinopenia occurs due to pyogenic infections and in response to exogenous steroids, estrogens, and epinephrine.

Circulating eosinophils adhere to the vascular endothelium by rolling and enter the interstitium by passing in between the endothelial cells and then migrate to the site of inflammation under the influence of certain cytokines and chemokines. They are primed by cytokines such as IL-5, platelet activating factor, and complement fragment of C5a resulting in the release of various mediators by piecemeal degranulation that include MBP, ECP, and other mediators.

Normal limits of eosinophils and defining limits of eosinophilia vary in different clinical syndromes (**Box 1**). HES is defined when the count is abnormally high lasting at least for 6 months along with lack of evidence for known causes of eosinophilia and signs and symptoms of organ involvement/dysfunction.

PULMONARY EOSINOPHILIC DISORDERS

A holistic approach to pulmonary eosinophilic disorders involves understanding the epidemiology. In recent years, a significant evolution in classification and differentiation has taken place. Broadly, eosinophilic disorders are divided into the following categories:

- Hypereosinophilic syndromes previously considered idiopathic for which the causes are now known.
- Organ-restricted eosinophilic syndromes—pulmonary eosinophilic disorders and eosinophilic gastrointestinal disorders
- Syndromes in which eosinophilia and eosinophil-associated pathogenesis are central to the diagnosis—CSS.
- Hereditary disorders characterized by eosinophilia

Pulmonary eosinophilic disorders may occur with or without a known cause or as an association of known lung disease (**Box 2**).

LÖFFLER SYNDROME

The original description by Löffler in 1932 was of a syndrome consisting of no to minimal respiratory symptoms along with fleeting pulmonary opacities and peripheral eosinophilia. A similar syndrome may be seen secondary to drug reactions. The clinical picture is characterized by an acute, self-limiting disease comprising of low-grade fever, dry cough, dyspnea, and occasionally, hemoptysis. Moderate to marked eosinophilia is seen in the peripheral blood and respiratory secretions. The chest X-ray will show transient, migratory, nonsegmental interstitial, or alveolar infiltrates on chest roentgenography. Symptoms generally resolve within a short period of 1–2 weeks.

BOX 1 Normal and abnormal limits of eosinophilia.

- **Normal eosinophil counts:**
  - Differential: ≤5%
  - AEC: ≤0.5 × 10^9/L
- **Eosinophilia:**
  - Mild: AEC 0.5–1.5 × 10^9/L
  - Moderate: AEC 1.5–5.0 × 10^9/L
  - Severe: AEC > 5.0 × 10^9/L
- **Hypereosinophilic syndrome (HES):**
  - AEC: >1.5 × 10^9/L lasting for 6 months

(AEC: absolute eosinophil count)

ACUTE EOSINOPHILIC PNEUMONIA

Acute eosinophilic pneumonia (AEP) is characterized by acute onset of fever, respiratory symptoms, and respiratory failure in a previously healthy subject. It is rapidly progressive.

PRESENTATION

AEP commonly occurs more frequently in men at a median age of 30 years. The exact cause in the majority of individuals is not known but it is more commonly associated with unusual activities such as *cave exploring* and *wood working*.

BOX 2 Some important causes of pulmonary eosinophilia.

- **Primary:**
  - Predominant involving lung:
    - Acute eosinophilic pneumonia
    - Chronic eosinophilic pneumonia
  - Systemic disease with lung involvement:
    - Eosinophilic granulomatosis with polyangiitis (Churg–Strauss syndrome)
    - Idiopathic hypereosinophilic syndrome
- **Pulmonary eosinophilia secondary to a known cause:**
  - Parasitic infestations due to transient passage through the lungs (Löffler syndrome): *Ancylostoma, Ascaris*, and strongyloides
  - Tissue resident parasites: Paragonimiasis and echinococcosis
  - Heavy hematogenous seeding by the parasites: *Trichinella*, visceral larva migrans, disseminated strongyloidiasis, and schistosomiasis
  - Fungal infections: Coccidioidomycosis and histoplasmosis
  - Other infections: Tuberculosis and brucellosis
  - Tropical pulmonary eosinophilia
  - Allergic bronchopulmonary aspergillosis
  - Hypersensitivity pneumonia
  - Drugs, toxins, and radiation
- **Eosinophilia associated with different lung disorders:**
  - Interstitial lung diseases; sarcoidosis, idiopathic pulmonary fibrosis, organizing pneumonia, Langerhans cell histiocytosis, and connective tissue diseases
  - Bronchial asthma
  - Neoplastic disorders: Hematological malignancies and solid organ tumors
  - Postlung transplant

Recently, it is reported with an increased frequency in *people who smoke e-cigarettes* or are exposed to passive smoking. E-cigarette smoking or vaping has been promoted as an alternative to smoking which has been thought to be safer. However, an increasing number of cases of electronic cigarette or vaping product use-associated lung injury have been noted. Though the most common pathological patterns are organizing pneumonia or diffuse alveolar damage, AEP has also been noted.

Acute eosinophilic pneumonia often presents with fever, cough, myalgias, dyspnea, and pleuritic chest pain that may rapidly progress to frank respiratory failure. Characteristically, there is no multisystem involvement despite severe respiratory failure. A possibility of AEP should always be kept in mind during the evaluation of any patient with acute respiratory distress syndrome (ARDS).

DIAGNOSIS

Typically there is leukocytosis with initial absence of peripheral blood eosinophilia. However, a recent study demonstrated that up to 28% of patients may have peripheral blood eosinophilia at presentation; also it may be associated with a better prognosis as compared to patients without initial eosinophilia. Bilateral patchy reticular infiltrates that progress rapidly to an ARDS-like picture are seen on chest radiography. The computed tomography (CT) scan may show ground glass opacities and/or consolidation which may be diffuse in nature; smooth interlobular septal thickening distributed in a random manner without any zonal predominance may sometimes be seen. Bilateral pleural effusions may be seen in some cases with pleural fluid analysis showing marked eosinophilia and high pH. Bronchoalveolar lavage (BAL) shows marked eosinophilia along with variably elevated levels of beta-D-glucan and many cytokines such as IL-5 and IL-18. Pulmonary function tests during the acute phase show a restrictive defect with reduced diffusing capacity of the lung for carbon monoxide (DLCO).

Pathologically, the main finding is that of *a diffuse alveolar damage syndrome*, with marked eosinophilic infiltration in the interstitium and in the alveolar spaces. Fibrinous membranes are commonly seen; airway involvement with mucus plugs has also been described. AEP is not characterized by either formation of granulomas or by alveolar hemorrhage. Pleural eosinophilic infiltration has been noted in 10% of cases. Despite its severe clinical presentation, AEP is *highly responsive to corticosteroids*. Mechanical ventilation may be required for severe cases, with ventilation strategies as for ARDS. Mortality rate is low if prompt treatment is instituted.

IDIOPATHIC CHRONIC EOSINOPHILIC PNEUMONIA

Idiopathic chronic eosinophilic pneumonia (ICEP) may occur at any age with the peak incidence between the ages of 30 and 40 years. Patients are *generally nonsmokers with a female preponderance*. Antecedent atopy, allergic rhinitis, or nasal polyps are present in one-third to half of the patients. Adult onset asthma is present in about two-thirds of patients.

The disease generally has an insidious onset and indolent course with predominant symptoms of low-grade fever, night sweats, and weight loss. Cough, dyspnea, and wheezing are the other common symptoms. Dyspnea is generally mild, but at times may progress to a point that mechanical ventilation may be required. Extrapulmonary manifestations which may be seen sometimes include arthralgias, joints pain, and heart failure. In fact, presence of significant extrapulmonary symptoms should necessitate a search for other systemic disorders such as vasculitis or HES.

DIAGNOSIS

The peripheral blood examination commonly reveals normocytic-normochromic anemia, mild to moderately elevated erythrocyte sedimentation rate, moderate leukocytosis, and an elevated eosinophil count; the platelet count may also be elevated. BAL fluid also shows marked eosinophilia with raised serum immunoglobulin E (IgE) levels. Pulmonary function testing may either be normal or show an obstructive or restrictive defect.

Radiologically, infiltrates are dense, patchy, bilateral, peripheral, and symmetrical, involve the upper and mid zones, and are progressive in nature. The characteristic "photographic negative of pulmonary edema" is seen in <25% of cases. Pleural effusions are uncommon. Histopathology reveals interstitial and alveolar infiltration by eosinophils, and other inflammatory cells. There is disruption of the local architecture and features of proliferative bronchiolitis obliterans, microangiitis, and microabscesses.

MANAGEMENT

Response to corticosteroids in CEP is often dramatic with symptoms decreasing within 6–48 hours and radiological clearing within 2 months. Oral steroids with dose ranging from 0.5 to 1 mg/kg/day can be used and treatment in low doses is maintained for at least 6 months to 1 year or longer. Relapse may occur in half to two-thirds of treated patients. Relapse can usually be controlled by reinstitution of steroids which may need to be given for prolonged periods of time; the dose of oral steroids can be brought down by the addition of inhaled corticosteroids.

The use of omalizumab, an anti-IgE antibody, has been described recently as a steroid sparing agent in CEP with good results. Use of agents acting against IL-5 has also been described. Mepolizumab and reslizumab are agents that prevent the binding of IL-5 with eosinophils and prevent degranulation and release of chemokines. Benralizumab, another agent, acts by binding to the IL-5 receptor and also by inducing antibody-dependent cell-mediated cytotoxicity and apoptosis of target cells. Only scattered case reports of use of these agents are available, with good results.

EOSINOPHILIC GRANULOMATOSIS WITH POLYANGIITIS (EGPA)

Churg–Strauss syndrome was first described as a separate entity in the early 1950s. The nomenclature was recently revised and it has now been renamed as eosinophilic granulomatosis with polyangiitis (EGPA). It has now been defined as an eosinophil-rich and necrotizing granulomatous inflammation often involving the respiratory tract, and necrotizing vasculitis predominantly affecting small to medium vessels, and associated with asthma and eosinophilia. The diverse clinical presentation and the difficulty in differentiating the disease often lead to a delay in the diagnosis. It is 2–10 times less common than the other antinuclear cytotoxic antibodies (ANCA)-associated vasculitis with an incidence of 0.5–3.7 per million and a prevalence of 2–22 per million population. It can affect any age group with peak incidence between 30 and 50 years.

The underlying pathology is believed to be an immune hypersensitivity, accounting for the presence of ANCA and nearly universal finding of an atopic state in these individuals. The presence or absence of ANCA allows the differentiation of these patients into two subgroups. The group with ANCA positivity has more frequent mononeuritis multiplex, glomerulonephritis, purpura, and alveolar hemorrhage while the ANCA negative group has more frequent cardiomyopathic features and lung infiltrates. This has also been supported by a recent genome-wide association study which suggests the presence of two distinct EGPA groups, corresponding to ANCA status.

Eosinophilic granulomatosis with polyangiitis has been described in association with the use of leukotriene inhibitors, montelukast more than zafirlukast. The onset of the disease is variable from 2 days to 12 months after the initiation of therapy and it occurs almost exclusively as corticosteroids are being tapered off. This is considered to be an unmasking of the underlying disease rather than the result of drug use. There have also been reports of EGPA occurring after the use of omalizumab.

CLINICAL FEATURES

Eosinophilic granulomatosis with polyangiitis is commonly diagnosed when a patient with long-standing asthma develops symptoms suggestive of vasculitis, i.e., mononeuritis multiplex, purpura, along with peripheral eosinophilia and lung infiltrates. Three stages have been described clinically:

1. *Prodromal stage:* Presence of late onset atopic states such as allergic rhinitis, nasal polyposis, and asthma.
2. *Eosinophilic stage:* Eosinophilic infiltration of various tissues such as the skin, gastrointestinal tract (GIT), and lungs.
3. *Vasculitic stage:* Clinical onset of constitutional symptoms; histological presence of eosinophilic infiltration, vasculitis, and granulomatous infiltration

The clinical course can be variable and may not strictly adhere to the mentioned stages. The respiratory manifestations of EGPA include upper respiratory tract disease, asthma, pleural effusions, and Löffler-like syndrome. The upper respiratory tract involved in about 75–85% of cases manifests as allergic rhinitis, sinusitis, and nasal polyposis. Usually, there is no necrosis is seen in EGPA.

Asthma is the predominant feature of EGPA. It may be present for many years before the diagnosis of EGPA is made. It is usually predominant in the prodromal and eosinophilic stages of the disease and may subside with the onset of the vasculitic phases. A short interval between the onset of asthma and that of vasculitis is considered a sign of increased severity.

DIAGNOSIS

Diagnosis is established on the basis of clinic-radiological features and hematological examination described earlier. Overall, about 40% of patients have ANCA positivity; this is generally perinuclear (pANCA) with specificity against myeloperoxidase. However, only 25% of patients with EGPA who have no renal disease are ANCA positive, while ANCA is positive in 75% of patients with any renal disease and in 100% with documented necrotizing glomerulonephritis. The titers of ANCA do not have utility as a marker of disease activity on follow-up examinations.

TREATMENT

There is no stratified treatment schedule available in EGPA as in other ANCA-associated vasculitis. The choice of treatment is based on the presence of systemic involvement. *The five-factor score (FFS) is the most commonly used guide for treatment initiation.* The five factors are: (1) proteinuria > 1 g/24 h; (2) serum creatinine level > 140 mmol/L; (3) myocardial involvement; (4) severe gastrointestinal involvement; and (5) central nervous system involvement. Presence of ≥1 of these factors is indicative of a higher risk of morbidity and mortality; if the FFS is ≥1, treatment is started with both *steroids and immunosuppressive agents* while steroids alone would suffice with a FFS of 0. Oral prednisolone may be started at a dose of 1 mg/kg/day and continued for 6–12 weeks followed by a gradual taper to a maintenance dose, which might be continued for a year or more.

Indications for the use of *cytotoxic chemotherapy* include nonresponsiveness to steroids and severe systemic disease including cardiac, GIT, and renal disease (proteinuria > 1 g/day or renal insufficiency). Pulse cyclophosphamide is probably the immunosuppressive treatment of choice in an acute phase, whereas azathioprine may be useful for maintenance. Pulse steroids may also be used in acute settings. Other immunomodulators such as high-dose intravenous Ig and interferon-alpha in standard dose have also been used in severe disease and so have been plasma exchange.

Mepolizumab, an anti-IL-5 humanized monoclonal antibody, has been also been evaluated in a double-blind, placebo-controlled randomized trial. In this trial, relapsing and refractory patients were randomized to additional mepolizumab versus standard care alone. Patients on mepolizumab remained in remission longer and had a higher chance of remission. This effect was more pronounced in the group of ANCA negative patients rather than in patients with ANCA positivity. Other agents active against IL-5 (benralizumab and reslizumab) are also been investigated in EGPA.

The use of *rituximab, an anti-CD-20 agent,* has expanded tremendously in other ANCA-associated vasculitides. However, its use in EGPA has been less extensively evaluated. Expert panel guidelines from the European League Against Rheumatism (EULAR) and the British Society for Rheumatology have recommended the treatment of EGPA similar to that of other ANCA-associated vasculitides. Rituximab has emerged as an alternative induction and remission maintenance agent in all forms of ANCA-associated vasculitis.

PROGNOSIS

The use of corticosteroids has dramatically reduced the mortality rate. Long-term remissions are usually achieved, though relapses may occur. The current cumulative survival rates are 88–97% and 78–89% at 5 and 10 years, respectively. The use of steroids and immunosuppressive agents may cause significant morbidity though, in the form of infections, osteoporosis, solid organ malignancies etc.

HYPEREOSINOPHILIC SYNDROME

Also known as Löffler endocarditis and eosinophilic leukemia, HES is a disorder which predominantly affects males, more common in age groups of 20–50 years and characterized by multisystem involvement. The cause of this disorder is unknown but the organ damage occurs as a result of eosinophilic infiltration and/or thromboembolic phenomena.

CLINICAL FEATURES

Hypereosinophilic syndrome is a heterogeneous disease. Its clinical manifestations are highly variable in the terms of duration, severity, and organ involvement. The symptoms most often are indolent; include fever, weight loss, fatigue, anorexia, night sweats, skin rash, hepatosplenomegaly, angioedema, and other system involvement. Respiratory system is involved in approximately 40% of cases, manifested predominantly by nocturnal cough wheezing and dyspnea. Occasionally, the disease can progress to ARDS. Pleural effusion, pulmonary hypertension, and thromboembolism may develop over a period of time.

The cardiovascular system is common involved with an eosinophilic infiltration of the endocardium and myocardium, endocardial fibrosis, and mitral regurgitation. Intracardiac thrombus formation occurs, leading to pulmonary thromboembolism. Associated peripheral arterial or venous thrombosis has also been reported. Neurological manifestations include encephalopathy, neuropsychiatric disturbances, memory loss, visual changes, and cerebrovascular accidents secondary to thromboembolism.

DIAGNOSIS

Blood examination shows anemia, leukocytosis (10,000–50,000/mm^3) with 30–70% eosinophils; associated may be blood and or bone marrow neutrophilia, basophilia, and eosinophilic dysplasia. Circulating immune complexes are occasionally found. Bone marrow shows an increase in eosinophils and eosinophil precursors. Eosinophilic blast transformation has been noted in 28–51% of patients. Eosinophilic infiltration of other organs is also demonstrable on histopathological examination.

Hypereosinophilic syndrome should be differentiated from other eosinophilic disorders like CEP, CSS, AEP, tropical pulmonary eosinophilia (TPE), fungal infections and parasitic infestations etc. Different laboratory criteria are used for the differential diagnosis of lymphoproliferative and myeloproliferative variants.

TREATMENT

Treatment depends upon the symptomatology and presence of end-organ dysfunction.

Asymptomatic peripheral eosinophilia can be followed up every 3–6 months without any treatment. Steroids constitute the first line of therapy; prednisone, in a dose of 1 mg/kg/day for 1–2 months is followed by a slow taper to a maintenance dose, which can be continued for 1 year or longer as required. In refractory cases, treatment can be tried with hydroxyurea, vincristine, chlorambucil, cyclosporine, or interferon-α. The anti-IL-5 antibody, mepolizumab has also been used in patients with high IL-5 levels.

Patients with myeloproliferative variant do not respond well to steroids. Use of tyrosine-kinase inhibitors such as imatinib and dasatinib results in a gratifying response.

Steroids should be added to imatinib in patients with evidence of myocarditis on echocardiography, electrocardiography, or biochemical parameters (elevated serum troponin).

In the last few years, novel agents acting against IL-5 have been tried. These include mepolizumab, benralizumab, and reslizumab. Mepolizumab, an IL-5 antibody, was tested in a double-blind, placebo-controlled phase 2 trial in 85 PDGFRA-negative patients at a higher dose that in other hypereosinophilic syndromes and was found to be safe and effective as a steroid sparing agent. Benralizumab and reslizumab have been tested in smaller studies while further larger studies are ongoing.

The causes of death in HES include refractory congestive cardiac failure, renal failure, hepatic failure, venous thromboembolism, gut perforation, and infections. However, proper treatment leads to a mean survival of >10 years.

OTHER EOSINOPHILIC LUNG DISEASES

LANGERHANS CELL GRANULOMATOSIS

Langerhans cell granulomatosis or histiocytosis X includes three closely related disorders: (1) LCH, (2) Letterer–Siwe disease, and (3) Hand–Schüller–Christian disease. Also known as eosinophilic granuloma of the lung, primary pulmonary histiocytosis X is almost exclusively seen in smokers, during the third and fourth decades of life with an equal male to female distribution.

Langerhans cell histiocytosis may present with respiratory symptoms, fever, wheezing, and weight loss. Recurrent, often bilateral pneumothorax is a characteristic feature. Patients may also develop diabetes insipidus and bony disease. Chest X-ray shows involvement of the upper and middle zones with sparing of the costophrenic angles, reticulonodular changes, cystic lesions, and bullae that may rupture to cause recurrent pneumothorax. Microscopically, the lesion consists of a granulomatous infiltrate of histiocytes, eosinophils, and other cells. The histiocyte is a large cell with an indented nucleus that has Birbeck granules on electron microscopy.

Smoking cessation is an important component of therapy. Treatment, based on the severity of the disease, primarily consists of corticosteroids with other drugs such as vincristine, cyclophosphamide, and fludarabine.

SARCOIDOSIS

It is a multisystem granulomatous disease primarily with pulmonary involvement. Constitutional symptoms such as fever, malaise, and weight loss are common. Pulmonary manifestations consist of bilateral mediastinal and hilar lymphadenopathy with or without interstitial lung infiltrates.

Characteristically, the histological lesions consist of noncaseating epithelioid granulomas and absence of caseation necrosis. The incidence of eosinophilia in sarcoidosis may range from 10 to over 60%.

NEOPLASTIC DISORDERS

Eosinophilia may occur in association with both hematological malignancies and solid organ tumors. Depending upon the underlying disorder, eosinophilia may or may not indicate an adverse prognosis. Hematological disorders associated with eosinophilia include systemic mastocytosis (in approximately 20%), nodular sclerosing Hodgkin's disease (15%), B-cell non-Hodgkin's disease, T-cell leukemia, and Sézary syndrome. Eosinophilic leukemia is also a known variant of acute myelomonocytic leukemia (M4). Solid organ malignancies usually associated with eosinophilia include large cell cancer of the lung, squamous cell carcinomas of cervix, skin, nasopharynx, and bladder transitional cell carcinoma.

TROPICAL PULMONARY EOSINOPHILIA

Tropical pulmonary eosinophilia should always be considered whenever there is a marked eosinophilia. It commonly occurs in tropical regions due to filarial parasitic infestation. The disease frequently presents with fever, chills, and rigors along with respiratory symptoms of cough, wheezing, and breathlessness. Diagnosis is suspected on the basis of clinical picture and presence of marked eosinophilia in a patient belonging to an endemic area. Peripheral eosinophil count is frequently $>3 \times 10^9$/L. Serum *IgE* levels are elevated (>1,000 kU/L). Common causes of eosinophilia must be excluded before labeling a patient as TPE. Chest radiology may show bilateral micro- or miliary nodules and reticulation. Pulmonary hypertension may be present in chronic cases. Microfilariae can sometimes be seen on peripheral blood smear examination besides the increased titers of *antifilarial antibodies*.

Tropical pulmonary eosinophilia is treated with antifilarial drugs such as *diethylcarbamazine*. The response is often dramatic and almost confirms the diagnosis. Diethylcarbamazine (6 mg/kg/day in three divided doses) is usually administered for 21 days. It is a well-tolerated drug but headache, fever, pruritus, and gastrointestinal upset may sometimes be seen. The eosinophil count often falls within 7–10 days of starting treatment.

INFECTIONS

Eosinophilia may be seen in the presence of systemic and pulmonary infections due to different bacterial, fungal, and parasitic microorganisms. Sometimes, tuberculosis may be associated with an undulating pattern of eosinophilia. Eosinophilia in tuberculosis correlates with a good prognosis while eosinopenia points to a fulminant or miliary disease. Eosinophilia is also seen in chronic brucellosis and fungal infection such as coccidioidomycosis, histoplasmosis, and cryptococcosis.

BOX 3 Drugs causing eosinophilic lung disease.

- **Antitubercular drugs:**
  - Streptomycin and isoniazid
  - Para-amino salicylic acid
- **Antimicrobials:**
  - Nitrofurantoin
  - Penicillin and sulfonamides
  - Tetracycline and minocycline
  - Dapsone + pyrimethamine
- **Antineoplastic and immunosuppressives:**
  - Bleomycin and methotrexate
  - Melphalan and azathioprine
- **Anti-inflammatory drugs:**
  - Beclomethasone, penicillamine, and gold salts
  - Nonsteroidal anti-inflammatory drugs (NSAIDs): Aspirin, naproxen, piroxicam, nimesulide, and phenylbutazone
- **Cardiovascular:**
  - Amiodarone, hydralazine, and thiazides
- **Antidiabetics:**
  - Clofibrate and sulfonylureas
- **Neurological and psychotropic agents:**
  - Carbamazepine and phenytoin
  - Dantrolene and methylphenidate
  - Imipramine
  - Cocaine or heroin exposure
- **Miscellaneous:**
  - Iodinated contrast media, L-tryptophan

DRUG AND TOXIN INDUCED

Eosinophilic lung disease is seen after use of various drugs and toxins (**Box 3**). The signs and symptoms of disease may manifest anywhere from a few minutes after exposure to weeks afterward. Nitrofurantoin is one of the more common drugs which cause acute, subacute, and chronic reactions. Typical symptoms include low-grade fever, cough, and dyspnea with or without wheezing. Chest examination is nonspecific, might show wheezing and crackles. Chest radiology may reveal diffuse or patchy pulmonary infiltrates; bilateral consolidation and ground-glass opacification, both of which may be peripheral. Spirometry may either be normal, or show a mild restrictive defect. Similarly, DLCO may be normal or reduced. The clinical features usually disappear after discontinuation of the responsible drug. Corticosteroids are not always beneficial, though their use may hasten recovery, especially in sick patients.

In conclusion, pulmonary eosinophilia is neither a disease nor even a syndrome. It helps to identify a broad group of diseases characterized with eosinophilic pulmonary infiltration with or without peripheral blood eosinophilia. It is important to diagnose the cause of the underlying disease-state with relevant investigations and treat accordingly.

RECOMMENDED READINGS

1. Varma S, Jindal A. Pulmonary Eosinophilic Disorders. In: Jindal SK (Ed). Textbook of Pulmonary and Critical Care Medicine, Vol 2. New Delhi: Jaypee Brothers Medical Publishers; 2017. pp. 1061-73.
2. Simon D, Simon HU. Eosinophilic disorders. Current reviews of allergy and clinical immunology. J Allergy Clin Immunol. 2007;119:1291-300.
3. Wechsler ME. Pulmonary eosinophilic syndromes. Immunol Allergy Clin North Am. 2007;27(3):477-92.
4. Varma N, Varma S, Marwaha N, Dash S. Hypereosinophilic syndrome: the spectrum of clinical, haematological and morphological features. J Assoc Physicians India. 1994;42(3):242-4.
5. Vaglio A, Buzio C, Zwerina J. Eosinophilic granulomatosis with polyangiitis (Churg–Strauss): State of the art. Allergy. 2013;68(3):261-73.
6. Klion AD, Bochner BS, Gleich GJ, Nutman TB, Rothenberg ME, Simon HU, et al. Approaches to the treatment of hypereosinophilic syndromes: a workshop summary report. J Allergy Clin Immunol. 2006;117(6):1292-302.
7. Renston JP, Goldman ES, Hsu RM, Tomashefski Jr JF. Peripheral blood eosinophilia in association with sarcoidosis. Mayo Clin Proc. 2000;75(6):586-90.
8. Rothenberg ME, Klion AD, Roufosse FE, Kahn JE, Weller PF, Simon HU, et al. Treatment of patients with the hypereosinophilic syndrome with mepolizumab. N Engl J Med. 2008;358(12):1215-28.
9. Gotlib J. World Health Organization-defined eosinophilic disorders: 2017 update on diagnosis, risk stratification, and management. Am J Hematol. 2017;92:1243-59.
10. Barnes PJ. Inflammatory endotypes in COPD. Allergy. 2019;74(7):1249-56.
11. Allen J, Wert M. Eosinophilic pneumonias. J Allergy Clin Immunol Pract. 2018;6(5):1455-61.
12. Woolnough K, Wardlaw AJ. Eosinophilia in pulmonary disorders. Immunol Allergy Clin North Am. 2015;35(3):477-92.
13. Zimmermann N, Wikenheiser-Brokamp KA. Hypereosinophilic syndrome in the differential diagnosis of pulmonary infiltrates with eosinophilia. Ann Allergy Asthma Immunol. 2018;121(2):179-85.
14. Rose DM, Hrncir DE. Primary eosinophilic lung diseases. Allergy Asthma Proc. 2013;34(1):19-25.

CHAPTER 216

Pulmonary Vasculitides

Kavitha Venkatnarayan, Uma Mohan Krishnaswamy

ABSTRACT

The pulmonary vasculitides encompass a spectrum of disorders characterized by inflammation of large, medium, or small vessels mediated by immune processes and augmented by genetic, epigenetic, environmental, and infectious influences. These disorders are characterized by hemoptysis with or without accompanying extrapulmonary involvement; the most common organs involved being the kidneys, skin, upper respiratory tract, peripheral nerves, and heart. These diseases often present acutely but can have an insidious presentation. Disease course can be relentlessly progressive or relapsing-remitting. Common differential diagnoses include infections and malignancy.

An assiduous syndromic approach is invaluable in suspecting pulmonary vasculitis; however, there can be considerable overlap in the clinical presentation of various entities. Although immunological tests coupled with histopathological confirmation of vasculitis are gold standard tests, obtaining tissue biopsies may not be feasible in severely ill patients. Thus, diagnosis is based on a combination of immunological, radiological, and biochemical tests. Therapeutic options are centered around three endpoints namely, suppression of the dysregulated immune response, maintenance of remissions, and management of target organ dysfunction. Broad treatment modalities include corticosteroids, immune-suppressant medications, monoclonal antibodies, plasmapheresis, and supportive therapies like renal replacement, blood transfusions, and antibiotics. In addition to maintaining disease remission, monitoring for drug side-effects is an important component of follow-up.

Prognosis is dependent on the severity at presentation, extent and number of organs involved, response to immune suppression, and occurrence of intercurrent secondary infections. Timely diagnosis and institution of treatment along with regular follow-up are cornerstones in reducing mortality and morbidity related to pulmonary vasculitides.

"Medicine is a science of uncertainity and an art of probability"

—William Osler

INTRODUCTION

Pulmonary vasculitides are intrathoracic manifestations of a heterogeneous group of systemic disorders characterized by unifying histopathological features of vasculitis (inflammation and necrosis of the blood vessel wall). In view of the wide spectrum of clinical and radiological manifestations, variable extrapulmonary features and similarities in their clinical presentation with infections and malignancies, a high index of suspicion is vital for their diagnosis. Some of the clinical presentations which should prompt the consideration of vasculitides as a diagnostic possibility are enumerated in **Box 1**.

Eliciting a comprehensive history and performing a meticulous clinical examination with special attention to pulmonary, dermatologic and neurological signs aided by laboratory analysis (urinalysis and autoantibody profile) and radiological findings help in diagnosing probable vasculitis which can be further confirmed by tissue biopsies.

BOX 1 Clinical manifestations that should induce a high suspicion for vasculitides.

- Alveolar hemorrhage
- Tracheal or subglottic stenosis
- Pulmonary nodules or cavities (once malignancy and infection have been excluded)
- Glomerulonephritis
- Destructive or ulcerating upper airway disease
- Mononeuritis multiplex
- Retro-orbital mass
- Palpable purpura
- Unexplained ischemic events
- Severe or refractory maturity-onset asthma

PATHOPHYSIOLOGY

The pathophysiological basis of vasculitides is complex and is yet to be completely understood. Some of the well-established mechanisms are depicted in **Figure 1** and briefly detailed below:

- *Antineutrophil cytoplasmic antibodies (ANCA)* (***Fig. 1 A***): Genetic, epigenetic, environmental, and infective [bacterial superantigens like *Staphylococcus aureus* in granulomatosis with polyangiitis (GPA)] triggers are postulated to incite the production of antibodies. These triggers result in translocation of proteins from primary granules of neutrophils [proteinase 3 (PR3) and myeloperoxidase] to the surface resulting in loss of immune tolerance and production of ANCA. Proinflammatory effects of ANCA lead to increased neutrophil adhesion to endothelium, release of reactive oxygen species, and proteolytic enzymes thus leading to endothelial injury.
- *Immune complex mediated* (***Fig. 1 B***): Immune complex deposition is a widely accepted mechanism in vasculitis. The antigen in the immune complex is identified in a few of them like hepatitis B antigens in polyarteritis nodosa and hepatitis C antigens in cryoglobulinemic vasculitis. Such deposition leads to complement activation, neutrophil chemoattraction, and increased permeability finally leading to vessel injury and inflammation.
- *T lymphocyte-mediated granuloma formation* (***Fig. 1 C***): Activation of CD4 and CD8 T cells by antigen-presenting cells leads to release of cytokines which initiate a granulomatous inflammation.

Endothelial injury and vessel inflammation that ensue due to the above mechanisms lead to vessel thrombosis and tissue ischemia or aneurysms.

The most widely accepted nosology for these disorders is as defined in the International Chapel Hill Consensus Conference 2012 and is based on the size of the vessels involved (**Table 1**).

Among the vasculitides mentioned above, pulmonary involvement is predominantly seen in the small vessel vasculitides of which ANCA-associated vasculitis is pivotal.

ANCA-ASSOCIATED VASCULITIDES

ANCA-associated vasculitides (AAV) are necrotizing vasculitides, with few or no immune deposits, predominantly affecting small vessels (i.e., capillaries, venules, arterioles, and small arteries). They include three clinicopathologic conditions:

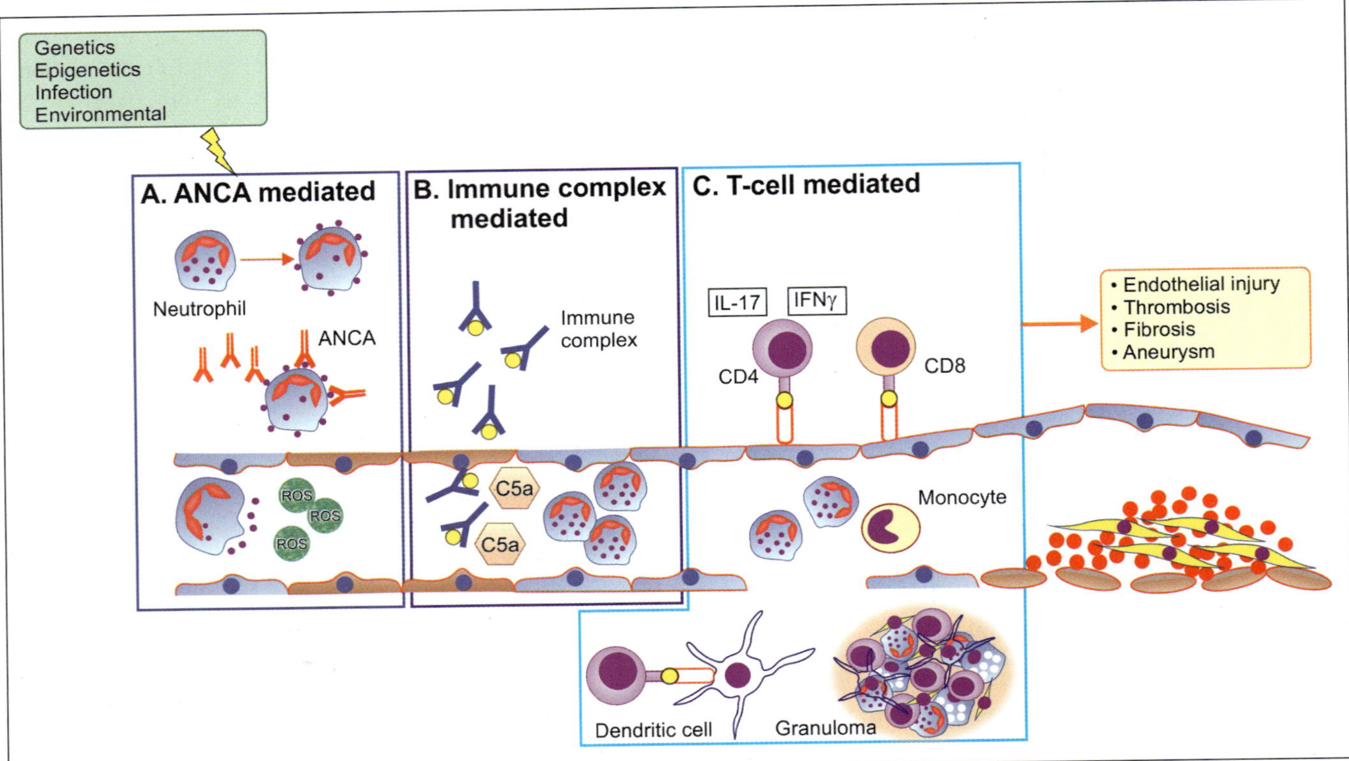

(ANCA: antineutrophil cytoplasmic antibodies)

FIGURE 1: Pathophysiology of vasculitides.

TABLE 1 Nomenclature of vasculitides based on the size of vessels involved (CHCC 2012).

Vessel involvement	Nomenclature
Large vessel vasculitis	• Takayasu's arteritis • Giant cell arteritis
Medium vessel vasculitis	• Polyarteritis nodosa • Kawasaki disease
Small vessel vasculitis (SVV)	Antineutrophil cytoplasmic antibody-associated vasculitis (AAV): • Microscopic polyangiitis • Granulomatosis with polyangiitis (formerly Wegener's granulomatosis) • Eosinophilic granulomatosis with polyangiitis (Churg–Strauss syndrome) Immune complex SVV: • Antiglomerular basement membrane disease • Cryoglobulinemic vasculitis • Immunoglobulin A vasculitis (Henoch–Schönlein purpura)
Variable vessel vasculitis	• Behçet's disease • Cogan's syndrome

(CHCC: International Chapel Hill Consensus Conference)

1. Granulomatosis with polyangiitis (GPA), formerly Wegener's granulomatosis
2. Microscopic polyangiitis (MPA)
3. Eosinophilic GPA (EGPA), formerly Churg–Strauss syndrome

This group of syndromes are characterized by the presence of ANCA. ANCA are autoantibodies directed against cytoplasmic antigens in the primary azurophilic granules of neutrophils. Although indirect immunofluorescence (IIF) is the usual initial screening test performed, high quality immunoassays [enzyme-linked immunosorbent assay (ELISA)] are now recommended for screening. Based on the staining pattern on IIF, two types of ANCA have been identified:

1. c-ANCA with cytoplasmic staining pattern reacting against the enzyme proteinase-3 (anti-PR3); predominant antibody in GPA
2. p-ANCA with a perinuclear staining pattern reacting against the enzyme myeloperoxidase (anti-MPO); predominant antibody in MPA and EGPA

Antineutrophil cytoplasmic antibody by IIF may also be positive in infections like tuberculosis, infective endocarditis, *Pseudomonas aeruginosa* infection, ulcerative colitis, other autoimmune diseases (rheumatoid arthritis, systemic lupus erythematosus), and malignancies. A positive ANCA by IIF should always be confirmed by ELISA. There is mounting evidence to suggest that grouping based on ANCA status as PR3-ANCA positive, MPO-ANCA positive, or ANCA negative vasculitis may yield more homogeneity with respect to organ involvement, treatment

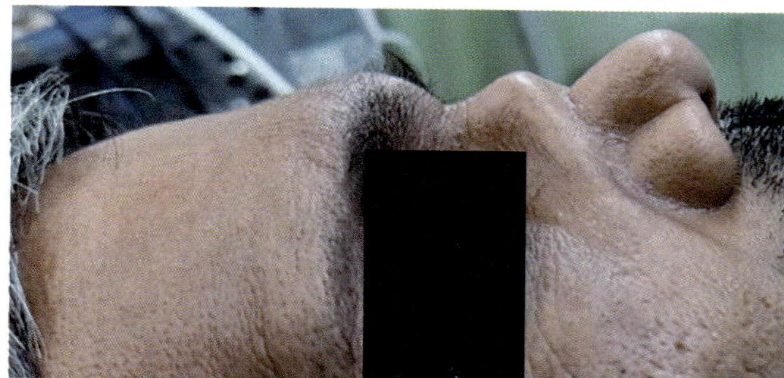

FIGURE 2: Saddle nose deformity.

response, and prognostic implications rather than the traditionally followed phenotypic classification mentioned above.

Granulomatosis with polyangiitis: Granulomatosis with polyangiitis is a systemic disease characterized by necrotizing granulomatous inflammation usually involving the upper and lower respiratory tract, and necrotizing vasculitis affecting predominantly small to medium vessels usually presenting as glomerulonephritis. Usual presentation is in the fifth decade with no gender predilection and clinical manifestations include:

- *Upper respiratory tract*: It is involved in nearly 90% of GPA patients in the form of nasal mucosal ulceration causing epistaxis and purulent nasal discharge, nasal septal perforation, saddle nose deformity due to ischemia of nasal cartilage (**Fig. 2**), chronic serous otitis media, or gingival hyperplasia.
- *Lower respiratory tract*: Lungs are involved in approximately 80% of patients. Airway involvement in the form of subglottic stenosis or bronchostenosis may cause stridor, wheezing, or postobstructive pneumonia. Parenchymal involvement may present with dyspnea, cough, and hemoptysis with radiological features of parenchymal nodules and masses which may undergo cavitation or consolidation (**Figs. 3 A** to **D**). Histopathological examination of lung biopsy specimens shows characteristic necrotizing granulomatous inflammation with vasculitis.
- *Renal*: Glomerulonephritis is seen in roughly 40% of patients at presentation and develops in 80% over the course of the illness. It is diagnosed by the presence of an active urinary sediment, proteinuria, or hematuria and may progress to renal failure. Renal biopsy is of diagnostic and prognostic value and shows characteristic pauci-immune glomerulonephritis on direct immunofluorescence.
- *Other manifestations*: Apart from nonspecific systemic symptoms like fever, malaise, and weight loss, ocular involvement may occur in the form of scleritis, corneal ulceration, uveitis, retinal vasculitis, and retro-orbital pseudotumors. Cardiac manifestations include cardiomyopathy with regional wall motion abnormalities in a noncoronary distribution. Neurological manifestations like CNS vasculitis, pachymeningitis and mononeuritis multiplex, and skin lesions in the form of palpable purpura which show leukocytoclastic vasculitis may provide important diagnostic clues.

Microscopic polyangiitis: Microscopic polyangiitis is indistinguishable from GPA as there is a significant clinical and histopathological overlap between the two entities. It occurs predominantly in males in their sixth decade with predominant renal involvement characterized by rapidly progressive glomerulonephritis (RPGN). MPA is the most frequent cause of pulmonary renal syndrome with diffuse alveolar hemorrhage (DAH) secondary to pulmonary capillaritis. Pulmonary fibrosis is a well-established feature of MPA with the "usual interstitial pneumonia" pattern being the most common manifestation. Other features include skin lesions like palpable purpura, gastrointestinal bleeding, abdominal pain, and mononeuritis multiplex.

Diagnosis is usually based on renal biopsy showing pauci-immune glomerulonephritis. In contrast to GPA, granulomatous inflammation is rarely found in MPA.

Eosinophilic granulomatosis with polyangiitis: Eosinophilic granulomatosis with polyangiitis is characterized by eosinophil-rich and necrotizing granulomatous inflammation often involving the respiratory tract, with the necrotizing vasculitis predominantly affecting small to medium vessels. It is distinctively associated with asthma and eosinophilia. Three distinct phases of the disease are described:

1. Allergic phase: It may last for many years and characterized by presence of asthma.
2. Eosinophilic phase: Characterized by peripheral blood and tissue eosinophilia
3. Vasculitic phase: Showing evidence of systemic vasculitis

Pulmonary involvement includes fleeting infiltrates in a peripheral distribution similar to that seen in eosinophilic pneumonia. In contrast to GPA and MPA, DAH and renal involvement are rare. Peripheral nerves are more frequently involved in the form of mononeuritis multiplex. Presence of ANCA is associated with active disease and renal involvement. In contrast, cardiac involvement is more common with ANCA negativity. EGPA has been discussed in detail in the previous chapter no. 215.

DIAGNOSIS OF AAV

ANCA-associated vasculitis should be strongly suspected in patients with unexplained systemic symptoms not explained by infections or malignancy. When armed with a strong clinical suspicion, ANCA assay helps make a probable diagnosis of AAV. ELISA is the preferred modality for ANCA assay rather than IIF. In the presence of characteristic clinical and radiological findings and corroborative ANCA, biopsy may be deferred in a few patients. However, presence of ANCA should be used as an adjunct to diagnosis and not as a substitute for tissue biopsy. ANCA positivity varies between the three AAV as follows:

1. GPA—95% ANCA positive with nearly 75% of them being PR3-ANCA

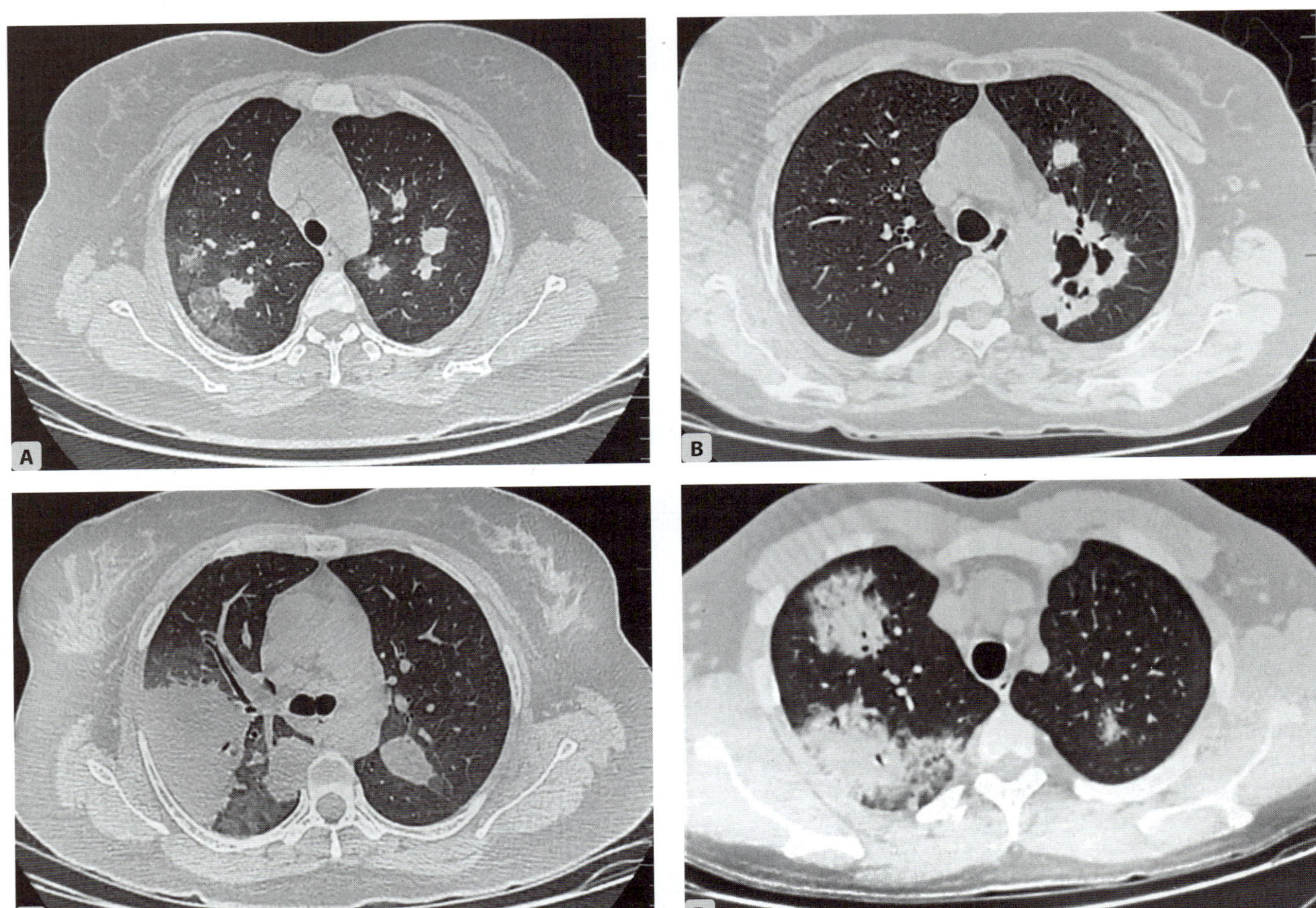

(AAV: ANCA-associated vasculitides)

FIGURES 3 A to D: Radiological findings in AAV: (A) Bilateral lung nodules; **(B)** Cavitating nodules; **(C and D)** Consolidation.

2. MPA—90% ANCA positive with nearly 70% of them being MPO-ANCA
3. EGPA—45% ANCA positive with predominant MPO-ANCA

The diagnosis is established by appropriate tissue biopsies based on the organ involved. Demonstration of pauci-immune glomerulonephritis or necrotizing vasculitis in the involved tissue remains the gold standard for diagnosis of AAV. Diagnostic yield depends on the organ involved and is highest with renal biopsies (90%) and upper airway biopsies (60%). Open lung biopsies provide a higher diagnostic yield than transbronchial biopsies.

TREATMENT OF AAV

The natural history of AAV is marked by varying degrees of disease severity (**Table 2**) with possible life- and organ-threatening manifestations, disease remissions and relapses complicating the disease course.

Management of AAV is complex and entails long-term follow up of patients for maintenance of remission, prompt diagnosis and treatment of relapses, management of disease, and drug-related complications. It is hence advisable to be done in liaison with or in centers with such expertise. Treatment of AAV can be divided into two phases:

TABLE 2 European Vasculitis Study (EUVAS) disease categorization of AAV.

Category	Definition
Localized	Upper and/or lower respiratory tract disease without any other systemic involvement or constitutional symptoms
Early systemic	Any, without organ-threatening or life-threatening disease
Generalized	Renal- or other organ-threatening disease, serum creatinine < 500 µmol/L (5.6 mg/dL)
Severe	Renal or other vital organ failure, serum creatinine > 500 µmol/L (5.6 mg/dL)
Refractory	Progressive disease unresponsive to glucocorticoids and cyclophosphamide

(AAV: ANCA-associated vasculitides)

(1) induction of remission and (2) maintenance of remission (**Table 3** and **Flowchart 1**).

The mainstay of induction therapy includes glucocorticoids with other immunosuppressants decided based on the severity of disease and presence of organ- or life-threatening manifestations. Cyclophosphamide

TABLE 3 Management of AAV based on severity of disease manifestation (EULAR recommendations 2016).

Severity	Induction therapy	Maintenance therapy
Organ- or life-threatening disease	• Glucocorticoids (1 mg/kg/day, maximum 80 mg) AND • Rituximab (375 mg/m^2 of body surface area, once a week for four infusions) OR • Cyclophosphamide (oral 2 mg/kg/day, maximum 200 mg OR intravenous 15 mg/kg every 2–3 weeks) for 3–6 months	• Target glucocorticoid dose of 7.5–10 mg at 3–6 months of therapy AND Either of the following: • Azathioprine (2 mg/kg/day) • Rituximab (500 mg every 6 monthly) • Methotrexate (20–25 mg once a week) • Mycophenolate mofetil (1 g twice a day) • To be continued for at least 24 months after attaining a sustained remission • *Pneumocystis jirovecii* prophylaxis with trimethoprim/sulfamethoxazole (800/160 mg on alternate days or 400/80 mg daily) to be continued for all patients receiving steroids with any other immunosuppressant drug
Non-organ-threatening disease*	• Glucocorticoids AND • Methotrexate (20–25 mg once a week) OR • Mycophenolate mofetil (1 g twice a day)	
Major organ/life-threatening relapse	• Glucocorticoids AND • Cyclophosphamide OR • Rituximab • Rituximab preferred in PR3-ANCA positive patients with relapse	
Non-organ-threatening relapse	• Increase glucocorticoid dose • Intensification/modification of maintenance immunosuppressant	
• Rapidly progressive renal failure • Diffuse alveolar hemorrhage	• Methylprednisolone 500–1,000 mg pulse for 3 days followed by 1 mg/kg/day AND • Rituximab OR cyclophosphamide • CONSIDER plasma exchange	
Refractory disease	• Rule out alternative diagnoses • Rule out complications like infections and malignancies • Switch from cyclophosphamide to rituximab or vice versa • Consider intravenous immunoglobulin therapy	

*Should not be used in meningeal involvement; retro-orbital disease; cardiac involvement; mesenteric involvement; acute-onset mononeuritis multiplex; pulmonary hemorrhage of any severity.

(AAV: ANCA-associated vasculitides; ANCA: antineutrophil cytoplasmic antibodies; EULAR: European League Against Rheumatism)

and rituximab are the preferred immunosuppressants for severe organ/life-threatening disease. Intravenous cyclophosphamide is preferred over oral therapy owing to reduced cumulative dose and drug toxicity with comparable remission induction and overall survival. Rituximab is favored in patients who wish to preserve reproductive function and has been found to be superior in relapsing and refractory disease.

Once disease remission is achieved, glucocorticoids should be tapered to the lowest required doses. Maintenance of remission is achieved by continuing immunosuppressant therapy with azathioprine or methotrexate. Mycophenolate mofetil is an alternative in patients intolerant to azathioprine. A close watch for relapse and therapy-related complications like adverse drug reactions and secondary infections is warranted.

Plasma exchange was hitherto used in life-threatening DAH and RPGN. Its role has become controversial and doubtful after the results of a recent trial showed no significant benefit.

Management of AAV is directed by several pivotal randomized trials as summarized in **Table 4**. Commonly used pharmacological agents and the anticipated side effects are summarized in **Table 5**.

Newer treatment modalities: Mepolizumab (anti-IL-5 antibody) has been found to be useful in patients with non-life-threatening EGPA. As depicted earlier the role of complement pathway in the pathogenesis suggests the possibility of using them as therapeutic targets. Drugs that inhibit C5a (eculizumab) and C5aR (Avacopan) are being studied as therapeutic options in clinical trials.

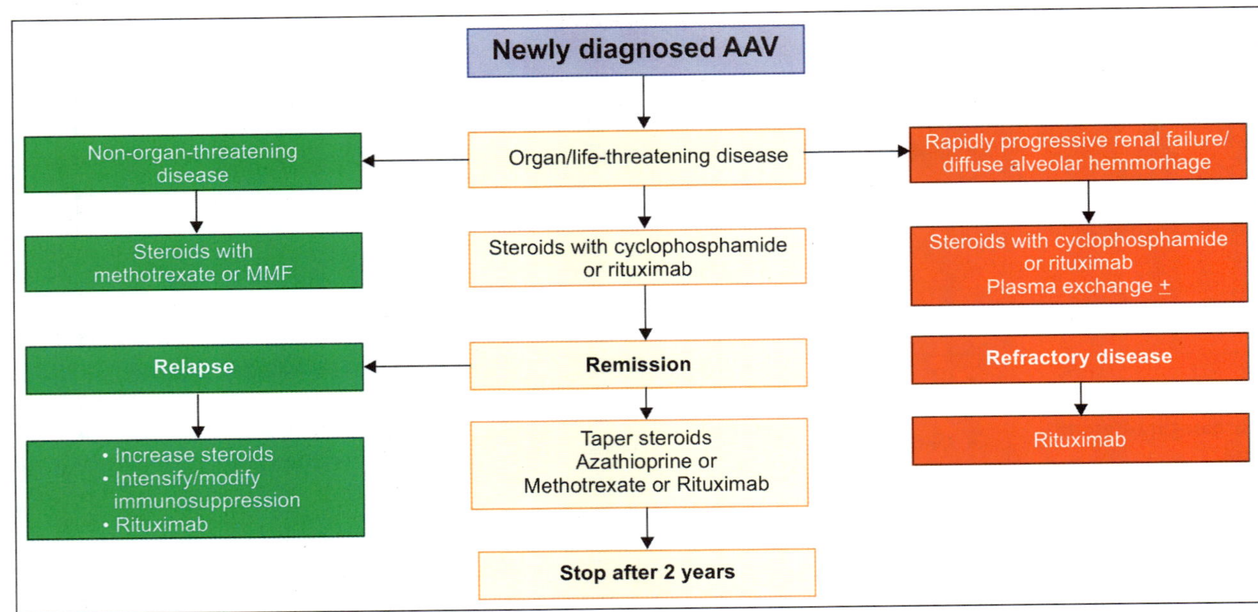

(AAV: ANCA-associated vasculitides; MMF: mycophenolate mofetil)

FLOWCHART 1: Management of AAV.

TABLE 4 Landmark trials in AAV.

Trials	Intervention	Primary outcome
Induction therapy		
CYCLOPS	IV vs. oral CYC with GC	IV CYC—noninferior for remission induction; reduced cumulative dose; more relapse on long-term with IV CYC
RAVE	RTX vs. oral CYC followed by AZA	RTX noninferior to CYC; RTX better in relapsing disease
RITUXVAS	• 2 doses of IV CYC; • RTX vs. IV CYC	Similar outcomes
MYCYC	IV CYC vs. MMF	MMF—noninferior for remission induction; increased relapse with MMF
NORAM	MTX vs. oral CYC	MTX—noninferior for remission induction; MTX less effective for extensive/pulmonary disease
Maintenance therapy		
CYCAZAREM	Oral CYC vs. AZA	Similar relapse rates
WEGENT	AZA vs. MTX	Similar relapse rates
MAINRITSAN	RTX (500 mg, every 6 months) vs. AZA	Higher relapse with AZA
IMPROVE	MMF vs. AZA	More relapse with MMF
RITAZAREM	RTX (1 g every 4 months) vs. AZA	RTX superior to AZA
Plasma exchange		
MEPEX	• CYC + GC • PLEX vs. methylprednisolone pulse	PLEX—lesser dialysis dependence at 3 months; long term—similar
PEXIVAS	• CYC/RTX + GC • PLEX vs. No PLEX	PLEX not superior

(AAV: ANCA-associated vasculitides; AZA: azathioprine; CYC: cyclophosphamide; GC: glucocorticoids; MTX: methotrexate; MMF: mycophenolate mofetil; PLEX: plasma exchange; RTX: rituximab)

DIFFUSE ALVEOLAR HEMORRHAGE

Diffuse alveolar hemorrhage is *a catastrophic syndrome* characterized by a constellation of features which include hemoptysis, anemia, diffuse pulmonary infiltrates, and respiratory failure. Hemoptysis may be absent in a third of these patients. Although DAH is usually associated with a known underlying systemic disease process, it can occasionally be the presenting manifestation.

TABLE 5 Common pharmacological agents used for treatment of AAV.

Drug	Adverse effects	Practical points
Cyclophosphamide	• Periodic intravenous pulse therapy favored over oral therapy • Metabolite acrolein toxic to urothelium—hemorrhagic cystitis and transitional cell carcinoma • Monitor blood counts for leukopenia • Associated with reduced ovarian reserve, ovarian failure, and male infertility	• Antiemetics to be used regularly • Encourage plenty of fluid intake • Oral or intravenous 2-mercaptoethanesulfonate sodium (MESNA) • *Pneumocystis jirovecii* prophylaxis • Periodic urinalysis for hematuria and transitional cell carcinoma lifelong
Rituximab	• Preferable in patients who wish to preserve reproductive potential • Infusion reactions • Reactivation of hepatitis B • Hypogammaglobulinemia	• Premedication • Immunoglobulin levels prior to each dose • Screen for hepatitis B
Methotrexate	Watch for cytopenias	Coadminister folic acid 1 mg/day or folinic acid 5–10 mg once a week on the day following methotrexate
Azathioprine	Watch for cytopenias	Consider thiopurine methyltransferase (TPMT) enzyme assay
Mycophenolate mofetil	Watch for cytopenias, uremia	Increased risk of lymphoma

(AAV: ANCA-associated vasculitides)

Typical *radiographic findings* include bilateral alveolar infiltrates in a bat-wing pattern but nonspecific focal infiltrates can also be seen on CT scans. Diagnosis is generally based on the clinical constellation with bronchoalveolar lavage showing increasingly bloody return in sequential aliquots and presence of hemosiderin laden macrophages on cytopathology (**Figs. 4 A** to **C**). *Diagnosis* is further reinforced by ancillary investigations like autoimmune serology, urinalysis, and renal functions. Histopathology is variable with pulmonary capillaritis being the most common finding. Pulmonary capillaritis is inflammation of pulmonary arterioles, capillaries, and venules with fibrinoid necrosis of blood vessel, neutrophilic interstitial infiltrate with leukocytoclasis. However, performing lung biopsies in these patients may be challenging and restricted to noncritically ill patients given the nonspecificity of pathological findings in obtaining an etiological diagnosis.

Irrespective of the etiology, *treatment* includes high-dose steroid pulse usually followed by cyclophosphamide or rituximab with continued steroids. Plasmapheresis is pivotal in anti-glomerular basement membrane (GBM) disease but its role in AAV is controversial given the results of a recent clinical trial. An approach to a patient with DAH is summarized in **Flowchart 2**.

ANTI-GBM DISEASE

Anti-GBM disease predominantly affects male smokers and results from autoantibodies against collagen antigens in the basement membrane of vessels. Both the lungs and kidneys are involved in majority of patients with the presenting features being DAH and RPGN (Goodpasture syndrome). Diagnosis is usually established by serological testing for anti-GBM antibodies and demonstration of crescentic glomerulonephritis on renal biopsy with immunofluorescence showing linear deposition of immunoglobulin G (IgG) antibodies along the GBM.

Treatment includes plasmapheresis, steroids, and cyclophosphamide with smoking cessation being of utmost importance.

OTHER VASCULITIDES

A detailed review of all the other vasculitides is beyond the scope of this chapter. Hence a brief overview of the pulmonary manifestations is provided below.

GIANT CELL ARTERITIS

Giant cell arteritis (GCA) or temporal arteritis involves inflammation of medium and large-sized vessels, predominantly branches of the carotid artery specifically the temporal artery. Presenting symptoms may include fever, myalgia, headache with claudication of jaw and tongue and polymyalgia rheumatica. A high ESR in a patient with typical symptoms in their sixth decade should prompt a suspicion for GCA. In about 5% of patients, GCA may involve other vessels with pulmonary manifestations like lung nodules and cavities. Biopsy reveals pathognomonic giant cells with necrotizing vasculitis.

TAKAYASU'S ARTERITIS

Takayasu's arteritis is inflammatory disease having a predilection for the aortic arch and its branches. The diagnosis should be suspected in young females presenting with absent peripheral pulses or discrepancies in blood pressure measured in different limbs. Pulmonary arteries may be involved in the form of pulmonary artery stenosis and pulmonary hypertension presenting with dyspnea, hemoptysis, and chest pain.

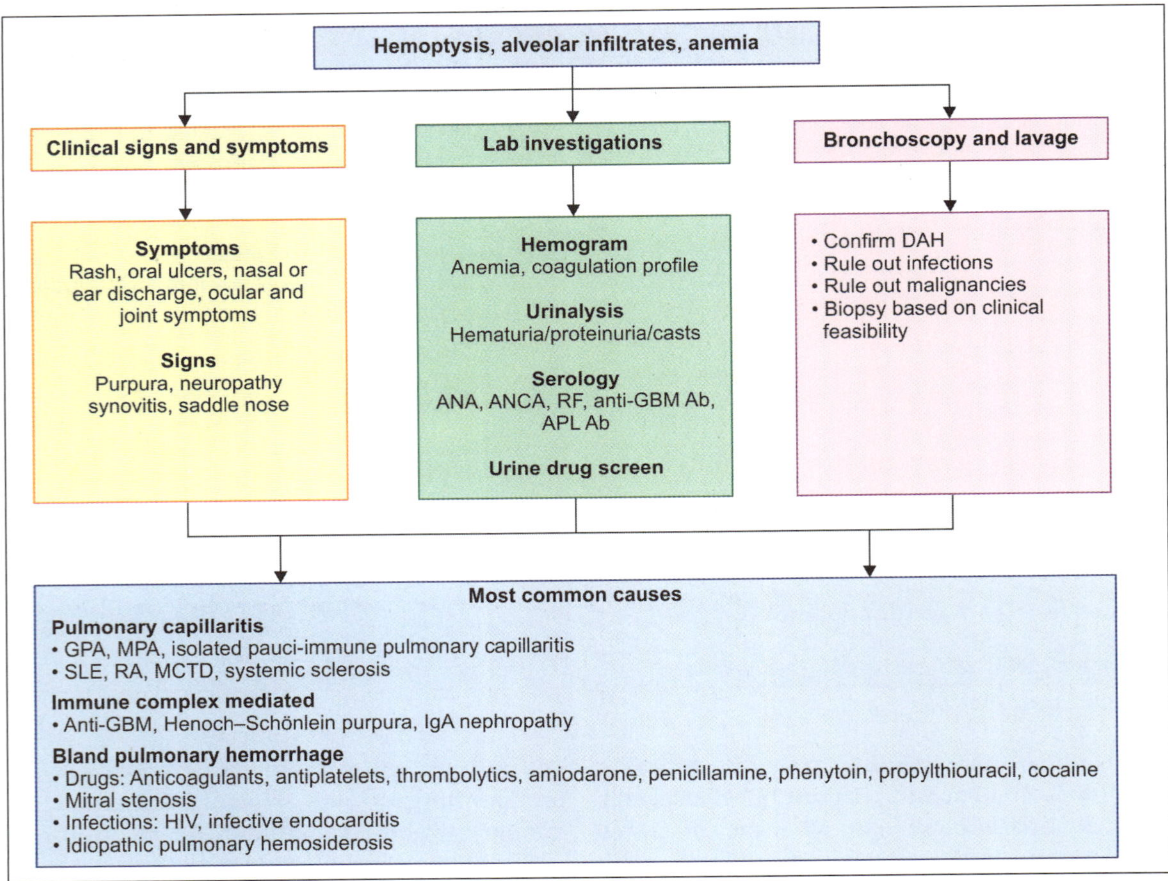

(ANA: antinuclear antibody; ANCA: antineutrophil cytoplasmic antibodies; DAH: diffuse alveolar hemorrhage; GBM: glomerular basement membrane; GPA: granulomatosis with polyangiitis; MCTD: mixed connective tissue disease; MPA: microscopic polyangiitis; RA: rheumatoid arthritis; SLE: systemic lupus erythematosus)

FLOWCHART 2: Diagnostic algorithm for diffuse alveolar hemorrhage.

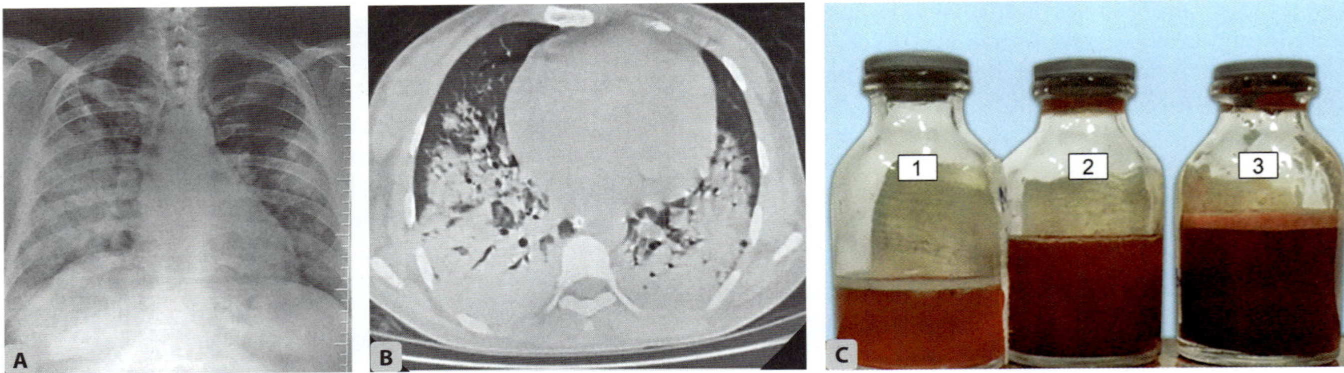

FIGURES 4 A to C: (A) Chest radiograph showing bilateral alveolar infiltrates; **(B)** CT chest showing extensive alveolar filling; **(C)** Bronchoalveolar lavage (BAL) from the patient showing characteristically increasing bloody return in sequential aliquots.

BEHÇET'S DISEASE

Behçet's disease is immune complex-mediated vasculitis which can affect vessels of any caliber. Venous involvement may lead to thrombosis which is not preventable by anticoagulation and needs antiplatelet therapy. Pulmonary arteries are involved with characteristic aneurysm formation which may present with fatal hemoptysis. Inflammation of the bronchial mucosa can lead to bronchostenosis causing recurrent pneumonia.

DRUG-INDUCED VASCULITIS

Drug-induced vasculitis (DIV) usually presents with small vessel vasculitis and is invariably ANCA positive. Commonly implicated drugs include propylthiouracil, hydralazine, sulfasalazine, levamisole adulterated cocaine, and phenytoin amongst others. Clinical and radiological presentation is indistinguishable from the other AAV. However, cutaneous manifestations are more likely to occur rather than pulmonary and systemic features. A detailed review of medications and drugs used in the past 6 months is important to identify the inciting agent. An atypical staining pattern of ANCA on IIF with dual positivity for p- and c-ANCA with multiple antigenic specificities is highly suggestive of DIV. Treatment is similar to that given in AAV and is based on the severity of disease. In limited disease, discontinuation of the offending agent will suffice.

SECONDARY VASCULITIS

Vasculitis can be seen as a part of other autoimmune diseases like systemic lupus erythematosus, rheumatoid arthritis, and sarcoidosis. Infections like tuberculosis, syphilis, and aspergillosis are also known to present with features of vasculitis.

CONCLUSION

Pulmonary vasculitides present with varied and nonspecific clinical and radiological manifestations and need a strong clinical suspicion to arrive at a diagnosis. Prompt diagnosis is usually made based on the clinical constellation of symptoms supported by radiology and serological tests showing presence of autoantibodies. A tissue biopsy is the gold standard for diagnosis but may not be feasible in patients presenting with severe disease. Glucocorticoids are the mainstay of therapy with appropriate immunosuppressants. The importance of close follow up for disease relapse, secondary infections, and adverse drug events cannot be over emphasized.

RECOMMENDED READINGS

1. Callahan SJ, Sturek JM, Richard RP. Pulmonary Vasculitides: A Review. Clin Pulm Med. 2019;26(1):10-7.
2. Geetha D, Jefferson JA. ANCA-Associated Vasculitis: Core Curriculum 2020. Am J Kid Dis. 2020;75(1): 124-37.
3. Kitching AR, Anders HJ, Basu N, Brouwer E, Gordon J, Jayne DR, et al. ANCA-associated vasculitis. Nat Rev Dis Primers. 2020;6(1):71.
4. Bossuyt X, Cohen Tervaert JW, Arimura Y, Blockmans D, Flores-Suárez LF, Guillevin L, et al. Revised 2017 international consensus on testing of ANCAs in granulomatosis with polyangiitis and microscopic polyangiitis. Nat Rev Rheumatol. 2017;13(11):683-92.
5. Yates M, Watts RA, Bajema IM, Cid MC, Crestani B, Hauser T, et al. EULAR/ERA-EDTA recommendations for the management of ANCA-associated vasculitis. Ann Rheumat Dis. 2016;75(9):1583-94.
6. Greco A, De Virgilio A, Rizzo MI, Gallo A, Magliulo G, Fusconi M, et al. Microscopic polyangiitis: Advances in diagnostic and therapeutic approaches. Autoimmun Rev. 2015;14(9):837-44.
7. Furuta S, Iwamoto T, Nakajima H. Update on eosinophilic granulomatosis with polyangiitis. Allergol Int. 2019;68(4):430-6.
8. Lara AR, Schwarz MI. Diffuse Alveolar Hemorrhage. Chest. 2010;137(5):1164-71.

CHAPTER 217

Pulmonary Vascular Diseases

Mohammad Azizur Rahman, Pajanivel Ranganadin, Ketaki Barve Utpat

ABSTRACT

Pulmonary vascular diseases (PVD) are a category of disorders characterized by involvement of pulmonary vascular bed by heterogeneous mechanisms. They can be broadly classified into pulmonary hypertension (PH), pulmonary thromboembolism (PTE), pulmonary vasculitis, and pulmonary arteriovenous malformation (PAVM). Pulmonary vasculitis is a heterogeneous group of diseases characterized by the inflammation and destruction of vessel walls that compromises the blood flow into tissues. These diseases are classified as per the size of the vessels involved. Vasculitides can be primary or secondary to connective tissue disease, infection, neoplasm, or hypersensitivity phenomena. Both PH and pulmonary vasculitides are discussed in details in separate chapters of the book.

Venous thromboembolism (VTE) can clinically present as deep venous thrombosis (DVT), PTE which can be acute or chronic thromboembolic pulmonary hypertension (CTEPH). The essential investigations involve computed tomography pulmonary angiography (CTPA) or a ventilation–perfusion scan (VQ scan). Pretest probability scores help in triaging patients and deciding appropriate line of further workup. Therapy involves thrombolysis or anticoagulation depending on the time of presentation and the severity.

Pulmonary arteriovenous malformations are uncommon pulmonary vascular connections that bypass the normal pulmonary capillary bed, hence establishing an intrapulmonary right-to-left shunt. The spectrum of PAVMs extends from tiny lesions incidentally diagnosed radiologically to huge aneurysmal connections that can distressing symptoms.

"The biggest risk a person can take is to do nothing"

—Robert T Kiyosaki

PULMONARY THROMBOEMBOLISM

INTRODUCTION

- Venous thromboembolism can clinically present as deep venous thrombosis or DVT or PTE also called as pulmonary embolism (PE)
- Pulmonary thromboembolism is globally the third most frequent acute cardiovascular syndrome after myocardial infarction and stroke.
- The overall age and sex-adjusted annual incidence of VTE is approximately 1–2 cases per 1,000 persons.

RISK FACTORS

Major risk factors, both genetic and acquired, are as given in **Box 1**.

BOX 1 Major risk factors for venous thrombosis.

- Advancing age
- Arterial disease (carotid and coronary disease)
- Personal or family history of VTE
- Recent surgery, trauma, or immobility, including stroke
- Congestive heart failure
- Chronic obstructive pulmonary disease
- Acute infection
- Air pollution
- Long-haul air travel
- Pregnancy, oral contraceptive pills, or postmenopausal hormone replacement therapy
- Pacemaker, implantable cardiac defibrillator leads or indwelling central venous catheter

Hypercoagulable states:

- Factor V Leiden resulting in activated protein C resistance
- Prothrombin gene mutation 20210
- Antithrombin deficiency
- Protein C deficiency
- Protein S deficiency
- Antiphospholipid antibody syndrome

PATHOPHYSIOLOGY

- Acute PTE interferes with both circulation and gas exchange.
- Right ventricular (RV) failure due to acute pressure overload
- Anatomical obstruction and hypoxic vasoconstriction
- Decrease in arterial compliance.

DIAGNOSIS

Clinical:

- The clinical signs and symptoms of acute PE are nonspecific.
- In most cases, PE is suspected in a patient with dyspnea, chest pain, presyncope or syncope, or hemoptysis; Well's scoring is used for risk stratification to estimate the probability for acute pulmonary embolism (**Table 1**).
- Dyspnea may be acute and severe in central PE; in small peripheral PE, it is often mild and may be transient. Chest pain is a frequent symptom of PE and is usually caused by pleural irritation due to distal emboli causing pulmonary infarction.

TABLE 1 Original and simplified Wells scores.

	Original Wells score (points)	Simplified Wells score (points)
Clinical signs of lower-extremity DVT	3	1
Alternative diagnosis less likely than PE	3	1
Heart rate > 100 beats/min	1.5	1
Surgery or immobilization within 4 weeks	1.5	1
Previously objectively diagnosed PE or DVT	1.5	1
Hemoptysis	1	1
Active cancer	1	1
Classification:		
• PE unlikely	≤4	≤1
• PE likely	>4	>1

(DVT: deep venous thrombosis; PE: pulmonary embolism)

Diagnostic tests: These include nonimaging and imaging methods. To decide appropriate diagnostic test for confirmation/exclusion following algorithm is useful in a suspected PE (**Flowchart 1**).

Nonimaging diagnostic tests:

- *D-dimer*: The presence of D-dimer in plasma is due to endogenous fibrinolysis of clot and can be estimated by enzyme-linked immunosorbent assay (ELISA). This is a

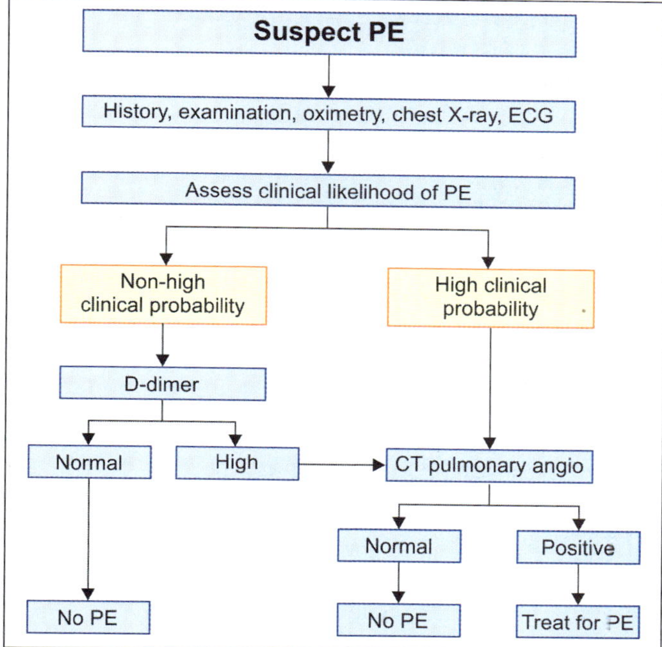

FLOWCHART 1: Diagnostic approach for pulmonary embolism (PE).

sensitive test but has low specificity as plasma D-dimer level is elevated in various systemic illnesses including sepsis, myocardial infarction, and cancer. Normal D-dimer test virtually rules out VTE.

- *Electrocardiography*: ECG findings include sinus tachycardia, ST-T abnormalities, S1Q3T3 pattern or right bundle branch block. T-wave inversion in V_1 to V_3 suggests RV dysfunction and carries poor prognosis.

Imaging methods:

- *Chest radiography*: It is often normal in PE. Abnormal findings that can be observed include focal oligemia (Westermark's sign) in the lung field, peripheral wedge-shaped opacity above the diaphragm (Hampton's hump and enlarged descending pulmonary artery (Palla's sign). Fleischner sign: enlarged pulmonary artery, pleural effusion, knuckle sign; Chang sign: dilated right descending pulmonary artery with sudden cut-off.
- *Ultrasonography*: Ultrasonography of deep veins not only helps to diagnose venous thrombosis by demonstrating thrombus in situ, lack of compressibility, and apposition of vessel wall due to passive distension by the thrombus but also to exclude other conditions. Compression ultrasonography (CUS) has a sensitivity >90% and a specificity of approximately 95% for proximal symptomatic DVT.
- *Computed tomographic pulmonary angiography (CTPA):* Multidetector CTPA is the method of choice for imaging the pulmonary vasculature in patients with suspected PE. It allows adequate visualization of the pulmonary arteries down to the subsegmental level. Taken together, the available data suggest that a negative CTPA result is an adequate criterion for the exclusion of PE in patients with low or intermediate clinical probability of PE. Acute emboli may be occlusive or nonocclusive, the latter is seen with a thin stream of contrast adjacent to the embolus. Chronic thromboembolic are often complete occlusions or nonocclusive filling defects in the periphery of the affected vessel which form obtuse angles with the vessel wall. Features noted with chronic pulmonary emboli include: Webs or bands, intimal irregularities, abrupt narrowing or complete obstruction of the pulmonary arteries, and "pouching defects."
- *Magnetic resonance imaging*: Gadolinium-enhanced magnetic resonance angiography (MRA) is useful when contrast-enhanced CT (CECT) chest is contraindicated due to contrast allergy or nephrotoxicity. It is less sensitive than CT but has advantage of nonexposure to ionizing radiation. It can assess RV size and function.
- *Echocardiography*: It is not reliable for diagnosing PE. It helps to detect RV enlargement and wall motion abnormality associated with PTE. McConnell's sign-hypokinesia of RV free wall with normal motion of RV apex is best known indirect sign of PE.
- *Ventilation–perfusion lung scan:* Lung scanning is less often used, and its value is now relegated to those cases who cannot tolerate intravenous (IV) contrast. Presence of two or more segmental perfusion defects with normal ventilation is diagnostic in 90% of cases with high probability of PE.
- *Invasive pulmonary angiography*: Invasive pulmonary angiography which was once gold standard diagnostic modality due to potential risks has been virtually replaced by chest CT with contrast and is reserved for cases in whom catheter-directed thrombolysis, mechanical clot fragmentation, or suction embolectomy is planned.

TREATMENT

Aim of the therapy of PE is to restore patency of pulmonary artery and perfusion. This can be achieved by primary therapy consisting of thrombolysis or removal of clot by embolectomy. Anticoagulants are used to prevent clot formation.

Anticoagulation:

- Effective anticoagulation to prevent clot formation is the foundation therapy for all cases of DVT and PE unless contraindicated due to active bleeding.
- It should be initiated immediately and continued with close monitoring of prothrombin time and international normalized ratio (INR).
- Anticoagulation is achieved initially with heparin and later a long-term basis by oral anticoagulants.
- Both unfractionated as well as fractionated heparin can be used. Unfractionated heparin has short half-life and therefore useful in cases who require endovascular interventions. Low-molecular-weight heparin (LMWH) has greater bioavailability, longer half-life, and predictable dose response. Various LMWHs in use are enoxaparin, dalteparin, nadroparin, and reviparin.
- Anticoagulation therapy needs strict monitoring for preventing bleeding risks and ensuring therapeutic

efficacy with proper dosage. However, caution is required while using anticoagulants in cases with a high risk of bleeding such as in elderly and in history of gastrointestinal bleeding.

- The mainstay of therapy for anticoagulation has been vitamin K antagonist therapy bridged with parenteral anticoagulants. The recent approval of new oral anticoagulants (NOACs) like apixaban, dabigatran, and rivaroxaban has generated significant interest in their role in managing VTE especially PE due to their improved pharmacokinetic and pharmacodynamic profiles, predictable anticoagulant response, and lack of required efficacy monitoring.

Thrombolysis:

- Thrombolysis restores patency of occluded vessels—both pulmonary and deep veins—by dissolution of the clot.
- Currently, preferred fibrinolytic agent is recombinant tissue plasminogen activator which is indicated and approved by FDA in cases with massive PE, this is recommended in cases with hemodynamic instability with no major bleeding risk. FDA has approved alteplase in a dose of 100 mg as a continuous infusion for 2 hours.
- In India, considering the cost factor streptokinase (STK) is commonly used. STK is initially given in a dose of 250,000 units IV over 30 minutes followed by 100,000 units/hr for 24 hours as a continuous infusion.
- Thrombolysis therapy can be initiated up to 14 days of onset of PE.

Inferior vena cava filter:

- If anticoagulant therapy is contraindicated and/or ineffective, or to prevent new emboli from entering the pulmonary artery and combining with an existing blockage, an inferior vena cava (IVC) filter may be implanted.
- Use of IVC filter has the inherent risk of providing nidus for thrombus formation; filter may fail to prevent passage of small-to-medium-sized clots and paradoxically facilitate passage of large clots through collaterals that develop following insertion of the filter.

Pulmonary embolism interventions:

- These include catheter-directed mechanical clot fragmentation or clot pulverization, percutaneous rheolytic thrombectomy, and pigtail rotational catheter embolectomy.
- Catheter procedures are risky and can result in mechanical hemolysis, macroembolization and microembolization.

Surgical embolectomy:

- This procedure is done under cardiopulmonary bypass and has a better outcome if performed before the onset of cardiogenic shock.
- Indications include massive PE with RV dysfunction in whom thrombolysis is contraindicated or refractory.

PULMONARY ARTERIOVENOUS MALFORMATIONS

INTRODUCTION

- Pulmonary arteriovenous malformations are infrequent vascular structures that connect a pulmonary artery to a pulmonary vein.
- They thereby bypass the normal pulmonary capillary bed and culminate in an intrapulmonary right-to-left shunt.
- The spectrum of severity PAVMs extends from minute lesions radiologically detected to lesions that cause significant symptoms due to profound hypoxemia.
- The other names for PAVM include pulmonary AV fistulas or hemangiomas.

CLASSIFICATIONS AND CAUSES

- The most common cause for PAVM is congenital.
- The frequent associations are hereditary hemorrhagic telangiectasia (HHT) or Osler–Weber–Rendu syndrome (OWRS). Generally, a higher incidence of PAVM is noted in HHT1 than in HHT2.
- Acquired causes of PAVM are uncommon and include postoperative after chest surgery, trauma, infections like actinomycosis and schistosomiasis, hepatic cirrhosis-related hepatopulmonary syndrome (HPS), and metastatic carcinomas.

CLINICAL FEATURES

- The magnitude of clinical manifestations depends on the degree of right to left shunting.
- The common symptoms include hypoxemia, fatigue, dyspnea, and cyanosis.
- A pathognomonic clinical feature of PAVM is the worsening hypoxia in the upright position also termed as orthodeoxia and worsening of dyspnea in the upright position termed as platypnea. This occurs because of the common location of PAVMs in the lower lobes, which worsens the ventilation–perfusion mismatch in the upright position.
- Some patients can present with various neurologic manifestations like infarction, abscess, and seizure due to paradoxical embolization.
- An association between PAVM and PAH has also been reported.
- Rupture of PAVM can have manifestations like hemoptysis of varying intensity or clinical features suggestive of a pleural disease due to hemothorax.

DIAGNOSTIC TESTS

- The screening test commonly employed includes transthoracic contrast echocardiography (TTCE).
- Bedside tests involve measurement of arterial oxygen saturation (SpO_2) by pulse oximetry and arterial blood gas (ABG) analysis measurement of partial pressure of oxygen in arterial blood (PaO_2).

- The imaging modalities employed are CECT and CTPA. The hallmark feature is the presence of a feeding artery and a draining vein coursing to and from the abnormal communication. In the case it constitutes a microscopic telangiectasia, ground-glass opacity (GGO) may be seen in the area on enhancing focus.
- Pulmonary arteriovenous malformations are broadly classified into simple and complex types depending on the number of the feeding arteries. The simple types are more common and account for 80% of these lesions.
- The source of origin of the feeding artery is in majority of the cases the pulmonary arteries however infrequently the feeders could arise from the systemic arteries.
- The venous drainage of the PAVMs is usually through a pulmonary vein, but rarely through the inferior vena cava and the left atrium.

TREATMENT

- Asymptomatic and small PAVM not associated with HHT may be observed with interval imaging monitoring.
- *Embolization*: Transcatheter embolization (TCE) is the treatment modality of choice recommended for all PAVMs with a feeding artery size >3 mm as they have a high risk of rupture. It can be done with balloons, coils, or vascular plugs. It is a safe and effective procedure and prevents recurrence and rupture.

RECOMMENDED READINGS

1. Guyatt GH, Akl EA, Crowther M, Schünemann HJ, Gutterman DD, Lewis SZ. Introduction to the ninth edition: Antithrombotic Therapy and Prevention of Thrombosis, 9th edition. American College of Chest Physicians Evidence-Based Clinical Practice Guidelines. Chest. 2012;141:48S-52S.
2. Barco S, Ende-Verhaar YM, Becattini C, Jimenez D, Lankeit M, Huisman MV, et al. Differential impact of syncope on the prognosis of patients with acute pulmonary embolism: a systematic review and meta-analysis. Eur Heart J. 2018;39:4186-95.
3. Agarwal R, Gulati M, Mittal BR, Jindal SK. Clinical profile, diagnosis and management of patients presenting with symptomatic pulmonary embolism. Indian J Chest Dis Allied Sci. 2006;48:111-4.
4. Parakh R, Kakkar VV, Kakkar AK. Venous Thromboembolism (VTE) Core Study Group. Management of venous thromboembolism. J Assoc Physicians India. 2007;55:49-70.
5. Casal A, Díaz-Garel J, Pereiro T, Toubes ME, Ricoy J, Valdés L. Pulmonary vasculitis. J Thorac Dis. 2018;10(9):5560-75.
6. Saboo SS, Chamarthy M, Bhalla S, Park H, Sutphin P, Kay F, et al. Pulmonary arteriovenous malformations: diagnosis. Cardiovasc Diagn Ther. 2018;8:325-37.

CHAPTER

218

Lung Cancer

Srinivas Rajagopala, Saurav Verma, Navneet Singh

ABSTRACT

Lung cancer is an important cause of cancer-related morbidity and mortality globally. Tobacco smoking remains the most important etiological factor while environmental tobacco smoke (ETS) exposure (passive smoking) and other environmental as well as occupational exposures (both indoor and outdoor) continue to have an ever-increasing role in the etiopathogenesis of this disease. Clinical features and radiological findings of lung cancer are not always specific and may overlap with several other infectious and noninfectious pulmonary disorders as well as with systemic disorders having pulmonary involvement.

Hence, obtaining tissue for making/confirming the diagnosis is mandatory and the first step in management of suspected lung cancer. The attempt should be to get maximum tissue by the least invasive method from the most easily accessible site as tissue is needed not just for confirming the diagnosis of lung cancer but also for histological subtyping and molecular testing—both of which are of paramount importance in deciding treatment. Accurate staging is a key step following confirmation of diagnosis. Noninvasive staging (largely imaging based) may need to be followed by invasive staging (preferably by endoscopic methods) for potentially resectable early-stage disease in whom surgical resection is being contemplated and forms the mainstay of treatment.

Locally advanced non-small-cell lung cancer (NSCLC) not amenable to surgical resection is treated with a combination of chemotherapy and thoracic radiation. Metastatic NSCLC treatment is largely determined by the histological subtype (squamous vs. adenocarcinoma) and the molecular profile [presence or absence of oncogenic drivers as well as programmed death-ligand 1 (PD-L1) expression]. Targeted therapies remain the cornerstone of treatment for oncogene-driven metastatic NSCLC while non-oncogene-driven metastatic NSCLC is managed by chemotherapy and/or immunotherapy. There is limited role of surgical resection and targeted therapies, as of now, in small-cell lung cancer (SCLC) treatment which is managed by either chemoradiation (limited stage) or chemotherapy +/– immunotherapy (extensive stage). Palliative and supportive care are an integral part of the management of lung cancer at all time points during the course of the patient's illness.

"The first step is to establish that something is possible; then – probability will occur"

—Elon Musk

EPIDEMIOLOGY

Lung cancer has been the most common cause of cancer-related mortality worldwide now for decades with an estimated 2.2 million cases (11.4% of all cancers) and 1.8 million deaths (18% of all deaths) annually. Linked to falling prevalence of smoking, the incidence of lung cancer has been falling in developed countries, with a lag in women. However, in developing countries including India, the ongoing high prevalence of smoking and poor air quality have contributed to a projected increase in the incidence of lung cancer based on GLOBOCAN data (2020). While there is substantial heterogeneity in the incidence and type of cancer geographically within India and by gender, lung cancer is now the most common cancer in males in India and this is especially true in urban areas and South India. About 98,278 cases of lung cancer are projected to occur in 2020; this includes 26,490 cases in women. About 44% of cases in men and 47% of the cases in women presented with distant metastases at diagnosis and this highlights the challenges in the management of lung cancer in India.

RISK FACTORS

- **Smoking:** Exposure to tobacco smoke is the most common risk factor for lung cancer, with risk increasing according to the intensity and duration of exposure to cigarettes. A variety of other formulations such as *beedi, hookah, chhutta, dhumti,* or *chillum* are more commonly used in India in addition to several smokeless tobacco formulations. *Beedi* is a cheap handmade dried, rectangular piece of *temburni* leaf (*Diospyros melanoxylon*) with 0.15–0.25 g of sun-dried, flaked tobacco. It is filled into a 4.0–7.5 cm conical shape and the roll is secured by a thread. It is the most common formulation used, especially in rural areas and contributes to 40% of all tobacco consumed. It is estimated that 14% of the population smoke (23.5% men and 2.5% in women) and that 130 million aged more than 15 years have exposure to tobacco smoke. Several regulations have contributed to a reducing prevalence of smoking in India; India is party to the World Health Organization (WHO) framework convention on tobacco control, the Cigarette and Other Tobacco Product Act (COTPA, 2003) banning advertisement for tobacco products, smoking being banned in several cities and public places, pictorial warnings on tobacco products and higher taxation on tobacco products are some of them.
- **Environmental tobacco smoke exposure (passive smoking):** Previous data from India suggested that 33.5% of households had second-hand exposure to tobacco products. Despite the implementation of COTPA and ban on smoking in public spaces, data from the Global Adult Tobacco Survey I and II has not shown a reduction in exposure to second-hand smoke
- **Occupational exposures and environmental exposures** to asbestos, silica, and radon have been associated with an increasing risk of lung cancer. Radon is a naturally occurring radioactive gas emanating from uranium present in all rocks and soils.
- **Air pollution:** India has 21 of the 30 most polluted cities in the world. There are several sources of both indoor and outdoor air pollution in India; refuse and biomass burning at both outdoors and indoors for cooking/heating, vehicles, power plant emissions and industrial sources. Air pollution contributes to poor lung function and is also increasingly being recognized as a cause of lung cancer.

There is an increase in the recognition of lung cancer in never smokers, especially in North India. Some series report up to 45–55% of their cancers in never smokers. In the largest series till date, 23.7% were never-smokers. Air pollution, environmental tobacco smoke, and genetic causes have been associated with lung cancers in never smokers but more research is needed in this area. When compared to lung cancers in smokers, nonsmokers are younger, more likely to be women (47.8 vs. 7%, $p < 0.005$), have higher education level, have adenocarcinoma on histology (62.3%, $p < 0.001$), harbor epidermal growth factor receptor (*EGFR*) mutations and have longer median survival.

SCREENING

Only 13.9–17% of all lung cancers present with localized disease in India (GLOBOCAN 2020) and this affects lung cancer survival. Screening using low-dose computed tomography (LDCT) has shown to reduce mortality by 20% from the seminal National Lung Screening Trial (NLST) (2013) and has the potential to detect earlier disease; this trial enrolled 53,439 ex-smokers or current smokers between 55 and 74 years of age with at least 30 pack-years exposure to annual LDCT for 3 years.

Refinement of the NLST algorithm has occurred from data of the NELSON trial (2020) and nodule management using Lung-RADS (lung imaging reporting and data system) and nodule volume-based strategy. Substantial problems in implementation of a screening program exist in India. These include appropriate definition of the target group given the large proportion of *beedi*-smokers, never smokers, and women in our population; nodule management algorithms given the higher incidence of granulomatous lung disease in our population; infrastructure for LDCT, nodule evaluation, and radiological reporting; development of smoking cessation clinics; and integration with lung cancer screening and reimbursement of costs.

WHO CLASSIFICATION

The WHO Classification of Tumors of the Lung, Pleura, Thymus and Heart was published in 2015 (**Box 1**). This update includes significant changes to the classification of lung cancers with substantial changes to the classification of adenocarcinomas and recommendation on the routine use of immunohistochemistry (IHC) and genetic markers to classify lung tumors. One major change includes discontinuation of the term bronchoalveolar carcinoma and usage of the term "lepidic" with extent of invasion in completely resected specimens forming various categories (adenocarcinoma-in-situ, minimally invasive, and invasive mucinous adenocarcinoma). Terminologies for small biopsy specimens have also been separately provided and this is different from that of resected specimens.

CLINICAL PRESENTATION

Clinical symptoms are often nonspecific and variable, contributing to the substantial delays in diagnosis. In one study of 1,370 patients from AIIMS Delhi, 94.5% of patients with NSCLC presented with advanced disease. There was a delay of a median of 101 [interquartile range (IQR), 56–168] days to definitive diagnostic study, 107 (IQR, 60–173) days for diagnostic confirmation, and 126 (IQR, 85–196.8) days before treatment initiation. This delay was substantially worse in those days for treatment initiation. This was significantly worse in those with prior radiological tuberculosis (187 vs. 113 days, $p < 0.0001$). Most of the delays were prior to evaluation in a specialty clinic and this service did not reduce delays.

Symptoms can be classified into (1) symptoms of local tumor, (2) effects of extension into the thoracic cavity, and (3) symptoms related to distant metastases and paraneoplastic syndromes.

A change in the character of cough with an increase in intensity can be seen in 8–75% of patients. Chest pain can be present in 25–50% of patients and can indicate parietal pleura involvement and mediastinal or chest wall invasion. Breathlessness can be seen in 50% and is present in lung cancer due to a variety of reasons: Endobronchial obstruction with tumor, extrinsic compression of the airway by tumor, postobstructive pneumonia, malignant pleural effusion, pulmonary embolism, phrenic nerve palsy and diaphragmatic weakness, superior vena cava (SVC) syndrome, deconditioning, worsening of airway disease by a large tumoral mass, and hemoptysis. Hemoptysis in a smoker can be the first symptom of lung cancer and is seen in 6–35%. Occasionally, it can be massive. Weight loss and anorexia in the setting of suspected lung cancer indicate advanced presentation and is associated with poorer outcomes.

BOX 1 2015 WHO histologic classification of lung tumors.

In resected specimens

- Adenocarcinomas:
  - Variants: Lepidic, acinar, papillary, micropapillary, solid
  - Invasive mucinous adenocarcinoma: Mixed invasive mucinous and nonmucinous
  - Colloid, fetal, enteric
  - Minimally invasive adenocarcinoma: Mucinous, nonmucinous
  - Preinvasive lesions: Atypical adenomatous hyperplasia, adenocarcinoma-in-situ
- Squamous cell: Keratinizing, nonkeratinizing, basaloid, preinvasive (in situ)
- Adenosquamous carcinoma
- Neuroendocrine:
  - Small-cell carcinoma
  - Large cell neuroendocrine carcinoma
  - Carcinoid tumors; typical, atypical
  - Preinvasive: Diffuse idiopathic pulmonary neuroendocrine cell hyperplasia
- Large-cell carcinoma
- Sarcomatoid carcinomas:
  - Pleomorphic, spindle cell, giant cell, carcinosarcoma, pulmonary blastoma
- Other and unclassified carcinomas:
  - Lymphoepithelioma-like carcinoma, NUT Carcinoma

Small biopsy/cytology terminology

- Adenocarcinoma (with description of identifiable patterns):
  - Adenocarcinoma with lepidic pattern (if pure, invasion cannot be excluded in small biopsy)
  - Invasive mucinous adenocarcinoma (patterns describe additional lepidic pattern)
  - Adenocarcinoma with colloid features
  - Adenocarcinoma with fetal features
  - Adenocarcinoma with enteric features
- NSCC favor adenocarcinoma (when diagnosis supported only by IHC and not morphology)
- Squamous cell carcinoma
- NSCC favor squamous cell carcinoma
- NSCC NOS; when no clear morphology or staining pattern
- Small-cell carcinoma
- NSCC with NE morphology and positive NE markers. Possible LCNEC
- NSCC with NE morphology (stains negative for NE markers)

(NE: neuroendocrine; NSCC: non-small-cell carcinoma; NOS: not otherwise specified; IHC: immunohistochemistry; WHO: World Health Organization; LCNEC: large-cell neuroendocrine carcinoma)

TABLE 1 Common paraneoplastic syndromes associated with lung cancer.

Musculoskeletal	Clubbing, hypertrophic osteoarthropathy, polymyositis, osteomalacia
Cutaneous	Dermatomyositis, acanthosis nigricans, erythema multiforme
Endocrinologic	SIADH, hypercalcemia, carcinoid syndrome, Cushing's syndrome
Neurologic	Peripheral neuropathy, encephalopathy, myelopathy, cerebellar degeneration, Lambert–Eaton myasthenic syndrome
Vascular/Hematologic	Thrombophlebitis, arterial thrombosis, red cell aplasia. Eosinophilia and leukemoid reaction
Miscellaneous	Cachexia, hyperuricemia, and nephrotic syndrome

(SIADH: syndrome of inappropriate secretion of antidiuretic hormone)

Local invasion can present with localized or radiating radicular chest pain, hoarseness, dysphagia, drooping of eye lids, and shoulder and arm pain.

Symptoms suggesting distant metastases are often absent but may include weakness, bony pains or fractures, and abdominal pain.

A wide variety of paraneoplastic syndromes are reported with lung cancer (**Table 1**) and can be seen in 10–20%. In general, these are hormonal, neurologic, hematologic, or other remote effects of cancer not related to the direct invasion, obstruction, or metastatic effects of the tumor.

FUNCTIONAL CLASSIFICATION

Performance status is a measure of a subject's ability to perform the activities of daily living and this information predicts survival in cancer and is used to decide the therapeutic approach to cancer. Karnofsky Performance Status (KPS) scale and Eastern Cooperative Oncology Group (ECOG) scale are the most commonly used performance status tools worldwide for patients with cancer. The KPS scale is an 11-point numerical scale, with scores ranging from 100 (normal functional status) to 0 (death), in decremental steps of 10. The ECOG PS scale is a 6-point numerical scale, with scores ranging from 0 (normal functional status) to 5 (death) in incremental steps of 1. A large retrospective study from PGIMER, Chandigarh showed that 10–40, 50–60, 70, 80–90, and 100 in the KPS are equivalent to ECOG PS categories of 4, 3, 2, 1, and 0, respectively.

STAGING

An accurate staging of lung cancer is crucial for correct choice of treatment and also has significant prognostic implications (see below). Staging is based on the Tumor-Node-Metastases classification (TNM 8, 2017). The current staging system is based on information from a global database of 94,708 patients receiving a diagnosis between 1999 and 2010 from 35 sources and 16 countries. Staging assessments can be clinical, pathological, restaging, at the time of recurrence, or at autopsy. *The TNM staging applies to both NSCLC and SCLC.* A simplified version is also employed in SCLC where patients are classified into "limited disease" (LD) (disease limited to one hemithorax, including supraclavicular and mediastinal lymph nodes) and "extensive disease" (ED) (any disease outside the hemithorax). Patients with malignant pleural effusion and LD are treated as "extensive disease" as they have the survival similar to this group even if disease is confined to one hemithorax.

The *T-staging component* is based on size (of the maximum dimension of the solid component on imaging and invasive component on pathology), degree of local invasion including the trachea, and additional tumor nodules relative to the primary lesion (**Table 2**). The categories of nodes in the N staging remain unchanged from the seventh edition; there are 14 stations and station 10 is hilar, stations 11–14 are intrapulmonary nodes, stations 2–9 are mediastinal nodes and station 1 includes low cervical, supraclavicular, and sternal notch nodes. The American Joint Committee on Cancer/ Union for International Cancer Control (AJCC/UICC) staging system recommends that at least six nodes are removed during surgical resection, including three from N1 and three from N2 groups. The *grouping of the nodal system* has undergone a slight change (**Table 2**). The analysis shows differences between p-stage tumors with single versus multiple N1 or N2 station involvement, but no differences between multiple N1 stations and a single N2 skip metastasis (no N1 involvement). This subgrouping was not included in the stage classification (**Table 3**). The *M staging components* have undergone change (**Table 2**) and the resultant stage groupings are described (**Table 3**). Staging has significant implications for management (see below) and for prognosis (**Table 4**).

Once the diagnosis is confirmed, a clinician performs imaging to place the patient in one of the stage groupings. This can sometimes be the same step as obtaining a tissue diagnosis when the patient presents with distant metastases; however, a complete staging even in this circumstance can have important implications while on therapy to assess response. Staging can be accomplished by noninvasive and invasive studies and the choice is based on the least invasive and acceptable option applicable to the patient.

Noninvasive staging: Computed tomography (CT) of the chest is available in most cases even before the diagnosis is established by histology. The next step is typically to review the lung windows for additional nodules and local invasion,

TABLE 2	Definitions for T, N, and M descriptions in the 2017 TNM 8 staging system of lung cancer.
T (Primary tumor)	**Description**
T0	No primary tumor
Tis	Carcinoma in-situ (squamous or adenocarcinoma)
T1	Tumor ≤ 3 cm
T1a (mi)	Minimally invasive adenocarcinoma
T1a	Superficial spreading tumor in the airway
T1a	Tumor ≤ 1 cm
T1b	Tumor > 1 cm but ≤2 cm
T1c	Tumor > 2 cm but ≤3 cm
T2	Tumor > 3 cm but ≤5 cm or tumor involving visceral pleura, main bronchus (but not carina) and atelectasis to hilum
T2a	Tumor > 3 cm but ≤4 cm
T2b	Tumor > 4 cm but ≤5 cm
T3	Tumor > 5 cm but ≤7 cm or invading chest wall, pericardium, phrenic nerve or separate tumor nodule(s) in the same lobe
T4	Tumor > 7 cm or invading mediastinum, diaphragm, heart, great vessels, recurrent laryngeal nerve, carina, trachea, esophagus, spine or tumor nodule(s) in a different ipsilateral lobes
N	*Regional lymph node*
N0	No regional node metastases
N1	Metastases in ipsilateral pulmonary or hilar nodes
N1a	Single-station N1 involvement
N1b	Multiple-station N1 involvement
N2	Metastases in ipsilateral mediastinal/subcarinal nodes
N2a1	Single-station N2 without N1 (skip)
N2a2	Single-station N2 with N1 involvement
N2b	Multiple-station N2 involvement
N3	Metastases in contralateral mediastinal/hilar, or supraclavicular nodes
M	*Distant metastases*
M1a	Malignant pleural/pericardial effusion or pleural/pericardial nodules or separate tumor nodule(s) in contralateral lobe
M1b	Single extrathoracic metastases
M1c	Multiple extrathoracic metastases (≥1 organ)

Note: Pleural effusions are excluded that are cytologically negative, nonbloody, transudative, and clinically judged not to be due to cancer.

mediastinal lymphadenopathy, contour of the pleural and pericardial surface including any effusion, bony erosions or lesions and available abdominal cuts for liver, and adrenal metastases. A lymph node > 1 cm in diameter is the most widely accepted criteria for significant lymphadenopathy. The pooled sensitivity for CT to stage the mediastinum was 51% and the pooled specificity was 86%; CT can neither rule in nor rule out a suspicious nodule and this should always be confirmed histologically before aggressive therapy is denied to an otherwise eligible patient. CT staging of the mediastinum is especially limited and 5–15% of those with no nodes on CT will have lymphadenopathy on surgical staging and 40% of those with nodes detected by CT will have benign nodes. CT of the abdomen and pelvis and head along with bone scan for occult bony secondaries completes noninvasive staging.

Positron emission tomography (PET): PET is a metabolic imaging technique based on the function of a tissue as indicated by its cellular uptake of glucose; the rate of uptake of ^{18}F-fluorodeoxyglucose (FDG) by neoplastic tissues can be imaged by a PET detector and this can be compared to normal tissues. A standard uptake value (SUV) > 2.5 or greater than mediastinal background activity is used as a cutoff to define abnormal uptake.

PET can upstage nearly 20% more patients than conventional CT-based staging; however, false positives can occur due to infections and granulomatous processes and false negatives can occur due to lesions < 1 cm on CT and PET findings should always be confirmed histologically before aggressive therapy is denied to an otherwise eligible patient. PET-CT can also stage bones and distant sites for secondaries. Given intense background brain activity on FDG, magnetic resonance imaging (MRI)-brain or high-slice CT-head (than available on a hybrid scanner) is still needed to complete staging after PET-CT. Conventionally, PET-CT hybrid scanners allow both anatomical and functional imaging to be performed at the same time and help with better staging.

Invasive staging: Invasive mediastinal staging is prompted by the presence of anatomically enlarged nodes on CT or uptake by PET scans. Accurate mediastinal staging is crucial for correct categorization of patients into one of the TNM groups (**Table 3**) in early lung cancer. As pointed out earlier, invasive staging is necessary to confirm that the enlarged nodes are involved by cancer and not by unrelated pathologic processes. However, in India, the majority present with local-regional and distant metastases and endobronchial ultrasound (EBUS) is often needed only to confirm involvement.

Endobronchial ultrasound-guided fine-needle aspiration (EBUS-FNA) is increasingly being undertaken worldwide as the initial procedure of choice for mediastinal staging. When combined with endoscopic ultrasound-guided fine-needle aspiration (EUS-FNA), which helps image paraesophageal and pulmonary ligament nodes and sample other stations not accessible by EBUS-FNA. EUS-FNA has replaced mediastinoscopy as the initial procedure of choice for mediastinal staging. However, given the false-negative rates of 15–20%, negative nodes will still need to be evaluated by mediastinoscopy prior to definitive surgery.

Physiologic evaluation for surgical resection: Lung cancer often develops in patients with prior lung disease

TABLE 3 The AJCC/UICC staging of lung cancer grouping (8th edition).

T/M	Subgroup	N0	N1	N2	N3
T1	T1a ≤ 1 cm	IA1	IIB	IIIA	IIIB
	T1b > 1–2 cm	IA2	IIB	IIIA	IIIB
	T1c > 2–3 cm	IA3	IIB	IIIA	IIIB
T2	T2a*	IB	IIB	IIIA	IIIB
	T2a > 3–4	IB	IIB	IIIA	IIIB
	T2b > 4–5	IIA	IIB	IIIA	IIIB
T3	T3 > 5–7	IIB	IIIA	IIIB	IIIC
	T3 invasion	IIB	IIIA	IIIB	IIIC
	T3 satellite nodules	IIB	IIIA	IIIB	IIIC
	T4 > 7 cm	IIIA	IIIA	IIIB	IIIC
T4	T4 invasion	IIIA	IIIA	IIIB	IIIC
	T4 ipsilateral nodules	IIIA	IIIA	IIIB	IIIC
	M1a contralateral nodule	IVA	IVA	IVA	IVA
M	M1a pleural dissemination	IVA	IVA	IVA	IVA
	M1b single	IVA	IVA	IVA	IVA
	M1c multi	IVB	IVB	IVB	IVB

* T2 as per other descriptors; size unknown or not >4 cm.

(AJCC: American Joint Committee on Cancer; UICC: Union for International Cancer Control)

TABLE 4 Expected 5-year survival (%) for the TNM stage groups (adapted from the AJCC/UICC statement).

Type	IA1	IA2	IA3	IB	IIA	IIB	IIIA	IIIB	IIIC	IVA	IVB
Clinical	92	83	77	68	60	53	36	26	13	10	0
Pathologic	90	85	80	73	65	56	41	24	12	–	–

(AJCC: American Joint Committee on Cancer; UICC: Union for International Cancer Control)

and while it may be anatomically resectable, patients may not be functionally able to undergo resection. The first step is to calculate the predicted postoperative FEV_1 (forced expiratory volume in 1 second) and DLCO (diffusing capacity of the lung for carbon monoxide) (preoperative FEV_1/DLCO × remaining segments/18). Further testing is needed if either of this value is <60% predicted (**Flowchart 1**)

OVERVIEW OF TREATMENT MODALITIES

The current paradigm of lung cancer treatment care is achieved in a multidisciplinary setting. Various treatment modalities include surgery, radiotherapy, systemic therapy (chemotherapy, targeted therapy, and immunotherapy), and palliative care. Treatment depends on multiple disease factors such as histology, stage; and host factors such as age, performance status, and the presence of comorbidities.

SURGERY

Surgery is the standard of care for early-stage lung cancer, i.e., stage I and II NSCLC. It has a role in multimodality management of stage III NSCLC. Various surgical procedures include wedge resection, segmentectomy, lobectomy, sleeve resection, and pneumonectomy. Less invasive techniques such as video-assisted thoracoscopic surgery (VATS) have improved perioperative outcomes. Surgery has a limited role in SCLC, except in selected patients with stage I disease.

CHEMOTHERAPY

Systemic chemotherapy can be used in a neoadjuvant (before surgery), adjuvant (after surgery in stages IB to IIIA), concurrent (along with radiotherapy), and palliative setting. The goal of chemotherapy in advanced disease is prolongation of survival and relief of symptoms. Various agents in NSCLC include platinum compounds (cisplatin, carboplatin), taxanes (paclitaxel, docetaxel), vinorelbine, gemcitabine, pemetrexed, and irinotecan. Usually, a combination of agents is chosen and selection of chemotherapy combinations are largely histology driven. Standard chemotherapy regimen for NSCLC is a platinum doublet typically cisplatin or carboplatin in combination with either a taxane/gemcitabine or pemetrexed (latter restricted to nonsquamous histology). For SCLC also, the standard chemotherapy regimen is a platinum doublet. However, the nonplatinum compound here is typically etoposide or irinotecan. Other drugs with (largely historical) activity against SCLC include cyclophosphamide, doxorubicin, ifosfamide, and topotecan.

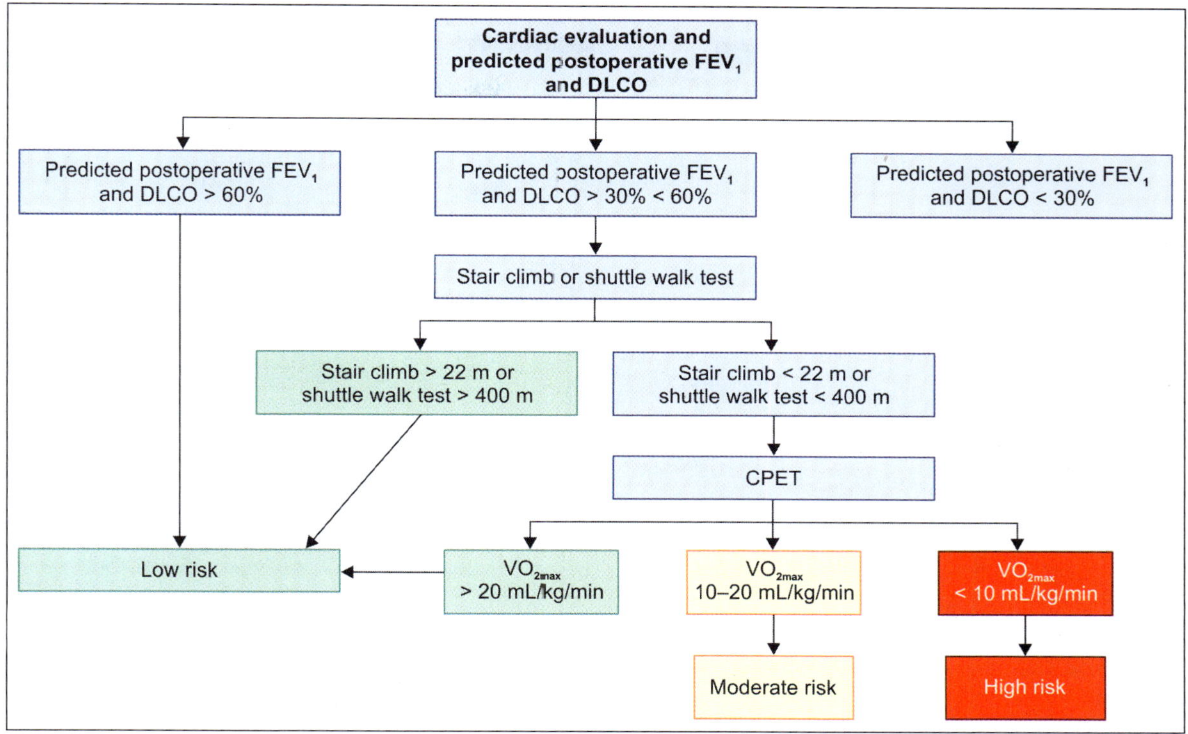

(DLCO: diffusing capacity of the lung for carbon monoxide; CPET: cardiopulmonary exercise testing; FEV_1: forced expiratory volume in 1 s)

FLOWCHART 1: Functional cardiopulmonary evaluation of a patient for eligibility for surgical resection.

RADIATION

The techniques of radiotherapy have evolved over time and recent techniques provide more precise radiation delivery and less toxicity. Radiotherapy has a role in patients with stage I and II NSCLC who are not candidates of surgery. It is also used in stage III NSCLC along with chemotherapy (concurrent chemoradiotherapy). Radiotherapy is also used to palliate the symptoms in advanced stage disease, particularly for SVC syndrome, hemoptysis, and bone and brain metastasis. Survivors may have toxicities such as radiation pneumonitis, pulmonary fibrosis, esophagitis, cardiac toxicity, and rarely brachial plexopathy.

TARGETED THERAPY

Over the last one decade, a better molecular characterization of disease has resulted in identification of new targets and eventually personalized treatment. We now understand that lung cancer, especially NSCLC, is a heterogeneous disease driven by specific molecular alterations. This has led to development of agents that target the specific molecular pathway.

It is imperative to test for the most commonly occurring oncogenic drivers [EGFR mutations and anaplastic lymphoma kinase (ALK) rearrangements] in all patients with stage IIIC/IV NSCLC. The list of potentially targetable oncogenic drivers has now expanded and includes at least three other mutations (a *BRAF* especially *V600E*; *MET* especially exon 14 skipping; *HER2* (*ERBB2*) and three other fusions/rearrangements (ROS1, RET, NTRK).

If any of these oncogenic drivers is detected, patients can be offered the appropriate targeted therapy as this approach is not only associated with better clinical outcomes but also reduced toxicity compared to conventional chemotherapy (**Table 5**). Most common toxicities of EGFR tyrosine kinase inhibitors (TKIs) are skin rash and diarrhea while other gastrointestinal, pulmonary, hepatic, and ocular toxicities are observed less commonly. Common toxicities of ALK TKIs include gastrointestinal toxicities such as nausea, vomiting, diarrhea, dysgeusia; transaminitis, fatigue, and visual disorders (with crizotinib). Bevacizumab, a monoclonal antibody against vascular endothelial growth factor (VEGF) is sometimes used along with chemotherapy in advanced nonsquamous NSCLC. A phase I trial recently showed good encouraging anticancer activity of sotorasib (AMG 510) in NSCLC patients harboring *KRAS p.G12C* mutation.

IMMUNOTHERAPY

Immunotherapy has changed the landscape in treatment of lung cancer patients, especially those with stage III and IV disease (**Table 6**). Immune checkpoint inhibitors (ICIs) block inhibitory interactions between tumor cells and immune cells. This results in enhanced T-cell antitumor activity. Response rates of ICIs in advanced disease are 20–45%. Interestingly, patients who respond to immunotherapy have a durable response. ICIs are now approved as monotherapy or in combination with chemotherapy in advanced NSCLC and as consolidation treatment after definitive chemoradiation in stage III disease.

TABLE 5 Molecular alterations with approved targeted therapy in advanced NSCLC.

Molecular alteration	Frequency	Technique	Agents
***EGFR* mutation**	25–30%	PCR	1st generation: Gefitinib, Erlotinib
		NGS	2nd generation: Afatinib, Dacomitinib
			3rd generation: Osimertinib
***ALK* rearrangement**	9–11%	FISH	1st generation: Crizotinib
		IHC	2nd generation: Ceritinib, Alectinib, Brigatinib
		NGS	3rd generation: Lorlatinib
***ROS1* rearrangement**	1–2%	FISH NGS	Crizotinib, Ceritinib, Entrectinib and Lorlatinib
***BRAF* mutation**	1%	PCR NGS	Dabrafenib with Trametinib

(FISH: fluorescence in-situ hybridization; IHC: immunohistochemistry; NGS: next-generation sequencing; NSCLC: non-small- cell lung cancer; PCR: polymerase chain reaction)

TABLE 6 Immune checkpoint inhibitors (ICIs) in advanced NSCLC.

Target	ICIs
CTLA-4	• Ipilimumab
PD-1	• Nivolumab • Pembrolizumab
PD-L1	• Atezolizumab • Durvalumab

(CTLA-4: cytotoxic T-lymphocyte-associated protein 4; NSCLC: non-small-cell lung cancer; PD-1: programmed death 1; PD-L1: programmed death-ligand 1)

NSCLC MANAGEMENT AS PER STAGE

STAGE I/II

Surgical resection: Surgical resection is the mainstay of treatment for patients who can tolerate the procedure. Lobectomy is superior to wedge resection in patient with stage IA lung cancer. Pneumonectomy is reserved for patients with central tumors and should be performed only in patients with an excellent pulmonary reserve. Accurate pathological staging requires mediastinal lymph node dissection. The 5-year survival rates are 60–80% for patients with stage I NSCLC and 50–60% for patients with stage II NSCLC.

Radiation therapy: Patients who cannot tolerate surgery can be treated with definite radiation with curative intent with improved techniques such as stereotactic body radiation therapy (SBRT). Cryoablation is also an option for peripheral tumors < 3 cm. Postoperative radiation therapy is used in stage II NSCLC with positive margins.

Chemotherapy: There is no recommendation for adjuvant chemotherapy in patients with resected stage IB (except those with negative prognostic factors, i.e., larger tumor size > 4 cm, tumor differentiation, vascular invasion, and histologic features) NSCLC. Adjuvant chemotherapy is not recommended for completely resected stage IA tumors. Adjuvant chemotherapy is best applied in patients with resected stage II NSCLC. Adjuvant chemotherapy improves survival in resected NSCLC by 4% as compared to surgery alone. Cisplatin-based combinations are preferred.

STAGE III

Stage III is a heterogeneous group of patients and hence treatment requires multidisciplinary approach. After careful evaluation of distant metastasis and invasive mediastinal staging, T3N1 and T4N0/1 tumor may be considered for surgery followed by adjuvant chemotherapy. For incidental stage IIIA (N2 disease found intra- or postoperatively), postoperative chemotherapy with or without sequential radiotherapy is recommended. For patients with discrete N2 disease on imaging, a thorough imaging to rule out distant metastases and invasive mediastinal staging should be done. Confirmed N2 disease can be treated by either definitive chemoradiotherapy (CRT) or preoperative therapy (chemotherapy or CRT) followed by surgery. Concurrent CRT is preferred for those with multistation N2 or bulky (>3 cm) lymph nodes. The latter option of induction chemotherapy followed by surgery may be chosen in selected cases with single-station N2 disease that was <3 cm prior to induction therapy. For those with N3 disease, concurrent CRT is the standard approach. For patients with stage III disease who received concurrent chemoradiation, adjuvant immunotherapy with durvalumab is recommended as it improves progression-free survival (PFS). Various chemotherapy options during CRT include, etoposide-platinum (EP), carboplatin plus paclitaxel or cisplatin plus pemetrexed (in nonsquamous NSCLC).

STAGE IV (METASTATIC NSCLC)

The goal of therapy in advanced NSCLC is to improve quality of life and survival. The choice of therapy depends on histology (squamous vs. nonsquamous), molecular alterations, age, ECOG PS (performance score), comorbidities, and patient preferences. Besides systemic treatment, adequate control of symptoms should be considered (painful bone metastasis, cord compression,

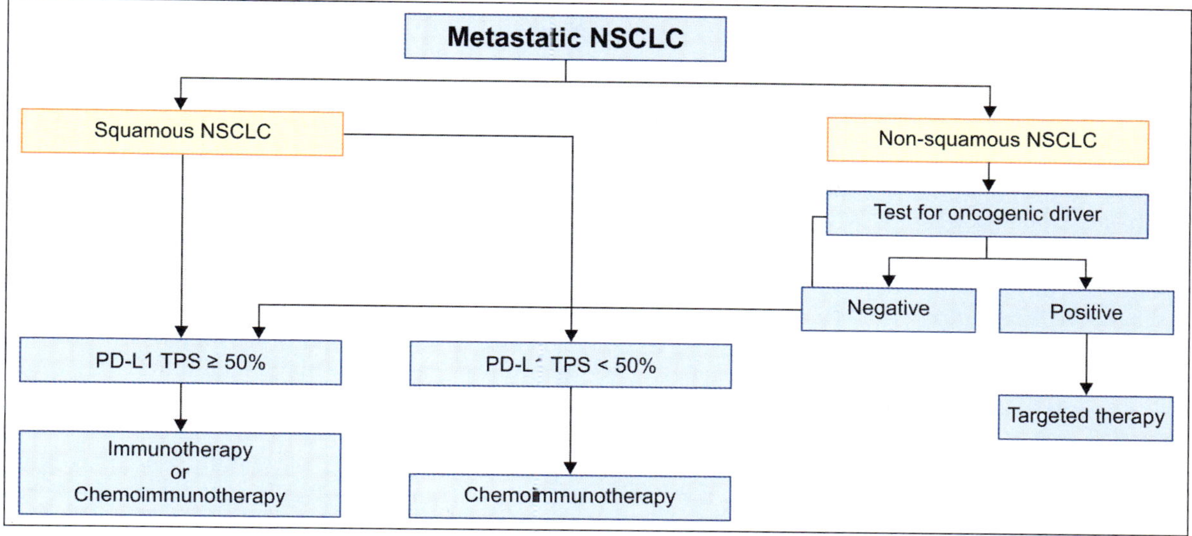

(NSCLC: non-small-cell lung cancer; PD-L1: programmed death-ligand 1; TPS: tumor proportion score)

FLOWCHART 2: Approach to advanced NSCLC.

CNS symptoms, or uncontrolled hemoptysis). Early referral for palliative care is recommended. The systemic treatment options are generally offered to patients with Eastern Cooperative Oncology Group performance status (ECOG-PS) of 0–1 and some patients with ECOG-PS of 2. Those with ECOG-PS 3–4 are usually offered best supportive care, unless eligible for targeted/immunotherapy which have a better tolerability profile. The general approach to management of stage IV lung cancer is depicted in **Flowchart 2**.

Patients with advanced lung adenocarcinoma should be tested for at least *EGFR* mutations and *ALK* rearrangements (and depending upon resources available, other potentially targetable oncogenic drivers described earlier). Molecular testing should also be offered to other nonsquamous NSCLC histological types or even squamous histology wherein clinical characteristics indicate the possibility of a mixed histological type (e.g., if the patient is a female OR nonsmoker). If an oncogenic driver is detected, patients should be offered treatment with the appropriate targeted drug (**Table 5**). If no oncogenic driver is detected, the preferred initial treatment consists of conventional chemotherapy and immunotherapy (**Table 6**). PD-L1 expression (tested with IHC) helps further in guiding the treatment (**Flowchart 2**). For patients with high PD-L1 (≥50%), immunotherapy (with pembrolizumab) is an appropriate first-line treatment option. Patients with PD-L1-negative tumors and those with PD-L1 ≥ 1% and < 50% are treated with combination of immunotherapy and chemotherapy (± bevacizumab). The chemotherapy generally consists of a platinum-based doublet. For those with nonsquamous histology, the preferred regimen consists of platinum plus pemetrexed while for those with squamous histology, the platinum drug is combined either with paclitaxel/nab-paclitaxel or gemcitabine.

Relapsed metastatic NSCLC: For a patient who has progressed on first-line therapy, docetaxel and gemcitabine are an appropriate option as a subsequent single-agent chemotherapy. Pemetrexed can be given to patients with nonsquamous histology if not given previously. Similarly, immunotherapy-naïve patients can benefit with ICIs. Patients with targetable mutation should be evaluated for resistant mechanisms and treated accordingly.

SCLC TREATMENT

Small-cell lung cancer is a highly aggressive disease and grows rapidly. It shows a dramatic response to chemotherapy and radiotherapy. The classification of disease into limited or extensive is largely based on feasibility of encompassing the disease in a single radiation portal. Systemic treatment is important even in LD because of the presence of occult micrometastases. More recently, the TNM staging system (7th and current 8th editions) have been validated and are being used for SCLC also.

LIMITED DISEASE

Patients with LD-SCLC are treated with concurrent chemoradiation with four cycles of EP and 45-Gray twice-daily radiotherapy, followed by prophylactic cranial irradiation (PCI) in patients who had a response to chemotherapy. The exception is patients with stage I disease who might be candidates for resection followed by adjuvant chemotherapy with EP for four cycles. The response to first-line therapy is around 80% and the cure rate is 20–25%. Despite response to first-line therapy, majority of patient relapse.

EXTENSIVE DISEASE

Patients with ED-SCLC should be treated with 4–6 cycles of systemic chemotherapy with carboplatin-etoposide (CE) along with immunotherapy (atezolizumab or durvalumab). Those with a favorable response to systemic therapy may be considered for thoracic irradiation. Both PCI and surveillance with a brain MRI are an option for those who respond to systemic therapy. In case of symptomatic brain metastases, upfront whole brain radiotherapy (WBRT) is advised. The median survival for patients with ED is 8–13 months.

PROPHYLACTIC CRANIAL IRRADIATION

As mentioned above, all SCLC patients who had a good response to initial therapy are candidates for PCI (25-Gray in 10 fractions). A meta-analysis including LD-SCLC patients showed improved overall survival in patients who had a complete response to initial therapy. In ED-SCLC, a trial showed reduced incidence of symptomatic brain metastasis in patients who received PCI after an initial response. However, radiotherapy to brain is associated with long-term toxicities (cognitive diminution), and therefore decision to go ahead with PCI should be taken after a discussion of risks and benefits with the patient.

RELAPSED AND REFRACTORY DISEASE

Patients who relapse after 6 months of initial treatment are said to have a sensitive disease while those who relapse earlier are said to have a refractory disease. Patients with sensitive disease can be rechallenged with the first-line regimen while those with refractory disease can be treated with second-line chemotherapy (e.g., topotecan) or immunotherapy. Palliative radiotherapy has a role in refractory disease.

IMMUNOTHERAPY

Immunotherapy improves survival in ED-SCLC. Both atezolizumab and durvalumab are approved for treatment in ED-SCLC along with chemotherapy (four cycles of EP) followed by immunotherapy maintenance. Nivolumab and pembrolizumab are an option for second-line therapy in patients with refractory disease.

SPECIAL SITUATIONS

SUPERIOR VENA CAVA SYNDROME

Lung cancer accounts for 75–85% of all cases of SVC syndrome of malignant origin. NSCLC is a more frequent cause of SVC syndrome (largely because it has 4–5 times greater incidence than SCLC). However, the likelihood of developing SVC syndrome is more common with SCLC than with other histological types. Symptoms and signs include facial or upper extremity edema, chest pain, dyspnea and, neurologic manifestations. Endovenous intervention is recommended for life-threatening symptoms. In stable patients, treatment is individualized based on histological diagnosis and symptoms. Patients with SCLC respond rapidly to chemotherapy. Patients with NSCLC are treated with radiotherapy and systemic therapy after endovenous stenting.

PANCOAST TUMOR

Pancoast tumors are those tumors that invade the structures of the thoracic inlet. They typically present with arm pain and/or Horner syndrome. The treatment for localized tumors is concurrent chemoradiation followed by resection.

PLEURAL/PERICARDIAL EFFUSION

Asymptomatic effusions may not require any treatment. Symptomatic effusions may require a thoracentesis/pericardiocentesis for immediate relief, and respond to systemic therapy. If symptoms occur within 2 weeks, a chest tube drainage is required. For recurrent effusions, pleurodesis (most commonly using talc or doxycycline or povidone-iodine) can be attempted. Medical thoracoscopy is a procedure wherein the pleural fluid can be drained, pleural biopsy taken under direct vision and pleurodesis attempted in the same setting.

BONE METASTASIS

Analgesic optimization improves pain control. Radiation therapy helps in palliation of painful bone metastases, stabilization of impending pathologic fractures, and treatment or prevention of spinal cord compression. Surgical intervention is a mainstay of treatment for pathologic fractures. Bisphosphonates relieve malignant bone pain and delay skeletal progression.

LEPTOMENINGEAL METASTASIS

Leptomeningeal metastasis is a serious complication of advanced NSCLC (3–5%). The diagnosis is established on neurological, radiographic, and cerebrospinal fluid findings. Survival is dismal with conventional therapy; though patients with oncogenic drivers tend to do better when treated with appropriate targeted therapies that have good CNS activity and good penetration across the blood-brain barrier.

SUPPORTIVE CARE

There have been advances in supportive care which has made more aggressive treatment possible leading to better patient outcomes. It includes management of anemia, febrile neutropenia, venous thromboembolism and other side effects of therapy. Early integration of palliative care, including aggressive pain, and symptom control, improves patient's quality of life and outcomes.

Patients with lung cancer often have coexisting comorbidities such as cardiovascular disease and COPD. These should be addressed with treatment optimization and correction of reversible problems such as anemia,

TABLE 7 Stagewise 5-year survival rates in non-small- and small-cell lung cancer.

Non-small-cell lung cancer	5-year OS (%)
IA1/IA2/IA3	92/83/77
1B	68
IIA	60
IIB	53
IIIA	36
IIIB	26
IVA/IVB	10/0
Small-cell lung cancer	**5-year OS (%)**
Limited stage	15–25
Extensive stage	<5

(OS: overall survival)

electrolyte and fluid disorders, infections, cardiac disease, and arrhythmia. Smoking cessation should be encouraged in all patients.

OUTCOMES

The 5-year outcomes of lung cancer, as per stage, are outlined in **Table 7**.

RECOMMENDED READINGS

1. Singh N, Aggarwal AN, Behera D. Management of advanced lung cancer in resource-constrained settings: a perspective from India. Expert Rev Anticancer Ther. 2012;12(11):79-95.
2. International Association for the Study of Lung Cancer (IASLC). In: Rami-Porta R. Staging Handbook in Thoracic Oncology, 2nd edition. North Fort Myers, FL, United States: Editorial Rx Press; 2016.
3. Vachani A, Sequist LV, Spira A. AJRCCM: 100-year anniversary. The shifting landscape for lung cancer: past, present, and future. Am J Respir Crit Care Med. 2017;195(9):1150-60.
4. Reck M, Rabe KF. Precision diagnosis and treatment for advanced non–small-cell lung cancer. N Engl J Med. 2017;377(9):849-61.
5. Hirsch FR, Scagliotti GV, Mulshine JL, Kwon R, Curran WJ Jr, Wu YL, et al. Lung cancer: current therapies and new targeted treatments. Lancet. 2017;389(10066):299-311.
6. Rolfo C, Mack PC, Scagliotti GV, Baas P, Barlesi F, Bivona TG, et al. Liquid biopsy for advanced non-small cell lung cancer (NSCLC): a statement paper from the IASLC. J Thorac Oncol. 2018;13(9):1248-68.
7. Kalemkerian GP, Narula N, Kennedy EB, Biermann WA, Donington J, Leighl NB, et al. Molecular testing guideline for the selection of patients with lung cancer for treatment with targeted tyrosine kinase inhibitors: American Society of Clinical Oncology endorsement of the College of American Pathologists/International Association for the Study of Lung Cancer/Association for Molecular Pathology clinical practice guideline update. J Clin Oncol. 2018;36(9):911-9.
8. Yatabe Y, Dacic S, Borczuk AC, Warth A, Russell PA, Lantuejoul S, et al. Best practices recommendations for diagnostic immunohistochemistry in lung cancer. J Thorac Oncol. 2019;14(3):377-407.
9. Mohan A, Garg A, Gupta A, Sahu S, Choudhari C, Vashistha V, et al. Clinical profile of lung cancer in North India: A 10-year analysis of 1862 patients from a tertiary care center. Lung India. 2020;37:190-7.
10. Saxena P, Singh PK, Malik PS, Singh N. Immunotherapy alone or in combination with chemotherapy as first-line treatment of non-small cell lung cancer. Curr Treat Options Oncol. 2020;21(8):69.
11. Hanna NH, Schneider BJ, Temin S, Baker S Jr, Brahmer J, Ellis PM, et al. Therapy for stage IV non–small-cell lung cancer without driver alterations: ASCO and OH (CCO) joint guideline update. J Clin Oncol. 2020;38(14):1608-32.
12. Hanna NH, Robinson AG, Temin S, Baker S Jr, Brahmer JR, Ellis PM, et al. Therapy for stage IV non-small-cell lung cancer with driver alterations: ASCO and OH (CCO) joint guideline update. J Clin Oncol. 2021; 39(9):1040-91 (Epub ahead of print; DOI: 10.1200/JCO.20.03570).

CHAPTER 219

Pleural Diseases

Javid Ahmad Malik

ABSTRACT

Pleura is a double-layered smooth, serous and elastic lubricating membrane that covers the outer surface of lungs and mediastinum and inner surface of thoracic wall. It primarily decreases the friction between lungs and thoracic wall generated during respiratory cycle. The outer layer of pleura covers inside of thoracic cavity is called parietal pleura and the inner layer of pleura covers outside of lungs and is known as visceral pleura. The wet potential space between the two layers of pleura that behaves like a stretchable elastic bag is known as pleural cavity. Normal pleural cavity contains about 5–15 mL of fluid.

Various pleural disorders include accumulation of abnormal quantity of fluid in pleural cavity known as pleural effusion, accumulation of air within the pleural cavity called pneumothorax, and pleural tumors which can arise primarily from pleura itself like mesothelioma or could be metastatic deposits from lung cancer or extrathoracic cancers. Importantly in developing countries like India, pleural surface gets frequently infected particularly with *Mycobacterium tuberculosis*. Accumulation of pus within pleural cavity is known as empyema and is usually a complication of pneumonia or septicemia. Various connective tissue disorders particularly systemic lupus and rheumatoid arthritis also tend to involve pleura at some stage in the course of the disease. Pleura involvement can also be a consequence of adverse drug effect.

"When you can't breathe, nothing else matters"

—Canadian Lung Association

PLEURAL EFFUSION

Pleural effusion results from either excess fluid formation in pleural space or decreased absorption by pleural lymphatics. Normally 0.13 mL/kg of body weight of fluid is present in pleural space. This small amount of fluid acts as a lubricant to allow the smooth sliding of parietal and visceral pleura during respiration. Normal amount of fluid is maintained by the critical balance between hydrostatic plus oncotic pressures of pleural capillaries and intrapleural pressure plus oncotic pressure of pleural fluid. Any imbalance of the above mechanism will lead to excess fluid accumulation in pleural space, i.e., pleural effusion.

DIAGNOSTIC APPROACH

For optimal outcome it is important for any clinician to keep in mind various causes of trasudative and exudative pleural effusions (**Box 1**) so as to individualize further diagnostic and therapeutic options. Congestive heart failure is the most common condition to produce transudative pleural effusion followed by hepatic hydrothorax. Nephrotic syndrome and hypoproteinemia are also common causes.[3] Common causes of exudative effusion include tuberculosis (TB), parapneumonic effusion, viral infections, and malignancy.

Imaging studies like chest radiograph, ultrasound, and often a contrast computed tomography (CT) scan thorax are the essential components of evaluation of pleural effusion.

On **chest radiograph**, pleural effusion is usually seen as an area of homogeneous opacity with ill-defined margins with tracking along the lateral chest wall. If the fluid is small (up to 50 mL) lateral chest radiograph is better than posteroanterior chest X-ray. CT is usually required to quantify the fluid and to identify loculations along with the presence of parenchymal and mediastinal abnormalities which may be missed on the standard radiograph. **Ultrasonography** of chest recently gained more importance in diagnosis of pleural effusion and it is more sensitive than chest radiograph. It is safe, there is no radiation, and has the benefit of repeatability. It can be used to identify the loculations and septations in pleural cavity. It can also be used to guide aspiration and choose site of insertion of intercostal chest tube.

Once pleural effusion is confirmed on imaging, **diagnostic aspiration** is essential to classify it as transudate or exudate (**Table 1**) which requires measurement of protein and lactate dehydrogenase (LDH) levels in the fluid. In exudative effusions, laboratory tests that are performed to arrive at a specific diagnosis include total leukocyte count, differential count, and biochemical tests such as proteins, glucose, LDH, amylase, microbiological examinations such as AFB stain, Gram stain, culture sensitivity in addition to adenosine deaminase (ADA) levels, and cytopathology. Additional investigations such as triglycerides and chylomicrons are requested depending on the clinical situation. **Closed pleural biopsy** is indicated, if ADA levels are low there is suspicion of TB or malignancy. Thoracoscopy is a highly sensitive tool for evaluation of undiagnosed exudative pleural effusions. Two diagnoses that commonly obtained with thoracoscopic pleural biopsy are TB and malignancy.

TUBERCULAR PLEURAL EFFUSION

Tuberculosis is a global health problem and it is evident from the World Health Organization (WHO) Global TB report of 2016 that the TB epidemic is larger than previously estimated, with an estimated 10.4 million new cases and 1.4 million deaths. This document further reports an additional 0.4 million deaths from TB disease among patients coinfected with HIV. Pulmonary TB is the most common form of TB with extrapulmonary TB (EPTB) accounting for approximately 15% of cases but this estimate increases to nearly 50% in high HIV prevalence settings. Tuberculosis pleural effusion (TPE) is the second most common site of EPTB.

Tubercular pleural effusion is the most common cause of exudative pleural effusion in the developing countries like India. It is usually associated with pulmonary TB. The mechanism of tubercular pleural effusion formation involves a hypersensitivity reaction by pleural membranes to the tubercular protein.

Clinical presentation includes fever, chest discomfort, cough, dyspnea, and weight loss. Diagnosis in majority of the patients is established by pleural fluid examination. Effusion is lymphocyte predominant exudate with high concentration of tubercular markers like ADA > 40 IU/L or interferon gamma > 140 pg/mL.

In a recent Indian study that addressed the clinical and etiological profile of an exudative pleural effusion found *pleural fluid ADA levels highly sensitive with good specificity for the diagnosis of tubercular effusions.* In some but not all patients, diagnosis is confirmed by mycobacterial culture or gene Xpert in the pleural fluid.

In any exudative pleural effusion when TB markers are low and malignancy cannot be confidently excluded, pleural biopsy is indicated. Blind pleural biopsy is done conventionally by Abraham's needle or True-Cut needle though in higher institutions it is usually performed under image guidance by CT scan or ultrasound. Thoracoscopic pleural biopsy is performed if pleural fluid reports are equivocal and if some other concomitant procedure like ahesiolysis or pleurodesis is required to be performed in the same setting (**Figs. 1 A** and **B**). Pleural tissue is not only examined for presence of caseating granulomas but the yield of MTB culture is also high compared to pleural fluid itself.

A recent study by DJ Christopher et al. from CMC Vellore revealed that thoracoscopic pleural biopsy improves yield of Xpert MTB for diagnosis of pleural TB. These authors demonstrated an increase in diagnostic sensitivity when the Xpert test is performed on pleural tissue obtained by thoracoscopic biopsy and yield exceeds pleural fluid Xpert and mycobacterial culture.

BOX 1 Differential diagnosis of pleural effusion.

Transudative pleural effusion:

- CHF
- Chronic liver disease
- Nephrotic syndrome
- SVC obstruction
- Myxedema

Exudative pleural effusion:

- Infectious causes:
  - Tuberculosis
  - Bacterial infections
  - Viral infections
  - Fungal infections
  - Parasitic infections
- Neoplastic causes:
  - Metastatic disease
  - Mesothelioma
- Pulmonary thromboembolism
- Collagen vascular diseases:
  - SLE
  - Rheumatoid arthritis
  - Sjögren syndrome
  - Granulomatosis with polyangiitis (Wegner's)
  - Churg–Strauss syndrome
  - Immunoblastic lymphadenopathy
- Gastrointestinal causes:
  - Pancreatitis
  - Esophageal rupture
  - Abdominal abscess
  - Diaphragmatic hernia
  - Postvariceal sclerotherapy
- Drugs:
  - Dantrolene
  - Nitrofurantoin
  - Bromocriptine
  - Methysergide
  - Dasatinib
  - Amiodarone
  - Procarbazine
- Hemothorax and chylothorax
- Postcardiac injury syndrome and post-CABG
- Asbestos exposure
- Radiation therapy
- Meigs syndrome
- Uremia
- Sarcoidosis
- Yellow nail syndrome

TABLE 1 Classification of pleural fluid as exudate vs. transudate.

Rule	Criteria
Light's criteria	PF/S > 0.5 or PF/S LDH > 0.6 or PF LDH > two-thirds upper limit of laboratory's normal serum LDH
Rule that does not require serum tests	PF protein > 2.9 g/dL or PF cholesterol > 45 mg/dL or PF LDH > 0.45 times upper limit of laboratory's normal serum LDH

Source: Pack AI, Elias JA, Fishman JA, Grippi MA, Kotloff R, Robert M (Eds). Fishman's Pulmonary Diseases and Disorders, 5th edition, volume 2. McGraw-Hill Education; 2015. p. 1164.

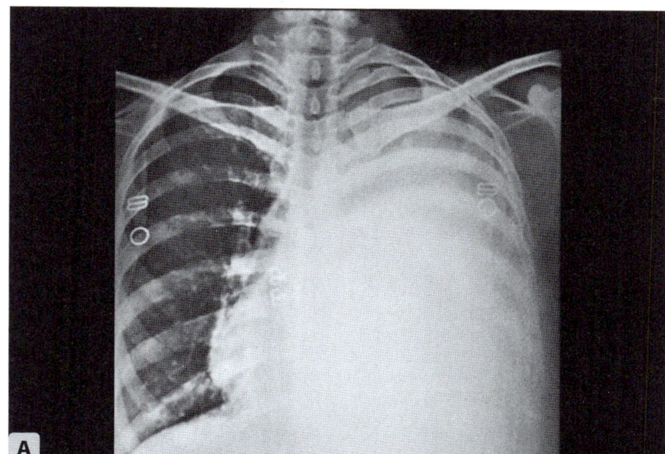

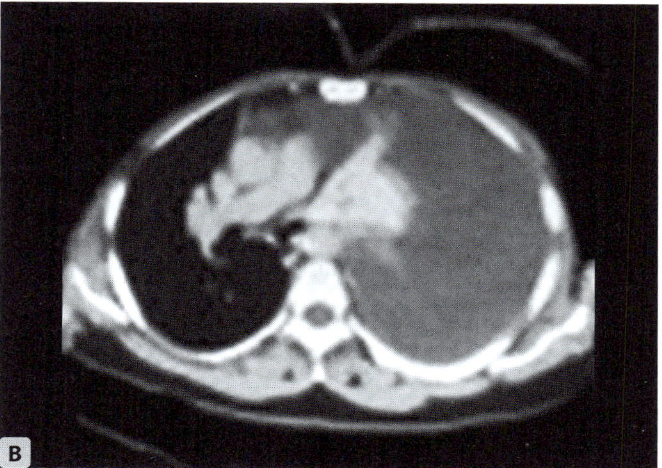

FIGURES 1 A & B: Massive left-sided pleura effusion with contralateral mediastinal shift. This 34-year-old female had exudative pleural effusion with low adenosine deaminase and cytology negative for malignancy. Thoracoscopic pleural biopsy revealed tuberculosis on both histopathology and culture. Patient responded to tuberculosis drugs and radiograph normalized on follow-up.

Pharmacological treatment of pleural TB is same as of pulmonary TB.

PARAPNEUMONIC EFFUSION AND EMPYEMA

Pleural effusion that sometimes complicates bacterial pneumonia, lung abscess, or bronchiectasis is called parapneumonic effusion. Grossly purulent effusion is called empyema. **Thoracic empyema** continues to be an important cause of morbidity especially in developing countries. Pulmonary infections including community acquired pneumonia, bronchiectasis, and lung abscess are the most common cause of empyema in the Western countries followed by surgical trauma. In contrast, studies from India reveal that TB accounts for a large number of empyema cases (38.6–65%).

These patients usually have fever, chest pain, and productive cough. Neutrophilic leukocytosis is often present. Lateral decubitus radiograph, ultrasound, or CT scan of chest is needed for evaluation. More than 10 mm free fluid that separates the lung from chest wall is an indication for therapeutic thoracentesis. *Intercostal drainage* by chest tube or a pig-tail catheter is usually indicated if the pleural fluid reveals any of the following on analysis:

- Gross pus
- Gram stain or culture positivity
- Glucose < 60 mg/dL
- pH < 7.2
- Loculated pleural fluid

Intrapleural fibrinolysis is carried out with instillation of tissue plasminogen activator (10 mg) in combination with deoxyribonuclease (5 mg) via chest tube. If this combination fails, medical thoracoscopy is used to breakdown loculations with complete drainage of fluid from the pleural cavity. For adhesilysis rigid thoracoscope is preferred over semirigid thoracoscope. If all these measures do not yield adequate results, services of thoracic surgeon for *video-assisted thoracoscopic surgery (VATS) or conventional decortication* should be evaluated as a last resort.

Somenath K et al. in a study on adult thoracic empyema concluded that TB is an important cause of empyema in the young population of India. Tuberculous empyema patients have a protracted duration of illness, a significant incidence of bronchopleural fistula formation necessitating complicated drainage including surgical drainage. These patients have a relatively poor outcome compared to patients with nontuberculous empyema.

VIRAL PLEURAL EFFUSION

Diagnosis of viral pleural effusion is mostly a presumption in a given clinical scenario. Approximately 15–20% of exudative pleural effusions remain undiagnosed even after extensive work-up and tend to resolve spontaneously on follow-up. It is pertinent to mention that majority of these viruses do not have specific markers in pleural fluid or blood and viral culture facilities are lacking in most of the centers. If patient is clinically improving and imaging study reveals resolution of exudative pleural effusion, there is no need to expand investigations except for a chest radiograph on follow-up.

CONGESTIVE HEART FAILURE RELATED

Left ventricular failure is the most common cause of pleural effusion and effusion is usually bilateral. Diagnostic thoracentesis is indicated under the following circumstances:

- Unilateral effusion
- Asymmetrical bilateral effusion
- Pleuritic chest pain
- Fever

Diagnosis of heart failure-related pleural effusion is confirmed by pleural fluid level of >1,500 pg/mL of N-terminal pro-brain natriuretic peptide (NT-pro-BNP).

PULMONARY EMBOLISM RELATED

Though pulmonary embolism is one of the most common causes of exudative pleural effusion, it is commonly not suspected and hence not investigated for (**Fig. 2**). Suspicion should be high in any patient with deep venous thrombosis. Dyspnea and chest pain are the main symptoms. Uncommonly patient may have hemoptysis. Spiral CT scan or pulmonary arteriography is essential to confirm the diagnosis. Plasma D-dimer levels are usually elevated to more than 500 mg/dL. Pleural effusion in this setting does not need any specific treatment and resolves with the treatment of pulmonary emboli.

HEMOTHORAX

Hemothorax is defined as pleural fluid hematocrit more than one-half of peripheral blood. Hematocrit measurement is ordered if pleural fluid is bloody on diagnostic thoracentesis. Etiology of hemothorax is depicted in **Box 2**.

Management of hemothorax involves urgent placement of an intercostal chest tube which in addition to symp-

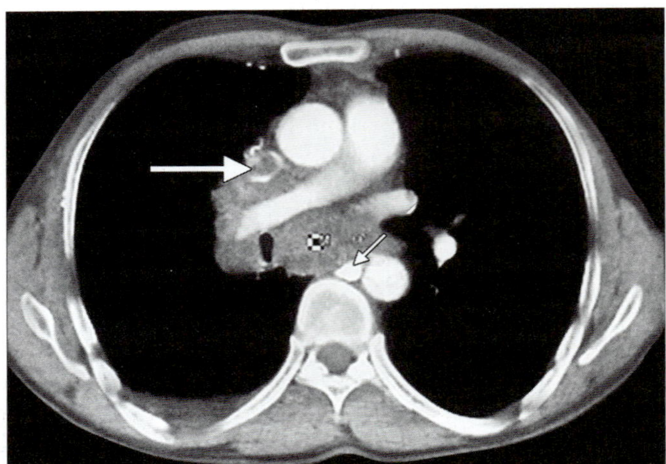

FIGURE 2: Contrast computed tomography scan of chest of a patient of small cell carcinoma showing a thrombus in superior vena cava (short arrow). Enlargement of right hilar, subcarinal and azygoesophageal recess lymph nodes is also seen. Note pleural effusion on right side and dilated azygos vein (long arrow) due to blood diversion.

BOX 2	Causes of hemothorax.
Common causes:	
• Trauma	
• Coagulopathy and bleeding diatheses	
• Pneumothorax and ruptured lung bullae	
• Neurofibromatosis	
• Arteriovenous malformations	
• Aneurysms	
Rare causes:	
• Connective tissue diseases	
• Ehlers–Danlos disease	
• Extramedullary hematopoiesis	
• Endometriosis	
• Exostoses	
• Postpartum	

Source: Pack AI, Elias JA, Fishman JA, Grippi MA, Kotloff R, Robert M (Eds). Fishman's Pulmonary Diseases and Disorders, 5th edition, volume 2. McGraw-Hill Education; 2015. p. 1170.

tomatic relief allows a clinician to quantitate bleeding. Thoracoscopy or thoracotomy is considered if bleeding exceeds 200 mL/h.

CHYLOTHORAX

Accumulation of chyle in pleural space due to rupture of thoracic duct is known as chylothorax. Various causes leading to chylothorax formation are summarized in **Box 3**.

Chylothorax patients present with dyspnea and chest radiograph and CT scan reveal moderate to massive pleural effusion. Fluid is milky in appearance. Biochemical hallmark is triglyceride level >110 mg/dL in an exudative effusion. Lymhpangiogram is sometimes required to clinch the diagnosis. Octreotide administration and chest tube insertion constitute treatment of choice. Prolonged chest tube drainage should be discouraged as it can lead to immunological incompetence and malnutrition. In nonresponders pleuroperitoneal shunt is placed provided patient does not have concomitant chylous ascites. Ligation of thoracic duct and percutaneous transabdominal thoracic duct blockage are viable alternative treatment options.

HEPATIC HYDROTHORAX

Hepatic hydrothorax complicates approximately 5% of liver cirrhosis and ascites. It occurs more frequently on right side compared to left. Hepatic hydrothorax occurs due to the upward movement of peritoneal fluid through small holes in the diaphragm. Effusion is usually moderate to massive leading to shortness of breath.

MALIGNANT PLEURAL EFFUSION

In developing countries like India where the incidence of infections particularly TB is high malignant pleural effusion (MPE) is the second most common cause of exudative effusions. Whereas MPE is the most common cause of exudative pleural effusion in developed countries with 75% being caused by lung carcinoma, breast carcinoma, and lymphoma (**Figs. 3 A** and **B**). Germ cell tumors, sarcomas, and prostatic carcinoma account for 10% of MPE whereas in the remaining 7–15% the primary source of malignancy remains unknown. Metastatic MPE is 25 times more common than mesothelioma. Among lung cancer patients 15% have pleural effusion at the time of diagnosis and half of them develop it during the course of disease.

Breathlessness and chest discomfort are the usual symptoms. Neck and axillary lymph node enlargement may be evident on clinical examination. The important predictors of survival include performance status of the patient, site of primary tumor, and stage of underlying cancer.

Contrast CT scan of chest should include upper abdomen to assess for possible hepatic and adrenal metastasis. The presence of pleural nodularity, parietal pleural thickening of more than 1 cm, and circumferential and mediastinal pleural thickening on CT scan are highly suggestive of malignancy.

Approximately 50% of MPEs are nonhemorrhagic and around 20% have pleural sugar levels below 60 mg/dL. Pleural fluid cytology usually confirms the diagnosis of MPE in 60% of the patients. Cytology smear analysis and cell-block enable immunohistochemistry thereby enhancing the diagnostic yield. In patients with negative cytology pleural biopsy is indicated. Blind pleural biopsy by Abraham's needle has a yield of 40–75% because pleural involvement

BOX 3	Causes of chylothorax.
• **Traumatic chylothorax:**	
○ Traumatic 50% thoracic surgery most cause	
○ Central venous catheter insertion	
○ Pacemaker insertion	
○ Traction injury to chest and neck	
○ Abrupt intrathoracic pressure changes related to labor, sneezing, and vomiting	
• **Nontraumatic chylothorax:**	
○ Lymphomas and other mediastinal tumors	
○ SVC syndrome	
○ Constrictive pericarditis	
○ Lymphangiectasis	
○ Lymphangioleiomyomatosis	
○ Granulomatous infections	
○ Intrathoracic goiter	
○ Downs syndrome	
○ Yellow nail syndrome	
○ Noonan's syndrome	
• **Idiopathic chylothorax**	

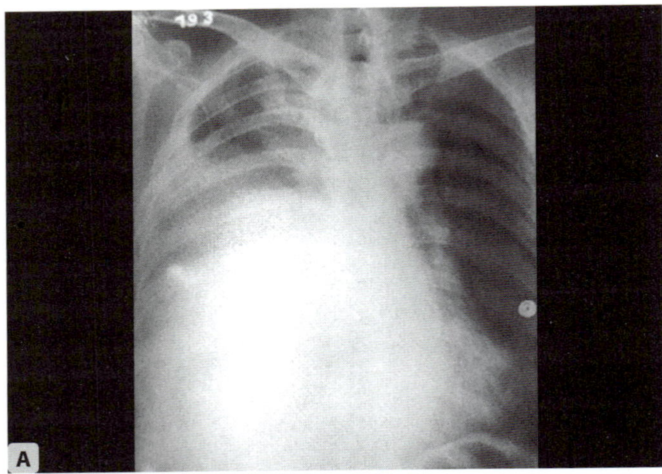

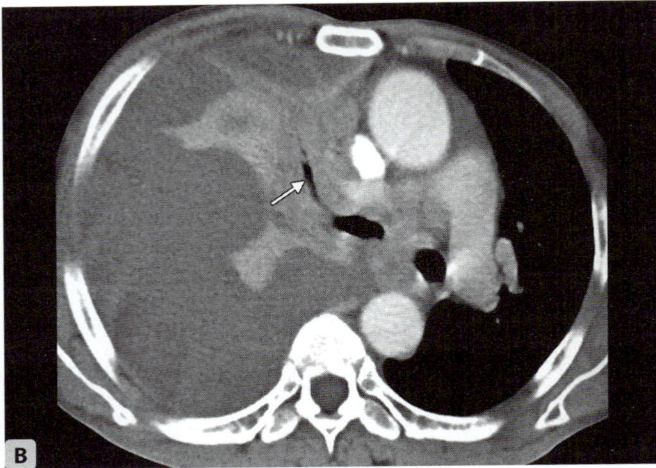

FIGURES 3 A & B: Malignant pleural effusion. (A) Chest X-ray: Massive pleural effusion on right side. **(B)** Contrast-enhanced computed tomography scan of chest: Massive pleural effusion causing compression of right upper lobe bronchus (arrow) and collapse of the underlying lung along with displacement of mediastinal structures to the left. Bronchoscopy in this 70-year-old male revealed an endobronchial growth and pleural fluid cytology confirmed metastatic nonsmall cell lung cancer.

by malignancy is usually patchy. Pleural biopsy specimen is also obtained by ultrasound or CT-guided procedure. The diagnostic yield of both CT-guided biopsy and thoracoscopic biopsy is around 87%. Thoracoscopic pleural biopsy is preferred if pleurodesis is also planned to be performed simultaneously.

Management: Management of MPE is mostly guided by the underlying tumor which guides the clinician about chemo-radio or hormonal therapies. Therapeutic options include:

- *Therapeutic pleural fluid aspiration*: It is indicated in all patients of MPE with dyspnea. Usually no more than 1,500 mL of pleural fluid is aspirated in one session because of risk of reperfusion pulmonary edema.
- *Intercostal chest tube drainage*: Chest tube is a more effective drainage procedure. It is a safe procedure usually inserted blindly by resident doctors of medical as well as surgical sides. Procedure is sometimes done under ultrasound guidance.
- *Pleurodesis*: Pleurodesis is a procedure aimed to affect symphysis of two pleural membranes. Purpose of pleurodesis is to prevent recurrence of MPE and is performed either by chemical or mechanical means. It is done with tube thoracostomy or thoracoscopy through which a chemical agent is introduced into the pleural cavity to induce intense inflammation and subsequent fusion of parietal and visceral pleural membranes resulting in obliteration of pleural space. Various chemical agents used for pleurodesis include talc, parenteral preparation of tetracycline (35 mL/kg) or doxycycline 10 mg /kg or 20 mL of 10% iodopovidone and 80 mL normal saline. Other rare agents that have been used for pleurodesis include transforming growth factor beta, silver nitrate, quinacrine, corynebacterium parvum etc. Currently graded talc as poudrage or slurry is most effective and most widely used agent used for pleurodesis.
- *Long-term ambulatory pleural drainage*: In situations where pleurodesis is not appropriate like trapped lung or when pleurodesis fails, placement of a tunneled pleural catheter is the best management option. Its one-way valve allows drainage into a vacuum bottle at regular intervals and prevents air from entering the pleural cavity.

MESOTHELIOMA

Tumor that originates from mesothelial cells lining the pleural cavity is known as mesothelioma. Any form of injury to these mesothelial cells results in the release of growth factors which induce proliferation. Asbestos exposure is usually present in all patients. Simian virus 40 (SV40) and radiation therapy have also been found to be associated with subsequent development of mesothelioma in rare cases.

Malignant pleural mesothelioma (MPM) starts as multiple small nodules on parietal pleura which coalesce to form a thick rind of tumor that eventually fuses together the two layers of pleura. Histologically mesothelioma is of three types:

1. Epitheloid
2. Sarcomatoid
3. Mixed (biphasic)

These tumors commonly present between 40 and 70 years of age with dyspnea and chest discomfort. Pleural effusion is a rare presentation. Various paraneoplastic syndromes associated with mesothelioma include:

- Migratory thrombophlebitis
- Disseminated intravascular coagulation
- Thrombocytosis
- Hpercalcemia
- Hypoglycemia
- Coomb's positive hemolytic anemia

Poor prognostic factors in a patient of mesothelioma include:
- Male sex
- Age > 75 years
- Symptomatic for > 2 months before diagnosis
- Poor performance status
- Chest pain
- Nonepithelioid histology
- Advanced stage disease

Diagnostic imaging modalities include a radiograph and CT scan both of which reveal pleural thickening and nodularity in addition to effusion. Tissue diagnosis is made by pleural biopsy obtained by ultrasound or CT-guided procedure because closed pleural biopsy usually does not provide sufficient material for a confident diagnosis of MPM. Thoracoscopic pleural biopsy if available is also a preferred option to achieve diagnosis.

Though their role has not been well established the two tumor markers found in the serum of mesothelioma patients include:
1. Serum mesothelin-related protein (SMRP)
2. Osteopontin

Various immunohistochemical markers important in the diagnosis of malignant mesothelioma include:
- Calretinin
- EMA
- WTI
- Cytokeratin 5/6
- HBME-1
- Mesothelin

Aggressive surgical interventions in malignant mesothelioma are precluded by advanced age at presentation, comorbidities, and locally advanced disease. The surgical options include pleurectomy and extrapleural pneumonectomy and are usually palliative and rarely curative. Thus surgical option is considered generally as a part of multimodality approach in combination with chemotherapy and radiotherapy. Pleurodesis either by tube thoracostomy or thoracoscopy is one significant palliative option in mesothelioma-related effusion.

Malignant mesothelioma is generally resistant to radiotherapy; however, local radiation can be given for palliative purposes. Decision regarding administration of chemotherapy has to be individualized after thorough discussion with the patient considering risk-benefit ratio of this treatment modality. Cisplatin is the cornerstone of combination chemotherapy in malignant mesothelioma. It can be combined with:
- Pemetrexed
- Gemcitabine
- Vinca alkaloids or
- Anthracycline

PNEUMOTHORAX

Presence of air in pleural space is called pneumothorax. *Various types of pneumothorax include:*
- **Traumatic pneumothorax:** It is a consequence of chest injury and can result from any one of the following:
  - Direct trauma to chest
  - Indirect trauma to chest
  - Iatrogenic pneumothorax: It is a consequence of diagnostic or therapeutic procedure.
- **Spontaneous pneumothorax:** It occurs without trauma to the chest and is of two types:
  1. Primary spontaneous pneumothorax (PSP): It occurs in absence of underlying lung disease.
  2. Secondary spontaneous pneumothorax (SSP): It occurs in presence of underlying lung disease.
- **Tension pneumothorax:** Any pneumothorax in which intrapleural pressure is positive throughout respiratory cycle is known as tension pneumothorax. It can complicate either traumatic or spontaneous pneumothorax.
- **Closed pneumothorax:** It is one in which alveolar-pleural communication is sealed.
- **Open pneumothorax:** It communicates with the atmosphere.
- **Catamenial pneumothorax:** It is seen in 3% of women with PSP.

TRAUMATIC PNEUMOTHORAX

Both penetrating and nonpenetrating chest trauma can result in pneumothorax. Chest tube should be immediately inserted to drain the air. If there is hemopneumothorax insertion of two chest tubes is indicated, lower one to drain blood and the upper tube to drain air.

Traumatic pneumothorax that occurs due to thoracentesis, insertion of central venous catheter or pacemaker catheter is called iatrogenic pneumothorax. Most cases of iatrogenic pneumothorax settle with oxygen and aspiration but chest tube drainage is indicated in nonresponders.

PRIMARY SPONTANEOUS PNEUMOTHORAX

It is exclusively a disease of smokers and 50% have recurrence in future. Though by definition it occurs in people without underlying lung disease, most often apical pleural bleb rupture is responsible for the occurrence of PSP. Blebs can be found in more than 75% patients undergoing thoracoscopic treatment for primary PSP but it is not clear that how often are these blebs actually the sites of air leakage.

Male patients with PSP are usually taller and thinner. In women smoking and body shape are less relevant in the development of PSP. PSP usually occurs at rest rather than during exertion and is common between 20 and 40 years of age. Acute pleuritic chest pain localized to the side of pneumothorax is the most common presentation.

Upright posteroanterior chest radiograph with demonstration of pleural line confirms the diagnosis in majority of the cases. Radiograph shows collection of lucent gas with absent pulmonary vascular markings between outer margin of visceral pleura (lung) and parietal pleura (chest wall). Lateral decubitus radiograph is superior to erect or supine radiograph and is as sensitive as CT scan in detection of pneumothorax.

BOX 4	Treatment options for primary spontaneous pneumothorax.
• Observation with oxygen supplementation	
• Simple needle aspiration	
• Small catheter drainage	
• Chest tube drainage	
• Medical thoracoscopy and pleurodesis with talc poudrage or pleural abrasions	
• VATS with blebectomy, bullectomy, pleural abrasion, or pleurectomy	
• Thoracotomy	

Treatment options for PSP depend upon extent of pneumothorax, clinical status of the patient, and presence or absence of underlying lung disease (**Box 4**). Aspiration is the initial recommended treatment. Thoracotomy or thoracoscopy for stapling of blebs and pleural abrasion is indicated if lung does not expand with simple aspiration or if there is recurrence of pneumothorax.

SECONDARY SPONTANEOUS PNEUMOTHORAX

Almost all lung diseases predispose an individual to SSP although the most common cause is TB in India and COPD in the Western countries. Due to limited pulmonary reserve these, patients are at higher risk of respiratory failure.

Most of the patients with SSP in India are between 40 and 50 years of age. The recurrence risk of 40–80% in SSP is higher than that of PSP. Immediate tube thoracostomy is the initial treatment of choice. Thoracotomy or thoracoscopy for stapling of blebs and pleural abrasion is indicated in most of these patients. Pleurodesis with doxycycline or talc is reserved for those patients who are unfit for surgery or refuse surgery.

TENSION PNEUMOTHORAX

In tension pneumothorax, the intrapleural pressure is positive throughout the respiratory cycle. The intrapleural pressure rises in proportion to volume of air in the pleural cavity and once it is above atmospheric pressure, it is called tension pneumothorax. **It is a life-threatening emergency** because of severe respiratory compromise coupled with decreased cardiac output due to reduced venous return to heart. It usually occurs during mechanical ventilation or resuscitation.

Tension pneumothorax should be suspected if there is significant tachycardia, cyanosis, hypotension, or electromechanical dissociation. Profound hypoxemia and hypotension are the hallmarks of tension pneumothorax with contralateral mediastinal shift.

No time should be wasted in inserting a *large-bore needle into the pleural space* through the second intercostal space anteriorly which should be removed only after the insertion of chest tube.

PLEURODESIS

Pleurodesis is a procedure aimed to affect symphysis of two pleural membranes. Purpose of pleurodesis is to prevent recurrence in both PSP and SSP. It is done with tube thoracostomy or thoracoscopy through which a chemical agent is introduced into the pleural cavity to induce intense inflammation and subsequent fusion of parietal and visceral pleurae resulting in obliteration of pleural space. Various chemical agents used for pleurodesis include talc, parenteral preparation of tetracycline (35 mL/kg) or doxycycline (10 mg/kg), iodopovidone (20 mL of 10% mixed with 80 mL normal saline), silver nitrate etc. Recurrence rates can be reduced from 40% to 25% by pleurodesis and to just 5% by thoracoscopic blebectomy and pleural abrasion demonstrating a clear edge of thoracoscopy.

RECOMMENDED READINGS

1. Diaz-Guzman E, Dweik RA. Diagnosis and management of pleural effusions: A practical approach. Compr Ther. 2007;33:237-46.
2. Noppen M. Normal volume and cellular contents of pleural fluid. Curr Opin Pulm Med. 2001;7:180-2.
3. Chetty KG. Transudative pleural effusions. Clin Chest Med. 1985;6:49-54.
4. Collins TR, Sahn SA. Thoracocentesis. Clinical value, complications, technical problems, and patient experience. Chest. 1987;91:817-22.
5. Froudarakis ME. Diagnostic work-up of pleural effusions. Respiration. 2008;75:4-13.
6. Lau JS, Yuen CK, Mok KL, Yan WW, Kan PG. Visualization of the inferoposterior thoracic wall (VIP) and boomerang signs: novel sonographic signs of right pleural effusion. Am J Emerg Med. 2018;36:1134-8.
7. Light RW. Diagnostic principles in pleural disease. Eur Respir J. 1997;10:476-81.
8. World Health Organization. Global tuberculosis report 2016. Geneva: World Health Organization, 2016. [online] Available from https://apps.who.int/iris/handle/10665/250441
9. Light RW. Update on tuberculous pleural effusion. Respirology. 2010;15:451-8.
10. Wares F, Balasubramanian R, Mohan A, Sharma SK. Extrapulmonary tuberculosis: management and control. In: Agarwal SP Chauhan LS (Eds). Tuberculosis Control in India. New Delhi: Elsevier; 2005. pp. 95-114.
11. Reddy SL, Varaprasad K, Narahari N, Bhaskar K, Varma GR, Paramjyothi GK. Clinical and Etiological Profile of an Exudative Pleural Effusion in a Tertiary Care Center. Indian J Respir Care. 2019;8(1):22-6.
12. Christopher DJ, Dinakaran S, Gupta R, James P, Isaac B, Thangakunam B. Thoracoscopic pleural biopsy improves yield of Xpert MTB/RIF for diagnosis of pleural tuberculosis. Respirology. 2018;23:714-7.
13. Malhotra P, Aggarwal AN, Agarwal R, Ray P, Gupta D, Jindal SK. Clinical characteristics and outcome of empyema thoracis in 117 patients. A comparative analysis of tubercular vs. non tubercular aetiologies. Respir Med. 2007;101:423-30.
14. Kundu S, Mitra S, Mukherjee S, Das S. Adult thoracic empyema: A comparative analysis of tuberculous and

nontuberculous etiology in 75 patients. Lung India. 2010;27:196-201.
15. Banga A, Khilnani GC, Sharma SK, Dey AB, Wig N, Banga N. A study of empyema thoracis and role of intrapleural streptokinase in its management. BMC Infect Dis. 2004;4:19.
16. Doerr CH, Allen MS, Nicholas FC 3rd, Ryu JH. Etiology of chylothorax in 203 patients. Myo Clin Proc. 2005;80:867-70.
17. Roberts ME, Nevile E, Berrisford RG, Antunes G, Ali NJ. Management of a malignant pleural effusion. British Thoracic Society pleural disease guideline 2010. Thorax. 2010:65;ii32-ii40.
18. Lumb AB, Pearl RG (Eds). Nunn's Applied Respiratory Physiology, 6th edition. Elsevier Limited. 2005.
19. Makhija Z, Marrinan M. A case of Catamenial pneumothorax with diaphragmatic fenestrations. J Emerg Med. 2012;43(1):e1-3.

CHAPTER

220

Mediastinal Anatomy and Disorders

Priya N, Balamugesh T

ABSTRACT

Mediastinum is a potential space between the pleural cavities which is bounded in all sides by various vital structures. The mediastinum is divided into three compartments and each of these compartments comprises blood vessels, organs, nerves, and lymphatics and hence the involvement of these vital structures can cause myriad of symptoms due to compression of these vital structures. The diagnosis, radiology, and the treatment of these mediastinal diseases are very challenging. Also the lymphatics in the mediastinum are interconnected and hence their involvement forms the key in the staging of bronchogenic carcinoma.

One of the most common conditions involving the mediastinum is the pneumomediastinum which is diagnosed as the presence of air in the mediastinum due to rupture of alveoli and tracking of air in the fascial planes. The management being the treatment of the cause and supportive therapy. There are other benign conditions involving the mediastinum like the fibrosing mediastinitis, acute and chronic mediastinitis. There are various neoplastic conditions involving each of the compartments of the mediastinum, which are being classified as cysts and tumors involving the mediastinum. Cysts include the bronchogenic cyst, thymic cyst, pericardial cyst, and neuroenteric cysts. Tumors include thymoma, germ cell tumor (GCT), seminoma, and lymphomas. The clinical presentation, the diagnosis, radiology, and the management are dealt in detail.

"Careful evaluation of information that is portrayed as fact is critical"

—Steven Redhead

OVERVIEW

NON-NEOPLASTIC DISORDERS

- Mediastinal anatomy and compartments
- Imaging of mediastinum
- Pneumomediastinum
- Mediastinitis and mediastinal fibrosis

NEOPLASTIC DISORDERS

- Tumors and cysts of mediastinum

INTRODUCTION

Mediastinum is defined as the potential space between the two pleural cavities, which is surrounded anteriorly by the sternum, posteriorly by the vertebral column, superiorly by the thoracic inlet, and the diaphragm being in the inferior aspect. Mediastinum is interestingly an area where there is myriad of many vital structures and hence the diseases of each of the structures have distinct clinical and radiological presentations and hence mediastinal evaluation makes a daunting and challenging task.

NON-NEOPLASTIC DISORDERS

MEDIASTINAL ANATOMY AND COMPARTMENTS

The well-known classification proposed by Shield's in 1972 divides mediastinum into three compartments: (1) Anterior, (2) middle, and (3) posterior (**Fig. 1**).

The boundaries of anterior compartment are comprised of the sternum, the first rib, and an imaginary curved line

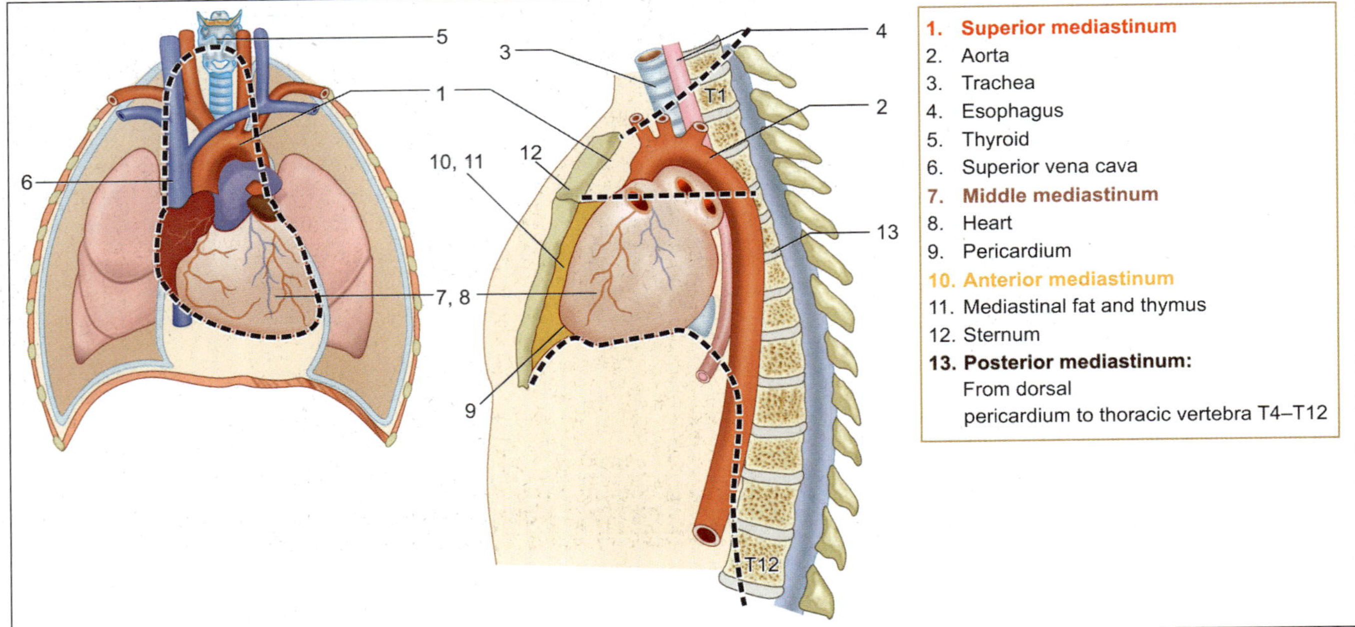

FIGURE 1: Mediastinal anatomy: The three compartments and their components.

Courtesy: Dr Abu Arif.

along the anterior heart border and brachiocephalic vessels from the diaphragm to the thoracic inlet. The extension of the middle mediastinum is from the posterior limit of the anterior compartment to the anterior surface of the vertebral columns and then to the thoracic inlet. The posterior compartment spans from the anterior surface of the vertebral column to the anterior surface of the paravertebral ribs. The mediastinum communicates with both the neck and the retroperitoneum, and these communications can also function as pathways of egress from the mediastinum. Fascial planes connect the neck, mediastinum, and retroperitoneum and thus facilitate movement of air or infection from one location to another. The contents of each of these compartments are explained in **Table 1**.

As with the three compartments of mediastinum, the lymphatics are interconnected and hence spread of malignancy and other infections is extremely common and hence the division of the lymph node stations by Naruke in 1978 is important to be known and it forms the cornerstone of staging of bronchogenic carcinoma, which helps in prognosis and further management (**Fig. 2**).

TABLE 1 Contents of mediastinal compartments.

Anterior	Middle	Posterior
• Pericardial fat • Thymus gland • Substernal extensions of thyroid and parathyroid glands • Lymph nodes • Connective tissue	• Heart and pericardium • Trachea, main bronchus, and hila • Innominate veins and superior vena cava and • Aortic arch and great vessels • Phrenic and vagus nerves • Lymph nodes • Connective tissue	• Azygos vein • Hemiazygos veins • Esophagus • Descending aorta • Sympathetic trunk • Lymph nodes • Connective tissue

IMAGING OF MEDIASTINUM

Chest radiography: Conventional chest radiography posteroanterior (PA) view is usually the first step in the evaluation of any respiratory symptom and any mediastinal pathology. 40% of mediastinal masses may be detected during the chest radiography. Radiography with PA and lateral views will give us a clear picture of the mediastinum. Radiologically, there is a line formed when certain conditions are met: Where there is a difference in density between adjacent tissues, the beam hits this surface tangentially, there occurs reflection of the lungs on the mediastinum, forms lines known as mediastinal lines. If the line has a double interface, it may be called as stripe. In a normal mediastinum, the lines are intact and if distorted, then it means there is a space-occupying lesion in the mediastinum. Chest radiography is able to always indicate the presence and site of mediastinal disease, but it cannot define the characteristics of the lesion, infiltration, and the origin of the lesion. Hence, it requires further investigations.

Computerized tomography: Axial imaging usually avoids the problem of overlapping tissues of similar density and hence demonstration of all mediastinal structures and also helps in guided biopsy procedures.

Magnetic resonance imaging: Magnetic resonance imaging (MRI) is used less frequently than CT in the mediastinal evaluation. But it holds good for posterior mediastinal masses and also to look for infiltration of the adjacent soft tissue structures especially during the preoperative evaluation.

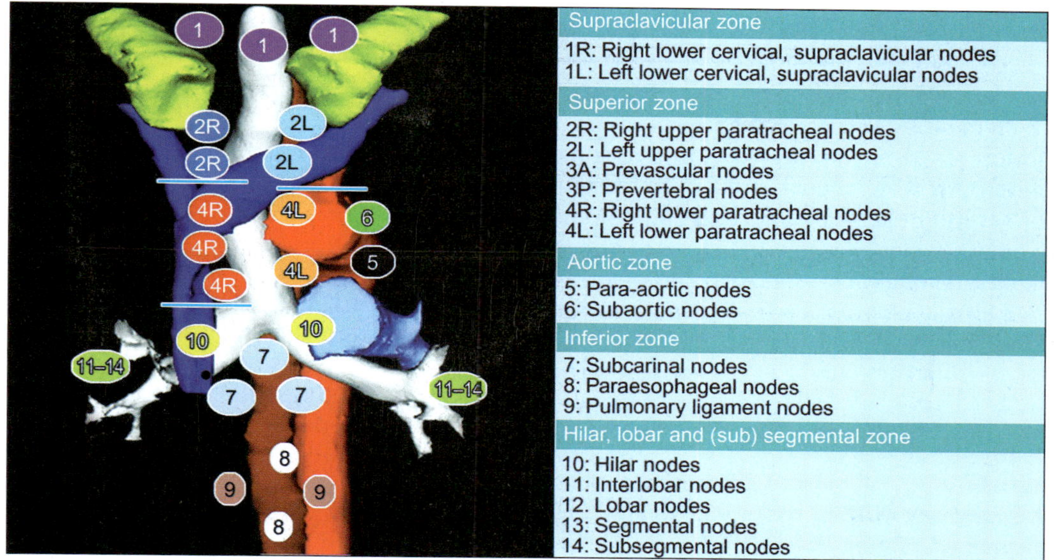

FIGURE 2: Lymph node stations.

Courtesy: Dr Robin Smithuis, Department of Radiology, Rijnland Hospitals, Netherlands; from Radiology Assistant.

Ultrasonography: Endobronchial ultrasonography (EBUS) helps in mediastinal evaluation of the various lymph node stations and also helps in sampling from the lymph nodes. Compared to mediastinoscopy, the EBUS is as effective in determining the pathologic lymph node state in patients with potentially resectable lung cancer. It cannot access the prevascular and paraesophageal lymph nodes.

Radionuclide Imaging: The modern positron emission tomography (PET) cameras are hybrid systems in which a PET camera is combined with either a CT or MRI camera. So the PET CT imaging is more precise for tumor node metastasis and for staging. Usually a metabolic tracer with glucose analog fluorodeoxyglucose (FDG) is used.

PNEUMOMEDIASTINUM

Free air detected in the mediastinum on any form of thoracic imaging is pneumomediastinum (mediastinal emphysema). It can be spontaneous without any surgical or medical procedures or trauma. Secondary pneumomediastinum occurs more commonly as in barotraumas especially in mechanically ventilated patients and any injury or surgery in upper and lower airways and esophagus.

Pneumomediastinum is usually associated with other forms of extra-alveolar air as in pneumothorax, pneumopericardium, pneumoperitoneum, subcutaneous emphysema, and pulmonary interstitial emphysema. Macklin in 1944 designed a theory based on an experimental cat model where he found that the theory of progression of extra-alveolar air following alveolar rupture. The key point to understanding lies in the recognition of the common fascial planes that unite these areas as in **Figure 3**. Pneumomediastinum usually results from a ruptured alveolus due to a Valsalva maneuver or mechanical ventilation. There are many other possible sources, however,

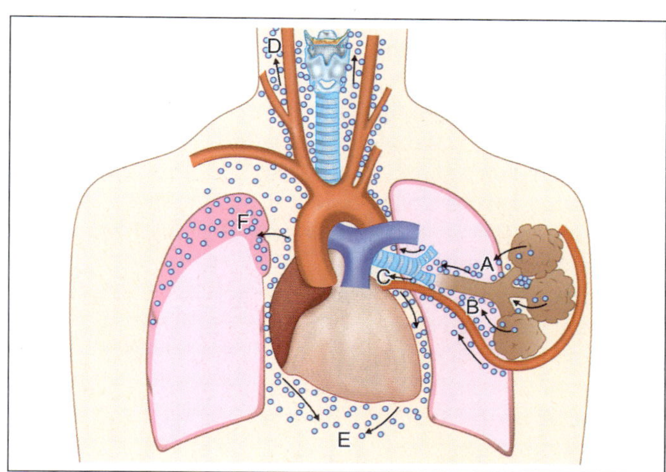

FIGURE 3: Schematic diagram showing the tracking of air in pneumomediastinum. **A**-Alveolus, **B**-Pulmonary interstitium, **C**-Hila of lung, **D**-Deep cervical fascia, **E**-Retroperitoneum, **F**-Pneumothorax

that must be considered when the physician has to manage a patient with pneumomediastinum.

In the neck, the deep cervical fascia encases trachea and esophagus and the same fascial plane continues into the mediastinum—fascial plane continues into the hilum of the lung into the bronchovascular sheath and encloses the terminal bronchioles, veins, and arteries and then extends around the pericardium also.

So after alveolar rupture as seen in **Figure 3**, the air from alveolus (A) enters the pulmonary interstitium (B) and then tracks along the bronchovascular sheath which encloses the terminal bronchioles, arteries and veins, and moves along the hila of lung in the mediastinum (C). After which, it escapes into the neck through the deep cervical fascia (D) or in the subcutaneous spaces into the pericardium and then retroperitoneum (E) and into the pleura causing pneumothorax (F) when the pleura is ruptured.

SPONTANEOUS PNEUMOMEDIASTINUM

Idiopathic or spontaneous pneumomediastinum was first described by Hamman which is a rare self-limiting condition, characterized by spontaneous airway rupture, due to forceful increase in airway pressure, due to some predisposing conditions which cause sudden increase in lung volumes or severe increase in volumes with forceful conditions like vomiting, coughing, or exercising and during marijuana smoking, inhaling of cocaine, or during a seizure (**Fig. 3**). Localized airway obstruction from tumor, foreign bodies, and asthma can also cause alveolar rupture. Getting an accurate history from the patient is very important to find the etiology.

Clinical features are:
- Usually presents with substernal pain, chest pain, bloating, change in voice, dyspnea, dysphagia, odynophagia, and dysphonia.
- Palpable crepitations, cardiac crunch on auscultation, and the Hamman's sign (click or crunch-like sound heard over the pericardium which is synchronous with the heartbeat)
- Esophageal rupture should be suspected if there is history of retching/forceful vomiting/any esophageal instrumentation.
- Usually esophageal rupture presents with other features like shock, left-sided pleural effusion.

Radiologically seen in chest X-ray as a translucent line usually along the aortic knob and also CT imaging is more sensitive and accurate in localizing the air around the thoracic structures (**Fig. 4**).

Treatment is usually supportive care and reassurance. Also needs the prompt management of pneumothorax if present by tube thoracostomy. Timely diagnosis and management of the treatable causes like asthma, foreign body obstruction, or tumor obstruction has to be done. Oxygen supplementation is found to hasten the absorption of the air, but still it is not necessary many times. There is no definite evidence for other measures like needle aspiration, subcutaneous incisions, and prophylactic tube thoracostomy. Pneumopericardium presenting with massive tamponade is more common in neonates and rare in adults. So in neonates, usually, drainage with subxiphoid tube is done.

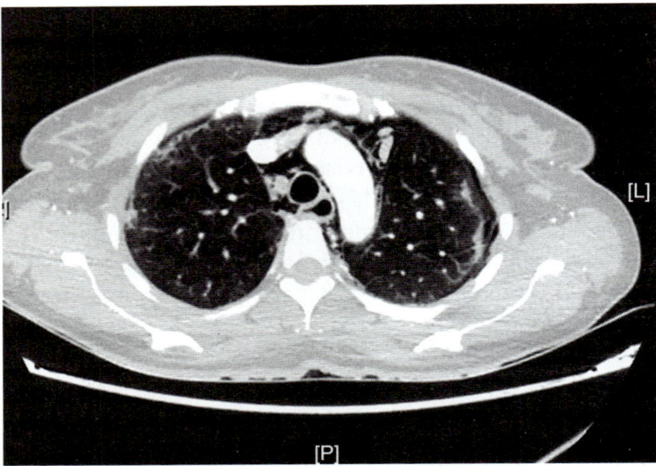

FIGURE 4: A case of spontaneous pneumomediastinum in a 28-year-old lady with antisynthetase syndrome-associated interstitial lung disease—nonspecific interstitial pneumonia pattern with subpleural cyst, which ruptured causing pneumothorax and pneumomediastinum.

SECONDARY PNEUMOMEDIASTINUM

Secondary pneumomediastinum occurring in mechanically ventilated patients may be very catastrophic as usually they present with sudden deterioration due to tension pneumothorax. So the intensivist should have high clinical suspicion in patients on mechanical ventilation, when there is sudden hypotension and elevated pulmonary pressures on the ventilator. Typical factors which predispose to pneumomediastinum in an ICU setting are delivering high tidal volumes, high levels of positive end-expiratory pressure (PEEP), and "fighting" the ventilator due to asynchrony between the patient and the ventilator. Air trapping due to the development of intrinsic PEEP is many times missed out as a cause of barotrauma in an ICU setting. Prophylactic tube thoracostomy is controversial, at the minimum, the chest tube insertion tray should be kept ready and the nursing staff should be aware of those warning signs of tension pneumothorax.

MEDIASTINITIS

ACUTE MEDIASTINITIS

Acute mediastinitis is a life-threatening condition which has a high mortality and is associated with infection of all the three mediastinal compartments. Anterior mediastinum is most commonly affected after sternotomy for cardiac surgery, the middle compartment usually from esophageal perforation, and the posterior compartment from direct extension from the neck, lung, or spine.

Acute mediastinitis usually occurring after esophageal perforation is rapid with usually shock, tachypnea, tachycardia, and subcutaneous emphysema, usually in the cervical region. Water-soluble contrast esophagogram should be performed immediately when the diagnosis is suspected, knowing that this study also has a false negative rate of about 10%. A chest CT scan is the next best study in a patient in whom esophageal perforation is suspected but who has a negative esophagogram.

Immediate appropriate management includes surgical repair or closure with appropriate initiation of broad-spectrum antibiotics with anaerobic coverage and the maintenance of proper nutrition by parenteral feeding. Mortality is <10% if the leak is recognized and repaired within 24 hours, but the mortality increases up to 40% if there is delay >24 hours. The mortality rises even higher in elderly patients.

Mediastinitis rarely also develops after severe deep head and neck infections that originate from the oropharynx or hypopharynx. *Streptococcus* and *Bacteroides* species are the most common organisms involved. Other etiologies are tracheo-bronchial perforations, necrotizing mediastinitis from pancreatitis from retroperitoneum, and anthrax mediastinitis.

CHRONIC MEDIASTINITIS

It includes a spectrum of mediastinal involvement like mediastinal granuloma, fibrosing mediastinitis, and vascular or structural compression syndromes arising from fibrosing mediastinitis.

Mediastinal granuloma or granulomatous mediastinitis is usually a group of diseases wherein there is disease and infection of the mediastinal lymph nodes by tuberculosis and histoplasmosis. So the caseous lymph nodes usually form a large nodal mass in the right paratracheal station, which usually moves into a spectrum of diseases, which may lead on to form a mediastinal granuloma and then to mediastinal fibrosis over 2 year period. These caseous mediastinal lymph nodes may also rupture and communicate into esophagus with a fistulous communication also as shown in **Figure 5**.

FIBROSING MEDIASTINITIS

Fibrosing mediastinitis is either an idiopathic condition where there is fibrosis, and many compression syndromes appear due to the compression of vital structures in the mediastinum (**Fig. 6**).

It is usually caused by infections like histoplasmosis, fungal, tuberculosis, other lung conditions like silicosis, sarcoidosis, drug-induced by methysergide, and other autoimmune disorders. There is an accepted theory that this could be due to the hypersensitivity reaction to the above antigens.

Symptoms are usually due to compression of the vital structures with superior vena cava (SVC) obstruction, subcarinal fibrosis can cause narrowing of esophagus and also tracheobronchial tree and the pulmonary artery branches. Contrast-enhanced CT is the diagnostic imaging modality which shows fibrotic tissue with variable enhancement.

The treatment is only supportive. Other treatment options like anti-inflammatory, antifungals, and antifibrotic are controversial.

Compression syndromes can occur secondary to mediastinal fibrosis, the most common being the SVC obstruction in about 20–50% cases of mediastinal fibrosis. Other manifestations like tracheobronchial compression, esophageal compression causing dysphagia or fistulous communication, compression of pulmonary arteries and veins, and presenting like a pulmonary veno-occlusive disease have also been reported. Management is mainly supportive. Consider SVC stenting, Y stenting in case of tracheobronchial compression, esophageal dilatation, and surgical closure of the fistulous communication as appropriate.

Spontaneous mediastinal hemorrhage is rare. Mediastinal hemorrhage due to aortic dissection, contained rupture of a thoracic aortic aneurysm, or iatrogenic vascular injury is much more common.

NEOPLASTIC DISORDERS

CYSTS OF MEDIASTINUM

In the case series of mediastinal masses reported so far, the mediastinal cysts comprise about 10–25% with similar incidences in male and female population. Bronchogenic cysts account for the majority of the mediastinal cysts of about 40%, while pericardial cysts (35%), enteric (10%), and nonspecific cysts are seen in about 15%. The etiology and distribution of cystic mediastinal masses are different in children and adults, as pericardial cysts are more common in adults whereas the simple foregut cysts are mainly seen in the pediatric age group.

Bronchogenic cyst: Cysts abutting the trachea, carina, or hilum are termed *mediastinal bronchogenic cysts* and they rarely maintain communication with the respiratory tract. Occasionally, these lesions are found within the pulmonary

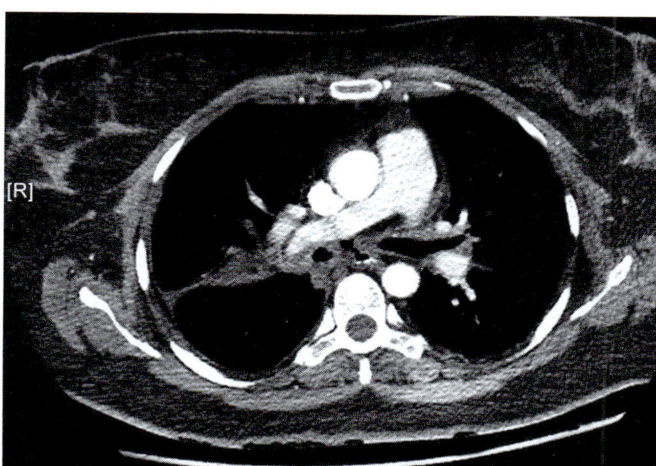

FIGURE 5: A case of tuberculosis in a 38-year-old lady, with inadvertent use of steroids for asthma, who presented with acute mediastinitis as evidenced by contrast leak is seen from the esophagus into the cavitating enlarged subcarinal lymph node—esophageal perforation and leak.

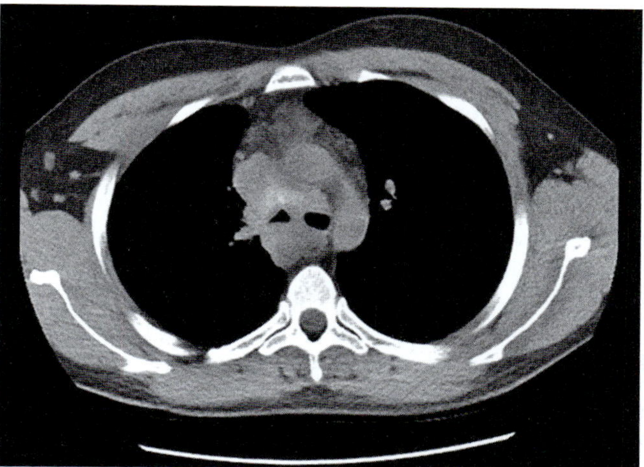

FIGURE 6: A case of idiopathic mediastinal fibrosis who presented as superior vena cava obstruction.

Courtesy: Dr Santiago, Radiopaedia.org.

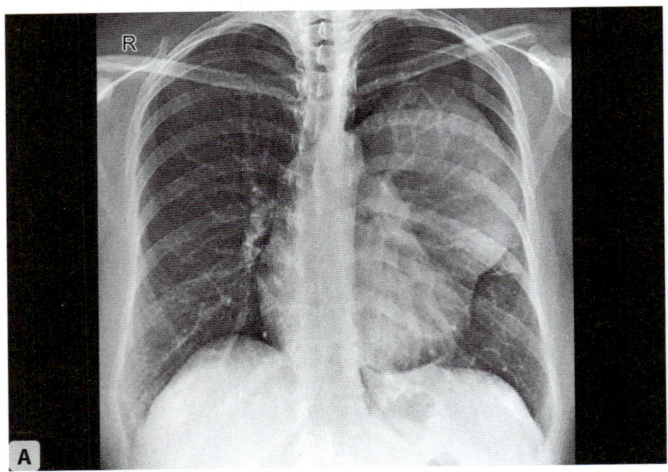

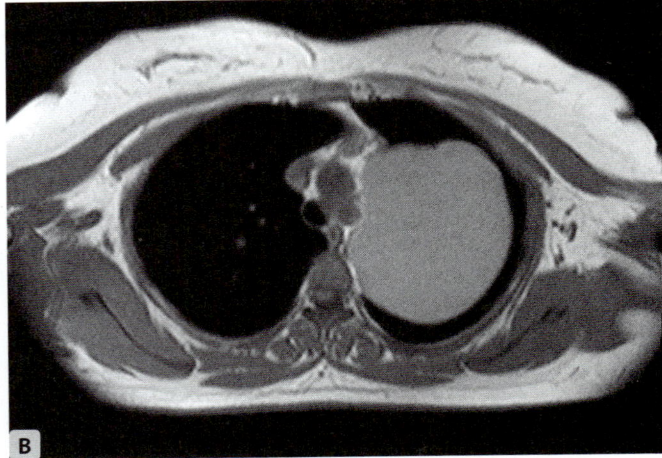

FIGURES 7 A & B: A 31-year-old lady with mediastinal mass lesion, suggestive of bronchogenic cyst. **(A)** Chest X-ray, **(B)** MRI thorax.

parenchyma, most commonly located in the lower lobes and are termed *intrapulmonary bronchogenic cysts*. Sometimes they may be seen in the neck, esophageal wall, pleura and diaphragm, and, rarely, in the skin.

Clinically, it usually presents as wheezing and stridor in the pediatric population. Radiologically, it appears as a 2- to 10-cm ovoid, smooth, homogeneous mass that abuts the mediastinum or hilum or splays the carina. Presence of air–fluid level denotes either persistent bronchial communication or secondary infection of the cyst. Prenatal diagnosis of bronchogenic cyst is also possible with ultrasonography (**Figs. 7 A** and **B**).

Treatment is always complete excision of the cyst either by open surgery or video-assisted thoracoscopic surgery (VATS). In case of asymptomatic cases, excision is controversial.

Enterogenous cysts: Enterogenous cysts are also termed *esophageal duplications* which are formed as a result of failure of normal recanalization. They arise from the elongating esophagus, which separates from the respiratory tract at about the 5th week of gestation. Usually, they present before 16 years of age and mostly asymptomatic in adults, noted incidentally in thoracic imaging. Esophageal duplications appear as smooth-walled, posterior mediastinal lesions at the base of the right hemithorax.

Radiologically, they look like the bronchogenic cysts except that the wall may be thicker and in closer contact with the esophagus. Endoesophageal ultrasound (EUS) has been a very safe tool to investigate these lesions and to allow sampling of cyst contents to confirm that the lesion, in an otherwise asymptomatic patient, is benign. Excision is recommended in all these patients even if asymptomatic, as it can lead to complications like infection.

Neuroenteric cysts: It usually presents before 1 year of life. It is a rare cyst, presents usually with a triad of symptoms of neurological, airway, and spinal abnormalities. They present with back pain, gait disturbances, and motor deficits of lower limbs. They are usually diagnosed by imaging. In about 50% of the affected patients, CT scans have shown vertebral abnormalities and is also useful to define bony abnormalities and to demonstrate extension of the cystic lesion into the spinal canal. MRI also helps to rule out extension into the spinal cord and to exclude a meningocele. Complete excision is the treatment of choice.

Other cysts like thymic cyst develop due to incomplete development of third pharyngeal pouch leading to thymic cyst which usually forms about 2–3% of the anterior mediastinal masses. They have to be differentiated from other thymic neoplasms and anterior mediastinal tumors. Pericardial cysts are smooth-walled cystic lesions that are commonly located at the lateral basal region of the pericardium, where it fuses with the diaphragm at the right cardiophrenic angle. They are called as "spring water cysts" as they appear as thin-walled translucent cysts and they are usually benign and nonmalignant. Hence if asymptomatic these cysts do not need excision.

MEDIASTINAL TUMORS

Mediastinal tumors are mainly incidentally detected on chest radiography or CT scan done for other purposes. The incidence of these tumors varies. *Thymoma (26.5%) is the most commonly diagnosed*, followed by the neurogenic tumors (20%), followed by the GCTs and lymphomas (13% each) among the adults. Among the *pediatric population, it is predominantly the neurogenic tumors (41%)* followed by the GCTs and other cysts. About 60% of the mediastinal masses are incidentally detected, and those presenting with symptoms are usually malignant and they present with complaints of dyspnea, and cough due to airway involvement, or dysphagia due to esophageal compression, invasion of the recurrent laryngeal nerve causing hoarseness, facial swelling due to SVC compression, and pleural effusion. Constitutional symptoms like night sweats and weight loss usually occur in lymphomas and myasthenic symptoms occur in thymoma.

The most common mediastinal tumors like thymoma, lymphomas, and GCTs are explained in detail in this section.

Thymoma: Thymomas are the most common anterior mediastinal tumors. They are usually considered as benign tumors but could metastasize to the pleura, pericardium,

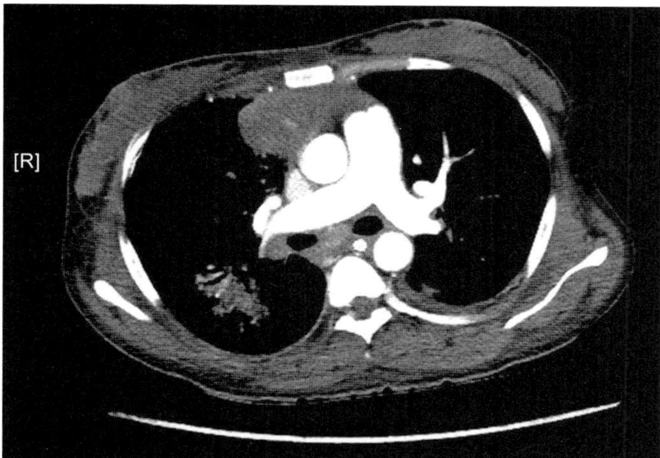

FIGURE 8: Thymoma in a 28-year-old lady as a lobulated lesion in the anterior mediastinum.

and (less commonly) distant sites. It presents in age group between 34 and 70 years with an average age of 54 years. Usually the treatment of thymoma is best to proceed with surgical excision without needle biopsy. Radiologically, it presents as a well-circumscribed mass without any areas of solid/cystic structures, which is suggestive of teratoma and there are no clinical features of constitutional symptoms, which can occur in lymphomas (**Fig. 8**).

Surgical biopsy using needle biopsy is to be considered only if the mass shows invasion and other forms of therapy like chemotherapy or radiation therapy are being planned or if there is a strong suspicion of lymphoma. If the patients have clinical features of myasthenia gravis, it requires preoperative evaluation with two positive confirmatory tests among pharmacologic (Tensilon test), serological [anti-acetylcholine receptor (AChR) antibodies], and electrodiagnostic (EMG) studies. Also, it requires preoperative stabilization by a neurologist with medications like a combination of cholinesterase inhibitors, steroids to prevent myasthenic crisis in the postoperative period, plasmapheresis, and immunoglobulin therapy. The Masaoka classification system has prognostic value and permits stratification for adjuvant therapy. Stage 1–3 can be treated with complete en bloc excision with the preferred approach being the medial sternotomy approach.

Germ cell tumors: Germ cell tumors are derived from the gonadal tissue. Usually, it occurs in the younger age group between 20 and 40 years. GCTs account for 15% of all anterior mediastinal masses in adults (85% of which are benign mature GCTs) and 25% of anterior mediastinal masses in children (essentially all of which are benign). The benign and the malignant GCTs and their classification are as given in **Box 1**.

Teratomas are defined by the presence of tissue from more than one of the three primitive germ cell layers. Mature (benign) teratomas are composed of well-differentiated elements such as fat, muscle, and cartilage (mesoderm); hair, skin, and teeth (ectoderm); and intestinal tissue (endoderm). Mature teratomas can be symptomatic or asymptomatic upon presentation. Symptoms include chest pain, dyspnea, cough, or fever (if they become infected). Occasionally, the tumor may erode into an airway and a patient may cough up hair (trichophytosis).

BOX 1 Classification of germ cell tumors (GCTs).

Benign GCTs:
- Mature teratoma

Malignant GCTs:
- Immature teratoma
- Teratomas with malignant component:
  - Type I: With an associated GCT (seminoma etc.)
  - Type II: With another epithelial malignancy (squamous, adenocarcinoma etc.)
  - Type III: With sarcomatous component (rhabdomyosarcoma, osteosarcoma etc.)
  - Type IV: A combination of any of the above
- Seminoma
- Nonseminomatous GCTs:
  - Yolk sac tumor (endodermal sinus tumor)
  - Embryonal carcinoma
  - Choriocarcinoma
  - Combined GCT without teratomatous component

Malignant teratomas usually occur in males of the 20–40 year age group and usually present with chest pain and cough. Bilateral testicular examination must be done in all these cases of GCTs to look for testicular involvement.

Tumor markers such as β-human chorionic gonadotropin (hCG) and alpha-fetoprotein (AFP) should be measured and will not be elevated in benign teratoma. However, in malignant GCTs, among the seminomatous GCTs, there is mild elevation of the beta-hCG levels <100 mIU/mL, while higher levels indicate it is either mixed tumor or nonseminomatous GCTs (NSGCT). Elevated AFP levels exclude the diagnosis of seminomatous GCTs and denotes that the tumor is usually NSGCT or mixed type.

Computed tomography imaging of the thorax with contrast is the diagnostic modality where the GCTs are usually seen as bulky large tumor masses with bulky lymphadenopathy (**Fig. 9**).

Usually these tumors, in 60–70% of the patients, will metastasize to local structures at the time of diagnosis. CT-guided percutaneous needle biopsy could help in diagnosis. Chemotherapy with first-line cisplatin-based regimens has found to have a better survival rates.

Lymphomas: Mediastinal masses are present in 50–60% of Hodgkin's lymphomas and only 20% of the non-Hodgkin's lymphomas. They are usually diagnosed with needle biopsies and treated with chemotherapy regimens (**Fig. 10**). Surgery has no role in lymphomas.

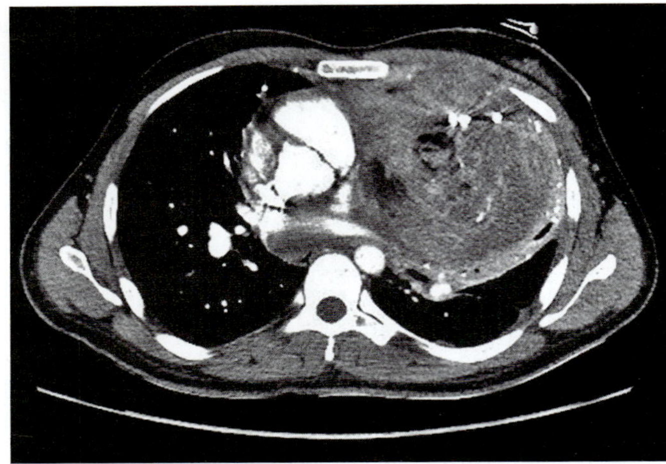

FIGURE 9: Mediastinal teratoma in a 34-year-old gentleman—seen as an anterior mediastinal mass lesion containing fluid, enhancing septae, fatty lobules, and calcific foci.

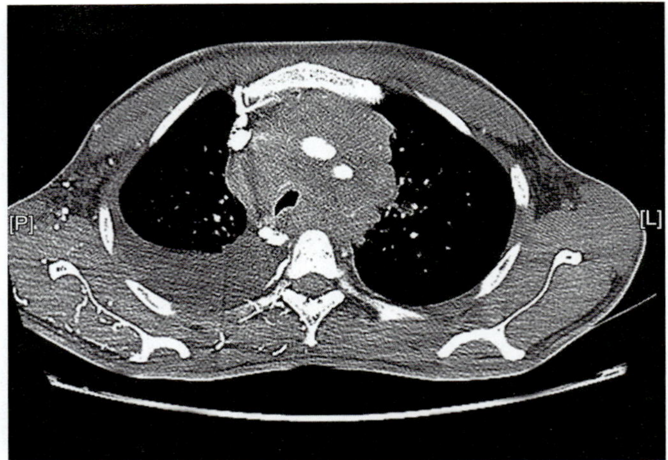

FIGURE 10: T-cell lymphoma in a patient presenting as mediastinal mass lesion with right-sided pleural effusion.

RECOMMENDED READINGS

1. Carter BW, Marom EM, Detterbeck FC. Approaching the patient with an anterior mediastinal mass: a guide for clinicians. J Thorac Oncol. 2014;9:S102-9.
2. Davis RD, Oldham HN, Sabiston DC. Primary cysts and neoplasms of the mediastinum: Recent changes in clinical presentation, methods of diagnosis, management and results. Ann Thorac Surg. 1987;44(3): 229-37.
3. Macklin MT, Macklin CC. Malignant interstitial emphysema of the lungs and mediastinum as an important occult complication in many respiratory diseases and other conditions: an interpretation of the clinical literature in the light of laboratory experiment. Medicine. 1944;23:281-358.
4. Hamman L. Spontaneous mediastinal emphysema. Bull Johns Hopkins Hosp. 1939;64:1-21.
5. Czarnecka-Kujawa K, Yasufuku K. The role of endobronchial ultrasound versus mediastinoscopy for non-small cell lung cancer. J Thorac Dis. 2017;9(Suppl 2):S83-S97.
6. Dines DE, Payne WS, Bernatz PE, Pairolero PC. Mediastinal granuloma and fibrosing mediastinitis. Chest. 1979;75:320-4.
7. Mole TM, Glover J, Shepard MN. Sclerosing mediastinitis: a report on 18 cases. Thorax. 1995;50:280-3.
8. Logerstrom CF, Mitchell HG, Graham BS, Hammon JW Jr. Chronic fibrosing mediastinitis and superior vena caval obstruction from blastomycosis. Ann Thorac Surg. 1992;54:764-5.
9. Toonkel RL, Borczuk AC, Pearson GD, Horn EM, Thomashow BM. Sarcoidosis associated fibrosing mediastinitis with resultant pulmonary hypertension: a case report and review of the literature. Respiration. 2010;79:341-5.
10. Hasegawa K, Ohno S, Takada M, Ogino H, Shiotsu S, Takumi C, et al. Sarcoidosis complicated with major pulmonary arteryobstruction and stenosis. Intern Med. 2012;51:2775-80.
11. Peikert T, Colby TV, Midthun DE, Pairolero PC, Edell ES, Schroeder DR, et al. Fibrosing mediastinitis: clinical presentation, therapeutic outcomes, and adaptive immune response. Medicine (Baltimore). 2011;90:412-23.
12. Azarow KS, Pearl RH, Zurcher R, Edwards FH, Cohen AJ. Primary mediastinal masses: a comparison of adult and pediatric populations. J Thorac Cardiovasc Surg. 1993;106:67-72.
13. Benjamin SP, McCormack LJ, Effer DB, Grover LK. Primary tumors of the mediastinum. Chest.1972; 62:297-303.
14. Bower RJ, Kiesewetter WB. Mediastinal masses in infants and children. Arch Surg. 1977;112:1003-9.
15. Donahue J, Nichols F. Primary mediastinal tumors and cysts and diagnostic investigation of mediastinal masses. In: Shields T, Locicero J, Reed C, Feins R (Eds). General Thoracic Surgery, 7th edition. Philadelphia, PA: Lippincott Williams and Wilkins; 2009. p. 2195.
16. Mullen B, Richardson JD. Primary anterior mediastinal tumors in children and adults. Ann Thorac Surg. 1986;42:338-45.
17. Moran CA, Suster S. Primary germ cell tumors of the mediastinum: I. Analysis of 322 cases with special emphasis on teratomatous lesions and a proposal for histopathologic classification and clinical staging. Cancer. 1997;80:681-90.

CHAPTER
221

The Chest Wall

Priya N, Balamugesh T

ABSTRACT

The chest wall is comprised of bony thoracic cage and muscles functioning in various phases of respiration. Abnormalities of the chest wall can cause extraparenchymal restriction leading on to abnormalities in pulmonary functions, alveolar hypoventilation, ventilation–perfusion mismatch, and finally respiratory failure. Abnormalities in spine include kyphoscoliosis which may be congenital or idiopathic or it may be secondary to underlying systemic diseases. Abnormalities of the sternum present as pectus excavatum/carinatum which also causes ventilatory restriction in severe cases. Flail chest which occurs due to trauma is caused by a segment of deformed chest wall due to multiple rib fractures, and this can cause respiratory failure by various pathogenic mechanisms. Morbid obesity (MO) can have a deleterious effect on ventilation by various mechanisms. Ankylosing spondylitis (AS) is a condition which causes restriction in ventilation due to the considerable reduction in spinal and rib joints mobility. These abnormalities are dealt in detail with in this chapter.

"The preservation of health is easier than the cure of the disease"

—Anonymous

INTRODUCTION

The chest wall comprises the bony thoracic cage and the soft tissue structures, the muscles which take part in various phases of respiration. Disorders of the chest wall generally cause restrictive ventilatory defect by limiting the chest wall motion or causing dysfunction. They have similar pathophysiological mechanisms by reduced chest wall compliance, ventilation-perfusion imbalance, alveolar hypoventilation, pulmonary hypertension, and finally respiratory failure. Kyphoscoliosis has the maximum impact on respiration, while pectus excavatum has the least.

KYPHOSCOLIOSIS

The term kyphoscoliosis refers to the group of disorders characterized by excessive spinal curvature in the lateral plane (scoliosis) and sagittal plane (kyphosis) along with rotation of the spinal axis. Kyphoscoliosis is considered as the most common spinal abnormality, which is classified as in **Box 1**. The idiopathic type, being the most common form, has the estimated prevalence of 0.47–5.2%. Idiopathic kyphoscoliosis usually presents in late childhood or early adolescence, females being more involved than males with a ratio of 4:1.

Diagnosis of kyphoscoliosis is done by inspection of the chest wall, usually in severe cases, it is visualized as dorsal hump, which is due to the angulated ribs and shoulder asymmetry with hip tilt, which is related to the spinal rotation. In mild cases, Adam forward bending test is used in the clinical diagnosis of kyphoscoliosis, in which the patient is asked to bed forward and he is viewed along the horizontal plane for the spine symmetry and for any angulation of ribs or hump as in **Figure 1**.

Radiological diagnosis of kyphoscoliosis is based on upright PA and lateral view, where **Cobb's angle** is used to confirm the diagnosis and to assess the severity. This angle is formed by the intersection of two lines, each of which is parallel to the top and bottom vertebrae of the scoliotic or kyphotic curves (**Fig. 2**). A spinal deformity with a Cobb angle >10° is considered scoliosis. The greater the Cobb angle, the more severe the deformity (**Figs. 3** and **4**).

Cobb angles <60°—not associated with ventilatory impairment, >100° are invariably associated with respiratory symptoms, >120° with respiratory failure.

RESPIRATORY MECHANICS

The main pathophysiology in kyphoscoliosis is the inability of the chest wall to distend during respiration, resulting in more pressure needed to expand than in a normal individual. So the functional residual capacity (FRC) is reduced significantly with increased work of breathing. Respiratory muscle strength, as reflected in measurements of maximal static inspiratory (PImax) and expiratory pressures (PEmax), is usually normal in individuals with idiopathic kyphoscoliosis.

There may be mild to moderate reductions in PImax and PEmax with Cobb angles measuring >50°. The reductions in PImax with idiopathic kyphoscoliosis may be attributed to mechanical disadvantage of the respiratory muscles coupled to an angulated rib cage. However, in patients with secondary kyphoscoliosis, reductions in PImax are related to intrinsic respiratory muscle weakness. In these patients, the

BOX 1 Classification of kyphoscoliosis.

- **Idiopathic**
  - Multigene condition with autosomal or sex-linked inheritance with variable phenotype expression
  - Genetic defect in the chromatin remodeling gene family, *CHD7*, and several other genetic loci are associated with susceptibility to idiopathic kyphoscoliosis
- **Paralytic or secondary**
  - Neuromuscular disorders:
    - Poliomyelitis
    - Muscular dystrophy
    - Cerebral palsy
    - Friedreich ataxia
    - Charcot-Marie-Tooth disease
  - Disorders of connective tissue:
    - Marfan syndrome
    - Morquio syndrome
    - Ehler–Danlos syndrome
  - Vertebral diseases:
    - Osteoporosis
    - Osteomalacia
    - Tuberculous spondylitis
    - Spina bifida
    - Vitamin D-resistant rickets
  - Post-thoracoplasty
- **Congenital:**
  - Due to spinal/vertebral anomalies at birth
  - It occurs 1 in 1,000 newborns and is much less common than idiopathic scoliosis

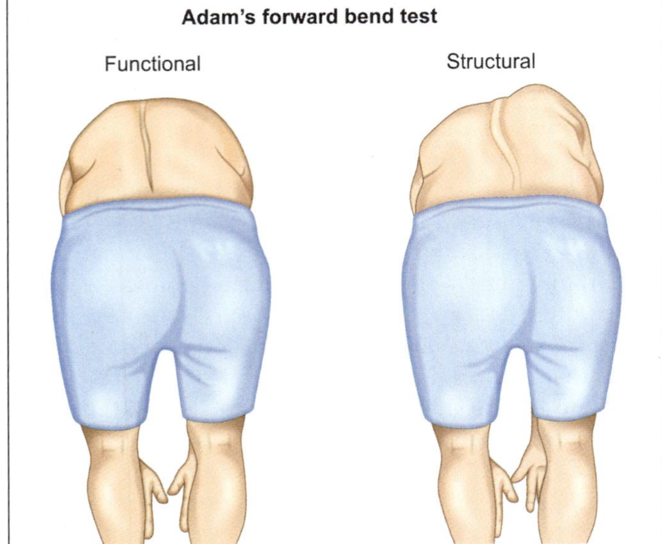

FIGURE 1: **Adam's forward bending test in scoliosis.**

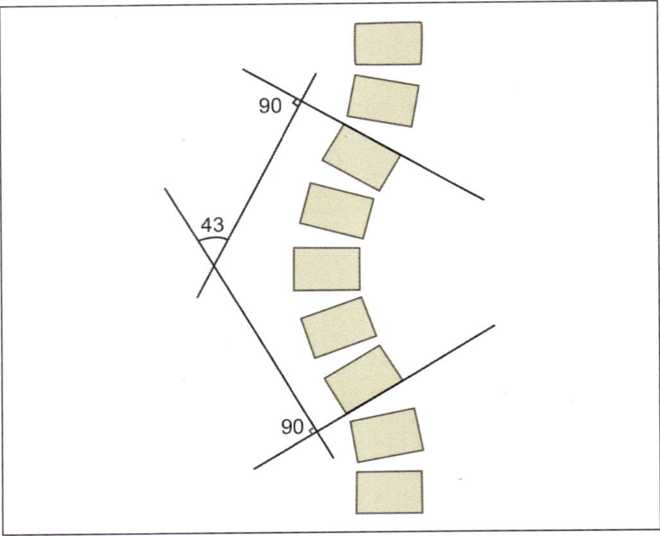

FIGURE 2: **Schematic description of Cobb's angle in a posterior–anterior film—43°.**

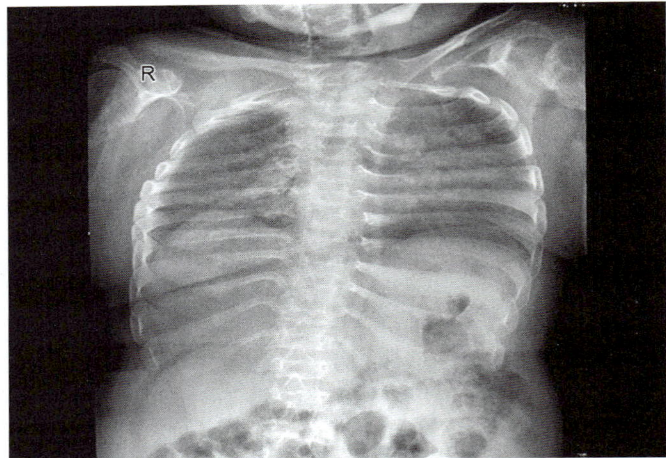

FIGURE 3: **Kyphoscoliosis with skeletal dysplasia** in a 33-year-old lady with Morquio syndrome.

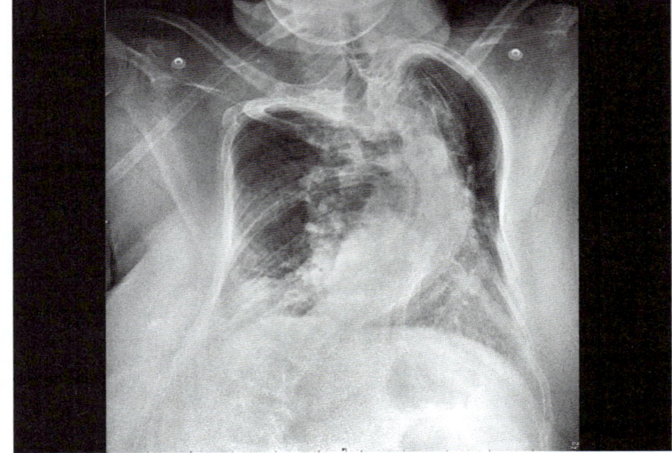

FIGURE 4: **Congenital severe kyphoscoliosis with restrictive ventilatory defect.**

combined effect of the weakened inspiratory muscles and a poorly compliant respiratory system will lead to profound reduction in vital capacity (VC) and predispose these individuals to respiratory failure. Indirect measurements of the neural drive to the respiratory muscles, such as mouth occlusion pressure at 100 ms (P0.1), are usually elevated in these individuals and it correlates positively with the degree of scoliosis.

SLEEP DISORDERED BREATHING

During sleep, the neural inspiratory drive is lost and hence in kyphoscoliosis patients during rapid eye movement (REM) sleep, they depend mainly on diaphragm to maintain their alveolar ventilation. Hence inspiratory muscle weakness may lead to further nocturnal hypoventilation in patients with kyphoscoliosis.

The presence of persistent nocturnal desaturation and chronic hypercapnia may further weaken the respiratory muscles, lead to pulmonary hypertension and eventually cor pulmonale. Obstructive sleep apnea, which has a similar prevalence in kyphoscoliosis to that of the general population, also may complicate nocturnal hypoventilation.

PROGNOSIS

Idiopathic kyphoscoliosis usually has a benign course. In general, if the kyphoscoliosis appears in early life (0–8 years), it is generally progressive with increasing Cobb's angle leading on to progressive ventilatory impairment and cardiorespiratory failure. Consequently, individuals with severe idiopathic kyphoscoliosis, especially those with a Cobb angle >110°and VC of <45% of predicted, should be monitored for respiratory compromise as age advances. Pregnancy is poorly tolerated when the VC is <1 L usually when the patient requires supplementary oxygen and noninvasive ventilation (NIV), they worsen and may have death within 1 year.

TREATMENT

Surgical correction has a role when done early in life. Nonspecific measures like vaccination with pneumococcal and influenza vaccinations to prevent infection, rehabilitation measures to prevent physical deconditioning, maintaining the ideal body weight, smoking cessation, prompt treatment of respiratory infections and also supplementary oxygen when needed and during exercise are the other aspects of management.

Noninvasive ventilation via full face mask or nasal mask with or without supplemental oxygen should be offered to all the patients with kyphoscoliosis and those who are in respiratory failure. Long-term NIV significantly reduces the number of hospitalizations for respiratory failure and the length of hospital stay. Survival benefit of kyphoscoliosis patients treated with NIV and supplemental oxygen over those patients treated with just oxygen has been demonstrated by comparative and observational studies. Indications of NIV are given in **Box 2**.

BOX 2	**Indications of NIV initiation in patients with restrictive lung diseases.**
	Symptoms of hypercapnia (e.g., fatigue, morning headaches, and dyspnea)
	Or
	Signs of cor pulmonale
	And one of the following:
	• Daytime arterial PCO_2 ≥45 mm Hg
	• Nocturnal oxygen saturation ≤88% for 5 consecutive minutes
	• Progressive neuromuscular disease with maximal inspiratory pressure (PImax) <60 cm H_2O or FVC <50% of predicted

(FVC: forced vital capacity; NIV: noninvasive ventilation)

Source: Adapted from Chest Consensus Conference. 1999.

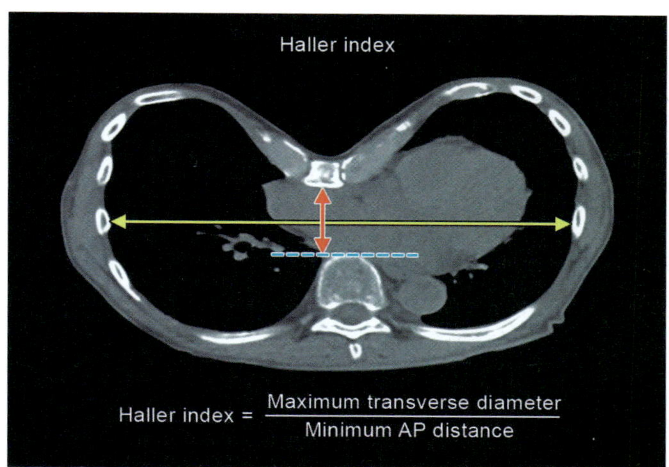

(AP: anterior–posterior)

FIGURE 5: Haller index.

Courtesy: Copyright permission from Dr Jan Frank Gerstenmaier, radiopaedia.org.

PECTUS EXCAVATUM

Pectus excavatum, or funnel chest, is a congenital deformity that is associated with characterized by shallow inward depression of the sternum, thereby caving of the adjacent ribs. It is hypothesized to be due to defective collagen in the cartilage, thereby a resultant abnormal chest wall. The pathogenesis is unknown but found to have higher prevalence in patients with Marfan syndrome. Usually the patients are asymptomatic and even in severe cases, it produces only mild restriction.

Computed tomography thorax is the best modality to diagnose pectus excavatum. The ratio of the transverse to anterior–posterior (AP) diameters of the rib cage at the level of the deepest sternal depression (Haller index) can easily be measured using this technique (**Fig. 5**). Haller index—normal ratio is about 2.5. Index more than 3.25 is suggestive of significant sternal depression.

Chest X-ray shows right paracardiac opacity due to parasternal soft tissue and should not be mistaken for middle lobe infiltrates. Electrocardiogram may show abnormalities such as T inversion in right-sided chest leads, right axis deviation, P wave inversion, and qR or rsr pattern V_1. This is due to the distortion of the right ventricular geometry by the sternal compression. Severe cases may have exercise limitation. The explanation for the limited exercise tolerance in this group of patients is due to a reduction in venous return to heart associated with right ventricular compression due to sternal depression.

TREATMENT

Surgical repair is only done if really indicated for respiratory compromise only. The optimal age to repair is around 10–14 years of age or at the earliest if there is significant cardiopulmonary compromise. Individuals selected for repair typically have a Haller index >3.25. Named techniques such as Ravitch procedure, Nuss procedure and sternochondroplasty are performed for pectus excavatum.

PECTUS CARINATUM

Pectus carinatum results from anterior protrusion of the sternum and occasionally is associated with severe childhood asthma or ventricular septal defect. It is probably due to excessive growth of the ribs or costal cartilages. The respiratory effects are minimal and surgery is indicated only for cosmetic reasons.

ANKYLOSING SPONDYLITIS

Ankylosing spondylitis is a chronic multisystem disorder associated with human leukocyte antigen-B27 (HLA-B27), which is characterized by inflammation of the joints of the axial skeleton, leading on to the ankylosis of the vertebral and rib joints and hence only the diaphragm performs inspiration in these patients. There is considerable reduction in the spinal column mobility and rib cage expansion.

Typically, patients present in late adolescence or early adulthood with chronic back pain and typical worsening of symptoms in morning or after prolonged periods of rest. Chest expansion measured at the level of 4th intercostal space <2.5 cm in a young adult with back pain should raise the suspicion of AS. Exercise intolerance and dyspnea are uncommon, unless there is associated underlying lung fibrosis, diaphragmatic dysfunction, or cardiac manifestations. Total lung capacity and VC are slightly reduced. The immobility of thoracic cage leads to atrophy of intercostal muscles and hence maximal inspiratory and expiratory pressures are reduced.

Some patients have associated apical fibrobullous lung disease which has been postulated due to a variety of causes including diminished upper lobe ventilation due to chest wall rigidity, mechanical strain because of bamboo-like spine, and impaired cough related to recurrent lung infection. Rarely patients can have cricoarytenoiditis which presents as hoarseness of voice or stridor due to upper airway obstruction. Chest X-ray may show characteristic "bamboo spine" appearance due to calcification of paraspinal ligaments (**Fig. 6**). Sleep-disordered breathing may also coexist as many patients usually present with fatigue and hence screening for OSA should also be considered.

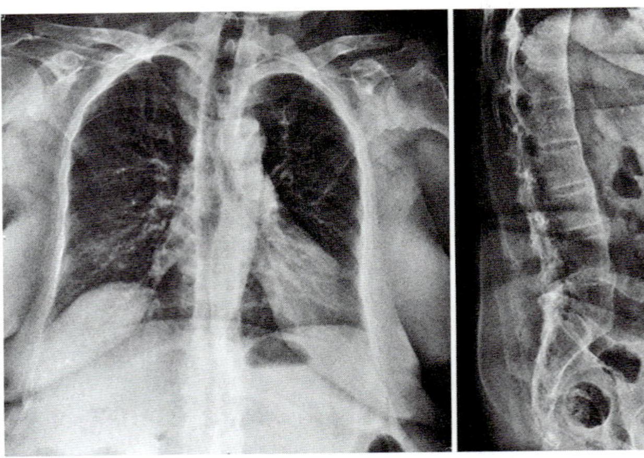

FIGURE 6: Bamboo spine and scoliosis in a patient with ankylosing spondylitis causing restrictive defect.

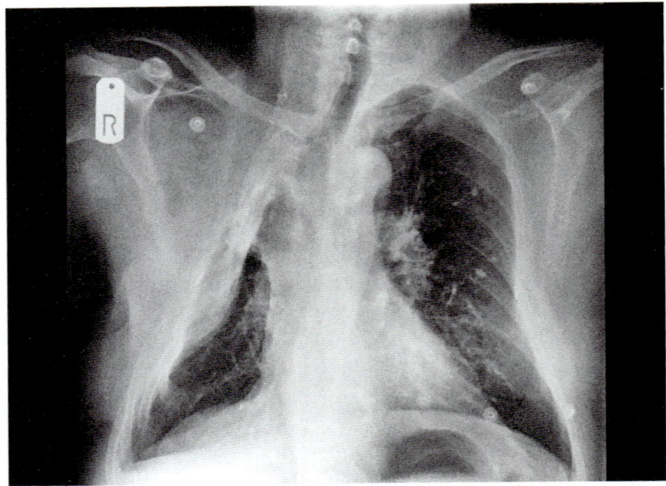

FIGURE 7: Post-thoracoplasty ventilatory defect.
Courtesy: With permission from Dr Ian Bickle from radiopaedia.org.

Treatment is mainly physical therapy exercises that promote rib cage expansion to alleviate pain and to enhance spinal mobility. Smoking cessation and baseline chest radiographs and spirometry are obtained tumor necrosis factor alpha (TNF-α) antagonists have revolutionized the treatment of AS. But the main complication of these medications is reactivation of tuberculosis (TB). So, all patients with AS should undergo screening for latent TB before initiation of treatment.

THORACOPLASTY

Pretreatment era, before the advent of antituberculosis therapy (ATT), the standard approach was surgery to control tuberculosis with techniques like rib removal, rib fracture, phrenic nerve resection, or lung compression with objects like ping pong balls as in **Figure 7**. The intercostal and shoulder girdle muscles are directly damaged by the surgery while the distortion of the rib cage and the development of scoliosis results in an additional mechanical disadvantage for the inspiratory muscles. Diaphragmatic excursion is reduced, particularly on the side of the thoracoplasty. This can also lead to restrictive ventilatory defects similar to those in kyphoscoliosis leading to dyspnea and exercise limitation, and then to ventilator compromise and cor pulmonale. Treatment is with supplementary oxygen and prompt treatment of respiratory infections and NIV care. In the modern era, thoracoplasty is rarely done.

FLAIL CHEST

Flail chest refers to a segment of deformed chest wall during respiration, due to multiple rib fractures. For a flail chest to manifest, there should be at least two sets of three or more adjacent ribs fractures or the combined sternal as well as rib fractures. It can result in a subsequent respiratory failure. Most common causes of flail chest are due to high velocity injuries or following aggressive resuscitation techniques, or rarely in multiple myeloma.

Clinically, it is diagnosed by visualizing the paradoxical movement of the affected cage. However, in assisted or mechanically ventilated patients, the diagnosis might be obscured. In these patients, CT thorax helps in the diagnosis. The flail segment is commonly noticed in the lateral aspect of the rib cage.

The mechanism of respiratory failure in flail chest is complex. Associated respiratory muscle dysfunction and pulmonary parenchymal changes contribute to respiratory failure. Specifically:

- Flail chest usually causes considerable pain, which can impair the cough effectiveness, hence can cause regional atelectasis, rib cage muscle spasm, and therefore the pattern of respiratory activation is altered.
- Flail chest may increase the elastic load imposed on the respiratory muscles through development of regional (near the flail segment) or generalized atelectasis (due to splinting and pain). The mortality rate in a patient with chest wall trauma without flail segment ranges between 7% and 14%. When chest wall trauma is complicated by flail chest, the mortality rate further increases. This can be attributed to other pulmonary complications, such as pulmonary contusion, hemothorax, or pneumothorax, which can coexist in patients with flail chest.

TREATMENT

In most cases, supportive therapy with adequate pain relief and maintaining oxygenation is effective. Stabilizing the flail segment by external strapping is not very successful. Those with respiratory failure require positive pressure ventilation to achieve "pneumatic splinting" of the flail segment. Recently NIV together with regional anesthesia has been found to reduce morbidity and avoid complications.

OBESITY

Obesity is one of the major noncommunicable diseases which is of increasing prevalence in the world. In India, more than 150 million were affected by overweight/obesity. ICMR-INDIAB study had shown the prevalence of obesity varies between 12% and 36% across various Indian states. The severity of obesity is assessed by calculating the BMI (Body Mass Index) = weight (in kg)/Height (in cm^2). BMI between 23 and 24.9 kg/m^2 is overweight, and a BMI >25 kg/m^2 is considered obese; BMI >40 kg/m^2 is considered morbid obesity (MO).

There is significant respiratory compromise in terms of morbidly obese subjects, and it increases exponentially with increasing BMI. Obesity alters lung functions by decreasing lung volumes, poor respiratory muscle strength, and reducing the respiratory drive. Respiratory impairment associated with obesity can be broadly classified into three groups:

1. Simple obesity (SO): With minimal respiratory compromise
2. Morbid obesity: Eucapnic individuals with compromised pulmonary function
3. Obesity hypoventilation syndrome (OHS) with daytime hypercapnia

Obstructive sleep apnea can coexist with any of these.

In SO, there is reduction in the expiratory reserve volume (ERV) and the FRC due to the increase in thoracic and abdominal fat which decreases the chest wall compliance.

In MO and eucapnic patients, there is increase in the airway resistance due to reduction in lung volume and small airways obstruction and hence exhibit expiratory airflow limitation with development of intrinsic positive end-expiratory pressure (PEEP), resulting in orthopnea.

In OHS patients, the hypercapnia during wakefulness is the most defining characteristic feature. It occurs primarily due to alveolar hypoventilation, which in turn reduces the partial pressure of O_2 with raise in the partial pressure of CO_2 in the alveoli. Also, the ventilation-perfusion mismatch widens the alveolar-arterial oxygen gradient, which in turn causes worsening of the hypoxemia. In individuals with OHS, there is blunted ventilatory response to both hypoxia and hypercapnia; however it is much more blunted to hypoxia. Hyperleptinemia, in severely obese individuals, is associated with decreased respiratory drive. Respiratory muscle strength is preserved in SO, but due to deconditioning and fatty infiltration of muscles, it is decreased in OHS. To attain the requisite levels of ventilation and minimize the work of breathing, the obese individuals adopt a rapid shallow breathing pattern with breathing frequency about 40% higher than that of nonobese individuals. The pathogenesis of OHS leading to chronic hypercapnia is explained in **Flowchart 1**.

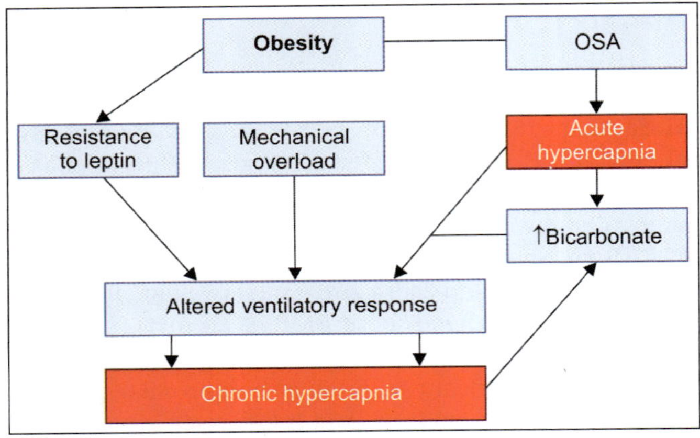

(OSA: obstructive sleep apnea)

FLOWCHART 1: Pathogenesis of obesity hypoventilation syndrome.

TREATMENT

Weight loss induced by either diet or surgery improves hypoxia in patients with OHS. However, losing weight and maintaining weight loss can be difficult. In patients with OHS, NIV helps to improve gas exchange and daytime symptoms. Bariatric surgeries play an important role in weight reduction especially in morbidly obese patients.

RECOMMENDED READINGS

1. Konieczny MR, Senyurt H, Krauspe R. Epidemiology of adolescent idiopathic scoliosis. J Child Orthop. 2013;7(1):3-9.
2. Giampietro PF, Blank RD, Raggio CL, Merchant S, Jacobsen FS, Faciszewski T, et al. Congenital and idiopathic scoliosis: clinical and genetic aspects. Clin Med Res. 2003;1(2):125-36.
3. Cobb JR. Outline for the study of scoliosis. AAOS Instruct Course Lect. 1948;5:261-75.
4. Shneerson JM, Simonds AK. Noninvasive ventilation for chest wall and neuromuscular disorders. Eur Respir J. 2002;20(2):480-7.
5. Kafer ER. Idiopathic scoliosis. Mechanical properties of the respiratory system and the ventilatory response to carbon dioxide. J Clin Invest. 1975;55(6): 1153-63.
6. Leech JA, Ernst P, Rogala EJ, Gurr J, Gordon I, Becklake MR. Cardiorespiratory status in relation to mild deformity in adolescent idiopathic scoliosis. J Pediatr. 1985;106(1):143-9.
7. Szeinberg A, Canny GJ, Rashed N, Veneruso G, Levison H. Forced vital capacity and maximal respiratory pressures in patients with mild and moderate scoliosis. Pediatr Pulmonol. 1988;4(1):8-12.
8. Inal-Ince D, Savci S, Arikan H, Saglam M, Vardar-Yagli N, Bosnak-Guclu M, et al. Effects of scoliosis on respiratory muscle strength in patients with neuromuscular disorders. Spine J. 2009;9(12):981-6 .
9. Ramonatxo M, Milic-Emili J, Prefaut C. Breathing pattern and load compensatory responses in young scoliotic patients. Eur Respir J. 1988;1(5):421-7.
10. Guilleminault C, Kurland G, Winkle R, Miles LE. Severe kyphoscoliosis, breathing, and sleep: the "Quasimodo" syndrome during sleep. Chest. 1981;79(6):626-30.
11. Pehrsson K, Bake B, Larsson S, Nachemson A. Lung function in adult idiopathic scoliosis: a 20 year follow up. Thorax. 1991;46(7):474-8.
12. McKim DA, Road J, Avendano M, Abdool S, Cote F, Duguid N, et al. Home mechanical ventilation: a Canadian Thoracic Society clinical practice guideline. Can Respir J. 2011;18(4):197-215.
13. Consensus Conference. Clinical indications for non-invasive positive pressure ventilation in chronic respiratory failure due to restrictive lung disease, COPD, and nocturnal hypoventilation - a consensus conference report. Chest. 1999;116(2):521-34.
14. Narayan RL, Vaishnava P, Castellano JM, Fuster V. Quantitative assessment of right ventricular function in pectus excavatum. J Thorac Cardiovasc Surg. 2012;143(5):e41-2.
15. Kelly RE Jr. Pectus excavatum: historical background, clinical picture, preoperative evaluation and criteria for operation. Semin Pediatr Surg. 2008;17(3):181-93.
16. Nuss D, Kelly RE Jr, Croitoru DP, Katz ME. A 10-year review of a minimally invasive technique for the correction of pectus excavatum. J Pediatr Surg. 1998;33(4):545-52.
17. Thai D, Ratani RS, Salama S, Steiner RM. Upper lobe fibrocavitary disease in a patient with back pain and stiffness. Chest. 2000;118(6):1814-6.
18. Ahirwar R, Mondal PR. Prevalence of obesity in India: A systematic review. Diabetes Metab Syndr. 2019;13(1):318-21.
19. Sampson MG, Grassino AE. Load compensation in obese patients during quiet tidal breathing. J Appl Physiol Respir Environ Exerc Physiol. 1983;55(4):1269-76.
20. Wanek S, Mayberry JC. Blunt thoracic trauma: flail chest, pulmonary contusion, and blast injury. Crit Care Clin. 2004;20(1):71-81.

CHAPTER
222
Respiratory Sleep Disorders

Avishek Kar, Khushboo Saxena, Abhishek Goyal

ABSTRACT

Respiratory sleep disorders are a spectrum of sleep-related breathing disorders (SBDs) which includes obstructive sleep apnea (OSA), central sleep apnea (CSA) syndromes, and sleep-related hypoventilation disorders. OSA is common and its prevalence is increasing with rising obesity in population. Pathophysiology involves narrowing of upper airway mainly in retropalatal and retroglossal areas. Daytime sleepiness is among the most common symptoms, but many patients with OSA are asymptomatic and can even have insomnia as presenting complaint. Risk factors for OSA include male sex, older age, postmenopausal, increased neck circumference (>17 inches in male, >16 inches in female), obesity [body mass index (BMI) > 30 kg/m^2], and craniofacial abnormalities to name a few. OSA is associated with a two- to three-fold increased risk of cardiovascular and metabolic disease.

Gold standard for diagnosis is laboratory-based fully attended polysomnography (level I PSG), though home sleep testing is more popular. Home sleep apnea testing (HST) may be used to support, but not to rule out, the diagnosis of OSA. Apnea–hypopnea index (AHI) is used to grade the severity of OSA. Continuous positive airway pressure (CPAP) is considered first-line therapy for symptomatic or moderate-to-severe OSA. Other modalities are weight reduction, surgery, and oral appliances. Recommended lifestyle modifications include weight-loss counseling in overweight and obese patients, avoiding medications and substances that promote relaxation of the upper airway (e.g., alcohol, benzodiazepines, and narcotics), and increasing awareness of and providing countermeasures for the risk of drowsy driving. Treatment with CPAP improves symptoms and reduces complications associated with OSA.

"Sleep is the golden chain that binds health and our bodies together"

—Thomas Dekkar

Sleep-related breathing disorder is characterized by presence of abnormal respiratory events during sleep. As per International Classification of Sleep Disorders-3 (ICSD3), there are eight major categories of sleep disorders and SBD is one of them. SBD is further classified into different categories (**Box 1**).

The most commonly encountered SBD is OSA. In this chapter we will mainly focus on OSA and discuss in detail the various aspects of it.

OBSTRUCTIVE SLEEP APNEA

Obstructive sleep apnea is a highly prevalent condition characterized by episodic collapse of the upper airway during sleep, resulting in periodic reductions or cessations in ventilation with consequent hypoxia and/or arousals during sleep. OSA is responsible for increased sleepiness or insomnia leading to poor quality of life, poor work performance, and increased motor vehicle accidents risk. Patients with OSA are also at higher risk for cardiovascular and metabolic complications. The signs, symptoms, and consequences of OSA are a direct result of derangements that occur due to repetitive collapse of upper airway viz. sleep fragmentation, hypoxemia, hypercapnia, marked swings in intrathoracic pressure, and increased sympathetic activity.

HISTORICAL BACKGROUND

It is in the last few decades that understanding of this medical entity has started evolving, although it was reported as early as 1837 in "Posthumous papers of the Pickwick Club" written by Charles Dickens where he described a "fat boy named Joe". This character was extremely obese and always sleepy. Thus, the term "Pickwickian syndrome" was earlier used for patients with obesity hypoventilation syndrome; although this term is no longer preferred. In 1965, Gastaut et al. showed that cessation of respiration was due to upper airway obstruction and thereby OSA came to be a known as an entity.

EPIDEMIOLOGY

Obstructive sleep apnea increases with age and is twice as common in males than in females.

Obstructive sleep apnea is associated with overweight and obesity. Among individuals aged 30–49 years with a BMI <25 kg/m^2, the prevalence of OSA among men is 7.0% and among women is 1.4%, compared with 44.6% among men and 13.5% among women with a BMI of 30–39.9 kg/m^2. It is also worthwhile to note that as many as 50% of subjects with OSA are nonobese.

In one of the landmark epidemiological studies (HypnoLaus Study), the prevalence of moderate-to-severe

BOX 1	Classification of sleep-related breathing disorders (International Classification of Sleep Disorders-3).

Obstructive sleep apnea (OSA) disorders:

- OSA, adult
- OSA, pediatric

Central sleep apnea syndromes:

- Central sleep apnea with Cheyne–Stokes breathing
- Central sleep apnea due to a medical disorder without Cheyne–Stokes breathing
- Central sleep apnea due to high altitude periodic breathing
- Central sleep apnea due to a medication or substance
- Primary central sleep apnea
- Primary central sleep apnea of infancy
- Primary central sleep apnea of prematurity
- Treatment-emergent central sleep apnea

Sleep-related hypoventilation disorders:

- Obesity hypoventilation syndrome
- Congenital central alveolar hypoventilation syndrome
- Late-onset central hypoventilation with hypothalamic dysfunction
- Idiopathic central alveolar hypoventilation
- Sleep-related hypoventilation due to a medication or substance
- Sleep-related hypoventilation due to a medical disorder

OSA (which is defined as ≥15 obstructive breathing events per hour of sleep) is 23% among women and 50% among men in the general population in the age group of 40–85 years. In the United States, the Wisconsin Sleep Cohort Study also reported increase in prevalence of moderate to severe OSA by 14–55% over the past two decades. This marked increase in prevalence of OSA is due to increasing obesity in general population, advancement in diagnostic techniques, and relaxation of diagnostic criteria for scoring hypopneas.

Data regarding prevalence of OSA in India is scarce and has been derived largely from community-based study and is 13.7% overall prevalence with 19.7% in males and 7.4% among females. Prevalence of OSA among Indian school going children (aged 5–10 years) in Bhopal was found to be 9.8%.

PATHOPHYSIOLOGY

Obstructive sleep apnea has multifactorial pathophysiology. Pathogenesis involves an *anatomical compromise* viz. a narrow, crowded, and collapsible upper airway and *nonanatomical contributors* like ineffective pharyngeal dilator muscle function during sleep, a low threshold for arousal to airway narrowing during sleep, and unstable control of breathing (high loop gain).

The upper airway extends from the posterior margin of the nasal septum to the larynx and lacks a rigid bony support thereby making it prone to collapse during sleep in the retropalatal or retroglossal area or both (**Figs. 1** and **2**).

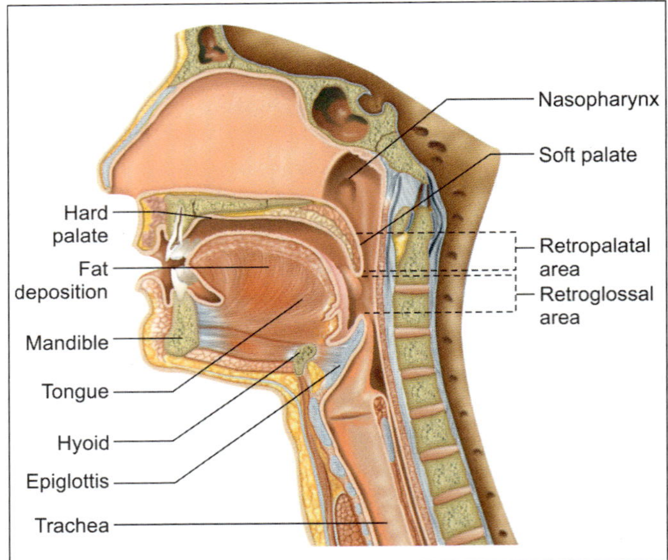

FIGURE 1: Figure illustrates **upper airway anatomy of humans.** Retroglossal and retropalatal area are the sites for anatomical as well as physiological narrowing of airway responsible for obstructive sleep apnea.

Collapse of the upper airway reduces its intraluminal diameter and increases resistance leading to apneas and hypopneas which defines OSA. Most of the existing therapies are directed towards reversal of this anatomical problem (e.g., CPAP, dental devices, and upper airway surgery).

People with OSA have *reduced cross-sectional area of the upper airway* due to either excessive fat deposition around the soft tissues of neck (tongue, soft palate, and lateral pharyngeal walls) or defective craniofacial anatomy or both. During inspiration, there is generation of negative intrathoracic pressure in the airway which promotes airway closure; however, action of pharyngeal dilator muscles (genioglossus and tensor palatini) maintains patency. The activity of these muscles decreases during sleep but is adequate enough to maintain patency in healthy individuals. In subjects with OSA, the *action of the pharyngeal dilators is insufficient* to prevent narrowing or closure of the upper airway. This sleep state-dependent change is the major contributor leading to an obstructed upper airway. In addition, patients with OSA have decreased muscle responsiveness and muscle effectiveness thereby making them blunt to respiratory stimuli like CO_2 and pharyngeal pressure changes. During rapid eye movement (REM) sleep there is further reduction in phasic and tonic activity of these muscles leading to more pronounced apneas and hypopneas. In addition some people have unstable ventilatory control (high loop gain) which also contributes to the pathogenesis.

Mechanism of termination of apnea/hypopnea is controversial. Termination may occur with or without associated arousal which can be at either cortical or subcortical level. Cortical arousals are detectable by EEG. Although arousals are not required for termination of all obstructive events but patients with OSA have decreased arousal threshold thereby making them prone to sleep

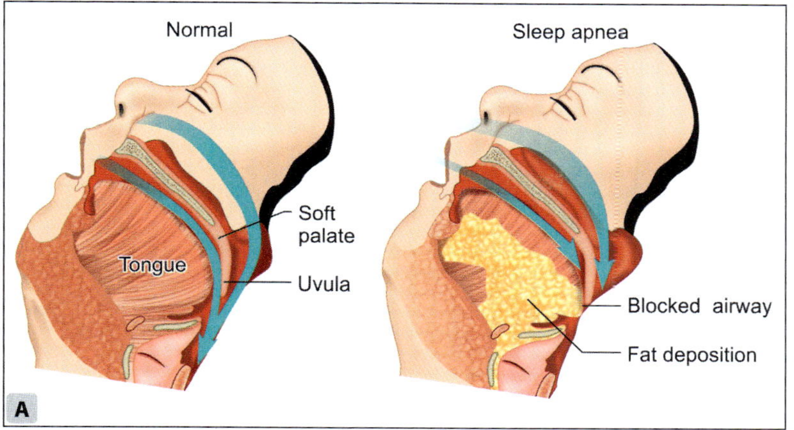

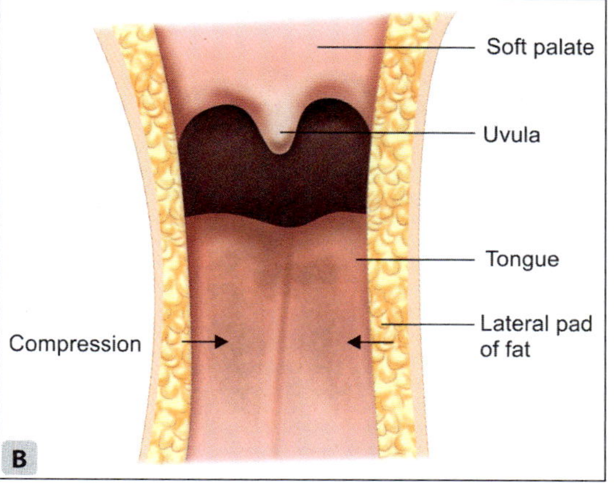

FIGURES 2 A & B: Figure **(A)** illustrates the narrowing and blocked airway leading to obstructive sleep apnea (OSA). There is increased fat deposition in tongue of patients with OSA leading to obstruction of airway during sleep; **(B)** Coronal section image shows compression or airway leading to decreased cross sectional area of upper airway as a result of increased fat deposition in the soft tissue structures around neck.

fragmentation which leads to increased daytime sleepiness. These obstructive events are often exaggerated in REM sleep. As the obstructive events progresses, the patient becomes more hypoxemic. The degree of desaturation depends on the severity of OSA as well as baseline oxygen saturation of the patient, lung volumes, and comorbid conditions of the lung. Hypercarbia also occurs mainly in those with chronic obstructive pulmonary disease (COPD), neuromuscular diseases, kyphoscoliosis, and obesity hypoventilation syndromes.

Patients with OSA have *elevated levels of circulating inflammatory mediators* related to repeated episodes of oxygen desaturation and increased sympathetic activity. These changes are contributory to development of systemic hypertension and other cardiovascular complications relating to OSA. The major predisposing factors in the development of OSA are summarized in **Box 2**.

BOX 2	Predisposing factors.
• Obesity	
• Central body fat distribution	
• *Sex*: Male > female; postmenopausal female are at higher risk as compared to premenopausal females	
• *Anthropometric factors*: Increased neck circumference (>17 inches in males, >16 inches in females)	
• Familial/genetic factors	
• Craniofacial abnormalities like micrognathia, retrognathia, and narrow hard palate	
• Higher Mallampati grade (3 or 4)	
• Tonsillar enlargement (especially in children)	
• Endocrine abnormalities like hypothyroidism, acromegaly, and polycystic ovarian syndrome	
• Alcohol, hypnotics, and sedatives	

ASSESSMENT AND DIAGNOSIS

Questions for assessment of sleep apnea in subjects should include:

- Night-time symptoms (snoring, breathing pauses at night, nocturnal choking spells, unrefreshing sleep, nocturia, and sleep quality or insomnia).
- Daytime symptoms [excessive fatigue or sleepiness throughout the day, memory impairment, irritability, depression, sexual dysfunction like erectile dysfunction and decreased libido, morning headache, and systemic complaints like gastroesophageal reflux disease (GERD)]
- History of diabetes, hypertension, hypothyroidism, coronary artery disease, and other comorbidities should be enquired.
- Approximately 40% of patients with OSA have hypersomnia and 30% have insomnia as presenting complaints. Approximate 30% patients do not have any sleep complaints ands these patients present late with cardiovascular complications.

Questionnaires available for assessment of OSA risk are Berlin questionnaire, STOP-Bang, and NoSAS. The Epworth Sleepiness Scale is a widely used tool to assess sleepiness but has low sensitivity for OSA (**Table 1**).

Physical examination findings are not specific to OSA although it is more prevalent in the obese and overweight population. Clinical examination findings suggestive of OSA are shown in **Box 3**.

If the clinical evaluation is suggestive of OSA, diagnostic confirmation in the form of overnight PSG, in-laboratory or home-based, is warranted. Based on the number of parameters monitored, PSG can be divided into four types (**Table 2**).

DIAGNOSTIC CRITERIA

Obstructive sleep apnea is diagnosed if it meets (**A and B**) **or C** criteria (according to ICSD3):

A. Presence of one or more of following symptoms:
   1. Daytime sleepiness, unrefreshing sleep, insomnia
   2. Observed apneic spells, gasping and choking events during sleep
   3. Habitual snoring, breathing interruptions

TABLE 1 Different questionnaires used for screening OSA and sleepiness and their interpretation scores.

Questionnaire	Description	Interpretation	Sensitivity %	Specificity %
Berlin questionnaire	11 items grouped in 3 domains: Snoring/apneas Fatigue/sleepiness Obesity/hypertension	A score of ≥2, in two or more categories	41 (37–45)	81 (79–83)
STOP-Bang	8 items assessing Snoring, Tiredness, Observed apneas, Hypertension, BMI, Age, Neck girth, Gender	• Range: 0–8 • Score ≥3 indicates risk of OSA	94 (91–96)	40 (37–43)
NoSAS	Neck circumference, Obesity, Snoring, Age and Sex	• Range: 0–17 • Score ≥8 indicates high probability of OSA	79 (75–82)	69 (65–72)
Epworth Sleepiness Scale	Self-administered assessment of sleep tendency in 8 common situations	• Range: 0–24 • Score >10 indicates excessive sleepiness	47 (35–59)	62 (56–68)

Source: Adopted from "HypnoLaus" study.

TABLE 2 Levels of polysomnography (PSG).

Level of PSG	Neuro channels (EEG, EOG, EMG)	Respiratory channels (nasal flow, thoracoabdominal belts and oxygen saturation)	Technician present during study
I	Yes	Yes	Yes
II	Yes	Yes	No
III (HST)	No	Yes (3 or more channels)	No
IV (HST)	No	Yes (1 or 2 channels)	No

BOX 3 Physical examination findings suggestive of OSA.

- Neck circumference >16 inches (40.6 cm) in females; >17 inches (43.2 cm) in males
- BMI ≥ 30 kg/m^2
- Modified Mallampati score 3 or 4
- Upper airway examination findings such as micrognathia, retrognathia, high-arched palate, enlarged tonsils, deviated nasal septum, or nasal abnormalities

4. If patient is diagnosed case of systemic hypertension, diabetes mellitus, coronary artery disease, congestive cardiac failure, atrial fibrillation, mood disorder, stroke, and cognitive dysfunction

B. Polysomnography showing AHI ≥ 5 obstructive events per hour, OR

C. Polysomnography showing AHI ≥ 15 events per hour.

Polysomnography (i.e., level I PSG) remains gold standard for diagnosis of OSA. But it is costly and labor intensive. HST or level-III PSG is gaining popularity now-a-days because of low cost and convenience of patient and physician. The sensitivity and specificity of HST are 79% (95% CI; 71–86%) and 79% (95% CI; 63–89%). However in patients with high probability of OSA, a negative home sleep study should be followed up by laboratory-based PSG.

Apnea-hypopnea index is currently the most accepted marker used for stratification of severity of OSA and is categorized as:

- Mild: ≥5 AHI <15
- Moderate: ≥15 AHI <30
- Severe: ≥30 AHI

DEFINITIONS USED IN POLYSOMNOGRAPHY

Apnea: It is defined as cessation of breathing or airflow for 10 seconds or longer in a PSG study. It is of three types:

1. Obstructive apnea: There is no airflow at nose or mouth but with persistent respiratory efforts (**Fig. 3 A**).
2. Central apnea: There is no airflow at nose or mouth without any respiratory effort as well (**Fig. 3 B**).
3. Mixed apnea: An apnea can be defined as mixed if it meets criteria of apnea along with absent respiratory efforts during some part of event but efforts are present in another part of the event (**Fig. 3 C**).

Hypopnea: It is defined by reduction in amplitude of airflow by ≥30% of pre-event baseline using nasal pressure for ≥10 seconds which is either followed by an arousal or 3% desaturation or both.

Respiratory effort-related arousal (RERA): It is defined as an arousal from sleep that follows a 10 second or longer sequence of breaths characterized by increasing respiratory effort or by flattening of inspiratory portion of flow signal which does not meet the criteria of apnea or hypopnea.

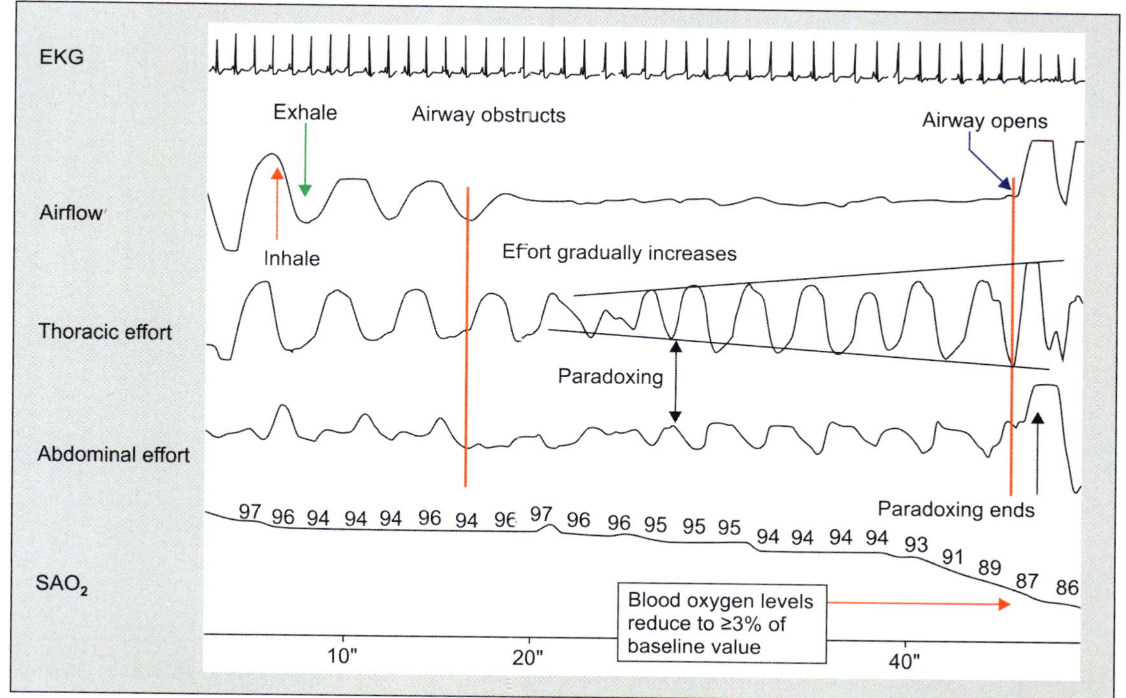

FIGURE 3 A: Polysomnogram of a patient with obstructive sleep apnea. Airflow is grossly decreased/absent leading to apnea with increasing thoracic effort leading to airway opening. Thoracoabdominal paradox is seen. Oxygen saturation has also dropped to >3% from baseline following an episode of obstructive apnea.

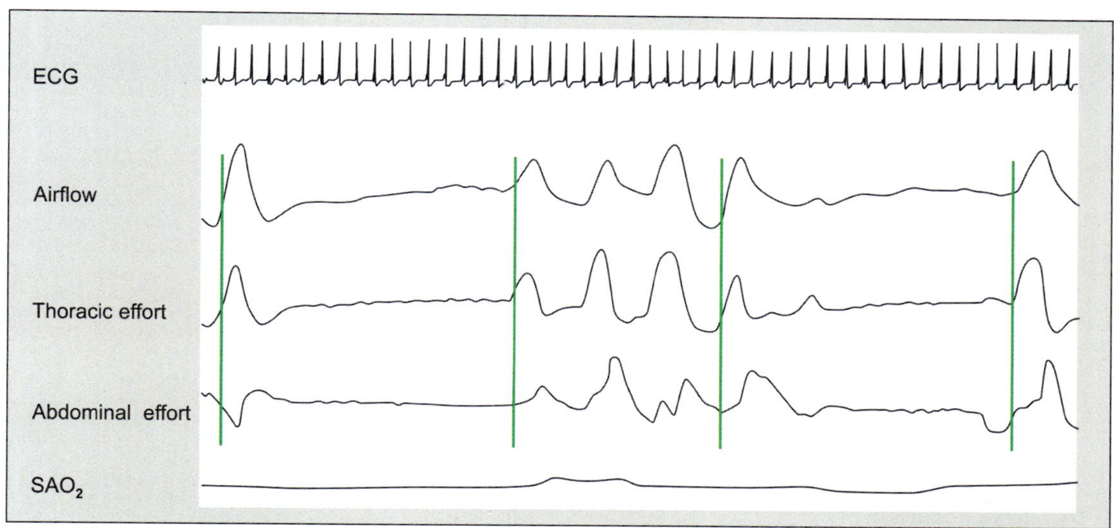

FIGURE 3 B: Polysomnogram of central sleep apnea which is evident by absent airflow along with absent thoracic and abdominal flow. If the changes persist for 10 seconds or more it is called central apneic event.

Apnea–hypopnea index: Calculated as number of apneas and hypopneas per hour of sleep.

Respiratory disturbance index (RDI): It is the number of apneas, hypopneas, and RERAs per hour of sleep, which is confirmed by EEG.

Cheyne–Stokes breathing: It is defined as:

- Three consecutive events of central apnea separated by crescendo-decrescendo pattern of breathing in a total cycle length of 40 seconds or more.

And

- There are five or more such pattern of central apneas with crescendo-decrescendo breathing per hour of sleep recorded for 2 or more hours of sleep.

Obesity hypoventilation syndrome *(earlier called as Pickwickian syndrome)*: It is defined by the presence of obesity (BMI ≥ 30 kg/m^2), sleep-disordered breathing with daytime hypercapnia (awake $PaCO_2$ ≥ 45 mm Hg) in the absence of any other known cause of hypoventilation.

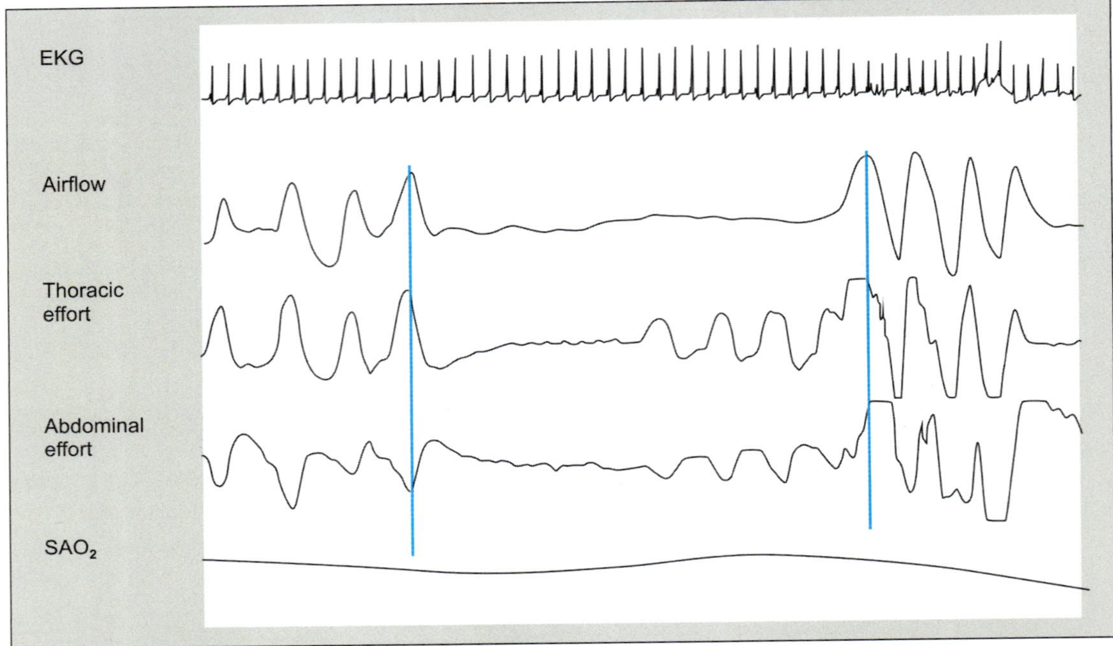

FIGURE 3 C: Polysomnogram of mixed apnea where it meets criteria of apnea along with absent respiratory efforts during first part of event but efforts are present in later half of the event.

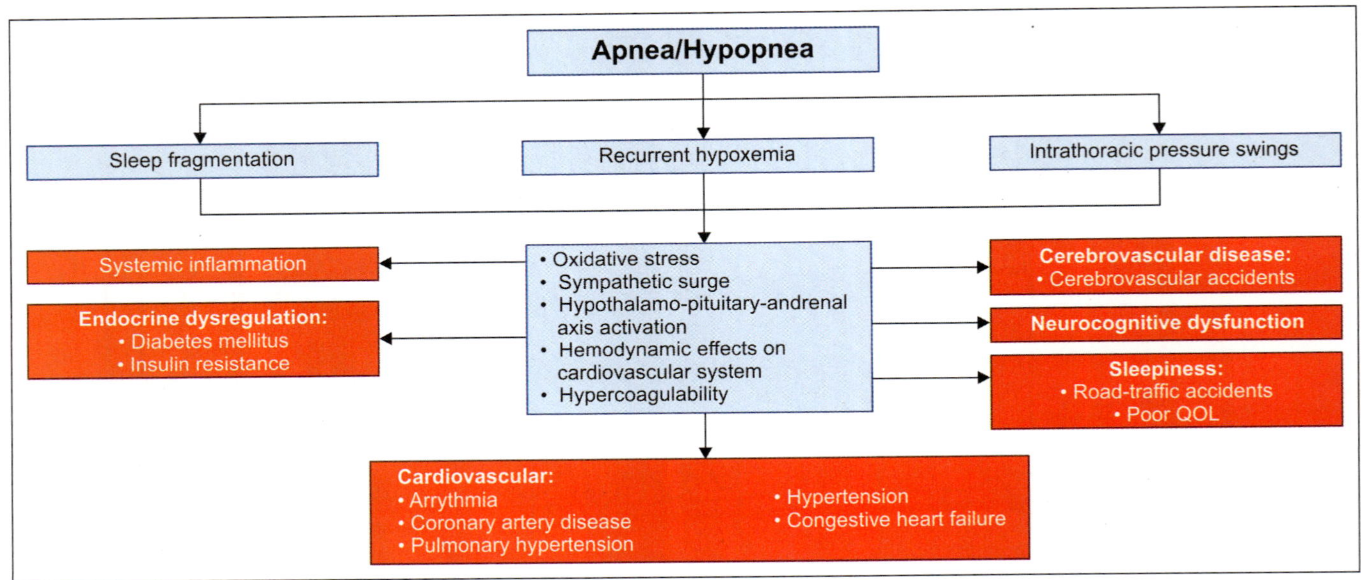

(OSA: obstructive sleep apnea; QOL: quality of life)

FLOWCHART 1: Pathophysiological consequences and their clinical manifestations are represented in this flowchart. OSA causes multisystem involvement with varied manifestations which occurs as a result of apneas/hypopneas.

Overlap syndrome: The co-occurrence of both COPD and OSA in the same individual is termed as overlap syndrome.

CONSEQUENCES OF OSA (FLOWCHART 1)

- **Mortality:** Severe OSA is associated with 3- to 4-fold risk for all-cause mortality and more so with cardiovascular mortality.
- **Cardiovascular disease:**
  - OSA and hypertension: OSA is an independent risk factor for systemic hypertension. Prevalence of hypertension in OSA is approximately 60% whereas OSA is present in approximately 30% of subjects with hypertension. OSA is seen in 83% of subjects with refractory hypertension. The odds of developing hypertension are 1% for every 1 event of SDB per hour and every 10% decrease in nadir oxygen saturation. OSA is now also considered as one of the modifiable risk factors for new onset HTN.
  - OSA and coronary artery disease: Independent association has been found between OSA and CAD with increasing prevalence.

- OSA and arrhythmias: Nocturnal arrhythmias are found in up to 50% of OSA patients. Atrial fibrillation, nonsustained ventricular tachycardia, sinus arrest, and 2° atrioventricular (AV) conduction block are more commonly seen in patients with OSA.
- OSA and heart failure: OSA is found in 10–37% of patients with heart failure. In addition about 30% patients of heart failure have CSA.

- **Cerebrovascular accident:** OSA has poorer functional outcome in stroke patients along with increased length of hospital stay and increased mortality. Patients of severe OSA have increased risk of stroke.
- **Diabetes mellitus:** OSA causes intermittent hypoxemia and sleep fragmentation leading to insulin resistance and glucose intolerance which further leads to peripheral neuropathy and abnormal ventilatory and upper airway control thus perpetuating the vicious cycle.
- **Cancer:** Increased overnight hypoxia as a surrogate of OSA severity was associated with increased cancer incidence. This association seems to be limited to men and patients younger than 65 years of age.
- **Excessive daytime sleepiness (EDS):** Sleep fragmentation due to frequent cortical arousals leads to EDS. EDS is responsible for increased motor vehicle accidents, increased work-related accidents, poor job performance, depression, family discord, and poor quality of life.
- **Neurocognitive function:** Forgetfulness, impaired concentration, slow thought process, and decreased workplace performance are associated with OSA.
- **Metabolic syndrome (MS) and syndrome Z:** MS consists of central obesity, hypertriglyceridemia, low high-density lipoprotein (HDL) cholesterol, hyperglycemia, and hypertension. The combination of MS and OSA is syndrome Z. In a study conducted at our center in central Indian population, MS was seen in 72% of OSA patients and prevalence of MS in nonobese patients with OSA (with BMI < 25 kg/m^2) was 34%.

DIFFERENTIAL DIAGNOSIS

Patients with isolated snoring with no obstructive events should be excluded with PSG. OSA must be differentiated from other causes of sleepiness like narcolepsy, idiopathic hypersomnia, insufficient sleep, restless leg syndrome, drugs, and depression.

Approach to a case of obstructive sleep apnea is described in **Flowchart 2**.

TREATMENT

Behavioral interventions:

- Weight loss: Remains a highly effective method. 10–15% reduction in weight can lead to approximately 30–40% reduction in sleep apnea severity in moderately obese male patients.

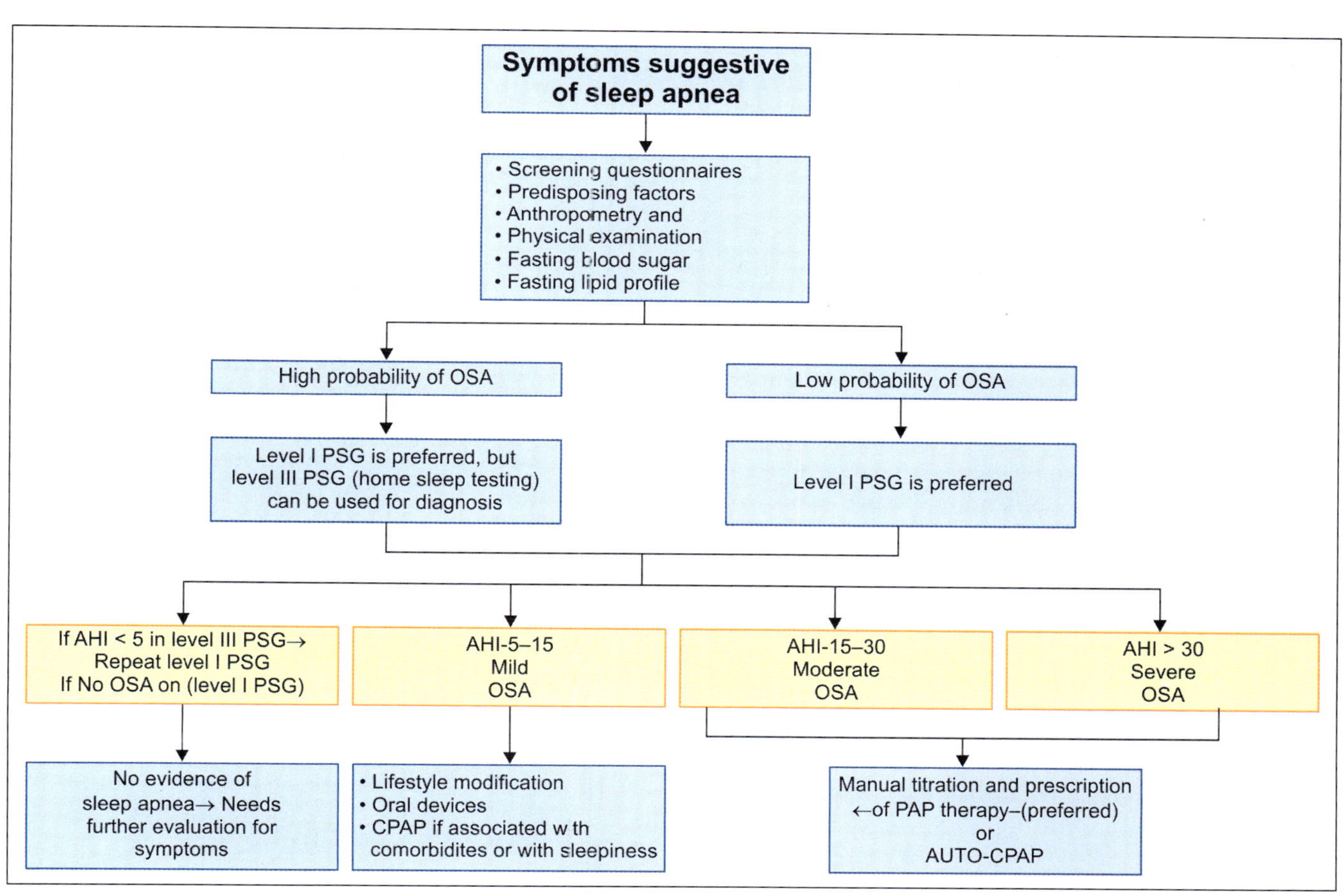

(CPAP: continuous positive airway pressure; OSA: obstructive sleep apnea; PSG: polysomnography)

FLOWCHART 2: Algorithm for approach to and management of obstructive sleep apnea.

- Avoidance of consumption of alcohol, sedatives, and nicotine
- Positional therapy—position-dependent OSA (POSA) is defined as a difference of 50% or more in AHI between supine and nonsupine position. Positional therapy to reduce POSA can be done by various methods like positional sleep trainer devices, tennis ball technique.
- Counseling regarding sleep hygiene practices:
  - Spend adequate time in bed and maintain fixed sleep timing
  - Reduce physical activity shortly before bedtime
  - Avoid stimulants such as caffeine in the evening
  - Minimize annoying noise, light, or extremes of temperature
  - Exercise regularly for at least 20 minutes, preferably 4–5 hours before bedtime
  - Do not try harder and harder to fall asleep. If you are unable to sleep, do something.

Positive airway pressure: It acts as splint to upper airway and thus keep it patent during sleep. It is the preferred mode of treatment for OSA.

- Continuous positive airway pressure: This is the preferred mode and has shown to decrease complications associated with OSA.
- Automatic positive airway pressure (APAP): This is most commonly used mode because of ease of prescription. It has been shown to be noninferior to CPAP mode in terms of adherence and outcome. APAP is not superior to CPAP for most OSA patients.
- Bi-level positive airway pressure (BiPAP): This mode is used in patients who require high pressures due to various reasons like severe obesity, severe OSA, and associated COPD. BiPAP is not superior to CPAP for most OSA patients.
- Average volume assured pressure support (AVAPS): It has been found useful in patients with hypercapnic hypoventilation like OSA-COPD overlap, obesity hypoventilation syndrome.
- Adaptive servo ventilation (ASV): It is used in patients with CSA who do not respond to CPAP. It is currently contraindicated in patients with ejection fraction <45%.
- Oral appliances (mandibular repositioning appliances and tongue retaining appliances) and dental appliances (mandibular advancement devices): These are recommended for patients with mild OSA, upper airway resistance syndrome (UARS), and snoring. It holds the lower jaw forward, thereby increasing the space in the oropharynx.

PAP therapy:

Advantages:

- Continuous positive airway pressure is the treatment of choice for patients with moderate and severe OSA (AHI >15/h). Randomized controlled trials have confirmed that compared to intraoral devices and lifestyle changes alone, CPAP treatment is more effective in reducing apneas, improving symptoms of sleepiness, and improving quality of life in patients with moderate to severe OSA. Regular use of CPAP for the duration of sleep has been shown to reduce systemic BP and improve lipid profile. Use of CPAP is associated with a reduction in road traffic accidents by 83% caused due to sleepiness in patients with OSA.
- Continuous positive airway pressure device consists of a unit that generates airflow and is connected to either a nasal (preferred) or full-face mask via a tube. A pressure is generated which splints the pharynx open by exerting positive airways pressure, thus preventing the airway from collapsing. Continuous positive airway pressure also increases end-expiratory lung volume, which stabilizes the upper airway through caudal traction. A fixed CPAP device delivers air at a constant pressure throughout the night and the pressure required for each patient can be determined by an overnight titration study. Autotitrating devices, which continually adjust the pressure delivered throughout the night, are more comfortable and better tolerated, but are more expensive. There is no evidence that their use results in a better outcome or adherence than fixed PAP devices. CPAP has substantial benefits for some patients but adherence is roughly 60–70% (**Fig. 4**).

Disadvantages of PAP device:

- *Mask-related issues*: Mask discomfort, leakage, difficulty in exhalation, claustrophobia, nasal skin abrasions, nasal congestion, rhinorrhea, nasal dryness, and sinus pain
- Bed partner intolerance

Pharmacological management: Wake promoting agents like modafinil and armodafinil. Currently, it is recommended to be used only in patients who have residual sleepiness even after adequately controlled OSA on CPAP. The residual AHI should be <5 per hour on download report and patient should use CPAP throughout sleep.

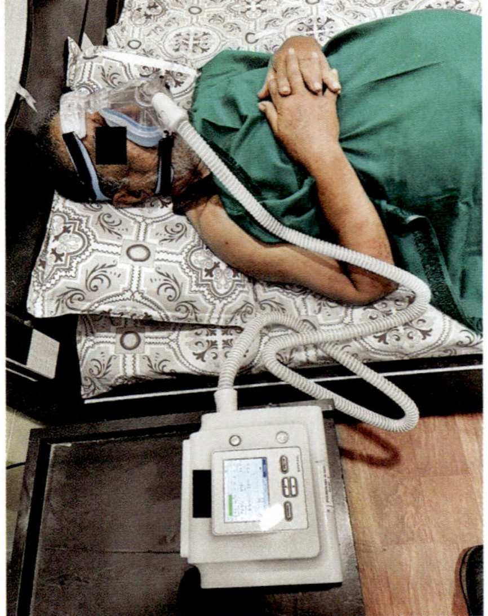

(OSA: obstructive sleep apnea; CPAP: continuous positive airway pressure)

FIGURE 4: A patient with OSA on CPAP therapy. Patient is wearing a full face oronasal mask.

These agents should not be routinely used without adequate treatment of OSA.

Surgical management:

- Maxillomandibular advancement osteotomy: This surgery has been done in patients with jaw abnormalities like retrognathia and micrognathia with good results.
- Tonsillectomy ± adenoidectomy is the preferred mode of treatment in pediatric OSA and is first line of treatment in children.
- Other surgeries (septoplasty, uvulopalatopharyngoplasty, and radiofrequency volumetric tissue reduction) have been tried with varying success. Data for success in Indian population is not available to support its efficacy.
- Bariatric surgery: It is indicated in patients with BMI > 40 kg/m^2. After significant weight loss, studies have shown improvement in daytime sleepiness, severity of OSA, and quality of life. It is also associated with decrease in PAP pressure requirement.

PREVENTION

Although many risk factors for OSA are fixed; weight loss and avoidance of cigarettes, alcohol, and other muscle relaxant drugs is beneficial. OSA resolved in 63% of patients with mild disease after significant weight reduction in one study from Europe. Weight reduction by means of bariatric surgery is also helpful. But only weight loss is not helpful in patients with severe OSA specially in Indian population because of coexisting craniofacial anatomical factors contributing to OSA.

CENTRAL SLEEP APNEA

It is characterized by diminished central drive for ventilation during sleep without any upper airway obstruction. Symptoms are similar as that of OSA like EDS, nocturnal dyspnea, and insomnia. Diagnosis of CSA requires both subjective symptoms and objective evidence of disease state in polysomnogram. PSG shows absence of airflow and thoracoabdominal movements during central sleep apneic events (**Fig. 3 B**).

Central sleep apnea is diagnosed when predominant apneic-hypopneic events (>50% of total AHI) are central during diagnostic PSG. CSA can be hypercapnic or hypocapnic/eucapnic. It is of various types (**Table 3**).

Central sleep apnea-Cheyne–Stokes breathing (CSA-CSB): It is characterized by recurrent central apneas or hypopneas alternating with a respiratory phase exhibiting a crescendo-decrescendo pattern of flow. The majority of patients with CSA-CSB have either systolic or diastolic heart failure. Patients typically have normal or low daytime arterial PCO_2. Some patients may have a mixture of both obstructive and central apneas. In these patients the central apneas may increase only after elimination of obstructive apneas on positive pressure therapy. Arousals do occur in central apnea resulting in sleep fragmentation; however patients mainly complain of disturbed sleep or nocturnal dyspnea rather than daytime sleepiness. These symptoms may be missed in view of heart failure symptoms. Studies have indicated that approximately 60% of patients with heart failure have some form of sleep apnea, so high index of suspicion is indicated for diagnosis.

Central sleep apnea-Cheyne–Stokes breathing is seen in individuals older than 60 years with a male predominance in those with heart failure. The most important predisposing factors of CSA-CSB are presence of congestive heart failure (CHF), stroke, and possibly renal failure. Risk factors of CSB pattern in sleep are: Male gender, age > 60 years, and atrial fibrillation. CSA with CSB arises because of ventilator instability (loop gain) relating to high ventilatory drive and delay in chemoreceptor response to gaseous changes. Hyperventilation occurs mainly due to increased central and peripheral chemoreceptor responsiveness as a result of increased sympathetic tone and vagal stimulation. The crescendo-decrescendo pattern of tidal volume mainly occurs due to increased lung-to-chemoreceptor circulatory delay resulting in gradual buildup and sudden falloff of ventilator stimuli.

- **Primary CSA:** It can be distinguished from CSB pattern by the absence of crescendo-decrescendo pattern in between apneas and history of heart failure or stroke.
- **CSA due to high altitude periodic breathing:** CSA which only occurs in high altitude (typically >1,500 m) and is not associated with systemic disease.
- **CSA due to substance:** Patients with CSA due to drug or substance have a history of use of such type of drugs (opioids) along with an ataxic breathing pattern. If periodic breathing is present also, the cycle length is decreased (<40 s). Drugs commonly implicated are opioids prescribed for chronic pain.
- **CSA due to a medical or neurological disease:** Patients with central neurological causes (like space occupying lesion in CNS or recent CNS surgery) can have CSA without Cheyne–Stokes morphology.
- ***Ondine's curse*** is a congenital form of CSA due to abnormal development of the neural crest.

TABLE 3 Various types of central sleep apnea (CSA).

Hypercapnic CSA	Hypocapnic/eucapnic CSA
Seen in	**Seen in**
• Defects in brainstem/impaired brainstem output, brainstem tumors	• Congestive cardiac failure
• Congenital central hypoventilation syndrome	• High altitude periodic breathing
• Obesity hypoventilation syndrome	• Cheyne–Stokes pattern of breathing is a type of hypocapnic CSA
• Can also be seen in impaired respiratory motor response, e.g., various neuropathies like myasthenia gravis, poliomyelitis	

Preferred mode of treatment in CSA is continuous positive pressure therapy after manual titration. In cases where ejection fraction is >45%, ASV can be tried.

NARCOLEPSY

Narcolepsy is a rare disorder of hypersomnolence which is primarily characterized by EDS and signs of REM-sleep dissociation, the most specific of which is cataplexy. EDS is the most disabling symptom; they experience repeated daily episodes of an irrepressible need to sleep. Most of them awaken refreshed after sleep but begins to feel sleepy again after some time. The disease is prevalent among young people with age of onset after 5 years of age typically between 10 and 25 years of age. Narcolepsy is of two types: type 1 and type 2.

Cataplexy is defined as more than one episode of generally brief (<2 min), usually bilateral symmetrical sudden loss of muscle tone with retained consciousness and is characteristic of narcolepsy type 1. Episodes are precipitated by strong emotions which are usually positive like laughter. Transient, reversible loss of deep tendon reflex during attack is diagnostic.

Narcolepsy is diagnosed by PSG (AHI < 5/h) and multiple sleep latency testing (MSLT) showing decreased sleep latency. It is usually treated by wake promoting drugs like modafinil, armodafinil, and sodium oxabate.

RECOMMENDED READINGS

1. International Classification Of Sleep Disorders-THIRD Edition (ICSD-3) [Online] Available from https://journal.chestnet.org/article/S0012-3692(15)52407-0/fulltext
2. AASM. (2020). AASM scoring Manual for the Scoring of Sleep and Associated Events, version 2.6. July 2020. [Online] Available from https://aasm.org/clinical-resources/scoring-manual/
3. Gottlieb DJ, Punjabi NM. Diagnosis and Management of Obstructive Sleep Apnea: A Review. JAMA. 2020; 323(14):1389-400.
4. Veasey SC, Rosen IM. Obstructive Sleep Apnea in Adults. N Engl J Med. 2019;380(15):1442-9.
5. Sharma SK, Katoch VM, Mohan A, Kadhiravan T, Elavarasi A, Ragesh R, et al. Consensus & Evidence-Based INOSA GUIDELINES (INdian initiative on Obstructive Sleep Apnea Guidelines) First Edition, 2014. Indian J Med Res. 2014;140(3):451-68.
6. Heinzer R, Vat S, Marques-Vidal P, Marti-Soler H, Andries D, Tobback N, et al. Prevalence of sleep-disordered breathing in the general population: the HypnoLaus study. Lancet Respir Med. 2015;3(4):310-8.
7. Sharma SK, Ahluwalia G. Epidemiology of adult obstructive sleep apnoea syndrome in India. Indian J Med Res. 2010;131:171-75.
8. Jordan AS, McSharry DG, Malhotra A. Adult obstructive sleep apnoea. Lancet. 2014;383(9918):736-47.

CHAPTER 223

Respiratory Failure

Surinder K Jindal

ABSTRACT

Respiratory failure is defined as impairment of lung function to maintain adequate oxygenation and carbon dioxide elimination. It is not a disease condition per se. It is diagnosed from the presence of hypoxemia with or without hypercapnia. There are two types of respiratory failure: (1) type I characterized by hypoxemia alone and (2) type II characterized by both hypoxemia and hypercapnia. It is also define as acute or chronic depending upon the duration of illness. Acute respiratory distress syndrome (ARDS) is the prototype of acute respiratory failure which usually occurs in patients without any antecedent lung disease following sepsis, trauma, or shock. Chronic respiratory failure occurs most commonly in patients with chronic lung diseases such as chronic obstructive pulmonary disease (COPD) and chronic interstitial lung diseases.

Diagnosis of respiratory failure is made on the basis of clinical history and blood gas examination. Treatment principles involve the maintenance of an intact airways, adequate oxygenation, and removal of carbon dioxide. Oxygen administration along with management of the underlying disease or other complications is adequate for mild and moderate respiratory failure. Severe respiratory failure such as due to ARDS characterized with refractory hypoxemia requires assisted respiratory support (ARS) with endotracheal intubation. Chronic respiratory failure in patients with COPD and hypercapnia can often be managed with noninvasive ventilation with the help of a tight fitting mask.

"In nothing do men more nearly approach the gods, than in giving health to men"

—Cicero

INTRODUCTION

Respiratory failure is defined by the presence of arterial hypoxia with or without hypercapnia as a result of impaired lung function failing in oxygenation and carbon dioxide elimination. Hypoxia (or hypoxemia) is defined as arterial oxygen tension (PO_2) of <60 mm Hg and hypercapnia as arterial carbon dioxide pressure (PCO_2) of >45 mm Hg at sea level, and with the patient at rest. In clinical practice, respiratory failure is defined as type 1 when it is characterized by the presence of hypoxia alone (hypoxemic), and type 2 (i.e., hypercapnic) when there is presence of both hypoxia and hypercapnia. It is an important cause of mortality and morbidity all over the world.

CAUSES

Respiratory failure can occur in both acute and chronic, progressive lung diseases, and sometimes due to nonrespiratory diseases. It can therefore be classified as acute or chronic depending upon the duration of condition. There is a long list of diseases which can be considered as responsible for causing respiratory failure (**Box 1**). There is failure of respiratory apparatus to deliver sufficient O_2 to pulmonary capillary blood resulting in arterial hypoxemia. But CO_2 excretion by the lungs is normal or even increased because of hyperventilation, therefore arterial PCO_2 is normal or low.

- **Acute respiratory failure:** This may occur in acute conditions such as severe pneumonia, cardiogenic or noncardiogenic pulmonary edema, pulmonary hemorrhage, or other causes of ARDS. Hypoxemia occurs due to severe ventilation/perfusion imbalance.
- **Chronic respiratory failure:** Chronic respiratory failure is frequently characterized by both hypoxemia and hypercapnia. This type of failure is seen whenever there is hypoventilation because of abnormalities in respiratory control, in the neuromuscular apparatus or in the chest wall. Common clinical examples include drug overdose, neuromuscular disease, chest wall abnormalities, and severe airway disorders (e.g., asthma and COPD). Chronic respiratory failure can also be classified as hypoxemic or hypercapnic respiratory failure. Low blood oxygen levels cause hypoxemic respiratory failure. High carbon dioxide levels cause hypercapnic respiratory failure.

BOX 1	Common causes of respiratory failure.
• **Acute respiratory failure:**	
○ Diffuse massive pulmonary infections—pneumonia	
○ Acute respiratory distress syndrome	
○ Inhalation of toxins and irritants	
○ Aspiration pneumonias	
○ Depression of respiratory drive—overdose of a narcotic and sedative	
○ Pulmonary edema	
○ Pulmonary hemorrhage	
• **Chronic respiratory failure:**	
○ Chronic obstructive pulmonary disease and poorly controlled asthma	
○ Interstitial pulmonary fibrosis	
○ Other chronic lung diseases: Tuberculosis, bronchiectasis, and cystic fibrosis	
○ Neuromuscular diseases: Respiratory muscle and chest wall weakness: Guillain–Barré syndrome, polio myelitis	
○ Severe kyphoscoliosis	

After management of acute exacerbation in the hospital, treatment for chronic respiratory disease is continued at home on long-term basis. *General principles of management* consist of the following:
- Maintenance drug treatment of the causative respiratory disease
- Adequate bronchial hygiene
- Maintenance oxygenation—domiciliary, long-term oxygen therapy
- *Respiratory rehabilitation*: Multidisciplinary supports which include regular exercise training, maintenance of nutrition, and psychosocial supports
- *Preventive measures*: Smoking cessation; vaccination against flu and pneumococcal infections
- Patient education

PATHOPHYSIOLOGY

There are three main pathophysiologic mechanisms of respiratory failure and hypoxemia:

1. **Hypoventilation:** $PaCO_2$, PaO_2, and alveolar-arterial PO_2 gradient (difference between the calculated oxygen pressure available in the alveolus and the arterial oxygen tension, measures the efficiency of gas exchange) are normal.
2. **Ventilation/perfusion ratio ($\dot{V}/\dot{Q}$ ratio or V/Q ratio):** V/P mismatch is the most common cause of hypoxemia. The V/Q ratio is used to assess the efficiency and adequacy of the matching of V (ventilation), i.e., the air that reaches the alveoli and Q (perfusion) the blood that reaches the alveoli via the capillaries. V/Q ratio is defined as the ratio of the amount of air reaching the alveoli per minute to the amount of blood reaching the alveoli per minute.
3. **Shunt:** It is defined as a pathological state in which the alveoli are perfused but not ventilated; hypoxemia will persist despite 100% O_2 inhalation. This is commonly seen in cases of pulmonary edema (cardiogenic or noncardiogenic), pneumonia, and atelectasis.

CLINICAL FEATURES

Clinical features of respiratory failure consist of symptoms and signs of the underlying disease as well as those attributable to the presence of hypoxia and hypercapnia which are often indistinguishable (**Table 1**).

TABLE 1 Clinical features of respiratory failure.

Due to underlying disease	Hypoxia	Hypercapnia
• Chronic cough, phlegm • Breathlessness on exertion • Weight loss and other constitutional symptoms • Signs of chronic lung disease: Chronic obstructive pulmonary disease, bronchiectasis, kyphoscoliosis etc.	• Tachypnea, tachycardia (terminally bradycardia) Sweating, restlessness, anxiety, and sleeplessness • Arrhythmias • High systolic blood pressure (later hypotension) • Cyanosis • Mental confusion, disorientation and incoordination, progressing to convulsions, coma	• Dilatation of cerebral vessels leading to increase in intracranial pressure • Headache • Sleep disturbances, personality changes, and disorientation • Pulse is fast, bounding, and collapsing with warm extremities • High systolic blood pressure • Flapping tremors (asterixis) • Papilledema • Coma

Acute hypercapnic respiratory failure develops within minutes to hours while the clinical picture of chronic respiratory failure is usually more insidious. Central cyanosis is the characteristic sign of hypoxia but may not be clinically appreciable in milder degrees of desaturation and in the presence of anemia. Hypoxic damage to other vital organs such as the brain, heart, liver, and kidneys may produce additional clinical manifestations. Severe untreated hypoxia is the frequent cause of death. Hypercapnia is always accompanied by hypoxia except for shorter periods following acute accidental inhalation of CO_2 or when high flow oxygen has been given to raise low PaO_2. Severe degree of CO_2 retention causes respiratory acidosis, cardiac arrhythmias, and arrest.

DIAGNOSIS

Diagnosis of respiratory failure is essentially made on blood gas examination. It is however suspected from the presence of the underlying disease and other risk factors considered to potentially responsible for the failure. Some of the important risk factors include the history of smoking, exposure to gases and fumes, presence of a chronic respiratory disease, severe pneumonia, sepsis, acute pancreatitis, and multiple trauma.

- **Clinical features:** A good clinical history and physical examination for an acute or chronic lung condition are helpful in making the diagnosis. The potential clinical symptoms and signs (**Table 1**) can frequently point to respiratory failure which may be either acute or chronic. A patient with chronic occult respiratory failure may also develop features of acute failure due to exaggeration of the underlying chronic condition, frequently referred to as "acute on chronic respiratory failure." The clinical markers of chronic hypoxemia, such as polycythemia or pulmonary hypertension suggest a long-standing disorder.
- **Blood gas and acid–base examination:** Measurement of oxygen and carbon dioxide levels is most important to establish the diagnosis. Arterial blood gases should be evaluated in all patients who are seriously ill or in whom respiratory failure is suspected. For noninvasive assessment, pulse oximetry and end-tidal breath capnometry are performed to measure arterial oxygen saturation (SaO_2%) and carbon dioxide pressure (ET pCO_2), respectively. Acute respiratory failure is characterized by abnormalities of arterial blood gases (hypoxemia and/or hypercapnia) and acid–base status. The distinction between acute and chronic hypoxemic respiratory failure cannot readily be made on the basis of arterial blood gases. Chronic respiratory failure develops over several days or longer, allowing time for renal compensation and an increase in bicarbonate concentration. Therefore, the pH usually is only slightly decreased.
- **Other investigations:** Hematological, biochemical, microbiological, and immunological investigations are required as needed for diagnostic assessments as well as to know the functional status of different organ systems. Chest radiography is almost always essential. It provides important information on lung parenchymal and pleural conditions such as consolidation, collapse, effusion, or pneumothorax. Electrocardiography provides useful information on the presence of any rhythm disturbance or underlying cardiovascular cause of respiratory failure. Echocardiography is not a routine but is sometimes useful to know of the cardiac status. Pulmonary functions tests (PFTs) such as spirometry and diffusion capacity are not required for the diagnosis of respiratory failure per se but are important for the diagnosis of the underlying respiratory disease such as the COPD, interstitial lung disease, and others. Other specific investigations may be needed to establish the diagnosis of the cause of respiratory failure.

ACUTE RESPIRATORY DISTRESS SYNDROME

Acute respiratory distress syndrome (ARDS) is a type of acute respiratory failure caused by damage to the alveolo-capillary membrane usually in patients with previously healthy lungs in the presence of severe sepsis, shock, trauma, and several other types of systemic or inhalational lung injuries. This is a type of inflammatory injury to the alveolo-capillary membrane causing increase in its permeability. Thus there is leakage of protein-rich fluid from pulmonary circulation into the lung parenchyma into the interstitium and alveolar sacs. The initial interstitial edema is followed by alveolar edema in the full blown picture of ARDS.

Some common conditions that may lead to this type of lung damage include:

- Inhalation of toxic gases and fumes
- Aspiration of the vomited material
- Severe blood infection—sepsis
- Severe pneumonia
- Acute pancreatitis
- Vehicular injury and multiskeletal trauma
- Sedative or drug over dosage.

Diagnosis: There is acute onset of respiratory distress characterized by hypoxemia which is usually oxygen-resistant accompanied by symptoms and signs of respiratory failure such as discomfort, dyspnea, and tachycardia (**Table 1**). Diagnosis is established on the basis of clinical history, chest X-ray, and blood gas examination. Chest X-ray in the early phases may be normal or show presence of reticular prominence due to interstitial edema. Bilateral fluffy lung consolidations due to bronchopneumonia are seen during the established ARDS after 24–48 hours of onset.

Lung inflammation and edema are frequently associated with similar changes in other systemic organs such as the liver, kidneys, and adrenals presenting with a picture of multiorgan dysfunction (MOD). These manifestations can be diagnosed from the presence of deranged liver, kidney, or adrenal function tests. Hematological and coagulation abnormalities are frequently present. There may be polymorphonuclear leukocytosis, low-platelet count, neutropenia, or pancytopenia. Disseminated intravascular coagulopathy (DIC) with bleeding from different sites is an important manifestation of MODS. In severe cases, there may be involvement of heart and brain causing cardiac arrhythmias, heart failure, encephalopathy, and other cerebral manifestations.

COMPLICATIONS

Complications related to different organ systems may occur during or subsequent to respiratory failure. Complications can occur due to the problems related to the underlying disease and/or respiratory failure per se because of the hypoxic damage.

- *Complications secondary to endotracheal intubation* (**Box 2**) and the use of mechanical ventilator related to barotrauma and/or volutrauma: Ventilator-associated pneumonias and pulmonary hemorrhage
- *Pulmonary*: Tracheobronchitis and bronchopneumonia, pulmonary thromboembolism, pleural effusion; pulmonary fibrosis is usually a late-stage complication which occurs during fibrous phase of ARDS.
- *Cardiovascular*: Hypotension, reduced cardiac output, cor pulmonale, arrhythmias, pericarditis, and acute myocardial infarction
- *Gastrointestinal*: Gastric hemorrhage and duodenal ulceration—caused by stress, gastric distention, paralytic ileus, diarrhea related to antibiotic use, pseudomembranous colitis, and pneumoperitoneum due to barotraumas
- *Infectious*: Nosocomial—pneumonia, urinary tract infection, and catheter-related sepsis. Central venous cannulation is another important site of nosocomial infections.
- *Renal*: Hypoperfusion and shock leads to acute renal failure; abnormalities of electrolytes and acid-base balance.
- Complications due to prolonged mechanical ventilation:
  - Nutritional deficiencies and malnutrition; anemia and other deficiencies of essential minerals; loss of fat and muscle mass
  - Complications due to parenteral or enteral nutrition—central venous thrombosis; complications associated with nasogastric tube—abdominal distention and diarrhea
  - Bed sores due to local ischemia of pressure points
  - *Psychological and neuropsychiatric complications*: Depression, acute psychotic episodes; critical illness neuropathy

BOX 2 Complications of endotracheal intubation.

- **During the procedure:**
  - Trauma to the teeth and oropharyngeal airways
  - Injury of the vocal cords, trachea, or esophagus
  - Bleeding
  - Esophageal placement of the tube
  - Temporary hoarseness
  - Barotraumas: Pneumothorax
- **Complications due to prolonged intubation:**
  - Pressure ulcer around adhesive tapes
  - Infections due to accumulation of secretions
  - Sinusitis
  - Aspiration of gastric content, atelectasis
  - Increased incidence of ventilator-associated pneumonia
  - Vocal cord paralysis
  - Tracheomalacia
  - Tracheoesophageal fistula
  - Laryngotracheal stenosis

Acute respiratory distress syndrome patients with previously healthy lungs fully recover within a period of few weeks or months. However, some patients are left with residual pulmonary fibrosis causing permanent respiratory disability. Other post ARDS sequelae include persistent muscle weakness and fatigue and impaired quality of life. Some of the patients may continue with a compromised mental health due to prolonged psychological trauma.

MANAGEMENT

Diagnosis of early, insipient respiratory failure is sometimes delayed. Arterial blood gas analysis is most important in the diagnosis and management. The dangerous levels of hypoxia, hypercapnia, and acidosis may vary with the underlying condition. It is however agreed that PO_2 below 40 mm Hg and pH below 7.2 are poorly tolerated.

Management essentially comprises of supportive measures and treatment of the underlying cause. Supportive measures include the airways management for adequate ventilation to maintain oxygenation and correction of the blood gases abnormalities. Some of the important steps of management are discussed as under:

CLEAR AIRWAYS AND ADEQUATE VENTILATION

Retention of secretions in the upper airways is an important problem which requires immediate and constant attention. Several factors are responsible for the presence and retention of secretions:

- Acute pulmonary disease causing excessive production due to infection and inflammation—chronic bronchitis, asthma, pulmonary contusion, bronchiectasis, tuberculosis, and others.
- Excessive bronchorrhea associated with organophosphates or other poisons, scorpion stings, and severe hypothermia
- Dehydration and drying of secretions which are difficult to cough out.
- Inadequacy or inability to cough due to muscular weakness and/or altered sensorium

Presence of thick, dry secretions leads to blocking of the airways, hypoventilation, hypoxemia, and increased work of breathing. Following steps may help to keep the airway clear and maintain a good bronchial hygiene:

- Adequate hydration
- Liquefaction of secretions through humidification of inspired air/gases and nebulization.
- Chest physical therapy to promote bronchial hygiene—chest percussion and vibration methods

OXYGENATION

Correction of hypoxemia is the most critical goal of management of respiratory failure. One aims to achieve an arterial oxygen tension of 60 mm Hg or arterial oxygen saturation of about 90% for purpose of adequate tissue oxygenation. High concentrations of inspired oxygen (FiO_2) are necessary in cases of acute respiratory failure with rapid hypoxemia. FiO_2 should be however reduced as soon as possible to avoid the risk of oxygen toxicity due to damage to the alveolo-capillary membrane.

There is no need to achieve a normal or even super normal PO_2 results in the O_2 content of the blood in the presence of chronic respiratory failure when the simplest method and the lowest inspired oxygen tension will achieve the desired result. Uncontrolled oxygen supplementation may end with oxygen toxicity. Moreover, any increase in arterial PO_2 carries significant risk of respiratory depression due to CO_2 narcosis in patients with chronic hypercapnia such as those of COPD. It is therefore important to adjust the inspired oxygen concentration at the lowest level, which is just adequate for tissue oxygenation.

Oxygen can be delivered with the help of the nasal cannula, simple face mask, non-rebreathing mask or high-flow nasal cannula. ARS and mechanical ventilation may be required if hypoxemia is persistent and nonresponsive to conventional oxygen administration. Extracorporeal membrane oxygenation may be needed in refractory cases.

CORRECTION OF HYPERCAPNIA AND RESPIRATORY ACIDOSIS

Presence of hypercapnia and respiratory acidosis generally indicates the presence of a chronic disease. This may also occur in acute conditions of hypoventilation due to respiratory depression or arrest or during an acute exacerbation of a chronic condition. Correction of hypercapnia is achieved by treating the underlying cause or providing assisted ventilatory support.

ASSISTED RESPIRATORY SUPPORT

Assisted respiratory support is required for management of respiratory failure if it does not improve with other treatments. There are three primary goals of ventilatory support:

1. Correction of hypoxemia
2. Correction of hypercapnia and acute respiratory acidosis
3. Providing rest to the ventilatory muscles

There are two main types of ARS which are available for these patients:

1. Noninvasive respiratory support (NIV): NIV is provided with the help of a tight-fitting face mask without tracheal intubation/via upper airway. There are different modes of NIV which include the bi-level positive airway pressure (BiPAP) and continuous positive airways pressure (CPAP) ventilation. It is essential that the patients should be conscious and have an intact airway with the presence of airway protective reflexes. NIV lowers the reduce complications rate, duration of ICU stay, and mortality in patients with mild to moderate respiratory failure. It is more effective in acute respiratory failure due to COPD than other causes.

2. Invasive respiratory support: Invasive respiratory support is provided with the help of endotracheal intubation. Intubation is associated with several complications (**Box 2**) and should therefore be undertaken only in the presence of the following situations:

- Persistent hypoxemia despite receiving maximum oxygen therapy
- Hypercapnia with impairment of consciousness
- Respiratory muscle fatigue

Ventilatory management: Different physiotherapeutic interventions have been used to increase the ventilatory function by removing excessive pulmonary secretions and prevent atelectasis in mechanically ventilated patients. Early physiotherapy is also shown to improve ventilator-related complications and help an early weaning. Body positioning (such as side-lying, semirecumbent or upright) is an important intervention which helps to improve ventilation/perfusion matching (V/Q), promote mucociliary clearance, and improve aeration via increased lung volumes. Overall, this will help to reduce the work of breathing. In particular, prone position in ARDS not only improves V/Q matching but also promotes redistribution of lung edema and increase functional residual capacity, thus causing an improvement in oxygenation.

Other physical measures which have been used to facilitate mucociliary clearance include the following:

- Chest percussion and postural drainage
- Repetitive suctioning
- Manual hyperinflation
- Manual shaking and vibration

Tracheostomy: Tracheostomy is performed whenever assisted ventilation gets prolonged beyond 7–10 days. Ventilation through the tracheostomy tube has its own advantages and disadvantages which have been discussed elsewhere in this book.

GENERAL MANAGEMENT

- **Management of fluids:** Adequate fluid balance is necessary for hemodynamic maintenance and adequate renal perfusion. Excess of fluid can lead to cardiac dysfunction and pulmonary edema.
- **Pharmacological treatment:** Drug treatment for the underlying diseases will continue as usual. Blood pressure and diabetes should be appropriately controlled. Nebulized bronchodilators are required to manage bronchospasm and airway hygiene.
  Other important medication includes the following:
  - Analgesics and sedatives to relieve pain and discomfort
  - Antibiotics to treat an infection: Choice of antibiotic and other antimicrobial drugs is an important decision. This will normally depend upon the hospital policy, culture and sensitivity reports of blood, endotracheal secretions, and/or other specimens and the local microbial epidemiology. Different hospitals normally follow the antibiotic-stewardship policy to prevent misuse and development of drug resistance.
  - Anticoagulant prophylaxis: For prevention of deep venous and pulmonary artery thromboembolism
- **Maintenance of nutrition:** It is important to maintain nutrition including the caloric intake, essential vitamins, minerals, and electrolytes. Regular monitoring is done for their levels and replacements given as per requirement. Caloric intake is similarly important for prevention of muscle mass and body weight.
- **Prevention of bed-sores:** Change in body position is frequently required to prevent the formation of pressure sores. Appropriate air mattresses are also helpful.
- **Care of bladder and bowels:** The bed-ridden patients often have urinary and/or fecal incontinence. Adequate attention should be given for their care. Urinary catheterization is necessary to take care of incontinence. Regular cleaning and change of bed sheets is also necessary. Bowel enema may be required in case of constipation.
- **Exercises:** It is important to maintain muscle tone and strength, joint mobility, and flexibility. Regular limb exercises (passive, active-assisted, and active) will reduce the effects of immobility as well as help to optimize oxygen transport. In addition, inspiratory muscle training will aid improvement of inspiratory muscle strength and facilitate weaning. Lastly, early mobilization should be encouraged as it improves overall body function and mobility.

PROGNOSIS

Prima facie, prognosis depends upon the cause of respiratory failure and associated complications. Advances in assisted ventilation and airway management have significantly improved prognosis. ARDS-related mortality rates have now been reduced to around 30–40% especially in the younger patients of <60 years of age. Mortality in cases of COPD and acute respiratory failure has significantly declined to 10% or so. Mortality in these patients is associated with antecedent comorbidities and poor nutritional status.

RECOMMENDED READINGS

1. Roussos C, Koutsoukou A. Respiratory failure. Eur Respir J Suppl. 2003;47:3s-14s.
2. Kaynar AM, Pinsky MR. Respiratory Failure. Drugs & Diseases > Critical Care. [online] Available from https://emedicine.medscape.com/article/167981
3. Paul AS, Agarwal R. Respiratory failure. In: Jindal SK (Ed). Textbook of Pulmonary and Critical Care Medicine, 2nd edition. New Delhi: Jaypee Brothers Medical Publishers; 2017. pp. 1479-87.
4. Keddissi JI, McCaffree DR. Acute respiratory distress syndrome. In: Jindal SK (Ed). Text Book of Pulmonary and Critical Care Medicine, 2nd edition. New Delhi: Jaypee Brothers; 2017. pp. 1488-500.
5. Rochwerg B, Brochard L, Elliott MW, Hess D, Hill NS, Nava S. Official ERS/ATS clinical practice guidelines: noninvasive ventilation for acute respiratory failure. Eur Respir J. 2017;50(2):1602426.
6. Agarwal R, Gupta R, Aggarwal AN, Gupta D. Noninvasive positive pressure ventilation in acute respiratory failure due to COPD vs other causes: effectiveness and predictors of failure in a respiratory ICU in North India. Int J Chron Obstrut Pulmon Dis. 2008;3(4):737-43.
7. Jindal SK, Aggarwal AN, Gupta D. Adult respiratory distress syndrome in the tropics. Clin Chest Med. 2002;23:445-55.
8. Jindal SK. Oxygen Therapy: Important considerations. Ind J Chest Dis Allied Sci. 2008;50:97-107.
9. Scala R, Pisani L. Noninvasive ventilation in acute respiratory failure: which recipe for success? Eur Respir Rev. 2018;27(149).
10. Calverley PM. Respiratory failure in chronic obstructive pulmonary disease. Eur Respir J Suppl. 2003;47:26s-30s.

CHAPTER

224

Pulmonary Rehabilitation

Deepak Talwar

ABSTRACT

Pulmonary rehabilitation (PR) can be defined as a structured multimodality program which includes aerobic exercise training and strength training in patients with chronic pulmonary diseases to improve exercise tolerance. It is not just exercise training but also disease-related education, nutritional advice and support, psychological mediations, as well as incorporating better self-care interventions to enhance their daily life activities. PR programs have grown considerably in recent years and demonstrate improvements in dyspnea, exercise performance, and quality of life (QoL) in individual patients. Most of research in PR has been done in chronic obstructive pulmonary disease (COPD), where it has become standard of practice to be a part of treatment regimen in B, C, and D group of patients. Recent research finds its benefits being seen in other chronic respiratory diseases, e.g., interstitial lung disease (ILD), chronic asthma, bronchiectasis, pre- and post-lung surgery, and chest wall disorders with common denominator being persistent respiratory symptoms especially breathlessness on exertion despite adequate and appropriate pharmacotherapy.

The programs are historically used for outpatients delivered in hospital, community centers, or at home for more severe patients with hospital-based programs being standardized with protocol of exercise training 2–4 times a week and single session lasting 1–2 hours which includes all interventions concurrently or sequentially for 9–12 weeks. Energy conservation breathing techniques, inspiratory muscle training (IMT), chest physiotherapy, postural drainage, and muscle kinetics augmenting measures. Scientific and evidence-based exercise training is the backbone of any successful PR program as it targets individualized clinically meaningful outcomes. Referred patients undergo assessments on the basis of clinical examination, laboratory data, exercise capacity, and health-related questionnaires by PR team which includes respiratory therapist who is essential for any PR activity. On the basis of baseline assessments, an individualized PR program with predefined goals is designed for every patient and constantly monitored throughout the program as it may require changes to achieve expected targets.

On completion of PR program, outcome assessments are done and further advice is given to patient to maintain lifestyle changing behavior and increased physical activity in order to achieve improved long-term health-related self-care. Beneficial effects of PR are lost over 6–12 months and require strategies to maintain sustained improvements. This may include repeat enrollment's in PR programs periodically or continue once a week maintenance PR visit or extending PR at home or community level. Despite guidelines, PR is being utilized by <1% of needy patients due to deficiencies in early referral, acceptance by patient, availability of PR services, travel issues, finances, and time constraints. In view of these limitations and World Health Organization (WHO) goal to provide "rehabilitation" to all, alternative modalities to deliver PR programs are being developed and home PR with or without tele-PR services is being studied. COVID pandemic opened doors for virtual platforms and PR is also being utilized as its becoming more acceptable to large population in India.

"All progress takes place outside the comfort zone"

—Michael J Bobak

INTRODUCTION

Pulmonary rehabilitation is an integral and essential component of clinical management and health maintenance of patients with chronic respiratory disease who remain symptomatic or continue to have decreased function despite standard medical treatment **(Fig. 1)**. PR is a complex multidisciplinary intervention with variable composition as per needs and requirements of an individual respiratory patient. Components of PR, e.g., breathing techniques, walking exercises, muscle training, bronchial hygiene, disease-related education, and respiratory medications including oxygen have been included for many centuries as a part of good medical care.

In 1974, American Collage of Chest Physicians gave its name and in 1981, American Thoracic Society (ATS) published first official statement on PR. 6-minute walk test and respiratory-related QoL questionnaires led to clinical trials demonstrating effectiveness in patients particularly in COPD. In 1991, Casaburi demonstrated dose-dependent effect of exercise training on physiological benefit in COPD and subsequently it was shown to improve exertional dyspnea. In 2001 on the basis of unequivocal impact of PR in COPD not only on exercise capacity and QoL but also

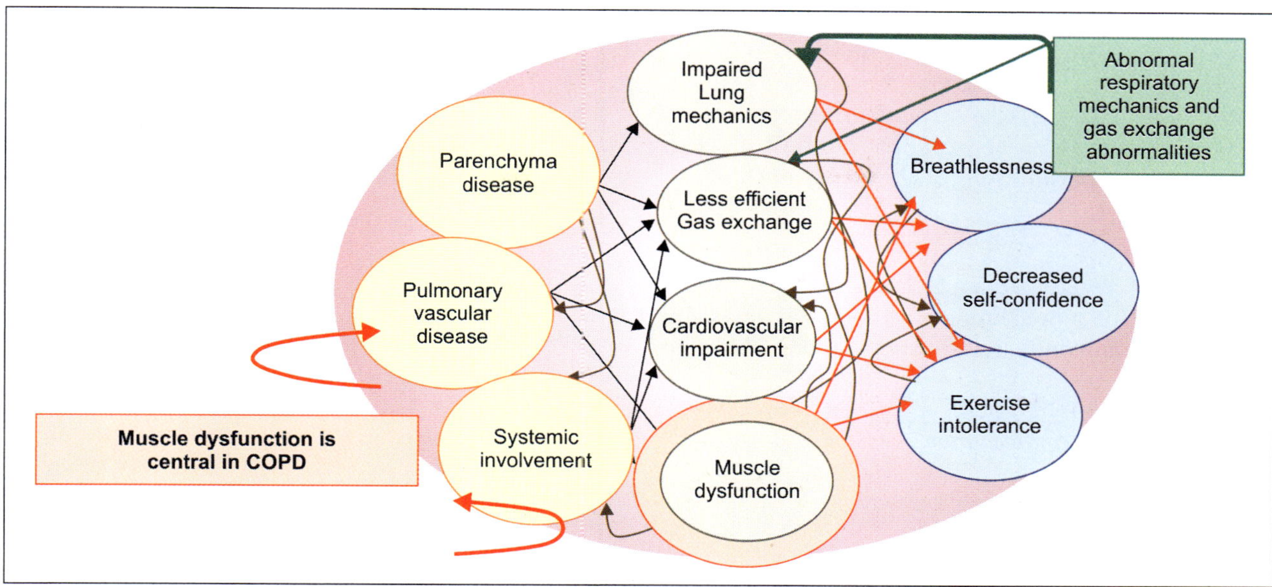

FIGURE 1: Breathlessness in chronic obstructive pulmonary disease (COPD) is multifactorial and muscle dysfunction is a key player which remains unaddressed in pharmacotherapy and is targeted in pulmonary rehabilitation.

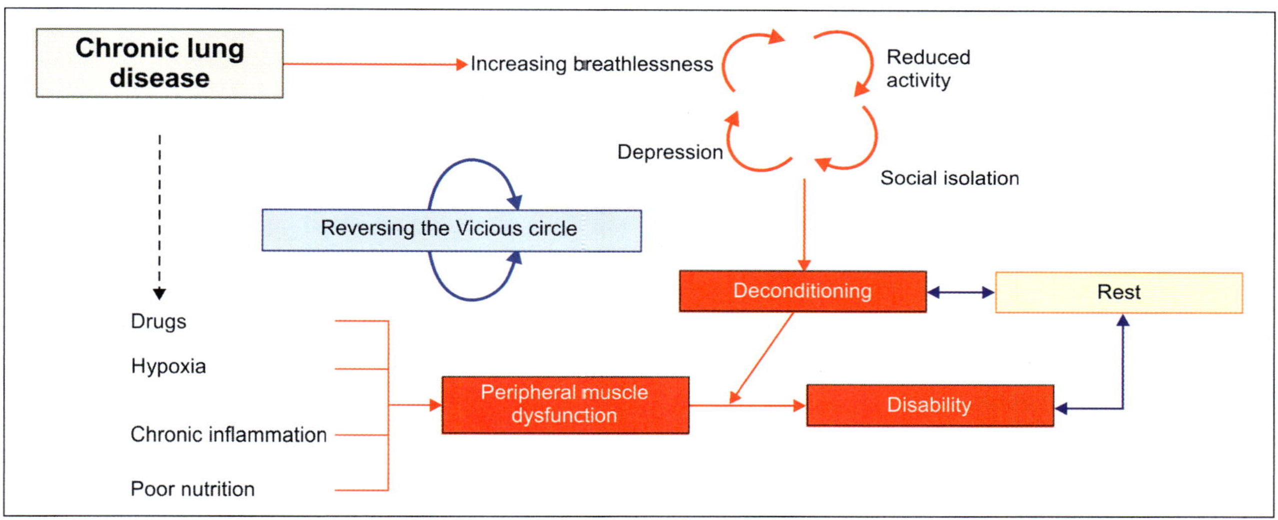

FIGURE 2: The relationship between chronic lung disease, muscle deconditioning, and disability.

on subsequent need for healthcare, it was recommended in management of COPD in Global Initiative for Chronic Obstructive Lung Disease (GOLD) 2–4 stages as an element of nonpharmacological treatment. Also, as physical inactivity is related to shortened survival and recurrent hospitalizations, PR targets in improving activity with collateral benefit (**Fig. 2**).

DEFINITION

In 2013, ATS/European Respiratory Society (ERS) statement on PR is closest to workable definition of PR. It is a comprehensive intervention based on a thorough patient assessment followed by patient-tailored therapies, which include, but are not limited to, exercise training, education and behavioral change, designed to improve physical and emotional condition of persons with chronic respiratory disease, and to promote the long-term adherence to health enhancing behaviors (**Fig. 3**). In short, PR is an entity on

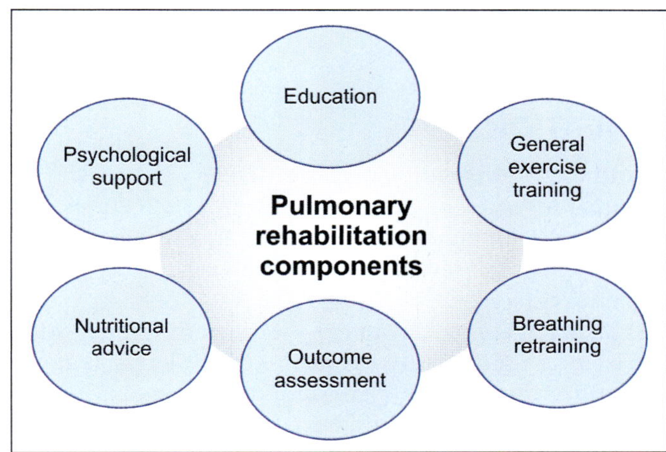

FIGURE 3: Pulmonary rehabilitation is a multifaceted program with essential component being exercise training but many other supports to overall improve quality of life.

its own though it combines different therapies delivered by different professionals with relevant expertise, e.g., respiratory physician, respiratory therapist, dietician, education counselor, exercise physiologist etc., also, PR as intervention is given to the patient at multiple times in disease trajectory of chronic lung disease.

GOALS

The goals of PR are dependent on patients' needs depending upon functional limitations and disabilities and hence have to be individualized for each patient. The main goals are to:

- Minimize symptom burden
- Maximize exercise performance
- Promote autonomy
- Increase participation in everyday activities
- Decrease psychological symptoms
- Improve health-related QoL

Hence, in effect PR targets to achieve long-term health-enhancing behavior change in an individual. However, primary goal remains to improve exercise capacity and there by enhance overall QoL of patients with chronic respiratory impairment.

TEAM

Pulmonary rehabilitation is implemented by a dedicated, interdisciplinary team, which includes generally following specialists depending upon availability and resource utilization:

- Respiratory physicians
- Exercise physiologists
- Respiratory therapists
- Physiotherapists
- Psychologists/Behavioral specialist
- Nutritionists
- Occupational therapists
- Social workers
- Patient educator or nurse practitioner

However, resources and availability of healthcare professionals limit most of PR programs and hence, some of the teammates play dual or more roles to fill in for nonavailable staff members.

INDICATIONS

Although conventionally any COPD patient who is symptomatic is to be referred to PR but indications are broadening with more research in this area with beneficial effects being reported in patients with various non-COPD respiratory diseases.

Pragmatic approach would be to refer any patient with persistent respiratory symptoms, e.g., dyspnea, fatigue, and/or functional impairment despite optimized available therapy and not restricting to COPD or obstructive lung diseases. Even, patients with restrictive lung diseases secondary to any cause including ILD with above said clinical indications should also be referred to PR.

TABLE 1 Indications and contraindications of pulmonary rehabilitation.

Indications	Contraindications
• Persistent respiratory symptoms, especially dyspnea • Limitation of functional status despite optimal medication • Impaired health-related quality of life • Decreased occupational performance • Psychosocial problems attendant on the underlying respiratory illness • Difficulty with medical regimen • Difficulty performing day-to-day activities • Nutritional depletion • Increased use of medical resources • Gas exchange abnormalities	• Conditions that substantially increase risk during rehabilitation, e.g., unstable angina • Conditions that substantially interfere with rehabilitative process • Uncontrolled diabetes • Psychiatric illness, e.g., dementia • Severe exercise-induced hypoxemia, not correctable with oxygen supplementation • Inability to exercise due to orthopedic or other reasons

Complementing these general recommendations, there are indications where PR should be prescribed without any hesitation, i.e., patients recently discharged from hospital with COPD-acute exacerbation (AE) and patients with Medical Research Council (MRC) grade 3 dyspnea or greater regardless of lung functions impairment. Patients with bronchiectasis, chronic bronchial asthma etc., are also referred to PR program.

Broadly absolute contraindication would be a completely demotivated patient or if exercise would be painful/potentially dangerous, but still risk versus benefit should be considered in each such case. Comorbidities are no longer considered as CI to PR and adaptation in PR may be required to address such issues, e.g., depression or anxiety by incorporating psychiatrist or psychologist or associated coronary artery disease (CAD) requiring physician for assessment and planning. Other concurrent conditions which may interfere with PR process or places patient at substantial risk during exercise should be stabilized prior to taking them in PR. Cases with orthopedic conditions may require modifications in exercise regimens in PR program (**Table 1**).

SELECTION CRITERIA

This depends upon the patients who are likely to benefit from PR and since results of rehabilitation may improve many dimensions, patient referral will vary. As improvement in exercise capacity is major positive outcome, any respiratory patient who is breathlessness on exertion, would be an ideal candidate for PR but challenge is to identify responders, which too will vary at different dimensions. Patients with reduction in functional capacity, QoL or occupational/daily activities-related performance, may indicate good responders as clear and achievable goals are known prior to initiation of PR. Generally, patients with preexisting skeletal muscle weakness, poor exercise capacity with better ventilator parameters and are relatively young, do better in PR. These points are useful as PR is labor intensive and time-consuming with financial implications.

PATIENT ASSESSMENTS

At the beginning of PR, it is crucial to have patient-physician interaction with clear dialog where patient is to be clarified about limitations of pharmacotherapy and goals to be set by chest physician on the basis of expectations by the patient and realistic outcomes possible as per the current knowledge of PR. Patient assessment is on-going process and done even if conducted on previous visits. Complete assessment of patient begins with checking medical history with particular reference to respiratory as well as neuromuscular and orthopedic problems, comorbidities, smoking, or other addictions as they may pose challenge during PR. Baseline literacy, hearing, vision, and cognitive ability require to be looked into as these would influence outcomes of PR. Symptom assessment of dyspnea, fatigue, cough, chest pain, or sputum allows PR team to know the burden of disease to set outcome expectations. Medication history is needed not only to see if it is optimized to the disease but also if any special care in PR to be provided, e.g., corticosteroids, bronchodilators or diuretics, insulin etc.

Physical examination findings of respiratory distress, breathing pattern, and oxygenation status are to be recorded as would need to be addressed during PR. Diagnostic test results to be reviewed include spirometry, oximetry, both at rest as well as at walk, chest X-ray (CXR) and if available 6-minute walk test, or cardiopulmonary exercise test report. It is important to note body mass index (BMI), serum albumin, fluids intake or restrictions, and detailed dietary history with fat-free mass estimation to target skeletal muscle strengthening in PR and baseline electrocardiogram (EKG) and echocardiogram (ECHO) to know cardiac limitations during PR if any. Exercise capacity assessment includes physical limitations if any, gait and balance, exercise tolerance and related hypoxia etc., factors which would influence exercise training plan in PR. Pain chest, limbs, or back is also worth noting as may become limiting factors in exercise program.

Finally, a brief history of activities of daily living (ADL) with reference to functional task performance, e.g., bathing, washing, changing clothes, leisure activities, and use of supplemental oxygen during day-to-day work. Some PR programs include questionnaire (SGRQ, SF36, BODE Index etc.) at baseline to document improvement at the end of the program. Anxiety or depression assessment using simple questionnaires (PHQ-2 and 3) is included to identify any significant psychological impairment which would require special assistance (**Fig. 4**).

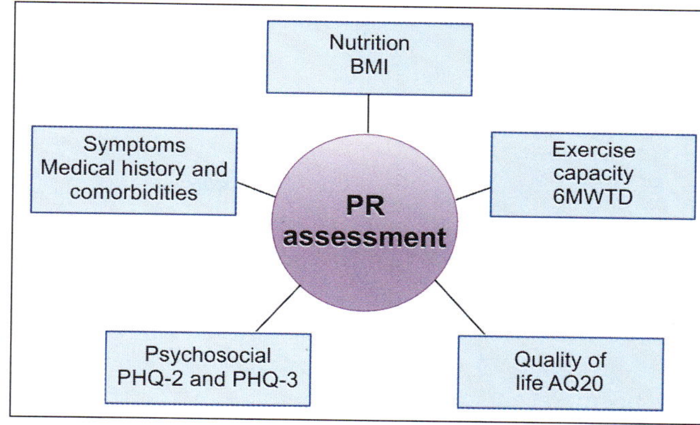

(AQ20: Airways Questionnaire 20; 6MWTD: 6-minute walk test distance; PHQ: patient health questionnaire)

FIGURE 4: Various assessments required prior to initiation of pulmonary rehabilitation in an individual patient.

At the end of this global assessment, depending upon rehabilitation potential PR team formulates goals both short term as well as long term which are individualized, measurable, patient centered and realistic, and being graded from excellent to poor.

It is sufficed to say that such exhaustive assessment would need multidisciplinary team work and coordination, as everything needs to be done in limited time with limited discomfort to the patient.

COMPONENTS

Pulmonary rehabilitation is not exercise training as includes many other aspects to improve overall functional capacity of the patients. A good PR program includes optimized medications and delivery, smoking cessation, education about disease and prognosis, self-management plan for AE and daily situations, nutritional support, energy conservation techniques, psychological counseling, behavior change, ADL training, home adaptation and aids, oxygen and noninvasive ventilation (NIV) therapy, mucus handling and bronchial hygiene, hormonal supplements, IMT etc.

DURATION

Ideally, rehabilitation should continue as long as gains are being made. There is no consensus on optimal duration of PR but it is ideally set by continued progress toward goals and optimization of benefit. In reality, it is also influenced by financial resources and traveling burden. Generally, longer programs are considered to produce greater gains and maintenance of benefits achieved on short term. But a minimum of 8 weeks is recommended to gain substantial benefit. Our study showed that as short as 3 weeks after discharge from hospital for COPD-AE is effective considering difficulties in sustaining long-term programs. Also, length of PR is also dependent on the setting, i.e., hospital based, community based, or home based and if one can be followed by the other as per convince and teams decisions. Two to three visits per week are recommended during PR.

LOCATION AND SETTINGS

Although programs have been conventionally developed where patient visits PR center in the hospital or clinic two or three times a week but PR has been shown to be effective inpatient settings too. Recently, successful PR programs have demonstrated to be delivered in other settings, e.g., primary care (physiotherapists clinic), home, or secondary care (community or nursing homes) and systemic review has confirmed beneficial effects of home-based PR but such programs are to be considered for most severely disabled provided supervision by experts is available which is rare.

PATIENT COMPLIANCE

As with any therapy in medicine, long-term compliance rate is not excellent in PR also. Nearly 23% dropouts are reported with primary issues related to travel, family, finances, or due to exacerbations or hospitalization related to primary disease or unrelated health problems.

PRINCIPLES OF EXERCISE TRAINING

This is one of the most important components of PR and is based on following principles in exercise training:

- *Intensity*: Higher intensity produces greater results (e.g., >60% of VO_{2max} or at 60–80% W_{max}).
- *Specificity*: Only muscles trained produce the desired effect.
- *Reversibility*: Stopping regular exercise training decreases the effect.
- Exercise regimen is to improve endurance, strength, or both.

Duration, frequency, mode, and intensity of exercise prescription are based on severity of disease, degree of conditioning, and initial exercise capacity. Aerobic endurance training whether given as high or low intensity would improve patient's ability to perform activities which require continuous effort for long periods, e.g., walking and optimal exercise plan would include cycle ergometry and treadmill walking. Generally biking induces less exercise induced hypoxia and hence more suitable for hypoxic patients. Interval training is an option for those who cannot sustain extended continuous high intensity exercise in the form of rest periods in between or alternating periods of high- and low-intensity exercises.

Strength or resistance training is used for explosive activities which require excessive strength in bursts for short period of time, e.g., sprinting, jumping, and lifting weights. Exercise targets local muscle groups with reduced mass and strength of peripheral muscles required to perform these activities and as collateral benefit improves bone mineral density. This training improves muscle mass and results in improved exercise tolerance as patient experiences less dyspnea. Training is done using free weights, squatting, stair climbing, elastic resistive bands, machine weights, or simply repeated sit and stand from chair. Lesser weights and more repetitions improve endurance and higher weights with fewer repetitions improve muscle mass.

Exercise plan targets both upper and lower limb muscles as upper limb muscles are required for daily activities like dressing bathing and performing house hold activities while lower limbs muscle dysfunction is main cause of exercise limitation in respiratory patients and provides best physiological gains in PR.

Inspiratory muscle training is needed as there weakness leads to more perception of dyspnea and hence impaired exercise tolerance. Training includes voluntary isocapnic hyperventilation, inspiratory threshold, or resistive loading. This is more useful, if patient has underlying COPD or reduced respiratory muscle strength demonstrated by measurement of maximum inspiratory pressures.

NUTRITIONAL SUPPORT

Weight as well as fat-free mass (FFM) estimates of the patient needs consideration in PR. Caloric supplementation is provided to meet the extra demands for energy from PR and if any deficit preexisting (BMI < 21 kg/m^2). Indian guidelines also recommend to monitor BMI periodically to see the effect of nutritional support, as it has also been shown to improve QoL.

PSYCHOLOGICAL SUPPORT

Prevalence of anxiety and depression in COPD is 36% and 40%, respectively and depression is known to increase the risk of AE and hospitalizations in COPD. Patient may be provided with vocational counseling, education strategies to cope stress, and involvement of family members to resolve conflicts. However, patients with severe psychological problems need formal evaluation by psychiatrist.

EDUCATION SUPPORT

Patient education is an important part of PR and topics include but not limited to, are, normal lungs structure and function, disease aspects, smoking cessation, avoidance of potential risk factors of irritants and allergens, clearance of secretions, energy conservation techniques, appropriate inhaler technique, breathing strategies, benefits of drugs prescribed and compliance, recognition of worsening of disease, and initial self-management plan.

OUTCOME ASSESSMENTS

Outcome of PR is done either on real time or during the course of the program or at the end of the program by recall. Generally, QoL, dyspnea indices, and functional status parameters (6 MWT, BODE index, CAT etc.) are evaluated.

LONG-TERM/MAINTENANCE

Benefits appear to diminish over 6–12 months after discontinuation of PR, and it is due to:

- Decrease in treatment adherence, especially to long-term regular exercise

- Progression of underlying disease
- Development of comorbidities
- Acute exacerbations

Benefits can be maintained by establishing ongoing communication of the patient with PR team through, weekly telephone calls and monthly reinforcement visits, or weekly supervised outpatient-based exercise plus unsupervised home exercise. Other strategies include: Continuous rehabilitation, maintenance programs, and repeated courses. It is not clear what form maintenance therapy should take or how it should be applied. More research in this area is needed. Repeating a course of rehabilitation does seem to have the ability to reproduce the short-term gain but without long-term advantage.

HOME-BASED PR

Home-based PR is an alternative model that could improve uptake and access. Initial reports suggested that home-based PR is safe and may improve clinical outcomes; however, these studies had limitations due to trial methods and protocols. As a result, there has been little uptake in clinical practice, with home-based PR offered in <5% of centers worldwide **(Fig. 5)**. Present pandemic has affected future research and also need for more home-based programs. A recent home-based PR program by Holland et al., using minimal resources and little direct supervision, has been shown to deliver short-term improvements in functional exercise capacity and health-related QoL that are at least equivalent to conventional center-based PR in COPD patients. QoL outcomes were also equivalent at 12 months following program completion. More work is being done to evaluate essential components as well as duration of such programs but appears to be a way forward in providing PR in India.

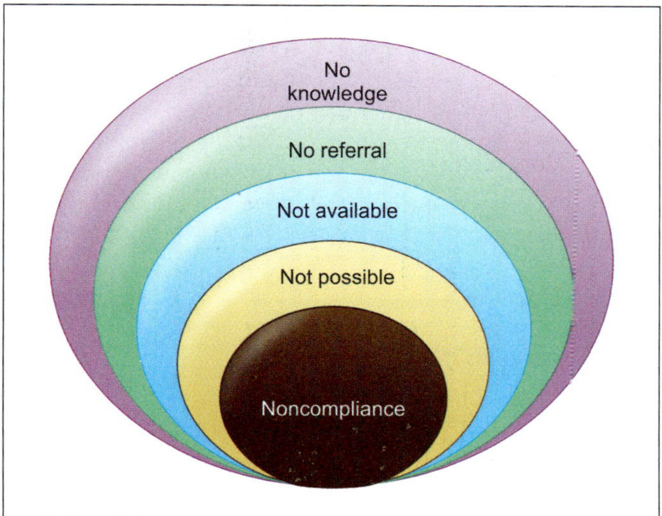

FIGURE 5: Barriers in implementing pulmonary rehabilitation (PR) from identifying patient for PR to referral, acceptance, availability, workability and managerial as well as long-term understandings of the process.

VIRTUAL PR

Considering limitations in providing PR to large number of needy patients and looking at vast geography of our country, need for novel alternative models of PR is required to improve both equity of access and patient-related outcomes. Present COVID times made tele- and video consultations acceptable and patient friendly and work is going on providing virtual PR services, which can reach majority of needy patients eliminating there need for visit to hospitals and rehabilitation centers. Preliminary data suggests that tele-PR is effective and needs more large scale studies to implement it on wide scale. But it would require support of sufficient trained staff to provide such guidance without compromising safety of the patients. However, it would be premature to conclude that virtually supervised home-based PR program may be the future of PR.

FUTURE PERSPECTIVE

Pulmonary rehabilitation addresses the systemic effects of chronic respiratory disease, which are complex and involve peripheral muscle dysfunction. Although in COPD role of PR has been established beyond doubt and has been shown to be far superior to any other therapy at patient-oriented multiple outcome areas, its role is in other chronic respiratory diseases is evolving. Recently role of PR has been extended from stable patients to patients in hospitals and immediately after discharge while being treated for exacerbation.

PR has also been recommended early in critical illness with neuromuscular stimulation started in mechanically ventilated patients. Also, data from pooled clinical trials in COPD showed that physical inactivity is also reported in mild and early COPD, PR is being recommended in these patients also. Realizing difficulties of traveling to PR centers, home-based and community-based programs are being developed to circumvent these problems and extend benefit to many more patients. Furthermore, the internet and telemonitoring have advanced scope of PR further where it can be assisted remotely.

RECOMMENDED READINGS

1. Casaburi R. A brief history of pulmonary rehabilitation. Respir Care. 2008;53:1185-9.
2. Zuwallack R. A history of pulmonary rehabilitation back to future. Pneumonol Alergol Pol. 2009;77:298-301.
3. Spruit MA, Singh SJ, Garvey C, ZuWallack R, Nici L, Rochester C, et al. ATS/ERS Task Force on Pulmonary Rehabilitation. An official American Thoracic Society/ European Respiratory Society statement: key concepts and advances in pulmonary rehabilitation. Am J Respir Crit Care Med. 2013;188(8):e13-64.
4. American Association of Cardiovascular and Pulmonary Rehabilitation. Guidelines for pulmonary rehabilitation programs, 3rd Edition. United States: Human Kinetics; 2004.

5. ZuWallack RL. Selection criteria and outcome assessment in pulmonary rehabilitation. Monaldi Arch Chest Dis. 1998;53:429-37.
6. Hornikx M, Van Remoortel H, Demeyer H, Marcal Camillo CA, Decramer M, Janssens W, et al. The influence of comorbidities on the outcomes of pulmonary rehabilitation programs in patients with COPD; a systematic review. Biomed Res Int. 2013;2013:146148.
7. Ali MS, Talwar D, Jain SK. The effect of a short-term pulmonary rehabilitation on exercise capacity and quality of life in patients hospitalised with acute exacerbation of chronic obstructive pulmonary disease. Indian J Chest Dis Allied Sci. 2014;56:13-9.
8. Mendes de Oliveira JC, Studart Leitão Filho FS, Malosa Sampaio LM, de Oliveira AC, Hirata RP, Costa D, et al. Outpatient vs. home based pulmonary rehabilitation in COPD: a randomized controlled trial. Multidiscip Respir med. 2010;5:401-8.
9. Nici L. Adherence to a pulmonary rehabilitation program: start by understanding the patient. COPD. 2012;9:445-6.
10. Gloecki R, Marinov B, Pitta F. Practical recommendations for exercise training in patients with COPD. Eur Respir Rev. 2013;22:178-86.
11. Smith K, Cook D, Guyatt GH, Madhavan J, Oxman AD. Respiratory muscle training in chronic airflow limitation: a meta-analysis. Am Rev Respir Dis. 1992;145:533-9.
12. Reis AL, Kaplan RM, Myers R, Prewitt LM. Maintenance after pulmonary rehabilitation in chronic lung disease; a randomized trial. Am J Respir Crit Care Med. 2003;167:880-8.

CHAPTER 225

COVID-19: Acute Respiratory Manifestations

Uma Mohan Krishnaswamy, Chitra Veluthat

ABSTRACT

COVID-19 infection, which is caused by the novel corona virus, has emerged as a pandemic over the past year and infected millions of people worldwide. The virus mainly spreads through droplets, aerosol, and contaminated surfaces. In 80% of patients, it presents in a "mild" form characterized by fever, sore throat, dry cough, and malaise. However, in 15–20% of patients, the disease manifests as "moderate" or "severe" pneumonia characterized by hypoxemic respiratory failure, multiorgan dysfunction, and a propensity for thrombotic events. Moderate and severe forms of disease are typically seen in the elderly and in those patients with comorbid illnesses like diabetes, ischemic heart disease, and chronic kidney disease as well as those on immunosuppressive medication.

Mild cases are advised symptomatic treatment and self-monitoring at home while moderate and severe cases are managed in a hospital setting. The mainstay of managing Coronavirus disease 2019 (COVID-19) is supportive and consists of symptomatic treatment, corticosteroids, thromboprophylaxis, and oxygen and ventilatory support; the last two modalities being reserved for moderate and severe cases. Antiviral agents, anti-interleukin-6 (IL-6) agents, and convalescent plasma are recommended on a case-by-case basis in moderate and severe cases.

Preventive measures include ensuring mask use, avoiding social gatherings, social distancing, and hand hygiene. Candidate vaccines are being trialed and are expected to be rolled out soon.

"Life is the art of drawing sufficient conclusions from insufficient premises"

—Samuel Butler

INTRODUCTION

Since the dawn of the 21st century, multiple outbreaks of viral illnesses transmitted from animal species to human beings have been reported. These include disease caused by the influenza virus and corona viruses [severe acute respiratory syndrome (SARS) and middle east respiratory syndrome (MERS)]. In the year 2020, nearly a century after the Spanish flu, yet another pandemic caused by a respiratory virus reared its ugly head and continues to hold the world in its vice-like grip. This pandemic, caused by a newly identified strain of the corona virus family, is known by the acronyms, COVID-19 or SARS-CoV-2 (Severe acute respiratory syndrome coronavirus 2) infection and is believed to have been transmitted to human beings from bats or pangolins.

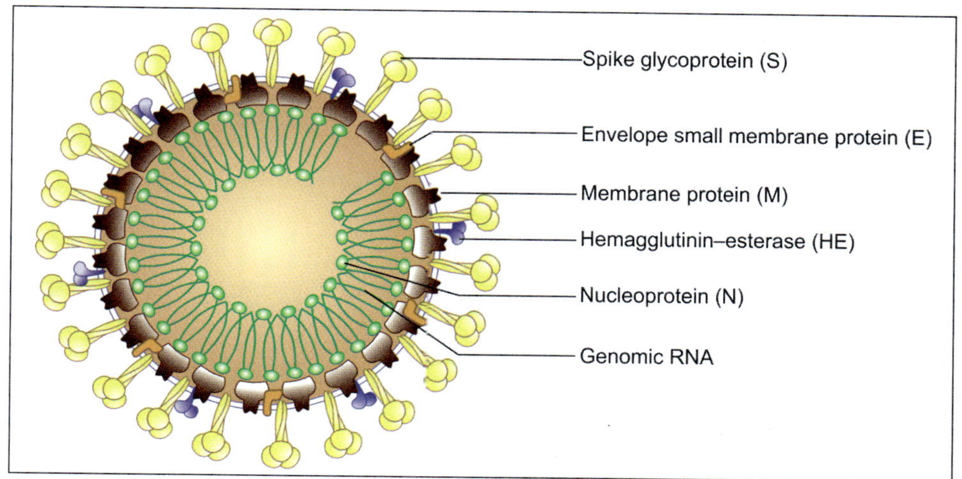

FIGURE 1: Structure of the SARS-CoV-2 virus.

Source: Adapted from Sous-vided L, Ghaderi S. Genotype and phenotype of COVID-19: Their roles in pathogenesis. J Microbiol Immunol Infect. 2020. Also available from https://doi.org/10.1016/j.jmii.2020.03.022

Although the virus enters through the upper respiratory tract, predominantly by droplet spread, it "homes" in the lower respiratory tract and can affect multiple organs other than its primary target, the lungs. In the following paragraphs, the pathophysiology, clinical presentation, and principles of management of the acute respiratory manifestations of COVID will be discussed.

VIROLOGY AND PATHOPHYSIOLOGY

Severe acute respiratory syndrome-corona virus 2 is a single-stranded enveloped RNA virus which belongs to the family of beta corona viruses (**Fig. 1**). It has four structural proteins—S (spike), M (membrane), E (envelope), and N (Nucleocapsid). The viral structural protein S (spike protein), a transmembrane trimetric glycoprotein, attaches to the angiotensin-converting enzyme 2 (ACE2) receptors present on the nasal epithelium and type 2 pneumocytes in the alveoli, where the expression of these receptors is high. Cleavage of the ACE2 receptor by TMPRSS2 (transmembrane protease) facilitates viral entry.

After viral entry into the alveolar epithelium, a release of inflammatory mediators [tumor necrosis factor (TNF)-alpha, IL-1, IL-6] occurs, resulting in a condition called cytokine response syndrome (CRS). The continued inflammatory response results in increased vascular permeability and hyaline membrane formation, which is similar to the pathophysiology of acute respiratory distress syndrome (ARDS).

In the later stages, the virus enters the pulmonary capillary endothelium resulting in endothelial injury, activation of the coagulation cascade, and thrombosis. Arterial thrombosis can also occur by a similar mechanism in COVID-19 infection.

The rapidly worsening respiratory failure in COVID-19 infection is attributable to the large surface area of lungs with type 2 alveolar epithelial cells which have an abundant expression of the ACE2 receptors. A dysregulated immune response to the infection as well as therapeutic modalities used to curb the inflammatory response can result in secondary infection severe sepsis and multiorgan dysfunction (**Flowchart 1** and **Fig. 2**).

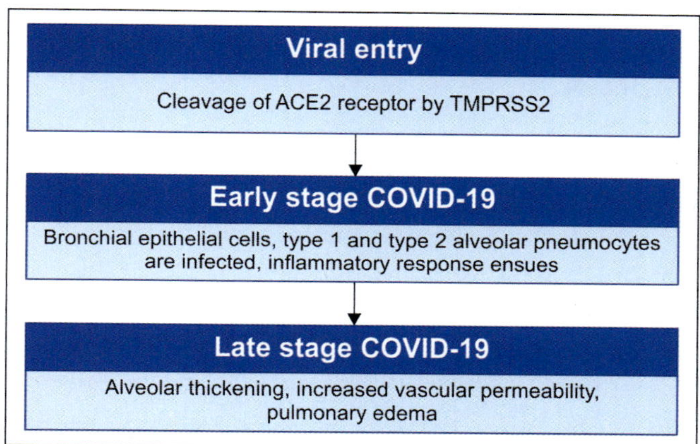

(ACE: angiotensin-converting enzyme; TMPRSS2: transmembrane serine protease 2)

FLOWCHART 1: Pathogenesis of COVID-19 disease.

CLINICAL PRESENTATION

Human-to-human transmission of COVID-19 occurs through droplets (coughing, sneezing, and sniffling) and rarely through touching contaminated surfaces. The mean incubation period is 5 days; however, it can vary from 2 to 11 days.

The clinical spectrum of COVID-19 infection varies from asymptomatic/presymptomatic to severe illness like ARDS and septic shock. Severity grading of COVID-19 pneumonia is depicted in **Table 1**.

Approximately 80% of patients present with mild symptoms. Fever (90%) is the most common presenting symptom followed by dry cough, shortness of breath, and fatigue. Some patients present with isolated gastrointestinal symptoms like vomiting and diarrhea. The other presentations

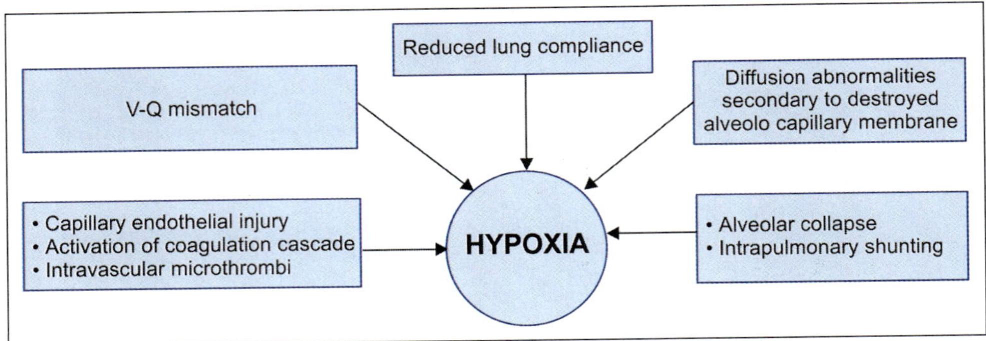

FIGURE 2: **Proposed mechanisms of hypoxia in COVID-19 infection.**

TABLE 1 Severity spectrum of COVID-19 infection.

Severity grade	Clinical features
Mild	• Uncomplicated upper respiratory tract infection • Normal room air saturation
Moderate	• Pneumonia, clinical features of dyspnea and/or hypoxia • SpO_2 90–94%, respiratory rate (RR) >24 breaths/min
Severe	Clinical signs of pneumonia and one of the following features: • RR >30 breaths/min • Severe respiratory distress • SpO_2 <90% • Acute respiratory distress syndrome • Sepsis • Septic shock

TABLE 2 Extrapulmonary manifestations of COVID-19 disease.

Heart	Myocarditis, cardiomyopathy, ventricular arrhythmias, and myocardial ischemia
Brain	Encephalopathy, acute cerebrovascular disease (8%)
Vascular complications	Arterial thrombi, deep vein thrombosis, and acute pulmonary thromboembolism (10–25%)
Liver	Elevated bilirubin, AST, and ALT
Kidney	Acute kidney injury
Dermatologic	Petechiae, erythematous rash, and vesicles

(ALT: alanine aminotransferase; AST: aspartate aminotransferase)

are fatigue, myalgia, sore throat, rhinorrhea, dizziness, anorexia, anosmia, and ageusia. Extrapulmonary manifestations are enumerated in **Table 2**.

A certain subset of patients progresses to severe illness due to coexistent risk factors, which include age (>65 years), diabetes mellitus, underlying cardiovascular disease, chronic lung or kidney disease, cancer, obesity, and use of immunosuppressive medications.

The clinical examination in patients with COVID-19 should focus on features of respiratory failure like tachypnea and cyanosis. Respiratory system examination may be normal in mild infection. The presence of localized findings like crepitations and bronchial breathing points toward pneumonia.

One should be aware of the entity, "Happy Hypoxia" in COVID-19, wherein a severely hypoxic patient with moderate-to-severe COVID pneumonia may not exhibit clinical symptoms or signs of respiratory distress and thus present late to the hospital.

Another complication to be considered in the presence of rapidly worsening hypoxia and hemodynamic instability is pulmonary thromboembolism, which can occur due to the procoagulant state triggered by the "cytokine storm" which occurs in severe COVID pneumonia. This "cytokine storm" occurs due to a dysregulated host immune response to the viral infection resulting in the release of cytokines [IL-1β, IL-6, IFN-γ, macrophage inflammatory protein-1 alfa (MIP-1α), and vascular endothelial growth factor (VEGF)].

DIAGNOSIS

The specimens collected for a definitive diagnosis of COVID-19 are upper and lower respiratory tract specimens (nasal, throat, nasopharyngeal swab, bronchoalveolar lavage, and tracheal aspirate). The samples collected are transported in an appropriate viral transport medium (VTM). The tests performed on the specimens as well as the utility of measuring serum antibody levels are discussed below.

Polymerase chain reaction: The diagnosis of COVID-19 infection is by identifying the viral RNA through reverse transcriptase-polymerase chain reaction (RT-PCR) from respiratory samples. The specimens collected are pharyngeal swab, nasopharyngeal swab, sputum, bronchoalveolar lavage, or tracheal aspirate. The sensitivity of the test varies (70–90%) with the highest sensitivity reported to be on the third day after the onset of symptoms.

Rapid antigen test: The rapid antigen detection test detects viral protein. However, is less sensitive than RT-PCR. If the pretest probability of COVID infection is high and rapid antigen test (RAT) is negative, it should always be followed by RT-PCR. The sensitivity of this test varies from 50 to 60%. In hospital settings the choice of testing is RT-PCR followed by RAT.

Antibody assay: Antibody assays, which are performed on serum samples, measure the host immune response to SARS-CoV-2 infection, wherein most of the antibodies are produced against the viral nucleocapsid (N) antigen. Enzyme-linked immunosorbent assay (ELISA)-based tests measuring immunoglobulin G (IgG) and IgM antibodies have a sensitivity of 96%. As antibodies start appearing in the serum after the first week of symptom onset, the assay is of use in patients suspected of having COVID infection but presenting more than a week after symptom onset.

Other tests: There are various serum inflammatory markers which are elevated in COVID-19 infection and are of prognostic value. These markers are enumerated in **Table 3**.

TABLE 3 Inflammatory markers in COVID-19 infection.

Test	Clinical significance
WBC count	• Lymphopenia—83% (seen in early infection) • ↑ NLR—neutrophil lymphocyte ratio (>3.3 is linked to disease severity and poor survival, low-cost marker)
D-dimer	Increased, associated with poor prognosis
Ferritin	Elevated, acute phase reactant, nonspecific
CRP	Increased, nonspecific
IL-6	Proinflammatory cytokine, potential therapeutic target
LDH	Increased in >50%, nonspecific
Procalcitonin	Normal or slightly elevated, if increased, secondary bacterial infection should be considered

(IL: interleukin)

Chest radiography: Chest radiograph will be normal in mild cases. In moderate pneumonia, bilateral peripheral and basal predominant infiltrates and airspace consolidation are seen. In severe pneumonia, the radiological presentation is like ARDS. The other radiological abnormalities seen are pneumomediastinum and pneumothorax. Pleural effusion is rare (**Figs. 3 A** and **B**).

Computed tomography thorax: In early stages of COVID pneumonia, computed tomography (CT) thorax may pick up abnormalities in up to 15% of cases despite chest radiography being normal. The typical findings in CT are peripheral, bilateral ground-glass opacities with or without consolidation or visible intralobular lines (crazy-paving) (**Figs. 4 A** to **D**).

Based on the recommendations of RSNA (Radiological Society of North America) along with Radiological Society of Netherlands, radiologists use the "CO-RADS" (COVID-19 Reporting and Data System) score to report the probability of COVID-19 pneumonia. CO-RADS 1 and 2 imply a very low suspicion of pneumonia, CO-RADS 3 being equivocal, and CO-RADS 4 and 5 being highly suspicious. The findings in a CO-RADS 5 CT include subpleural ground-glass opacities without fissural sparing and in a multifocal bilateral distribution. CT pulmonary angiogram will help in identifying pulmonary thromboembolism.

In addition to CO-RADS, there are CT severity scores which take into account the number of segments involved; these include the CT severity score (CT-SS) in which the total possible score is 25 and a score proposed by the RSNA, with a total possible score of 40. However, these severity scores require further validation.

MANAGEMENT

Multiple antivirals, anti-inflammatory, and immunomodulatory drugs have been used and subjected to the rigor of clinical trials since the beginning of the pandemic, but no drug has stood the test of time. In the initial stages of the pandemic, hydroxychloroquine has been used both for treatment and prophylaxis against the COVID-19

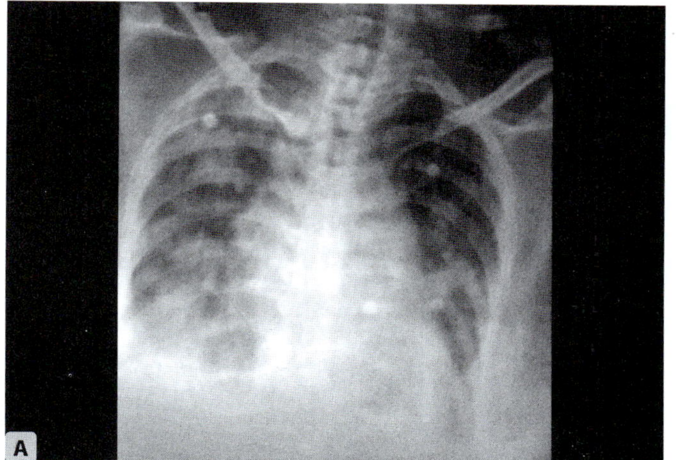

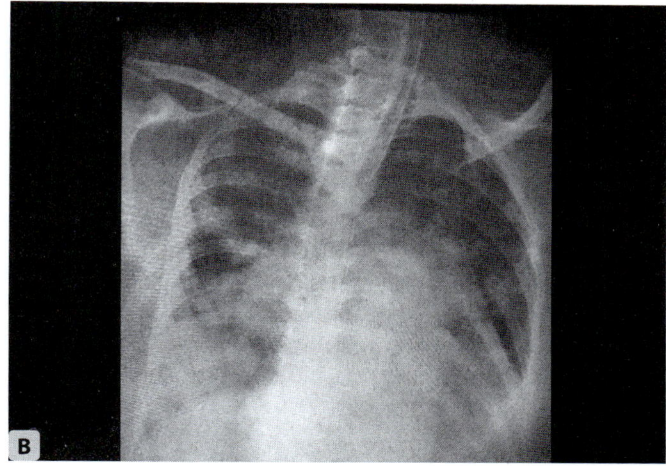

FIGURES 3 A & B: Chest radiograph in a patient with moderate and severe COVID-19.

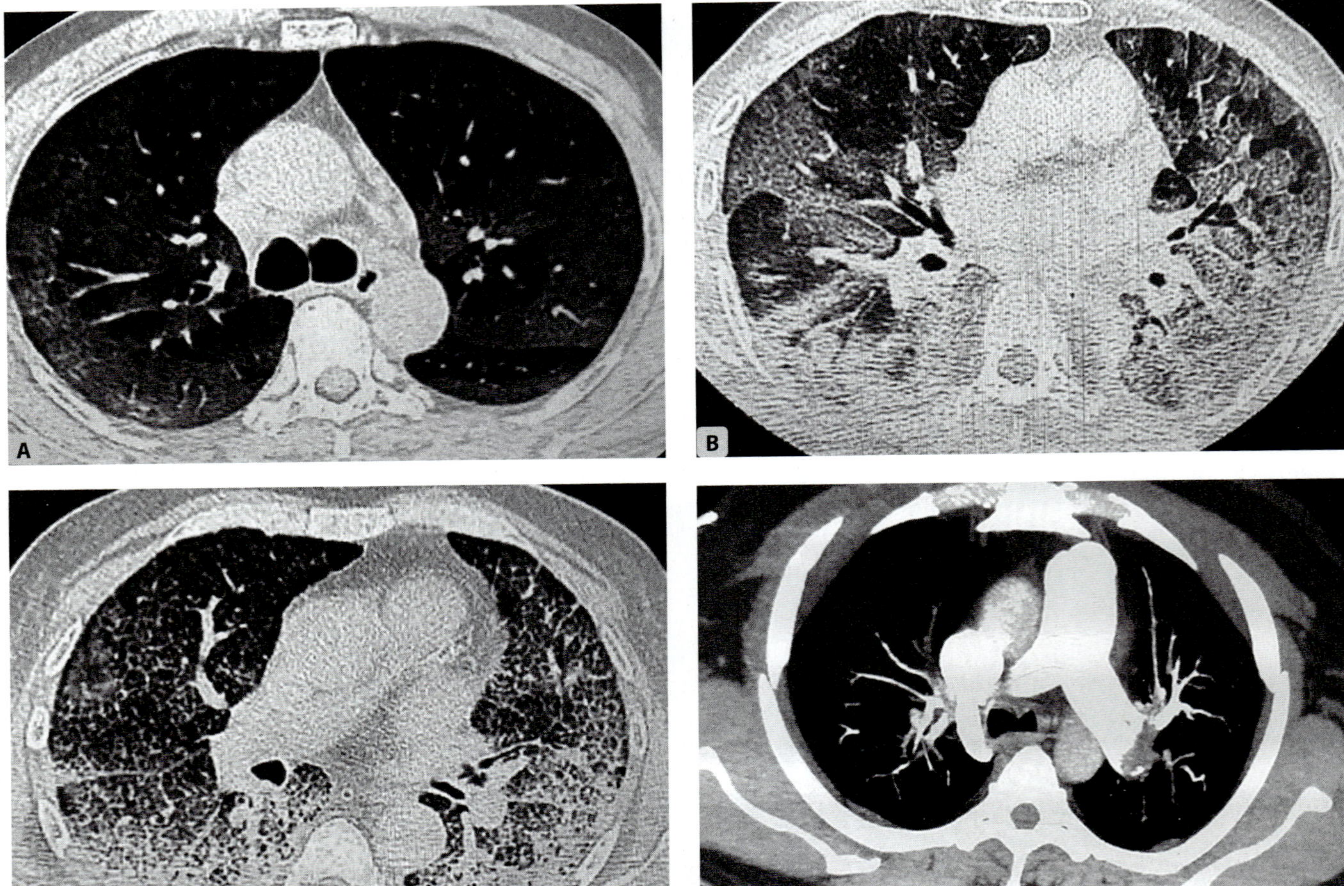

FIGURES 4 A to D: CT findings in COVID-19. (A and B) Bilateral peripheral ground-glass opacities. **(C)** Crazy paving pattern. **(D)** Filling defect in the left main pulmonary artery; pulmonary thromboembolism.

infection but was not found to confer a morality benefit in infected patients. Other drugs that received "Emergency Use Authorization" (EUA) are remdesivir, convalescent plasma, and tocilizumab. The next section covers current therapeutic options for COVID-19 infection.

GENERAL MEASURES

Oxygen therapy and supportive measures are the mainstay of COVID-19 treatment. Thromboprophylaxis with enoxaparin or unfractionated heparin (UFH) is recommended in all hospitalized patients with moderate and severe COVID-19 infection.

DRUGS USED IN THE MANAGEMENT

Systemic corticosteroids: The "RECOVERY" trial investigated the use of dexamethasone in the management of COVID-19 infection. Early institution of dexamethasone 6 mg once a day for 10 days was found to decrease the 28-day mortality in patients requiring supplemental oxygen. However, there was no survival benefit with dexamethasone in patients who presented with severe COVID and required mechanical ventilation. If dexamethasone is not available, other equivalent steroids like prednisolone or methylprednisolone can be used (**Table 4**).

TABLE 4	Drugs used in the management of COVID-19.
Steroids	Dexamethasone 6 mg intravenously (IV) once daily for 5–10 days (RECOVERY Trial)
Remdesivir	200 mg IV on day 1 followed by 100 mg IV od × 4 days. If no clinical improvement, total duration of 10 days
• Unfractionated heparin (UFH) or • Low-molecular-weight heparin	• Heparin 5,000 u subcutaneously (s/c) bid • Enoxaparin 40 mg s/c od UFH in ESRD (end-stage renal disease)

(RECOVERY Trial: The Randomized Evaluation of COVID-19 Therapy Trial)

Remdesivir: This is an intravenous nucleotide prodrug of an adenosine analogue. It inhibits viral RNA dependent RNA polymerase. It had shown inhibitory activity against SARS-CoV and MERS (**Table 4**).

Adaptive COVID-19 Treatment Trial (ACTT-1) is a double-blinded randomized controlled placebo trial which evaluated the efficacy of remdesivir in managing patients with COVID-19 infection. The drug, when compared to placebo, showed a benefit in the number of days to recovery in patients who required supplemental O_2.

In adults weighing >40 kg, the recommended dose is 200 mg intravenously once daily on day 1 followed by 100 mg intravenously for the next 4 days. If there is no clinical improvement after 5 days, the duration can be extended to a total of 10 days. For patients who are on mechanical ventilation or extracorporeal membrane oxygenation (ECMO), the recommended duration is 10 days. The drug is contraindicated in renal failure (eGFR <30 mL/min) and pregnancy.

Common side effects are nausea, vomiting, elevation in alanine aminotransferase (ALT) and aspartate aminotransferase (AST), hypersensitivity, and elevated prothrombin time. Hence monitoring of liver enzymes, renal function, and prothrombin time/international normalized ratio (PT/INR) is recommended prior to and during the administration of the drug.

Tocilizumab: This is an anti-IL-6 receptor monoclonal antibody which has been investigated in the treatment of COVID-19 infection. Preliminary data from trials failed to show any positive results for the use of tocilizumab. Off-label use of tocilizumab may be considered in patients with moderate disease with worsening oxygenation and mechanically ventilated patients who are not improving on steroids (Government of India guidelines). Secondary infections are known to occur after tocilizumab. It is recommended to test inflammatory markers [C-reactive protein (CRP), ferritin, IL-6] prior to administering tocilizumab. The dose of tocilizumab is a single dose of 8 mg/kg in 100 mL normal saline (NS) over 1 hour with dose ceiling of 800 mg.

Convalescent plasma: The plasma from patients recovered from COVID-19 was initially approved by FDA for EUA in the treatment of patients with COVID-19 infection. However, there are no clear-cut standards for screening plasma from the donors for neutralizing antibodies. Currently, in India off-label use of convalescent plasma is approved for those not improving on supplemental oxygen and systemic steroids.

However, results of large trials like PLACID and PlasmAr failed to show any positive results in patients administered convalescent plasma.

MANAGEMENT BASED ON SEVERITY

MILD COVID-19

The mainstay of treatment of mild infection is containment of infection and symptomatic treatment. This subset of patients may not require hospitalization; hence home isolation needs to be enforced with emphasis on adequate nutrition and appropriate hydration. It is also important to educate the patient regarding self-monitoring for worsening symptoms and hypoxia (**Table 5**).

MODERATE COVID-19

Hospitalization and isolation are recommended for moderate COVID-19 patients. "NEWS2" (**see Tables 2 and 3 in chapter 67**) score and "qSOFA" (quick sequential organ failure assessment) are the two scores which help in triaging patients with moderate COVID-19 pneumonia. NEWS2 consists of six simple physiological parameters that need to be monitored which helps in recognizing clinical deterioration and need for escalation of care. In qSOFA, three physiological parameters are measured as indicators of mortality, namely, respiratory rate >22, systolic BP <100 mm Hg and altered sensorium (**Table 5**).

TABLE 5 Management based on severity (Ministry of Health and Family Welfare, Government of India guidelines).

Severity category	Management
Mild	• Isolation • Symptomatic management • Adequate nutrition and appropriate hydration • Hydroxychloroquine may be considered in patients with comorbidities—in inpatient setting
Moderate	• Isolation • Investigations—Chest X-ray, complete blood count, and monitoring of vitals and SpO_2 • Target SpO_2 92–96% • Awake proning as indicated • Daily 12 lead ECG • Prophylactic anticoagulation • Steroids: Intravenous methylprednisolone 0.5–1 mg/kg or dexamethasone 0.1–0.2 mg/kg for 3 days (preferably within 48 h of admission or if oxygen requirement is increasing and if inflammatory markers are increased) • Control of comorbid conditions
Severe	Symptomatic management to continue • Adequate oxygenation • Intravenous steroids: Methylprednisolone 1–2 mg/kg or dexamethasone 0.2–0.4 mg/kg for 5–7 days • Prophylactic anticoagulation • Emergency use authorization Tocilizumab/convalescent plasma/remdesivir

Patients with respiratory failure (SpO_2 <94%) who do not require mechanical ventilation should be started on supplemental oxygen. The choice of oxygen delivery device can be made based on the requirement to achieve a target SpO_2 of >90%. The various oxygen delivery devices are nasal prongs, oxygen mask (full face, nonrebreathing mask, or venturi mask), and high-flow nasal cannula (HFNC). HFNC can be used when the patient's oxygen requirement is high. HFNC can provide oxygen at a flow rate as high as 60 L/min and a FiO_2 of 100%.

Noninvasive ventilation (NIV): When compared to HFNC offers benefit in patients with type 2 respiratory failure or when there are other indications for positive pressure ventilation like cardiogenic pulmonary edema. It is preferred to give NIV through a nonvented mask with a double limb circuit and an antiviral filter in the expiratory limb to reduce the risk of aerosolization and nosocomial spread of COVID-19.

Awake prone positioning: Awake prone positioning in COVID-19 is recommended in case of hypoxia to ventilate the dorsal part of lungs and open the collapsed alveoli. Contraindications to awake prone positioning are hemodynamic instability, severe hypoxia requiring mechanical ventilation, recent abdominal surgery or unstable spine.

Protocol for awake proning: The patient is advised to rotate position from prone to right and left lateral decubitus to sitting, each session of 30–120 minutes each.

Management of severe COVID-19 pneumonia: Patients who are in respiratory distress and not improving on NIV/HFNC should be electively intubated. Appropriate precautions for intubation are a must to prevent nosocomial spread. This includes intubation by the personnel skilled in airway management in a negative pressure room with minimum number of personnel for assistance and appropriate personal protective equipment. The ventilatory strategies in severe COVID-19 pneumonia are the same as that of ARDS and are based on the ARDSNet protocol. Low tidal volume (4–8 mL/kg) and high positive end-expiratory pressure (PEEP) targeting a plateau pressure of <30 cm H_2O are recommended. Prone position ventilation in case of severe hypoxia (PaO_2/FiO_2 <150 mm Hg) is also indicated for at least 12–16 hours per session.

Supportive measures in critically ill COVID-19 patients are like that of any other critically ill ARDS patient and include fluid management, appropriate antibiotics, thromboprophylaxis, and management of nonrespiratory organ dysfunction. Along with these measures, it is important to continue physiotherapy and nutrition in all patients. Management principles in critically ill COVID-19 patients are enumerated in **Figure 5**.

Infection control in the ICU

- Aerosol-generating procedures in the ICU–adequate PPE and negative pressure room

Hemodynamics

- Balanced crystalloids, monitoring with lactate and capillary refill time
- Noradrenaline—vasopressor of choice followed by vasopressin
- Low-dose corticosteroids in refractory shock

Ventilation

- HFNC preferred to NIV
- Lung protective ventilatory strategy—low TV and high PEEP, Pplat <30 cm H_2O
- Prone ventilation
- Veno venous ECMO

(ECMO: extracorporeal membrane oxygenation; HFNC: high-flow nasal cannula; NIV: noninvasive ventilation; PEEP: positive end-expiratory pressure; PPE: personal protective equipment)

FIGURE 5: Management principles in critically ill COVID-19 patients.

PROGNOSIS

Prognosis varies widely based on the level of care, modalities available, early case identification, and treatment initiation. Hospital mortality varies from 15 to 20%. Among those requiring ICU care, mortality is approximately 40%. In elderly aged between 80 and 90 years, the reported mortality is as high as 60%.

CONCLUSION

COVID-19 pandemic has resulted in worldwide morbidity and mortality, particularly among the elderly and patients with comorbidities. The containment of infection and prevention of complications are important for infection control. Treatment is mainly aimed at modulating inflammation and controlling viral load. Ongoing trials for vaccines against COVID-19 are promising. Social distancing, wearing masks in public places, and frequent hand hygiene can curtail the spread of infection.

RECOMMENDED READINGS

1. Wiersinga WJ, Rhodes A, Cheng AC, Peacock SJ, Prescott HC. Pathophysiology, Transmission, Diagnosis, and Treatment of Coronavirus Disease 2019 (COVID-19): A Review. JAMA. 2020;324(8):782-93.
2. Agarwal A, Mukherjee A, Kumar G, Chatterjee P, Bhatnagar T, Malhotra P, et al. Convalescent plasma in the management of moderate COVID-19 in adults in India: open label phase II multicentre randomised controlled trial (PLACID Trial). BMJ. 2020;371: m3939.
3. Beigel JH, Tomashek KM, Dodd LE, Mehta AK, Zingman BS, Kalil AC, et al. ACTT-1 Study Group Members. Remdesivir for the Treatment of COVID-19—Final Report. N Engl J Med. 2020;383(19):1813-26.
4. RECOVERY Collaborative Group, Horby P, Lim WS, Emberson JR, Mafham M, Bell JL, et al. Dexamethasone in Hospitalized Patients with COVID-19—Preliminary Report. N Engl J Med. 2021;384(8):693-704.

5. Clinical Management Protocol: COVID-19. Ministry of Health and Family Welfare Directorate General of Health Services (EMR Division) July 2020. [online] Available from https://www.mohfw.gov.in/pdf/UpdatedClinicalManagementProtocolforCOVID19dated03072020.pdf.
6. Clinical management of COVID-19 - WHO interim guidance 27 May 2020. [online] Available from https://www.who.int/publications/i/item/clinical-management-of-covid-19.
7. Alhazzani W, Møller MH, Arabi YM, Loeb M, Gong MN, Fan E, et al. Surviving Sepsis Campaign: guidelines on the management of critically ill adults with Coronavirus Disease 2019 (COVID-19). Intensive Care Med. 2020;46(5):854-87.

CHAPTER 226

Post-COVID Respiratory Complications

Surinder K Jindal

ABSTRACT

Post-coronavirus disease (COVID) pulmonary complications are common and may be seen up to several weeks and months after recovery from the acute illness. These are commonly observed in patients with severe illness. There are three main types of post-COVID syndromes: (1) long COVID symptoms, (2) impaired pulmonary function, and (3) pulmonary fibrosis. Of these, pulmonary fibrosis is most concerning, especially when diffuse and symptomatic. In view of large number of such cases, post-COVID pulmonary fibrosis will continue to be considered as an important cause of interstitial lung diseases (ILDs). Residual and diffuse fibrosis cause persistent breathlessness and cough. Diagnosis is established on the basis of clinical features, lung function tests, and chest roentgenography on high-resolution computed tomography (HRCT). Histocytological diagnosis is frequently not available. Patients are managed with oxygen supplementation and symptomatic therapy. Anti-inflammatory drugs such as corticosteroids are used in the presence of diffuse radiological infiltrates and hypoxemia. Use of antifibrotic drugs such as nintedanib or pirfenidone is under investigation.

The pandemic coronavirus disease-2019 (COVID-19) caused by infection due to severe acute respiratory syndrome coronavirus-2 (SARS-CoV-2) owes its origin to the Wuhan city of China which was first recognized in December 2019. Within a period of about a year, it has affected around 100 million cases and killed over a million people worldwide. The disease primarily involves the respiratory tract in humans. The infection starts off with mild flu-like symptoms or no symptoms, and further progress to severe symptoms. In the majority of the cases, i.e., 80% will exhibit mild symptoms, 14% will have pneumonia, 5% will suffer from septic shock and organ failure (mostly respiratory failure), and in 2% cases it will be fatal. COVID-19 with severe pneumonia and acute respiratory distress syndrome (ARDS) is characterized with acute lung injury and respiratory failure. A number of patients who recover from infection and survive an acute sever disease may continue to suffer from persistent symptoms or develop post-COVID complications. Patients with post-COVID manifestations are now recognized with greater frequency when the continued rise in the number of active cases is apparently under control after over a year.

"A wise man proportions his belief to the evidence"

—David Hume

POST-COVID SYNDROMES

Post-COVID syndromes involve different organ systems. Lungs are the most frequently involved organs. Post-COVID syndromes may be classified as acute or chronic depending upon the duration from the onset of first COVID symptoms:

- **Acute post-COVID 19:** It is defined as symptoms extending beyond 3 weeks from the onset of first symptoms. About 10% of patients who have tested positive for SARS-CoV-2 remain unwell beyond 3 weeks.
- **Chronic post-COVID-19:** It is defined as symptoms extending beyond 12 weeks; a smaller proportion may have symptoms for months.

Some of the common post-COVID pulmonary manifestations may be listed as under:

- Long COVID syndrome
- Impaired lung function
- Pulmonary fibrosis

A significant number of general systemic and neuropsychiatric symptoms may actually be attributed to an

BOX 1	High-risk groups for post-coronavirus disease-2019 (COVID-19) syndromes.
• Elderly patients (age > 60 years)	
• Presence of comorbidities (diabetes mellitus, hypertension, coronary artery disease, and chronic kidney disease)	
• Patients requiring domiciliary oxygen at discharge from COVID-19 admission facility	
• Patient who required noninvasive ventilation (NIV) or mechanical ventilation (MV) during COVID-19 management in the hospital	
• Patients with preexisting chronic respiratory diseases	

aggravated anxiety, fear, and other mental stresses. Some of the organs such as the lungs may suffer from residual pathological damage.

Even mild COVID-19 patients may be associated with long-term common symptoms. Post-COVID syndromes are more likely to occur in some high-risk groups in the presence of risk factors (**Box 1**).

CLINICAL MANIFESTATIONS

- **Long COVID syndrome:** Long COVID is a term used rather loosely to describe patients who either continue to persist with multiorgan symptoms between 4 and 12 weeks after the start of acute illness or develop new symptoms and complications after initial after recovery from acute infection and illness. The period of appearance of these symptoms is usually considered as 12 weeks after initial recovery. Symptomatology is highly variable but may be extensive such as chronic cough, shortness of breath, chest tightness or pain, muscle pains, and extreme fatigue. Gastrointestinal upset, rashes, metabolic disruption, thromboembolic phenomena, depression and other psychological disturbances, mental confusion, cognitive dysfunction, headaches, and anosmia are other common symptoms. Long COVID is also termed as post-COVID-19 syndrome. The National Institute for Health and Care Excellence (NICE) guidelines recommend clinical assessment for level of breathlessness, heart rate, and O_2 saturation and investigations as below for all such patients presenting with new or ongoing symptoms 4 weeks or later after acute infection:
  - Total and differential blood count
  - Kidney and liver function tests
  - C-reactive protein estimation
  - Chest X-ray for patients with respiratory symptoms at 12 weeks after acute infection

  It should be however kept in mind that the guidelines with reference to COVID-19 in general and post-COVID syndromes in particular may change in view of the a rapidly changing scenario of this pandemic.

  Long COVID symptoms are managed with symptomatic treatment. Most of these symptoms are likely to disappear with time. Antitussive agents and antihistaminics are generally enough for management of chronic cough. Inhalational treatment with corticosteroid and/or bronchodilator inhalers is required in some patients. Appropriate assessment of preexisting asthma, chronic obstructive lung disease, or other disorders is important for long-term management.
- **Lung function impairment:** Some degree of impairment of lung function has been shown to persist at 3 months after discharge from an intensive care unit (ICU) in about half of the patients who recover from critical COVID-19 patients. The loss of lung function is usually proportional to the extent of radiological lung involvement.

  Impairment of lung function is commonly seen with measurements of spirometric indices and diffusion capacity of carbon monoxide (DLCO):
  - *Spirometry*: Typically, spirometry is restrictive in nature even though small airway obstruction may be present in some cases. As per current guidelines, abnormalities of spirometric capacities such as forced vital capacity (FVC) and forced expiratory volume in 1 second (FEV1) are expressed against the lower limit of normal (LLN); restrictive pattern is defined by reduced FVC (FVC > LLN) and normal or increased FEV1/FVC ratio (FEV1/FVC ratio > LLN).
  - *Impaired diffusion capacity*: DLCO, a more sensitive marker of lung function impairment in patients with ARDS is reduced in about 40–50% of patients at 1 month after discharge. This is consistent with earlier observations in survivors of SARS-CoV-1 and Middle East respiratory syndrome (MERS).
  - *Other pulmonary function tests (PFTs)*: There are limited data in post-COVID patients on other tests which are reported to reduce in survivors of ARDS from other causes. The results are inconsistent on respiratory muscle strength measurements and 6-minute walk distance test (6MWDT) which are likely to reduce. Similarly, the data on dyspnea scale and quality of life measures is limited.
  - *Oximetry*: Monitoring of arterial oxygen saturation (SaO_2) with the help of finger oximetry is an important measure of oxygen desaturation and hypoxia. Persistence of oxygen desaturation points to the presence of impaired gas exchange function of the lungs. Frequently, SaO_2 is normal at rest and appears only after exertion. Exercise-induced desaturation is almost characteristic of interstitial and parenchymal lung disease.

    Presence of persistent lung function impairment may in fact indicate either the occurrence of residual parenchymal lung fibrosis or a preexisting lung disease. Diagnosis is required to be made from a good past history, radiological assessment, and other relevant investigations. Management will depend upon the cause of impairment.
- **Post-COVID pulmonary fibrosis:** There are increasing reports on varying degrees of post-COVID pulmonary

fibrosis among survivors of COVID-ARDS. These patients are often left with severe respiratory disability. Taking cue from data of SARS-CoV-1 infection survivors, it can be estimated that about one-third of ARDS survivors of COVID-19 are likely to suffer from pulmonary fibrosis.

PATHOLOGY OF LUNG FIBROSIS

Pathologically during an acute infection, lungs are affected by COVID-19 with different mechanisms which may include the following:

- Pulmonary consolidation
- Diffuse destruction of alveolar epithelium
- Formation of hyaline membrane
- Diffuse pulmonary microvascular thrombosis
- Capillary endothelial damage
- Proliferation of alveolar septa
- Alveolar and vascular remodeling leading to pulmonary fibrosis

It is highly likely that several of residual lesions may persist even after the recovery from acute illness. This is particularly in cases of severe infection. Pulmonary fibrosis is a healing process—a natural consequence of lung injury due to SARS-CoV-2 virus, which damages type 2 pneumocytes. Impairment of cell function and cellular death (apoptosis) result depending on the effects of viral replication and the release of proinflammatory cytokines. The different stages of damage and healing sequentially include the occurrence of pulmonary edema and desquamation of pneumocytes to formation of hyaline membranes, diffuse alveolar damage, inflammation, and organization. Finally, there occurs interstitial remodeling and lung fibrosis.

MECHANISM OF PULMONARY FIBROSIS

The pathogenic mechanism of pulmonary fibrosis is not fully understood. SARS-CoV-2 is likely to cause pulmonary fibrosis with similar molecular mechanism as described in the past for SARS-CoV-1 infection. There is upregulation of cytokines such as transforming growth factor beta-1 (TGF-beta-1) and downregulation of angiotensin-converting enzyme-2 (ACE-2) which normally has a protective antifibrotic role. There is increased myofibroblast activation and deposition of extracellular matrix—collagen and fibronectin leading to fibrosis.

In addition, there are other mechanisms/factors which are also considered to be responsible for promotion of fibrosis:

- Airway inflammatory viral damage
- Increased oxidative stress
- Intra-alveolar thrombosis
- *Iatrogenic factors—oxygen toxicity and ventilator-induced lung injury*: Almost all patients who develop fibrosis are likely to have received prolonged periods of high concentrations of oxygen while many might have remained on mechanical ventilation. Both these factors are known to independently cause pulmonary fibrosis.

PREDICTORS

Fibrosis is more likely in the following categories of patients:

- Disease severity—the severe the illness, the greater the chances of residual fibrosis
- Age—more common in elderly patients
- Prolonged hospital and ICU stay—patients who have received high concentrations of oxygen and on mechanical ventilation
- History of smoking and chronic alcoholism
- Some of the inflammatory markers [higher levels of C-reactive protein, lactate dehydrogenase (LDH), and interleukin-5 (IL-5)] and treatment factors (treated for prolonged periods with pulse doses of corticosteroids and/or antiviral drugs) are also considered as predictors of fibrosis. Presence of these markers may in fact indicate the severity of disease.

CLINICAL FEATURES

Breathlessness and distressing cough are the most common symptoms. Cough is usually dry although it may be accompanied with frothy and mucoid sputum. Breathlessness is directly proportional to the extent of fibrosis and lung function impairment. Even slight degree of exertion may precipitate dyspnea and oxygen desaturation. Patients with bilateral, diffuse, and extensive fibrosis may find it difficult to move and remain confined to the bed. Chest tightness, fatigue, restlessness, and palpitation are other common symptoms.

There are no characteristic physical signs except tachypnea and tachycardia. Localized or diffuse Velcro crackles may be heard on auscultation, but not necessarily present as are typically described for pulmonary fibrosis associated with other etiologies or when idiopathic in origin. Pulmonary hypertension may develop due to increased right ventricular overload.

DIAGNOSIS

Diagnosis is suspected from the onset of clinical symptoms as above following the history of COVID-19 infection. It has been described to occur any time following the recovery from the illness. Most patients persist with continued symptoms after recovery though some may develop after 8–12 weeks afterwards.

Baseline investigations are done to assess general status of the patient as well as the presence of concomitant diseases such as diabetes mellitus, hypertension, and liver or renal dysfunction. Mild-to-moderate leukocytosis is generally seen, although there may be leukopenia and/or thrombocytopenia. Other markers of inflammation which are typically raised during the acute infection such as the C-reactive protein, LDH, serum ferritin, and creatinine may be high or normal. High D-dimer level may point to the propensity of thromboembolic tendency. Cardiac involvement is assessed with electrocardiogram (ECG) and chest X-ray, which should be routinely done in all cases. Echocardiography is often required for detection of pulmonary arterial hypertension and other cardiac lesions.

PULMONARY FUNCTION TESTS

Pulmonary function tests are done to assess the severity of impairment of the respiratory involvement as well as to follow the treatment and determine the prognosis. It also helps to detect airflow obstruction that may be present due to coexisting emphysema. Spirometry is the basic standard test, since it is easy to perform and is reproducible. All post-Covid patients should undergo resting spirometry for a reasonable assessment of disease severity. Airflow obstruction is determined by the ratio of FEV1 to the FVC. Restrictive defect is suggested if the FEV1/FVC ratio is normal, but the FVC is below the LLN. The severity of restrictive defect can be graded as mild (>70% of the predicted), moderate (50–70% of the predicted), and severe (<50% of the predicted) depending on the FVC values. Generally, there is a restrictive defect on spirometry; FVC is used to assess the efficacy of various treatments. Decline in FVC is also a predictor of mortality.

Other PFTs which help in the overall assessment of ILDs include the following:

- Lung volumes
- DLCO
- Exercise testing
- Pulse oximetry and arterial blood gas analysis

Lung volume testing: It is helpful to confirm the restrictive defect, especially when the clinicoradiologic picture is not consistent with spirometric parameters. Lung volume measurement helps to identify mixed obstructive-restrictive defect as well as to quantify the restrictive defect. DLCO helps to determine abnormal gas exchange, especially in early disease, when spirometry may be normal. Further, spirometry may show normal FVC but disproportionately low DLCO in combined pulmonary fibrosis and emphysema (CPFE). However, standardization across different laboratories is difficult since the reproducibility and accuracy of DLCO estimation are low as well as the intraindividual variability may be high. DLCO is a more reliable indicator of outcome than other resting lung function indices. DLCO level of <40% indicates advanced disease.

Exercise testing: It provides a more global assessment of patient's disability than lung function testing alone, but it is affected by the presence of comorbidities (such as obesity) and disease complications (such as pulmonary hypertension). A 6-minute walk test (6MWT) is a simple method for assessment of the exercise capacity as well as for identification and quantification of exercise-induced desaturation in these patients. Desaturation during the 6MWT at presentation is a better predictor of prognosis than resting lung function.

Pulse oximetry: It is useful to identify hypoxia in patients with advanced disease and to assess oxygen desaturation following exercise. Typically, the patient gets desaturated after an exertional activity. SaO_2 of <92% measured on pulse oximetry is considered as indicative of hypoxemia. Hypoxemia in the resting state indicates the presence of an advanced disease. SaO_2, which can be repeated as required, is routinely helpful for disease-monitoring. Arterial blood gas analysis, which requires an arterial puncture, is not done as a routine procedure. It is needed to document partial pressure of oxygen in the arterial blood in patients with resting hypoxia with pulse oximetric saturation <90%. Blood gas analysis also helps to identify the presence of hypercarbia in the presence of significant airflow obstruction.

RADIOLOGICAL FEATURES

Radiology is the most important step in each case to establish the diagnosis while histopathology is required whenever there is a doubt. Imaging techniques comprise of conventional chest radiographs and the HRCT of the thorax.

The abnormal radiological findings on CT thorax are classified as linear or reticular opacities, nodules, consolidation or ground glass opacity (GGO), cystic, and as areas with decreased attenuation (**Box 2**). Generally, there is a combination of findings with one abnormality being predominant. To characterize the disease the distribution of the abnormality should also be considered (upper or lower lung regions, involvement of subpleural region around the peribronchovascular region and others). The presence of GGO can represent interstitial inflammation, infiltration or fibrosis or the presence of cells or fluid in the alveolar spaces. The etiology of GGO is dependent on the duration of symptoms (acute, subacute, or chronic).

PATHOLOGICAL ASSESSMENT

Bronchoscopy to obtain bronchoalveolar lavage fluid (BALF) for cytological assessment and lung biopsy are rarely required. BALF is needed to exclude infection when strongly suspected. A confirmed diagnosis after lung biopsy is certainly helpful, but one must weigh the option of moving ahead with an uncertain diagnosis against the potential risks and benefits of lung biopsy. Biopsy is not recommended if

BOX 2 Typical lesions on lung high-resolution computed tomography scan suggestive of pulmonary fibrosis.

- Reticular or linear opacities
- **Nodules:** Centrilobular, perilymphatic (along the peribroncho-vascular structures or interlobular septa or subpleural region), and random, i.e., diffusely distributed
- **Parenchymal opacities:** Increased lung opacity (attenuation), i.e., ground-glass opacity or consolidation
- **Decreased attenuation:** Includes mosaic attenuation pattern and air trapping
- **Honeycomb cyst:** Clustered cystic air spaces that are 3 mm to 1 cm in size and have a well-defined wall; generally represents advanced disease and fibrosis

the patient is not fit for the procedure, or a treatment plan can be devised through less invasive assessments, or if the clinician feels that making a confirmed diagnosis is unlikely to alter the therapeutic plan, it may not be advisable to proceed further.

Lung biopsy can be performed through conventional transbronchial lung biopsy (TBLB), lung cryobiopsy, or video-assisted thoracic surgery (VATS). The choice of procedure(s) depends upon the differential diagnosis, available infrastructure and personnel, and physician expertise and comfort with specific procedures. TBLBs yield small tissue specimens that are usually inadequate. Lung cryobiopsy is safer when performed in experienced hands.

MANAGEMENT

The major proven therapeutic options include the use of immunosuppressive and antifibrotic agents. Supportive therapy with oxygen and other drugs for symptomatic relief is required in all patients.

- **Corticosteroids:** Active pulmonary inflammation and edema respond well to corticosteroids. Use of corticosteroids has been shown to be definitely useful in patients with hypoxemia and radiological evidence of diffuse lung disease in the active stage of the illness. In the RECOVERY trial, dexamethasone in a dose of 4–6 mg per day for about 10 days has been shown to accelerate recovery. There are no data however to say that the steroids help to reduce or reverse an established pulmonary fibrosis. Methylprednisolone or prednisolone may be used as alternatives to dexamethasone. It is desirable that the drug is tapered off within a period of 3–4 weeks. Excessive use of corticosteroids is unlikely to benefit and may be harmful due to associated complications. Steroid-induced hyperglycemia and proximal myopathy may in fact delay the recovery from the illness.
- **Antifibrotic drugs:** Antifibrotic drugs such as nintedanib and pirfenidone are indicated primarily for the management of idiopathic pulmonary fibrosis (IPF). There is evidence from the recent studies regarding their beneficial use for other progressive and fibrosing illnesses. This has encouraged physicians to exploit the use for post-COVID fibrosis, both for prevention and treatment. Nintedanib is a tyrosine kinase inhibitor that causes suppression of several signaling receptors such as fibroblast growth factor, vascular endothelial growth factor, and platelet-derived growth factor. Its use in IPF has been shown to reduce the rate of lung function decline and incidence of acute exacerbations. Pirfenidone is a pyridine derivative that has anti-inflammatory, antioxidant, and antifibrotic properties. It inhibits fibroblasts and collagen synthesis, although its precise mechanism of action in IPF is not clear. There is emerging but conflicting data from different centers on the efficacy of these drugs for post-COVID fibrosis.
- **Supportive therapy**: Oxygen supplementation is required to manage hypoxia both during admission in the hospital and at home after discharge. Antibiotics are not required unless there is definite evidence of infection. Mild-to-moderate leukocytosis, elevated erythrocyte sedimentation rate, and levels of other inflammatory markers are common in these patients and should not be considered in favor of infection. Anticoagulant drugs are recommended for thromboprophylaxis since the patients are bed-ridden and at high risk of clotting complications.

  Pulmonary rehabilitation is important for patients with poor functional reserve. It should be initiated as early as possible.
- **Lung transplantation:** There are a few reports on lung transplantation done for advanced end-stage disease. This is the last option which is considered when the condition is refractory to all other forms of treatment. There are however several limitations such as the costs, technical feasibility, and availability of organs.

PREVENTION

Considering the seriousness of diffuse post-COVID fibrosis, it is important that preventive strategies are adopted during the active stage of the illness. Besides the general approach for effective prevention of the spread of the virus and inhibition of virus replication it is important to contain the inflammatory response and initiate treatment to prevent fibrosis at an early stage. It should be however kept in mind that the injudicious use of anti-inflammatory and/or antifibrotic drugs may be harmful.

RECOMMENDED READINGS

1. George PM, Wells AU, Jenkins RG. Pulmonary fibrosis and COVID-19: the potential role for antifibrotic therapy. Lancet Respir Med. 2020;8:807-15.
2. Truffaut L, Demey L, Bruyneel AV, Roman A, Alard S, De Vos N, et al. Post-discharge critical COVID-19 lung function related to severity of radiologic lung involvement at admission. Respir Res. 2021;22:29.
3. Spagnolo P, Balestro E, Aliberti S, Cocconcelli E, Biondini D, Casa GD, et al. Pulmonary fibrosis secondary to COVID-19: a call to arms? Lancet Respir Med. 2020;8:750-2.
4. Udwadia ZF, Tripathi AR, Nanda VJ, Joshi SR. Prognostic Factors for Adverse Outcomes in COVID-19 Infection. J Assoc Physicians India. 2020;68(7):62-6.
5. Mo X, Jian W, Su Z, Chen M, Peng H, Peng P, et al. Abnormal pulmonary function in COVID-19 patients at time of hospital discharge. Eur Respir J. 2020;55:2001217.
6. Lechowicz K, Drożdżal S, Machaj F, Rosik J, Szostak B, Zegan-Barańska M, et al. COVID-19: The Potential Treatment of Pulmonary Fibrosis Associated with SARS-CoV-2 Infection. J Clin Med. 2020;9(6):1917.

7. Ojo AS, Balogun SA, Williams OT, Ojo OS. Pulmonary Fibrosis in COVID-19 Survivors: Predictive Factors and Risk Reduction Strategies. Pulm Med. 2020;2020: 6175964.
8. Vasarmidi E, Tsitoura E, Spandidos DA, Tzanakis N, Antoniou KM. Pulmonary fibrosis in the aftermath of the COVID-19 era (Review). Exp Ther Med. 2020; 20(3):2557-60.
9. Li J. Rehabilitation management of patients with COVID-19: lessons learned from the first experience in China. Eur J Phys Rehabil Med. 2020;56(3):335-8.
10. Tale S, Ghosh S, Meitei SP, Kolli M, Garbhapu AK, Pudi S. Post-COVID-19 pneumonia pulmonary fibrosis. QJM. 2020;113(11):837-8.

MULTIPLE CHOICE QUESTIONS

To access the multiple choice questions of this Section online, kindly scan the QR code.

CHAPTER 227

Approach to a Patient with Musculoskeletal Complaints

Rohini Handa

ABSTRACT

The approach to a patient who presents with musculoskeletal (MSK) pain is overwhelmingly clinical. History and physical examination go a long way in pointing toward the diagnosis. Rheumatic diseases exhibit characteristic patterns, and pattern recognition enables diagnosis. Laboratory investigations including radiology are corroborative and seldom, if ever, pathognomonic. Patterns may evolve over time. Periodic clinical evaluation becomes necessary in such cases.

"To simplify complications is the first essential of success."

—George Earle Buckle

INTRODUCTION

Musculoskeletal complaints are common in outpatient practice. The underlying conditions range from simple tendonitis or bursitis to more complex multisystem connective tissue diseases (CTDs). Patient history followed by MSK examination plays a vital role in arriving at a diagnosis. The first task of the clinician is to distinguish "arthralgias" from "arthritis". Nonspecific arthralgias are common in a variety of illnesses like hypothyroidism, after strenuous exertion, or after viral fevers. While the joint examination is unremarkable in "arthralgias", features of inflammation like joint swelling and tenderness are evident in "arthritis". However, raised temperature and visible redness are uncommon in chronic arthritides like rheumatoid arthritis (RA) or spondarthritis (SpA). It is only acute conditions like gout or septic arthritis that may exhibit the classical features of inflammation by way of color change and raised temperature in addition to joint pain and swelling.

All pains around a joint may not originate from the joint. The periarticular structures such as bone, ligaments, tendons, bursae, or muscles may be responsible. History and examination help determine the source of pain. Articular pains tend to be diffuse, deep-seated, and increase on both active and passive movements. Bursitis is characterized by point tenderness over the anatomical site while tendonitis exhibits a linear, tender swelling of the tendon sheath. The pain in bursitis or tendonitis is more on active than passive movements. Enthesitis is pain at the tendon insertion site. Bone pains tend to be deep-seated while muscle pains are diffuse and poorly localized. Fibromyalgia is associated with chronic widespread pain with or without tender points.

PATTERN RECOGNITION

Pattern recognition incorporates several features like inflammatory or noninflammatory nature, onset, number of joints affected, distribution, type of joints affected, the sequence of involvement, associated features etc., as outlined in **Table 1**.

Inflammatory rheumatic diseases, like RA, SpA etc., are characterized by stiffness after rest and improvement on moving the joint. The morning stiffness is more pronounced. In contrast, noninflammatory joint diseases like osteoarthritis (OA) have pains that improve with rest and worsen on moving the joint. The morning stiffness is typically <30 minutes. Of note, even patients with inflammatory joint disease can develop mechanical symptoms, for example, secondary OA of knees in a patient with RA.

Arthritides are divided into monoarthritis (involvement of 1 joint), oligoarthritis (involvement of 2, 3, or 4 joints) (also known as pauci-articular disease), and polyarthritis (involvement of 5 or >5 joints). The number of joints affected helps in the differential diagnosis (**Tables 1** and **2**). Unexplained monoarthritis is treated as an infection unless proven otherwise. Joint aspiration and synovial fluid analysis are recommended in most such instances. The SpA constitutes the vast chunk of oligoarthritides encountered in clinical practice. It is a big group of interrelated conditions where ankylosing spondylitis is the prototypic illness. Other disease entities in SpA include reactive arthritis, psoriatic arthropathy (PsA), arthritis associated with inflammatory

TABLE 1 Pattern recognition in musculoskeletal (MSK) diseases.

Characteristic	Clinical information provided
Mode of onset: Acute or insidious	Acute onset is seen with septic arthritis, reactive arthritis, viral arthritis, or gout. Arthritides like RA and SpA are gradual in onset
Duration: Acute or chronic	Based upon duration, MSK complaints are traditionally classified into acute (lasting <6 weeks) or chronic (lasting >6 weeks). Patients with acute, self-limited conditions like viral arthritis require minimal investigations. However, patients with a symptom duration >6 weeks often need detailed evaluation
Number of affected joints: Monoarthritis (1 joint), oligoarthritis (2–4 joints), or polyarthritis (>5 joints)	*Monoarthritis*: Joint infection and gout are important differentials. *Oligoarthritis* is the hallmark of SpA. *Polyarthritis* is typical of RA, PsA, and CTDs
Symmetry: Symmetrical or asymmetrical	RA, SLE, SSc, and nodular OA of hands are typical examples of symmetric polyarthritis. Gout and SpA are typically asymmetric
Distribution: Lower limbs vs. upper limbs	RA and PsA affect both upper and lower limbs. SpA and gout preferentially affect lower limb joints. Hemochromatosis preferentially affects joints of upper limbs
Type of joints affected: Small vs. Large joints	RA and PsA involve both small and large joints. In contrast, SpA affects large joints much more than smaller joints
Specific joints	• Distal interphalangeal (DIP) joint involvement is characteristic of nodular OA and PsA while DIP joints are spared in RA. The involvement of the first carpometacarpal joint is typical of OA, while ankle, elbow, and shoulder are rarely involved in primary OA • Spinal involvement other than the cervical spine is rare in RA. Inflammatory low back pain is a characteristic feature of SpA
Extra-articular features	These include fever, mucocutaneous lesions, eye involvement, and presence or absence of nodules. Details discussed in the text
Sequence of involvement: Intermittent, additive or migratory	*Intermittent arthritis* is asymptomatic periods in between the episodes. Examples include gout, Behcet's syndrome, reactive arthritis, and palindromic rheumatism. *Additive arthritis* is one where more and more joints are picked up with time. This is seen with RA, SpA, psoriasis, OA etc. *Migratory polyarthritis* is a pattern wherein pain and swelling in a specific joint starts rapidly and subsides in 24–36 h; arthritis then picks up new joints. The migratory pattern is seen in rheumatic fever and gonococcal arthritis. Treatment often alters these textbook patterns
Type of joint swelling: Sausage digit vs. fusiform swelling	Sausage digit or dactylitis refers to diffusely swollen digit and is seen in reactive arthritis or PsA. In contrast, in RA only the joint gets swollen giving rise to a fusiform or spindle-shaped swelling (**Figs. 1 A** and **B**)

Note: Psoriasis can cause asymmetric oligoarthritis or symmetric polyarthritis. Gout is typically monoarticular, occasionally oligoarticular, and rarely polyarticular.

(CTD: connective tissue disease; OA: osteoarthritis; PsA: psoriatic arthritis; SpA: spondyloarthritis; SSc: systemic sclerosis)

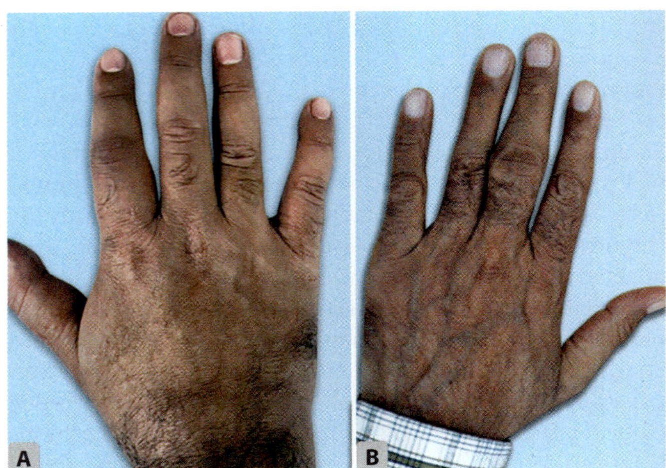

FIGURES 1 A & B: Dactylitis of psoriatic arthritis vs. fusiform swelling of rheumatoid arthritis. **(A)** Right second finger dactylitis (cylindrical) in psoriatic arthritis; **(B)** Left third PIP joint synovitis (fusiform or spindle shaped) in rheumatoid arthritis.

TABLE 2 Differential diagnosis based on the number of joints affected.

Monoarthritis	Oligoarthritis	Polyarthritis
• Infections • Crystals	• SpA	• RA • PsA • CTD • Nodular OA

(CTD: connective tissue disease; OA: osteoarthritis; PsA: psoriatic arthritis; RA: rheumatoid arthritis; SpA: spondyloarthritis)

bowel disease, and nonradiographic SpA. Inflammatory low back pain and enthesitis (pain along tendinous insertion sites) are typical of SpA. Polyarthritis may be due to inflammatory causes like RA, PsA, CTDs like systemic sclerosis (SSc) or systemic lupus erythematosus (SLE) etc. Noninflammatory causes like nodular OA of hands can have polyarticular involvement.

The extra-articular features play an important role in disease characterization. Fever accompanying arthritis is seen in SLE, systemic-onset JIA (Still's disease), vasculitis, infective endocarditis, rheumatic fever, and adult-onset Still's disease. Fever of moderate to high grade is unusual in RA and should necessitate a search for other causes. Prominent mucosal or cutaneous lesions in the setting of inflammatory arthritis draw attention to SLE. Other dermatoarthritides include psoriasis, Behcet's syndrome, reactive arthritis, SSc, erythema nodosum, vasculitides, and gonococcal arthritis. Eye involvement varies with the type of arthritis. RA usually causes keratitis or scleritis in contrast to uveitis seen in SpA. Arthritides associated with nodules include RA, OA (Heberden and Bouchard nodes), tophaceous gout, rheumatic fever, multicentric reticulohistiocytosis, sarcoidosis, erythema nodosum etc.

Different rheumatic diseases give rise to typical phenotypes that permit disease identification. For example, inflammatory polyarthritis in a young woman with fever and malar rash is highly likely to be lupus. Similarly, an insidiously developing arthritis associated with Raynaud's phenomenon and skin thickening and tightening suggests a diagnosis of SSc. Some of the typical phenotypes are illustrated in **Figures 2** to **6**. However, at times, the symptoms and signs may not fit into any one pattern. The term "undifferentiated" arthritis is used in such situations. Over a period of time, the disease may resolve, evolve into a definitive entity, or stay "undifferentiated."

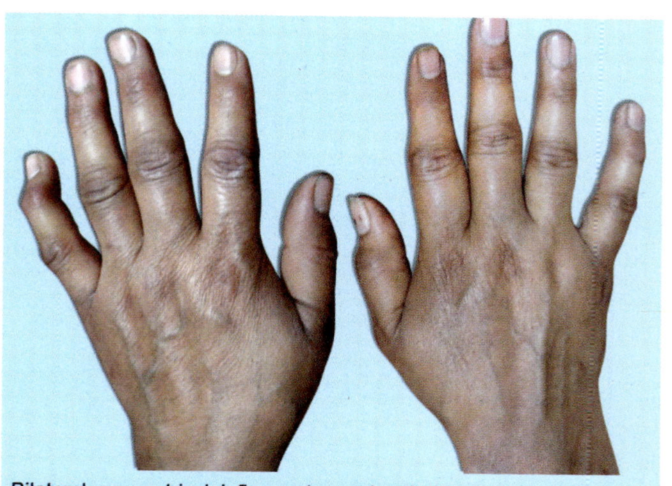

Bilateral, symmetrical, inflammatory polyarthritis of small and large joints, especially hands and feet. DIP joints typically spared. Joint swelling is boggy

(DIP: distal interphalangeal)

FIGURE 2: Typical pattern of rheumatoid arthritis.

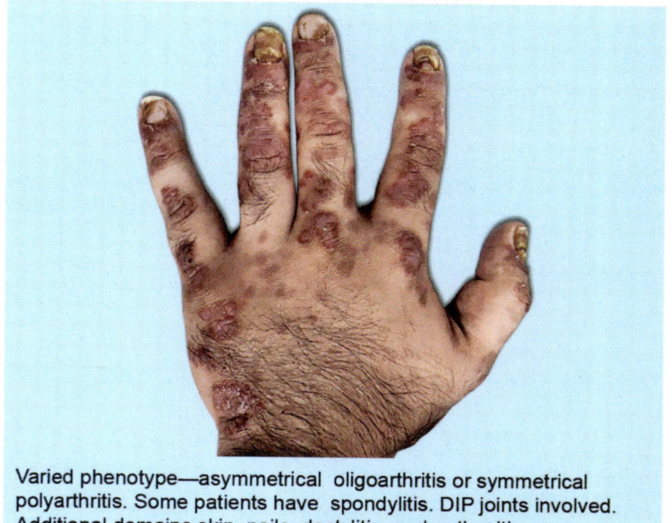

Varied phenotype—asymmetrical oligoarthritis or symmetrical polyarthritis. Some patients have spondylitis. DIP joints involved. Additional domains skin, nails, dactylitis, and enthesitis

(DIP: distal interphalangeal)

FIGURE 4: Typical pattern of psoriatic arthritis.

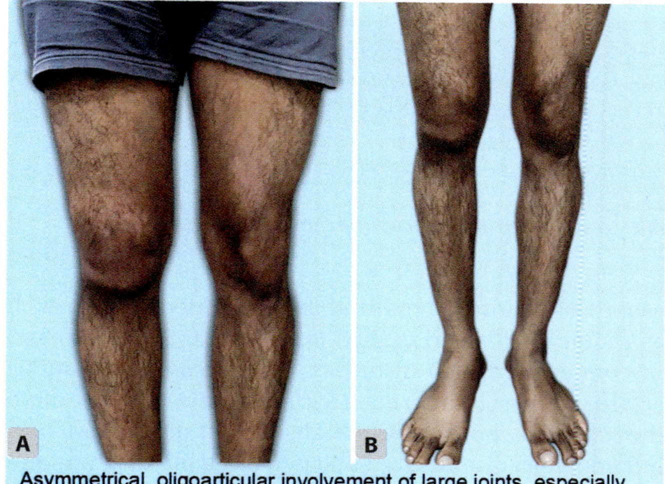

Asymmetrical, oligoarticular involvement of large joints, especially of lower limbs with inflammatory low back pain

Note: Right knee effusion and right ankle arthritis.

FIGURES 3 A & B: Typical pattern of spondyloarthritis.

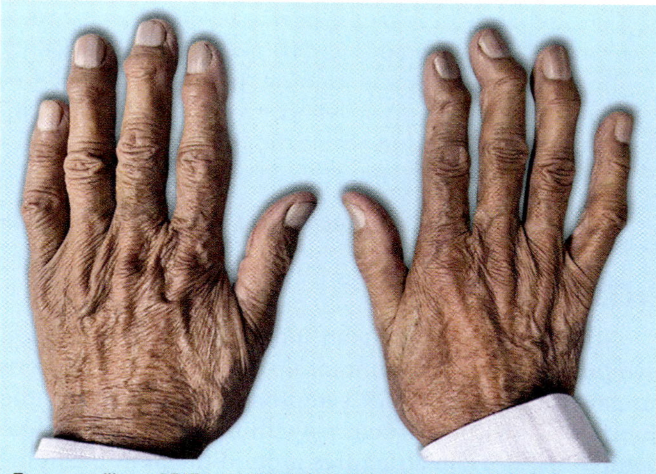

Bony swelling of PIP and DIP joints (Bouchard and Heberden nodes) To be differentiated from boggy swelling (synovitis) in RA. Wrists and MP joints are spared (unlike RA)

(DIP: distal interphalangeal; MP: metacarpophalangeal; PIP: proximal interphalangeal; RA: rheumatoid arthritis)

FIGURE 5: Typical pattern of nodular osteoarthritis.

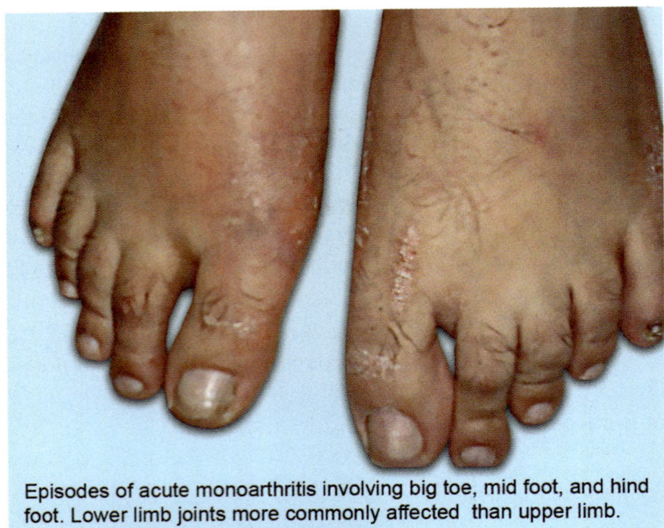

Episodes of acute monoarthritis involving big toe, mid foot, and hind foot. Lower limb joints more commonly affected than upper limb. Affected joint may be red and hot

FIGURE 6: Typical pattern of gouty arthritis.

CONCLUSION

The approach to MSK complaints is predominantly clinical and relies on pattern recognition. History and physical examination provide nearly 80% and 15% of diagnostic information, respectively. The laboratory investigations contribute only about 5% to the making of a diagnosis in rheumatology. The evolution of distinct patterns may take time. Periodic reassessment and symptomatic treatment are recommended in such instances.

RECOMMENDED READING

1. Handa R. Basic considerations of rheumatology. In: Kamath SA (Eds). API Textbook of Medicine, 11th edition. Mumbai: Publisher Association of Physicians of India; 2019. pp. 485-88.

CHAPTER 228

Soft Tissue Rheumatism

SJ Gupta

ABSTRACT

Soft tissue rheumatism (STR) refers to musculoskeletal (MSK) symptoms arising from structures around the joints and not from the joints themselves. These symptoms are not associated with any systemic features and are most often localized. The structures responsible are: Ligaments, tendons, fascia, entheses, tendon sheaths, bursae, muscles, and soft tissue. Though the origin of pain is not from the joint itself, patients may attribute their symptoms to nearby joints and complain of "hip pain," "shoulder pain," etc. These structures may occasionally be the cause of symptoms as part of a more generalized inflammatory arthritis and this distinction is important. This chapter will attempt to provide an overview to the management of some of the more common soft tissue rheumatic problems.

"Being able to walk pain free is a blessing. Being able to walk without showing the pain is a skill"

—Kylie Mc Pherson

INTRODUCTION

Musculoskeletal pain or "joint pain" is a common symptom and may account for up to 30% of consultations in general practice. MSK symptoms can arise from the joint itself or from structures within the joint (articular symptoms) or from structures around the joint including soft tissues (extra-articular) (**Fig. 1**). Symptoms due to extra-articular structures are called STR or nonarticular rheumatism (NAR). The various articular and extra-articular structures and their potential problems are enumerated in **Table 1**. These structures may sometimes be involved as part of a more generalized inflammatory arthritis such as rheumatoid arthritis (RA) or spondarthritis (SpA) and in connective tissue disorders (CTDs) such as systemic sclerosis or scleroderma (SSc). However, more often they cause symptoms in the absence of any generalized inflammatory disease. The etiology is thought to be stress and strain of the soft tissues or muscles, as with long-standing overuse or repetitive low-grade trauma. Though the origin of symptoms is not from the joints themselves, patients with STR may attribute their problems to nearby joints, such as "hip pain," "shoulder pain" etc. When evaluating a patient

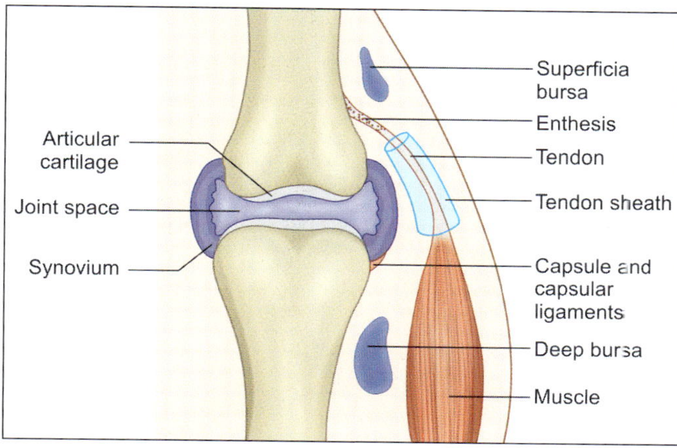

FIGURE 1: Structures that can cause joint/musculoskeletal pain.
Source: SKF Slide Atlas of Rheumatology. Gower Medical Publishing; 1986.

TABLE 1 Articular and extra-articular structures responsible for musculoskeletal pain.

Articular structures	Extra-articular structures
• *Articular cartilage*: As in osteoarthritis • *Synovium*: As in inflammatory joint disorders such as rheumatoid arthritis	• *Tendon*: Tendonitis • *Tendon sheath*: Tenosynovitis • *Enthesis*: Enthesitis • *Bursa*: Bursitis • *Muscle*: Myofascial pain • *Capsule*: As in adhesive capsulitis or frozen shoulder

with joint pain, it is important therefore to ascertain if: (A) the symptoms are arising from within the joint or are extra-articular in origin and (B) if extra-articular, whether they are isolated (STR) or part of a more generalized inflammatory joint disorder. One would consider the patient to have STR or NAR if the cause is periarticular and there is no evidence of a generalized inflammatory joint disease.

CLINICAL PRESENTATION

Soft tissue rheumatism may present clinically in two main forms: (1) Localized pain syndromes and (2) Diffuse pain syndromes.

LOCALIZED PAIN SYNDROMES

Localized soft tissue rheumatic problems may be due to:

- **Involvement of individual periarticular structures:** Tendonitis, bursitis, fasciitis, and enthesitis.
- **Structural disorders:** These may be congenital, developmental, or acquired; resulting in abnormal joint movement and/or stability. Even mild or subtle disorders may result in significant problems. Examples of some structural disorders include: Genu valgus or varus; femoral anteversion with internal rotation of the hip, malalignment of the patellae, and external tibial torsion. Structural disorders such as these may predispose to overuse or sports injuries. Early recognition and appropriate management with supports, splints, braces, and surgical correction where indicated, would be important.
- **Entrapment disorders:** Due to compression of nerves at specific sites due to a variety of reasons. A typical example is carpal tunnel syndrome at the wrist.
- **Myofascial pain syndrome (MPS).** MPS is a localized muscle pain characterized by acutely sensitive thickening in the muscle-trigger points. The cause is often physical activity that results in strain or injury to a particular muscle group. Common areas for MPS are neck, back, shoulder, or hip. Management includes education, advice on adequate rest and physical activity, and the recognition and treatment of any psychosocial factors. Analgesics, nonsteroidal anti-inflammatory drugs (NSAIDs) both topical and systemic, and topical local anesthetic patches may be helpful. Needling or trigger point injections may be helpful in persistent symptoms.
- **Complex regional pain syndrome (CRPS):** CRPS refers to a characteristic collection of clinical features that are localized to a particular region of the MSK system. This is distinct from diffuse pain syndromes that invariably have widespread pain. CRPS is often triggered by some injury, often in the context of workplace-related injury and compensation. Its severity and impact on day-to-day functioning vary amongst individuals and contributing factors include central sensitization, referred pain, and emotional distress. Management involves early recognition and diagnosis, adequate counseling, advice on appropriate mobilization and exercises, drugs such as tricyclic antidepressants, and pregabalin.

Some of the more commonly seen localized soft tissue problems caused by periarticular structures are enumerated in **Box 1**; and a few of these will be discussed in more detail.

DIFFUSE PAIN SYNDROMES

Hypermobility syndrome (HMS): It is also known as hypermobility spectrum disorder or joint HMS. HMS is an inherited CTD, resulting in joint and ligament laxity leading to overuse and strain of the joints, ligaments, and soft tissues. Symptoms include inability to walk, joint and soft tissue pain on exertion, tiredness, and depression. The diagnosis is based on recognizing joint hypermobility in at least 4 out of 9 joints (Beighton score) along with other features such as skin laxity or striae, joint dislocation, arthralgia etc. Management includes appropriate counseling and avoidance of stress and strain at joints and soft tissues, use of splints or supports to maintain joint alignment, and the use of analgesics or NSAIDs when required.

Fibromyalgia (FM): This is a clinical syndrome comprising chronic widespread pain, fatigue, and a number of other clinical features. This will be discussed further.

BOX 1	Some common localized soft tissue problems.

Region and clinical problem(s):

- ***Head and neck:*** Temporomandibular joint pain, carotodynia, occipital neuralgia, and thoracic outlet syndrome
- ***Chest:*** Costochondritis
- ***Wrist:*** De Quervain's tenosynovitis (first ETS), carpal tunnel syndrome
- ***Hip:*** Trochanteric bursitis, ischial bursitis, meralgia paresthetica, and adductor tendonitis
- ***Shoulder:*** Rotator cuff lesion, adhesive capsulitis, bicipital tendonitis, subacromial bursitis
- ***Elbow:*** Epicondylitis and olecranon bursitis
- ***Hand:*** Stenosing tenosynovitis—trigger finger or thumb, Dupuytren's contracture
- ***Knee:*** Prepatellar bursitis, pes anserine bursitis, collateral ligament strain, and popliteal (Baker's) cyst
- ***Ankle/Foot:*** Plantar fasciitis, Achilles tendonitis; metatarsalgia; retrocalcaneal bursitis

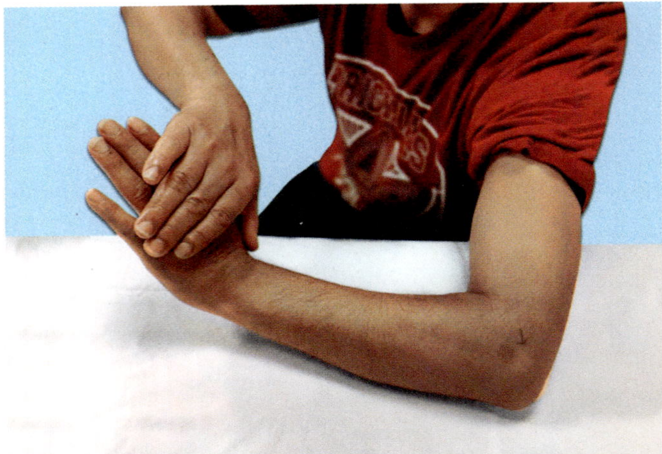

FIGURE 2: Tennis elbow: Demonstrating resisted extension of the wrist (lateral epicondyle marked by arrow).

CLINICAL APPROACH

The approach to a patient with MSK pain and STR, as indeed for all clinical problems, is a systematic approach, aimed at excluding systemic causes and establishing a diagnosis. In most situations a good history and physical examination will enable an accurate diagnosis. The pain or discomfort of STR is usually diffuse over a wide area and the patient may attribute the symptoms to a neighboring joint, such as "hip pain" for trochanteric bursitis (TB) or "elbow pain" for lateral epicondylitis (LE) (tennis elbow). However, in STR there will be no joint swelling and the tenderness will be localized to the area of interest and not at the joint line; that is, over the lateral epicondyle in tennis elbow and over the greater trochanter in TB.

Specific movement or maneuvers, such as resisted extension of the wrist for tennis elbow (**Fig. 2**), will aggravate the pain. A detailed history and careful examination will enable a diagnosis of STR to be reached with some confidence. However, appropriate investigations might be required to confirm a diagnosis and more importantly, to exclude systemic inflammatory conditions. **Table 2** outlines differentiating clinical features of STR and inflammatory joint disease and **Table 3** enumerates some "typical" constellation of symptoms that patients with STR may complain of and the possible diagnosis to be considered for each.

TABLE 2 Clinical features of inflammatory and noninflammatory MSK symptoms.

Clinical feature	Noninflammatory (STR)	Inflammatory (articular)
Pain	Diffuse with local tenderness	Localized, over joint line
Swelling	Absent	Joint swelling present
Stiffness	Absent or not significant	Present, with EMS ≥ 30 min
Movement	Aggravated by specific movement; rest helps	Gentle movement helps; stiffness aggravated by rest
Inflammatory markers (ESR/CRP)	Not elevated	Elevated
Imaging	Plain radiographs are usually normal or may reveal structural abnormalities if present; MRI may confirm specific problem	May reveal changes of specific IJD—sacroiliitis in SpA or typical erosions of RA

(EMS: early morning stiffness; IJD: inflammatory joint disease; MSK: musculoskeletal; SpA: spondarthritis; STR: soft tissue rheumatism)

SPECIFIC LOCALIZED PAIN SYNDROMES

It is important to re-emphasize that a generalized inflammatory disorder might present with localized symptoms predominantly, such as a patient of SpA, presenting with an enthesopathy. The patient might not connect his/her back or other systemic symptoms and may complain of the symptom that his troubling him/her the most at that time—the localized pain. A detailed history and examination should, however, reveal the correct clinical picture. In localized regional pain syndromes due to STR, symptoms will be diffuse, over the region or area involved; the pain will be aggravated by specific movements or posture and localized tenderness may be elicited over the structure causing symptoms. There will be an absence of generalized or systemic features. It would be beyond the scope of this chapter to review all possible localized syndromes in detail. However, a few common localized conditions and FM will be reviewed, along with the general principles of management.

SHOULDER

The commonly encountered localized soft tissue problems around the shoulder are enumerated in **Box 1** and

TABLE 3 Some "typical" symptoms and possible diagnosis.

Symptom complex	*Possible diagnosis to consider
Pain and paresthesia at hand—mainly thumb and three fingers; increased at night	Think of carpal tunnel syndrome
Pain in the finger with sticking or "triggering" on flexion or extension	Possible tenosynovitis
Lateral thigh pain, increased on exertion and by lying on affected side	Possible trochanteric bursitis
Anterior thigh pain, associated with dysesthesia and aggravated by prolonged standing or pressure on inguinal ligament	Consider meralgia paresthetica
Shoulder pain; restriction of active and passive abduction and rotation	Think of adhesive capsulitis
Shoulder pain; restricted active abduction and internal rotation	Consider rotator cuff lesion
Diffuse forearm pain aggravated by gripping or lifting	Consider lateral or medial epicondy itis

*These would need to be confirmed by further evaluation and appropriate investigations.

the important muscles and structures that are responsible for these problems are illustrated in **Figures 3** and **4**. This region possibly accounts for most of the STR problems.

Rotator cuff lesion: Tendons of the three main muscles that comprise the rotator cuff: (1) supraspinatus, (2) infraspinatus, and (3) subscapularis—are illustrated in **Figure 3**. The subacromial bursa is in close vicinity to these tendons. The patient will typically complain of "shoulder pain" or pain in the shoulder region. This pain is aggravated by active shoulder abduction (usually between 30° and 120°) and by rotation. The cause could be tendonitis of either of these muscles or subacromial bursitis, resulting from mild trauma or low-grade muscle "strain" or overuse. Passive movements are usually possible, unlike in adhesive capsulitis (AC), where both active and passive movements are restricted. Localized tenderness at either of these tendons or the subacromial bursa, if elicited, may identify the specific cause. Often, the tenderness is more diffuse and a more general diagnosis of "rotator cuff lesion" is made. Inflammatory markers and plain radiographs are usually normal. Magnetic resonance imaging (MRI) will often reveal the soft tissue inflammation and may be required if traumatic injury to tendons is suspected or to rule out other causes.

Management comprises analgesics and NSAIDs with appropriate counseling to avoid active movements of the affected shoulder. If symptoms persist a local steroid injection into the subacromial bursa or a tendon sheath may prove to be helpful. Physiotherapy, with local application of ultrasound to the tender point, may also be helpful. However, active exercises would need to be avoided. A torn rotator cuff apparatus or the shoulder impingement

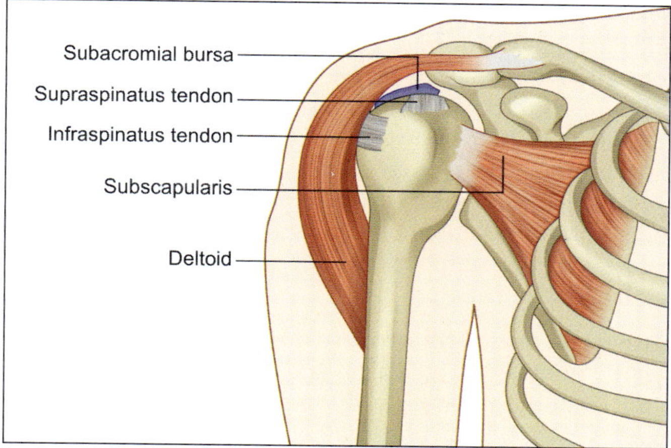

FIGURE 3: Muscles around the shoulder comprising rotator cuff.
Source: SKF Slide Atlas of Rheumatology. Gower Medical Publishing; 1986.

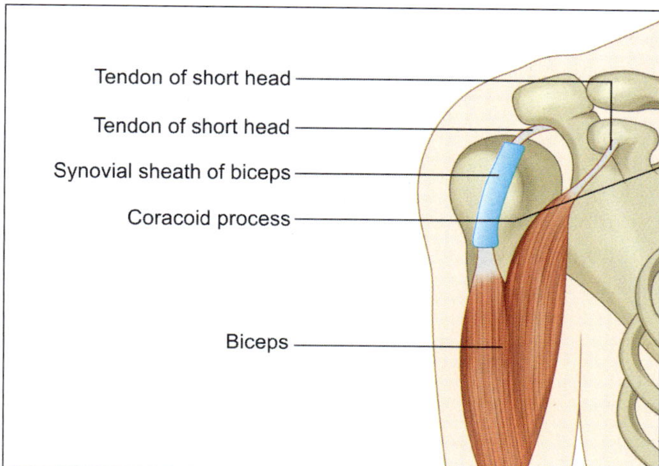

FIGURE 4: Biceps tendon: Long and short head.
Source: SKF Slide Atlas of Rheumatology. Gower Medical Publishing; 1986.

syndrome may also cause similar clinical problems and would warrant appropriate referral to an orthopedic/arthroscopic specialist for specialist management.

Bicipital tendonitis: Figure 4 illustrates the biceps muscle and the insertion of the two heads of the muscle; short head into the coracoid process and the long head passing through the intertubercular groove (or bicipital groove) of the humerus into the supraglenoid tubercle of the scapula. Distally, the two heads form a single muscle and are attached to the radial tuberosity. Thus the biceps traverses both the shoulder and the elbow joints. A strain of the biceps tendon may follow weight lifting or similar mechanical stress, involving overhead movements. The patient complains of anterior shoulder pain and occasionally pain at the cubital fossa. Flexion at the elbow may be painful as is abduction of the shoulder; and sometimes a "click" may be palpated or even audible, as the biceps tendon moves in the bicipital groove. Localized tenderness over either of the two heads of the muscle and in particular, over the bicipital groove and sometimes at the radial tuberosity distally, may be elicited, enabling a diagnosis.

Treatment involves appropriate counseling, with avoidance of active movements that aggravate the discomfort. Analgesics and NSAIDs may be helpful. Physiotherapy with local application of ultrasound over the tendon/tendon sheath may help; however, active exercises should be avoided. A local steroid injection into the tendon sheath or at the site of tendon insertion may be required if symptoms persist. More severe injuries, which might result in muscle or tendon tears, might require appropriate surgical advice and management.

Adhesive capsulitis (frozen shoulder): AC is a rather poorly understood condition and is characterized by pain and gradual limitation of generalized movement at the shoulder, both active and passive. There are usually no significant radiological findings, other than occasionally osteopenia. AC may be primary or secondary. It is seen more commonly in diabetics and in thyroid disorders, dyslipidemia, and prolonged immobilization. It may occur as a secondary problem following shoulder injury or surgery. The pathogenesis of AC is poorly understood. The initiating process is thought to be inflammation around the axillary fold of the joint capsule, which spreads to other areas and is followed by fibrosis and adhesions. There is no consensus as yet on whether AC is essentially an inflammatory or fibrotic condition. AC is generally a self-limiting condition, but improvement may occur rather slowly and over weeks and months.

Analgesics and NSAIDs may help the pain and in the painful stage, appropriate rest to the shoulder is advised. Injection of steroid in the subacromial space might help the pain and gradual mobilization of the shoulder should be undertaken once the pain settles. It may take several months for movements to improve however.

Differential diagnosis: One should bear in mind, the other localized conditions that may simulate the conditions discussed, such as shoulder girdle injury, acromioclavicular joint syndrome, glenohumeral instability, osteoarthritis of the shoulder, and brachial neuralgia. In addition, inflammatory conditions need to be ruled out, such as polymyalgia rheumatica; inflammatory arthritis and infective arthritis of the shoulder.

ELBOW

The two most common regional pain syndromes around the elbow are: (1) Epicondylitis—lateral (tennis elbow) and medial (golfer's elbow) and (2) Olecranon bursitis.

Lateral and medial epicondylitis: An enthesitis or strain of the common extensor tendon of the wrist is responsible for LE and of the common flexor tendon for medial epicondylitis (ME). The patient will complain of pain and discomfort in the forearm, with radiation into the hand and occasionally, even up to the shoulder. Common day-to-day tasks involving gripping, become difficult. The history is fairly suggestive and the diagnosis may be confirmed, by eliciting tenderness at the lateral and medial epicondyles respectively, on resisting movements of the common extensor and flexor muscles of the wrist. Thus, painful resisted extension of the wrist will confirm a tennis elbow (**Fig. 3**) and painful resisted flexion of the wrist will confirm golfer's elbow.

A strain or enthesitis of the distal common biceps tendon, which inserts into the radial tuberosity, and a strain or enthesitis of the triceps tendon, which inserts into the posterior olecranon, are two other local pain syndromes at the elbow that might cause diagnostic confusion with epicondylitis. However, both will cause pain and discomfort at the cubital fossa or on resisted elbow flexion.

Management includes rest, avoiding active painful movements, analgesics, and NSAIDs. An appropriate splint particularly over the lateral epicondyle (tennis elbow splint) may also help. In addition, local application of ultrasound over the epicondyle at the site of tendon insertion may help and with persistent symptoms, a local steroid injection at that site may be of additional benefit.

Olecranon bursitis: The olecranon bursa (OB) is situated posterior to the olecranon process of the ulna and is rather superficial. Causes of OB include: Trauma—acute or mild chronic trauma; inflammatory disorders—RA or gout; or infection. Symptoms are pain, swelling with redness overlying the olecranon process (**Fig. 5**) and in addition, one may elicit a history suggestive of the underlying primary cause. These typical clinical features will enable a diagnosis of OB; though a detailed history and examination would be required to rule out any systemic causes.

Initial management is with rest, analgesics, and NSAIDs. Aspiration of the bursa with examination of the aspirated fluid is essential to exclude gout or infection. Septic bursitis would require treatment with appropriate antibiotics and may require repeated aspiration or incision and drainage. The primary condition—RA or gout—would require specific management. With persistent symptoms and once infection can be excluded, an injection of steroid into the bursa can be very helpful.

HIP

There are a number of conditions that can cause pain around the hip region and these may be categorized

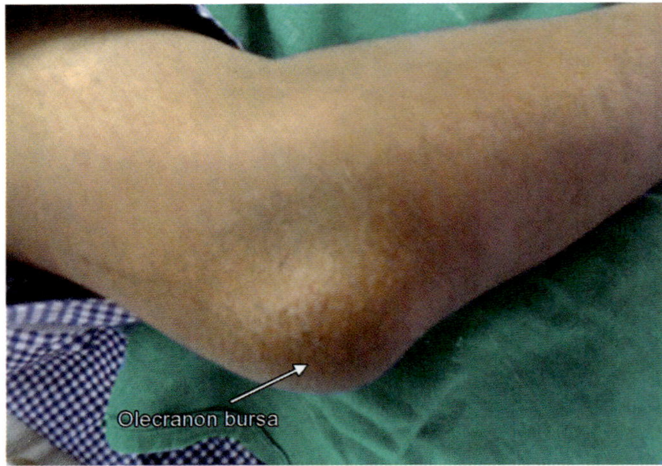

FIGURE 5: Olecranon bursitis.

according to the site of the symptoms—anterior groin, lateral trochanteric, or posterior buttock pain.

- Anterior groin pain may be caused by: (A) Hip joint disease such as with osteoarthritis, osteonecrosis, hip dysplasia, avascular necrosis, or inflammatory arthritis; (B) Soft tissue problems such as adductor tendonitis, pubic symphysitis, enthesitis of rectus abdominis and rectus femoris, or iliopsoas bursitis; and (C) Inguinal or femoral hernia.
- Lateral trochanteric pain may be caused by: (A) TB and; (B) Meralgia paresthetica (MP).
- Posterior buttock pain may be caused by: (A) Referred pain from the back; (B) Sacroiliitis; (C) Systemic conditions such as polymyalgia rheumatica; (D) Ischiogluteal bursitis; and (E) Vascular insufficiency.

The more commonly seen problems around the hip are TB, AT, and MP.

Trochanteric bursitis: The trochanteric bursa is situated on the greater trochanter (**Fig. 6**). Tendons of the gluteus medius and minimus muscles are also in close proximity. Inflammation of the trochanteric bursa or tendonitis of the gluteus medius or minimus muscles can cause lateral hip pain with tenderness on lying on the affected side, with tenderness being elicited over the affected greater trochanter. This is referred to as TB or greater trochanteric pain syndrome (GTPS) which is currently the favored term for this condition. GTPS or TB is seen more often in females, with risk factors being obesity, weak gluteals, and pelvic floor muscles and chronic low back pain. The diagnosis is clinical, based on the features as described. An ultrasound or MRI may help to confirm the diagnosis and exclude any other cause; and an X-ray of the pelvis will exclude hip disease.

Initial management is with rest, avoiding movements that exacerbate the pain, analgesics, and NSAIDs. Physiotherapy with muscle strengthening and gradual stretching exercises may be helpful. With persistent symptoms, a local steroid injection can be beneficial.

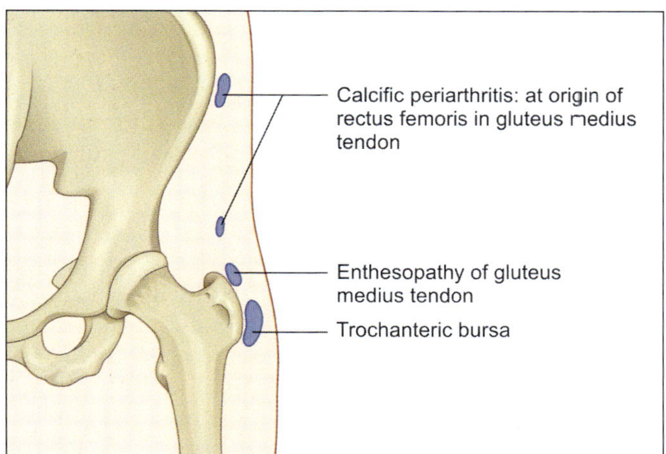

FIGURE 6: Greater trochanter showing trochanteric bursa and gluteus medius insertion.

Source: SKF Slide Atlas of Rheumatology. Gower Medical Publishing; 1986.

Adductor tendonitis: It refers to injury or strain of the adductor muscles of the hip. This results in pain and discomfort over the adductor muscles at the thigh with painful resisted adduction of the hip and tenderness over the muscles or their point of insertion, i.e., at the pubic symphysis which is the insertion of adductor longus. The diagnosis is usually made on clinical grounds. Radiographs, ultrasound, or MRI may be required for confirmation or to rule out other causes.

Management includes: Rest, ice packs, limb elevation, NSAIDs, or analgesics as required, with gradual mobilization. Local steroid injections may be needed for more persistent symptoms.

Meralgia paresthetica: It refers to the sensory symptoms of pain, paresthesia, and dysesthesia over the anterolateral thigh, resulting from compression of the lateral cutaneous nerve of the thigh as it exits from the abdomen under the inguinal ligament. Risk factors include: Obesity, old age, pregnancy, pendulous abdomen, diabetes, and tight garments around the belt area. The diagnosis is based on clinical symptoms, demonstrating sensory loss in the distribution of the lateral cutaneous nerve at the anterior thigh and excluding other causes. Nerve conduction studies may help in confirming the diagnosis. MP is often benign and self-limiting.

Management: Initially, analgesics and advice on how to reduce pressure on the lower abdomen may suffice. With more persistent symptoms, a local steroid injection at the exit point of the nerve under the inguinal ligament may help and occasionally one might need drugs like carbamazepine, phenytoin, or gabapentin.

KNEE

Common conditions at the knee include: Prepatellar bursitis (PB), pes anserine bursitis (PAB), and popliteal cyst (PC).

Prepatellar bursitis: Inflammation of the prepatellar bursa, which is situated anterior to the knee, between the patella and subcutaneous tissue, is known as prepatellar bursitis also referred to as "housemaid's knee." Repetitive kneeling is the most important risk factor. However, other causes include infection and inflammation due to crystals as in gout. Aspiration and examination of the fluid is essential to rule out infection or crystal inflammation.

Management includes rest, avoidance of aggravating movement, ice compression, analgesics, and NSAIDs. In more persistent symptoms and once infection is excluded, a local steroid injection may be helpful.

Pes anserine bursitis: The pes anserine bursa is situated at the upper, medial aspect of the tibia, beneath the tibial tubercle and deep to the insertion of the tendons of gracilis, sartorius, and semitendinosus muscles (GST) (**Fig. 7**). PAB occurs due to overuse or friction at the bursa due to valgus or rotatory stress at the knee or may occur as a result of direct injury. The patient complains of anteromedial knee pain. The discomfort will be distal to the knee joint however

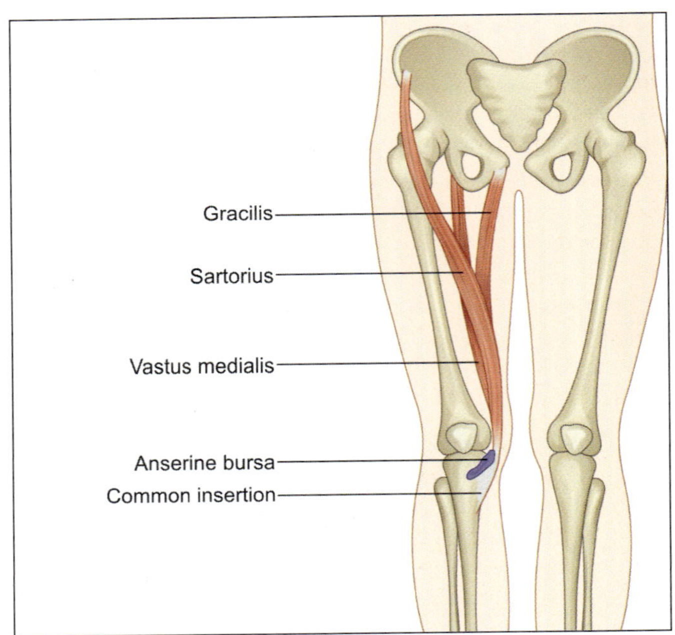

FIGURE 7: Pes anserine bursa and insertion of semitendinosus, gracilis, and sartorius muscles.

Source: SKF Slide Atlas of Rheumatology. Gower Medical Publishing; 1986.

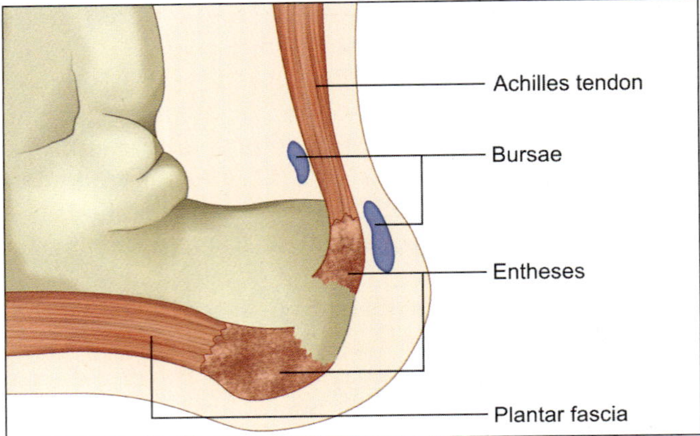

FIGURE 8: Bursae in relation to Achilles tendon and insertions of Achilles tendon and plantar fascia.

Source: SKF Slide Atlas of Rheumatology. Gower Medical Publishing; 1986.

and tenderness on palpation can be elicited over the PAB. An enthesitis of the common insertion of GST muscles can cause very similar symptoms. Risk factors include obesity, long distance runners, and underlying knee joint disease such as in osteoarthritis or RA.

Initial management is with rest, analgesics, and NSIADs. A well-placed local steroid injection can be very helpful.

Popliteal cyst: PC or baker's cyst is an inflammation of the bursa between the semimembranosus (SM) and medial head of gastrocnemius muscles at the medial aspect of the popliteal fossa. The PC communicates with the knee joint with a one way valve-like mechanism that allows movement of synovial fluid from the knee into the cyst but not vice versa. Most often, a PC will develop secondary to inflammatory disorders at the knee such as with RA or it could be a more gradual process. The patient will complain of a painful swelling in the popliteal fossa which will appear cystic on palpation. As the cyst enlarges, it may occasionally rupture, causing acute swelling and discomfort at the calf with discoloration of the overlying skin, which may simulate deep venous thrombosis (DVT). The diagnosis is often made on clinical grounds, though an ultrasound/Doppler study of the knee and calf may be required to rule out other causes such as DVT, aneurysms, ganglion, or meniscal cysts.

Initial management is with rest, ice packs, analgesics, and NSAIDs. Associated knee inflammation will need to be managed and this may alleviate the PC. Intra-articular injection of steroid for inflammatory joint disorders often results in resolution of the PC. For persistent PC associated with noninflammatory knee joint disease such as OA, aspiration of the cyst directly, preferably under ultrasound guidance, with injection of steroid, can be very helpful.

ANKLE OR FOOT

Plantar fasciitis (PF) and Achilles tendonitis are two common localized STR conditions seen around the ankle and foot.

Achilles tendonitis: Figure 8 illustrates the insertion of the Achilles tendon and plantar fascia into the calcaneus and the bursae in relation to the Achilles tendon. Conditions such as high intensity running, previous trauma, use of high heels, or treatment with quinolones or systemic steroids or associated inflammatory conditions such as SpA or RA, may predispose to the development of Achilles tendonitis. The patient will complain of pain at the back of the heel and local tenderness can be elicited at the point of insertion of the tendon into the calcaneus. An acute rupture of the tendon may occur due to sudden high intensity activity and is extremely painful. Palpating the length of the tendon may elicit tenderness and a gap at the point of rupture.

Initial management is conservative, with rest, ice packs, splint or brace, analgesics, and NSAIDs. Physiotherapy with local ultrasound application and gradual mobilization and strengthening exercises can be helpful. Rupture of the tendon may require surgical repair or appropriate immobilization. Local steroid injections may be considered for chronic AT; however, they should be undertaken with extreme caution and preferably under ultrasound guidance, to avoid injecting steroid into the tendon and causing an iatrogenic tendon rupture.

Plantar fasciitis: The plantar fascia is a thick, fibrous, collagenous tissue (or aponeurosis) that originates proximally from the medial tubercle of the calcaneus (**Fig. 8**) and then fans out over the sole distally, to be inserted at the base of each proximal phalanx. PF occurs due to chronic, degenerative enthesitis at the proximal end of the plantar fascia. Conditions such as deformities of the foot—pes cavus and pes planus, use of inappropriate foot wear, and limb length inequality may predispose to the development of PF. The patient typically complains of pain at the medial aspect of the heel, which is worse in the morning. Clinical examination will reveal tenderness on palpation of the medial aspect of the heel and also with passive dorsiflexion of the ankle and toes.

Management is conservative and includes rest, heel cushions and arch supports where indicated, analgesics, and NSAIDs. Physiotherapy with local ultrasound application and gradual stretching may be helpful. With more persistent symptoms, local steroid injections may be helpful.

DIFFUSE PAIN SYNDROMES

FIBROMYALGIA

Fibromyalgia is a clinical syndrome, characterized by persistent, diffuse pain, or chronic widespread pain in the body. This is typically described by the patient as "pain all over the body" including joints, muscles, and spine. However, there is no clinical discernible evidence of inflammation at any of these sites. This is more commonly seen in middle-aged women and the pain is accompanied by a number of other symptoms including: Fatigue, depressed mood, sleep disturbance, headaches, and social isolation. The incidence of some disorders, such as migraine or irritable bowel syndrome, is higher in individuals with FM.

Diagnosis: The diagnosis of FM is based essentially on recognizing the core clinical features of generalized pain, fatigue, and sleep disturbance, present for at least 3 months duration and in the absence of any other explanation for these symptoms. Amongst the first classification criteria for FM was brought out by the American College of Rheumatology in 1990 (**Box 2**) and was based on widespread pain of at least 3 months duration and tender points being elicited in at least 11 out of 18 sites. Attempts have been made to refine these criteria, recognizing the practical difficulties in correctly interpreting tender points on examination. Revisions to the criteria were made in 2010 and 2011, where physical examination and recording of tender points were not required and instead were based on painful body regions assessed by the widespread pain index (WPI) and the severity of symptoms-based symptom severity scale (SSS). The most recent revision on similar lines was in 2016 (**Box 3**).

Considering the rather wide range and nonspecific somatic symptoms, sometimes the diagnosis may be confusing. However, the constellation of diffuse, generalized body pain, sleep disturbance, clinical multiple tender points, and absence of clinical and examination features to suggest inflammation, should strongly suggest the diagnosis. It is important, however, to carefully examine each patient, to look for any clinical signs that might suggest an alternative diagnosis. There are no specific investigations for FM and the diagnosis rests on excluding other conditions and the typical clinical features. **Table 4** summarizes the main differential diagnoses for FM and some key investigations to exclude these.

Management of FM depends upon a systematic approach aimed at alleviating symptoms and allaying anxiety. Both pharmacologic and nonpharmacologic measures are important. Successful management will need to take into consideration both nonpharmacological and pharmacological measures.

BOX 2	Classification criteria for fibromyalgia (American College of Rheumatology 1990).
A.	**History of widespread pain for at least 3 months. Widespread pain defined as being present in:**
•	Left side of body; right side of body; above the waist; below the waist; axial skeleton
B.	**Pain on digital palpation in at least 11 of the following 18 sites (bilateral):**
1.	Occiput at suboccipital muscle insertion
2.	Low cervical region: At anterior aspect of C5 to C7
3.	Trapezius: At midpoint of anterior border
4.	Supraspinatus: At origin, above scapular spine, near middle border
5.	Second rib: At second costochondral junction
6.	Lateral epicondyle: 2 cm distal to the epicondyle
7.	Gluteal: Upper outer quadrant of buttock in anterior fold of muscle
8.	Greater trochanter: Posterior to trochanteric prominence
9.	Knee: At medial fat pad proximal to the joint line
Patients will be considered to have fibromyalgia for the purposes of classification, if both criteria A and B are satisfied	

BOX 3	Fibromyalgia criteria 2016 revision.
Criteria:	
A patient satisfies modified 2016 fibromyalgia criteria if the following three conditions are met:	
1.	Widespread pain index (WPI) ≥ 7 and symptom severity scale (SSS) score ≥ 5
	OR WPI 4–6 and SSS score ≥ 9
2.	Generalized pain, defined as pain in at least 4 of 5 regions, must be present. Jaw, chest, and abdominal pain are not included in generalized pain definition
3.	Symptoms have been generally present for at least 3 months
4.	A diagnosis of fibromyalgia is valid irrespective of other diagnoses. A diagnosis of fibromyalgia does not exclude the presence of other clinically important illnesses
WPI recorded in five regions; score 0–19	
(Regions: Left upper region; right upper region; left lower region; right lower region; axial region)	
SSS score: Three symptoms: (1) fatigue, (2) waking unrefreshed, and (3) cognitive symptoms. Each of these three symptoms graded 0–3; plus 1 point each, for the following three symptoms: Headache, pain/cramps in lower abdomen, depression	
SSS score 0–12:	
Fibromyalgia severity (FS) scale = WPI + SSS score	

TABLE 4 **Differential diagnosis and possible investigations for fibromyalgia.**

Disease/Condition	Investigations
Inflammatory conditions such as: • Rheumatoid arthritis (RA) • Systemic lupus erythematosus (SLE) • Polymyalgia rheumatica, inflammatory myositis	• ESR, CRP, RF, anti-CCP antibody, ANA, CPK, LDH • Complete blood count
Noninflammatory conditions: Osteoarthritis and joint hypermobility	• Radiology of affected joints • Clinical assessment for hypermobility
Endocrine disorders: Hypothyroidism and metabolic bone disease	• T3, T4, and TSH • Calcium, phosphate, serum PTH, alkaline phosphatase, and vitamin D level
Others: Steroid withdrawal, myeloma, malignancy, and statin ingestion	Based on history and where indicated: Cortisol levels, bone scan, serum protein, electrophoresis, CPK, LDH etc.

(CCP: cyclic citrullinated peptide)

Nonpharmacological measures: These will include the following:

- *Patient education and information*: This is a crucial aspect of management. Patients need to be explained the nature of the disease and that there is often a dichotomy between symptoms and physical findings. It should be stressed that there will be no permanent disability and there is no need for an aggressive drug regime.
- *Graded physical exercises*: A suitable program of graded exercises can be very helpful in maintaining adequate mobility and improving functional capacity.
- *Psychobehavioral management*: It can also help and these might comprise psychotherapy, hypnotherapy, and relaxation response therapy, where available.

Pharmacological measures: Some drug therapy will need to be part of the management regime and is often helpful in the overall treatment. The drugs that might be useful are:

- *Analgesics and NSAIDs*: Simple analgesics (paracetamol and tramadol) might be adequate for mild pain. NSAIDs, either nonselective (conventional) or the Cox-II selective (Coxibs), might be helpful for more persistent aches and pains.
- *Local injection*: For one or two very troublesome tender points not responsive to analgesics or NSAIDs, a local steroid injection may often be helpful.
- *Antidepressants*: Tricyclic antidepressants such as amitriptyline and cyclobenzaprine may be useful adjuncts in the drug treatment of FM and may alleviate pain, fatigue, and poor sleep. The selective serotonin reuptake inhibitors (SSRIs) like fluoxetine, citalopram, and paroxetine and the serotonin norepinephrine inhibitors (SNRIs) like duloxetine and milnacipran may be more helpful. They are best used in combination with an NSAID and it is important to remember, that this combination may take several weeks to show any clinical benefit.
- Some antiepileptic drugs have been found useful in these situations. Gabapentin and pregabalin that bind to the $\alpha_2\delta$ subunit of calcium channels have also been shown to be beneficial in the management of FM, particularly when combined with an antidepressant or analgesic/NSAID.

SUMMARY

Soft tissue MSK problems are fairly common. Early recognition and appropriate management are crucial to reduce the patient's pain and discomfort and minimize disability. Most of these disorders can be diagnosed by a detailed history and examination. It is important to rule out systemic or inflammatory joint conditions, for which appropriate investigations might be required. Management includes patient counseling, avoidance of aggravating activities, judicious use of analgesics and NSAIDs, physiotherapy as indicated, and local steroid injections. Surgical options might need to be considered if initial management is not successful.

RECOMMENDED READINGS

1. Kushner I. Overview of Soft Tissue Rheumatic Disorders. [online] Available from https://www.uptodate.com/contents/overview-of-soft-tissue-rheumatic-disorders.
2. Gupta SJ. Soft tissue rheumatism. In: Shah SN (Ed). API Text Book of Medicine, 8th edition. New Delhi: Association of Physicians of India; 2008.
3. Hubbard JM, Hildebrand BA, Battafarano MM, Battafarano DF. Common soft tissue musculoskeletal pain disorders. Prim Care Clin Office Pract. 2018;45(2):289-303.
4. Littlejohn G. Regional pain syndrome: clinical characteristics, mechanisms and management. Nature Clin Prac Rheumatol. 2007;3(9):504-11.
5. Goldenberg DL. Clinical Manifestations and Diagnosis of Fibromyalgia in Adults. [online] Available from https://www.uptodate.com/contents/clinical-manifestations-and-diagnosis-of-fibromyalgia-in-adults.
6. Wolfe F, Clauw DJ, Fitzcharles MA, Goldenberg DL, Häuser W, Katz RL, et al. 2016 Revisions to the 2010/2011 Fibromyalgia Diagnostic Criteria. Semin Arthritis Rheum. 2016;46(3):319-29.

CHAPTER
229

Low Back Pain

Molly Mary Thabah, Ved Chaturvedi

ABSTRACT

Low back pain is a leading cause of disability worldwide. Low back pain is acute if the duration is <6 weeks, subacute if the duration is from 6 to 12 weeks, and chronic if the duration of low back pain is persisting >12 weeks. Most acute low back pain resolve spontaneously, in only 10% it becomes chronic. For this very reason imaging of the spine is not recommended for acute low back pain unless there are compelling indication such as constitutional symptoms, weight loss, glucocorticoid use, cauda equina syndrome, or suspicion of infections or malignancy or it persists for >6 weeks. The etiology of low back pain is identifiable in only 10% cases, while in the remaining 90% no definite structural abnormalities is identified. This group is known as nonspecific low back pain. Genetic factors could be a risk to development of nonspecific low back pain. Degenerative spine disease is an important cause of low back pain with or without neurologic involvement. The diagnosis of spondyloarthritis needs to be considered in young people who present with chronic low back pain. Management is directed at the etiology of back pain. In nonspecific low back pain with a high risk of progression to chronic pain, the treatment consists of cognitive behavioral therapy, physical therapy, and structured exercises.

"Take care of your body. It's the only place you have to live"

—Jim Rohn

INTRODUCTION

Low back pain refers to pain that is localized between the costal margins (below the 12th rib) and the inferior gluteal folds. It is one of the most common musculoskeletal disorders in the community and is a common reason that brings a patient to hospital. A survey sponsored by Indian Council of Medical Research (ICMR) on the prevalent musculoskeletal conditions in three Indian cities revealed that up to 37% respondents had complaints of back pain/ spine pain. Back pain appeared to occur in the same frequency in urban and rural population, but slightly more prevalent in women compared to men. There are plenty of small community-based studies among Indian population that has consistently shown that low back pain is a highly prevalent symptom in adult men, adult women, and adolescents.

On a global level, the 2019 Global Burden of Disease study estimated that low back pain is among the top 10 diseases and injuries that account for the highest number of disability adjusted life years (DALYs) and years lived with disability (YLDs), in the age groups from 10 to 24 years, 25 to 49 years, and 50 to 74 years. Studies from industrialized nations show that the lifetime prevalence of low back pain ranges from 60% to 70%. In those who suffer from acute low back pain >90% recover, while in about 10% it can become chronic.

The Institute for Clinical Systems Improvement defines low back pain as acute when duration of symptoms is from 0 to 6 weeks, as subacute from 6 to 12 weeks, and as chronic >12 weeks.

APPROACH

There are numerous causes of low back pain (**Table 1**). Some causes of low back pain are serious conditions that merit prompt investigation and treatment.

HISTORY

A good history to identify "red flags" helps to narrow down the differential diagnosis, and plan investigations accordingly (**Table 2**). For example, a patient with back pain, fever, night sweats, and weight loss could be having infective etiology such as tuberculosis. Diskitis due to brucellosis is also well described in the literature. An elderly person presenting with back pain, and anemia will need workup for multiple myeloma. History of spontaneous fractures mandates one to rule out multiple myeloma. In those patients with a known history of malignancy, and recent back pain one must rule out metastasis.

If there is history of long-term glucocorticoid intake, or history of trivial trauma that precipitated low back pain, especially in an older individual vertebral (spinal) fracture must be ruled out. A systematic review has shown that the red flags with the highest posttest probability for detection of fracture were older age, prolonged use of corticosteroid drugs, severe trauma, and presence of a contusion or abrasion. Probability of spinal fracture is higher when multiple red flags are present.

If there is no fever or weight loss or other prominent constitutional symptoms, or malignancy in the history, it is useful to ask whether the back pain is inflammatory in

TABLE 1 Major causes of low back pain.

Causes	Clue to diagnosis
Infectious: • Tuberculosis of spine • Brucellosis • Others	• Fever, weight loss, lymphadenopathy, respiratory symptoms, and other supporting evidence of tuberculosis • History of consumption of raw milk and close contact with cattle is a risk factor for brucellosis
Malignancy related: • Direct involvement • Metastasis • Plasma cell dyscrasias	• Weight loss • History of cancer, receiving chemotherapy • History of new onset low back pain in an older individual • Nocturnal pain • Presence of anemia suggests multiple myeloma
Inflammatory *low back pain*: Spondyloarthritis	Patients with spondyloarthritis are young, in the age group <40 years. There can be other clues to spondyloarthritis such as presence of lower limb peripheral large joint arthritis, history of red eye or psoriasis
Mechanical *back pain*: • Spinal injuries • Vertebral compression fracture (spinal fracture) • Degenerative: ▪ Lumbar spondylosis/ osteoarthritis of the facet joints ▪ Lumbar spondylolisthesis ▪ Intervertebral disk prolapse ▪ Spinal canal stenosis • Diffuse idiopathic skeletal hyperostosis (DISH)	• History of significant trauma is present in cases of spinal injuries • Risk factors for vertebral (spinal) fracture include older age, chronic steroid use, and trauma • Intervertebral disk prolapse that is significant enough to cause impingement on the nerve root exits results in neurological symptoms. • Similarly, spinal canal stenosis if severe results in neurological symptoms
Pregnancy-related: • Pregnancy-related low back pain • Osteitis condensans ilii	• Low back pain with onset during pregnancy • Osteitis condensans ilii is seen in multiparous women. The onset of pain is pregnancy or postpartum period. Diagnosis is based on imaging and is characterized by sclerosis of the iliac side of the sacroiliac joint
Referred pain	In clinical practice low back pain can sometimes be referred pain from abdominal viscera. For example, a patient with kidney stones or a diabetic patient with pyelonephritis may complain of low back pain

TABLE 2 Red flags in patients who present with low back pain.

Red flag	Likely diagnosis
Unintentional weight loss	Malignancy or infections
Fever	Infections or malignancy
Anemia	Myeloma, other malignancies
Immunosuppression	Infections
History of cancer	Vertebral body metastasis
History of chronic glucocorticoid intake	Vertebral fracture
History of trivial trauma in an older person	Vertebral fracture
History of severe trauma or lifting heavy weights	Vertebral fracture
Inflammatory back pain in a young person	Spondyloarthritis
Low back pain not responding to treatment	Spinal canal stenosis
Acute retention of urine, overflow incontinence, and fecal incontinence	Cauda equina syndrome
Weakness of lower limbs or saddle anesthesia	Cauda equina syndrome

nature. Low back pain lasting >3 months in young adults can be due to spondyloarthritis.

Inflammatory back pain: It is a major presenting feature of axial spondyloarthritis (ankylosing spondylitis). But not all patients with inflammatory back pain will have spondyloarthritis. In a seminal study involving 170 individuals who satisfied the European Society Study Group (ESSG) criteria for spondyloarthritis (the ESSG criteria was developed in the 1990s to classify spondyloarthritis), only 114 individuals (67%) had spondyloarthritis confirmed on imaging and human leukocyte antigen B27 (HLA-B27) positivity. In this study the other causes for inflammatory back pain were other inflammatory, infectious, or degenerative disease.

The main characteristics of inflammatory back pain that are relevant for diagnosing axial spondyloarthritis are age at onset of back pain ≤35 years, improvement by exercise, improvement with nonsteroidal anti-inflammatory drugs (NSAIDs), waking up in the second half of the night, and alternating buttock pain.

There are many criteria used to classify inflammatory back pain (**Box 1**). The criteria for inflammatory back pain according to the Assessment of Spondyloarthritis International Society (ASAS) are able to correctly identify 92% inflammatory back pain (not for diagnosis of axial spondyloarthritis).

BOX 1 Inflammatory back pain.

Inflammatory back pain according to Calin et al. (1977)	
• Insidious onset • Age at onset <40 years • Duration >3 months • Morning stiffness • Relieved with exercise • *Requires the presence of four out of five	
Newer criteria for inflammatory back pain	
• *Berlin criteria (2006)*	• *Assessment of Spondyloarthritis International Society (ASAS 2010)*
• Morning stiffness >30 min duration • Alternating buttock pain • Nocturnal awakening (second half of the night because of pain) • Improvement in back pain with exercise but not with rest	• Insidious onset • Age at onset <40 years • Pain at night (with improvement on getting up) • Improvement with exercise • No improvement with rest
*The sensitivity is 70% and specificity 81% if two of the four criteria are fulfilled for classification of inflammatory back pain	*If at least four out of five parameters are present, sensitivity is 77.0% and specificity is 92% for presence of inflammatory back pain

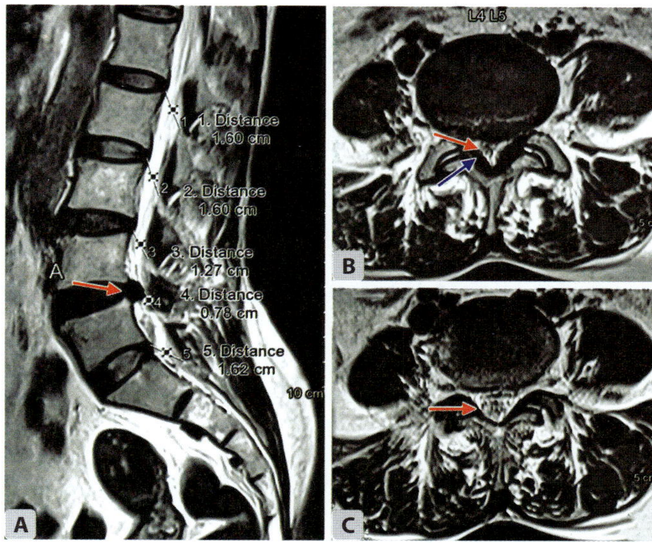

FIGURES 1 A to C: (A) Sagittal T2-weighted MRI image of lumbosacral spine shows L4–L5 disk herniation causing thecal sac indentation; **(B)** Axial T2-weighted MRI image at L4–L5 level shows narrowing of the spinal canal (red arrow). The blue arrow shows a markedly thickened ligamentum flavum. Compare this with axial images **(C)** at L3–L4 level showing a relatively preserved spinal canal (red arrow). These images are of a 48-year-old woman who presented with low back pain radiating to left buttock and the left leg for 1 month.

Mechanical low back pain: It arises as a consequence of functional abnormality or degenerative changes in structures of the spine, namely the vertebral bodies, the intervertebral disks, the facet joints, and soft tissues. In the absence of red flags (**Table 2**), majority (90% or more) cases of low back pain are mechanical in nature.

Mechanical low back pain is typically described as a diffuse pain in the low back that worsens on activity and is often relieved with rest or recumbent position. It is more common in people above the age of 30 years with slight female predominance.

Radiation of pain down the back of the thigh and leg, means that there is entrapment of the sciatic nerve due to intervertebral disk herniation at L4/L5 level or a spinal canal stenosis (**Figs. 1 A to C**). Whereas pain of the thigh and anterior calf would suggest impingement of L2/L3 or L3/L4 level nerve roots. The pain is often described as shooting or sensation of electric current. Pain can be exacerbated by movements that increase intradiskal pressure such as coughing or urinating.

In spinal canal stenosis apart from low back pain, the patient will have pain in the lower limbs that is precipitated by walking or standing (neurogenic claudication) and relieved by sitting down or bending forward. Sometimes pain in the leg may be unilateral, but the pain is not of a "shooting" quality unlike sciatica.

History should include enquiry for bowel or bladder involvement. Presence of urinary symptoms, namely retention of urine, difficulty in initiation of urination, overflow incontinence, and fecal incontinence should strongly arouse the suspicion of cauda equina syndrome. The cauda equina syndrome arises as a result of compression of the lower part of the spinal cord, i.e., the cauda equina by lumbar disk herniation at the L4/5 and L5/S1 level. Predisposing factors for a cauda equina syndrome are degenerative changes of the intervertebral disk, facet joints, and the thickening of ligamentum flavium overall contributing to spinal canal stenosis. There are other causes of cauda equina syndrome as well, for example traumatic injury and malignancy.

EXAMINATION

A focused physical examination is indicated to rule out systemic causes of low back pain, namely infections and malignancy. In case anemia is present, look for hepatomegaly and/or splenomegaly.

Neurologic examination is important to diagnose cauda equina syndrome and radiculopathies of L3–L5, and S1 nerve roots. Particularly look for presence of motor weakness in the ankle and foot, loss of sensations in the area of distribution of lumbar nerve roots (L2 to L5), and sacral nerve roots (S1 to S5). Also look out for the deep tendon reflexes as they help to localize the lesion. Absent knee jerk indicates involvement of L4 nerve root, while absent ankle jerk indicates involvement of L5 and S1 nerve root.

After completing neurological examination proceed to local examination of the spine. Inspect the spine for any deformities such as kyphosis, scoliosis, and gibbus. Palpate for tenderness or paraspinal muscle spasm. Movements of the cervical spine, forward and lateral lumbar flexion are limited in ankylosing spondylitis. The modified Schober's test is used to look for forward lumbar movement in ankylosing spondylitis.

Straight leg raising (SLR) test is performed with the patient lying supine on the examination couch. The examiner elevates the patient's leg, with knee extended. If the patient experiences sharp pain going down the leg below the knee, the test is positive. It indicates entrapment of the L5 and S1 nerve root. Pain usually occurs at about 30–70° hip flexion. Further if dorsiflexion of the ankle exacerbates the pain felt on SLR, it suggests spinal nerve compression due to disk herniation at L4–L5 and L5–S1 level. This test is also called Lasegue's sign. On SLR test elicitation of pain on the back of the thigh and knee should not be considered positive test, as it is due to hamstring tightness.

In the crossover sign, the examiners perform an SLR test on the nonaffected side. The patient experiences pain on the limb that is at rest. Positive test again indicates spinal nerve compression due to disk herniation at L4–L5 and L5–S1 level. It is supposed to be more specific than the SLR test.

In another test called the *femoral stretch test*, patient lies prone on the examination couch, then the examiner flex the knee. If there is pain in the anterior thigh the test is positive and indicates tension of nerve roots L2–L4.

IMAGING

Imaging in the evaluation of low back pain is primarily to rule out serious diseases. The American College of Radiology does not recommend imaging for acute, subacute, or chronic uncomplicated low back pain or radiculopathy in the absence of red flags unless back pain persists despite six weeks of treatment. This is because degenerative findings on plain radiographs and magnetic resonance imaging (MRI) spine are also seen in a large number of asymptomatic individuals. There is good evidence to suggest that *routine imaging does not have clinically meaningful benefits* and is associated with high cost.

A systematic review of 33 papers reporting on imaging findings of spinal degeneration in asymptomatic individuals, found that a large number of the study participants have features of spinal degeneration on MRI. This review found that disk degeneration was present in as many as 37% symptomatic 20-year-old individuals and in up to 96% of 80-year-old individuals. The prevalence of disk bulge and disk protrusion was found in 30% and 29% among the 20-year-old and up to 84% and 43% of 80-year-old age group, respectively.

A prospective cohort study involving >5,200 individuals older than 65 years who visited primary care for low back pain showed that early imaging is not helpful. In this study 1,174 had early radiographs, and 349 had early MRI or computed tomography (CT). At the end of 1 year the disability scores were not significantly different between those who had imaging by plain radiograph or CT/MRI versus those who did not undergo imaging.

However in those patients with low back pain and radiculopathy with "red flags" such as presence of one or more of the following features, namely trauma, osteoporosis, elderly, or chronic intake of glucocorticoids, where vertebral fracture is most likely pathology it is appropriate to proceed with plain radiograph of the lumbar spine or CT lumbar spine or MRI lumbar spine without contrast.

Similarly in those patients where there is suspicion of malignancy or infection, or those who are on immunosuppression MRI lumbar spine with or without contrast or CT lumbar spine is indicated.

Plain radiography of the lumbar spine is a reasonable initial choice of imaging and is adequate to diagnose fracture. *But MRI is the investigation of choice* for assessing soft tissue abnormalities, diskitis, vertebral foraminal narrowing, spinal canal stenosis, assessing the facet joints, spinous processes, and other finer details.

DIFFERENTIAL DIAGNOSIS

Given below is a discussion on the identifiable causes of low back pain. The conditions listed below is not exhaustive. Clinical judgement is useful to decide whether to investigate further or to classify the patient as chronic nonspecific low back pain.

DEGENERATIVE SPINE DISEASE

Degeneration of the spine is an important cause of mechanical low back pain. The cervical spine and lumbar spine are the most susceptible part of the spine to degenerate because of high mobility in these areas. Degenerative spine disease can be in several forms, namely disk bulge, disk herniation/protrusion/prolapse, and disk rupture whereby there is rupture of the nucleus pulposus.

Lumbar disk herniation: The first event to probably happen in disk herniation is an age-related dehydration of the nucleus pulposus, micro-tears in the annulus, followed by weakening of the annulus, all contributing to disk herniation into the extradural spinal canal. Other factor that contributes to disk herniation is calcification of the vertebral end plate with advancing age. Most of the time disk herniation occurs posterolaterally rather than central or extraforaminal. In the lumbar spine disk herniation most often occurs at L4–L5 levels (**Figs. 1 A** to **C**) or L5–S1 levels. A Schmorl's nodes is herniation of the nucleus pulposus through the vertebral end plate into the adjacent vertebral body. Schmorl's nodes are incidental imaging findings and do not correspond to back pain.

Initial symptoms of lumbar disk herniation are low back pain, and radicular pain involving buttocks and lower limb. The onset can be acute or gradual. Pain can be worsened by coughing or sneezing and is sometimes relieved by flexing the hip. Impingement on the L5 and S1 nerve root (because of L4–L5, or L5–S1 disk herniation) produces sensory loss in the area of distribution of L5 and S1 respectively, with absent ankle jerk in the latter. Sensory findings are more predominant than motor findings. Lumbar spine MRI helps in clearly delineating the lesion. Majority of the cases improve with conservative management alone, few become chronic.

Lumbar spondylosis: Lumbar spondylosis also known by other names such as *spinal osteoarthritis and spondylosis deformans is a degenerative spine disease.* It is characterized by osteophytes at the anterior, lateral, and less commonly posterior margins of the vertebral body. Osteophytes often occur secondarily to disk degeneration. The other component of lumbar spondylosis is facet joint osteoarthritis. As the disease progress, osteophytes grow inward and cause spinal canal stenosis and sometimes disk bulge. It usually occurs in older people and majority patients are above 40 years of age. The imaging findings of lumbar spondylosis characterized by osteophytes of the vertebral bodies, thickened ligamentum flavum, and narrowing of the disk space occur quite commonly in the general population. Lumbar spondylosis is usually asymptomatic. If symptomatic the symptoms are low back pain, that worsens with hyperextension of spine, and neurogenic claudication if there is spinal stenosis. The patient usually feels better with rest. If there is associated symptomatic facet joint osteoarthritis the pain radiates to buttocks and thighs and worsens on lateral flexion to the involved side.

Lumbar spondylolisthesis: Spondylolisthesis is when one vertebral body including its pedicle and associated articular facet slips over another vertebral body (**Figs. 2 A** and **B**), while its posterior elements are left behind. Spondylolisthesis can be anterior or posterior. The various causes of spondylolisthesis are trauma, infections, spondylosis, and degenerative disk disease. Spondylolisthesis due to spondylosis and degenerative disk disease usually occurs at L4–L5 level (**Fig. 2 A**).

Lumbar spondylolisthesis is a prominent cause of low back pain. It can cause radiculopathy, spinal canal stenosis (**Fig. 2 B**), and severe cases result in cauda equina syndrome. When the condition is advanced one can feel "step off" on palpation in the lumbosacral region.

Lumbar spondylolysis: While spondylosis is seen in older people, *lumbar spondylolysis is seen in young people who are athletes by profession.* It can also occur secondary to trauma. Lumbar spondylolysis is a defect in the posterior segments of the vertebra especially the pars interarticularis region also called isthmus of the vertebra. It is most common in L5 vertebra followed by L4. Professional gymnasts are at risk to spondylosis as hyperextension movement of the spine creates a stress fracture in the isthmic region. Those individuals with bilateral spondylolysis are also at risk of associated lumbar spondylolisthesis. It often seen in the general population as an asymptomatic condition, but it can also present with low back pain and radiculopathy. Diagnosis by CT or MRI is more sensitive than by plain radiography.

Lumbar canal stenosis: Lumbar canal stenosis is a prominent cause of low back pain, radiculopathy, and neurogenic claudication. Patients often present with neurogenic claudication that gets relieved on sitting or bending forward. Usually there is no bladder involvement. Lumbar canal stenosis can be congenital, idiopathic, or acquired. It can also be a manifestation of metabolic bone diseases such as renal osteodystrophy and Paget's disease.

Usually degenerative pathology such as facet joint osteoarthritis, thickening of the ligamentum flavum, disk bulge, disk herniation, and spondylolisthesis all pool together to cause acquired lumbar canal stenosis (**Figs. 2 A** and **B**). The stenosis can be central or in the lateral recess. Lumbar canal stenosis is absolute when the midsagittal diameter of the central spinal canal is <10 mm or relative if it is between 10 mm and 13 mm. Initial treatment consists of analgesics and an attempt to reduce the inflammation and edema with epidural steroids. In cases where there is significant spondylolisthesis surgical decompression by laminectomy or laminectomy is the preferred treatment option.

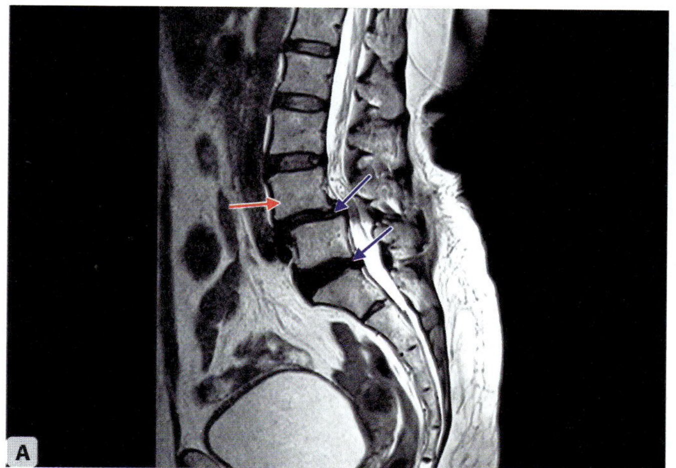

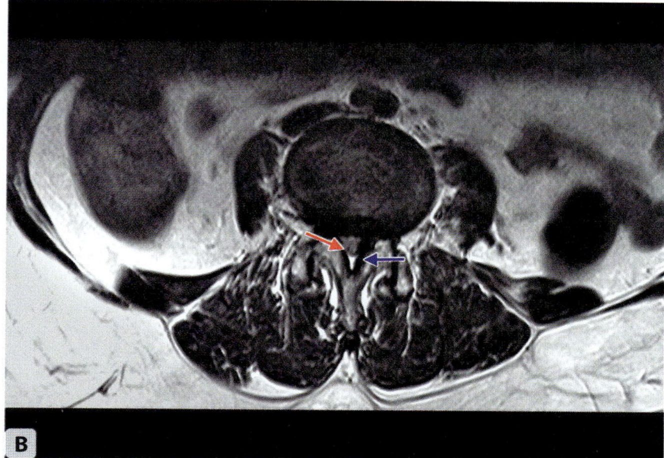

FIGURES 2 A & B: (A) Sagittal T2-weighted MRI image of lumbosacral spine shows bilateral pars plana defect of L3 with grade 1 anterolisthesis of L3 over L4 (red arrow). L4–L5 shows diffuse disk bulge causing thecal sac indentation (blue arrows); **(B)** Axial images show diffuse bulge of the L3–L4 disk causing spinal canal stenosis (red arrow), with thecal sac, traversing and exiting nerve rot compression. Disk bulge is also causing bilateral neural foraminal narrowing. There is bilateral mild ligamentum flavum thickening (blue arrow) at L3–L4, and L4–L5. These images are of a 46-year-old woman who has low back pain and radiculopathy since 1 year. Conservative management was advised.

CAUDA EQUINA SYNDROME

Cauda equina syndrome is compression of the lumbosacral nerve roots within the spinal canal distal to the termination of spinal cord leading to back pain, acute onset urinary retention, overflow incontinence, fecal incontinence due to decrease anal tone, and asymmetrical weakness of the lower limbs.

The syndrome occurs when there a compressive lesion of the cauda equina usually due to ruptured or herniated intervertebral disk. The other types of compressive lesions are fracture of spine due to trauma, and hematoma in spinal canal. The signs are asymmetrical lower limb motor weakness, absent knee, and ankle reflex, with saddle anesthesia. Vertebral disk pathology resulting in a cauda equina syndrome needs to be urgently attended and an urgent surgery is recommended. The procedure generally involves partial laminectomy with excision of prolapsed disk (diskectomy).

INFECTIONS

Vertebral osteomyelitis is usually caused by *Staphylococcus aureus*. Other organisms involved are *Escherichia coli*. Diabetics, alcoholics, and patients on immunosuppression are at risk for developing vertebral osteomyelitis and diskitis. Posterior extension of the infection can result epidural abscess. More often times than not there is a focus of primary infection in the skin and soft tissue, or urinary tract or endocarditis. The clinical features of infections are low back pain, fever, leukocytosis, and high inflammatory markers. The back pain is usually present continuously and has no relation with activity nor posture. MRI will characterize the site of abscess and can be used to guide local drainage procedures.

Tuberculosis and brucellosis are two chronic infections that can involve vertebral bodies and the intervertebral disk causing infectious diskitis. In tuberculosis apart from back pain, patients will have fever, weight loss, and involvement of the respiratory system. Many of these patients will have evidence of tuberculosis elsewhere. In tuberculosis the diskitis can progress to cause soft tissue swelling that compresses the spinal cord and result in neurological impairment such as paraplegia. Examination of the spine may reveal a spinal deformity called gibbus. CT of the spine helps in clearly differentiating tuberculosis from brucellosis, while tuberculosis is associated with destruction of vertebral components, brucella causes sclerotic vertebral bodies, can involve the sacroiliac joint sometimes mimicking ankylosing spondylitis.

OSTEOPOROSIS

Osteoporotic vertebral fracture is a differential diagnosis of back pain in elderly women. The most common site of osteoporotic vertebral fracture is the mid thoracic and thoracolumbar junction (T12–L1). Osteoporosis is typically painless, and vertebral fractures occurring slowly over time are often incidentally detected on plain radiography, but sometimes vertebral compression fractures can occur acutely precipitated by a mild trauma or the patient can have sudden onset of low back pain after lifting a weight or bending forward. Vertebral compression fractures involving upper dorsal spine or accompanied by fever and weight loss need further evaluation. Management is conservative with analgesics like NSAIDs or opioids.

Spondyloarthritis is discussed in a separate section of the book.

OTHER CONDITIONS

Traumas from road traffic accidents are obvious reasons for injury to the spine resulting in low back pain. Other traumas due to fall from height can lead to direct injury to the spine causes anterior wedging and compression fractures. Others with history of lifting heavy weights can predispose to listhesis in an already degenerative spine. When neurological impairment is present, early surgical intervention is indicated. Neck and back need to be immobilized with spine board until diagnosis is achieved and treatment is planned.

Malignancy can be considered in the differential diagnosis if red flags such as weight loss, nocturnal pain, and pain that does not get relieved with rest are present. Other red flags are a history of malignancy, in which case metastatic deposits from breast, prostate, and lung can occur.

Diffuse idiopathic skeletal hyperostosis (DISH) is often incidentally detected on plain radiographs. DISH can be considered in the differential diagnosis of back pain in older individuals especially if there is diabetes and hypertension. The anterior longitudinal ligament is ossified, together with large bridging osteophytes gives the appearance of flowing wax on plain lateral view radiographs of the dorsolumbar spine. In individuals with chronic kidney disease renal osteodystrophy can be a cause of low back pain.

CHRONIC (NONSPECIFIC) LOW BACK PAIN

In >90% cases of low back pain no serious pathology nor major anatomic issue is identified. This is the major chunk of low back pain seen in primary care and the general population. Such patients are classified as chronic nonspecific low back pain. Sometimes the word "lumbago" or "lumbar sprain" or lumbar strain" is used to indicate this group. Ensure there are no red flags before assigning patient in this category. Just like there are red flags to identify serious conditions of low back pain, "yellow flags" (**Table 3**) are psychological risk factors that predict progression of acute low back pain to become chronic, further leading on to work disability, absenteeism, and presenteeism at work.

As mentioned in the imaging section, findings of degenerative spine disease are seen quite commonly in the general population without any symptoms at all. On the other hand there are those patients with nonspecific low back pain who have disabling pain that even leads to loss of productivity at work but the source of pain cannot be identified on spine imaging. This disconnect between imaging findings and low back pain has led to research on role of genetics in low back pain. In fact recent twin

TABLE 3 Yellow flags are psychological risk factors for chronic low back pain.

Yellow flag	Example
Beliefs, appraisals, and judgment	• Unhelpful beliefs about pain: Indication of injury as uncontrollable or likely to worsen • Expectations of poor treatment outcome • Delayed return to work
Emotional response	• Distress not meeting criteria for diagnosis • Worry • Fears • Anxiety
Pain behaviors and pain coping strategies	• Avoidance of activities due to expectations of pain and possible reinjury • Overreliance on passive treatments (hot packs, cold packs, and analgesics)

Source: Adapted from Nicholas MK, Linton SJ, Watson PJ, Main CJ; "Decade of the Flags" Working Group. Early identification and management of psychological risk factors ("yellow flags") in patients with low back pain: a reappraisal. Phys Ther. 2011;91(5):737-53. With permission from Oxford University Press.

studies, single candidate gene analysis, and Genome-Wide Association Studies (GWAS) data are also available that have identified a possible link between low back pain and heritability.

To identify the low back pain patient who is likely to progress to chronic low back pain screening tools have been developed. An example is the online STarT Back calculator that is available at https://startback.hfac.keele.ac.uk/training/resources/startback-online/. This questionnaire-based calculator has nine questions relating to radicular pain, neck pain or shoulder pain, difficulty in walking due to pain, difficulty in dressing, other questions relating to worry, and fear avoidance and emotional distress. A score of 4 or more suggest high risk of progressing to chronic low back pain. Another questionnaire is the Örebro Musculoskeletal Pain Screening Questionnaire (OMPSQ) short form originally developed by Linton et al. in 1997 and revised in 2011. This questionnaire can predict absenteeism and identify those who are likely to have delay in returning to work.

The management of chronic nonspecific low back pain can be done either by the stepped approach or by risk stratification approach. In the stepped approach treatment depends on the duration of low back pain. Those with acute or subacute pain (duration of back pain <12 weeks) are advised self-management, superficial heat therapy, massage, and acupuncture. Those with chronic pain (duration >12 weeks) are advised exercises, spinal manipulation, and cognitive behavioral therapy.

The risk stratification approach classifies patients into those with a low risk and those with a moderate-high risk of having chronic low back pain. This approach is an attempt to prevent development of chronic pain in those who are at risk. Risk assessment is done by the OMPSQ short form or the StarTBack screening tool. Moderate to high risk individuals are given structured exercises, cognitive-based therapy, and other psychological therapies. Low risk individuals are given manual therapy, i.e., spinal manipulation, and/or group exercises. Needless to say, physical therapists and psychologists have a major role in the management of chronic nonspecific low back pain. In both the approaches pharmacological therapy using NSAIDs, opioid analgesics, and skeletal muscle relaxants is advised if nonpharmacological therapy is not helpful.

CONCLUSION

Low back pain is a major problem in the general population. Clinical approach to such a patient involves *identification of red flags that would suggest an underlying serious condition*. Once these are ruled out, identify those patients with significant neurological deficits, namely cauda equina syndrome. These patients will need urgent surgical intervention. Next are those patients with radiculopathy and duration of pain that is <6 weeks, for these patients conservative management is advised. If spinal canal stenosis is suspected, those with severe symptoms will need early MRI and surgical consultation, otherwise if symptoms are mild, conservative care is advised, followed by imaging if symptoms persist beyond 6 weeks. Patients with nonspecific low back pain require physical therapy, structured exercise program, and cognitive behavioral therapy for a good outcome, apart from pharmacological treatment.

RECOMMENDED READINGS

1. Sharma R (Ed). Epidemiology of Musculoskeletal Conditions in India. New Delhi, India: Indian Council of Medical Research (ICMR); 2012.
2. GBD 2019 Diseases and Injuries Collaborators. Global burden of 369 diseases and injuries in 204 countries and territories, 1990-2019: a systematic analysis for the Global Burden of Disease Study 2019. Lancet. 2020;396(10258):1204-22.
3. Safiri S, Kolahi AA, Cross M, Hill C, Smith E, Carson-Chahhoud K, et al. Prevalence, deaths and disability adjusted life years (DALYs) due to musculoskeletal disorders for 195 countries and territories 1990-2017. Arthritis Rheumatol. 2021;73(4):702-14.
4. Downie A, Williams CM, Henschke N, Hancock MJ, Ostelo RW, de Vet HC, et al. Red flags to screen for malignancy and fracture in patients with low back pain: systematic review. BMJ. 2013;347:f7095.
5. Braun A, Saracbasi E, Grifka J, Schnitker J, Braun J. Identifying patients with axial spondyloarthritis in primary care: how useful are items indicative of inflammatory back pain? Ann Rheum Dis. 2011;70(10):1782-7.
6. Brandt J, Bollow M, Häberle J, Rudwaleit M, Eggens U, Distler A, et al. Studying patients with inflammatory back pain and arthritis of the lower limbs clinically and by magnetic resonance imaging: many, but not

all patients with sacroiliitis have spondyloarthropathy. Rheumatology (Oxford). 1999;38(9):831-6.
7. Markman JD, Czerniecka-Foxx K, Khalsa PS, Hayek SM, Asher AL, Loeser JD, et al. AAPT Diagnostic criteria for chronic low back pain. J Pain. 2020;21(11-12):1138-48.
8. Chou R, Qaseem A, Owens DK, Shekelle P. Diagnostic imaging for low back pain: Advice for high-value health care from the American College of Physicians. Ann Intern Med. 2011;154(3):181-9.
9. Brinjikji W, Luetmer PH, Comstock B, Bresnahan BW, Chen LE, Deyo RA, et al. Systematic literature review of imaging features of spinal degeneration in asymptomatic populations. AJNR Am J Neuroradiol. 2015;36(4):811-6.
10. Jarvik JG, Gold LS, Comstock BA, Heagerty PJ, Rundell SD, Turner JA, et al. Association of early imaging for back pain with clinical outcomes in older adults. JAMA. 2015;313(11):1143-53.
11. Vlaeyen JWS, Maher CG, Wiech K, van Zundert J, Meloto CB, Diatchenko L, et al. Low back pain. Nat Rev Dis Primers. 2018;4(1):52.
12. Patel ND, Broderick DF, Burns J, Deshmukh TK, Fries IB, Harvey HB, et al. ACR Appropriateness Criteria Low Back Pain. J Am Coll Radiol. 2016;13(9):1069-78.
13. Linton SJ, Hallden K. Can we screen for problematic back pain? A screening questionnaire for predicting outcome in acute and subacute back pain. Clin J Pain. 1998;14(3):209-15.
14. Nicholas MK, Linton SJ, Watson PJ, Main CJ, "Decade of the Flags" Working Group. Early identification and management of psychological risk factors ("yellow flags") in patients with low back pain: a reappraisal. Phys Ther. 2011;91(5):737-53.
15. Almeida M, Saragiotto B, Richards B, Maher CG. Primary care management of nonspecific low back pain: key messages from recent clinical guidelines. Med J Aust. 2018;208(6):272-75.

CHAPTER 230 Osteoarthritis

Renu Saigal, Amit Kansal, Vikramraj Jain

ABSTRACT

Osteoarthritis (OA) is the most prevalent, age-related, multifactorial degenerative disease of joints. Age, obesity, trauma, and genetic factors play an important role in pathogenesis. The whole of the joint is involved in OA. Loss of articular cartilage leads to joint space narrowing, subchondral sclerosis, subchondral cyst formation, and osteophyte formation. Treatment includes nonpharmacologic measures such as exercise, weight loss, and bracing. Pharmacologic treatment includes topical capsaicin and nonsteroidal anti-inflammatory drugs (NSAIDs), and if the patient is unresponsive, systemic NSAIDs and duloxetine are given. In selected indications, intra-articular injection of corticosteroids may be preferred. Various disease-modifying osteoarthritis drugs are in the pipeline. Failure of pharmacologic therapy and functional disability requires surgery.

"My message is - keep moving. If you do, you'll keep arthritis at bay"

—Donna Mills

INTRODUCTION

Osteoarthritis is the most prevalent, age-related, multifactorial degenerative disease of joints. The disease process is slowly progressive and destroys articular cartilage irreversibly, and affects the whole joint. As inflammation too plays an important role in pathogenesis, so the term osteoarthritis is justified.

The disease poses health problems in the elderly population. Early diagnosis, therapeutic intervention, and physiotherapy can slow down the degenerative process.

RISK FACTORS

AGE

Incidence and prevalence of OA increase with age especially after 50 years. With age, extracellular matrix (ECM) and cells of the joint also undergo senescence. With increasing age, articular cartilage thinning because of reduced hydration and proteoglycan content and accumulation of advanced glycation end products (AGEs) make the collagen more brittle.

Aging also leads to mitochondrial dysfunction, reduced autophagy, and reduced response to anabolic factors, e.g., insulin-like growth factor (IGF)-1, transforming growth factor-beta (TGF-β), thus repair processes lag behind destructive process mediated by proinflammatory mediators and proteases.

SEX HORMONES

Apart from aging, loss of estrogen is contributing to the increased occurrence of post-menopausal OA among women.

OBESITY

Mechanical overloading is a key factor in the pathogenesis of OA. Intra-articular stress leads to initiation and later destruction of joints. Obesity may add inflammatory risk in OA joints by increased levels of adipokines such as leptin and adiponectin secreted by adipose tissue. Macrophages within adipose tissue also produce proinflammatory cytokines interleukin-6 (IL-6) and tumor necrosis factor-α (TNF-α). Besides weight-bearing joints such as knee and hip joints, this inflammatory process also involves hand joints viz. first carpometacarpal joint (CMC) and distal interphalangeal (DIP) joints.

TRAUMA

Osteoarthritis may develop after surgical or nonsurgical trauma to menisci, cartilage, ligaments, capsule, and subchondral bone. Occupations involving frequent squatting, kneeling, and stair climbing lead to microtrauma and OA. Heavy repetitive labor and knee bending (e.g., in farming, construction industry etc.) is a risk factor for OA. A sports injury in high-impact sports (e.g., football) can lead to anterior cruciate ligament (ACL) injury, nearly half of whom develop radiographic knee OA in 10–15 years.

GENETICS

Rare mutation of collagen type II, IX, or XI may cause hereditary form of OA, which may start in adolescence and is usually severely destructive. Twin studies have shown that a less severe form of OA also has a genetic risk of approximately 40%. *GDF-5, ADAM12, CLIP, COL11A2, IL10,* and *MMP3* are susceptibility genes that lead to increased collagen degradation.

DEFECTS IN CARTILAGE METABOLISM

Chondrocyte metabolism is dependent on various growth factors—TGF-β, Wnt-β catenin, bone morphogenic protein-2 (BMP-2), nitric oxide (NO) metabolism etc. Human OA cartilage overexpresses proteins of the Wnt pathway, matrix metalloproteinase (MMP) 13, and a disintegrin and metalloproteinase with thrombospondin motifs (ADAMTs). Loss of TGF-β expression is seen in human OA.

SECONDARY OSTEOARTHRITIS

Cartilage damage secondary to systemic diseases:

- **Hereditary diseases:** Alkaptonuria, hemochromatosis, and Wilson's disease
- **Bone diseases:** Paget's disease and avascular necrosis
- **Charcot's joints:** Loss of proprioception and joint laxity makes the joint more susceptible to destruction as in diabetes, syringomyelia, and aging
- **Hemoglobinopathies:** Sickle cell disease and thalassemia
- **Acromegaly:** Cartilage thickening due to excess growth hormone (GH) and IGF-1 followed by damage
- **Infection:** Septic arthritis causing cartilage and subchondral bone destruction
- **Congenital or developmental anatomic aberrations:** Epiphyseal dysplasia, slipped capital femoral epiphysis, Legg–Calve–Perthe disease, and congenital dislocation, leading to biomechanical injury
- **Inflammatory arthritis:** Rheumatoid arthritis, spondyloarthritis, crystal arthritis, e.g., calcium pyrophosphate dihydrate disease (CPPD) and gout

PATHOGENESIS

Normal joint consists of articular cartilage consisting of chondrocytes, surrounded by ECM of collagen and proteoglycans. Cells of synovial membrane, i.e., synoviocytes form synovial fluid (SF) by ultrafiltration of serum, which has noncellular component hyaluronic acid (a glycosaminoglycan) and proteoglycan 4. SF provides nutrition to the avascular articular cartilage and provides viscosity and elasticity to the joint during movements.

PATHOLOGY

Articular cartilage, subchondral bone, synovium, and SF all are affected in OA. Loss of cartilage results in joint space narrowing especially at areas of highest loads. In the knee joint, mainly medial tibiofemoral (TF) space is reduced though lateral TF and patellofemoral (PF) space may also be reduced. After the destruction of cartilage, subchondral bone is exposed and vascular invasion occurs resulting in thickening of subchondral bone because of increased cellularity, and it is called eburnation, which occurs at areas of pressure. Cyst formation may occur at subchondral bones because of the intrusion of SF. These cysts are also known as subchondral cysts or geodes, range from 2 to 20 mm in size. Osteophytes form at the insertion of tendons and ligaments.

The pathophysiological process of OA (**Flowchart 1**) can be divided into three overlapping stages:

1. ECM network damage/alteration at a molecular level
2. Impaired chondrocyte response to tissue damage
3. Failure to restore cartilage leads to its progressive loss

ROLE OF INFLAMMATION

Synovial inflammation is present in OA joints; macrophages are present in SF in contrast to T and B cells in rheumatoid arthritis. In response to joint injury, several proinflammatory cytokines and chemokines are liberated. As a result of inflammation, proteolytic enzymes are produced, which degrade ECM and destroy joint tissue especially the articular cartilage.

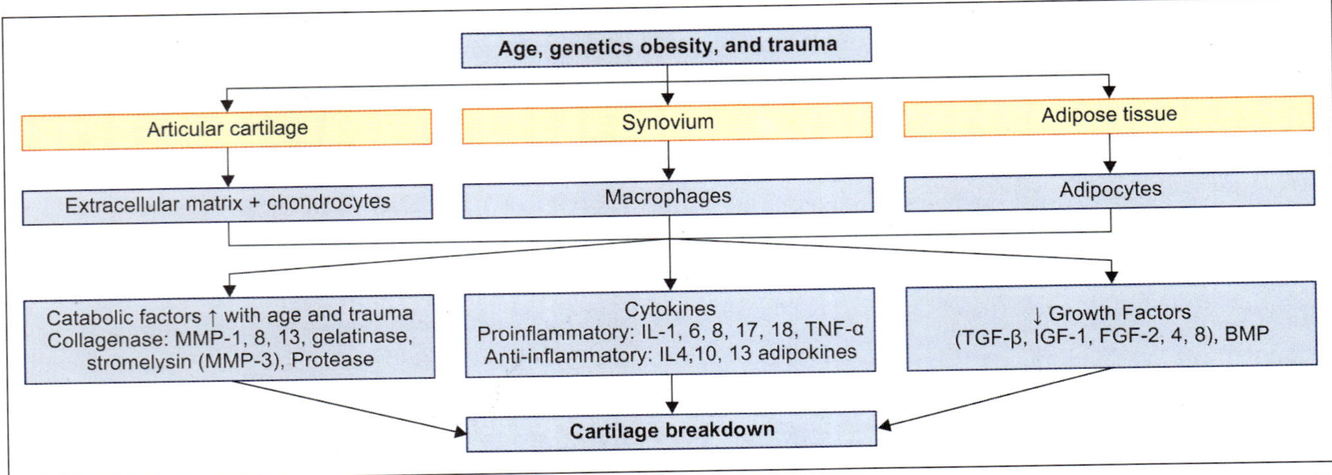

(MMP: matrix metalloproteinase; IL: interleukin; TGF: transforming growth factor; IGF: insulin-like growth factor; BMP: Bone morphogenetic protein; FGF: fibroblast growth factor)

FLOWCHART 1: Pathogenesis of osteoarthritis.

Cytokines that are found in high concentration are IL-6, macrophage chemotactic protein (MCP)-1, interferon-induced protein (IP)-10, and monokine induced by interferon (MIG). Various other cytokines are secreted by articular chondrocytes or meniscal cells, which attract macrophages into the joint and promote matrix degradation.

Chondrocytes also secrete various proteases, e.g., MMPs, cysteine proteinases including cathepsin K and serine proteinases. Cartilage resiliency provided by aggrecans (a proteoglycan) is degraded by aggrecanases—ADAMTS 4 and 5. Type II collagen, which gives tensile strength to cartilage, is degraded by collagenases like MMP 13.

Articular cartilage does not exhibit adequate repair response probably due to avascularity, so irreversible matrix damage occurs.

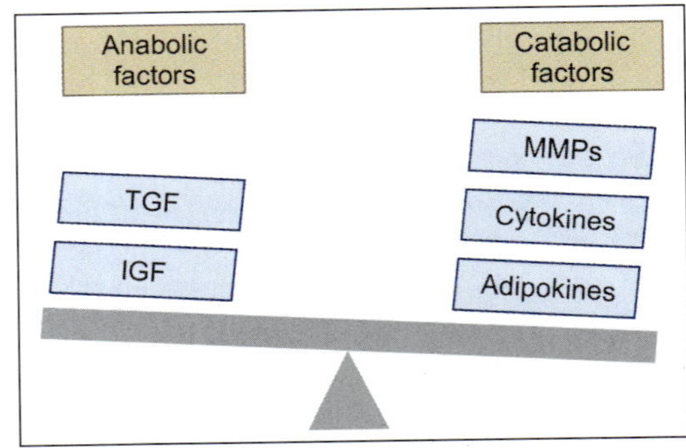

(MMP: matrix metalloproteinase; TGF: transforming growth factor; IGF: insulin-like growth factor)

FIGURE 1: The imbalance between catabolic and anabolic factors in the articular cartilage.

ROLE OF INFRAPATELLAR FAT PAD

Infrapatellar fat pad (IFP) is located underneath the patella, between the patellar tendon, femoral condyle, and tibial plateau. The IFP contains large numbers of adipocytes, fibroblasts, macrophages, leukocytes, and other immune cells capable of producing inflammatory cytokines. Neutrophils produce cytokines such as IL-1, IL-8, and MMP-8, which contribute to cartilage breakdown. Adipocytes are responsible for the secretion of the adipokines, such as leptin and adiponectin. While leptin stimulates the production of IL-1β and MMPs, adiponectin induces the production of IL-6 and MMP-1.

In summary, in OA, there is an imbalance between the catabolic and anabolic processes in the articular cartilage with low-grade inflammation in the cartilage, bone, and synovium, leading to joint dysfunction (**Fig. 1**).

FACTORS CAUSING PAIN

- Synovial membrane inflammation and nociceptor activation
- Increased intraosseous pressure in the subchondral bone because of increased vascularity
- Periosteal elevation because of osteophytes
- Stretching of the joint capsule because of effusion
- Bursitis in the periarticular region
- Muscle spasm around joint
- Central pain sensitization
- Psychological factors
- Meniscal tearing

CLINICAL FEATURES

- Deep joint pain aggravated by activity with either no early morning stiffness (EMS) or EMS of <30 minutes known as gelling.
- In some patients, pain is of burning, i.e., neuropathic quality around the joint suggestive of associated fibromyalgia.
- In patients with associated CPPD, signs of inflammation such as redness and swelling may be present.
- Tenderness along the joint line with bony enlargement may be palpated.
- Decreased range of movements and crepitus, a crunchy sensation, on palpation of the knee may be present.

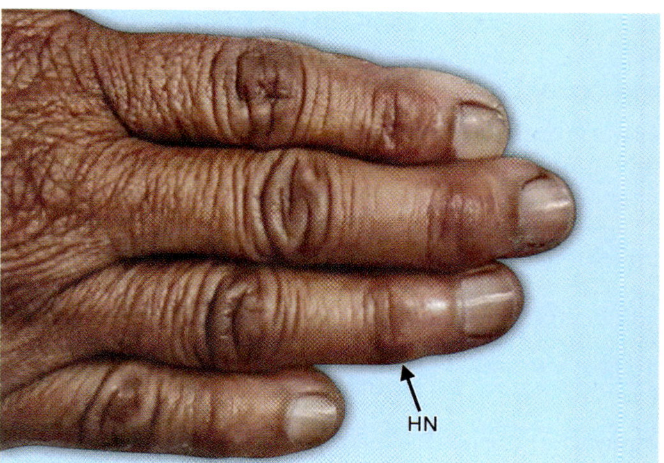

FIGURE 2: Heberden's node (HN).

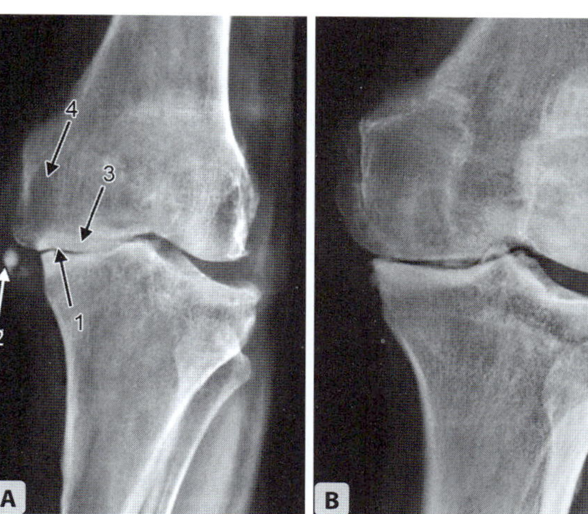

FIGURES 3 A & B: Weight-bearing X-ray of knee joint antero-posterior (AP): **(A)** 1—tibiofemoral joint—joint space narrowing grade IV; 2—loose body in joint cavity; 3—subchondral sclerosis (eburnation); 4—subchondral cyst. **(B)** 5—osteophytes.

- Joint deformity, e.g., squaring of hand and subluxation of thumb may occur because of advanced damage to the 1st CMC joint. Genu varus deformity may occur because of damage to the TF joint.
- Joint instability may be seen because of muscle weakness and altered patellar tracking (with lateral patellar tracking), giving rise to true joint instability and patients may fall.
- *Hand OA*: First CMC joint (over snuffbox) is painful and tender. Both proximal interphalangeal (PIP) and DIP joints may be involved with the bony enlargement at these sites called Bouchard's and Heberden's nodes (**Fig. 2**), respectively. Joint involvement is usually symmetrical.
- *Missouri syndrome*: Second and third MCP may be involved in OA in the elderly occurring due to physically demanding occupation.
- Erosive OA targets DIP joints more frequently than PIP joints. Symptoms persist longer and functional impairment is more in erosive than in nonerosive OA.
- Rapid progression of OA is seen in patients with high body mass index, varus deformity, older age, and multiple joint involvements.

DISTRIBUTION OF JOINTS

Joints affected in primary OA are knees, hips, PIP and DIP joints, first CMC joints, first MTP joints, and apophyseal (facet) joints of the lower cervical and lower lumbar spine (L3, 4, and 5).

DIAGNOSIS

Imaging is not usually required to make the diagnosis in typical OA. In the atypical presentation, it may be done to confirm the diagnosis or make alternative or additional diagnoses.

CONVENTIONAL RADIOGRAPHY

In knee joints, weight-bearing and PF radiological views are recommended.

TABLE 1 **Kellgren–Lawrence grading system.**

Grade	Description
Grade 1	Doubtful joint space narrowing (JSN) and possible osteophytic lipping
Grade 2	Definite osteophytes and possible JSN
Grade 3	Moderate osteophytes, definite JSN, some sclerosis, possible bone-end deformity
Grade 4	Large osteophytes, marked JSN, severe sclerosis, and definite bone ends deformity

Marginal osteophytes and joint space narrowing (a marker of cartilage loss) may be seen in affected joints with subchondral sclerosis (eburnation) or cyst formation (**Figs. 3 A** and **B**). **Table 1** shows the 4 grades of OA in X-rays.

MAGNETIC RESONANCE IMAGING

In early OA, conventional radiography (CR) may be normal, so to visualize early changes in cartilage, meniscus, ligaments, synovium, SF, and capsule MRI may be done. However, MRI is not recommended for routine clinical management of OA.

ARTHROCENTESIS

Synovial fluid is noninflammatory, with WBC count of <2,000 cells/mm^3 mononuclear cells. Usually, arthrocentesis is not required; it may be done to rule out infection or crystal arthropathy (gout and CPPD).

DIFFERENTIAL DIAGNOSIS

Gout, septic arthritis, inflammatory arthritides, and malignancy producing bone pain are few diseases with which OA may be confused. Signs of inflammation, clinical features, and laboratory investigations can clarify the picture.

MANAGEMENT

The goal of management: To minimize symptoms and optimize function are the aim and joint damage has to be modified, though no approved disease-modifying OA drugs (DMOAD) are yet available. Joint malalignment, muscle weakness, overweight and obesity, and concurrent depression have to be managed judiciously.

NONPHARMACOLOGIC MEASURES

These measures are the mainstay of management in OA (**Tables 2** and **3**).

Patient education: Patients should be educated regarding etiology, risk factors, management, and prognosis of OA and modification by lifestyle changes. Misconceptions are to be allayed.

TABLE 2 Nonpharmacologic measures: Strongly recommended.

Measures	Strongly recommended
Exercise	Muscle strengthening, walking, stationary cycling, and aquatic exercises
Weight loss	If overweight or obese
Cane	Assist walking, reduce pain, and increase mobility. To be used in the hand contralateral to the affected side
Tai Chi	Improved balance, reduction of pain, and improvement in depression were observed in studies
Self-management	Either individually or in groups especially exercise
Supportive devices	Knee braces for patellofemoral and tibiofemoral OA, 1st CMC orthosis, and tap turners

(CMC: carpometacarpal joint; OA: osteoarthritis)

TABLE 3 Nonpharmacologic measures: Conditionally recommended.

Measures	Conditionally recommended
Heat/Therapeutic cooling	With heat, beneficial short-term effects are observed. For flare in pain/swelling, cold compresses may be useful
Cognitive behavioral therapy (CBT)	For coping with pain or psychological symptoms, weight loss, and exercise
Acupuncture	By releasing endorphins may reduce pain, however, results are equivocal
Knee and hand OA	Kinesio taping
Patellofemoral	Knee brace, Yoga, and radiofrequency ablation
For knee and hip OA	Balance training
For hand OA	Paraffin and hand orthoses

(OA: osteoarthritis)

Recommendations are different for hip, knee, PF joint, first CMC, or particular patient populations (e.g., those with erosive OA).

Exercise: Muscle strengthening and general aerobic fitness, irrespective of disability, comorbidity, and age are very important in the management of OA.

Starting with walking for 10 minutes, gradually increasing to 30 minutes thrice a week after 2–3 months. Aerobic and strengthening exercises improve pain and function.

Weight loss: In obese and overweight patients, body weight loss of 10% will reduce pain markedly.

Supportive devices: Walking aids and knee braces will improve pain in PF and TF OA. Splints are useful for hand joint arthritis at the base of the thumb.

PHARMACOLOGIC RECOMMENDATIONS

Failure of the nonpharmacological measures in a symptomatic patient requires pharmacological agents (**Table 4**). No agent till date has shown a disease-modifying effect.

Before prescribing drugs, comorbid conditions, hypertension, chronic kidney disease, cardiovascular disease, and gastrointestinal bleed risk have to be considered.

Topical NSAIDs and capsaicin: Topical NSAIDs are strongly recommended for knee joints, while in hand joint, topical NSAIDs are conditionally recommended. The risk of renal, cardiovascular, and gastrointestinal toxicity is much lower with topical NSAIDs than oral preparations.

For knee OA, topical capsaicin (0.025–0.1%) three to four times daily downregulates transient receptor potential vanilloid-1 (TRPV1) receptor activity on sensory neurons and depletes substance P (which produces pain). Local burning may occur in some patients, which improves with continued use.

Acetaminophen: The analgesic effect of this drug is clinically not significant, but it may be used if NSAIDs are not tolerated or are contraindicated, even in these conditions, episodic and short-term use is recommended. With a higher dose, hepatotoxicity, gastrointestinal bleed,

TABLE 4 Pharmacological measures.

Strongly recommended	• Topical NSAIDs and capsaicin • Oral NSAIDs • Intra-articular steroids for knee and hip OA: Image-guided for latter
Conditionally recommended	• Acetaminophen • Tramadol • Duloxetine • *Hand OA:* Topical NSAIDs, chondroitin sulfate and IA CS • Topical capsaicin in knee OA

(CS: corticosteroid; IA: intra-articular)

renal failure, and cardiovascular disease have been seen. Toxicity should be monitored by getting liver function and renal function tests done.

Oral NSAIDs: When topical NSAIDs or acetaminophen fails, oral NSAIDs are given. For the knee, hip, and hand OA, oral NSAIDs are strongly recommended in low doses for a short period on an as-needed basis, after ruling out the possible contraindications and monitoring the adverse effects. Cyclo-oxygenase-2 (COX-2) inhibitors, e.g., etoricoxib may be used, as they have fewer gastrointestinal side effects, nevertheless, proton pump inhibitors should be given along with NSAIDs.

Intra-articular corticosteroid (CS) injections: Knee and hip joints intra-articular CS injections are strongly recommended as an adjunct to core treatment for moderate-to-severe pain; in hand OA, it is conditionally recommended. Frequent intra-articular GC should be avoided, as it may lead to cartilage loss and progression of OA. In the hip joint, ultrasound guidance may be required since the joint is deep. Triamcinolone or methylprednisolone depot injections are recommended. Triamcinolone hexacetonide injection is less soluble so preferred because its effect is more prolonged than methylprednisolone depot injections. Local anesthetic is given along with intra-articular CS, as it provides instant relief from pain and reducing or eliminating postinjection flare.

Serotonin–norepinephrine reuptake inhibitors: In the knee, hip, and hand OA, duloxetine is conditionally recommended. It acts by modulating nociceptive processing in the spinal cord and periaqueductal area thus reducing pain and when given with oral NSAIDs, pain reduction was more as compared to oral NSAIDs given alone. Side effects such as dry mouth, constipation, nausea, reduced appetite, and fatigue may be seen. Newer agent milnacipran had superior efficacy because of better-balanced affinity for noradrenergic and serotonergic reuptake transporters.

Other centrally acting agents such as pregabalin, gabapentin, selective serotonin reuptake inhibitors, and tricyclic antidepressants have not shown as good effect as duloxetine.

Tramadol: In patients with contraindications to NSAIDs, failure of other therapies and, if surgery is not feasible, tramadol may be used. The addiction potential of tramadol should be considered, if used for longer than 1 year. Adverse effects such as nausea, drowsiness, and dizziness may occur.

HAND JOINT OSTEOARTHRITIS MANAGEMENT

The basic aim is to relieve pain and stiffness and maximize function and quality of life, by muscle strengthening and exercise. Patients should be educated and trained in ergonomic principles and the use of assistive devices such as splints. Orthoses should be considered for the relief of symptoms and long term use.

- *Topical NSAIDs:* Treatment of choice
- *Oral NSAIDs:* For limited duration for relief of symptoms
- *Chondroitin sulfate:* For pain relief and functional improvement
- *Intra-articular CS preferred* for painful interphalangeal joints, otherwise not recommended

Box 1 summarizes the management of mild-to-severe OA.

BOX 1	Management of mild-to-severe osteoarthritis (OA).
Mild OA:	
• Education of patient	
• Exercise	
• Weight reduction in an obese or overweight patient	
Patient reassessment, if the patient improves, this strategy is continued and the patient is monitored for progression of symptoms. If symptoms progress then:	
• Topical NSAIDs or capsaicin is recommended and the patient is monitored. If the patient improves then these measures are continued	
If symptoms are persistent or progress, then the diagnosis is re-evaluated or treated for moderate/severe OA	
Treatment of moderate/severe OA:	
Besides the measures mentioned in mild OA, the following measures are taken:	
• Knee braces for tibiofemoral or patellofemoral OA	
• Cane for walking	
• CBT for coping pain and psychological symptoms	
If symptoms persist or progress then:	
• Oral NSAIDs are added	
If symptoms progress or persist:	
• Oral duloxetine may be added	
If still, symptoms persist or progress:	
• Intra-articular CS may be tried in selected patients for short-term pain relief	
Adjunctive measures are to be employed and for persistent pain, surgery may be required	

(CBT: cognitive behavioral therapy; CS: corticosteroid)

EXPERIMENTAL/CONTROVERSIAL THERAPIES

Nutraceuticals (food substances that provide health benefits):

Glucosamine and chondroitin: These nutritional agents in doses of glucosamine 1,500 mg and chondroitin in 800 mg were not found to be unequivocally effective in various trials. Some trials showed relief of pain and delayed structural progression and some observed that these drugs were not better than placebo. Due to these uncertain data, these agents are not strongly recommended in various OA guidelines.

Curcumin (derived from turmeric) and Boswellia serrata: Low-quality evidence for pain relief in OA was observed. Two-thirds of these trials are industry-funded, so unbiased trials are needed.

Other nutritional supplements: Fish oil, vitamin D, diacerein, avocado soybean unsaponifiables, and undenatured type II collagen have been used but there is lack of clear evidence of the beneficial effect of these supplements. Vitamin D is given, if its deficiency exists.

Platelet-rich plasma: It is derived from autologous blood, contains growth factors, which help in matrix and collagen formation. By reducing NF-kappa-beta signaling, it decreases inflammatory cytokine activation and subsequent inflammation. Trials done so far lack standardization and so further standardized studies are required before its use in OA can be validated.

Intra-articular hyaluronans: Large double-blinded, high-quality trials show very small benefit in knee OA over intra-articular placebo, which was not relevant clinically. It may be associated with pain flare up and its cost is high. Currently, it is not recommended in various guidelines for the management of OA.

DISEASE-MODIFYING OSTEOARTHRITIS DRUGS

These are the drugs that reduce the structural progression in OA, relieve pain, and improve functional outcome. Numerous disease-modifying osteoarthritis drugs (DMOADs) are still under consideration (**Box 2**). No current drug is able to modify the progression of OA and prevent long-term disability.

NOVEL THERAPIES

Antibodies to nerve growth factor (NGF): Elevated levels of NGF were found in SF of OA patients; it modulates the expression of pain-related substances and sensitization of nociceptive neurons in response to inflammation. Phase III trials of anti-NGF drug, Tanezumab, showed significant relief in pain, function, and stiffness. Pain relief may lead to intensive use of compromised joints and subsequently increased damage to joints. Osteonecrosis is another concern with the use of Tanezumab.

Bradykinin receptor B2 antagonist: Bradykinin is a vasodilator and inflammatory peptide, induces angiogenesis, and promotes vessel permeability, growth, and remodeling through Bradykinin B_2 receptor. Studies are going on with fasitibant.

BOX 2	Disease-modifying osteoarthritis drugs (DMOADs) emerging drugs under trial.
• Aggrecanase inhibitor	
• MMP inhibitor	
• Cathepsin K inhibitor—MIV-711(O)	
• iNOS inhibitor	
• Transforming growth factor-β (I/A)	
• Recombinant human FGF18—sprifermin (I/A)	
• Senolytic drug—fisetin (O)	
• Wnt inhibitor—lorecivivint (I/A)	

(MMP: matrix metalloproteinase; FGF: fibroblast growth factor; iNOS: inducible nitric oxide synthase; O: oral; I/A: intra-articular)

REGENERATIVE THERAPIES

Repair and regeneration of cartilage are done by mesenchymal stem cells, which are obtained from adipose tissue, synovium, and bone marrow. Studies are going on in these therapies. Autologous chondrocyte implantation is an evolving surgical technique for early OA, especially in younger patients.

SURGERY

Arthroscopic lavage and debridement should only be done, if the patient of knee OA gives a history of locking and there is radiological evidence of loose bodies. Osteotomies (e.g., tibial osteotomy) are joint preserving surgeries aimed at restoring the biomechanics of the diseased joint. These are useful in a select subset of patients, especially younger patients with few comorbidities and good bone quality.

Arthrodesis (joint fusion) is another option for OA of the ankle, first MTP, and joints of the hand. Trapeziectomy for thumb base OA and arthroplasty with silicone implants are preferred for PIP joints except for PIP-2 for which arthrodesis may be done. For DIP joints also, arthrodesis is preferred to relieve pain but not for improving function.

For structural abnormalities and advanced knee and hip OA when medical therapies fail and there is pain, stiffness, and functional impairment, which is substantially affecting the quality of life, surgery such as knee or hip replacement may be done before there is established functional limitation and severe pain.

Surgery should *not* be deferred or contraindicated because of age, sex, smoking, obesity, or other comorbidities. Patients should be educated regarding the benefits and risks of surgery and rehabilitation after surgery. Postoperatively, some patients may have moderate to severe pain.

CONCLUSION

Osteoarthritis is most prevalent, age-related, degenerative disease, which involves all the tissues of joint and leads to irreversible loss of articular cartilage. Management includes modification of risk factors, pain relief, and physiotherapy. DMOADs are being tried and trials are going on but till date, no drug is yet approved.

RECOMMENDED READINGS

1. Kolasinski SL, Neogi T, Hochberg MC, Oatis C, Guyatt G, Block J, et al. 2019 American College of Rheumatology/Arthritis Foundation Guideline for the Management of Osteoarthritis of the Hand, Hip, and Knee. Arthritis Rheumatol. 2020;72(2):220-33.
2. Deveza AL, Hunter D, Curtis MR, UpToDate Inc. (2020). Overview of the management of osteoarthritis. [online] Available from https://www.uptodate.com/contents/overview-of-the-management-of-osteoarthritis.
3. National Institute for Health and Care Excellence (NICE). [2020]. Osteoarthritis overview. [online] Available from http://pathways.nice.org.uk/pathways/osteoarthritis.

4. Lozada CJ, Diamond HS. (2020). Osteoarthritis. [online] Available from https://emedicine.medscape.com/article/330487-overview.
5. Malfait AM, Schnitzer TJ. Towards a mechanism-based approach to pain management in osteoarthritis. Nat Rev Rheumatol. 2013;9(11):654-64.
6. Bajpayee AG, Grodzinsky AJ. Cartilage-targeting drug delivery: can electrostatic interactions help? Nat Rev Rheumatol. 2017;13(3):183-93.
7. Latourte A, Kloppenburg M, Richette P. Emerging pharmaceutical therapies for osteoarthritis. Nat Rev Rheumatol. 2020;16:673-88.
8. Kapoor M, Mahomed NN. Chapter: Pathogenesis of osteoarthritis. Osteoarthritis: Pathogenesis, Diagnosis, AvailableTreatments, Drug Safety, Regenerative and Precision Medicine. Switzerland: Springer International Publishing; 2015.

CHAPTER 231

Gout and Other Crystal-related Arthritides

Binoy J Paul, Reeta James

ABSTRACT

The crystal-related arthropathies represent a heterogeneous group of disorders in which minerals get deposited in musculoskeletal tissues and result in pathological changes. Intra-articular crystals can cause acute and chronic inflammation and joint damage via biomechanical and biochemical pathways. The most common crystal-related arthropathies are gout, calcium pyrophosphate (CPP) dihydrate disease (pseudogout), basic calcium phosphate (BCP) crystal deposition disease, and calcium oxalate arthropathy. Other substances, which may lead to crystal-induced arthropathy, include xanthine, cholesterol, cystine, aluminium phosphate, Charcot–Leyden crystals and possibly others. The recent advances in imaging modalities have made a welcome change in the rapidity and specificity of diagnosis of these conditions and extensive research has yielded newer drugs, which have revolutionized the treatment thereby reducing the associated morbidity and improved the quality of life of people suffering from these arthropathies.

"Nobody can take away your pain, but don't let pain take away your happiness"

—Mariska Hargitay

GOUT

When serum uric acid levels remain persistently above the saturation threshold of urate (about 7 mg/dL), monosodium urate (MSU) crystals get deposited in the joints or soft tissues such as cartilage or renal parenchyma, resulting in the clinical syndrome of gout. In the joints, this leads to inflammatory changes whereas in other sites, inflammation does not occur.

Uric acid is the end product of purine metabolism. Purines are derived partly from the diet and partly from endogenous metabolism. In the liver, nucleic acids and purine nucleotides are degraded to form the purine bases, *xanthine*, and *hypoxanthine*, which are oxidized to form uric acid by the enzyme *xanthine oxidase*. This urate circulates in the plasma to be excreted mainly by the kidneys. A smaller amount is secreted into the gut. In normal men taking purine-free diets, the daily urinary excretion of uric acid is 350–500 mg.

Plasma levels of uric acid vary from 2 to 7 mg/dL (0.12–0.42 mmol/L) in health. The term hyperuricemia denotes values above 7 mg/dL (0.42 mmol/L) in men and 6 mg/dL (0.36 mmol/L) in women. Hyperuricemia may result either from underexcretion (85–90% cases) or overproduction (10–15% cases). Though hyperuricemia is a biochemical precursor of gout, not everyone with high urate levels develop gout.

The genetic basis of the disease is poorly understood. Urate transport genes—*SLC2A9* and *ABCG2*; the gene encoding the renal transporter of uric acid (SLC17A1) and gene encoding the anion exchanger URAT1 (SLC22A12) are thought to be the major genes involved. GLUT-9 (glucose transporter-9) transports uric acid along with glucose and fructose and so explains the pivotal role of dietary glucose and fructose in hyperuricemia. So, gout is now considered to be more of a transportopathy.

Gout is seen predominantly in men during middle life. The male-female ratio is 7:1 to 9:1. Onset of gout is usually in the third decade of life. Early onset should raise the possibility of other metabolic disorders of purine metabolism such as hypoxanthine–guanine phosphoribosyltransferase (*HGPRT*) deficiency.

SECONDARY HYPERURICEMIA

Here, hyperuricemia results from a demonstrable disorder, leading either to overproduction or defective excretion of uric acid (**Table 1**).

PATHOGENESIS

The pathological hallmark of gout attack is the *neutrophil influx into synovium and joint fluid* triggered by the interaction between MSU crystals and synovial lining cells. MSU crystals are phagocytosed by macrophages triggering formation of inflammasomes, which results in formation of proinflammatory cytokines, especially interleukin (IL)-1β. Inflammasomes are multimeric cytoplasmic protein complexes, which act as molecular platforms for activation of inflammatory caspases following stimulation by foreign agonists. Enhanced MSU crystal-induced superoxide production by neutrophils, driven by the subclinical inflammatory cytokine environment, combined with hyperuricemia contributes to elevated neutrophil IL-8 production and survival in the absence of direct crystal stimulation.

Crystals are demonstrable in the synovium and articular cartilage in the stage of acute arthritis. In the chronic stage, erosion of articular cartilage, proliferation of synovial membrane, pannus formation, cystic erosions of bones, and secondary osteoarthritic changes develop.

CLINICAL FEATURES

Gout passes through four clinical stages:

1. Asymptomatic hyperuricemia
2. Episodes of acute gouty arthritis
3. Asymptomatic intervals (intercritical gout)
4. Chronic gouty arthritis

Acute gout: Gout classically presents as "podagra"—acute onset of pain with erythema and swelling in the first metatarsophalangeal joint (**Fig. 1**) in 75% of patients. This may be mistaken for septic arthritis. Up to 3–14% may have polyarticular involvement at presentation. This may be associated with fever and other constitutional disturbances. The initial attack subsides with treatment or spontaneously to recur periodically, due to precipitating factors such as dietary excess, alcoholic bouts, infections, trauma, undue physical exercise, surgery, or withdrawal of urate-lowering drugs.

Intercritical (interval) gout: The interval between two gouty attacks is called intercritical gout. The patient will be totally asymptomatic, but uric acid crystals can be demonstrated by aspiration of synovial fluid (SF) from previously inflamed joint. Progressive bony erosions can also develop during this period, which can be demonstrated by serial radiographs of the affected joint. The duration of intercritical gout varies. Without diet control, lifestyle modification, or drugs, most patients experience a second episode of arthritis within 2 years and thereafter, more frequently.

Chronic tophaceous gout: The acute attacks do not remit completely and the joints become constantly painful and swollen. Tophi develop as subcutaneous nodular masses around the joints and on tendons (**Fig. 2**). Histologically, these consist of MSU crystals surrounded by mononuclear cell infiltration and foreign-body giant cells. They are soft and small initially but later on become hard and may reach up to very large sizes (**Fig. 2**). These lead to osteoarthritic changes, ankylosis of joints, and tissue destruction. They may ulcerate discharging the chalky material. Most common sites for tophi are around the olecranon, ankles, tendoachilles, helix of the ear, and over other joints. Osteoarthritis and ankylosis supervene.

Atypical forms may develop in addition to the typical gouty arthritis. Subacute polyarthritis similar to rheumatoid disease or isolated joint lesions may occur. Sometimes, the

TABLE 1 Causes of secondary hyperuricemia.

Increased urate production	Decreased renal clearance
• Inherited enzyme defects: ▪ HGPRT deficiency (Lesch–Nyhan syndrome) ▪ Glucose-6-phosphatase deficiency (G6PD) ▪ Phosphoribosyl pyrophosphate synthetase overactivity • Myeloproliferative disorders • Psoriasis • Hemolytic diseases • Malignancies • Tumor lysis syndrome • High-purine diet • Alcohol	• *Renal:* Chronic kidney disease, polycystic kidney disease, lead nephropathy • *Endocrine:* Hyperparathyroidism, hypothyroidism, diabetes insipidus (DI) • *Metabolic:* Lactic acidosis, starvation ketoacidosis, severe dehydration • *Metabolic syndrome:* Obesity, dyslipidemia, hypertension • *Drugs:* Diuretics, low-dose aspirin, pyrazinamide, cyclosporine, ethambutol • *Miscellaneous:* Sarcoidosis, toxemia of pregnancy, Down syndrome

(HGPRT: hypoxanthine-guanine phosphoribosyltransferase)

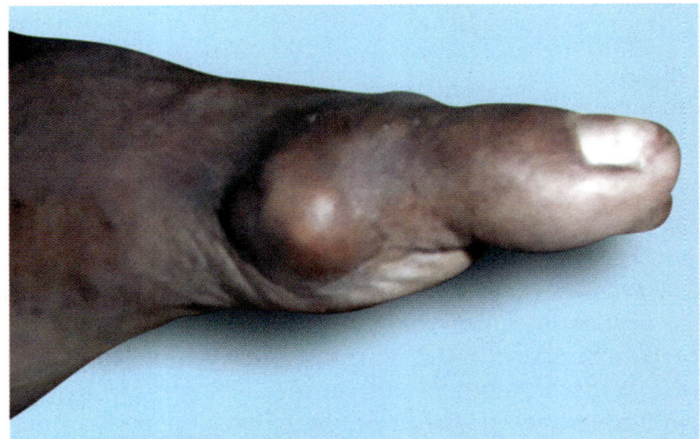

FIGURE 1: Acute gouty arthritis of first metatarsophalangeal joint.

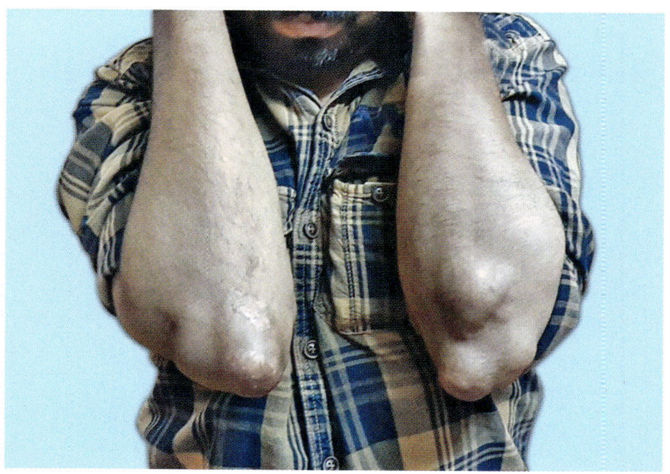

FIGURE 2: Bilateral olecranon bursitis with tophi in a patient with gout.

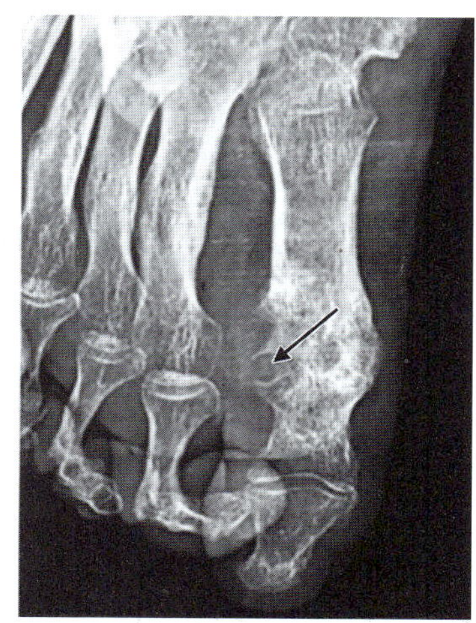

FIGURE 3: X-ray foot in gout.

Note: The punched out lytic lesions with overhanging margin (arrow) on the proximal phalanx of big toe.

initial presentation may be with soft tissue involvement such as Achilles tendinitis or olecranon bursitis (**Fig. 2**). Tophi may also be seen in organs such as the cornea, heart, tongue, bronchi, and pleura.

COMPLICATIONS

Renal damage: Persistently, high-uric acid level can lead to urolithiasis and urate nephropathy. Urolithiasis precedes the onset of gouty arthritis in many patients with hyperuricemia. The uric acid may act as a nidus on which other crystals such as calcium oxalate can precipitate. Uric acid stones can develop in individuals without other manifestations of gout, only 20% of whom are hyperuricemic. Urate nephropathy (urate nephrosis) is a late manifestation of severe hyperuricemia due to deposition of MSU crystals in the medullary interstitium and pyramids leading to chronic renal insufficiency. Untreated hyperuricemia patients may develop uric acid nephropathy, if severe dehydration or acidosis develops.

Other systems: There is higher incidence of hypertension and ischemic heart disease in gouty subjects. Gout is associated with insulin resistance also.

DIAGNOSIS

Strong clinical suspicion is required to make prompt diagnosis. Gout should be considered in all cases of obscure monoarticular or polyarticular disease. Presence of positive family history, hyperuricemia, and radiological findings strengthen the diagnosis.

Clinical picture:

- Typically, acute monoarthritis especially involving first metatarsophalangeal joint, though it may involve mid tarsal joint, ankle, knee, wrist or elbow
- Shoulders, hips, spine, and sacroiliac joints are rarely involved.
- Inflammation peaks in 24 hours.
- May remit spontaneously in few days but recurs in coming days
- Rapid response to colchicine or ice pack
- Recovery typically associated with desquamation of skin overlying the joint

Serum uric acid: Whereas hyperuricemia is often present in chronic gout, the serum uric acid may be normal or low in 30% during an acute attack due to uricosuric action of stress-induced adrenocorticotropic hormone (ACTH) and cortisol and disease-induced cytokines such as IL-1.

Synovial fluid examination: Demonstration of MSU crystals in SF is the gold standard for diagnosis of gout. Diagnostic arthrocentesis during acute gout is a safe procedure with low frequency of adverse events. SF should not be taken in formalin, as it dissolves the MSU crystals.

- *Light microscopy*:
  - MSU crystals are seen as needle-shaped crystals.
- *Compensated polarized light microscopy (CPLM)*:
  - Urate crystals can be demonstrated from synovial fluid or tophi as intracellular, needle-shaped, yellow (negatively birefringent) crystals.
- *Raman spectroscopy*:
  - Allows better detection of MSU crystals by utilizing a processing technique, which involves digestion of hyaluronic acid and organic debris in the synovial fluid.
  - May be used in conjunction with CPLM to detect MSU crystals at clinically relevant concentrations of 0.1 μm/mL

Radiological changes: Radiological changes occur in chronic recurrent gout. In well-developed chronic gout, *plain X-ray* shows periarticular small punched out erosions with overhanging margins (**Fig. 3**). In the late phases, there will be osteoarthritic changes and destruction and subluxation of joints.

Ultrasonography: Monosodium urate crystals within the synovial fluid give a *"snowstorm appearance"*. MSU crystal deposition on the superficial articular cartilage is seen as a hyperechoic band causing the *"double contour* *sign"* (**Fig. 4**). Tendon and ligament MSU depositions are also commonly seen in ultrasound. Tophi are seen as hypoechoic, hyperechoic, or mixed echogenicity nodules.

Magnetic resonance imaging: It helps in detection of joint effusion, synovitis, tendon abnormalities, tophus, cartilage disorder, and bone edema in gout.

Computed tomography: It may reveal discrete tophi at multiple sites adjacent to bone and within soft tissues. It also helps in scoring of bone erosions.

Dual energy computed tomography: Dual energy computed tomography (DECT) is a new technique, which can demonstrate MSU crystal deposition at rare locations (**Figs. 5 A** and **B**). It uses two different energies at orthogonal angles to each other and the software assigns different color codes to materials with different spectral profiles. This enables to differentiate low-density urate deposition from other denser materials such as calcium.

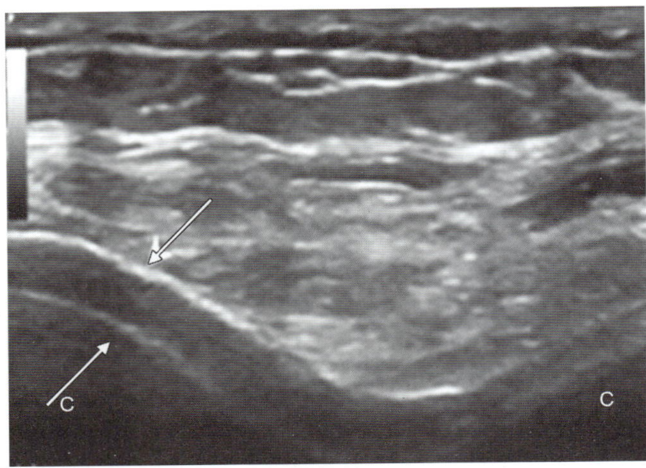

FIGURE 4: Ultrasonography (USG) knee—double contour sign (white arrows).

TREATMENT

Treatment of gout has to be considered under two heads:
1. Treatment of the acute attack
2. Management of chronic tophaceous gout

Management of the acute attack:
- *Nonpharmacological*:
  - Immobilization of the affected part with a splint and bandage
  - Ice pack
  - Adequate hydration
- *Nonsteroidal anti-inflammatory drugs (NSAIDs)*:
  - First choice, if diagnosis is fairly certain
  - *Indomethacin*: 25 mg thrice daily initially and then reduced to a maintenance dose
  - Naproxen or etoricoxib may also be used
- *Colchicine*:
  - Preferred when diagnosis is uncertain, as it is more effective in gout than in other arthritides.
  - Latest recommendation is an initial dose of 1 mg orally followed by 0.5 mg after 1 hour and an additional 0.5 mg after 12 hours, if required. Colchicine is then continued at 0.5 mg thrice a day until the acute attack resolves. This drug is freely available in India at present.
- *Glucocorticoids*:
  - Used when there is a contraindication for NSAIDs or colchicine
  - Oral prednisolone 30–40 mg daily or equivalent parenteral preparations are used and tapered over 7–10 days
  - Intra-articular steroids are highly useful in resistant monoarticular involvement. Dose of the drug and volume of the injection depends on the joint affected. The injection can be given as an outpatient procedure.
- *Corticotropin (ACTH)*:
  - Stimulates glucocorticoid secretion by adrenals and also stimulates melanocortin-3 receptors

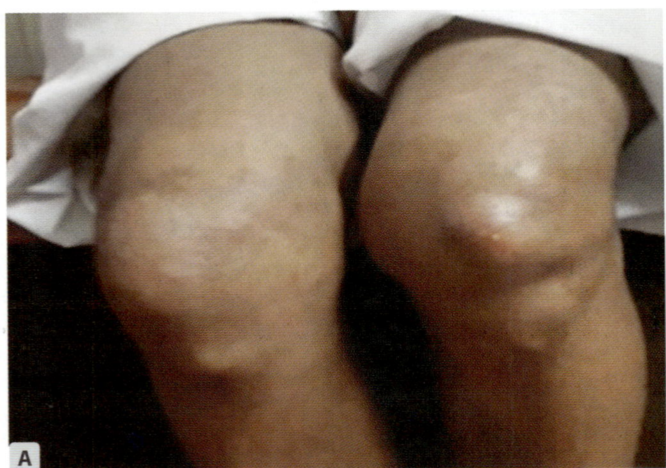

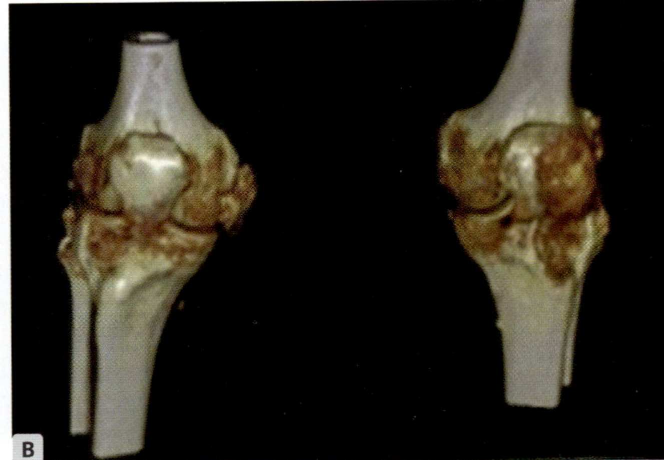

FIGURES 5 A & B: **(A)** Tophi at both knees; **(B)** Dual energy computed tomography (DECT) of same joints showing thick urate crystal deposition.

- Useful option in postsurgical and post-transplant patients
- Single injection of 60 IU IM is more effective than corticosteroids

- *IL-1 inhibitors*:
  - Novel concept based on the fact that IL-1β secretion by MSU-triggered inflammasomes is pivotal in the pathogenesis of gout
  - Effective first-line therapy in situations where NSAIDs, colchicine, and steroids are contraindicated, ineffective, or not tolerated. But it is not yet available in India
  - Especially beneficial in patients with ≥3 attacks in a year.
  - Anakinra, canakinumab, and rilonacept are the drugs used clinically.

Treatment of chronic gout: It aims at long-term reduction of serum urate well below the normal range (<6 mg in nontophaceous gout and <5 mg in presence of tophi) in order to eliminate acute gouty attacks, reduce tophi, and prevent ongoing joint or organ damage.

During acute attacks, urate-lowering therapy (ULT) is better avoided, as it can cause further flare-up of arthritis. If the patient is already on urate-lowering agents, it may be continued in the same dosage throughout the acute phase.

- *Diet and lifestyle changes*:
  - Maintain ideal body weight
  - Smoking cessation
  - Reduction or stoppage of alcohol
  - Avoid precipitating factors
  - Control of comorbid illnesses such as hypertension and dyslipidemia
  - Adequate hydration

Acute attacks can be avoided by omitting purine rich diets such as red meat, liver, testes, seafoods, and alcohol. Though vegetarian articles of diet such as lentils, peas, beans, spinach, mushrooms, cauliflower, and oatmeal are rich in purines, they generally do not provoke acute attacks. Obese individuals should reduce their weight gradually.

- *Drugs*: The drugs used for chronic gout can be divided in three categories:
  i. *Uricostatic drugs*: Allopurinol and febuxostat
  ii. *Uricosuric agents*:
     - *Primary uricosurics*: Probenecid, benzbromarone, sulfinpyrazone
     - *Secondary uricosurics*: Losartan, amlodipine, fenofibrate
  iii. *Uricolytic drugs*: Uricase, rasburicase, polyethylene glycol-uricase (pegloticase)

*Uricostatic drugs (**Table 2**)*:

- *Allopurinol*: It inhibits *xanthine oxidase* and also helps in urinary elimination of urates. The advantages of this drug are its low toxicity and sustained therapeutic effect even in the presence of renal disease or diuretic therapy. The starting dose is 100 mg daily and may be increased up to 800 mg/day, if required, to achieve the effect and later reduced to a maintenance level. Dose-dependent toxic effects include hypersensitivity reactions such as fever, eosinophilia, dermatitis, hepatic dysfunction, renal failure, and vasculitis.
- *Febuxostat*: Nonpurine xanthine oxidase inhibitor with high oral absorption (85%) and high affinity to serum proteins (**Box 1**). It has a half-life of 4–9 hours. It is metabolized by liver and renal excretion is insignificant. It selectively inhibits both oxidized and reduced forms of xanthine oxidase without inhibiting other enzymes in purine metabolism. The initial dose of febuxostat is 40 mg/day taken with or without food, which may be increased up to 80–120 mg/day. It can be safely given without dosage reduction in patients with renal impairment and moderate hepatic impairment.

Uricosuric agents: Uricosuric agents are useful in hyperuricemia due to inadequate renal excretion of urates. The drugs are contraindicated, if there is a history of urolithiasis or if there is oliguria. They are less effective in presence of renal disease with low glomerular filtration rate (GFR).

Probenecid inhibits URAT1, a transporter at the apical brush border of proximal nephron**.** *Benzbromarone* and *sulfinpyrazone* are well-tolerated uricosuric agents but are not freely available in India. *Losartan*, an angiotensin-2 receptor blocker, has moderate uricosuric properties by

BOX 1 Indications for febuxostat in gout.

- Patients with renal impairment
- Patients allergic to allopurinol
- Allopurinol failure (as a second-line drug)
- Concomitant use of oral anticoagulants such as warfarin

TABLE 2 Side effects of allopurinol and febuxostat.

Drug	Side effects	Contraindications
Allopurinol	• Diarrhea and dyspepsia • Skin rashes • Elevated hepatic transaminases • Allopurinol hypersensitivity syndrome including Steven–Johnson syndrome and toxic epidermal necrolysis • Drug rash, eosinophilia, and systemic symptoms (DRESS)	• Patients sensitive to sulfonamides • Patients taking ampicillin or thiazides • Patients on azathioprine
Febuxostat	• Nausea • Dizziness • Hepatic transaminase elevation	Patients on azathioprine, mercaptopurine or theophylline (as these are metabolized by xanthine oxidase)

decreasing the renal tubular reabsorption of uric acid. It inhibits URAT1 and GLUT9 and is particularly useful as an adjunct therapy in patients with gout and hypertension. It is also useful to control the hyperuricemia caused by thiazides. The usual dose needed is 50 mg/day. *Amlodipine* given in a dose of 5–10 mg/day is also found to be useful in reducing the urate levels in patients with cyclosporine-induced hyperuricemia. *Fenofibrate*, the lipid-lowering agent, increases the renal urate clearance by inhibiting URAT1. Up to 25–30% reduction of uric acid level is possible with a dose of 200 mg/day and is a good choice in patients with gout and dyslipidemia.

Uricolytic agents: Humans are prone to hyperuricemia due to lack of functional *uricase (urate oxidase)*, unlike lower animals. Biosynthesized recombinant *Aspergillus flavus uricase (rasburicase)* is available in the United States of America for tumor lysis syndrome in patients allergic to allopurinol, but is highly antigenic. PEG-uricase is another potentially powerful agent for treating refractory gout in those who are unable to tolerate other drugs. Pegylation has the advantages of prolonging the drug half-life and decreasing antigenicity. It has been tried in debulking tophi in advanced gout before switching over to other agents for maintenance treatment (**Table 3**).

ASYMPTOMATIC HYPERURICEMIA

There are many individuals with uric acid levels higher than normal (>7 mg in males and 6 mg in females) who are detected incidentally but are totally asymptomatic. Few of them may have musculoskeletal pain but not directly related to hyperuricemia. Mere presence of hyperuricemia is not an indication for specific uric acid-lowering treatment (**Box 2**). In >70% of hyperuricemia patients, an underlying cause such as metabolic syndrome, renal and thyroid diseases, alcoholism, or drugs can be readily found out by history, physical examination, and a few investigations. Correction of the underlying cause often brings back the uric acid values to normal levels. Currently, there is no evidence of benefit from treating sustained asymptomatic hyperuricemia unless indicated.

TABLE 3 Newer drugs for hyperuricemia.

Class	Drugs
Urate transporter (URAT1) inhibitors	Lesinurad, verinurad, arhalofenate, tranilast
Purine nucleotide phosphorylase (PNP) inhibitors	Ulodesine, topiroxostat
Melanocortin-3 receptor agonists	γ-MSH
Oral IL-1 inhibitors	AC201
Caspase inhibitors	Pralnacasan and emricasan
Uricosuric agents	Levotofisopam, canagliflozin
Uricases	Pegsiticase, SEL-212
Urate transporters to intestinal lumen	ABCG2 activators

(IL: interleukin; MSH: melanocyte-stimulating hormone)

OTHER CRYSTAL RELATED ARTHRITIS

CPP CRYSTAL DEPOSITION DISEASE (PSEUDOGOUT)

Calcium pyrophosphate crystals are derived from articular cartilage and seen in synovial fluid. Processes that lower solubility of the CPP crystals lead to their precipitation and deposition in hyaline cartilage and fibrocartilage, the latter being affected more. The condition may be familial, sporadic, or caused by metabolic disorders such as hyperparathyroidism, hemochromatosis, hypothyroidism, hypomagnesemia, hypophosphatasia, and others. The menisci of the knees, articular discs of distal radioulnar joints, acetabulum, symphysis pubis, and annulus fibrosus of lumbar and dorsal intervertebral discs are sites of predilection. Men above 50 years are more affected though both sexes are susceptible (**Fig. 6**).

Though many cases may be silent, some present with recurrent attacks of subacute inflammation and progressive degeneration of joints. Once the degenerative process starts, it proceeds relentlessly, despite treatment.

The presentation may resemble gout, rheumatoid arthritis (RA), osteoarthritis, or neuropathic joints.

Differential diagnosis includes all other types of monoarthritis or polyarthritis, depending upon the presentation. X-ray of the joints reveals calcification in

BOX 2 Indications for treatment of asymptomatic hyperuricemia.

- Previous history of recurrent gouty arthritis
- Presence of tophi
- Presence of uric acid stones or urate nephropathy
- Serum uric acid >9 mg/dL with other risk factors
- During chemotherapy of cancer to prevent tumor lysis syndrome
- Inherited enzyme defects

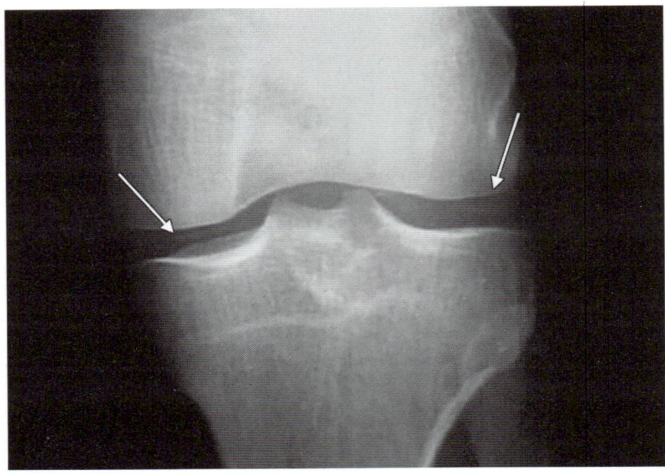

FIGURE 6: X-ray of knee showing chondrocalcinosis (arrows) in calcium pyrophosphate crystal deposition (CPPD) disease.

distinctive locations, which is diagnostic. Microscopy of the synovial fluid is confirmatory.

Management: During acute attacks, NSAIDs may be tried. Colchicine is also very effective. Aspiration of synovial fluid and injection of microcrystalline cortisone (cortisone acetate) gives rapid relief.

BCP CRYSTAL ARTHROPATHY

It is also known as calcium apatite deposition disease or as Milwaukee shoulder/knee syndrome. This condition affects elderly persons, mostly women. BCP crystals (hydroxyapatite and octacalcium phosphate) are present in the joint fluid and get deposited at sites of trauma or tissue damage, primarily on the matrix vessels. The shoulder or knee may be affected. Many cases may be asymptomatic. Symptoms include pain in the shoulders or knees after exertion and at night. Progressive destruction of joints occurs. The term *Milwaukee shoulder* refers to the arthritis (sometimes, destructive) of the shoulder seen in elderly patients caused by BCP crystals (**Fig. 7**). *Treatment* is symptomatic.

CALCIUM OXALATE ARTHROPATHY

This is a complication occurring in renal failure when the serum creatinine levels exceed 8 mg/dL, especially so in patients undergoing dialysis. Also, this is seen in those with primary oxalosis. Crystals of calcium oxalate may be deposited in joints, skin, blood vessels, and other tissues. Joint manifestations include subacute, chronic, or acute painful episodes.

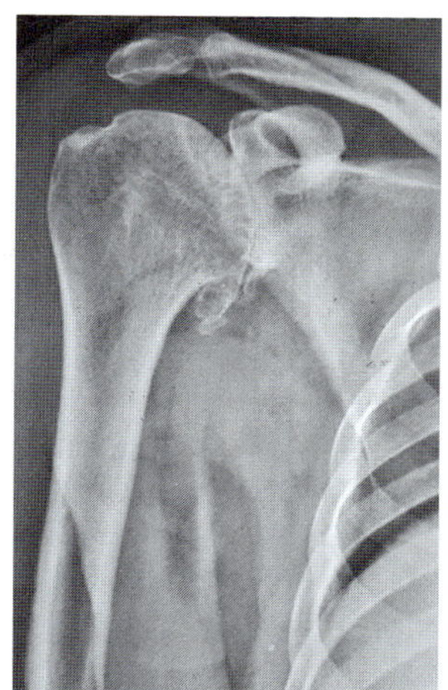

FIGURE 7: X-ray in Milwaukee shoulder. Note the joint space narrowing, subchondral sclerosis, and cyst formation.

RECOMMENDED READINGS

1. Paul BJ, James R. Gout: An Asia Pacific update. Int J Rheum Diseases. 2017;20(4):407-16.
2. Zell M, Zhang D, FitzGerald J. Diagnostic advances in synovial fluid analysis and radiographic identification for crystalline arthritis. Curr Opin Rheumatol. 2019;31(2):134-43.
3. Paul BJ. Crystal arthritis: Past, present and future. JK Science. 2006;8(4):232-34.
4. Paul BJ, Anoopkumar K, Krishnan V. Asymptomatic hyperuricemia: is it time to intervene? Clin Rheumatol. 2017;36(12):2637-44.

CHAPTER 232

Rheumatoid Arthritis

Ashok Kumar, Kushagra Gupta

ABSTRACT

Rheumatoid arthritis (RA) is the most common chronic inflammatory arthritis in adults. It is characterized by bilaterally symmetrical involvement of joints typically affecting metacarpophalangeal (MCPs), wrist, and proximal interphalangeal (PIPs). Prevalence of RA is estimated at 0.28–0.75% in India, with the disease primarily affecting middle-aged females, 40–60 years of age. There is a complex interplay between environmental, genetic, and immunological factors, which leads to breakdown of immune tolerance resulting in synovial inflammation. HLA-DRB1 is strongly associated with RA and smoking further amplifies the risk of developing anti-citrullinated protein antibody (ACPA)-positive disease.

Classical symptoms include pain, swelling, and stiffness in affected joints associated with early morning stiffness (EMS) lasting >30 minutes. Extra-articular manifestations such as interstitial lung disease (ILD), anemia, rheumatoid nodules, and sicca symptoms are frequently seen in patients with RA. Diagnosis is made clinically with laboratory features showing evidence of chronic inflammation and autoantibodies, namely rheumatoid factor (RF) and ACPA. Cardiovascular causes are the leading cause of mortality in RA.

Treatment strategy relies on making an early diagnosis, following a "treat-to-target" approach using composite disease activity scores and achieving early disease remission. Appropriate use of disease-modifying antirheumatic drugs (DMARDs) (conventional, biological, and targeted synthetic) along with steroids has significantly improved overall prognosis of this disease by preventing deformities, disability, and cardiovascular complications.

"I am not seeking out drugs, I am seeking relief"

—Anonymous

INTRODUCTION

Rheumatoid arthritis is a chronic inflammatory disorder primarily affecting the synovial joints. It is the most common cause of inflammatory arthritis in adults. It results in destruction of the articular cartilages and joints leading to functional disability. To prevent the damage, it is important to diagnose and treat it early. Increased risk of atherosclerosis due to widespread inflammation can lead to reduction in life expectancy by 6–7 years, if not treated.

EPIDEMIOLOGY

Rheumatoid arthritis affects approximately 0.5–1% of population in the West (Indian figures: 0.28–0.75%). Incidence of RA has been gradually decreasing in recent decades with overall prevalence remaining unchanged due to increased survival. *Females are three times more commonly affected than males.* Median age of onset of RA in India is 33 years as opposed to 50 years in the Western population. Onset of RA after 65 years of age is termed as late-onset RA or "LORA".

PATHOGENESIS

There is a complex interplay between environmental, genetic, and immunological factors, which leads to breakdown of immune tolerance resulting in synovial inflammation. Twin studies have estimated that contribution of heritability in the causation of RA is 60%. A family history, however, can only be obtained in about 5% of patients. This underscores the importance of environmental factors in RA. Activation of innate immunity upon environmental exposure seems to be the earliest step leading to citrullination of self-antigens and presentation to T cells. T cells, in turn, activate B cells, which lead to development of autoantibodies (RF and ACPA), years before the onset of clinically apparent disease. This stage is known as "pre-RA". Autoantibodies have been seen up to 14 years before the onset of RA.

GENETIC RISK FACTORS

Genes play a role in susceptibility as well as severity of RA. Genetic risk in RA is associated with the following factors:

- Human leukocyte antigen (HLA) genes [major histocompatibility complex (MHC) class II molecules]
- Non-HLA genes
- Epigenetic changes

Most of the genetic associations have been seen in ACPA-positive individuals.

Human leukocyte antigen association: It accounts for 30% of the genetic susceptibility in RA. HLA genes encode MHC class II molecules, present on antigen-presenting cells. The antigen is presented in combination with HLA class II molecule to the T cells to initiate an immune response. HLA-DRB1 shows the strongest association with RA. There are several alleles of HLA-DRB1, which share a common amino acid sequence (at position 70–74 in the third hypervariable region), which has been termed as "shared epitope" (SE). A strong association has been observed between SE and risk of RA.

Nonhuman leukocyte antigen association: More than 100 different genes have been identified using genome-wide association studies (GWAS). Some of the major polymorphisms include genes involved in T-cell signaling (such as PTPN22 and STAT4) and tumor necrosis factor (TNF) signaling (such as TNFAIP3). These genes, however, provide only a modest contribution to the genetic risk of RA.

Epigenetic changes: Epigenetic changes (e.g., DNA methylation, histone acetylation, and deacetylation) play an important role. They affect the expression of cytokine, chemokines, and matrix metalloproteinases (MMPs), thereby affecting RA pathogenesis. Environmental factors such as smoking have been shown to decrease DNA methylation.

ENVIRONMENTAL FACTORS

Table 1 summarizes the various environmental risk factors. Smoking is the most important risk factor for RA. Risk of developing RA positively correlates with the number of "pack years". In an individual with SE, smoking can

TABLE 1 Environmental risk factors associated with RA.

Predisposing factors	Protective factors
• Tobacco smoke (ACPA +ve) • Periodontal disease (*Porphyromonas gingivalis*) (ACPA+ve) • Coffee consumption (ACPA +ve) • Exposure to mineral oils (ACPA+ve) • Silica dust, pollution, and tobacco smoke (ACPA+ve) • Old age at menarche (>15 years) • Multiparity	• Alcohol consumption (ACPA +ve) • Younger age at menarche • Oral contraceptive use

(ACPA: anti-citrullinated peptide antibody; RA: rheumatoid arthritis)

increase the risk of developing ACPA-positive RA by up to 21-folds. Smoking has been shown to promote citrullination and inflammation, which may be how it contributes to RA pathogenesis. Exposure to mineral oils and silica also increases the risk for RA.

Interaction between human microbiome (oral cavity, gut, and lungs) and immune system is being increasingly studied. Dysbiosis (overgrowth of pathogenic bacteria and lack of "commensals") may be responsible for the development of RA. *Porphyromonas gingivalis* (involved in periodontitis) uniquely expresses a bacterial form of peptidylarginine deiminase (PAD), which can citrullinate peptides, generating self-antigens. An abundance of *Prevotella copri* with loss of *Bacteroides* has been demonstrated in the stool of patients with new onset RA. Gut dysbiosis correlates with disease activity while treatment with DMARDs results in its partial resolution.

AUTOANTIBODIES

A large number of antibodies targeting self-antigens (collagen type II, calreticulin, cathepsin) have been found in RA but no single arthritogenic autoantigen is known. Exact role of autoantibodies in RA pathogenesis is not understood but they do serve as diagnostic markers.

Rheumatoid factor: RF is an autoantibody targeting Fc portion of immunoglobulin G (IgG) in patients with RA. Commercial tests mostly detect RF of IgM class in the serum. However, IgG and IgA RF are also found in RA sera. RF is, however, less specific for RA and can be found in other infectious and autoimmune diseases as well.

Anti-citrullinated protein antibody: Citrullination is a process in which arginine residues are modified post-translationally by an enzyme PAD. Citrullination is a physiological process necessary for degradation of intracellular proteins during apoptosis. Antibodies directed against citrullinated proteins (fibrinogen, vimentin) are called ACPA. Presence of ACPA predicts progression and severity of RA. ACPA has been directly implicated in the development of erosions in RA.

Other autoantibodies: Other newly discovered antibodies include anticarbamylated antibodies (anti-CarP antibodies), antimalondialdehyde-acetaldehyde antibodies, and antiacetaldehyde antibodies.

INFLAMMATORY CELLS

T cells, B cells, and macrophages are the most important cells involved in the pathogenesis of RA.

- **T cells:** They are the most abundant cells in RA synovium. They play a vital role of initiating inflammation in synovium by stimulation of other immune cells.
    - T-helper 1 (Th1) cells stimulate macrophages and fibroblast-like synoviocytes via release of interferon-γ (IFN-γ).
    - T-helper 1 and T-helper 2 (Th2) cells activate B cells via release of interleukin-2 (IL-2), propagating autoantibody production.
    - Recognition of antigens by naïve T cells requires costimulation, i.e., interaction of CD28 (expressed on T cells) and CD80/86 [expressed on antigen-presenting cells (APCs)]. In the absence of costimulation, T cells undergo anergy. As expected, costimulation blocker (abatacept) is an effective treatment in RA.
    - Recent studies have implicated a direct role of Th17 cells in the pathogenesis of RA via release of IL-17 and IL-21. IL-17 acts in synergy with IL-1 and TNF-α in promoting inflammation. However, therapeutic blockage of IL-17 has not yielded significant results.
- **B cells:** B-cell activation occurs early in disease course as evident by the presence of autoantibodies in pre-RA stage. Apart from this, B cells act as APCs and stimulate T cells.
- **Macrophages:** They are central to driving and maintaining chronic inflammation. They are the major source of proinflammatory cytokines (IL-1, IL-6, and TNF-α), cartilage degrading enzymes (MMP-9 and MMP-12), and growth factors such as granulocyte-macrophage colony-stimulating factor (GM-CSF) in the synovium. They also act as APCs presenting antigens to T cells.

SYNOVIAL PATHOLOGY

Hallmarks of synovial pathology include synovial proliferation, inflammatory cell infiltration, neoangiogenesis, and focal bone erosions. *As a result of inflammation, synovial lining undergoes hypertrophy* (up to 15-cell thick) containing fibroblast-like synoviocytes. The underlying connective tissue gets infiltrated with T cells, B cells, macrophages, dendritic cells, plasma cells, and mast cells. T cells constitute 30–50% of cells and are distributed diffusely or may organize to form lymphoid follicles and rarely granulomas. To meet the demands of growing synovium, new blood vessels are formed in the connective tissue.

Inflamed synovium advances as an invasive "pannus" destroying the underlying cartilage and bone. Two important cell types involved in this process are: (1) synovial fibroblasts and (2) osteoclasts. Fibroblasts degrade the extracellular matrix in cartilage by secretion of MMPs and cathepsins. At the interface of pannus and bone, osteoclasts form resorption lacunae, which gradually progress to form erosions. Receptor activator of nuclear factor-kappa B ligand (RANKL), important for activation of osteoclasts, is expressed by T cells. Erosions are typically found at the site of attachment of synovial membrane to the bone. Another form of bone loss that occurs is periarticular osteopenia, which occurs due to bony trabecular thinning as a result of inflammation of bone marrow cavity.

CLINICAL MANIFESTATIONS

Rheumatoid arthritis typically presents as a polyarticular disease with gradual onset. Occasionally, patients may present with acute onset monoarticular disease.

Constitutional symptoms, such as fatigue, myalgia, and low-grade fever, may accompany articular symptoms.

ARTICULAR MANIFESTATIONS

Onset of RA is typically insidious with pain, stiffness, and swelling in multiple joints in a symmetrical distribution *primarily involving MCP, PIP, and wrist joints* (**Fig. 1**). It is associated with EMS and defined as "slowing or difficulty in moving joints after waking up". EMS lasting >30 minutes is typical of inflammatory arthropathies.

Other joints such as elbow, shoulder, knees, and ankles are often involved, but less specific for RA. Occasionally, disease may start as mono- or oligoarthritis gradually evolving into polyarthritis. Flexor tenosynovitis may cause decreased range of motion, reduced grip strength, and trigger finger.

Ulnar deviation of fingers due to subluxation of MCPs (**Fig. 2**) and "*swan-neck deformity*" due to hyperextension of PIPs and flexion at distal interphalangeal (DIPs) (**Fig. 3**) are typically seen in RA. Flexion of PIP and hyperextension at DIP cause "*boutonniere deformity*". Subluxation of first MCP with hyperextension of PIP results in "*Z-line deformity*". Subluxation of the distal ulna may lead to "*piano key sign*". In advanced cases, atlantoaxial instability may lead to compressive myelopathy of the cervical cord.

EXTRA-ARTICULAR MANIFESTATIONS

Extra-articular manifestations may be seen in up to 40% of patients with RA. Seropositive individuals with history of smoking and high disease activity are more at risk. Common extra-articular manifestations include sicca symptoms, ILD, rheumatoid nodules, and anemia. They have been summarized in **Table 2**.

Ocular: Sicca symptoms due to secondary Sjögren's syndrome can be seen in up to 10% of patients with RA. Episcleritis and scleritis may be occasionally seen. Episcleritis is associated with rapid onset of localized redness in eyes with no pain or discharge whereas scleritis is painful and can lead to perforation and blindness.

Hematological: Anemia of chronic disease commonly presents as normocytic or microcytic anemia. It results from defective release of iron from macrophages despite normal iron reserves. Neutropenia combined with splenomegaly is the hallmark of Felty's syndrome. It is less often seen nowadays due to more effective treatment regimes.

Pulmonary: Rheumatoid arthritis may affect the pleura, lung parenchyma, small and large airways, and occasionally pulmonary vasculature itself. Involvement of pleura leads to exudative pleural effusion. Occasionally, there may be associated fibrosis, fistula, or a pneumothorax due to rupture of underlying nodule. Parenchymal involvement commonly manifests as ILD (prevalence: 5–30%). Most common pattern is usual interstitial pneumonia (UIP), which is characterized by progressive fibrosis of lung seen as honeycombing on CT. Nonspecific interstitial pneumonia

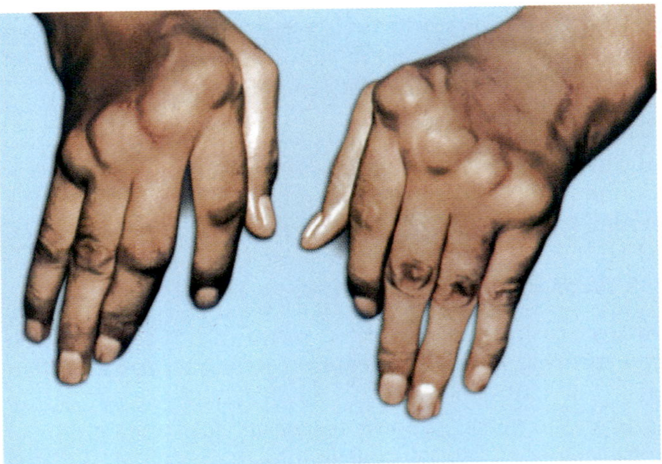

FIGURE 2: Advanced RA with bilateral MCP joint subluxation and ulnar deviation of fingers.

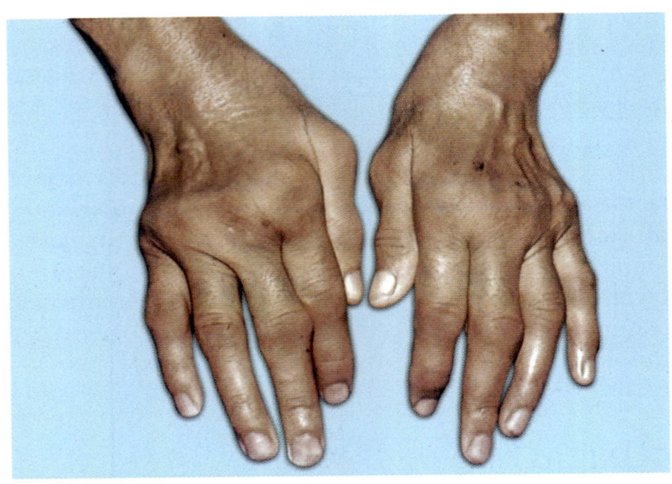

(MCP: metacarpophalangeal joints; PIP: proximal interphalangeal joints; RA: rheumatoid arthritis)

FIGURE 1: A case of severe RA with bilateral symmetrical arthritis of MCP and PIP joints.

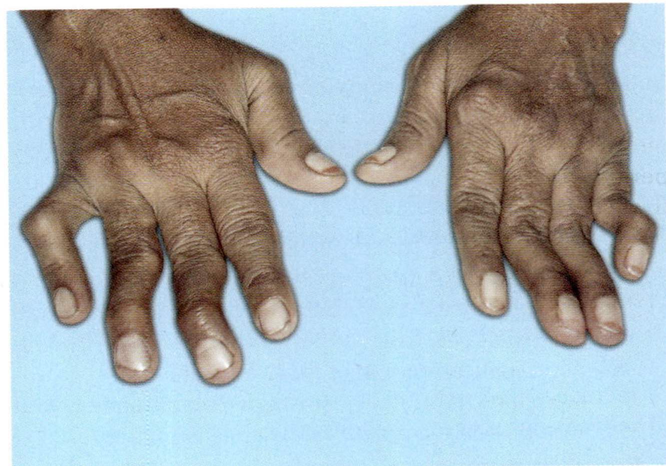

FIGURE 3: Advanced case of rheumatoid arthritis (RA) with typical "swan-neck" deformities.

TABLE 2	Extra-articular manifestations of rheumatoid arthritis (RA).
Hematological	• Anemia • Thrombocytosis (acute phase response) • Neutropenia and thrombocytopenia (Felty syndrome)
Pulmonary	• Interstitial lung disease • Pulmonary nodules • Pleural effusion • Bronchiectasis • Fibrosing alveolitis • Pneumoconiosis (Caplan syndrome) • Pulmonary arterial hypertension (rare)
Cardiac	• Pericarditis • Pericardial effusion • Valvular abnormalities • Conduction abnormalities
Ocular	• Keratoconjunctivitis sicca • Episcleritis • Scleritis
Neurological	• Nerve entrapment: Carpal tunnel syndrome • Cervical myelopathy (atlantoaxial subluxation) • Neuropathy: Peripheral neuropathy or mononeuritis multiplex
Cutaneous	• Subcutaneous nodules • Pyoderma gangrenosum • Vasculitic rashes • Leg ulceration • Amyloidosis
Renal	• Secondary amyloidosis • Membranous nephropathy
Vasculitis	• Purpuric lesions • Leg ulceration • Digital gangrene (rare) • Peripheral neuropathy • Mononeuritis multiplex

(NSIP) is the second most common pattern associated with diffuse ground-glass opacities predominantly in basal and peripheral distribution. NSIP carries a better prognosis than UIP. Pulmonary rheumatoid nodules are a common presentation usually associated with subcutaneous nodules and positive RF. They are usually asymptomatic. Calcified pulmonary nodules along with pneumoconiosis are typical features of Caplan syndrome. Bronchiectasis occurs in up to 50% of patients with RA. Bronchiectasis predisposes to increased risk of infections, especially with the use of immunosuppressive medication.

Cardiac manifestations: Pericarditis is the most common presentation usually with concomitant pleuritis. It usually subsides with control of disease activity. Other manifestations are rare.

Vasculitis: Small-vessel vasculitis can rarely be seen in patients with long-standing RA. It may manifest as purpuric spots on legs progressing to cutaneous ulcers, paraesthesias, mononeuritis multiplex, and rarely digital gangrene.

In addition to extra-articular manifestations, several conditions associated with RA contribute to morbidity. Cardiovascular diseases are the leading cause of mortality in RA patients. Chronic inflammation in RA predisposes to increased risk of atherosclerosis leading to increased cardiovascular morbidity. Patients with RA also show an increased risk for developing osteoporosis with increased incidence of vertebral and nonvertebral fractures as compared to general population. There is also a 2- to 4-fold increased risk of lymphoma seen in patients with RA, with diffuse large B-cell lymphoma being most common.

INVESTIGATIONS

LABORATORY FEATURES

- Patients with RA usually have evidence of inflammation in their blood.
  - Erythrocyte sedimentation rate (ESR) and C-reactive protein (CRP) are usually raised in the presence of active disease.
  - Anemia (with normal serum iron) and thrombocytosis also indicate inflammation in RA.

  Baseline liver and kidney function tests should be obtained before starting the patient on DMARDs.
- Specific antibody tests for RA include RF and ACPA.
  - Rheumatoid factor—it occurs in about 70% of patients with RA; however, it is not specific for RA. It can be found in other conditions such as Sjögren's syndrome, systemic lupus erythematosus (SLE), cryoglobulinemia, and infective endocarditis. It can be found in 1–5% of normal population as well. Titers above 50 IU/L have higher specificity for RA.
  - Anti-citrullinated protein antibody—it has similar sensitivity as RF, but it has a specificity reaching up to 95%. It can be helpful in differentiating RA from other causes of inflammatory arthritis. It can predict the development of RA in preclinical phase and is often associated with a severe disease phenotype.
- Synovial fluid analysis is usually not required, but if done, shows predominant neutrophilic infiltration with counts ranging from 5,000 to 50,000 white blood cell (WBC)/μL, as opposed to <2,000 WBC/μL seen in noninflammatory conditions such as osteoarthritis.
- Schirmer's test may be done to assess sicca symptoms in eyes.

IMAGING

- *Plain radiography*: It usually remains unremarkable in early disease course. Periarticular osteopenia around inflamed joint is one of the earliest changes to appear. In patients with long-standing disease, X-rays of hands, wrist, and feet can show erosions in MCPs, PIPs, and metatarsophalangeal (MTPs) usually at site where synovial membrane attaches to bone. Advanced cases may show loss of joint space (due to thinning of cartilage) with joint subluxation and damage.

- *MRI*: It offers high sensitivity for detecting synovitis, joint effusions, and bone marrow changes. MRI detects abnormalities before they appear on X-rays. Cost and availability are major limitations.
- *Ultrasound*: It is more sensitive than X-rays for erosions and synovitis. It can assess increased joint vascularity, which can be an early sign of inflammation. Limitations of ultrasound include its operator dependence and difficulty in evaluating deeper joints.
- High-resolution computed tomography (HRCT) of the chest and pulmonary function test (PFT) can be done for evaluation of ILD. PFT shows features of restrictive lung disease. A six-minute walk test (6MWT) is useful for monitoring disease progression and therapeutic response in ILD.

DIAGNOSIS

A diagnosis of RA is established on the basis of classical signs and symptoms along with characteristic laboratory features and serological markers. Classification criteria help in defining homogeneous groups of RA cases for research work. The American College of Rheumatology/European League Against Rheumatism (ACR/EULAR) classification criteria (**Table 3**) require a score of 6 to classify a case as RA. These criteria are aimed at early diagnosis of RA.

TABLE 3 2010 ACR/EULAR classification criteria for RA.

Domain	Parameters	Score
Joint involvement	1 large joint	0
	2–10 large joints	1
	1–3 small joints*	2
	4–10 small joints*	3
	>10 joints (at least 1 small)	5
Serology	Negative RF and anti-CCP	0
	Low positive RF or anti-CCP (<3 times of ULN)	2
	High positive RF or anti-CCP (>3 times of ULN)	3
Acute phase reactants	Normal ESR and CRP	0
	Elevated ESR or CRP	1
Duration of symptoms	<6 weeks	0
	≥6 weeks	1

This criterion is aimed at classification of new patients presenting with at least one joint with definite clinical synovitis. **A score of >6 fulfills the requirement for definite RA**.

*Small joints—metacarpophalangeal joint, proximal interphalangeal joints, thumb, metatarsophalangeal joints, and wrist.

(ACR: American College of Rheumatology; Anti-CCP: anti-cyclic citrullinated peptide; CRP: C-reactive protein; EULAR: European League Against Rheumatism; ULN: upper limit of normal)

MEASURING DISEASE ACTIVITY

Disease activity in RA can be assessed with parameters such as number of swollen and tender joints, pain assessment on visual analog scale (VAS), global assessment by both patients and physician, and inflammatory markers such as ESR and CRP. Composite scores have been developed, which combine these different parameters into a single score for easy assessment of disease. They have been summarized in **Table 4**. Meta-analyses have shown that guiding treatment based on these scores provides better control of disease.

TREATMENT

The treatment strategy in RA has evolved over the years. The goal of treatment today is to achieve early remission of disease, so that deformities are prevented and function is preserved. This has been made possible with the use of conventional DMARDs, biological/biosimilar drugs, and targeted synthetic DMARDs. Treatment strategy is based on *three principles*:

1. **Early diagnosis:** The ACR/EULAR classification criteria for RA have facilitated early recognition of RA. Ideally, a patient with joint swelling, having pain and stiffness of

TABLE 4 Composite disease activity scores in RA.

	DAS28*	CDAI**
Scoring parameters		
Tender joint count	✓	✓
Swollen joint count	✓	✓
ESR	✓	
CRP	✓	
Patient global assessment of disease activity	✓	✓
Physician global assessment of disease activity		✓
Disease activity (range)	0–9.3	0–76
Remission	≤2.6	≤2.8
Low	2.6 to ≤3.2	2.8 to ≤10
Moderate	>3.2–5.1	>10–22
High	>5.1	>22

*DAS28—28 joints are evaluated for tenderness and swelling in DAS28 (10 PIPs, 10 MCPs, two wrists, two elbows, two shoulder, and two knees). A calculator calculates the score using a complex formula after feeding the required parameters.

DAS28-ESR = [0.56 * sqrt (TJC)] + [0.28 * sqrt (SJC)] + [0.7 * ln (ESR)] + (0.014 * GH)

DAS28-CRP = [0.56 * sqrt (TJC28)] + [0.28 * sqrt (SJC28)] + [0.36 * ln (CRP + 1)] + (0.014 * GH + 0.96)

**CDAI—it is calculated by adding the sum total of tender joint counts, swollen joint counts, patient global assessment, and physician global assessment.

(CDAI: Clinical Disease Activity Index; MCP: metacarpophalangeal; PIP: proximal interphalangeal)

at least one joint, should be referred to a rheumatologist within 6 weeks to facilitate early diagnosis.

2. **Early control of disease activity:** Treatment should be started as soon as the diagnosis of RA is made with the aim of achieving remission within 6 months. Studies have shown that rate of progression of RA is highest during the early stage of disease, with up to 75% of patients developing erosions within the first 2 years.
3. **"Treat-to-target":** Development of composite indices such as DAS28 and CDAI has made assessment of disease activity convenient. Several randomized controlled trials (RCTs) and meta-analyses have shown that regular adjustment of DMARDs using disease activity measures, with an aim to achieve remission or low disease activity, is more effective than regular care.

Medications used in the treatment of RA can be broadly classified as:

- Nonsteroidal anti-inflammatory drugs (NSAIDs)
- Glucocorticoids
- Disease-modifying antirheumatic drugs

NONSTEROIDAL ANTI-INFLAMMATORY DRUGS

Nonsteroidal anti-inflammatory drugs can be used as analgesics and anti-inflammatory drugs in patients with RA for relief of symptoms. Trials have shown that all NSAIDs are equal in efficacy. Chronic use should be avoided to prevent peptic ulcer/gastropathy and renal insufficiency. NSAIDs are adjuvant therapies and do not alter the course of disease in RA.

GLUCOCORTICOIDS

Glucocorticoids, to some extent, have disease-modifying effect, but are not suitable for long-term therapy due to their adverse effects. They are usually employed as "bridge therapy" in RA, i.e., short-term, rapid control of disease before the full effect of conventional DMARDs comes into effect (~2–4 months). Glucocorticoids are similarly used for control of acute disease flares. Steroids may also be used as intra-articular injections, especially when inflammation is restricted to one or two joints. Low-dose steroids, i.e., <7.5 mg prednisolone equivalent are sometimes used for long-term treatment in patients refractory to other therapies. However, such patients are particularly at high risk for developing osteoporosis; hence, the risk-benefit ratio must always be justified.

DISEASE-MODIFYING ANTIRHEUMATIC DRUGS

Disease-modifying antirheumatic drugs have the ability to retard/stop the progression of disease. They have also been shown to improve cardiovascular outcomes in patients with RA, besides improving the long-term outcome of RA. The EULAR classifies DMARDs into two classes:

1. Synthetic DMARDs (sDMARDs)
2. Biological DMARDs (bDMARDs)

Synthetic DMARDs can be further categorized into conventional synthetic DMARDs (csDMARDs), which include methotrexate, leflunomide, sulfasalazine, and hydroxychloroquine and new targeted synthetic DMARDs (tsDMARDs), e.g., tofacitinib and baricitinib. bDMARDs include TNF inhibitors, B-cell-depleting agents, T-cell costimulation blocker, and therapies targeting IL-1 and IL-6. sDMARDs have the advantage that they can be administered by oral route whereas biologicals are large molecules which need to be administered parenterally. Studies have shown that bDMARDs and tsDMARDs are more effective in controlling disease activity in RA than conventional DMARDs. Their doses, mechanism of action, and adverse effects have been described in detail in **Table 5** and **Figure 4**. Although bDMARDs are expensive, their cheaper versions ("biosimilars") have largely overcome this limitation. Similarly, tsDMARDs have now become more affordable consequent to the expiry of patents of innovator molecules.

Conventional DMRDs: They are considered as the first-line therapy in RA with *methotrexate* being the DMARD of choice. It is the standard of treatment against which all new drugs are tested in clinical trials. Methotrexate has been shown to retard disease progression in RA. Leflunomide has an efficacy comparable to methotrexate. Both drugs can be used as monotherapy or as part of combination regimens. *Hydroxychloroquine* is used mostly as part of DMARD combinations. In addition to its disease-modifying effects, it reduces hepatotoxicity of methotrexate, improves the lipid profile, improves sugar control in diabetics, and has antiplatelet properties. *Sulfasalazine* also delays disease progression, but is more effective when used in combination. All these drugs are slow in onset and should be preferably combined with steroids when initiated. Older drugs such as gold salts, d-penicillamine, minocycline, azathioprine, and cyclosporine are not favored currently due to variable efficacy and unfavorable side effect profile.

Biological DMRDs: Biological disease-modifying antirheumatic drugs have revolutionized the treatment of RA over the past two decades. They are large molecules that require biological systems for production and they target cytokines and cell surface receptors. They are usually reserved for use as second-line agents after failure of conventional DMARDs. Anti-TNF agents were the first biologicals approved for treatment of RA. They target the proinflammatory cytokine TNF and are highly efficacious in controlling and delaying disease progression in RA. In Indian patients, they have a 10% risk of tuberculosis (TB) reactivation which is reduced to 1% by screening for and treatment of latent TB infection before starting anti-TNF agents. *Rituximab* is a chimeric monoclonal antibody which acts by depleting B cells which leads to reduction in the inflammatory response. It is more effective in seropositive patients. It is associated with infusion reactions, which can be prevented by premedicating with glucocorticoids and antihistamines.

Tocilizumab is directed against IL-6 receptor, thus blocking the action of IL-6 which is a major proinflammatory cytokine. IL-6 blockage controls RA, but it causes side effects such as neutropenia, hyperlipidemia, and gastrointestinal (GI) perforation. Abatacept blocks the costimulation signal (CD28 on T cells—CD80/86 on APCs

TABLE 5 DMARDs approved for the treatment of RA.

Drugs	Dose	Mechansim of action	Contraindications	Adverse effects	Screening
Conventional DMARDs					
Methotrexate	• 10–25 mg weekly • Oral or SC • Folic acid 5–10 mg/week after 48 h to reduce toxicity	Adenosine production, Reversible competitive inhibitor of DHFR	• Pregnancy (teratogenic) • CKD (dose titration) • HIV • Anemia (Hb < 7 g/dL) • Thrombocytopenia	• GI complains (nausea, diarrhea) • Hair loss, rash • Subcutaneous nodules • Hepatotoxicity • Myelosuppression • Infections (virus, opportunistic) • Interstitial pneumonitis	• Baseline CBC, liver function, creatinine, albumin, fasting glucose and lipid profile • Serology for HIV, HBV, HCV • Chest X-ray
Leflunomide	10–20 mg/day	Inhibits de novo pyrimidine synthesis	• Pregnancy • Breastfeeding	• Diarrhea • Weight loss • Hypertension • Hepatotoxicity • Myelosuppression (rare) • Infections (abscess)	Baseline CBC, liver enzymes, creatinine
Hydroxy-chloroquine	200–400 mg/day (<5 mg/kg/day)	Concenterates inside acidic cytoplasmic vacuoles and changes the pH, interfering with antigenic processing and hence modulating innate immune system	• Retinopathy • Allergy	• Anorexia, nausea, vomiting • Headache, dizziness • Rash, pruritis • Skin pigmentation • High risk of retinopathy in hepatic and renal dysfunction	• Baseline CBC, liver enzymes, creatinine • Baseline ophthalmological screening • ECG
Sulfasalazine	2–3 g/day in two divided doses (Gradually increase: 500 mg/week)	It is metabolized into sulfapyridine and 5-aminosalicylic acid (ASA). Sulfapyridine is the active agent, but its exact function is not known	• Hypersensitivity (sulfa allergy) • G6PD deficiency • Porphyria	• Nausea, pain abdomen • Headache, dizziness • Rash • Agranulocytosis • Reversible oligospermia • DRESS syndrome	Baseline CBC, liver enzymes, creatinine
Anti-TNF					
Etanercept	50 mg SC once a week or 25 mg SC twice a week	IgG-Fc receptor fusion protein	• Active infection • History of demyelinating disease • Malignancy in last 5 years • NYHA grade III/IV heart failure • Recent live attenuated vaccines • Hypersensitivity	• Infusion site reactions • Transaminitis • Weight gain • Increased risk of bacterial, fungal infections • Activation of latent TB • Drug-induced lupus	• Laboratory tests for CBC, liver function, creatinine, lipid profile • Dental infections • Complete recommended vaccination • Serology for HIV, HBV and HVC • Exclude active or latent TB - Mantoux test, Quantiferon Gold test, chest X-ray PA view
Adalimumab	40 mg SC once in 2 weeks	Human monoclonal antibody			
Infliximab	3–5 mg/kg IV at W0-W2-W6 and then every 6–8 weeks	Chimeric monoclonal antibody			
Golimumab	50 mg SC once month	Human IgG1 monocolonal antibody			
Certolizumab pegol	400 mg SC at W0-W2-W4 and then 200 mg once in 2 weeks	Humanized monoclonal antibody (conjugated with PEG chain)			

Continued...

Continued...

Drugs	Dose	Mechansim of action	Contraindications	Adverse effects	Screening
Anti-CD20 antibodies					
Rituximab	• 1 g IV repeated 14 days later • Premedi-cation: Paracetamol 1 g, methyl-prednisolone 100 mg, and dexchlor-pheniramine 25 mg • In case of relapse, to be repeated after at least 6 months	Chimeric monoclonal Ab (anti-CD20)	• Hypersensitivity • Active infection • NYHA grade III/IV heart failure • Pregnancy (relative)	• Infusion reactions • Allergy (rash, fever) • Increased risk of infection • Hepatitis B reactivation	• Laboratory tests for CBC, liver function, creatinine, lipid profile • Complete recommended vaccination • Serology for HIV, HBV and HVC • Exclude active or latent TB - Mantoux test, Quantiferon Gold test, chest X-ray PA view
IL-6 receptor antagonist					
Tocilizumab	8 mg/kg IV every 4 weeks (minimum 480 mg and maximum 1.2 g)	Humanized monoclonal Ab that inhibits IL-6 receptor (membrane bound and soluble form)	• Hypersensitivity • Active infection • Pregnancy (relative) • History of diverticulitis	• Neutropenia, thrombocytopenia • Reversible transaminitis • Increased risk of infection • Hyperlipidemia • GI perforation (more in patients with diverticulitis)	Same as above
IL-1 antagonist					
Anakinra	100 mg SC daily	Recombinant IL-1 antagonist	• Hypersensitivity • Active infection • Pregnancy	• Infusion reactions • Increased risk of infection	Same as above
Costimulation blocker (CTLA4)					
Abatacept	10 mg/kg IV on D0-D15-D30, then every 30 days or 125 mg SC weekly	Recombinant fully human protein CTLA4- Ig inhibits lymphocyte costimulation	• Hypersensitivity • Active infection • Pregnancy (relative)	• Infusion reactions • Headache • Increased risk of infections	Same as above
JAK-STAT inhibitors					
Tofacitinib	5 mg oral twice daily	JAK1/JAK3 inhibitor	• Hypersensitivity • Active infection/TB • Severe hepatic insufficiency • Pregnancy	• Reversible transaminitis • Myelosuppression • Hyperlipidemia • Increased risk of infection/TB • Reactivation of herpes zoster • GI perforation (rare) • Thromboembolic events	• Laboratory tests for CBC, liver function, creatinine, lipid profile • Serology for HIV, HBV and HVC • Exclude active or latent TB - Mantoux test, Quantiferon Gold test, chest X-ray PA view • Varicella zoster serology if indicated
Baricitinib	2 mg or 4 mg oral once daily	JAK1/JAK2 inhibitor			

(CD: cluster of differentiation; CTLA4: cytotoxic T-lymphocyte-associated protein 4; DHFR: dihydrofolate reductase; DMARDs: disease-modifying antirheumatic drugs; DRESS: drug reaction with eosinophilia and systemic symptoms; G6PD: glucose-6-phosphate deficiency; JAK: Janus kinase; NYHA: New York Heart Association; PEG: polyethylene glycol; SC: subcutaneous; STAT: signal transducers and activators of transcription; TNF: tumor necrosis factor)

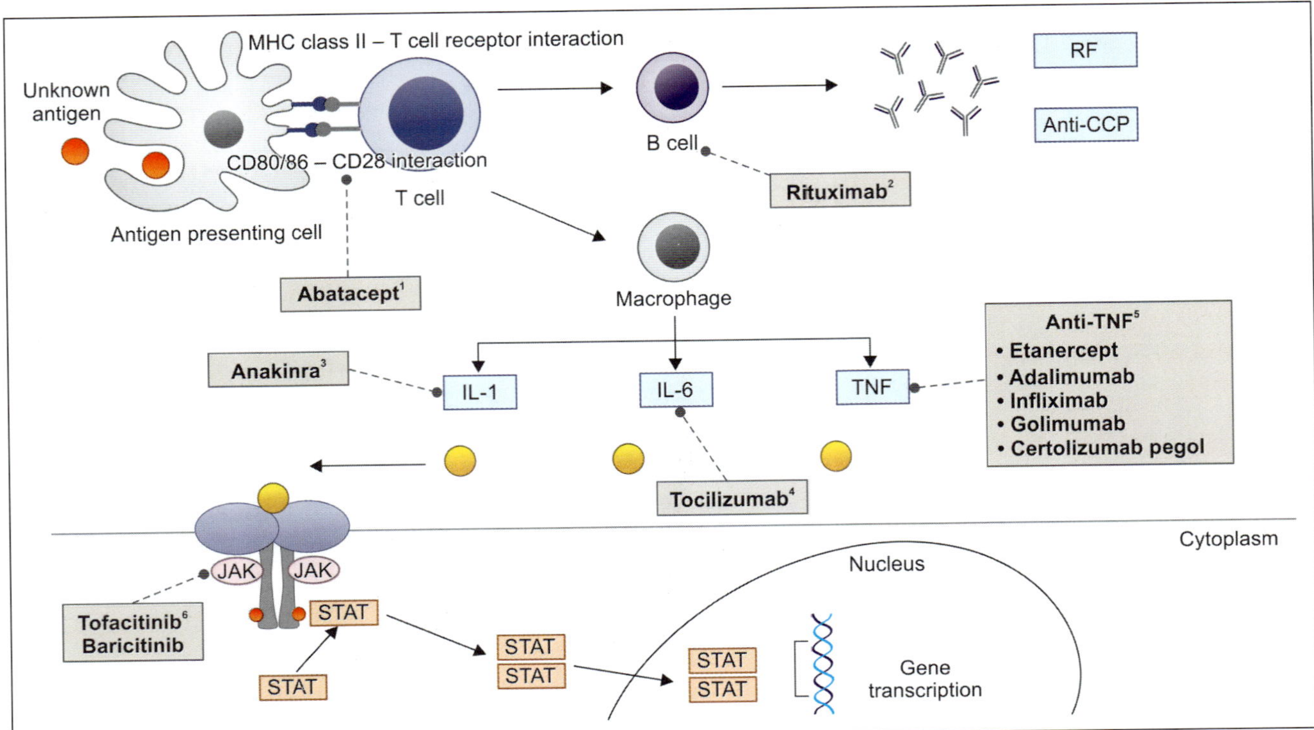

(APCs: antigen presenting cells; anti-CCP: anticitrullinated peptide antibody; CD: cluster of differentiation; IL, interleukins; JAK: janus kinase: MHC: major histocompatibility complex; STAT: signal transducer and activator of transcription)

FIGURE 4: Mechanism of action of bDMARDs and tsDMARDs. (1) Abatacept blocks the costimulatory interaction between CD80/86 and CD28. **(2)** Rituximab binds to CD20 on mature B cells and depletes them by causing apoptosis or immune-mediated lysis. **(3–5)** T cells also activate macrophages, which are the primary source of proinflammatory cytokines, i.e., IL-1, IL-6, and TNF. Anakinra binds to IL-1 receptor, tocilizumab binds to IL-6 receptor, and anti-TNF agents bind to TNF and inhibit their effects, respectively. **(6)** Tofacitinib diffuses across the cell membrane and blocks JAK receptors, preventing phosphorylation of STAT molecules, thus disrupting the JAK-STAT signal transduction pathway.

interaction) required for T-cell activation. In the absence of this signal, T cells undergo anergy and apoptosis. This leads to suppression of inflammation and control of disease activity. Abatacept has a similar risk of infections as other biologicals. Anakinra has the least efficacy among all biologicals in RA and its use in RA is restricted due to availability of better options. It is not available in India.

Targeted synthetic DMRDs: They are small molecules targeting the intracellular signaling pathways of cytokines, thus blocking their effect on cells. Tofacitinib and baricitinib are two drugs currently approved for use in RA. Tofacitinib inhibits JAK1 and JAK3 which mediate signaling of IL-2, IL-4, IL-7, IL-9, IL-15, IL-21, IFN-γ, and IL-6. Baricitinib is a JAK1 and JAK2 inhibitor. "Jakinibs" match the efficacy of bDMARDs and have similar side effect profile. They are approved for use in bDMARD-refractory RA and have the advantage of being administered orally. There is, however, an increased risk of herpes zoster reactivation that is seen with the use of this class of drugs.

Vaccinations: In view of increased risk of infections associated with the use of bDMARDs and tsDMARDs, vaccination against pneumococcus, influenza, and herpes zoster is routinely recommended for RA patients before starting these drugs.

CONCLUSION

Rheumatoid arthritis is the most common chronic inflammatory arthritis in adults. Its etiopathogenesis is not exactly understood, but recent research has shed light on some of the crucial pathways involved. Based on the modern understanding of this disease, significant therapeutic developments have taken place in the last 2–3 decades. These include biological agents (TNF inhibitors, rituximab, tocilizumab etc.) and targeted synthetic drugs (tofacitinib, baricitinib etc.). These advances have led to achievement of good control of disease activity and preservation of function leading to improved quality of life of patients. However, a cure of RA still eludes the scientific community and calls for continued efforts.

RECOMMENDED READINGS

1. Smolen JS, Landewé RBM, Bijilsma JWJ, Burmester GR, Dougados M, Kerschbaumer A, et al. EULAR recommendations for the management of rheumatoid arthritis with synthetic and biological disease-modifying antirheumatic drugs: 2019 update. Ann Rheum Dis. 2020;79:685-99.
2. Lau CS, Chia F, Dans L, Harrison A, Hsieh TY, Jain R, et al. 2018 update of the APLAR recommendations for treatment of rheumatoid arthritis. Int J Rheum Dis. 2019;22:357-75.

3. Horta-Baas G, Romero-Figueroa MS, Montiel-Jarquín AJ, Pizano-Zárate ML, García-Mena J, Ramírez-Durán N. Intestinal Dysbiosis and Rheumatoid Arthritis: A Link between Gut Microbiota and the Pathogenesis of Rheumatoid Arthritis. J Immunol Res. 2017;2017: 4835189.
4. Tracy A, Buckley CD, Raza K. Pre-symptomatic autoimmunity in rheumatoid arthritis: when does the disease start? Semin Immunopathol. 2017;39:423-35.
5. Markusse IM, Akdemir G, Dirven L, Goekoop-Ruiterman YPM, van Groenendael JHLM, Han KH, et al. Long-Term Outcomes of Patients With Recent-Onset Rheumatoid Arthritis After 10 Years of Tight Controlled Treatment: A Randomized Trial. Ann Intern Med. 2016;164:523-31.
6. Smolen JS, Aletaha D, McInnes IB. Rheumatoid arthritis. Lancet. 2016;388:2023-38.
7. Handa R, Rao URK, Lewis JFM, Rambhad G, Shiff S, Ghia CJ. Literature review of rheumatoid arthritis in India. Int J Rheum Dis. 2016;19:440-51.
8. Lau CS, Chia F, Harrison A, Hsieh TY, Jain R, Jung SM, et al. APLAR rheumatoid arthritis treatment recommendations. Int J Rheum Dis. 2015;18:685-713.

CHAPTER 233

Spondyloarthritis

Sakir Ahmed

ABSTRACT

Spondyloarthritis (SpA) is a group of diseases characterized by axial arthritis involving the sacroiliac joints and intravertebral joints and lower limb predominant oligoarthritis, enthesitis, and dactylitis. There is an overlap with recurrent acute anterior uveitis, inflammatory bowel disease (IBD), and psoriasis (PsO). Diseases included are ankylosing spondylitis (AS), axial SpA, psoriatic arthritis (PsA), reactive arthritis (ReA), and enteritis-associated arthritis. Common etiology includes gene such as *HLA-B27* and others, gut microbiota and mucosal infections, physical stress (mechanotransduction), male gender, and smoking. There is a dominant role of the innate immune cells, CD8-positive cells, and of cytokines such as tumor necrosis factor (TNF), interleukins-12, -17, and -23, and others that can be utilized for therapeutic targeting. Radiological characteristics include concomitant bone destruction (erosion, loss of joint space) and new bone formation (syndesmophytes and bony ankylosis). Uncontrolled disease is associated with multiple comorbidities such as accelerated atherosclerosis with increased cardiovascular events and osteoporosis.

Management is based on treat-to-target guided by various composite scores. The first line of therapy is exercise along with nonsteroidal anti-inflammatory drugs (NSAIDs). However, for PsA, first-line drugs include conventional disease-modifying antirheumatic drugs such as methotrexate. The choice for targeted therapy has greatly expanded in the last decade to include targeting of interleukin-17, interleukins-12/-23, and Janus kinase (JAK). Nevertheless, all subgroups of SpA respond differently to different drugs. Ultimately, the management of SpA is dependent on sound clinical knowledge and judgment and supported by good patient communication.

"Early diagnosis is central to avoiding prolonged suffering"

—Martindale J

INTRODUCTION

The word SpA implies an arthritis involving the vertebral column (spondylos = backbone). However, in true sense, it represents a spectrum of disorders inclusive of sacroiliitis, spondylitis, peripheral arthritis, skin involvement, enthesitis, dactylitis, uveitis, and IBD. Although, sacroiliitis is considered a defining feature, it can be absent in a significant proportion of patients. Historically, SpA was referred to as "*seronegative spondyloarthritis*" to emphasize the absence of antibodies [mainly rheumatoid factor, to differentiate from the more common rheumatoid arthritis (RA)]. Now, SpA is much better defined with clinical and imaging features and has been linked with certain antibodies. Hence, the "seronegative" descriptor is better left out.

This chapter aims to introduce the various SpA and principles of diagnosis and management. Numerous criteria and scoring systems are mentioned, so that the interested reader can follow them up. However, due to constraints of space, most have not been elaborated in the chapter.

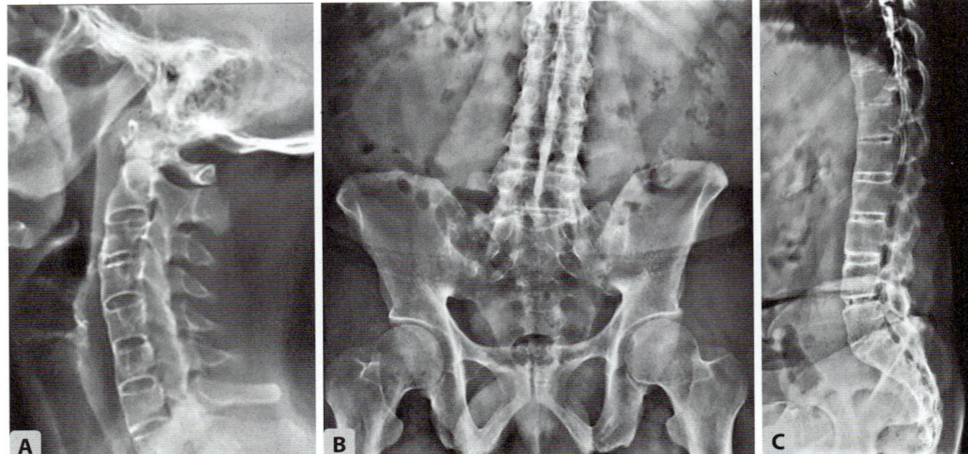

FIGURES 1 A to C: (A) Bridging syndesmophytes with fusion of apophyseal joints; **(B)** Obliteration (complete ankylosis) of the sacroiliac joint (grade 4 sacroiliitis) with calcification of the supraspinous ligament; and **(C)** Ankylosis of the lumbosacral spine ("bamboo spine").

Similarly, for complete treatment protocols, the reader can refer to various guidelines mentioned in the recommended reading.

SPECTRUM

AXIAL INVOLVEMENT

The classical involvement begins with sacroiliitis and gradually affects the spine in an ascending manner from the sacrum upward to the cervical spine. The characteristic lesion is bridging syndesmophytes (**Figs. 1 A** to **C**) leading to fusion or "ankylosis" of the spine. Syndesmophytes can be differentiated from osteophytes since the later have a marrow cavity. In addition to syndesmophytes, there can be involvement of the facet joints as well as of the intervertebral disk (see section on imaging). However, in case of PsA and ReA, the axial involvement may not follow an orderly caudocranial pattern and may have unilateral sacroiliitis.

INFLAMMATORY BACK PAIN

The clinical feature suggestive of axial involvement is inflammatory back pain (IBP). This is defined as summarized in **Box 1**. Only one-third of IBP is due to SpA. The remaining can be due to various causes such as herniation of intravertebral disks, infections (tuberculosis, brucellosis), pelvic inflammatory disease, endometriosis, malignancies, and others.

BOX 1	Features of inflammatory back pain (IBP).
• Age of onset <40 years	
• Worse in the morning at waking up	
• Associated night pain	
• Associated early morning stiffness (>30 minutes)	
• Improves with activity	
• Worsens with rest	
• Good response to nonsteroidal anti-inflammatory drugs	

RADIOGRAPHIC SACROILIITIS

Here the word "radiographic" refers to features of sacroiliitis that are seen on conventional radiographs and not sacroiliitis diagnosed on magnetic resonance imaging (MRI).

PERIPHERAL ARTHRITIS

The classic involvement is an oligoarthritis (two to five joints involved) predominantly affecting the lower limb joints (most commonly knees, ankles, and hips). Involvement of the sternoclavicular joint and subtalar or midfoot joints hint toward SpA and is rare in other arthritides such as RA.

SKIN INVOLVEMENT

Psoriatic arthritis is present in 9–41% of patients with PsO. The skin lesions present in chronic ReA [called keratoderma blennorrhagicum (**Fig. 2 A**) that starts often on the soles and can spread]. In widespread keratoderma blennorrhagicum, the lesions may be difficult to distinguish from PsO morphologically or histopathologically. The other pathognomonic rash for ReA is circinate balanitis, which is seen on the glans penis (**Fig. 2 B**).

ENTHESITIS

In addition to sacroiliitis, enthesitis is a defining feature of SpA. An enthesis is the site of attachment of a ligament or a tendon on the bone. The Achilles tendon is the most commonly affected. However, there are numerous entheseal sites in the body (**Table 1**) and various enthesitis indices use a different combination of the sites to document the burden of enthesitis (see management).

DACTYLITIS

This is another distinguishing feature of SpA that is pathologically characterized by tenosynovitis involving the flexor and extensor tendons. Diffuse painful swelling of digits (toes or fingers) is called dactylitis or colloquially referred to as "sausage digits" (**Fig. 3**).

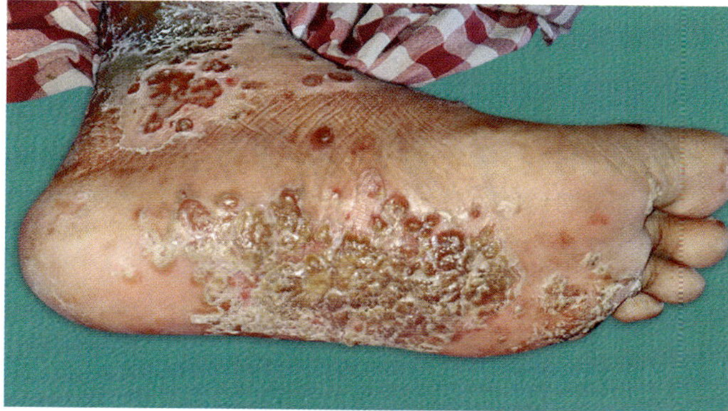

FIGURE 2 A: Keratoderma blennorrhagicum.
Courtesy: Dr Subhashree Madhual, SCB Medical College, Cuttack.

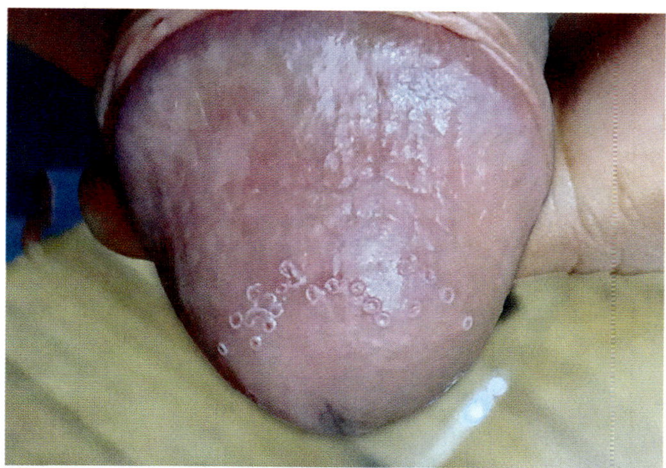

FIGURE 2 B: Circinate balanitis.
Courtesy: Abirami C, KIMS Medical College, Bhubaneswar.

TABLE 1 Common sites for enthesitis.

• Costochondral junctions	• Anterior-superior iliac spine
• Lateral epicondyle	• Greater trochanter
• Medial epicondyle	• Upper and lower poles of patella
• Tip of spinous process of vertebra	• Achilles tendon
• Iliac crest	• Plantar fascia

BOWEL DISEASE

5–10% of SpA have overlap with clinically symptomatic IBD. Nevertheless, asymptomatic bowel inflammation may be seen in up to 40–50% of SpA documented using ileal biopsies.

SPONDYLOARTHRITIS-ASSOCIATED UVEITIS

This is a nongranulomatous, recurrent, acute, and anterior uveitis. It is usually unilateral, but recurrence is common and can affect alternating eyes.

DISEASES WITHIN THE SPECTRUM

It should be remembered that if a patient has features of axial plus peripheral SpA, it is categorized under axial SpA. Peripheral SpA refers to only peripheral involvement [however, the Assessment of Spondyloarthritis International Society (ASAS) classification criteria allow for past history of IBP without changes on imaging or asymptomatic sacroiliitis on imaging]. **Figure 4** shows a schematic representation of overlap between the various diseases in the SpA spectrum.

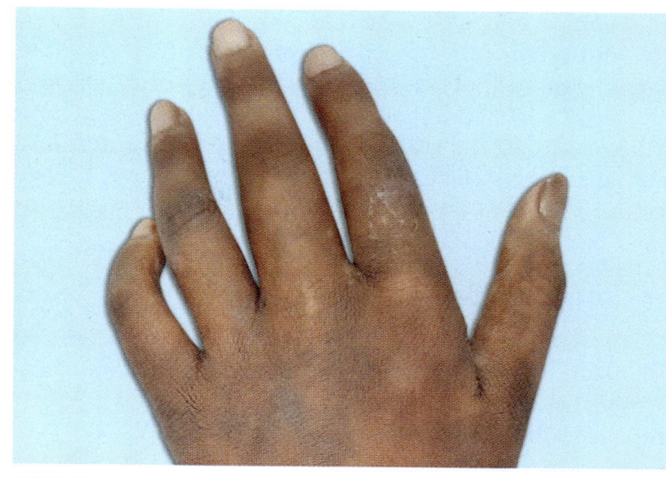

FIGURE 3: Dactylitis or sausage digit of the middle finger.

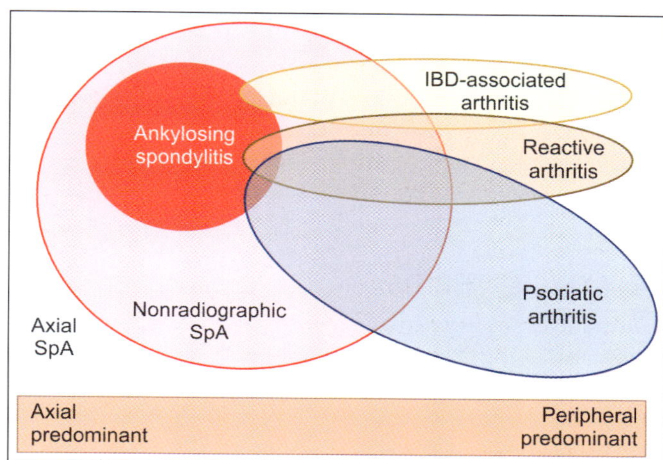

(IBD: inflammatory bowel disease; SpA: spondyloarthritis)

FIGURE 4: Schematic visualization of the overlap between different subgroups of SpA.

ANKYLOSING SPONDYLITIS

This is the prototypic SpA most well-known for its dreaded complication of "bamboo spine". The basis for AS diagnosis is radiographic sacroiliitis. For all practical purposes, AS is a diagnosis that can be made only on radiographs and not on MRI or clinical grounds. Not all patients of AS develop bamboo spine.

AXIAL SPONDYLOARTHRITIS

Since radiographic changes of AS take at least 7–8 years to develop, there was a very strong need to define early SpA for intervention and disease modification. Thus, in 2009, the ASAS defined criteria for "axial SpA". Axial SpA includes a spectrum of disease from nonradiographic SpA (NR-SpA) to define AS to a full-blown bamboo spine (**Fig. 4**). It also includes PsA or IBD with axial involvement. It is important to understand that possibly only a third of NR-SpA will evolve into AS and only third of these will evolve AS into bamboo spine. The presence of HLA-B27, male sex, and smoking are risk factors for more severe disease, but we cannot predict at an individual level who will progress to AS or to a complete bamboo spine.

PERIPHERAL SPONDYLOARTHRITIS

To complement axial SpA, the ASAS also defined criteria for peripheral SpA. This includes PsA (without axial involvement), ReA, IBD-associated arthritis, and a poorly defined undifferentiated form of peripheral SpA.

PSORIATIC ARTHRITIS

As mentioned earlier, PsA occurs in a subset of PsO patients but may rarely occur in the absence of PsO (PsA sans PsO). PsA is a faster progressing and more erosive disease as compared to RA. Without treatment, almost a half of PsA patients will develop an irreversible deformity within 2 years of disease onset. They are also more likely to develop *arthritis mutilans*, characterized by telescoping of digits.

REACTIVE ARTHRITIS

Acute onset of arthritis, with or without axial involvement, following a gut or urogenital infection, is known as ReA. To define classical ReA, certain bacteria must be demonstrated in stool, urine, or synovium (**Table 2**). In real life, such demonstration is less practical and not widely practiced. The triad of urethritis, uveitis, and arthritis had been given an eponym. This triad is not very frequently seen and the eponym is recommended not to be used since the person was a Nazi convicted of war crimes including unethical experiments on humans.

IBD-ASSOCIATED ARTHRITIS

As the name suggests, this is SpA developing in association with IBD.

JUVENILE IDIOPATHIC ARTHRITIS

This is the juvenile counterpart of SpA that has an onset before 16 years of age. It can present with high-grade fever (in contrast to adult disease) and other features of SpA such as enthesitis, axial involvement, and acute anterior uveitis.

EPIDEMIOLOGY

Depending on region of the world and methodology used, the prevalence of AS has been reported in between 1 and 5 per 1,000. Since axial SpA is a comparatively newly defined entity (and screening will need MRI and extensive investigations), data on prevalence is sparse. PsO occurs in around 0.5–2% of population and the prevalence increases with increase in median age of the population.

- **Genetics:** AS is known for a very strong genetic association with the B27 allele of human leukocyte antigen (HLA). The prevalence of *HLA-B27* genes in various SpA is summarized in **Table 3**. Apart from *HLA-B27*, other genes are also associated with SpA, the most important of which is endoplasmic reticulum aminopeptidase 1 (*ERAP1*) and interleukin-23 receptor

TABLE 2 Braun criteria for reactive arthritis (ReA).

Definite ReA	**Both major + one minor criteria**		
Probable ReA	**Both major but no minor criteria**		
Major criteria	(1) At least two of these should be present	Asymmetric arthritis	
		Predominantly lower limb	
		Oligoarthritis	
	(2) Arthritis should be preceded by	Diarrhea for >1 day	Between 3 days to 6 weeks before the onset of arthritis
		Dysuria or urethral discharge for >1 day	
Minor criteria	(1) Stool culture positive for specific organisms	• *Yersinia* • *Salmonella* • *Shigella* • *Campylobacter jejuni* Urogenital tract: • *Chlamydia trachomatis* • *Neisseria gonorrhoeae* • *Mycoplasma genitalium* • *Ureaplasma urealyticum*	**Less frequent agents:** • *Clostridium difficile* • *Campylobacter lari* • *Chlamydia psittaci* • *Chlamydia pneumoniae*
	(2) Positive urine ligase reaction	For *Chlamydia trachomatis*	
	(3) Proof from synovial biopsy	Positive immunohistology or polymerase chain reaction (PCR) for *Chlamydia*	

(*IL23R*) gene. However, it must be understood that SpA, including AS, can occur in absence of HLA-B27.

- **Age:** With the exception of PsA and possibly IBD-associated SpA, all others usually have onset below 40 years of age. The natural history is onset in second or third decade of life and usually the disease gradually dies out during the fifth or sixth decade. PsA can start late in life and last beyond the sixth decade.
- **Sex:** Though in AS, the *male to female ratio is around 2:1*, the ratio is reversed in NR-SpA. This might imply that females have less severe disease, while males progress to more severe disease with worse outcomes.

TABLE 3 Grading of sacroiliitis on radiographs.

Grades	Findings	Comment
0	Normal	Can consider MRI, if strong clinical suspicion
1	Suspicious	No definite changes CT may be helpful
2	Minimal sclerosis or joint irregularity	Joint can appear narrowed due to loss of articular cartilage
3	Unequivocal erosion, sclerosis, widening, narrowing, and/or partial ankylosis	Widening is due to multiple erosions
4	Complete ankylosis	Joint line is not visible

PATHOLOGY

The gut-joint axis represents a strong pathogenetic link in case of SpA. The connection is obvious in case of ReA in which the disease, by definition, is temporally related to a gut or urogenital infection. The presence of IBD-associated arthritis as well as the subclinical colitis present in almost a third of patients with AS provides strong evidence for the gut-joint ties. The complete set of microorganisms including nonculturable bacteria, fungi, and viruses constitute the gut microbiome. There is a strong relationship between the microbiome, innate immune cells, and SpA flares.

The clinically relevant cytokines in SpA include TNF-α, interleukin-17, interleukin-12, and interleukin-23. The significance of these cytokines is that blockade of these will lead to therapeutic effect with disease-modifying characteristics.

Figure 5 summarizes the currently knowledge about SpA pathology.

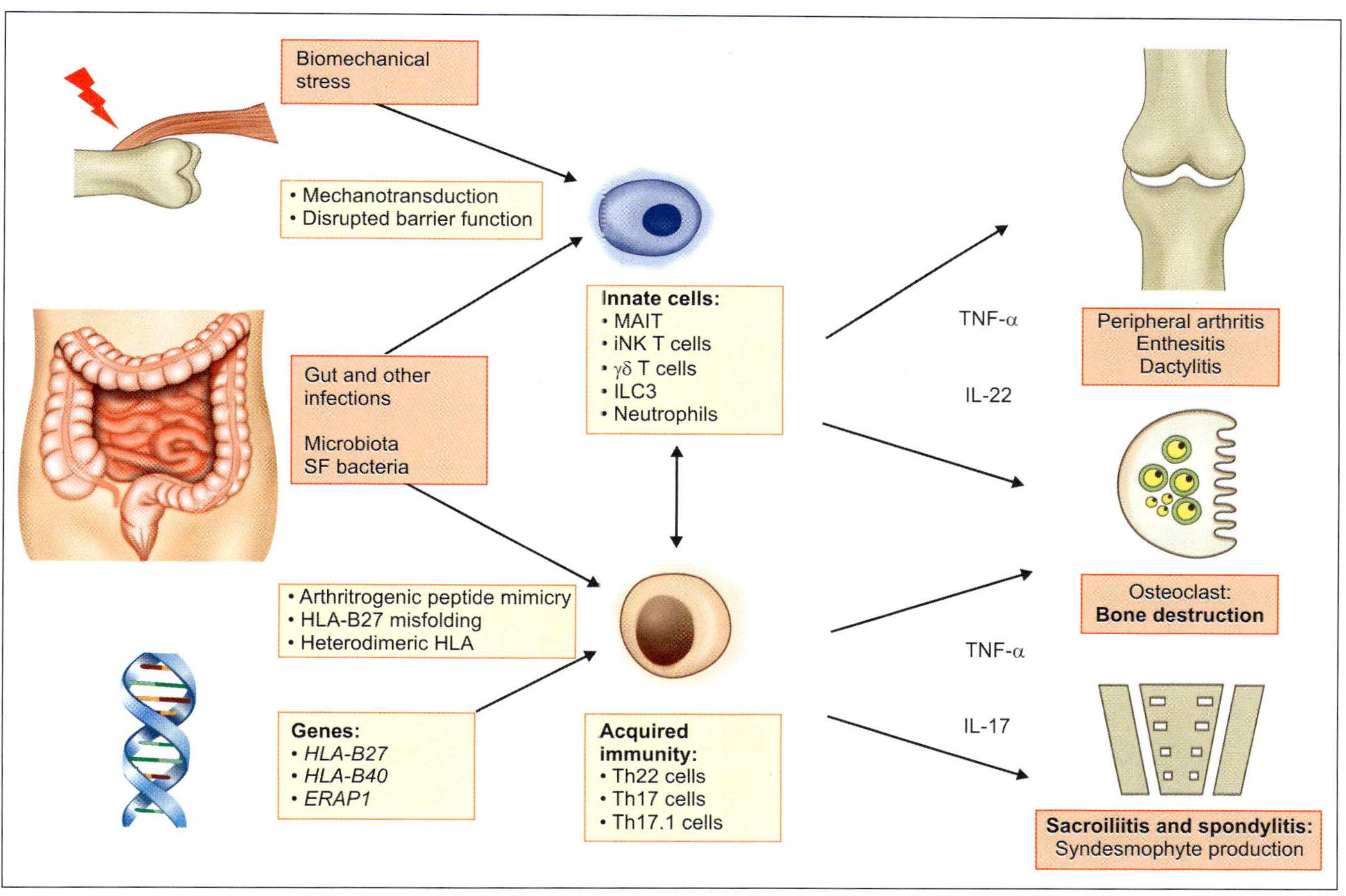

(ERAP1: endoplasmic reticulum aminopeptidase-1; HLA: human leukocyte antigen; IL-17: interleukin-17; ILC3: innate lymphoid cell 3; iNK: invariant natural killer; MAIT: mucosal-associated invariant T; SF: segmented filamentous; Th: T helper; TNF-α: tumor necrosis factor-α)

FIGURE 5: Pathogenesis of spondyloarthritis.

CLINICAL FEATURES

The typical description of axial SpA is that night pain gradually starts in the second half of the night and worsens toward early morning. *Pain and stiffness may awaken a patient from sleep*, the stiffness lasting for more than half an hour (one of the defining features of IBP), but in more severe cases can last the greater half of or even the whole day. Gradual activity and a shower using lukewarm water might help to reduce the stiffness. There can be restriction of spine movements due to both disease activity as well as damage or "ankylosis". Cervical spine can be assessed by rotation, lateral flexion, flexion, and extension. Thoracic spine mobility is assessed by chest expansion while lumbar mobility is measured by the *modified Schober test* and lateral lumbar flexion. For the modified Schober, the patient should be asked to stand straight and two points are marked in the midline on the back: at 10 cm above the line joining the two posterior superior iliac spines and at 5 cm below the same. Then, the patient is asked to bend forward, keeping knees straight and attempting to touch the floor. In this position, the distance between the points is measured and it should be >20 cm. Anything less implies restriction of lumbar spine mobility.

There can be chest pain due to involvement of costovertebral and costotransverse joints. Intermalleolar distance (between the medial malleoli in standing with knees extended) provides information about hip involvement while tragus-to-wall distance helps quantify cervical involvement. Peripheral arthritis, enthesitis, dactylitis, and uveitis can occur as described in the first section of this chapter.

Two common comorbidities are: (1) osteoporosis and (2) cardiovascular disease. Due to prolonged inflammatory state, there is accelerated atherosclerosis leading to premature cardiovascular events and mortality. Also, the spinal and periarticular inflammation and limitation of mobility of patients contribute to accelerated osteoporosis. Osteoporosis along with increased stiffness due to development of "bamboo spine" predisposes to spinal fractures, which represents one of the most dreaded complications in the advanced stages of the disease. Other common comorbidities that need to be addressed include depression, anxiety, and fibromyalgia.

Rarely, upper lobe lung fibrosis can be seen in patients with long-standing AS. Another complication of long-standing uncontrolled disease is amyloidosis leading to kidney failure. Immunoglobulin A (IgA) nephropathy can present with microscopic hematuria, proteinuria, and renal impairment.

INVESTIGATIONS

LABORATORY

Routine blood tests are useful only to monitor comorbidities and drug toxicities. Various acute phase reactants such as erythrocyte sedimentation rate (ESR), C-reactive protein (CRP), serum amyloid A (SAA), ferritin, or serum calprotectin may be elevated due to the ongoing inflammation. However, in clinical practice, only ESR and CRP are used for monitoring. A high CRP usually predicts a good response to therapy.

TABLE 4 MRI findings of SpA.

Sites	Feature of	Findings
Sacroiliac joint	Activity	Bone marrow edema
		Synovitis (of SI joint)
	Damage	"Backfill" or T1 fat infiltration
		Erosions
		Ankylosis
Spine	Activity	"Shiny corner" or Romanus sign
		Spondylodiskitis or Andersson sign
	Damage	Erosions
		Nonbridging and bridging syndesmophytes
		Ankylosis of facet joints
Others	Enthesitis/ Dactylitis/ Synovitis	Each has specific findings

(SpA: spondyloarthritis; SI: sacroiliac)

IMAGING

Spondyloarthritis is characterized by concurrent bone formation and destruction. Conventional radiography is the backbone for AS diagnosis. The grading of sacroiliitis on radiographs is mentioned in **Table 3**. Bony erosions and whiskering are at areas of entheseal attachment.

Ultrasound is helpful in delineating enthesis that can distinguish it from other forms of arthritis. It also has a role in therapeutic with the ease of guided injections to inflamed joints, bursae, and in tendon sheaths.

Computed tomography scores over conventional radiography are useful in demarcating sacroiliac joint erosions in doubtful cases. It is also useful in picking up spinal fractures: The ankylosed and osteopenic spine is at higher risks of fractures.

Magnetic resonance imaging is a current standard of care for diagnosis of axial SpA. The MRI features suggestive of SpA are mentioned in **Table 4**. The gold standard is the presence of erosion with demonstration of new bone formation. The minimum requirement for the ASAS MRI criteria is bone marrow edema (in at least two consecutive slices). Though this is a very sensitive marker, recent studies have shown that it is not at all specific. Hence, SpA should never be diagnosed based on MRI alone (without classical clinical features).

TABLE 5 The ASAS classification criteria for axial and peripheral SpA.

Axial SpA		Peripheral SpA	
Imaging criteria + One "clinical feature" **Or** **Two other "clinical features" in presence of HLA-B27**		**Peripheral arthritis and/or enthesitis and/or dactylitis Plus**	
"Imaging arm"	"Clinical arm"	One of the following features	Or two of the other following features
• Definite radiographic sacroiliitis • Active inflammation on MRI highly suggestive of sacroiliitis	• Inflammatory back pain • Arthritis • Enthesitis • Dactylitis • Uveitis • Psoriasis • Inflammatory bowel disease • Good response to NSA Ds • Family history of SpA • HLA-B27 • Elevated CRP	• Uveitis • Psoriasis • Inflammatory bowel disease • Preceding infection (urogenital or gut) • HLA-B27 • (Asymptomatic) sacroiliitis on imaging	• Arthritis • Enthesitis • Dactylitis • Family history of SpA • History of inflammatory back pain

(ASAS: Assessment of Spondyloarthritis International Society)

MANAGEMENT

The management varies as per the diagnosis and presence of comorbidities. The ASAS criteria (**Table 5**) are classification criteria to ensure a homogeneous group for trial or study purpose. Just meeting the classification criteria is not sufficient for a diagnosis, but the diagnosis should be a logical and clinical decision. On the other hand, the patient does not meet the criteria, a second opinion should be strongly considered before making a diagnosis of SpA. For diagnosis of PsA, another set of classification criteria called the CASPER criteria are available.

Table 6 mentions how different manifestations of SpA respond to various drugs. As an unwritten rule, axial SpA and AS are managed similarly while peripheral SpA including ReA- and IBD-associated arthritis can be managed similarly. PsA possibly has the widest range of available drugs. However, certain cases may be refractory to a majority of these drugs. The future is of personalized medicine that may help to predict which patient is best likely to respond to which drug.

UNIVERSAL APPROACH

In all SpA except PsA, the first-line therapy is physical exercises with NSAIDs (unless contraindicated). In case of failure of at least two NSAIDs given for optimum period (at least 2–4 weeks each) at optimum dose, patient should be given the option for biological disease-modifying antirheumatic drug (bDMARD) or targeted synthetic disease-modifying antirheumatic drug (tsDMARD). When peripheral joints are involved, NSAIDs are to be augmented by intra-articular injections of steroids. Oral steroids have very little effectiveness in SpA and should rarely be used.

Nonsteroidal anti-inflammatory drugs can possibly retard disease progression and are, hence, regarded as disease-modifying agents for SpA. In case of NSAIDs failure or contraindication, if the patient is unable to access bDMARDs or tsDMARDs, it is reasonable to try the various conventional synthetic disease-modifying antirheumatic drugs (csDMARDs). In PsA, patients are to be started on csDMARD from diagnosis. For all therapies, it is necessary to monitor the patient periodically for disease activity and drug toxicities (**Table 7**).

CLINICAL MONITORING

Just as diabetes mellitus is treated with individualized targets (fasting blood glucose, postprandial blood glucose, and glycosylated hemoglobin levels), SpA should be clinically monitored on various clinical, laboratory, and radiographic parameters for empowering treat-to-target approach. This objectifies escalation and de-escalation of therapy. Setting a target and choice of therapeutics should involve an informed decision between patient and physician as in chronic disease care; a good long-term outcome is determined by an adequate two-way communication between the patient and physician. **Table 8** mentions the common tools used to monitor different aspects of disease in SpA.

TABLE 6 Various drugs used for SpA.

Class of drug/ target	Names	Evidence for	Effective for	Comments
Nonsteroidal anti-inflammatory drugs	Various	• AS	• Spinal and peripheral arthritis • Less effective for enthesitis or dactylitis or AA uveitis	Recommended as first line for all SpA except PsA
csDMARD	Methotrexate	• PsA • AA uveitis	Skin manifestation, peripheral arthritis, possibly spinal arthritis	Evidence is limited in AS and axial SpA but is commonly used in India and other low- to medium-income countries
	Sulfasalazine	• Peripheral arthritis (AS) and PsA	Peripheral arthritis, possibly spinal arthritis	• Commonly used in India and other low- to medium-income countries • Not very effective in PsA or for dactylitis, enthesitis, or AA uveitis
	Leflunomide	• Limited evidence	Possibly peripheral arthritis and arthritis	Evidence is limited but when patients do not have access to targeted therapy, it may be a good alternative
Antitumor necrosis factor	Infliximab	• AS • PsA • PsO • AA uveitis • IBD	• Entire spectrum including dactylitis and enthesitis • Etanercept may worsen uveitis, PsO, and IBD	• For use of all anti-TNF agents, screening for both active and latent tuberculosis is must at baseline and then annually • For extra-articular manifestations, maximum evidence is for infliximab and adalimumab
	Etanercept (TNF receptor conjugated with immunoglobulin chain)	• AS		
	Adalimumab	• AS • PsA • PsO • AA uveitis • IBD		
	Golimumab	• AS • PsA • PsO		
	Certolizumab	• AS • Axial SpA		
Anti-interleukin-17A (IL-17A)	• Secukinumab • Ixekizumab	• PsO • PsA • AS • Axial SpA	• High efficacy against PsO/PsA • Efficacy may be less for Axial SpA	Increased risks for fungal infections
Anti-IL-17A and anti-IL-17F	Bimekizumab	• PsA	Emerging data	Superior to secukinumab
Anti-IL-12/anti-IL-23p40	• Ustekinumab • Briankizumab	• PsO • PsA	Emerging data	
Anti-IL-23p19	• Guselkumab • Tildrakizumab • Risankizumab • Brazikumab • Mirikizumab	• PsO • PsA	Remarkable efficacy for PsO and PsA	Emerging evidence for other indications
JAK inhibitors	• Tofacitinib • Baricitinib • Filgotinib • Upadacitinib	• PsO • PsA • AS	Emerging data	• Wide spectrum of mechanism of action • May have higher risk for infections mostly against various viruses

(csDMARD: conventional synthetic disease-modifying antirheumatic drug; JAK: Janus kinase; PsA: psoriatic arthritis; PsO: psoriasis; SpA: spondyloarthritis)

Note: Various other drugs, not mentioned in this table, are used for SpA in different parts of the world such as thalidomide, bisphosphonates, azathioprine, and others.

TABLE 7 Monitoring of SpA patients on drugs.

Minimum investigations	NSAIDs	csDMARDs	bDMARDs	tsDMARDs
Baseline	• Complete blood count (CBC) • Liver function test (LFT) • Creatinine • ESR/CRP • Chest radiograph • Spinal/pelvic radiograph	• CBC • LFT • Creatinine • ESR/CRP • Chest radiograph • Spinal/pelvic radiograph • Mantoux test • IGRA	• CBC • LFT • Creatinine • ESR/CRP • Chest radiograph • Spinal/pelvic radiograph • Mantoux test • IGRA	• CBC • LFT • Creatinine • ESR/CRP • Chest radiograph • Spinal/pelvic radiograph • Mantoux test • IGRA • Herpes vaccination
4 weeks after start of drug	• Hemoglobin • ALT • Creatinine	• CBC • ALT • Creatinine	• CBC • ALT • Creatinine	• CBC • ALT • Creatinine
Every 2–4 months	• Hemoglobin • ALT • Creatinine • ESR/CRP	• CBC • ALT • Creatinine • ESR/CRP	• CBC • ALT • Creatinine • ESR/CRP	• CBC • ALT • Creatinine • ESR/CRP
Annually	• CBC • LFTs • Creatinine • Acute phase reactants • Chest radiograph • Spinal/pelvic radiograph	• CBC • LFTs • Creatinine • Acute phase reactants • Chest radiograph • Spinal/pelvic radiograph • Mantoux test • IGRA	• CBC • LFTs • Creatinine • Acute phase reactants • Chest radiograph • Spinal/pelvic radiograph • Mantoux test • IGRA	• CBC • LFTs • Creatinine • Acute phase reactants • Chest radiograph • Spinal/pelvic radiograph • Mantoux test • IGRA

(bDMARDs: biological disease-modifying antirheumatic drugs; csDMARDs: conventional synthetic disease-modifying antirheumatic drugs; IGRA: interferon-gamma release assay; SpA: spondyloarthritis; tsDMARDs: targeted synthetic disease-modifying antirheumatic drugs)

TABLE 8 Various tools to monitor different dimensions of SpA manifestations.

Dimensions	Axial SpA (including AS)	Psoriatic arthritis
Disease activity	• Bath Ankylosing Spondylitis Disease Activity Index (BASDAI) • Ankylosing Spondylitis Disease Activity Score (ASDAS)	• Disease Activity Index for Psoriatic Arthritis (DAPSA) • Psoriatic Arthritis Response Criteria (PsARC) • Composite Psoriatic Disease Activity Index (CPDAI) • Psoriatic Arthritis Disease Activity Score (PASDAS) Axial involvement: • Same as for AS Skin involvement: • Psoriasis Area and Severity Index (PASI)
Functional status	• Bath Ankylosing Spondylitis Functional Index (BASFI) • Health Assessment Questionnaire Disability Index (HAQ-DI)	• GRACE index
Damage/Restrictions	• Bath Ankylosing Spondylitis Metrology Index (BASMI)	• PASI damage • BASMI
Radiographic damage	• Modified Stoke Ankylosing Spondylitis Spinal Score (mSASSS)	• Modified Sharp-van der Heijde (mSvdH) • Psoriatic Arthritis Ratingen Score (PARS)

Continued...

Continued...

Dimensions	Axial SpA (including AS)	Psoriatic arthritis
Quality of life	• Ankylosing Spondylitis Quality of Life (ASQoL)	• PsA Impact of Disease • PsA Quality of Life
Enthesitis	• Maastricht Ankylosing Spondylitis Enthesitis Score (MASES) • Mander Enthesis Index (MEI) • Spondyloarthritis Research Consortium of Canada (SPARCC) enthesitis score	• Leeds Enthesitis Index
Dactylitis	• Dactylitis Severity Score (DSS)	• Leeds Dactylitis Index

(AS: ankylosing spondylitis; SpA: spondyloarthritis)

RECOMMENDED READINGS

1. Rudwaleit M, van der Heijde D, Landewe R, Akkoc N, Brandt J, Chou CT, et al. The Assessment of SpondyloArthritis international Society classification criteria for peripheral spondyloarthritis and for spondyloarthritis in general. Ann Rheum Dis. 2011;70(1):25-31.
2. Ahmed S, Misra R. Human leukocyte antigen—HLAB*27: Unraveling the link to pathogenesis. Indian J Rheumatol. 2020;15(Suppl S1):13-8.
3. Machado PMMC, Landewé RBM, van der HEIJDE DM. Endorsement of Definitions of Disease Activity States and Improvement Scores for the Ankylosing Spondylitis Disease Activity Score: Results from OMERACT 10. J Rheumatol. 2011;38(7):1502-6.
4. Eriksson JK, Jacobsson L, Bengtsson K, Askling J. Is ankylosing spondylitis a risk factor for cardiovascular disease, and how do these risks compare with those in rheumatoid arthritis? Ann Rheum Dis. 2017;76(2):364-70.
5. Smolen JS, Schöls M, Braun J, Dougados M, FitzGerald O, Gladman DD, et al. Treating axial spondyloarthritis and peripheral spondyloarthritis, especially psoriatic arthritis, to target: 2017 update of recommendations by an international task force. Ann Rheum Dis. 2018;77(1):3-17.
6. Schoels MM, Braun J, Dougados M, Emery P, Fitzgerald O, Kavanaugh A, et al. Treating axial and peripheral spondyloarthritis, including psoriatic arthritis, to target: results of a systematic literature search to support an international treat-to-target recommendation in spondyloarthritis. Ann Rheum Dis. 2014;73(1):238-42.
7. Smolen JS, Braun J, Dougados M, Emery P, FitzGerald O, Helliwell P, et al. Treating spondyloarthritis, including ankylosing spondylitis and psoriatic arthritis, to target: recommendations of an international task force. Ann Rheum Dis. 2014;73(1):6-16.
8. Coates LC, Moverley AR, McParland L, Brown S, Navarro-Coy N, O'Dwyer JL, et al. Effect of tight control of inflammation in early psoriatic arthritis (TICOPA): a UK multicentre, open-label, randomised controlled trial. Lancet. 2015;386(10012):2489-98.
9. Dougados M. Treat to target in axial spondyloarthritis: From its concept to its implementation. J Autoimmun. 2020;110:102398.
10. van der Heijde D, Ramiro S, Landewé R, Baraliakos X, van den Bosch F, Sepriano A, et al. 2016 update of the ASAS-EULAR management recommendations for axial spondyloarthritis. Ann Rheum Dis. 2017;76(6):978-91.
11. Ward MM, Deodhar A, Gensler LS, Dubreuil M, Yu D, Khan MA, et al. 2019 Update of the American College of Rheumatology/Spondylitis Association of America/ Spondyloarthritis Research and Treatment Network Recommendations for the Treatment of Ankylosing Spondylitis and Nonradiographic Axial Spondyloarthritis. Arthritis Care Res. 2019;71(5):1285-99.
12. Coates LC, Kavanaugh A, Mease PJ, Soriano ER, Laura Acosta-Felquer M, Armstrong AW, et al. Group for Research and Assessment of Psoriasis and Psoriatic Arthritis 2015 Treatment Recommendations for Psoriatic Arthritis. Arthritis Rheumatol. 2016;68(5):1060-71.

CHAPTER 234

Systemic Lupus Erythematosus

Sarit Sekhar Pattanaik, Rudrarpan Chatterjee, Amita Aggarwal

ABSTRACT

Systemic lupus erythematosus (SLE), an autoimmune disease affecting young females, is associated with considerable morbidity and mortality. Interplay of host genetic susceptibility, environmental factors, and abnormal immune response trigger systemic autoimmunity, which leads to organ damage. The demonstration of autoantibodies in serum or immune complex deposition in tissues, along with multisystemic involvement, helps in diagnosis of patients. Constitutional symptoms and skin and articular involvement are seen in majority of cases. Nephritis, seen in 50–60% of patients, is the most common major organ involved and has impact on long-term outcome. Other systems such as hematological, central nervous system (CNS), cardiorespiratory, and gastrointestinal system can at times be the presenting manifestation of the disease.

Antinuclear antibodies are the hallmarks and are detected in nearly 98% of cases. Anti-Sm, anti-double-stranded DNA (dsDNA), and antiphospholipid antibodies are seen in 40–70% of patients. Serum complements such as C3 and C4 help to monitor disease activity. SLE is a relapsing-remitting disease, thus therapy must be tailored to attain low disease activity with minimal damage accrual and drug toxicity. Steroids along with immunosuppressive (IS) agents such as cyclophosphamide, mycophenolate mofetil, azathioprine, and calcineurin inhibitors are the mainstay of therapy in severe disease. Antimalarials should be used in all patients, as they prevent flares and reduce damage accrual. B-cell depleting agents (rituximab, belimumab), interferon-alpha axis inhibitors [anifrolumab, Janus kinase (JAK) inhibitors] and those targeting interleukin-6 (IL-6) and IL-17, and mammalian target of rapamycin (mTOR) pathway are showing encouraging results. The outcome of SLE has improved considerably over the last three decades with nearly 90% 10-year survival.

"Research is to see what everybody else has seen, and to think what nobody else has thought"

—Albert Szent-Gyorgyi

INTRODUCTION

Systemic lupus erythematosus is a multisystem autoimmune disease, *seen predominantly in women of childbearing age group.* The word "lupus" (Latin for "wolf") came from the erosive facial lesion seen in this disease that is reminiscent of a wolf's bite. SLE is characterized by presence of multiple autoantibodies including the most common antinuclear antibody (ANA). The estimated prevalence varies from 20 to 150 per 100,000 depending on race and gender. Afro-Americans and Asians have a higher prevalence as well as severity of SLE. Advances in immunology have helped us understand the pathogenesis of this complex disease better, leading to development of targeted therapies for SLE.

PATHOGENESIS

Systemic lupus erythematosus like other autoimmune diseases probably results from a complex interplay of genetic susceptibility, environmental factors, and abnormal immune response resulting in systemic autoimmunity.

GENETIC FACTORS

Recent genome-wide association studies have identified >60 susceptibility loci for SLE. Although, individually, these genes confer only a small risk for SLE with odds ratios of 1.5–3 SLE, but in combination, they account for about 20% of disease susceptibility. The major contributor to genetic risk is the major histocompatibility complex (MHC) locus. HLA-DRB1*0301 and HLA-DRB1*1501 are associated with SLE. Several non-HLA genes involved in innate and adaptive immune responses such as toll-like receptor 7 (TLR7) and BLK are associated with increased risk of SLE. Genes involved in clearance of apoptotic debris such as DNAse 1, neutrophil adherence [integrin alpha M (*ITGAM*)], and DNA repair [three prime repair exonuclease 1 (*TREX1*)] are also associated with SLE. Functional polymorphism in *STAT4* is associated with nephritis, high titers of anti-DNA antibodies, and antiphospholipid syndrome (APS). Similarly, *FcgRIIA* allele predisposes to nephritis. Rare single gene defects such as early complement (C1q, C1r, C1s; C2; C4) deficiency and a mutation in *TREX1* confer a very high risk for SLE.

In addition to genetic factors, epigenetic factors also modulate gene expression. DNA hypomethylation, histone acetylation, and various microRNAs regulate key gene expression in CD4+ T cells, B cells, and monocytes.

ENVIRONMENTAL FACTORS

Among the environmental factors, ultraviolet (UV) light, infections, and drugs are the key players. UV light by causing keratinocyte apoptosis leads to exposure of autoantigens triggering cutaneous and systemic flare. Epstein–Barr virus (EBV) by having sequence similarity with human spliceosomes can lead to generation of autoantibodies (molecular mimicry) and chronic B-cell activation induced by EBV can trigger disease in susceptible individual. Drugs such as hydralazine, procainamide, isoniazid (INH), and off-late antitumor necrosis factor-α (TNF-α) agents by generation of neoepitopes or epigenetic alterations have been associated with cutaneous disease. Tobacco smoking and crystalline silica exposure are also associated with increased risk of SLE.

HORMONAL FACTORS

The female predominance of SLE can be explained by hormonal factors, genes on the X chromosome, and epigenetic differences. Estradiol, binding to its receptors on T and B lymphocytes, increases activation and survival of these cells, leading to increased autoantibody production and heightened and sustained immune response. Presence of extra X chromosome as in XXY karyotype (Klinefelter syndrome) and differential silencing of genes on X chromosome predispose women to SLE.

THE PROCESS

In brief, genetic susceptibility acting in consort with environmental trigger leads to generation of nuclear debris and apoptotic cells which activate the innate immune cells such as plasmacytoid dendritic cells, macrophages, and neutrophils through sensors such as TLRs leading to production of multiple cytokines such as interferon-α (IFN-α), TNF-α, and the B-cell maturation/survival factors [(BLys/B-cell activating factor (BAFF)] and increased NETosis. These factors interact with autoreactive T and B cells, which are resistant to apoptosis, have altered metabolic requirements, and sustain the autoimmune response in a positive feedback loop. Apart from various immune cells, the tissue resident cells such as basal cells of the dermis, synovial fibroblasts, mesangial cells, podocytes and tubular epithelium in kidney, and endothelial cells throughout the body also participate in the inflammatory process (**Fig. 1**). Generation of autoantibodies leads to formation of immune complexes (ICs) and these ICs activate complement cascade and immune cells to produce proinflammatory mediators leading to tissue injury.

PATHOLOGY

Immune complex deposition occurs in small blood vessels as well as in tissues. Skin biopsy in SLE shows IC deposition at the dermal–epidermal junction, the so-called "lupus band" test. In addition, injury to basal keratinocytes with hydropic degeneration and mixed inflammatory infiltrate are seen at the dermoepidermal junction, around blood vessels and dermal appendages. Clinically unaffected

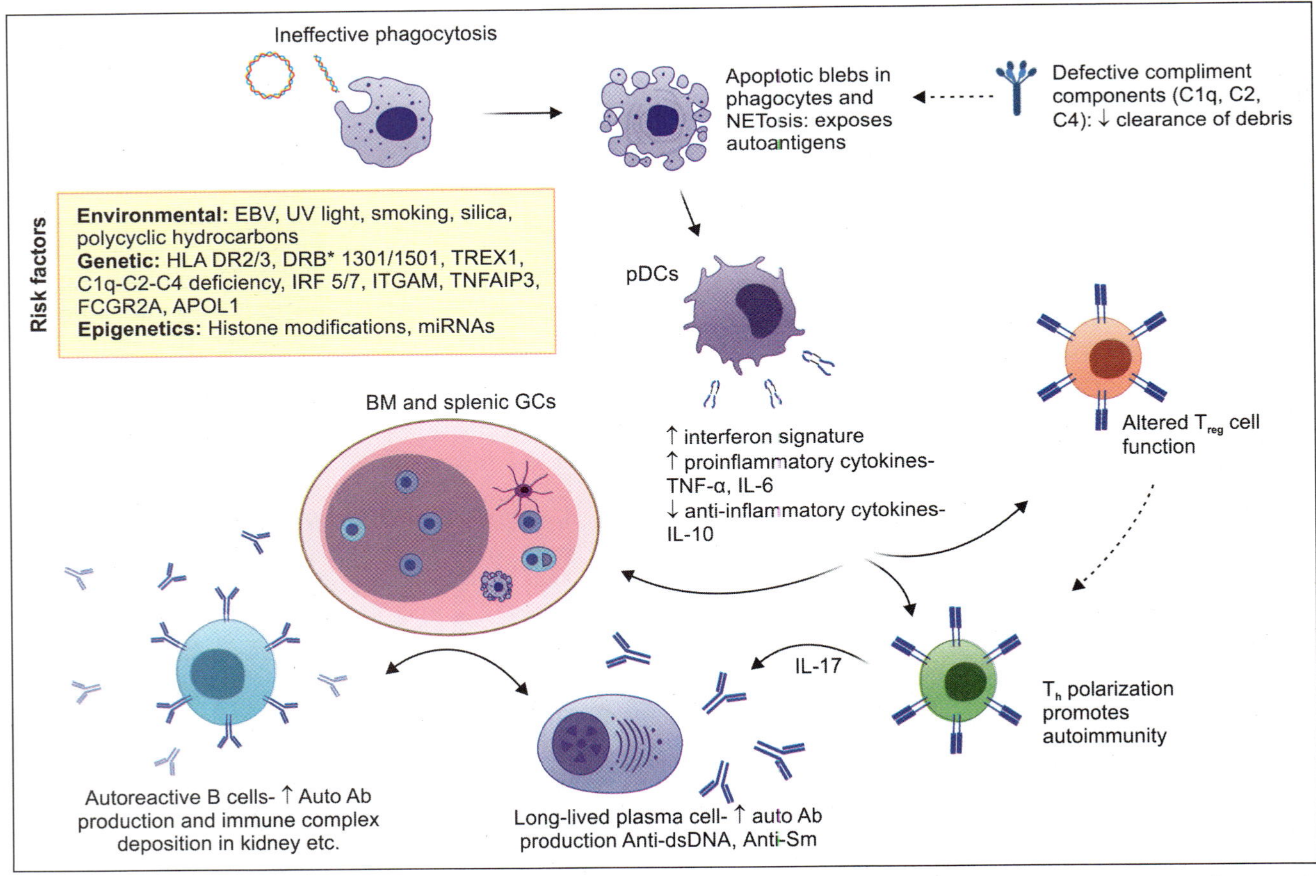

(Ab: antibody; dsDNA: double-stranded deoxyribonucleic acid; EBV: Epstein–Barr virus; GCs: germinal centers; IL-6: interleukin-6; pDCs: plasmacytoid dendritic cells; TNF-α: tumor necrosis factor-α)

FIGURE 1: Pathogenesis of lupus.

skin may also show IC deposition. Though these findings are not specific for cutaneous lupus, they are highly suggestive.

Kidney biopsy in patients with SLE helps both in diagnosis, treatment, and prognosis (**Figs. 2 A and B**). The International Society of Nephrology (ISN) and the Renal Pathology Society (RPS) classification is the most widely used (**Table 1**). This classification is focused on glomerular disease with less emphasis on tubulointerstitial and vascular compartments, although changes in tubulointerstitial compartment have also been associated with poor long-term prognosis and thus should be reported in detail.

Other tissues such as bowel, skin etc., may show features of leukocytoclastic vasculitis and mixed inflammatory infiltrate in the affected organ.

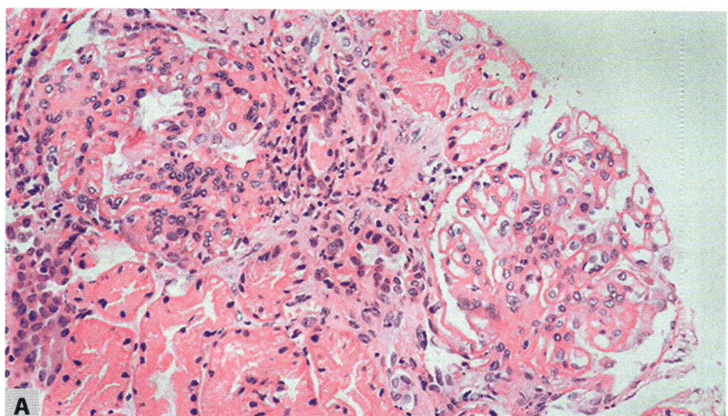

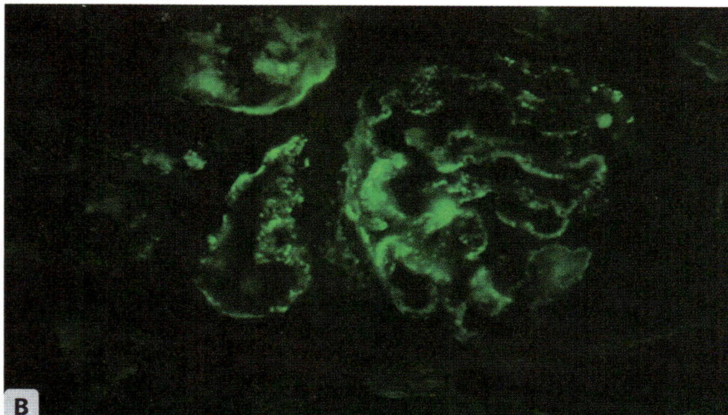

FIGURES 2 A & B: (A) Kidney biopsy showing diffuse proliferative glomerulonephritis with endocapillary proliferation in two glomeruli and; **(B)** Direct immunofluorescence shows immunoglobulin G (IgG) deposit in glomeruli and tubules.

TABLE 1 The ISN/RPS classification of lupus nephritis (modified 2018).

Class I: Minimal mesangial lupus nephritis

Normal glomeruli by light microscopy, but mesangial immune deposits by immunofluorescence

Class II: Mesangial proliferative lupus nephritis

Purely mesangial hypercellularity of any degree or mesangial matrix expansion by light microscopy, with mesangial immune deposits

Class III: Focal lupus nephritis

Active or inactive focal, segmental, or global endo- or extracapillary glomerulonephritis involving ≤50% of all glomeruli, typically with focal subendothelial immune deposits, with or without mesangial alterations

Class IV: Diffuse lupus nephritis

Active or inactive diffuse, segmental, or global endo- or extracapillary glomerulonephritis involving ≥50% of all glomeruli, typically with diffuse subendothelial immune deposits, with or without mesangial alterations

Class V: Membranous lupus nephritis

Global or segmental subepithelial immune deposits or their morphologic sequelae by light microscopy and by immunofluorescence or electron microscopy, with or without mesangial alterations. Class V lupus nephritis may occur in combination with class III or IV, in which case both will be diagnosed

Class VI: Advanced sclerotic lupus nephritis

≥90% of glomeruli globally sclerosed without residual activity

Modified National Institutes of Health (NIH) activity and chronicity index for severity and prognosis across all classes of lupus nephritis should be reported

Modified National Institutes of Health (NIH) activity and chronicity index

Activity index variables	Score
Endocapillary hypercellularity	0–3
Neutrophils/Karyorrhexis	0–3
Fibrinoid necrosis	0–3*
Hyaline deposits	0–3
Cellular/fibrocellular crescents	0–3*
Interstitial inflammation	0–3

Continued...

Continued...

Modified National Institutes of Health (NIH) activity and chronicity index	
Chronicity index variables	**Score**
Glomerular sclerosis	0–3
Fibrous crescents	0–3
Interstitial fibrosis	0–3
Tubular atrophy	0–3
0–3 is based on glomeruli involved. 1+ is <25% of glomeruli, 2+ is 25–50% of glomeruli, and 3+ is >50% of glomeruli.	
Total activity score is 24 and chronicity score is 12.	

*Multiplication factor of 2 is used.

(ISN: International Society of Nephrology; RPS: Renal Pathology Society)

DIAGNOSIS

Diagnosis of SLE is purely clinical, based on clinical findings and laboratory investigations including autoantibodies. The classification criteria over the years are meant to ensure homogeneous population of patients for research and clinical trials and should not be used in routine clinical practice.

The 1982 American College of Rheumatology (ACR) criteria, later modified in 1997, were in use for almost 4 decades worldwide and it had a high specificity (93%). In recent years, to pickup early cases and to improve sensitivity, the 2012 Systemic Lupus International Collaborating Clinics (SLICC) criteria were devised which require 4 of 17 points or presence of proliferative nephritis with ANA positivity for classifying a patient as SLE.

The proposed European League Against Rheumatism (EULAR)/ACR 2019 criteria have positive ANA as an entry criterion, weighted items within domains, and a common attribution rule of counting criteria for SLE only if there is no other likely alterative diagnosis (**Table 2**). The EULAR/ACR 2019 criteria have sensitivity similar to the SLICC criteria and specificity equal to that of the ACR criteria, but await external validation.

CLINICAL MANIFESTATIONS

The clinical presentation can be heterogeneous ranging from mild disease to life-threatening multisystemic involvement. Most patients have a relapsing-remitting course, with <1% of cases achieving long-term drug-free remission. Constitutional symptoms such as fever, fatigue, myalgia, and arthralgia are present in 90–95% of the patients at diagnosis and are often indicators of disease activity.

MUSCULOSKELETAL

Inflammatory symmetrical polyarthritis involving small joints of hands and feet, which is nondeforming and nonerosive, is seen in 60–70% of patients. Although rare erosive, deforming arthritis can be seen in nearly 10% of patients. Jaccoud's arthropathy with correctable deformities, avascular necrosis of femoral head, or other sites is seen rarely.

Though myalgias are common, significant muscle weakness involving proximal muscles with elevated muscle enzymes is seen in <10% of patients. The challenge is to differentiate from steroid-induced myopathy and rarely hydroxychloroquine and statin-induced myopathy.

SKIN

In SLE, skin involvement is seen invariably and can vary from alopecia to severe manifestation like toxic epidermal necrolysis. The skin manifestations can be grouped into lupus-specific and nonspecific types. The lupus-specific rashes include malar rash, generalized maculopapular rash, photosensitivity, diskoid lupus, subacute cutaneous lupus erythematosus (SCLE), and lupus profundus (LP). SCLE and LP are seen in <5% of patients. The nonspecific lesions include oral and nasal ulcers, Raynaud's phenomenon, nonscarring alopecia, bullous LE, palpable purpura, digital gangrene, nailfold infarcts etc. The most characteristic rash of lupus is malar rash. It is seen on cheeks and nasal bridge. It is erythematous, macular, and photosensitive and usually spares the nasolabial fold.

RENAL

Nephritis, seen in about 60–70% of patients with SLE during the course of disease, is one of the leading factors for poor outcome in SLE. The renal involvement can vary from asymptomatic urinary abnormalities to rapidly progressive renal failure. Thus, all patients should have a urine examination with 24-hour proteinuria estimation at diagnosis and simple urine examination on regular follow-up. Early renal biopsy has been shown to improve outcome, as it helps in planning treatment and knowing prognosis.

Patients with proliferative nephritis (ISN III and IV) usually have active urinary sediment [microscopic hematuria, leukocyturia, and red blood cell (RBC) cast] and proteinuria (>500 mg/24 h); approximately one-half develops nephrotic syndrome and most develop hypertension. Approximately, 15–20% of SLE patients with proteinuria (usually nephrotic) have pure membranous nephropathy. Apart from glomerulonephritis, tubulointerstitial disease, associated APS nephropathy, and lupus podocytopathy should be considered in a patient of SLE with renal disease with a normal glomerular histology.

TABLE 2 Different classification criteria for SLE.

ACR 1982	ACR 1997 modification	SLICC 2012	EULAR/ACR 2019
Cutaneous: • Malar rash • Diskoid rash		• Acute cutaneous or • SCLE • Chronic cutaneous	• Acute cutaneous-6 • SCLE-4 • Diskoid-4
Photosensitivity			
Oral ulcer		• Oral or nasal ulcer • Nonscarring alopecia	• Oral ulcer-2 • Nonscarring alopecia-2
Arthritis		Synovitis	Joint involvement-6
Serositis: • Pleuritis • Pericarditis		• Pleuritis or • Pericarditis	• Effusion-5 • Acute pericarditis-6
Renal: • Persistent proteinuria • Cellular casts		• Proteinuria or • RBC casts • Histology compatible with lupus nephritis	• Proteinuria-4 • ISN/RPS II/V-8 • ISN/RPS III/IV-10
Neurologic: • Seizures • Psychosis		Seizures, psychosis, acute confusional state, myelitis, mononeuritis multiplex, and peripheral or cranial neuropathy	• Seizures-5 • Psychosis-3 • Delirium-2
Hematologic: • Hemolytic anemia • Leukopenia • Lymphopenia • Thrombocytopenia		Hemolytic anemia • Leukopenia or lymphopenia • Thrombocytopenia	• Coombs positive hemolytic anemia-3 • Leukopenia-3 • Thrombocytopenia-4
Immunological disorder/ Autoantibodies • LE cell preparation • Anti-DNA • Anti-Sm • False-positive syphilis serology • ANA	• Anti-DNA • Anti-Sm • Antiphospholipid • ANA	• Anti-dsDNA • Anti-Sm • Antiphospholipid • Low complements • Coombs positive without hemolytic anemia • ANA	• Anti-dsDNA-6 • Anti-Sm-6 • Antiphospholipid-2 • Low complement • C3 or C4 low-3 • C3 and C4 low-4 • Entry criteria ANA
Fever-2 (New addition)			

(ACR: American College of Rheumatology; EULAR: European League Against Rheumatism; ISN: International Society of Nephrology; RPS: Renal Pathology Society; SCLE: subacute cutaneous lupus erythematosus; SLICC: Systemic Lupus International Collaborating Clinics)

Lupus nephritis tends to be an ongoing disease, with flares requiring retreatment or increased treatment over many years. If diffuse proliferative glomerulonephritis (DPGN) is inadequately treated, virtually all patients develop end-stage renal disease (ESRD) within 2 years of diagnosis. Therefore, early and effective IS treatment is usually indicated in these cases. For most people with lupus nephritis, apart from IS therapies, attention must be given to control of systemic inflammation, blood pressure, hyperlipidemia, and hyperglycemia as these increase risk of accelerated atherosclerosis. Despite the advances in treatment, about 20% of patients with lupus nephritis develop ESRD within 10 years of diagnosis.

NEUROLOGICAL

Systemic lupus erythematosus can affect any part of the nervous system including central and peripheral nervous system. In case of CNS involvement, a distinction needs to be made whether the clinical features are caused by a diffuse process (requiring immunosuppression) or a focal process due to vascular occlusion (requiring anticoagulation). Seizures of any type may be caused by lupus; treatment often requires both antiseizure and IS therapies, but whether to treat patients with a single seizure with no structural brain lesion is still debatable. Psychosis seen in 10–20% of patients often requires aggressive IS treatment along with antipsychotic treatment. It must be distinguished from glucocorticoid-induced psychosis as treatment of the two conditions is diagonally opposite. Vascular event leading to stroke or transient ischemic attack (TIA) can be seen in about 10% of patients with SLE; the most common cause is vasculopathy followed by vasculitis and embolization from carotid plaque or Libman–Sacks endocarditis. Most patients are treated with antiplatelet agents. In addition, anticoagulants are beneficial in patients with APS.

Cognitive dysfunction with difficulties with memory and reasoning, severe headaches, and nonresponsive to nonsteroidal anti-inflammatory drugs (NSAIDs) are also commonly seen. Aseptic meningitis and myelopathy are rare manifestations, which respond to high-dose IS therapy. Peripheral neuropathy and mononeuritis multiplex may be seen in about 5% of cases.

CARDIAC

All three layers of the heart can be involved in SLE with pericarditis being the most common manifestation and has a prevalence of 20–30%. Rarely, pericardial disease can lead to cardiac tamponade. Myocarditis usually presents with heart failure and tachycardia and occurs during active disease. Endocarditis can lead to mitral and aortic insufficiency as well as vegetations, which can cause embolic phenomenon. Myocardial infarction due to accelerated atherosclerosis is a common cause of late mortality in SLE.

PULMONARY

Pleurisy with or without pleural effusion is seen in about 30–50% of cases and usually responds to NSAIDs or IS treatment. Interstitial lung disease, diffuse alveolar hemorrhage, pulmonary arterial hypertension, and shrinking lung syndrome are all rare manifestations that often require aggressive IS therapy.

HEMATOLOGICAL

Anemia is the most common hematological manifestations, with anemia of chronic disease being the most important cause in 70% of cases. Nutritional deficiencies and autoimmune hemolytic anemia are other causes of cases. Lymphopenia is seen in about 50% of patients but by itself, it neither increases the risk of infection nor requires specific treatment, although its presence can be a clue to diagnosis of lupus. Thrombocytopenia is seen in about 15–20% of patients; however, bleeding is seen in <5% of patients. It can be recurrent and sometime difficult to manage. Lymphadenopathy, usually due to lymphoid hyperplasia and splenomegaly, can be seen in 10–15% of cases.

GASTROINTESTINAL

Diffuse abdominal pain caused by peritonitis, intestinal vasculitis, or acute pancreatitis can be life-threatening, if not managed timely with IS treatment and supportive care. Nausea, sometimes with vomiting, and diarrhea can be manifestations of lupus in up to 20% of cases. Lupoid hepatitis and autoimmune hepatitis have similar clinical presentation with elevated serum transaminases with or without jaundice but have subtle histologic differences. Both respond dramatically to immunosuppression. Gastrointestinal vasculitis can present with perforation, abdominal pain, bleeding, or distension.

OCULAR

Sicca syndrome and nonspecific conjunctivitis are common ocular symptoms seen in 10–15% of cases of SLE. In contrast, retinal vasculitis and optic neuritis are serious manifestations: Blindness can develop over days to weeks. Screening for cataracts, glaucoma, and visual field defects in patients on long-term steroids and hydroxychloroquine needs to done as per the accepted guidelines.

LABORATORY INVESTIGATIONS

Laboratory tests serve three primary purposes: (1) to establish the diagnosis, (2) to assess disease activity or organ damage, and (3) to identify adverse effects to drugs.

Screening tests include complete blood count, renal and liver function tests, urinalysis, and chest X-ray; these may detect abnormalities that contribute to the diagnosis and influence management decisions. *ANA by indirect immunofluorescence* is a screening test for SLE with 98% sensitivity (**Figs. 3 A** and **B**). If ANA comes negative, either an alternative diagnosis should be considered or the test should be repeated to exclude laboratory error. If ANA is still negative and clinical suspicion is high, then test for anti-Ro antibodies should be done. *Antibodies to dsDNA* are specific for SLE and can be seen in about two-thirds of patients. Other antibodies such as *antibodies to Sm, Ro, ribosomal P, and gamut* of other antibodies can be detected using line immunoassays or enzyme-linked immunosorbent assay (ELISA). But apart from established pathogenic role of anti-Ro antibodies in congenital heart block and neonatal lupus, other antibodies only support the diagnosis with an uncertain pathogenic role. Complement C3 and C4 levels and anti-dsDNA antibody level reflect disease activity and are, thus, useful in follow-up.

The levels of complement degradation products such as C3d and C4d, type I IFN signature in blood, urinary levels of neutrophil gelatinase-associated lipocalin-1, monocyte chemoattractant protein, TNF-like weak inducer of apoptosis (TWEAK), and host of other serum and urinary biomarkers are being investigated, but none has yet reached the clinic.

DISEASE ACTIVITY

Since SLE is a relapsing-remitting disease, measurement of disease activity is important at each visit to decide therapy. Several composite scores have been proposed for assessment of disease activity in lupus. The SLEDAI (Systemic Lupus Erythematosus Disease Activity Index) is a weighted score with 24 items and maximum possible score of 105. It is the most commonly used score. In resource-

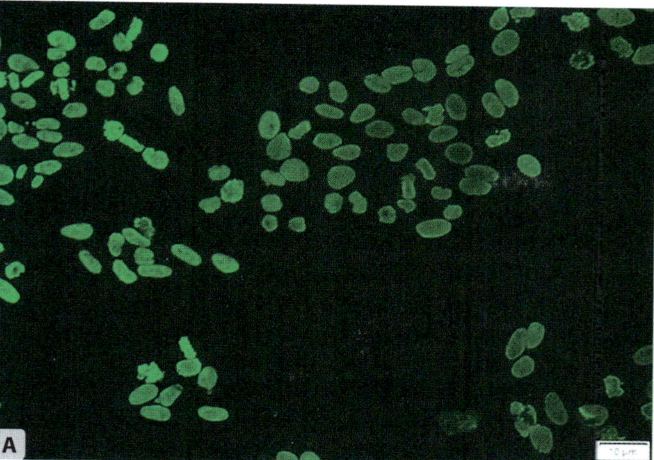

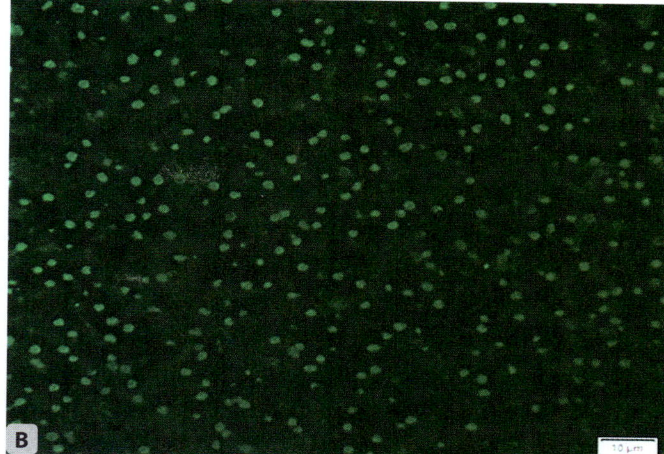

FIGURES 3 A & B: Antinuclear antibody using indirect immunofluorescence assay. Homogeneous pattern as seen on human epithelial type 2 (HEp-2) cells and liver substrate.

poor countries, MEX-SLEDAI that does not require laboratory parameters may be useful. The British Isles Lupus Assessment Group (BILAG) is a more extensive score accounting for organ involvement in a graded manner. The SLICC-ACR damage index is used to score irreversible organ damage due to disease or therapy. All these disease activity measure requires training for proper scoring and interpretation and anyone of them can be followed in day-to-day practice depending on the resources available.

TREATMENT

With no curative treatment and sustained remission difficult to achieve, therapy must be individualized by taking disease-specific and patient-specific aspects into consideration. The ultimate aim of therapy is to have low disease activity, prevent damage accrual, and have good quality of life with minimum drug toxicity. Studies have shown that more time the patient spends in low disease activity, the better is the long-term prognosis.

MINOR ORGAN DISEASE

Patients with predominant musculoskeletal involvement can be managed with *NSAIDs and antimalarials.* Antimalarials (hydroxychloroquine, chloroquine, and quinacrine) have proven beneficial role in reduction of number of flares, improving long-term prognosis, and having host of other beneficial metabolic effects. Although recent recommendations are for a judicious use of these drugs with dosage not to exceed 5 mg/kg/day with regular screening for visual field defects, there are studies that suggest that higher blood levels decrease the flare rates. A placebo-controlled prospective trial suggests that administration of *dehydroepiandrosterone* may reduce disease activity. If quality of life is unacceptable, despite these conservative measures, treatment with *low doses of systemic glucocorticoids* may be necessary.

Lupus-related skin disease should be managed with photoprotection, topical sunscreens, antimalarials, topical glucocorticoids, and/or tacrolimus. Simple measures such as full sleeve clothing, use of umbrella, and use of induction heater can help in photoprotection. If it is severe or unresponsive, *second-line agents* such as systemic glucocorticoids with or without *methotrexate, mycophenolate mofetil, azathioprine, or biologics* such as B-cell-depleting therapies may be considered. Belimumab may be considered in those with refractory disease, especially those with high disease activity, positive anti-dsDNA antibody, and low serum complement.

LUPUS NEPHRITIS

Therapy for proliferative nephritis is divided into induction and maintenance therapy. Steroids along with IS agents are the mainstay of therapy in proliferative lupus nephritis; glucocorticoids (0.5–1 mg/kg/day orally) or 500–1,000 mg of methylprednisolone and sodium succinate intravenous (IV) daily for 3 days followed by 0.5–1 mg/kg of daily prednisone or equivalent are the drug of choice.

Immunosuppressive agents such as cyclophosphamide (an alkylating agent) *or mycophenolate mofetil* (a relatively lymphocyte-specific inhibitor of inosine monophosphates) is part of the induction therapy. Cyclophosphamide is cost-effective, has better compliance, and is probably more effective in patients with crescentic glomerulonephritis or patients with high chronicity score on kidney biopsy. On the other hand, mycophenolate mofetil is an oral drug, thus has ease of administration, has similar efficacy to cyclophosphamide, and works better in Afro-Americans. Regarding toxicity, diarrhea is more common with mycophenolate mofetil; amenorrhea, leukopenia, and nausea are more common with high-dose cyclophosphamide. Importantly, rates of severe infections and death are similar with both agents. Two different regimens of IV cyclophosphamide are available. The low-dose cyclophosphamide (500 mg every 2 weeks for six total doses) followed by azathioprine or mycophenolate mofetil maintenance is as effective as standard high-doses cyclophosphamide (750 mg/m^2 monthly for 6 months) even at end of 10-year follow-up.

Calcineurin inhibitors (CNIs) such as tacrolimus has very good antiproteinuria effect, thus can be used in patients with membranous nephropathy. Newer CNIs such as voclosporin in combination with mycophenolate mofetil and rituximab or belimumab in combination with mycophenolate mofetil are being evaluated as alternate induction therapies, with a few studies showing favorable results. Response to therapy can take 6–9 months for complete response.

With the known adverse effects of steroids (e.g., infection, hyperglycemia, hypertension, osteoporosis), efforts are being made to reduce the duration of exposure, studies with frequent pulse steroids (125 mg with IV cyclosporin) and rapid taper of oral steroids in 4–6 weeks have shown comparative results with less adverse events. RITUXILUP, a trial evaluating combination of rituximab and mycophenolate mofetil with no steroids after induction pulse, uses a similar strategy with excellent remission rate.

For maintenance therapy, long-term follow-up studies have shown similar efficacy for mycophenolate mofetil and azathioprine with similar rates of progression to ESRD and toxicity. In addition to IS treatment, strict control of blood pressure, treatment of other comorbidities is important in the long-term management. Target of proteinuria < 0.5 g/day at 12 months of therapy has been associated with improved survival and maintenance therapy should be continued up to 3–5 years after complete remission.

EXTRARENAL SEVERE DISEASE

Glucocorticoids, at high dose, as in nephritis, are the mainstay of therapy; the evidence for use of IS agents is scarce, though they are often used for their steroid-sparing effect. Cyclophosphamide, mycophenolate mofetil, azathioprine, and rituximab can be used. Despite the failure of two randomized controlled trial of rituximab, several registry data showing real-world evidence support its use in organ-threatening disease. IV immunoglobulin and plasma exchange can be considered in specific circumstances such as diffuse alveolar hemorrhage, thrombotic thrombocytopenic purpura (TTP), disease activity in presence of infection etc.

NEWER DRUGS

Drugs targeting the interferon pathway (anifrolumab, sifalimumab, and rontalizumab) or drugs targeting the downstream signaling pathways (tofacitinib and baricitinib) are in various stages of development. The recent trials with anifrolumab showing promise in treatment of nonorgan-threatening disease have created a hope. Other targets are interferon-12 (IL-12)/IL-23 and IL-17 pathway, B cells, plasma cells, plasmacytoid dendritic cells, intermediary signaling molecules, and metabolic regulators such as metformin and rapamycin (mTOR inhibitor) are in the pipeline (**Fig. 4**) with a few showing promising results in

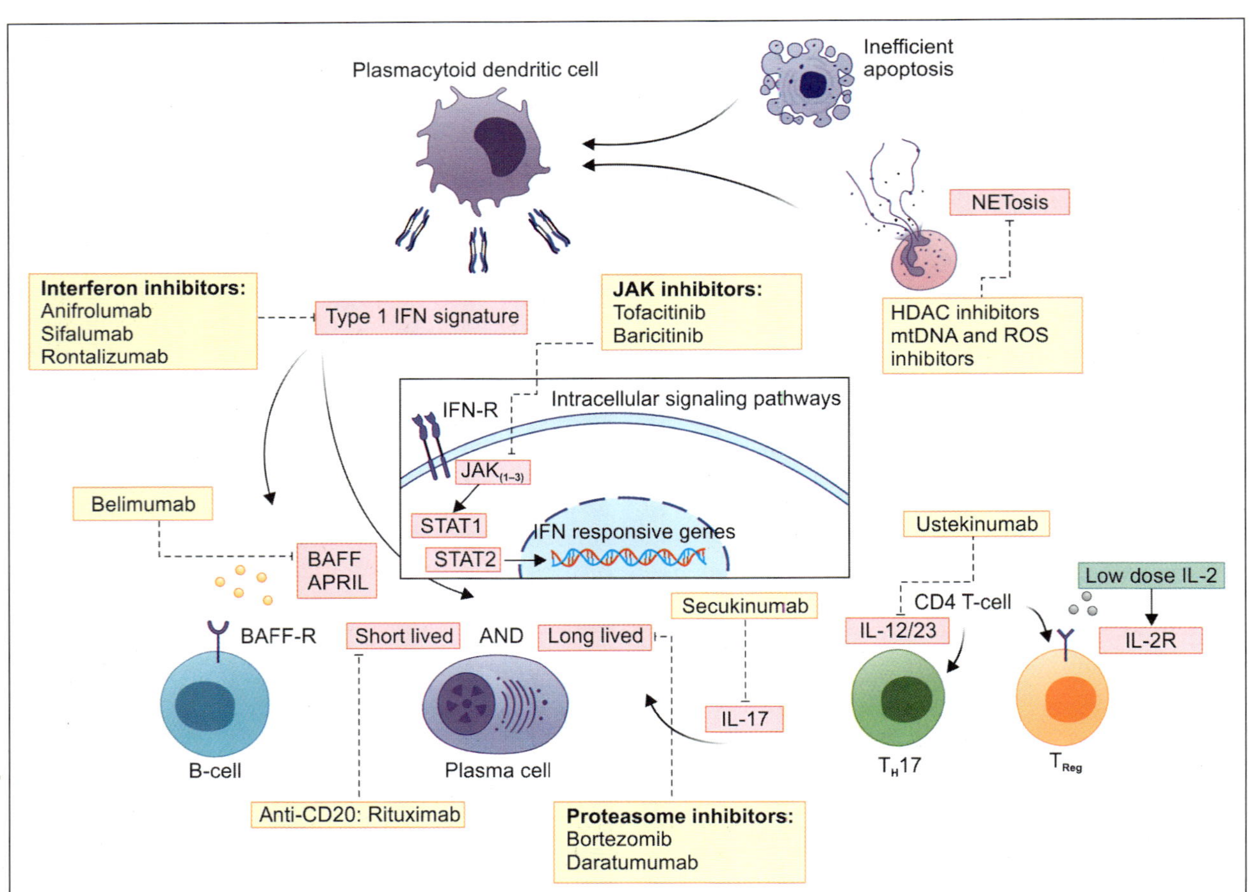

(HDAC: histone deacetylase; IFN: interferon; IL-2: interleukin 2; JAK: Janus kinase; ROS: reactive oxygen species)

FIGURE 4: Newer drug targets in SLE.

human trials. Lack of uniform disease activity measures, composite endpoints, heterogeneous clinical presentation, and ethical issues of not treating sick patients with standard of care make designing of clinical trials a daunting task.

In addition to IS agents, various preventive strategies such as vaccination against influenza, pneumococcus, and human papillomavirus (HPV), co-trimoxazole prophylaxis in those on high-dose corticosteroids, or cytotoxic therapies also improve outcome in patients with SLE. Screening for and appropriate treatment for osteoporosis and other comorbidities are essential to prevent long-term complications. As therapies have improved survival, screening for malignancies and atherosclerosis needs to be integrated into management. Addressing sociocultural issues related to patient, especially in developing countries, remains a challenge such as marriage, planning for pregnancy etc. Continuous patient counseling goes a long way in improving adherence to therapy, regular follow-up, planning of career, marriage, pregnancy, and ultimately, the long-term outcome.

PROGNOSIS

With increasing awareness, early diagnosis, and development in therapeutics, a 5-year and 10-year survival in lupus has increased over last three decades from 70 to 95% and 60 to 90%, respectively. Infections and high disease activity still are the two important causes of early deaths, while cardiovascular disease is an important cause of late death.

RECOMMENDED READINGS

1. Wallace DJ, Weismann MH. Clinical features of systemic lupus erythematosus. In: Hochberg MC, Gravallese EM, Silman AJ, Smolen JS, Weinblatt ME, Weisman MH (Eds). Rheumatology, 7th edition. Philadelphia: Elsevier; 2019. pp. 1103-15.
2. Bajema IM, Wilhelmus S, Alpers CE, Bruijn JA, Colvin RB, Cook H, et al. Revision of the International Society of Nephrology/Renal Pathology Society classification for lupus nephritis: clarification of definitions and modified National Institutes of Health activity and chronicity indices. Kidney Int. 2018;93:789-96.
3. Aringer M, Leuchten N, Johnson SR. New criteria for systemic lupus erythematosus. Curr Rheumatol Rep. 2020;22:18.
4. Dorner T, Furie R. Novel paradigms in systemic lupus erythematosus. Lancet. 2019;393:2344-58.
5. Tsokos GC. Systemic lupus erythematosus. N Engl J Med. 2011;365:2110-21.
6. Fanouriakis A, Kostopoulou M, Alunno A, Aringer M, Bajema I, Boletis AM, et al. 2019 update of the EULAR recommendations for the management of systemic lupus erythematosus. Ann Rheum Dis. 2019;78:736-45.
7. Porta S, Danza A, Saavedra MA, Carlomagno A, Goizueta MC, Vivero F, et al. Glucocorticoids in *Systemic Lupus Erythematosus*. Ten Questions and Some Issues. J Clin Med. 2020;9:2709.
8. Marder W. Update on pregnancy complications in systemic lupus erythematosus. Curr Opin Rheumatol. 2019;31:650-8.
9. Mosca M, Tani C, Aringer M, Bombardieri S, Boumpas D, Brey R, et al. European League Against Rheumatism recommendations for monitoring patients with systemic lupus erythematosus in clinical practice and in observational studies. Ann Rheum Dis. 2010;69:1269-74.
10. Lee YH, Choi SJ, Ji JD, Song GG. Overall and cause-specific mortality in systemic lupus erythematosus: an updated meta-analysis. Lupus. 2016;25:727-34.

CHAPTER 235

Antiphospholipid Syndrome

Sreejitha KS, Liza Rajasekhar

ABSTRACT

Antiphospholipid syndrome (APS) is an acquired autoimmune disease that manifests clinically as recurrent venous or arterial thrombosis and/or pregnancy loss, and serologically as antiphospholipid antibodies (aPLs). The aPL include anticardiolipin antibodies, anti-beta-2 glycoprotein I (anti-β2GPI) antibodies, and lupus anticoagulant (LAC). Thrombotic APS is treated by low-molecular-weight heparin (LMWH) and vitamin K antagonists. Low-dose aspirin (LDA) and heparin constitute the current standard of care for obstetric APS (OAPS).

"The biggest room in the world is the room for improvement."

—Helmut Schmidt

INTRODUCTION

The APS is an acquired immune prothrombotic state manifesting clinically with thrombosis and/or pregnancy morbidity and distinguished by the presence of antibodies commonly referred to as aPLs.

HISTORY

Syphilis, an important public health problem at the turn of the last century, led to screening of United States (US) army personnel and the general population with serologic assays developed for this purpose. Tissue from the hearts of neonates who had died of congenital syphilis and later tissue from beef cardiac muscle was used for the purpose. The antigen identified as cardiolipin, present on inner mitochondrial membrane, was purified and led to standardization of assays. Identification of false positive assays in the normal population and in infections was followed by reports of high prevalence in lupus patients. Subsequently case reports of lupus patients who presented with bleeding tendencies venous thrombosis and the association with pregnancy morbidity led to the association between these manifestations and the presence of the anticardiolipin antibodies being built up.

The term *lupus anticoagulant* came about to celebrate the association of bleeding tendencies in lupus patients with a factor which prolonged clotting times. The presence of thrombosis in such patients may not have received enough thought during the naming of the assay; however, the association of thrombosis, presence of LAC, and false positive tests for syphilis in a cohort of lupus led to syndrome being named antiphospholipid syndrome. Patients with no features of an underlying connective tissue disease (CTD) were labeled primary APS (PAPS) while those with features of CTDs usually systemic lupus erythematosus (SLE) were called secondary APS. In fact the first case series of APS was described in SLE patients. Even though a dichotomous distinction into PAPS and secondary APS is made emerging data suggests that PAPS and SLE with APS form part of the same spectrum of disease (Shoenfeld Y, 2009).

CLINICAL MANIFESTATIONS

Thrombosis, the defining feature of the aPL syndrome, can affect vessels of all sizes. Venous thrombosis is commoner than arterial thrombosis. Deep venous thrombosis (DVT), stroke, pulmonary embolism, superficial thrombophlebitis, and transient ischemic attacks are seen in decreasing order of frequency. DVT is the most frequently reported venous thrombotic event and cerebrovascular accidents are the most common arterial events.

Obstetric APS refers to women with only obstetric aPL-related complaints and no history of past or current thrombotic events at the time of diagnosis. Recurrent miscarriages, fetal losses, and stillbirths are the most common obstetric complications. Preeclampsia, eclampsia, and abruptio placentae are more common in pregnant patients with APS. An increasing awareness is there on infertility in APS patients.

Patients with *APS associated with SLE* have more episodes of arthritis, livedo reticularis (LR), thrombocytopenia, and leukopenia. Males with APS have more frequent myocardial infarction, epilepsy, and lower extremities arterial thrombosis and a later age of onset. Childhood onset APS patients tend to have more episodes of chorea and jugular vein thrombosis.

Livedo reticularis, a common cutaneous manifestation of APS, is characterized by transient or persistent, blotchy, reddish blue to purple, net-like cyanotic pattern on the skin and is a manifestation of disturbed cutaneous blood flow. A livid conical discoloration which is symmetric, irreversible, and composed of "broken" circular segments in a more generalized distribution is called livedo racemosa.

Noncriteria manifestations: Many manifestations came to be recognized in higher frequency in the patients with APS. Over time these came to be known as noncriteria manifestations.

They could be classified into obstetric and nonobstetric and are listed in **Table 1**.

Antiphospholipid syndrome nephropathy is associated with hypertension, uremia, occasional proteinuria, and focal cortical atrophy on imaging.

TABLE 1 Obstetric and nonobstetric criteria for APS.

Major	Minor
Nonobstetric	
• APS nephropathy • Heart valve disease • Livedo reticularis • Thrombocytopenia • Chorea • Longitudinal myelitis • Superficial vein thrombosis	• Amaurosis fugax • Brain MRI white matter lesions • Cognitive impairment • Coombs test positivity • Hemolytic anemia • Ischemic necrosis of bone • Migraine • Pseudomultiple sclerosis • Pulmonary hypertension • Raynaud's phenomenon • Seizures • Sensorineural hearing loss • Skin ulcers • Splinter hemorrhages
Obstetric	
• Late IUGR (after 34 weeks) • Late preeclampsia (after 34 weeks) • Placental abruption/ hematoma • Preterm birth (>34 to <37 weeks)	• Puerperal preeclampsia • Two or more unexplained in vitro fertilization failures • Two unexplained spontaneous abortions <10 weeks

(APS: antiphospholipid syndrome; MRI: magnetic resonance imaging; IUGR: intrauterine growth restriction)

CLASSIFICATION CRITERIA

Over time classification criteria were proposed to populate research cohorts with homogenous groups and to incorporate the transient nature of the antibodies already demonstrated in conditions as diverse as malaria. The original classification criteria were proposed by Sapporo and they were followed by the Sydney modification. The current classification criteria are referred to as the Miyakis criteria. A patient has to fulfill at least one clinical criterion and at least one laboratory criterion.

CLINICAL CRITERIA

Clinical criteria listed include:

Vascular thrombosis: One or more clinical episode of arterial, venous or small vessel thrombosis. To increase the specificity of the classification criteria it was deemed necessary to demonstrate thrombosis objectively and without inflammation of the vessel wall if there was histopathological confirmation.

Pregnancy morbidity: One or more unexplained death of a morphologically normal fetus ≥10 weeks of gestation; three or more ≥3 unexplained consecutive miscarriages at <10 weeks of gestation, with maternal and paternal factors (such as anatomical, hormonal, or chromosomal abnormalities) excluded or one or more premature delivery of a morphologically normal fetus <34 weeks gestation because of severe preeclampsia or eclampsia or recognized features of placental insufficiency.

LABORATORY CRITERIA

Laboratory criteria include: The detection of aPLs on at least two occasions 12 weeks apart and within 5 years of clinical manifestations. These could be one or more of either LAC in plasma or the immunoglobulin G (IgG) or IgM isotypes in medium to high titer of anticardiolipin antibodies [>40 IgG phospholipid (GPL) or IgM phospholipid (MPL), or >99th percentile] or anti-β2GPI antibodies (>99th percentile). The GPL and MPL are arbitrary units with 1 GPL or MPL referring to 1 µg of IgG or IgM antibody.

It was realized that many patients with clinical manifestation highly suggestive of APS did not meet the laboratory criteria. Research identified many other antigens to which antibodies could be identified in these patients. These included IgA anti-β2GPI and anticardiolipin (aCL) antibodies, and those against annexin A5, prothrombin, phosphatidylserine/prothrombin, phosphatidylethanolamine, phosphatidic acid, phosphatidylserine, phosphatidylinositol, and vimentin/cardiolipin complex. However, these are still not widely available. These are now being referred to as noncriteria laboratory tests.

Using this understanding there has been a recent attempt to classify patients with APS into following groups:

Seronegative APS (SN-APS): Patients with clinical manifestations fulfilling APS classification criteria, plus "noncriteria" manifestations with persistently negative aPL (at least two determinations 12 weeks apart) with exclusion of other thrombophilias that might justify the clinical presentation.

Clinical noncriteria APS: Patients with "noncriteria" manifestations–at least one obstetric or one major nonobstetric or two minor nonobstetric along with APS laboratory criteria.

Incomplete laboratory APS: Individuals with clinical manifestations fulfilling APS classification criteria, plus two or more determinations of aCL between the 95th and 99th percentiles (or below 40 GPL or MPL) and/or anti-β2GPI antibodies between the 95th and 99th percentiles.

Laboratory noncriteria APS: Patients with APS clinical criteria manifestations, negative or low titer laboratory criteria aPL, plus positive "noncriteria" aPL testing.

Vascular and obstetric APS: The clinical course of patients with PAPS tends to be stable over time with the occurrence of vascular events being infrequent in patients with pregnancy morbidity and vice versa. This has led to the terms of thrombotic and obstetric APS being coined.

Catastrophic APS (CAPS): A subset of the APS was reported in 1980s, the CAPS. This described a particularly devastating accelerated form of APS resulting in multiorgan failure characterized by clinical evidence of multiple organ involvement over a very short period of time accompanied by histopathological evidence of multiple small vessel occlusion with laboratory confirmation of aPLs often in high titer. Occurring in fewer than 1% of the APS cases the event is believed to be triggered by a precipitating factor like infection, surgical procedure, neoplasm, suboptimal anticoagulation, or its withdrawal, as an obstetric complication, during a lupus flare or by the use of oral contraceptives.

In patients who did not meet all the above criteria, probable CAPS could be considered in situations with only two organs targeted, or if small vessel occlusion could not be confirmed by histopathology or if the third event developed in more than a week but less than a month despite anticoagulation, or if a patient with positive aPL at the onset of the catastrophic APS could not have confirmed tests 6 weeks apart due to early death.

PATHOGENESIS

The role of β2GPI antigen: The discovery that (β2GPI), a member of the complement control family, was the target for antibody binding rather than phospholipid itself shifted the focus of laboratory testing to identify β2GPI-dependent aPLs. They are currently considered the main pathogenic autoantibodies of APS. In the fluid phase, β2GPI which is made of five domains has a circular conformation in which Domain 1 (D1) is bound to Domain 5 (D5) which blocks interaction of D1 with aPL. Membrane bound β2GPI has an exposed D1.

Differential expression of membrane bound β2GPI with higher concentrations present in decidual endothelial cells, syncytiotrophoblasts, and extravillous trophoblasts has been noted and may explain the clinical differences obstetric and vascular APS (Meroni P, 2018).

THROMBOTIC ANTIPHOSPHOLIPID SYNDROME

Normal endothelial cells lack bound β2GPI. Perturbed endothelial cells have membrane bound β2GPI critical for the formation of endovascular thrombi and providing the "first hit" in the pathogenesis of APS. A "second hit" like infection, mechanical trauma, or venous stasis may then trigger clot formation in thrombotic APS. β2GPI and its antibody binding lead to activation of platelets, endothelial cells, monocytes, and via toll-like receptor-2 (TLR2), LPR8, annexin A2, and activation of their intracellular signal transduction pathway, result in increased expression of tissue factor (TF) which is a procoagulant.

OBSTETRIC ANTIPHOSPHOLIPID SYNDROME

Obstetric APS can be initiated by a much lower concentration of aPLs and does not need a second hit, probably due to the high concentrations of β2GPI on the trophoblast and decidual endothelial cells. The finding of ischemic infarction of villi from thrombotic occlusions, though common is not specific to OAPS. Nonthrombotic mechanisms like impaired spiral artery remodeling may have a role in inducing defective placentation.

Inflammation almost undetectable in vascular APS has been documented in animal models of aPL-mediated fetal loss. This inflammatory response might interfere with the initial stages of implantation leading to early miscarriage.

TISSUE FACTOR

Increased TF mRNA (messenger ribonucleuc acid) expression and activity is seen in endothelial cells and monocytes treated with β2GP1 antibodies derived from patients. This combined with elevated plasma levels of vascular permeability factor/vascular endothelial growth factor (VPF/VEGF) leads to thrombosis.

ROLE OF COMPLEMENT

Hypocomplementemia is frequently found in patients with PAPS. There are associated high serum C3a and C4a levels which along with low C3 point to complement activation rather than complement deficiency. The factor H or factor I levels are not reduced, indicating that complement activation was not caused by their deficiency rather through enhanced immune complex formation. This immune complex formation might have a bearing on the anticoagulant potential of aPL, given the positive correlation between strong LAC and hypocomplementemia.

LABORATORY TESTS

The prevalence of aPLs in the general population ranges between 1% and 5% and increases with age. In those with a history of thrombosis prevalence of approximately 13% has been reported in individuals with stroke, 11% in those with myocardial infarction, and 9.5% with deep vein thrombosis.

Three conventional tests are employed for the detection of aPLs: Enzyme-linked immunosorbent assays (ELISAs) that measure aCL and anti-β2GPI and a functional clotting assay for LAC. The ELISAs measure IgG and IgM aPL, while the LAC test, being a functional assay, does not discriminate between antibody isotypes. IgG aPLs are present in a higher proportion of patients with APS than IgM or IgA antibodies and only IgG antibodies are associated with LAC positivity. Anti-β2GPI assays showed the best discrimination between APS and non-APS.

The ELISA for detection of β2GPI antibodies was conceived and developed by Balestrieri et al. in 1995.

LA assay: The LAC assay is considered positive for the presence of thrombotic antibodies if the following caveats are met:

- Prolongation of a PL-based clotting test, e.g., the activated partial thromboplastin time, prothrombin time, dilute Russell's viper venom test (dRVVT), and Kaolin clotting time.
- Confirmation of an inhibitor-like pattern in the clotting test by normalization of tests with normal sera.
- Confirmation of PL dependence in coagulation tests demonstrated by normalizing of prolonged clotting tests by addition of platelets which provide phospholipids, and
- Exclusion of a specific factor inhibitor.

Lupus-sensitive activated partial thromboplastin time and a dilute Russell's viper venom (which can spontaneously activate Factor Xa) time are used as screening tests (Marlar RA, 2008).

Proposed new tests include assays that measure IgA aPL and autoantibodies against domain I of β2GPI (DI). IgG, IgM, and IgA anti-DI (aDI) assays showed excellent specificity and with the exception of IgG aDI similar sensitivity for APS compared to anti-β2GPI. The presence of aDI increased the hazard ratio for APS by approximately 3–5-fold across all isotypes with the highest risk coming from presence of the IgA isotype. Also, positivity for IgG or IgA aDI increased the strength of association between aCL/anti-β2GPI and thrombotic manifestations. Hence DI could potentially be a more reliable source of antigen compared to whole β2GPI as the latter might depend on its conformation.

Importance of LAC as prognostic test for thrombosis: The risk for adverse pregnancy outcomes in patients with persistent positivity for LAC is extremely high. In addition to the high rate of fetal complications, mothers also frequently experienced severe and life-threatening pregnancy complications. The presence of LAC is a stronger thrombotic risk factor than either β2GPI or aCL with an odds ratio (OR) 5–16 times higher than controls which was independent of coagulation tests employed to detect them, site and type of thrombosis or the presence of concomitant SLE.

The risk of thrombosis increases with the number of positive tests both in APS patients and in asymptomatic carriers of persistent aPL. Triple positivity (LAC/aCL/anti-β2GPI) confers a higher risk for thromboembolic events with a cumulative incidence of thrombosis of 12.2%, 26.1%, and 44.2% after 1, 5, and 10 years of follow-up.

The presence of aCL is associated with an OR of 22.6% for recurrent miscarriage while that of anti-β2GPI antibodies increases the chance of recurrent miscarriage from 6.8% to 22.2% when compared with women positive for LAC or anticardiolipin.

The global APS score (GAPSS) which includes IgG/IgM aCL (five points), IgG/IgM anti-β2GPI (four points), LAC (four points), IgG/IgM anti-phosphatidylserine-prothrombin complex antibodies (three points), hyperlipidemia (three points), and arterial hypertension (one point) takes into account aPL profiles (criteria aPL and noncriteria aPL), as well as conventional cardiovascular risk factors and autoimmune antibody profiles attempts to predict risk of thrombosis.

TREATMENT

THROMBOTIC ANTIPHOSPHOLIPID SYNDROME

There are two aspects in the treatment of thrombotic APS—primary thromboprophylaxis and secondary thromboprophylaxis. *Primary thromboprophylaxis* describes the prevention of thrombosis in those without any previous history of thrombosis and *secondary thromboprophylaxis* is prevention of the recurrence of a clot following a thrombotic event.

Asymptomatic individuals having persistent high aPLs, triple positivity (presence of all three tests for APS), or additional cardiovascular risk factors can be considered for LDA (75–100 mg/day) or hydroxychloroquine (HCQ, 200 mg/day) though it is supported by low level of evidence. Primary thromboprophylaxis with hydroxychloroquine with or without LDA can be considered for individuals with SLE with persistent LAC or aPLs. The mainstay of treatment in thrombotic APS is anticoagulation. It is initiated with therapeutic dose of heparin [1 mg/kg every 12 h of LMWH, or 10,000–12,000 units of unfractionated heparin (UFH) in divided doses per day] followed by an oral anticoagulant. The prophylactic dose of heparin is 0.5 mg/kg/day of LMWH given as a once daily dose or 5,000 units twice daily of UFH.

The vitamin K-dependent oral anticoagulant warfarin forms the cornerstone of long-term anticoagulation. High-intensity warfarin therapy [international normalized ratio (INR) of >3] was not found to be more effective than moderate-intensity warfarin for the prevention of recurrent thrombosis and required an INR of only 2.0–3.0. This target range also resulted in lesser bleeding complications (Crowther, MA).

The anticoagulation is to be continued indefinitely in an unprovoked venous thrombosis and arterial thrombosis. It may be stopped after 6 months in a provoked venous event. The highest rate of recurrence is during the first 6 months after the discontinuation of anticoagulation therapy. The addition of LDA is considered in patients with recurrent arterial thrombosis while on anticoagulation. Currently there is no approved role for directly acting oral anticoagulants (DOAC) in APS.

OBSTETRIC ANTIPHOSPHOLIPID SYNDROME

In a recently concluded Cochrane database review, either form of heparin (LMWH or UFH) combined with aspirin was found to result in more live births in women with recurrent pregnancy loss due to aPL than treatment with aspirin alone. This thus informs the standard of care in obstetrical APS currently. Apart from its anticoagulant action, heparin promotes spiral artery remodeling by regulating extravillous trophoblast protein expression and function. It increases proliferation of primary placental villous cytotrophoblasts and cytotrophoblast-like cells, and also promotes endothelial function and angiogenesis. Through inhibition of C1q, it also inhibits the complement cascade, augments factor H, and inhibits the terminal lytic complement complex.

Aspirin blocks platelet cyclooxygenase and thromboxane production and promotes implantation in early pregnancy. LDA also stimulates interleukin-3, which has been found deficient during APS-associated abortion.

Low-dose aspirin along with prophylactic dose of heparin is initiated at confirmation of pregnancy, continued throughout the antenatal period and until 6 weeks into puerperium when the risk of thrombosis is high. Women with thrombotic APS have to be switched to therapeutic heparin during pregnancy and shifted back to oral anticoagulation once postpartum hemostasis is achieved. Vitamin K antagonists are safe while breastfeeding.

Intravenous Ig (IVIg) was not found to result in a better obstetric outcome in prospectively followed pregnancies compared to a combination of LMWH and aspirin.

The combination of anticoagulation, corticosteroids, and plasma exchange, with or without IVIg, is used in CAPS. Concomitant use of cyclophosphamide is indicated in APS associated with SLE.

IMMUNOMODULATORY APPROACH

This field is still evolving. By targeting the primary or first immunological hit they may provide alternatives to long-term anticoagulation. Other approaches include inhibition of TF, P38 mitogen-activated protein kinase, nuclear factor-κB, platelet glycoprotein receptor, β2GPI, and/or anti-β2GPI binding to target cells, complement, and B cell. Mouse models using HCQ and statins have also shown optimistic results. HCQ decreases aPL-induced platelet activation and hence thrombosis and prevents displacement of annexin A5 from phospholipids bilayers. Statins reverse aPL-induced endothelial cell activation and TF upregulation.

Eculizumab, humanized monoclonal antibody (mAb) blocking the complement C5 cleavage and activation to C5a, has been proven to be beneficial as an add-on therapy in improving patient survival in case reports of CAPS refractory to conventional therapy. This also provides confirmatory evidence of the pathogenic role of complement activation in APS.

Rituximab (RTX), a mAb against CD20 which results in B cell depletion, was proposed to have a role in APS given that B lymphocytes are responsible for aPL generation. There are reports of reduced titer or negativization of aPLs following administration of RTX. A pilot study by Erkan et al. found its efficacy in controlling noncriteria aPL manifestations like thrombocytopenia and skin ulcers which was thought to due to blockade of B cell effector functions independently of antibody production. A review of the CAPS registry showing 16 of 20 patients treated with RTX survived suggests a role of RTX in this less studied field.

PROGNOSIS

Mortality in patients with classic APS is approximately 5% at 5 years, with recurrent arterial thrombotic events—specifically stroke and myocardial infarction—identified as being the main causes of death. The previous 55% mortality in CAPS has fallen to 33% with current treatment strategies. Live birth is achieved in approximately 72.8% of OAPS with lesser incidence of prematurity and higher birth weights in patients receiving standard care of treatment.

RECOMMENDED READINGS

1. Shoenfeld Y, Meroni PL, Toubi E. Antiphospholipid syndrome and systemic lupus erythematosus: are they separate entities or just clinical presentations on the same scale? Curr Opin Rheumat. 2009;21(5):495-500.
2. Meroni PL, Borghi MO, Grossi C, Chighizola CB, Durigutto P, Tedesco F. Obstetric and vascular anti-phospholipid syndrome: same antibodies but different diseases? Nat Rev Rheumatol. 2018;14(7):433-40.
3. da Rosa GP, Bettencourt P, Rodríguez-Pintó I, Cervera R, Espinosa G. "Non-criteria" antiphospholipid syndrome: A nomenclature proposal. Autoimmun Rev. 2020;19(12):102689.
4. Alijotas-Reig J, Esteve-Valverde E, Ferrer-Oliveras R, Saez-Comet L, Lefkou Elmina, Mekinian A, et al. The European Registry on Obstetric Antiphospholipid Syndrome (EUROAPS): A survey of 1000 consecutive cases. Autoimmun Rev. 2019;18(4):406-14.
5. Hamulyák EN, Scheres LJ, Marijnen MC, Goddijn M, Middeldorp S. Aspirin or heparin or both for improving pregnancy outcomes in women with persistent antiphospholipid antibodies and recurrent pregnancy loss. Cochrane Database Syst Rev. 2020;5(5):CD012852.
6. Pericleous C, Ferreira I, Borghi O, Pregnolato F, McDonnell T, Garza-Garcia A, et al. Measuring IgA Anti-β2-Glycoprotein I and IgG/IgA anti-domain I antibodies adds value to current serological assays for the antiphospholipid syndrome. PLoS One. 2016;11(6): e0156407.
7. Sajjan VV, Lunge S, Swamy MB, Pandit AM. Livedo reticularis: A review of the literature. Indian Dermatol Online J. 2015;6(5):315-21.
8. Gebhart J, Posch F, Koder S, Quehenberger P, Perkmann T, Kuessel L, et al. High risk of adverse pregnancy outcomes in women with a persistent lupus anticoagulant. Blood Adv. 2019;3(5):769-76.
9. Balestrieri G, Tincani A, Spatola L, Allegri F, Prati E, Cattaneo R, et al. Anti-beta 2-glycoprotein I antibodies: a marker of antiphospholipid syndrome? Lupus. 1995;4(2):122-30.
10. Wat JM, Audette MC, Kingdom JC. Molecular actions of heparin and their implications in preventing pre-eclampsia. J Thromb Haemost. 2018;16(8):1510-22.
11. Crowther MA, Ginsberg JS, Julian J, Denburg J, Hirsh J, Douketis J, et al. A Comparison of Two Intensities of Warfarin for the prevention of recurrent thrombosis in patients with the antiphospholipid antibody syndrome. N Engl J Med. 2003;349(12):1133-8.
12. Oku K, Atsumi T, Bohgaki M, Amengual O, Kataoka H, Horita T, et al. Complement activation in patients with primary antiphospholipid syndrome. Ann Rheum Dis. 2009;68(6):1030-5.
13. Pierangeli SS, Erkan D. Antiphospholipid syndrome treatment beyond anticoagulation: Are we there yet? Lupus. 2010;19(4):475-85.
14. Espinosa G, Cervera R. Antiphospholipid syndrome: frequency, main causes and risk factors of mortality. Nat Rev Rheumatol. 2010;6(5):296-300.

CHAPTER 236

Systemic Sclerosis: An Update

Vineeta Shobha, Ramya Aithala

ABSTRACT

Scleroderma or systemic sclerosis (SSc) is a systemic multiorgan disorder characterized by autoimmunity, systemic inflammation, vascular injury, and tissue fibrosis. The pathogenesis of SSc encompasses interrelated yet distinct vascular, inflammatory, and fibrotic processes. Vascular injury is an early and primary event that results in obliteration of multiple small vessels and consequent tissue hypoxia. Inflammation and autoimmunity are prominent in early stage disease and fibrosis and vascular insufficiency dominate in late-stage disease. Interstitial and perivascular fibrosis occurs in the skin, lungs, heart, and many other internal organs. Considerable patient-to-patient variability exists in the relative contribution of these three pathomechanistic processes resulting in substantial clinical heterogeneity. Lung disease is the leading cause of mortality, and efforts at early detection of pulmonary arterial hypertension (PAH) and interstitial lung disease (ILD) are warranted.

Autoantibodies help to characterize disease subsets into limited or diffuse and risks of visceral involvement to some extent. These include anticentromere antibody (limited cutaneous SSc and risk of PAH), anti-topoisomerase antibody (diffuse cutaneous SSc and risk of ILD), and anti-RNA polymerase III antibody (diffuse cutaneous SSc and risk of renal crisis). Treatment of SSc is challenging, as advanced fibrosis of the lung and other major organs is frequently resistant to therapy and contributes to significant morbidity and mortality.

"You have an auto immune disease and its not pretty, but you can rebuild your life in a new way"

—Jennifer Esposito

INTRODUCTION

Systemic sclerosis (SSc), as the name indicates, is a chronic autoimmune disorder, which induces sclerosis or fibrosis of multiple organ systems in an ongoing manner. Hippocrates provided the first description of this illness as "thickened" skin texture around 400 BC followed by labeling of the skin as "wood-like" by Curzio. In 1836, Fantonetti used the term "scleroderma," derived from the Greek words skleros (hard or indurated) and derma (skin), to describe, skin and joint disease presenting with tightened dark-leathered skin resulting in impaired joint mobility. This disorder poses substantial challenges in both diagnosis as well as therapeutics.

It is characterized by three important features namely—small vessel vasculopathy, organ fibrosis and presence of specific autoantibodies. Fibroblast dysfunction resulting in excessive deposition of collagen and extracellular matrix (ECM) in the skin and many different internal organ systems such as lungs, heart, musculoskeletal system, gastrointestinal tract, and kidneys is one of key events in its pathogenesis. This results in vast heterogeneity in terms of clinical diversity as well as variable severity of organ dysfunction. The pattern and extent of internal organ system disease are the prime determinants of the outcome and survival. Skin, musculoskeletal, and gastrointestinal involvement frequently results in nonlethal manifestations, which have a major impact on quality-of-life.

DIAGNOSIS AND CLASSIFICATION

The purpose of disease classification is to facilitate reasonably accurate diagnosis and reliably predict prognosis. In 2013, the American College of Rheumatology (ACR) and European League Against Rheumatism (EULAR) published updated classification criteria. The previously available 1980 ACR classification criteria had poor sensitivity for early SSc and limited cutaneous SSc. This new validated criterion uses 23 weighted items arranged in a multicriteria additive point system with a threshold to classify cases as SSc (**Table 1**). Importantly, skin thickening of the fingers extending proximal to the metacarpophalangeal (MCP) joints is sufficient for the patient to be classified as limited SSc. Other items include skin thickening of the fingers, fingertip lesions, telangiectasia, abnormal nailfold capillaries, interstitial lung disease (ILD) or pulmonary artery hypertension (PAH), Raynaud's phenomenon, and SSc-related autoantibodies with varying weights.

TABLE 1 2013 American College of Rheumatology (ACR) European League Against Rheumatism (EULAR) classification criteria for systemic sclerosis (SSc).

Item	Subitem(s)	Weight/ Score*
Skin thickening of the fingers of both hands extending proximal to the metacarpophalangeal joints (sufficient criterion)		9
Skin thickening of the fingers (only count the higher score)	Puffy fingers Sclerodactyly of the fingers (distal to the MCPs but proximal to the proximal interphalangeal joints)	2 4
Fingertip lesions (only count the higher score)	Digital tip ulcers Fingertip pitting scars	2 3
Telangiectasia		2
Abnormal nailfold capillaries		2
Pulmonary arterial hypertension and/or interstitial lung disease (maximum score 2)	Pulmonary arterial hypertension Interstitial lung disease	2 2
Raynaud's phenomenon		3
SSc-related autoantibodies (maximum score 3)	ACA Scl-70 RNA pol	3

***The total score is calculated by adding the maximum weight/score in each category. A total score of ≥9 is classified as definite SSc.**

(ACA: anticentromere antibodies; MCP: metacarpophalangeal joint)

Even though this classification criterion had better sensitivity and specificity in the validation sample—0.91 and 0.92 than 0.75 and 0.72 for the 1980 ACR classification criteria, it is not useful for predicting outcomes.

Traditionally, SSc is classified as either limited or diffuse based on the extent of cutaneous involvement. Recently, the European Scleroderma Trials and Research (EUSTAR) group collated information for 24 clinical variables from 11,318 patients with SSc across 122 European referral centers in Europe. Using advanced computational methods such as unsupervised machine learning techniques and cluster analysis, EUSTAR group could classify SSc patients into six homogeneous subsets, which differ with regard to clinical features, autoantibody profiles, and survival. This is in contrast to traditional dichotomy of SSc into either diffuse or limited disease spectrum.

PATHOGENESIS

In recent years, the understanding of pathogenesis of SSc has improved considerably and it is no longer considered as a primarily fibrotic disease. Better understanding of the central role of endothelial damage, participation of immune response cells, inflammatory mediators, and components of ECM have changed the pathogenic modeling of this disease. There occurs a complex and dynamic interplay between these distinct processes resulting in initiation, amplification, and sustenance of disease process eventually resulting in tissue damage. Little is known about the triggering factors, which initiate or perpetuate the pathogenic process. It is hypothesized to manifest in a "genetically susceptible" individual following an encounter with an environmental or an infectious agent. The three key components of pathogenesis are—(1) vascular injury, (2) inflammation, and immune dysregulation, and (3) fibroblast activation resulting in fibrosis (**Fig. 1**).

VASCULOPATHY

An aberrant activation of the immune system after exposure to certain environmental influences seems to be the first step of the SSc disease process. Consistent with this notion, disease-specific autoantibodies are already present prior to the emergence of the first clinical symptoms associated with SSc, such as Raynaud's phenomenon, puffy fingers, and morning stiffness. The initial vascular insult results in endothelial cell (EC) injury and activation with reversible functional changes and increased expression of adhesion molecules resulting in perivascular inflammation. Damaged endothelium further induces platelet aggregation, thrombin, and reactive oxygen species (ROS) release. There also occurs an imbalance between vasodilator production such as nitric oxide (NO) and vasoconstrictors such as endothelin-1 (ET1).

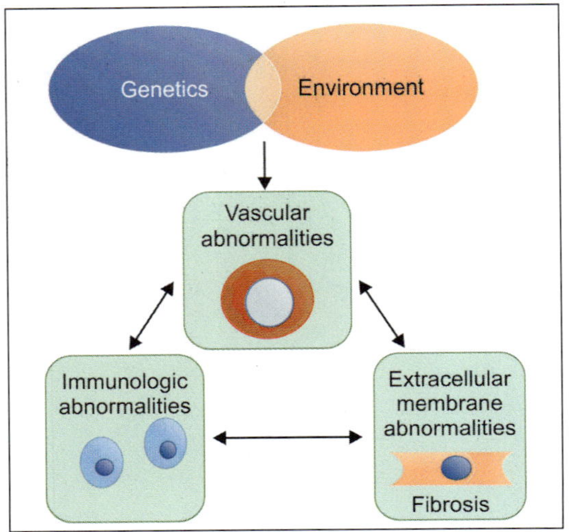

FIGURE 1: Overview of key pathogenic processes.

Recurrent episodes of ischemia-reperfusion promote oxidative stress with the generation of H_2O_2 and other oxygen-free radicals. Damaged microvessels show increased vascular permeability and injured ECs promote transendothelial leukocyte migration. Ongoing vasoconstriction and defective vasodilation aggravate vascular damage leading to irreversible progressive vascular remodeling, luminal occlusion, platelet aggregation, thrombosis, and subsequent tissue hypoxia. Additionally, there occurs loss of blood vessels partly due to inadequate vasculogenesis. Importantly, luminal thrombosis is also contributed by altered balance of coagulation/fibrinolysis system leading to impaired peripheral circulation, the induction of inflammation, and further activation of vascular cells (ECs and pericytes/vascular smooth muscle cells) and fibroblasts.

INFLAMMATION AND IMMUNE DYSREGULATION

The interaction of ECs with circulating immune cells through cell adhesion molecules and chemokine promotes the activation of inflammatory cells and their infiltration into the affected organs of SSc. Generally, the infiltration of T cells, macrophages, and mast cells is predominant in the skin, while lymphoid aggregates composed of B cells and T cells and macrophages are generally evident in the affected lung tissue of SSc ILD. Injury to vascular endothelium initiates another cascade of events, including release of proinflammatory mediators, growth factors, and a variety of chemokines.

Transition occurs from innate immune response (macrophages) to adaptive immune response, which is accompanied by T-cell activation and development of Th-2 (type-2 helper) and Th17 response. Th2 cytokines such as interleukin-4 (IL4), IL-5, and IL-13 exhibit profibrotic activity. Among Th17 cytokines, the expression levels of IL-17A, IL-21, and IL-22, but not of IL-17F, are increased in the lesional skin. It is believed that the T regulatory cells' (Treg) function is impaired in the active stage of SSc. The Tregs produce transforming growth factor-β (TGF-β) and suppress the effector T-cell function. B-cell stimulation leads to generation of specific autoantibodies that may directly contribute to tissue damage. Plasmacytoid dendritic cells (pDCs) produce excessive amounts of interferon-α (IFN-α) around small dermal vessels through the activation of TLR7 & -9 via the complex of self-DNA and LL-37 derived from ECs.

The direct role of SSc-related antinuclear antibodies (ANAs) such as antibodies against topoisomerase-I (TopoI), centromere, and RNA polymerase III (RNAP III) antigens in immunopathogenesis remains largely unknown. However, the close association of these antibodies with specific clinical manifestations suggests that altered B-cell phenotypes possibly correlate with the central abnormality driving the progression of the disease. Anti-topoisomerase-I antibody is demonstrated to react with nuclear antigens derived from ECs, and the immune subsets complex with nucleic acids, in particular RNA, thereby inducing IFN-α production from pDCs.

Additionally, many other autoantibodies are described in association with few subsets of SSc, which include anti-endothelial cell antibodies (AECA), antibodies against platelet-derived growth factor receptor (PDGFR), angiotensin II type 1 receptor (AT1R), and endothelin-1 type A receptor (ETAR). Overall, the continuous release of autoantigens from injured and senescent ECs and the failure to replace damaged endothelium from circulating endothelial progenitors are a fundamental fuel of SSc pathology, thereby perpetuating chronic inflammation.

FIBROSIS

Fibrosis in the skin and multiple internal organs is the distinguishing hallmark of SSc. The activation of fibroblasts is the final consequence of the SSc-specific disease cascade, which produces excessive amounts of collagen and ECM. Progressive build-up of biochemically and mechanically abnormal connective tissue disrupts the tissue architecture. A key growth factor involved in the activation of SSc fibroblasts is TGF-β, a potent inducer of ECM including fibrillar collagens constituting the dermis.

In the early stages of SSc, TGF-β also promotes inflammation by recruiting leukocytes through the regulation of cell adhesion molecules and by inducing various proinflammatory cytokines and other mediators. In the sclerotic phase, SSc dermal fibroblasts are constitutively activated into a profibrotic phenotype. Overall, SSc fibroblasts maintain their activated status through the self-activation system and the feed-forward loop by interacting with other cell types, eventually leading to the irreversible fibrotic remodeling of multiple organs.

SEROLOGIC FEATURES

Systemic sclerosis is characterized by the presence of several autoantibodies. Most patients have a positive ANA by indirect immunofluorescent assay, using HEp-2 cells as substrate. Most frequently, the ANA pattern is nucleolar. Positivity for anticentromere antibody is generally seen in patients with limited cutaneous SSc (lcSSc) (20–40%). Positivity for anti-Scl-70 antibody is associated with diffuse cutaneous SSc (dcSSc) and increased risk for the development of ILD. Those with anti-RNA polymerase III antibody have a worse prognosis, show extensive skin thickening with increased frequency of tendon friction rubs, and are more likely to develop scleroderma renal crisis (SRC), although they have a lower incidence of ILD. The Th/To antibody is associated with lcSSc and pulmonary hypertension. The U11/U12-RNP antibody is often associated with severe ILD.

CLINICAL FEATURES

The hallmark of clinical manifestations of SSc is diverse heterogeneity, both in terms of variety and severity (**Fig. 2**). The involvement and extent of major organ disease determines the outcome and survival. The burden of nonlethal manifestations has a major impact on their physical and emotional well-being.

SKIN

The most important and characteristic features of SSc is skin thickening. The extent of skin sclerosis is used to define limited (lcSSc) or diffuse disease (dcSSc); the proximal involvement defines diffuse disease. Three stages of skin changes may occur in patients with SSc. The initial stage is an inflammatory, edematous stage, which is associated with puffiness of the hands and fingers. This phase is frequently associated with pruritus. This initial inflammatory phase may last for months, and thereafter, induration and thickening of the skin begin to develop. In patients with dcSSc, diffuse skin changes involve the skin on the face, hands, forearms, arms, chest, abdomen, thighs, legs, and feet.

Those with lcSSc have skin changes limited to the face, neck, and distal extremities. Facial skin thickening occurs in both limited and diffuse cutaneous disease, frequently resulting in characteristic skin tightening and tethering in the perioral region causing a reduced oral aperture and *"Mauskopf" facies*. The front teeth may appear to be prominent because of lip and gum retraction, due to both fibrosis and atrophy of the mandible (**Figs. 3 A** and **B**). The extent of skin thickening can be assessed using the modified *Rodnan's skin score*. Pigmentary changes may occur throughout the course of illness. Depending on the patient's natural skin tones, the skin may become hypopigmented or hyperpigmented. Indian patients frequently develop areas of depigmentation, particularly of the scalp, chest, and upper back and over areas of pressure such as the dorsum of the hand or pretibial regions. These areas of vitiligo give the skin a "salt and pepper" appearance owing to perifollicular sparing of pigment loss.

Other skin manifestations include *telangiectasias, digital pits, and calcinosis*. Telangiectasias are dilated capillaries most commonly present on the face, hands, mucosal membranes, and chest. Digital pits are small areas of indentation on the distal finger pads caused by ischemic damage related to Raynaud's phenomenon. Subcutaneous calcinosis occurs in both limited and diffuse cutaneous disease but is more common in patients with limited disease, particularly those with an anticentromere antibody. It most commonly occurs over areas of trauma such as the

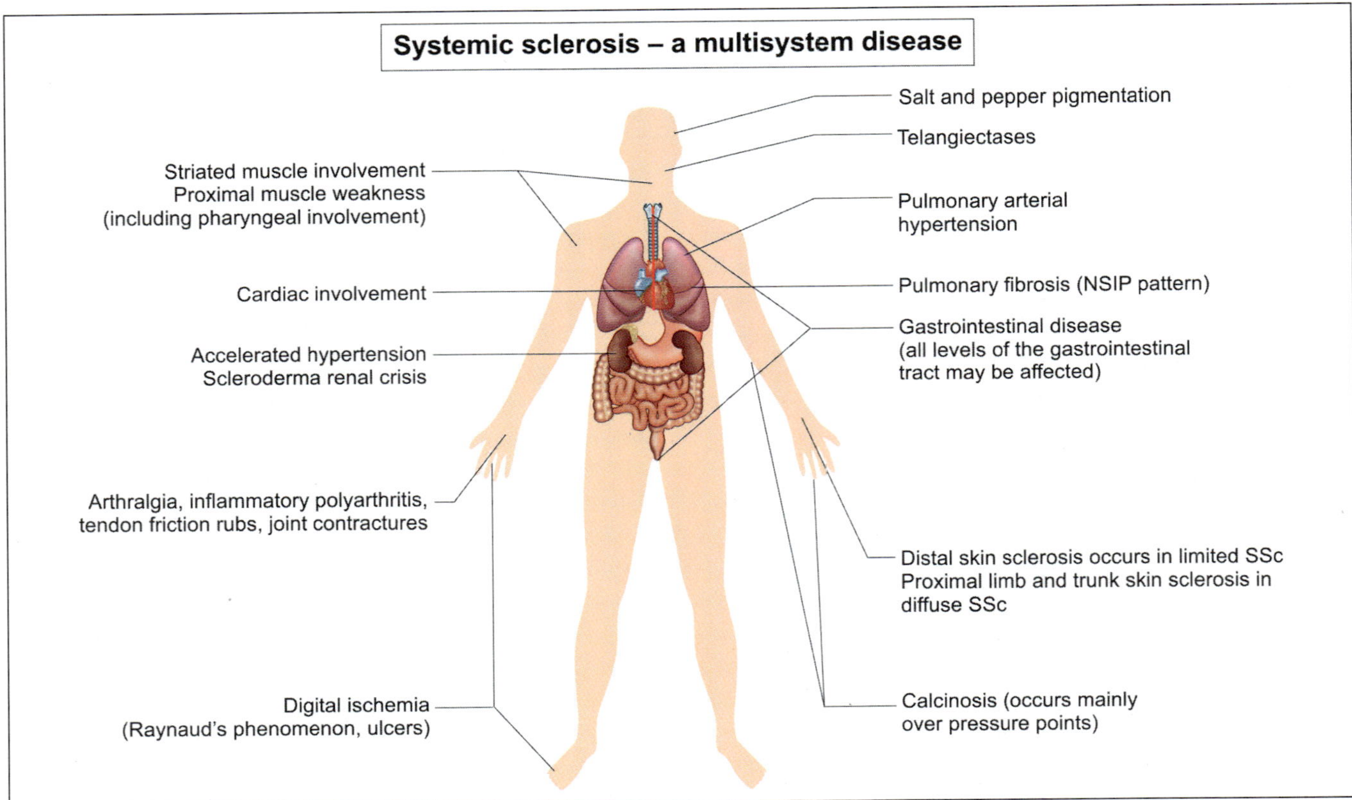

FIGURE 2: Overview of clinical features.

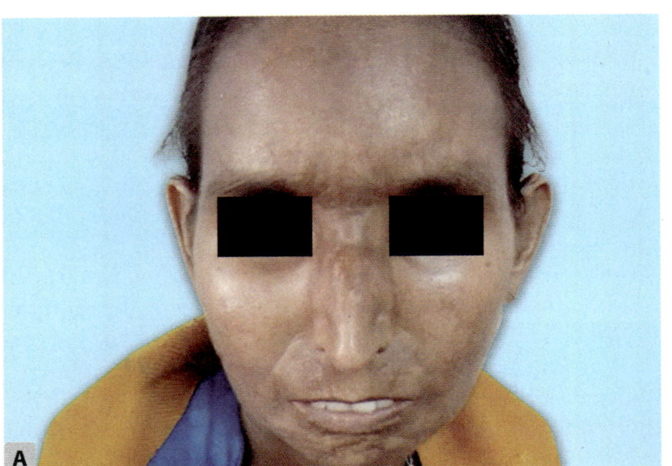

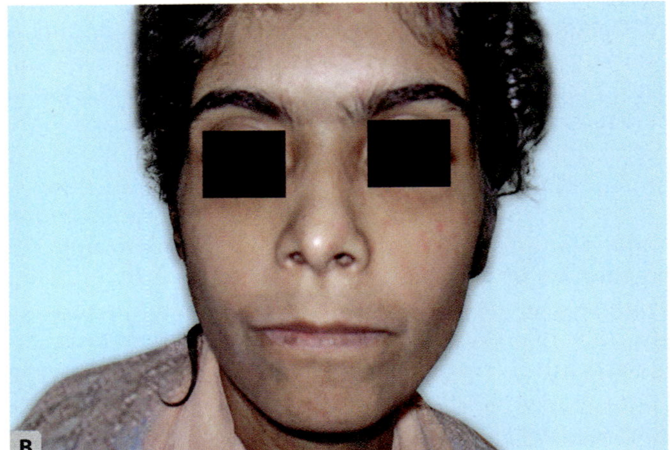

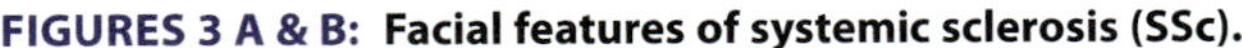

FIGURES 3 A & B: Facial features of systemic sclerosis (SSc).

extensor surfaces of the forearms and of the finger pads. Uncommonly, it may result in calcific periarthritis resulting in restricted movement and severe pain.

VASCULOPATHY

Raynaud's phenomenon is typically the earliest and most frequent symptom in patients with SSc in >95%. It is defined as cold-induced vasospasm of the digits (fingers > toes), rarely occurring in the ears, nose, or tongue. It is classically described as triphasic color change, an initial pallor, and a well-demarcated pale or white phase, which occurs in response to the vasospasm induced by cold exposure. This may be followed by a dusky discoloration due to ischemia and desaturation of hemoglobin; subsequently, reactive hyperemia occurs and the digits turn red. In addition to these color changes, patients often experience numbness, tingling, and discomfort.

In patients with lcSSc, Raynaud phenomenon typically begins many years before the onset of skin or visceral disease; while in dcSSc, the onset of Raynaud's phenomenon usually occurs simultaneously with or shortly after the onset of skin changes. However, in up to 20%, skin thickening may

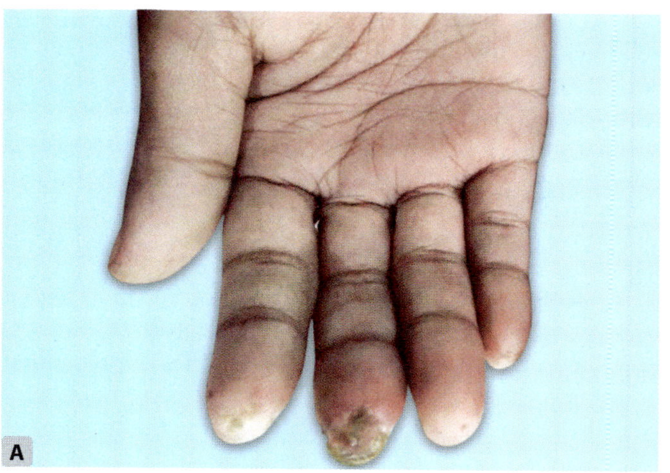

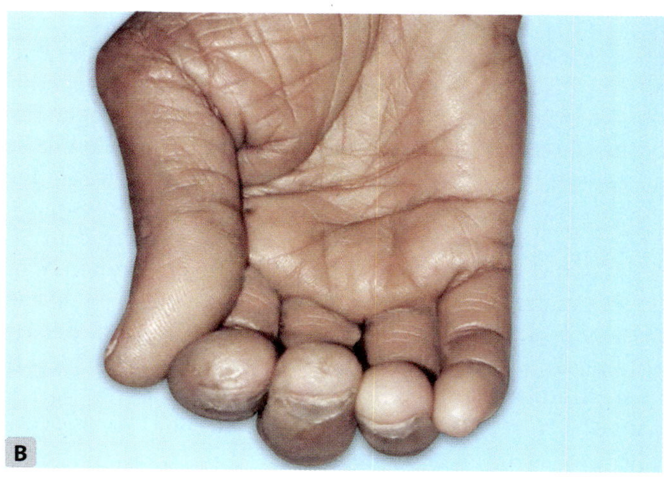

FIGURES 4 A & B: Vasculopathy: Digital pitted scars and cutaneous infarcts causing pulp-space resorption.

precede the development of Raynaud's phenomenon: this subgroup seems to be associated with the development of diffuse skin involvement and also of scleroderma renal disease. Raynaud's phenomenon may be complicated by development of digital pitted scars, fixed ischemic changes with threatened tissue loss, poorly healing digital ulcers, dry gangrene, and autoamputation. Digital pits, one of the SSc classification criteria, represent areas of ischemic insult to the distal fingertip (**Figs. 4 A** and **B**).

MUSCULOSKELETAL

Arthralgia and myalgia are quite frequent in SSc; some patients may develop true inflammatory arthropathy and metacarpophalangeal or myopathy as well. The joints most commonly involved are the proximal interphalangeal (PIP), MCP, wrist, and ankle joints. Because of overlying skin thickening, it may be difficult to appreciate the presence of joint swelling. Progressive skin changes can result in joint flexion contractures causing significant disability. Inflammation and fibrosis of the tendon may result in friction rubs overlying tendon sheaths, commonly at the finger, wrist, elbow, knee, and/or ankle joints. Tendon friction rubs are predictive of dcSSc and are manifested in approximately one-third of such patients. Muscle weakness and generalized fatigue are also prominent symptoms. Proximal muscle weakness may result from bland myopathy due to muscle fibrosis or an overlap syndrome of SSc with polymyositis or dermatomyositis with a true inflammatory myopathy.

GASTROINTESTINAL TRACT

Gastrointestinal involvement occurs in the majority of SSc. Its severity varies from asymptomatic to mild or severe and occurs in both limited and diffuse disease. The entire gastrointestinal tract may be involved from the oropharynx to the anus. Smooth muscle atrophy and fibrosis within the gastrointestinal mucosa play a role in gastrointestinal dysmotility; however, intimal proliferation similar to that seen in other vascular beds also occurs in the gastro-intestinal tract.

Oropharyngeal involvement includes reduced oral aperture from skin tightening, mandibular atrophy, and a shortened frenulum. Esophageal dysmotility occurs in nearly every patient with SSc owing to involvement of the distal two-thirds of the esophagus, which sometimes results in dysphagia. Reduced lower esophageal sphincter pressure may cause varying degrees of gastroesophageal reflux and dyspepsia. Barium esophagography may demonstrate esophageal dysmotility, including loss of primary and secondary peristalsis of the distal esophagus as well as esophageal strictures. Symptoms of gastric involvement include early satiety, bloating, nausea, emesis, anorexia, and weight loss. Delayed gastric emptying can exacerbate symptoms of gastroesophageal reflux and cause bloating. Early satiety and bloating may cause the patient to reduce caloric intake, which leads to weight loss.

Gastrointestinal blood loss may result from mucosal telangiectasia, gastritis, or, in more severe cases, gastric antral vascular ectasia, described endoscopically as a watermelon stomach. Intestinal dysmotility also causes bloating and cramping. Patients develop diarrhea alternating with constipation due to intestinal bacterial overgrowth. Pseudo-obstruction is a functional ileus, is a serious sequela of intestinal dysmotility, and manifests as abdominal pain, bloating, and emesis.

Large-intestinal mucosal muscular atrophy may result in wide-mouthed diverticula unique to SSc, typically occurring on the antimesenteric surface. Anorectal involvement due to decreased compliance and reduced anal sphincter tone may result in rectal prolapse and/or rectal incontinence. The liver is rarely primarily involved in SSc; however, an association exists between primary biliary cirrhosis (PBC) and SSc and a significant proportion of patients with PBC have an anticentromere antibody. Antimitochondrial antibodies occur in SSc patients with coexisting PBC.

LUNGS

Lung disease is the leading disease-related cause of mortality in SSc. Pulmonary disease most typically includes

ILD and/or PAH. Other less common lung manifestations include aspiration pneumonia, pleural disease, obstructive airway disease, alveolar hemorrhage, and cryptogenic organizing pneumonia. Characteristically, ILD begins as basilar pulmonary fibrosis and tends to be more common and more severe in patients with dcSSc than lcSSc. As many as 80% of patients may have evidence of pulmonary fibrosis on high-resolution computed tomography (HRCT) scans, although clinically evident disease is present in only approximately 40% of patients. The risk factors for ILD are presence of anti-topoisomerase I antibody (anti-Scl-70 antibody), disease onset within 4 years, and black males in their 5th and 6th decades. The presence of an anticentromere antibody or anti-RNA polymerase III antibody is associated with a reduced risk of the development of ILD.

Pulmonary function testing (PFT) with spirometry, measurement of lung volumes, and tests of gas exchange are the best screening methods for ILD. The most sensitive and earliest change is a reduction in diffusion capacity. PFT abnormalities may occur before the onset of clinical symptoms, and a reduction in lung volumes should prompt further evaluation for ILD. HRCT of the chest reveals ground-glass opacification that is indicative of active inflammation and/or early fibrosis. Other findings include thickening of the interlobular septa, subpleural nodules, honeycomb appearance, and traction bronchiectasis.

Pulmonary vascular disease may occur either as a primary vasculopathy or secondary to underlying cardiac disease, ILD, or, rarely, chronic thromboembolic disease. Isolated PAH occurs more frequently in patients with lcSSc, typically manifesting many years after the onset of Raynaud's phenomenon. However, patients with dcSSc can manifest isolated PAH relatively early in the disease course. Up to a quarter of patients with SSc may have undetected pulmonary hypertension, depending on the threshold value used for its diagnosis. Patients with SSc and pulmonary hypertension secondary to underlying ILD have a worse prognosis than patients with ILD without pulmonary hypertension. The presence of PAH is associated with high mortality.

HEART

Cardiac manifestations include pericardial disease, dilated cardiomyopathy, autonomic neuropathy, and arrhythmias. Pericardial disease can be manifested as either pericarditis or, as a pericardial effusion. Pericardial effusions, typically exudative if secondary to SSc, accumulate very slowly. Patients can also develop left or right ventricular systolic dysfunction and is usually a late occurrence. The presence of congestive heart failure has been associated with increased mortality in patients with SSc.

There seems to be a predilection for the development of either right or left ventricular diastolic dysfunction in SSc, which may be attributed to myocardial fibrosis and reduced ventricular compliance. Left ventricular diastolic dysfunction appears to occur with greater frequency than systolic dysfunction and is frequently observed in those with pulmonary hypertension. Higher frequency of atherosclerotic coronary artery disease occurs in patients with SSc, and postmortem studies reveal lesions that involve most commonly the small coronary arteries or arterioles. Fibrosis along with conduction pathways may cause arrhythmias.

RENAL

Scleroderma renal crisis (SRC) is one of the cardinal vascular manifestations of SSc. It classically presents with new-onset hypertension. Other clinical features include dyspnea, headache, visual disturbances, seizure, pulmonary edema, and fundoscopic changes quite like malignant hypertension. It is characterized by a microangiopathy with anemia and schistocytes on peripheral blood smear, along with thrombocytopenia, renal insufficiency, proteinuria, and urinary sediment. It is not an inflammatory process rather it is a high-renin state, and the pathologic changes in the blood vessels are similar to those seen in other vessels in patients with SSc.

It is estimated that 10% of patients with SSc develop SRC, which occurs almost exclusively in patients with dcSSc, usually within the first 3 years of disease. Risk factors for SRC include diffuse skin involvement, tendon friction rubs, anti-RNA polymerase III antibody, new-onset anemia, and pericardial effusion. Before the advent of angiotensin-converting enzyme (ACE) inhibitors, renal involvement was the leading cause of death in SSc.

Currently with early recognition and aggressive management, the outcome is much improved. Males, older age, and those with a serum creatinine concentration of > 3 mg/dL have the poorest outcome. A variant of SRC, termed normotensive SRC, is characterized by the typical laboratory abnormalities of SRC in the presence of a normal blood pressure and may progress to renal insufficiency and/or the need for dialysis. Normotensive renal crisis occurs most typically in patients who have previously been treated with glucocorticoids, particularly a prednisone dosage (or its equivalent) of >15 mg daily.

NEUROLOGIC

Although less frequent than other organ systems involvement, SSc can affect the nervous system in a variety of ways such as neuralgia, peripheral neuropathy, cranial neuropathy, and autonomic dysfunction. Intrinsic central nervous system pathology is extremely uncommon in SSc but vascular disease may occur. Significant neurologic complications can occur in context of SRC. Trigeminal neuralgia is the most common cranial neuropathy, frequently associated with anti-U1 RNP antibody.

SEXUAL DYSFUNCTION

Sexual dysfunction occurs in both men and women with SSc. Erectile dysfunction occurs in up to 80% of men with SSc and typically begins approximately 3 years after disease onset. A reduction in penile blood flow contributes to erectile dysfunction and is due to both endothelial changes in small arteries and corporal fibrosis from excessive collagen deposition. Altered penile blood flow occurs in the absence of atherosclerotic disease in SSc.

Sexual dysfunction is less well studied in women with SSc, but patients report symptoms of vaginal dryness, dyspareunia, and vaginal ulcerations. A significant relationship has been found between sexual dysfunction and gastroesophageal reflux and skin tightness in women with SSc. Decreased libido and decreased number and intensity of orgasms are also reported. Women with SSc experience an early menopause compared with control subjects.

EVALUATION AND TREATMENT

Effective evaluation and management of SSc largely depend on subset classification, extent of vasculopathy, and organ-based manifestations. It is necessary to take a systematic approach and evaluate each organ system involvement by symptom analysis and subsequent directed laboratory assessment (**Fig. 5**).

GENERAL PRINCIPLES

Many of the organ-based complications of SSc are treatable, if not curable. Management in scleroderma requires multiple strategies depending on the specific problems that are present for individual patients. A simplified algorithm is depicted in **Flowchart 1**. All patients with SSc should

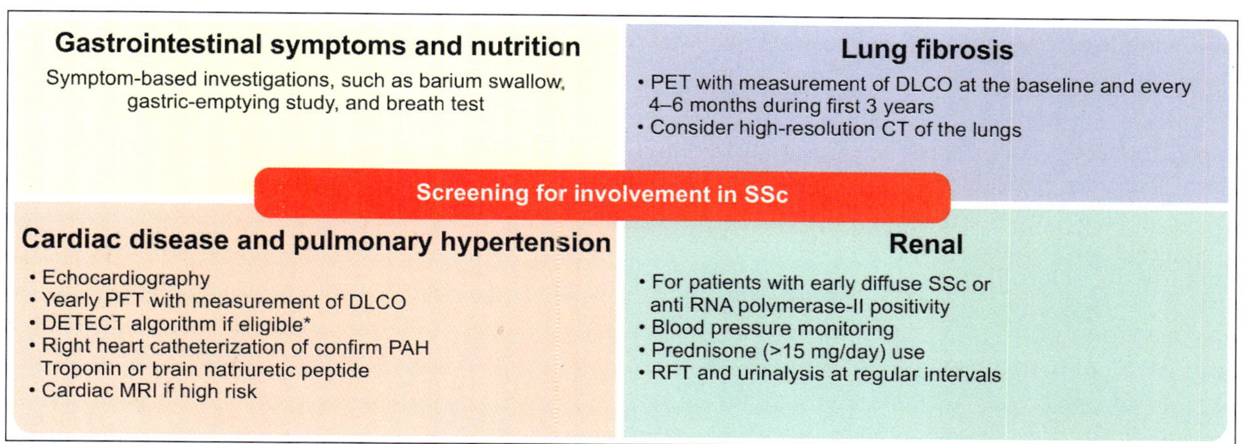

*The DETECT algorithm is a tool to identify asymptomatic PAH, by using clinical parameters, pulmonary function, immunological, biological, electrocardiographic, and echocardiographic parameters. www.detect-pah.com

(DLCO: diffusing capacity for carbon monoxide; SSc: systemic sclerosis)

FIGURE 5: Evaluation of organ systems.

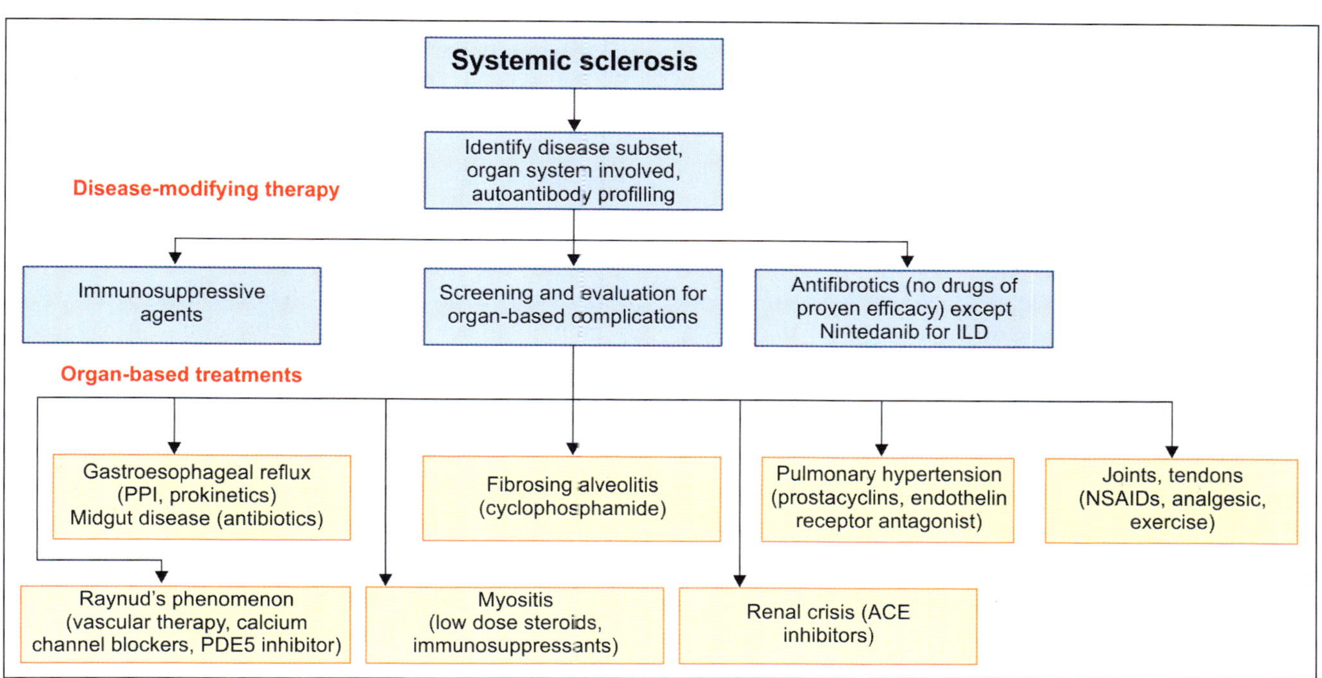

(PDE5: phosphodiesterase type 5)

FLOWCHART 1: Management strategies in systemic sclerosis.

preferably be managed as part of a specialist multidisciplinary team.

Optimal management of SSc requires the following key action items:

- Establishment of an accurate diagnosis at the earliest
- Analysis of disease status based on its onset, rate of symptom progression, determination of subset based on autoantibodies, and organ system involvement
- Institution of appropriate therapy, and aggressive intervention based on organ systems involved
- Patient education regarding lifestyle modification, risk factors, and prognosis

Clinical manifestations such as Raynaud's phenomenon, esophageal reflux, arthralgias, arthritis, fatigue, and sicca symptoms require treatment throughout the course of illness. Others such as lung or cardiac disease or renal involvement require treatment only, if affected.

Disease-modifying therapy: Few of the agents currently used as disease-modifying treatments for scleroderma spectrum disorders have undergone rigorous placebo-controlled evaluation. Cyclophosphamide has been reported to be effective for SSc-associated lung fibrosis. Recently, two major clinical trials evaluating cyclophosphamide in scleroderma-associated pulmonary fibrosis have shown advantage for cyclophosphamide over placebo, although clinical benefit was modest. Methotrexate is beneficial in patients with arthritis, inflammatory myositis, and also has a marginal role in improving skin fibrosis. Mycophenolate mofetil (MMF) is an antiproliferative immunosuppressive agent used in treatment of many autoimmune diseases including SSc related cardiac disease, lung, and skin fibrosis. Rituximab (RTX), a monoclonal anti-CD20 antibody, is also a promising therapeutic option especially for severe skin and lung fibrosis.

Vasodilatory therapy: Vascular-acting therapies are central to the management of SSc manifestations of Raynaud's phenomenon and digital ulcers. Lifestyle measures such as keeping warm and stopping smoking are essential in addition to pharmacologic therapy. These include calcium channel blockers (e.g., nifedipine) and phosphodiesterase type 5 (PDE5) inhibitors (tadalafil and sildenafil). The endothelin receptor antagonist bosentan is used for the prevention of digital ulcers in patients with severe/recurrent disease ulcer, but it does not impact on ulcer healing. Many pharmacological treatments such as PDE5 inhibitors and endothelin receptor antagonists are also used in the treatment of pulmonary hypertension. ACE inhibitors are the first-line pharmacological treatment for the SRC.

Antifibrotic agents: Therapeutic molecular targets of SSc—fibrosis are being actively researched. Nintedanib was found in a recent phase III trial to significantly reduce the annual rate of lung function decline (forced vital capacity), leading to its worldwide licencing for the treatment of SSc-associated ILD.

To summarize, the treatment of SSc remains a major medical challenge. A more formal stratified approach to management of SSc is needed, as it is a very heterogeneous disease with varied outcomes and different patterns of organ-based complications. Many controversies and uncertainties exist regarding the management of early as well as late disease and duration of treatment, which will probably be resolved in near future.

RECOMMENDED READINGS

1. Hochberg M, Gravallese E, Silman A, Smolen J, Weinblatt M, Weisman M. Rheumatology, 7th edition. Amsterdam, Netherlands: Elsevier; 2018.
2. Denton CP, Khanna D. Systemic sclerosis. The Lancet. 2017;390(10103):1685-99.
3. Furue M, Mitoma C, Mitoma H, Tsuji G, Chiba T, Nakahara T, et al. Pathogenesis of systemic sclerosis—current concept and emerging treatments. Immunol Res. 2017;65(4):790-7.
4. van den Hoogen F, Khanna D, Fransen J, Johnson SR, Baron M, Tyndall A, et al. 2013 classification criteria for systemic sclerosis: an American college of rheumatology/European league against rheumatism collaborative initiative. Ann Rheum Dis. 2013;72(11):1747-55.
5. Sobanski V, Giovannelli J, Allanore Y, Riemekasten G, Airò P, Vettori S, et al. Phenotypes determined by cluster analysis and their survival in the prospective EUSTAR cohort of patients with systemic sclerosis. Arthritis Rheumatol. 2019;71(9):1553-70.
6. Sobolewski P, Maślińska M, Wieczorek M, Łagun Z, Malewska A, Roszkiewicz M, et al. Systemic sclerosis—multidisciplinary disease: clinical features and treatment. Reumatologia. 2019;57(4):221-33.
7. Kowal-Bielecka O, Fransen J, Avouac J, Becker M, Kulak A, EUSTAR Coauthors, et al. Update of EULAR recommendations for the treatment of systemic sclerosis. Ann Rheum Dis. 2017;76(8):1327-39.
8. Goh NS, Hoyles RK, Denton CP, Hansell DM, Renzoni EA, Maher TM, et al. Short-term pulmonary function trends are predictive of mortality in interstitial lung disease associated with systemic sclerosis. Arthritis Rheumatol. 2017;69(8):1670-8.
9. Gabrielli A, Avvedimento EV, Krieg T. Scleroderma. N Engl J Med. 2009;360(19):1989-2003.
10. Mirsaeidi M, Barletta P, Glassberg MK. Systemic Sclerosis Associated Interstitial Lung Disease: New Directions in Disease Management. Front Med (Lausanne). 2019;6:248.
11. Hughes M, Allanore Y, Denton CP, Matucci-Cerinic M. Systemic sclerosis. EMJ Rheumatol. 2020;7(1):100-9.

CHAPTER

237

Sjögren's Syndrome

Ramakrishna Rao Uppuluri, Sripurna Deepti Challa

ABSTRACT

Sjögren's syndrome (SS) is an autoimmune disease characterized clinically by dryness of eyes, mouth, and other organs, pathologically by lymphocytic infiltration of the salivary, lacrimal, and other exocrine glands, and serologically by circulating antibodies such as anti-Ro/SSA and anti-La/SSB. It may occur alone as a primary SS or along with other autoimmune diseases such as rheumatoid arthritis (RA), systemic lupus erythematosus (SLE), systemic sclerosis, and polymyositis (secondary SS). It can occur at any age but seen more commonly between 40 and 60 years of age, predominantly in women.

Extraglandular features of primary SS include fatigue, polyarthritis, neuropathy, purpura, and interstitial lung disease (ILD). SS can be associated with autoimmune thyroiditis, autoimmune hepatitis, tubulointerstitial nephritis, and systemic vasculitis. It can have a stable course or present with serious systemic manifestations. There is an increased risk of developing B-cell non-Hodgkin lymphoma (NHL). Management of SS aims to provide symptomatic improvement in the clinical features. Control of extraglandular manifestations is brought out by the use of oral or biologic immunomodulatory drugs.

"The only limits of power are the bounds of belief"

—Harold Wilson

INTRODUCTION

Henrik Sjögren, a Swedish ophthalmologist, described dry eye syndrome—keratoconjunctivitis sicca (KCS) in 1933. Round cell infiltration and acinar loss in the lacrimal and salivary glands along with glandular enlargement characteristic to SS are also seen in Mikulicz disease. This syndrome arises from other disorders including lymphoma, leukemia, tuberculosis, immunoglobulin G4 (IgG4)-related disease, and sarcoidosis. Secondary SS was defined in 1965 as a triad of dry eyes, dry mouth, and RA or other connective tissue disease. Recent classification criteria (2016) for SS led to better understanding of the disease along with identification of anti-Ro/SSA and anti-La/SSB antibodies, minor salivary gland biopsy, salivary scintigraphy, and new ocular surface staining methods.

EPIDEMIOLOGY

Sjögren's syndrome is a worldwide disease with a female predominance often exceeding 10 times. It generally occurs between the ages of 40–60 years. Children, younger women, and older adults may also get SS. The annual incidence of primary SS in population-based studies ranges from 3.1 to 11.8 per 100,000 inhabitants, with the higher rates being noted in Asia. Current estimates of prevalence range from 0.1 to 4.6%. Up to 20% of patients with other autoimmune diseases such as RA, SLE, myositis, and scleroderma have features of secondary SS.

PATHOGENESIS

Sjögren's syndrome is an autoimmune disease mediated by the interaction of genetic, epigenetic, and environmental factors leading to immune dysregulation. SS is heterogeneous in terms of both clinical expression and severity.

GENETIC FACTORS

The major histocompatibility complex (MHC) class II genes, mainly human leukocyte antigen DQ (HLA-DQ) and HLA-DR, are major risk factors, with DR2 and DR3 haplotypes at the DRB1 locus.

Genes outside the MHC locus also influence susceptibility to SS. Single nucleotide polymorphisms (SNPs) have been identified in genes involved in the innate and adaptive immune response pathways. SNPs in the interferon regulatory factor 5 *(IRF5)* and signal transducer and activator of transcription 4 *(STAT4)* have been associated with SS.

ENVIRONMENTAL FACTORS

Viral infection may trigger autoimmune phenomenon in SS. The host immune response is initially directed against persistently infected cells, but becomes misdirected toward glandular tissue because of chronic antigen exposure. Ro52 is induced by interferons (IFNs) that are produced at high level during viral infection and enhanced autoantigen expression in tissues may trigger an autoimmune response. Similarly, Ro60 can bind RNA. Immune complexes containing this bound Ro60 induce type 1 IFN production. The predominance of SS in women during perimenopause points to a potential role for sex hormones in development of the disease.

IMMUNOINFLAMMATORY PATHWAYS

Interactions between several inflammatory pathways are identified in causing and sustaining inflammation and damage in SS (**Fig. 1**). Salivary gland epithelial cells are exposed to an exogenous insult such as a virus or radiation leading to cell death. Self-antigens, thus, released undergo endocytosis by dendritic cells (DCs) with subsequent processing and presentation on the cell surface for recognition by T cells.

Autoreactive T cells including T-helper 1 (Th1) and T-helper 17 (Th17) cells secrete proinflammatory cytokines, including interleukin-17 (IL-17) and IFN-γ. IFN-γ enhances antigen presentation by DCs and induces the expression of B-cell activating factor (BAFF) by salivary epithelial cells. BAFF induces the proliferation of autoreactive B-cells causing differentiation into autoantibody-secreting plasma cells. Autoantibodies form immune complexes which can coligate Fc receptors and toll-like receptors (TLRs) on plasmacytoid dendritic cells (pDCs) induce IFN-α production. IFN-α, in turn, induces autoantigen expression in epithelial cells, activates DCs, T-cell survival, and plasma cell differentiation. Cell signaling is mediated by surface receptors.

GLANDULAR PATHOLOGY

Lymphocytic infiltration of the salivary and lacrimal glands is associated with loss of acini and ducts in SS (**Fig. 2**). It is termed as focal lymphocytic sialadenitis. The infiltrates surround the striated ducts or blood vessels, which consist primarily of CD4+ T and B cells. Germinal centers or ectopic lymphoid follicles are present in 25% of labial gland biopsies from patients with SS. Histological feature of the major salivary gland involvement in SS is known as benign lymphoepithelial sialadenitis. Sometimes, it is a known precursor of mucosa-associated lymphoid tissue (MALT), an extranodal marginal zone lymphoma.

CLINICAL FEATURES

Clinical manifestations in SS depend upon the organ involved. In primary SS, glandular dysfunction is apparent initially. Systemic manifestations at the outset or during the progression of the disease appear in 25–75% of the patients.

GLANDULAR INVOLVEMENT

Ocular manifestations: The dry eye (KCS) symptoms are result of insufficient production of tears. They include

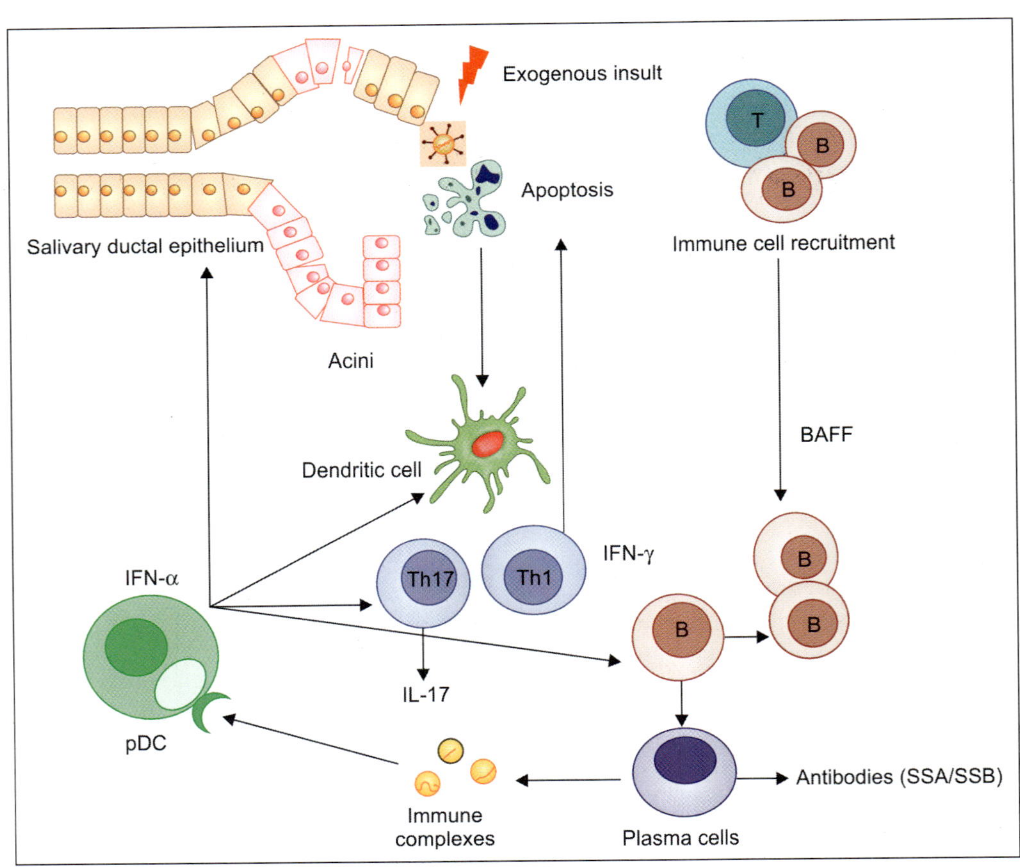

(BAFF: B-cell activating factor; IFN-γ: interferon-γ; IL-17: interleukin-17; pDC: plasmacytoid dendritic cells; SSA: Sjögren's syndrome A; SSB: Sjögren's syndrome B; Th1: T-helper 1; Th17: T-helper 17)

FIGURE 1: Pathogenesis of Sjögren's syndrome.

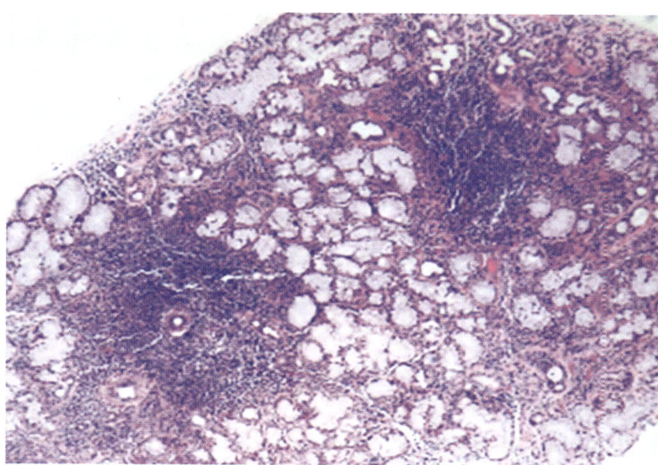

FIGURE 2: Histopathology of minor salivary glands showing multiple periductal lymphocytic infiltrates.

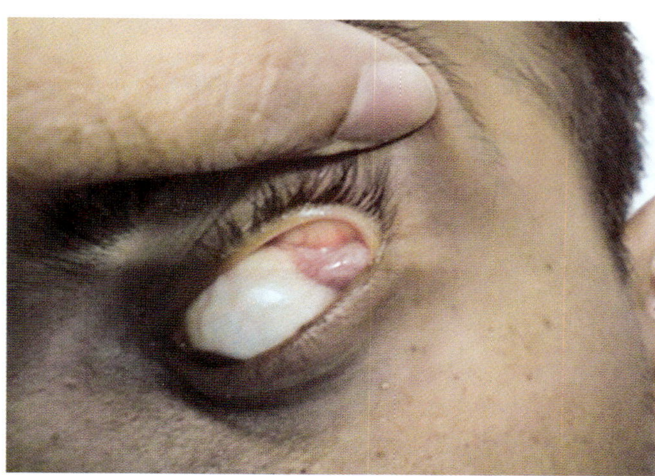

FIGURE 3: Lacrimal gland enlargement in Sjögren's syndrome.

burning, itching, foreign body sensation, and photophobia. The symptoms are often exacerbated by air movement, low humidity, continuous reading, and viewing a computer monitor. The tear film consists of three major layers—(1) the outer lipid layer, (2) the middle aqueous layer, and (3) the inner mucin layer. The middle aqueous layer is diminished in SS. Schirmer I test reveals a reduction in the tear flow.

Additional findings may include the absence of tears in the conjunctival sac, dilated bulbar conjunctival vessels, and thick mucus in inner canthus of the eye. After instillation of lissamine green dye or fluorescein onto the ocular surface, slit-lamp examination may expose devitalized cells or epithelial defects. Lacrimal gland enlargement may be seen rarely (**Fig. 3**). Apart from SS, dry eyes can be due to several other causes (**Box 1**). In advanced disease, conjunctivitis and corneal abrasion with bacterial infection may occur.

Oral manifestations: The dry mouth (xerostomia) symptoms are result of insufficient production of saliva. Apart from SS, there are other causes leading to dry mouth (**Box 2**). Patients report difficulty in chewing and swallowing dry food, speaking at length, and wearing dentures. They may also note impaired taste, thickened saliva, intolerance of acidic/spicy foods, burning sensation in the mouth/tongue, and dry lips. Dental decay and oral candidiasis often ensue in such patients. Parotid gland enlargement may be noticed clinically (**Figs. 4 A** and **B**). Apart from SS, there are several other causes for parotid gland enlargement (**Box 3**). Slowly progressive enlargement of the glands should raise concern for the presence of glandular lymphoma, particularly when asymmetric.

Involvement of other exocrine glands: Glandular hypofunction may affect the nasal passages (meatal obstruction by dried mucus), larynx (hoarseness), trachea (cough), vagina (dyspareunia), and skin (pruritus) producing symptoms of dryness.

BOX 1 Differential diagnosis of dry eyes.

Primarily evaporative:

- Eyelid and ocular surface disease
- Meibomian gland dysfunction
- Facial nerve paralysis
- Low blink rate (e.g., excess computer use)
- Extrinsic causes that enhance evaporation (e.g., hot/low humid)
- Trachoma
- Vitamin A deficiency
- Use of topical anesthetic drops
- Contact lens wear

Primarily aqueous deficient:

- Sjögren's syndrome
- Other forms of lacrimal gland disease
- Aging
- Inflammatory diseases (e.g., HIV, sarcoidosis, lymphoma, GVH disease)
- Lacrimal gland duct obstruction from various forms of cicatrizing
- Conjunctivitis
- Corneal surgery
- Diabetes mellitus
- Chronic contact lens wear
- Loss of lacrimal secretory motor function
- Drugs (e.g., antihistamines, beta-blockers, antispasmodics, diuretics)
- Central 7th nerve damage

(GVH: graft-versus-host)

BOX 2	Differential diagnosis of dry mouth.
• Drug side effects (drugs with anticholinergic, diuretic, anti-hypertensive, anxiolytic, or antihistamine effects)	
• Salivary gland diseases, including Sjögren's syndrome	
• Poorly controlled diabetes mellitus	
• Dehydration	
• Mouth breathing and nasal obstruction	
• Head and neck irradiation (including high doses of radioactive iodine for thyroid cancer)	
• Psychological factors	

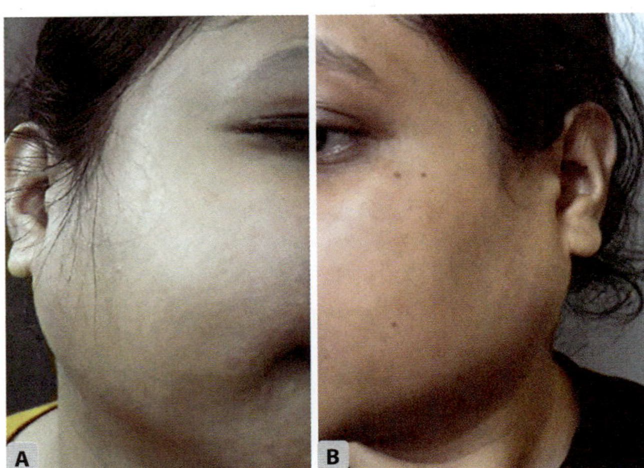

FIGURES 4 A & B: Parotid glands enlargement.

EXTRAGLANDULAR INVOLVEMENT

Extraglandular manifestations affect the majority of patients with SS which include fatigue, arthralgias, myalgias, and mild cognitive dysfunction. Clinically, significant involvement of nonglandular organ systems occurs in around 25% of primary SS. Dry skin (xerosis) and associated pruritus are common when skin is involved. Small-vessel vasculopathies are manifested by purpura (**Fig. 5**) and those of larger blood vessels by livedo reticularis and leg ulcers.

Nonerosive inflammatory polyarthritis: It occurs in up to 30% of patients with SS, mostly affecting the fingers, wrists, and ankles. Severe forms of arthritis may occur when SS overlaps with another systemic rheumatic disease such as RA (**Box 4**).

Pulmonary disease: It affects 10–20% of patients of SS. Both the upper and lower airways can be involved. Nonspecific, usual, and lymphocytic forms of interstitial pneumonitis [nonspecific interstitial pneumonia (NSIP), usual interstitial pneumonia (UIP), and lymphoid interstitial pneumonia (LIP)] and cryptogenic organizing pneumonia (COP) may be seen and are usually manifested as dyspnea and cough. Liver disease occurs in up to 20% of patients with SS; the usual forms being primary biliary cirrhosis and autoimmune hepatitis.

Tubulointerstitial nephritis: It is most common in patients with renal involvement in SS. It tends to occur in younger

BOX 3	Causes of salivary gland enlargement.
Infectious:	
• Viral infections (mumps, Epstein–Barr, hepatitis C, HIV)	
• Bacterial infections (suppurative parotitis, tuberculosis)	
• Fungal infections	
Autoimmune:	
• Sjögren's syndrome	
• Granulomatosis with polyangiitis	
Inflammatory:	
• IgG4-related disease	
• Allergic parotitis	
• Chronic recurrent parotitis	
• Kimura disease	
Metabolic:	
• Sialadenosis—soft, nontender, and bilaterally symmetric	
• Uncontrolled diabetes mellitus	
• Bulimia	
• Alcoholism with liver disease	
• Hyperlipoproteinemia	
Neoplastic:	
• Lymphoma	
• Leukemia	
• Warthin tumor	
Granulomatous:	
• Sarcoidosis	
Iatrogenic or occupational:	
• Radioactive iodine	
• Pneumoparotitis (wind instrument players, glass blowers)	

(IgG4: immunoglobulin G4)

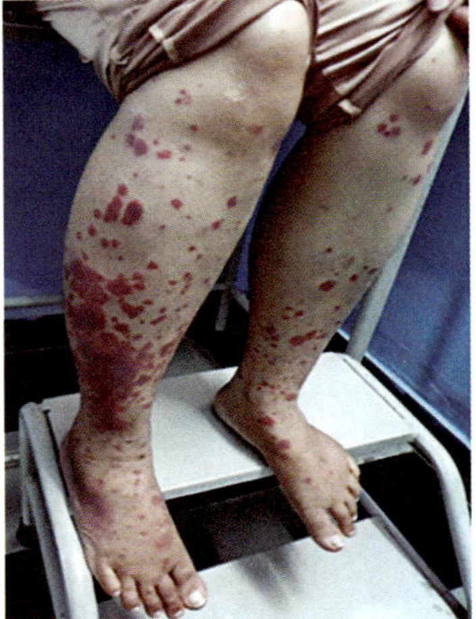

FIGURE 5: Palpable purpura in a patient of Sjögren's syndrome.

patients manifesting as polyuria, renal colic, or tubular proteinuria. Distal (type I) renal tubular acidosis can present with inability of the distal nephron to acidify the urine. Both central nervous system (CNS) and peripheral

BOX 4 Systemic manifestations of Sjögren's syndrome.

Constitutional:
- Fatigue
- Arthralgia

Musculoskeletal:
- Polyarthritis
- Myositis

Renal:
- Tubulointerstitial nephritis
- Glomerulonephritis

Neurologic:
- Peripheral neuropathy
- Neuromyelitis optica

Cutaneous:
- Vasculitis
- Subacute cutaneous lupus
- Annular erythema

Endocrine:
- Association with autoimmune thyroiditis

Hepatic:
- Association with primary biliary cirrhosis and autoimmune hepatitis

Pulmonary:
- Airway disease—bronchiolitis and bronchiectasis
- Interstitial pneumonitis

Lymphoproliferative lesions

Hematologic:
- Leukopenia, anemia, and thrombocytopenia
- Hypergammaglobulinemia and cryoglobulinemia
- Monoclonal gammopathy

nervous system involvement may occur in SS. Peripheral neuropathy is seen in approximately 10–20% of patients—most common being a pure sensory neuropathy. Axonal sensorimotor polyneuropathy is usually associated with systemic disease including vasculitis, monoclonal proteins, and lymphoma. CNS disease in SS is commonly characterized by memory loss, cognitive dysfunction, headache, or mood disorders.

Autoimmune thyroiditis: It is present in approximately 15–30% of patients with SS. Vasculitis affects 10% of patients with SS and most often involves small blood vessels of the skin, peripheral nerves, and kidneys. Biopsy specimens of purpuric or urticarial skin lesions show leukocytoclastic vasculitis. Cutaneous vasculitis is associated with anti-SSA antibodies. Anemia, leukopenia (usually neutropenia), and thrombocytopenia each occur in up to 20% of patients. Hypergammaglobulinemia is found in 20–40% in SS, which correlates with the presence of anti-Ro/SSA and anti-La/SSB antibodies. They may be at higher risk for B-cell lymphoma.

TABLE 1 ACR/EULAR classification criteria for primary Sjögren's syndrome.

Items	Weight/ Score
Labial salivary gland with focal lymphocytic sialadenitis and focus score of ≥one foci/4 mm	3
Anti-SSA/Ro positive	3
Ocular staining score ≥5 (or Van Bijsterveld score ≥4) in at least one eye	4
Schirmer test ≤5 mm/5 min in at least one eye	1
Unstimulated whole saliva flow rate ≤0.1 mL/min	1

(ACR: American College of Rheumatology; EULAR: European League Against Rheumatism)

LYMPHOMA

Patients with SS have a 6- to 19-fold increased risk for the development of B-cell NHL. MALT lymphoma, a marginal zone B-cell lymphoma, is the most common type. The risk is generally higher for secondary than for primary SS and exceeds that of any other autoimmune disease. The development of lymphoma is often heralded by persistent enlargement of the salivary or lacrimal glands or a new mass within one of the glands. Affected patients frequently have extraglandular features—splenomegaly, lymphadenopathy, neutropenia, cryoglobulinemia, or low C4. In a study, the prevalence of NHL was determined to be 4.3% with a median time of approximately 7.5 years from the diagnosis of primary SS.

CLASSIFICATION CRITERIA

The American College of Rheumatology (ACR) and European League Against Rheumatism (EULAR) jointly released a classification criteria for primary SS (2016), designed for classifying individuals for enrollment in clinical trials. The criteria had 96% sensitivity and 95% specificity for SS. The classification of primary SS applies to any individual who meets the inclusion criteria, does not have any of the conditions listed as exclusion criteria, and has a score of ≥4 when the weights from the five criteria items are summed (**Table 1**). SS in children can occur at any age. Persistent or recurrent parotitis and arthralgia are common symptoms; may not fulfill the 2016 classification criteria at the time of presentation.

INCLUSION CRITERIA

Inclusion criteria are applicable to any patient with at least one symptom of ocular or oral dryness, defined as a positive response to at least one of the following questions:

- Have you had daily, persistent, and troublesome dry eyes for >3 months?
- Do you have a recurrent sensation of sand or gravel in the eyes?
- Do you use tear substitutes more than three times a day?
- Have you had a daily feeling of dry mouth for >3 months?
- Do you frequently drink liquids to aid in swallowing dry food?

EXCLUSION CRITERIA

- History of head and neck radiation treatment
- Active hepatitis C infection (with confirmation by polymerase chain reaction)
- Acquired immunodeficiency syndrome (AIDS)
- Sarcoidosis
- Amyloidosis
- Graft-versus-host disease
- Immunoglobulin G4-related disease

DIAGNOSTIC EVALUATION

The diagnosis of SS is most often established with an objective measure of ocular dryness or salivary hypofunction along with the evidence of underlying autoimmunity. Antinuclear antibodies (ANAs) and rheumatoid factors (RFs) are positive in >50% of the patients with primary SS. ANA profile will show the presence of anti-Ro/SSA and anti-La/SSB antibodies (**Fig. 6**).

OPHTHALMOLOGIC EXAMINATION

The ophthalmologic examination includes an assessment of tear production (**Schirmer test**) and ocular surface staining. The latter offers the greatest utility for the diagnosis of dry eye disease and is typically performed with lissamine green (for the conjunctiva) and fluorescein (for the cornea). With a slit-lamp examination, the ophthalmologist can carefully examine the ocular surface evaluating for any signs of damage. The fluorescein dye stains corneal epithelium stroma revealing the defects, whereas lissamine green stains devitalized conjunctival cells. The Schirmer test measures the 5-minute wetting of a standardized strip of filter paper placed in the lower lateral fornix of the eyelid and serves as an indicator of basal (anesthetized) or stimulated (unanesthetized) tear flow (**Fig. 7**). The unanesthetized Schirmer test is supportive of SS when wetting measures 5 mm or less in either eye.

SALIVARY GLANDS

Measurement of salivary flow for glands hypofunction is done either with or without stimulation. The whole "unstimulated" saliva flow rate, relevant to oral health, correlates best with xerostomia. It arises primarily from the submandibular and sublingual glands. The patient should not have eaten chewed gum or drank water for the preceding 90 minutes. The saliva is emptied every minute into a preweighed cup for a period of 5–15 minutes. The volume of saliva is determined by weight, with the specific gravity assumed to be 1 g/mL and <0.1 mL/min being considered abnormal.

Saliva secretion after an olfactory, gustatory, or masticatory stimulus is larger in volume, involves the parotid glands, and facilitates eating. Whole "stimulated" saliva production can be measured by expectoration or suction of saliva produced after the patient chews gum for a period of 5–15 minutes or has taken pilocarpine 60 minutes earlier. Levels lower than 0.7 mL/min define salivary hypofunction. Latest imaging modalities to assess salivary gland structure include contrast-enhanced sialography, MRI, ultrasonography, and salivary gland scintigraphy.

LABIAL GLAND BIOPSY

Labial salivary gland biopsy is essential for definitive evaluation of patients with suspected SS who lack anti-Ro/anti-La antibodies. Additionally, it may provide useful prognostic information on all patients with SS and establish alternative diagnoses including amyloidosis, sarcoidosis, IgG4-related disease, and lymphoma. Focal lymphocytic sialadenitis is characteristic of SS and defined by the presence of tightly aggregated clusters or foci of lymphocytes containing 50 or more cells. The number of lymphocytic foci normalized to 4 mm^2 of glandular section area is termed the focus score. A score of 1 focus per 4 mm^2 or higher correlates strongly with SS.

Results from:

Antigen	Intensity	Class
RNP/Sm (RNP/Sm)	0	o
Sm (Sm)	0	o
SS-A native (60 kDa) (SSA)	76	+++
Ro-52 recombinant (52)	103	+++
SS-B (SSB)	10	(+)
Scl-70 (Scl)	1	o
PM-Scl100 (PM100)	1	o
Jo-1 (Jo)	1	o
Centromere B (CB)	0	o
PCNA (PCNA)	0	o
dsDNA (DNA)	4	o
Nucleosomes (NUC)	0	o
Histones (Hi)	0	o
Ribosomal-P-protein (RIB)	2	o
AMA-M2 (M2)	1	o
Control (Co)	88	+++
Label (La)		

Class	Explanation
o	Negative
(+)	Borderline
+	Positive
++	Positive
+++	Strong positive

(ANA: antinuclear antibody; dsDNA: double-stranded deoxyribonucleic acid)

FIGURE 6: ANA profile showing anti-Ro/SSA and Ro52 antibodies.

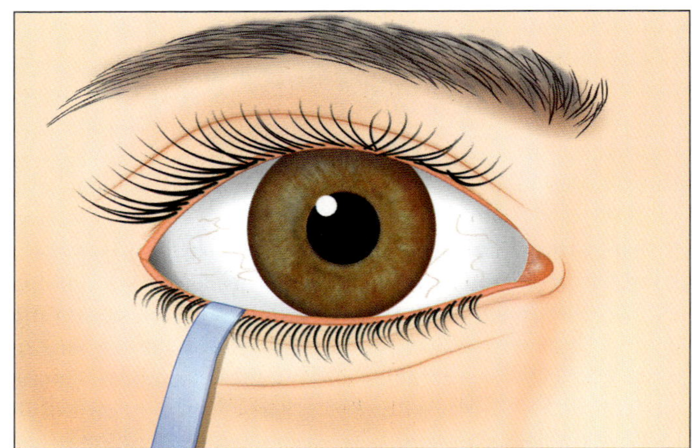

FIGURE 7: Schematic representation of Schirmer tear test.

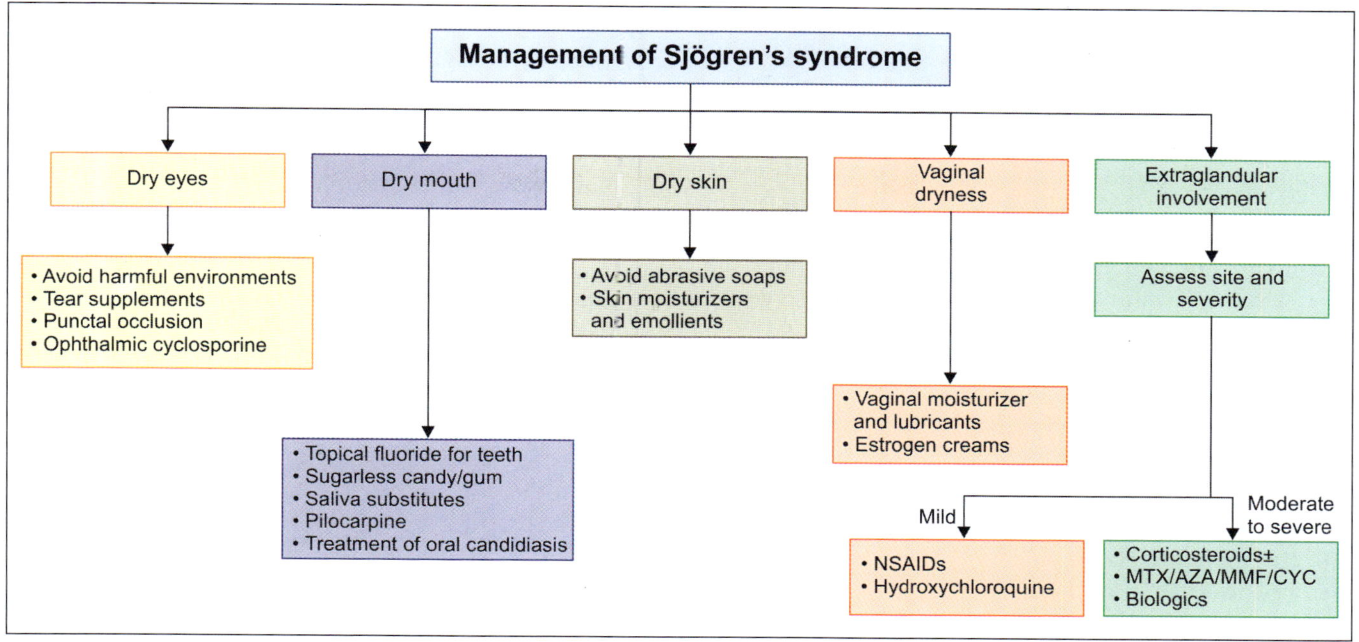

(AZA: azathioprine; CYC: cyclophosphamide; MMF: mycophenolate mofetil; MTX: methotrexate; NSAIDs: nonsteroidal anti-inflammatory drugs)

FLOWCHART 1: Flowchart for the management of Sjögren's syndrome.

MANAGEMENT

Management of primary SS requires multidisciplinary approach by ophthalmologist, pulmonologist, rheumatologist, dental surgeon, and family physician (**Flowchart 1**).

GLANDULAR DISEASE

Patients should maintain adequate hydration and avoid hot and dry environments. Smoking cigarettes is discouraged. The use of any drugs with anticholinergic properties should be minimized or replaced. For mild dry *eye disease*, preserved artificial tears up to four times and for more severe disease, preservative-free artificial tears more than four times along with topical gel or ointment at bedtime are advised. Ocular inflammation can be suppressed with short courses of topical steroids and prolonged use of topical cyclosporine. Punctal plugs or cauterization will preserve existing tears and systemic secretagogues may augment tear volume. Additional measures include autologous serum tears, scleral prostheses, moisture goggles, and rarely surgery such as partial tarsorrhaphy. Any infections in the eye should be treated promptly.

Patients with *dry mouth* are advised to sip water or sugar-free fluids frequently. Secretion of saliva can be stimulated by chewing sugar-free gum or xylitol-containing lozenges. Saliva replacement and oral lubrication can be achieved with artificial saliva, sprays, and gels. Pilocarpine, a muscaranic agonist, increases salivary flow rates and improves symptoms of oral and ocular dryness. Side effects may include sweating, nausea, and urinary frequency. It is contraindicated in patients with uncontrolled asthma, narrow-angle glaucoma, and iritis. Fluoride toothpaste may be used to prevent dental caries. Concomitant therapy with calcium and phosphate remineralizing agents may also be helpful. Treatment of oral candidiasis relieves intraoral burning and angular cheilitis. Oral fluconazole is one of the drugs of choice for the same.

Immunomodulating agents including hydroxychloroquine, azathioprine, IFN-α, cyclosporine, methotrexate, and mycophenolate mofetil had disappointing results in open trials. Glucocorticoids can be effective in treating parotid gland swelling, but their side effects discourage long-term use. Biologic agents have the potential to be clinically efficacious based on their mode of action. The tumor necrosis factor (TNF) antagonists—infliximab and etanercept—did not show benefit in short-duration placebo-controlled trials. Rituximab, a CD20 antibody, may augment salivary flow in patients with preserved gland function at baseline. Rituximab was effective in relieving marked salivary and lacrimal gland enlargement in a retrospective review. Vaginal dryness and dyspareunia are treated with lubricants and moisturizers.

EXTRAGLANDULAR DISEASE

Arthritis is initially treated with hydroxychloroquine with or without nonsteroidal antiinflammatory drugs (NSAIDs). More severe disease may require low-dose glucocorticoids, methotrexate, leflunomide, TNF antagonists, or rituximab. Fatigue is treated with attention to concomitant depression, fibromyalgia, and sleep disorders. Rituximab showed possible benefit in reducing fatigue in a randomized clinical trial and abatacept in an open-label trial.

Distal renal tubular acidosis (RTA) is treated with bicarbonate or citrate salts to control the acidosis and prevent the formation of renal stones. Glucocorticoids are the first-line treatment and may suffice for LIP or organizing pneumonia. Azathioprine, mycophenolate mofetil, and cyclophosphamide can be used as steroid-sparing agents. The nonvasculitic peripheral and cranial neuropathies are managed first with tricyclic antidepressants or antiepileptics (e.g., gabapentin, pregabalin, carbamazepine). Vasculitic neuropathies are usually treated with glucocorticoids, cyclophosphamide, or rituximab. Cutaneous vasculitis may not require pharmacologic treatment when manifested as mild intermittent purpura. Support stockings and avoidance of prolonged standing may suffice. More severe flares may require moderate dose of glucocorticoids.

CONCLUSION

Sjögren's syndrome is a common autoimmune disease affecting exocrine glands including lacrimal and salivary glands. Clinically, it is characterized by dry eyes and dry mouth and sometimes with extraglandular systemic manifestations. SS can be alone (primary SS) or can be associated with another autoimmune disease such as RA (secondary SS). Serologically, it is characterized by the presence of autoantibodies to anti-Ro/SSA and anti-La/SSB. Lymphocytic infiltration in the salivary gland biopsy is hallmark of the disease. Management includes symptomatic treatment for glandular disease and corticosteroids, disease-modifying immunomodulators, or biologics for systemic disease.

RECOMMENDED READINGS

1. Mariette X. Sjögren syndrome. In: Goldman L, Schafer A (Eds). Goldman-Cecil Medicine, 25th edition. Philadelphia: Elsevier Saunders; 2016. pp. 1785-8.
2. Shiboski CH, Shiboski SC, Seror R, Criswell LA, Labetoulle M, Lietman TM, et al. 2016 American College of Rheumatology/European League Against Rheumatism Classification Criteria for Primary Sjögren's Syndrome: A Consensus and Data-Driven Methodology Involving Three International Patient Cohorts. Arthritis Rheumatol. 2017;69:35-45.
3. Clair SW. Sjögren's syndrome. In: Firestein G (Ed). Kelley & Firestein's Textbook of Rheumatology, 10th edition. Philadelphia: Elsevier; 2017. pp. 1221-44.
4. Vivino F. Sjögren's syndrome: clinical aspects. Clin Immunol. 2017;182:48-54.
5. Porkodi R. Sjögren's syndrome. In: Chaturvedi V (Ed). Manual of Rheumatology, 5th edition. New Delhi: CBS Publishers & Distributors; 2018. pp. 391-7.
6. Baer A, Alevizos I. Sjögren syndrome. In: Hochberg M (Ed). Rheumatology, 7th edition. Philadelphia: Elsevier; 2019. pp. 1205-20.
7. Kumar U, Dasgupta S. Sjögren's syndrome. In: Kamat S (Ed). API Textbook of Medicine, 11th edition. New Delhi: CBS Publishers & Distributors; 2019. pp. 540-2.
8. Basiaga ML, Stern SM, Mehta JJ, Edens C, Randell RL, Pomorska A, et al. Childhood Sjögren syndrome: features of an international cohort and application of the 2016 ACR/EULAR classification criteria. Rheumatology (Oxford). 2020:keaa757 [Online ahead of print].

CHAPTER 238

Mixed Connective Tissue Disease and Overlap Syndromes

Debashish Mishra, Shefali K Sharma

ABSTRACT

Overlap syndromes are diseases with features of two or more defined rheumatic diseases in the same patient. Mixed connective tissue disease (MCTD) is the best defined overlap syndrome, having various classification criteria for its identification. Initially thought to be mild disease, current knowledge disregards this, as MCTD can have serious organ manifestations such as interstitial lung disease (ILD) and pulmonary arterial hypertension (PAH). Even arthritis and myositis can be disabling in these patients.

Similarly, there can be overlap between rheumatic diseases and other autoimmune diseases such as primary biliary cirrhosis, autoimmune hepatitis, Graves' disease, Hashimoto's thyroiditis etc. Multiple autoantibodies positivity can be seen in these patients, but, whether they are truly pathogenic or mere coexistent is still unknown. Some of these antibodies help to identify and define the underlying autoimmune disease.

Treatment decisions in these patients are based on organ involvement. Some features such as ILD, PAH, nephritic syndrome, and central nervous system (CNS) involvement require aggressive immunosuppression. Most of the clinical manifestations are treatment responsive; however, at times, it can be refractory as well.

"The art of simplicity is a puzzle of complexity"

—Douglas Horton

INTRODUCTION

Mixed connective tissue disease is an overlap syndrome with defined clinical and serological features. Organ involvement can be severe in MCTD requiring aggressive management. It is important to identify various overlap syndromes occurring in the patient for directed treatment.

Overlap connective tissue diseases or syndromes are the ones, which have clinical features of two or more different connective tissue diseases. The classic example of an overlap syndrome is MCTD which has features of different connective tissue diseases. MCTD has a defined set of criteria to classify for clinical research purposes; however, same is not true for other overlap syndromes which are mainly classified or diagnosed based on purely clinical and serological characteristics. In this chapter, a brief description is given on various overlap syndromes with special attention to MCTD in detail.

MIXED CONNECTIVE TISSUE DISEASE

First described by Sharp et al. in 1972 as an overlap disease with features of systemic lupus erythematosus (SLE), systemic sclerosis, inflammatory myositis, and rheumatoid arthritis (RA) with antibodies against U1 small nuclear ribonucleoprotein (U1 snRNP) particle. Initially thought to be a mild disease, MCTD has now been studied well and is no longer considered a benign disease. In some patients, MCTD can have major organ involvement such as lungs (ILD), heart [pulmonary hypertension (PH)], and kidneys (membranous nephritis) with guarded prognosis.

CLINICAL FEATURES

Raynaud's phenomenon (RP), arthritis, myositis, esophageal dysmotility, and fever are some of the common initial presentations of MCTD. On evaluation, clinically silent pulmonary/cardiovascular involvement can be identified in some patients.

RAYNAUD'S PHENOMENON

One of the most common clinical manifestations of MCTD is RP seen in >90% of patients. RP is triphasic color changes seen in pulp of fingers on cold exposure or with intense emotional stimulus. On cold exposure, initial vasoconstriction of cutaneous capillaries gives a whitish hue to the pulp of fingers (ischemic or pallor phase), followed by bluish (deoxygenated phase) and later on reperfusion, it becomes red (reperfusion phase). In Indian patients, all three color changes may not be appreciated. Presence of pallor phase is enough to suggest RP.

Raynaud's phenomenon can be divided into two types: (1) Primary and (2) Secondary (**Table 1**).

Although RP in MCTD is less severe than that seen in scleroderma, some of the patients can develop digital ulcers, pitted scars, or acro-osteolysis. Severity of RP can be an indicator to underlying systemic vasculopathy such as PH. Presence of anti-U1RNP is associated with such vasculopathic manifestations such as RP and PH. In patients presenting with RP as initial manifestation, nailfold capillaroscopy (NFC) can distinguish between primary and secondary RP. Abnormal NFC findings such as giant capillaries, capillary loss or dropouts, hemorrhages, and abnormal architecture, or in late stages, severe capillary loss with avascular areas is suggestive of secondary RP.

MUSCULOSKELETAL

The next most common manifestation in MCTD is arthritis seen in 75–95% of patients. It is polyarticular involvement with up to 50% showing erosive arthritis (unlike SLE). Patients can also develop deformities such as RA. Presence of anti-U1RNP, rheumatoid factor (RF), and HLA-DR4 increases the severity of arthritis.

Another important clinical manifestation of MCTD is myositis similar to idiopathic inflammatory myositis (more commonly dermatomyositis than polymyositis). It presents as proximal muscle weakness of subacute to chronic onset, without pain and tenderness in the muscle. The severity can vary from mild to severe (with oropharyngeal, neck flexors, or respiratory muscle involvement). Two-thirds of patients

TABLE 1 Differences between primary and secondary RP.

Points of difference	Primary RP	Secondary RP
Age of onset	15–30 years	More than 40 years
Frequency of attacks	Episodic	More frequent
Symmetricity	Symmetric involvement	Asymmetric involvement (may start with one finger and progress)
Sequelae	None	Digital ulcers, pitted scars, digital necrosis, gangrene, or autoamputation
Disease association	None	Mostly rheumatic diseases; others such as drug-induced, hematological, and vascular diseases. Can be occupational as well
Autoantibody	None	ANA positivity in rheumatic disease. Other extractable nuclear antigen such as U1RNP and anti-Ro/La can be positive as well in specific diseases
NFC	Normal	Abnormal

(RP: Raynaud's phenomenon; NFC: nailfold capillaroscopy)

with MCTD can have clinically evident myositis. Myositis in MCTD is more steroid responsive than idiopathic inflammatory myositis.

PULMONARY

Involvement of lung in MCTD is most commonly seen as ILD, which is clinically evident in 40–50% of patients; however, on high-resolution computed tomography (HRCT), up to 78% can have ILD. The most common ILD pattern seen in MCTD is nonspecific interstitial pneumonia (NSIP) followed by usual interstitial pneumonia (UIP) and lymphocytic interstitial pneumonia (LIP).

Pleuritis and pleural effusion can be other manifestations of MCTD in the lung.

CARDIOVASCULAR

Pulmonary hypertension is most important cardiovascular involvement in MCTD. Based on various cutoffs used to define pulmonary artery systolic pressure, the prevalence of PH in MCTD can vary from 3.4 to as high as 50%. Use of different diagnostic modalities (right heart catheterization vs. echocardiography) as well affects the prevalence rate reported.

Pulmonary hypertension in MCTD can be either group-1 due to PAH, group-2 due to preexisting left heart disease, group-3 due to underlying lung disease (ILD), group-4 due to chronic thromboembolic process, or group-5 due to multiple factors or undefined mechanisms. Currently, patients with right ventricular systolic pressure > 25 mm Hg on echocardiography are subjected to right heart catheterization for confirmation of PAH. Presence of anti-U1RNP, antiphospholipid antibodies, and antiendothelial cell antibodies are postulated to have pathogenic role in causing vasculopathy and PAH in MCTD. Presence of RP and abnormal NFC correlates with presence of PAH in MCTD. Prognosis of patients with PAH in MCTD is poorer as compared to those without PAH or other CTD [such as RA, SLE, or systemic sclerosis (SSc)] with PAH or those with idiopathic PAH. Screening of all patients with MCTD for PH is recommended.

Other cardiac involvement can be pericarditis, diastolic dysfunction, accelerated atherosclerosis, myocarditis, or rarely conduction disturbances.

CUTANEOUS

Apart from RP, other characteristic cutaneous features seen in MCTD are puffy fingers and thickening of skin over fingers (sclerodactyly) (**Figs. 1 A** to **C**). Sequelae of RP such as digital ulcers, pitted scars, gangrene, pulp loss, and acro-osteolysis can be seen as well.

Other cutaneous features such as photosensitive rash over trunk and extremities, malar rash, livedoid rash, calcinosis, vasculitic lesions etc., can also be seen in patients with MCTD.

ESOPHAGEAL

This is another common clinical feature in patients with MCTD presenting mostly as gastroesophageal reflux disease (GERD) due to lax lower esophageal sphincter. Esophageal dysmotility is also known to occur in these patients. Esophageal manometry is advised for early detection of dysmotility. Those with severe dysmotility and esophageal dilatation are at increased risk of ILD.

NEUROLOGICAL

Involvement of CNS or higher cognitive functions is rare in MCTD. The most common neurological involvement

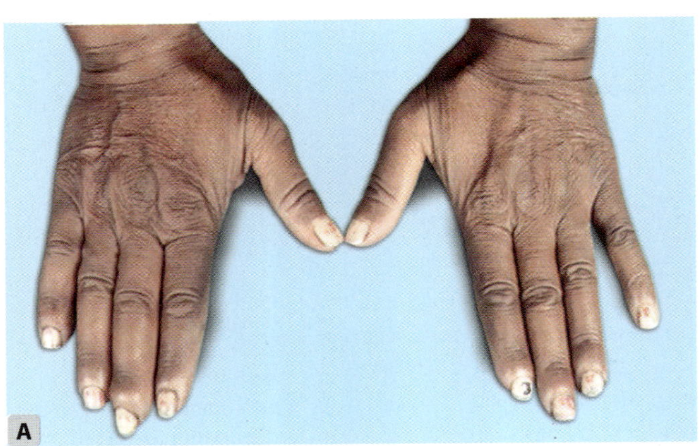

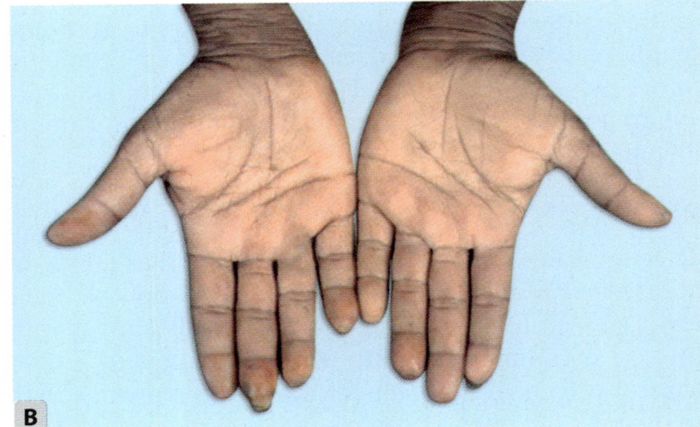

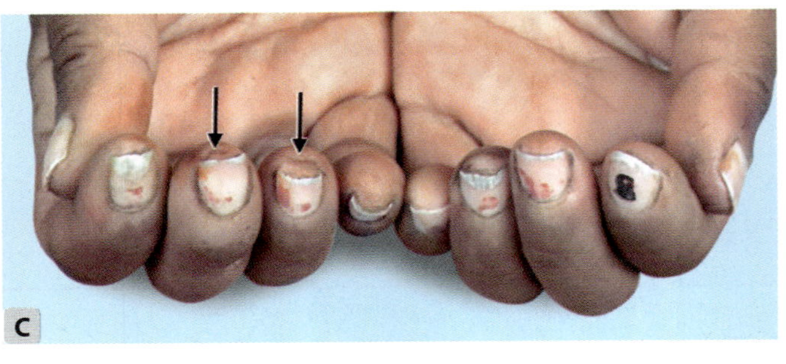

FIGURES 1 A to C: (A) Sclerodactyly in a patient with mixed connective tissue disease (MCTD) (note taut and glistening skin with tapered fingers); **(B)** Palmar aspect of same patient showing pulp loss and tapered digits; and **(C)** Fingertips of same patient showing pitted scars, which are sequelae of Raynaud's phenomenon (black arrows).

is trigeminal neuralgia. Apart from it, headache, seizure, aseptic meningitis, and peripheral neuropathy have been described with MCTD.

RENAL

Unlike SLE, presence of proliferative nephritis is rare in MCTD. Renal involvement in MCTD is commonly seen as membranous glomerulonephritis followed by mesangial glomerulonephritis.

HEMATOLOGICAL

Anemia, commonly seen in MCTD, could be hemolytic or nonhemolytic (due to chronic disease). Both Coombs positive as well as negative hemolytic anemia can occur in MCTD. Leukopenia and thrombocytopenia have as well been described in MCTD.

MISCELLANEOUS

As with other connective tissue diseases, fatigue, myalgia, fever (at times high grade), psychological distress, depression, and sleep disturbances have been described in MCTD.

INVESTIGATIONS

SEROLOGY

Antinuclear antibody (ANA) is positive in almost 100% of patients with MCTD. The most typical pattern of ANA seen is coarse speckled.

The characteristic antibody anti-U1RNP is seen in >90% of patients with MCTD; however, it is not specific to MCTD and is also seen with other connective tissue diseases such as SLE (20–40%), SSc (2–14%), and idiopathic inflammatory myositis (6–9%). Generally, the anti-U1RNP antibodies found in MCTD is immunoglobulin G (IgG) isotype and in high titers (in contrast to SLE where it is mostly IgM and low titers).

IMAGING

High-resolution computed tomography is advised to rule out ILD in patients with suggestive symptoms. The pattern and extent of involvement can as well be seen on HRCT (**Fig. 2**). Those with extensive involvement or fibrosis portend a grave prognosis.

Transthoracic two-dimensional (2D) echocardiography is recommended in all patients with MCTD to screen for PAH. Those having suspicion of PAH on echocardiography are further confirmed by right heart catheterization.

Barium swallow and esophageal manometry are means to diagnose and assess esophageal involvement in these patients. In patients with isolated RP, NFC can be done to look for capillaries structure and arrangement. Those with abnormal NFC need further evaluation to rule out connective tissue diseases.

Apart from above, routine hematological, biochemical, and urine analysis is done in all patients to look for various systemic involvement. Those with pulmonary involvement are also advised for spirometry to assess severity. Spirometry shows a restrictive pattern and serial assessments help to prognosticate patients.

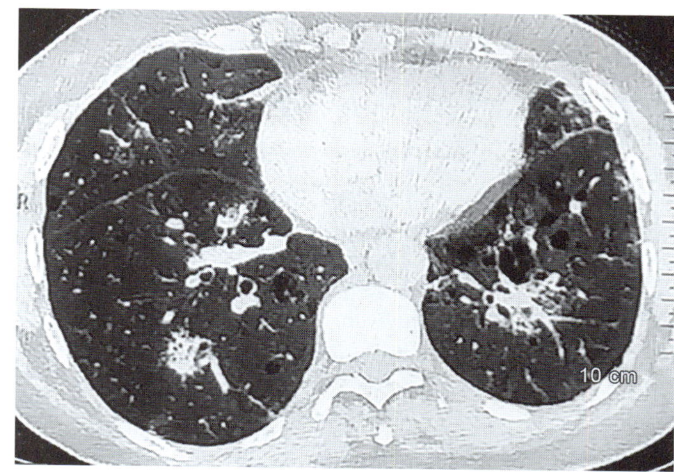

(HRCT: high-resolution computed tomography; MCTD: mixed connective tissue disease)

FIGURE 2: HRCT of the chest showing the presence of bilateral lung cysts and nodules with areas of patchy consolidation and ground-glass opacities suggestive of lymphocytic interstitial pneumonia (LIP) in a patient with MCTD.

CLASSIFICATION CRITERIA

The first set of criteria to classify and detect MCTD was given by Sharp et al. in 1987. After that, three more classification criteria have come. **Table 2** summarizes the Alarcón–Segovia and Kahn and Appeboom's criteria for MCTD. **Table 3** gives Kasukawa's criteria for MCTD.

Mixed connective tissue disease, being an overlap syndrome, needs follow-up to look for evolution into a defined CTD such as SLE or scleroderma. It is seen that on long-term follow-up, 17% evolve into SSc, 9% evolve into SLE, and 2.5% evolve into RA.

Studies from Indian cohorts of connective tissue diseases show that occurrence of MCTD is rare in India. However, use of different criteria to classify patients in a study also affects the prevalence. Study conducted by Lawrence et al. concluded that Kasukawa's criteria were most sensitive to diagnose MCTD. In their study, 16 patients out of 441 patients satisfied Kasukawa's criteria and at least one of the other two (Sharp's criteria or Alarcón–Segovia criteria). Another study by Dhir et al. described the clinical and serological profile of 41 MCTD patients. In their series, up to 50% patients were initially (mis)diagnosed as either RA, SLE, undifferentiated connective tissue disease (UCTD), myositis, or overlap syndrome. Apart from anti-U1RNP, they also reported up to 50% prevalence of anti-SSA and Ro52 antibodies in their cohort. Long-term follow-up data of Indian MCTD patients is lacking.

TREATMENT

Corticosteroids and immunosuppressive medications form the core of treatment armamentarium for MCTD. For

TABLE 2 Alarcón–Segovia and Kahn and Appeboom's criteria for MCTD.

Serology	Clinical	Diagnosis
Alarcón–Segovia criteria		
Positive anti-U1RNP at hemagglutination titer > 1:1600	• Edema of hands • Synovitis • Myositis (biopsy or laboratory proven) • Raynaud's phenomenon • Acrosclerosis	To make a diagnosis of MCTD, serology criteria are satisfied along with three or more clinical features (one of which must be synovitis or myositis)
Kahn and Appeboom's criteria		
High titers of anti-RNP antibodies corresponding to a speckled ANA titer of ≥1:2,000	• Raynaud's phenomenon • Swollen hands • Myositis • Synovitis	MCTD is diagnosed if serology criteria are present along with Raynaud's phenomenon and at least two other clinical features

(RNP: ribonucleoprotein)

TABLE 3 Kasukawa's criteria for MCTD.

Common symptoms	Symptoms of SLE, SSc, and PM	Serology
• Raynaud's phenomenon • Swollen fingers	**SLE:** • Polyarthritis • Lymphadenopathies • Malar rash • Serositis • Leukopenia and/or thrombocytopenia	Anti-snRNP antibodies
	SSc: • Sclerodactyly • Pulmonary fibrosis and/or restrictive changes and/or reduced DLCO on spirometry • Esophageal hypomotility or dilatation	
	PM: • Muscle weakness • Elevated muscle enzymes • Myogenic changes in EMG	
Diagnosis of MCTD if ≥1 common symptoms plus ≥1 manifestation in ≥2 of the defined connective tissue diseases such as SLE, SSc, or PM and the serologic criterion		

(DLCO: diffusing capacity for carbon monoxide; EMG: electromyogram; PM: polymyositis; RNP: ribonucleoprotein; SSc: systemic sclerosis)

arthritis and myositis, methotrexate is the first-line drug. If there is severe myositis, involvement of respiratory/oropharyngeal muscles or ILD intravenous cyclophosphamide pulses as induction can be given. Alternative to cyclophosphamide, mycophenolate mofetil, rituximab, or intravenous Ig can as well be given. After induction, patients have to be maintained for a relatively longer duration on methotrexate, azathioprine, or mycophenolate mofetil.

For management of PAH, apart from measures such as oxygen, diuretics etc., phosphodiesterase-5 (PDE-5) inhibitors (sildenafil, tadalafil), endothelin receptor antagonist (bosentan, ambrisentan), and prostanoids are needed. PAH associated with MCTD may respond to corticosteroids and immunosuppressant as well (unlike SSc). In case of severe PAH with functional limitations, operative measures such as atrial septostomy and lung transplant can be last resort.

Calcium channel blockers (nifedipine) are first-line treatment for RP. Other drugs such as PDE-5 inhibitors, prostacyclins, sympatholytic agent (prazosin), angiotensin II receptor type I blockers (losartan), selective serotonin reuptake inhibitor (fluoxetine), vasodilator (nitroglycerin), and pentoxifylline are used as add-on drugs (**Flowchart 1**). In refractory cases or with severe sequelae, selective digital sympathectomy can be tried.

Other manifestations such as esophageal dysmotility, acid reflux, trigeminal neuralgia, anemia, and constitutional symptoms need to be managed as in general cases.

PROGNOSIS

Initially thought to be a benign mild disease does not hold true for MCTD anymore. PAH is the leading cause of mortality in these patients. Other causes are ILD, coronary artery disease, infections, and malignancy. RP and esophageal dysmotility account for major morbidity in the initial years of disease onset. Later on, other organ involvement (ILD and PAH), treatment-related morbidities, and associated comorbidities (osteoporosis, fibromyalgia, and psychological distress) affect the quality of life. A holistic approach and multidisciplinary management can reduce most of these morbidities.

OVERLAP SYNDROMES

Apart from MCTD, there are other overlap syndromes which have defined clinical and/or serological features of two or more autoimmune diseases in the same patient. One-fourth of patients in the early stage have overlapping features, which on follow-up tend to progress to one of the defined CTD. Such overlap syndromes are also seen with autoimmune hepatic diseases such as autoimmune hepatitis, primary biliary cirrhosis, and primary sclerosing cholangitis.

At times, when the clinical features are not defined to suggest any CTD, the term "Undifferentiated" CTD or UCTD is used. Such patients also on follow-up develop a defined

First-line drugs: Dihydropyridine and CCBs (nifedipine, amlodipine) to start at low dose and titrate upward as per response Alternatives: PDE-5 inhibitors (tadalafil, sildenafil), ARB (losartan), SSRI (fluoxetine), and topical nitrate patch
↓
Second-line drugs: Add PDE-5 inhibitor or topical nitrate patch to CCBs Consider to add antiplatelet agent (low-dose aspirin), if there is digital ischemic lesions
↓
Third-line drugs: Prostanoids (iloprost, epoprostenol) or botulinum toxin injection or both for very severe RP with impending gangrene or refractory RP or repeated digital ischemic lesions Can also add ERA (ambrisentan, bosentan)
↓
Fourth-line drugs: Severe digital ischemia refractory to above treatments, consider selective digital sympathectomy

(ARB: angiotensin receptor blocker; CCBs: calcium channel blockers; ERA: endothelin receptor antagonist; PDE-5: phosphodiesterase-5; SSRI: selective serotonin reuptake inhibitor)

FLOWCHART 1: Management algorithm for Raynaud's phenomenon (RP).

Source: Adapted from Wigley FM, Flavahan NA. Raynaud's Phenomenon. N Engl J Med. 2016;375:556-65.

CTD or can remain as UCTD as well. Management in these cases is based on the clinical manifestations present.

MYOSITIS OVERLAP SYNDROME

This is one of the most common overlap syndromes seen with SSc or SLE. About 4–16% of SLE patients have myositis overlap. Antibodies present in such patients could be either myositis-associated autoantibodies (MAAs) or myositis-specific autoantibodies (MSAs). MSAs are important for classification and diagnosis of myositis. Other antibodies that can be present in myositis overlap syndromes are anti-U1RNP, anti-Ro/SSA, anti-La/SSB, anti-PM/Scl, anti-Ku, and anti-Th/To.

Myositis-specific autoantibodies are antisynthetase antibodies (anti-Jo-1, PL-7, PL-12, EJ, OJ, KS, Zo, and Ha), anti-MDA5, anti-TIF1γ, anti-NXP-2, anti-SAE, anti-Mi2, anti-SRP, and anti-HMGCR. MAAs can also coexist with MSAs.

SCLERODERMA OVERLAP SYNDROME

Overlap with scleroderma features such as skin thickening, sclerodactyly, and microstomia can occur with SLE, myositis, primary biliary cirrhosis, Hashimoto's thyroiditis, and very rarely with antineutrophil cytoplasmic antibody (ANCA) vasculitis. Patients with nucleolar ANA pattern generally have scleroderma overlap phenotype.

Another well-recognized overlap associated with limited type scleroderma is CREST (Calcinosis, Raynaud's phenomenon, Esophageal dysmotility, Sclerodactyly, Telangiectasia) syndrome and primary biliary cirrhosis (**Fig. 3**).

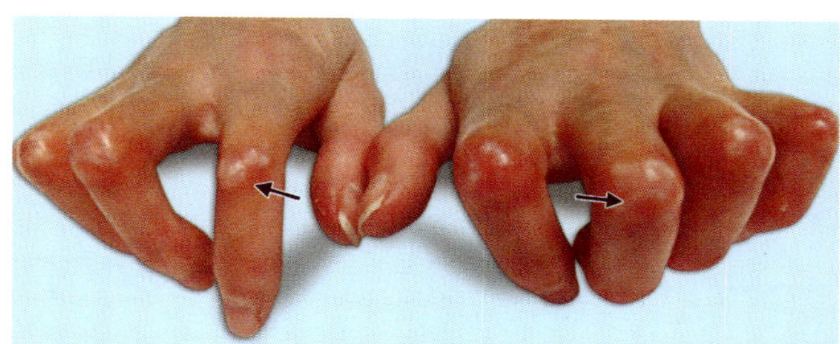

FIGURE 3: Contractures developed in a patient with Calcinosis, Raynaud's phenomenon, Esophageal dysmotility, Sclerodactyly, Telangiectasia (CREST) syndrome due to sclerodactyly. Also can be seen white calcinotic patches over proximal interphalangeal joints of both hands (black arrows).

SECONDARY SJÖGREN'S SYNDROME

Sjögren's syndrome is an autoimmune disorder primarily affecting lacrimal, salivary, and other exocrine glands. When it occurs solely, it is called primary and when associated with another rheumatic disease, it is called secondary. Very often, it is seen with RA, SLE, and SSc. Secondary Sjögren's syndrome is diagnosed based on clinical occurrence of subjective and objective evidence of dry eyes and mouth along with serological positivity for anti-Ro/La antibodies or histopathological confirmation of focus score ≥ 1 on minor salivary gland biopsy. The clinical relevance of anti-Ro/La antibodies does not lie on making a diagnosis of secondary Sjögren's syndrome because these antibodies are not specific for same. However, patients with these antibodies have higher chances of having fetuses with neonatal heart blocks. Hence, screening for same by fetal echocardiography is recommended after 18 weeks of gestation in patients with anti-Ro/La positivity. The chances of neonatal heart block increase with subsequent pregnancies, if one pregnancy is affected. Use of hydroxychloroquine has been only proven therapy to reduce occurrence of neonatal heart block.

RA AND SLE OVERLAP SYNDROME

The co-occurrence of RA and SLE has been termed as "rhupus". These patients have erosive arthritis (unlike SLE). Management depends, as with RA or SLE alone, on the organ involved by disease process.

OTHER OVERLAP SYNDROMES

Apart from the ones mentioned above, there can be other overlap syndromes as well like coexistence of primary biliary cirrhosis with SLE/CREST/RA/Sjögren's syndrome/polymyositis and also overlap between rheumatic diseases and autoimmune hepatitis.

CONCLUSION

Rheumatic diseases are very heterogeneous with varied clinical features and to complex this issue further, overlap syndromes manifest with two or more rheumatic diseases. It becomes crucial to address these overlapping features for wholesome treatment. Some of the features such as arthritis or myositis respond dramatically to treatment whereas some others such as ILD or PAH are refractory. Role of different autoantibodies, pathogenetic pathways, and genes is still unknown in overlap syndromes. Future may reveal many hidden mysteries in this unexplored area of rheumatic diseases.

RECOMMENDED READINGS

1. Chaigne B, Scirè CA, Talarico R, Alexander T, Amoura Z, Avcin T, et al. Mixed connective tissue disease: state of the art on clinical practice guidelines. RMD Open. 2018;4:e000783.
2. Ciang NC, Pereira N, Isenberg DA. Mixed connective tissue disease—enigma variations? Rheumatology. 2017;56:326-33.
3. Lawrence A, Aggarwal A, Misra R. MCTD: Is it rare in India? Clin Rheumatol. 2007;26:205-7.
4. Jury EC, D'Cruz D, Morrow WJ. Autoantibodies and overlap syndromes in autoimmune rheumatic disease. J Clin Path. 2001;54:340-7.
5. Iaccarino L, Gatto M, Bettio S, Caso F, Rampudda M, Zen M, et al. Overlap connective tissue disease syndromes. Autoimmun Rev. 2013;12:363-73.
6. Wigley FM, Flavahan NA. Raynaud's Phenomenon. N Engl J Med. 2016;375:556-65.

CHAPTER 239

Idiopathic Inflammatory Myopathies

Prithvi Sanjeevkumar Gaur, Latika Gupta

ABSTRACT

Idiopathic inflammatory myopathies (IIMs), popularly known as myositis, is a rare and relatively new rheumatic condition having multisystem involvement and a generalized presentation. This condition, being relatively new, lacks comprehensive literature; however, its increasing incidence in the world has piqued global interest. Multiple environmental and genetic predispositions have been hypothesized for this condition. It is classified in various ways based on its cutaneous manifestations, serum enzyme levels, and muscle involvement and biopsy findings. The patients commonly present with characteristic rashes, proximal muscle weakness, lung involvement, cardiac manifestations, malignancies, and esopharyngeal involvement in the form of dysphagia or hoarse voice.

The epidemiology studies show a bimodal prevalence of myositis. Further studies have uncovered the correlation of presence of various autoantibodies with its myopathic presentation. The various subtypes have different durations of onset and progressions. Dermatomyositis is said to have a slower progression rate than immune-mediated necrotizing myositis, which is said to be more acute. However, cases to prove otherwise have also been seen. Muscle biopsy findings are key to making an accurate diagnosis along with serum enzyme levels. MRI findings help to identify the muscle appropriate for a muscle biopsy. Generally, combination treatments of glucocorticoids (GCs) (prednisone: 1 mg/kg/day) along with other immunosuppressive agents such as azathioprine or methotrexate and intravenous immunoglobulins are adequate for remission. This chapter further discusses the epidemiology, classification, clinical features, diagnosis, and management of the disease.

"A disease causes two problems — a new disease and a newer disease"

—Anonymous

INTRODUCTION

Idiopathic inflammatory myopathies are a rare group of heterogeneous chronic systemic autoimmune disorders manifesting with muscle weakness accompanied by other organ system involvement, namely the lung, skin, heart, and joints. Wagner first documented myositis in 1863 with its cutaneous presentations. Later, the absence of skin manifestations in occasional cases with IIM was detected and reported. In 1891, Unverricht gave myositis its name describing its myopathy and dermatological involvement (**Fig. 1**).

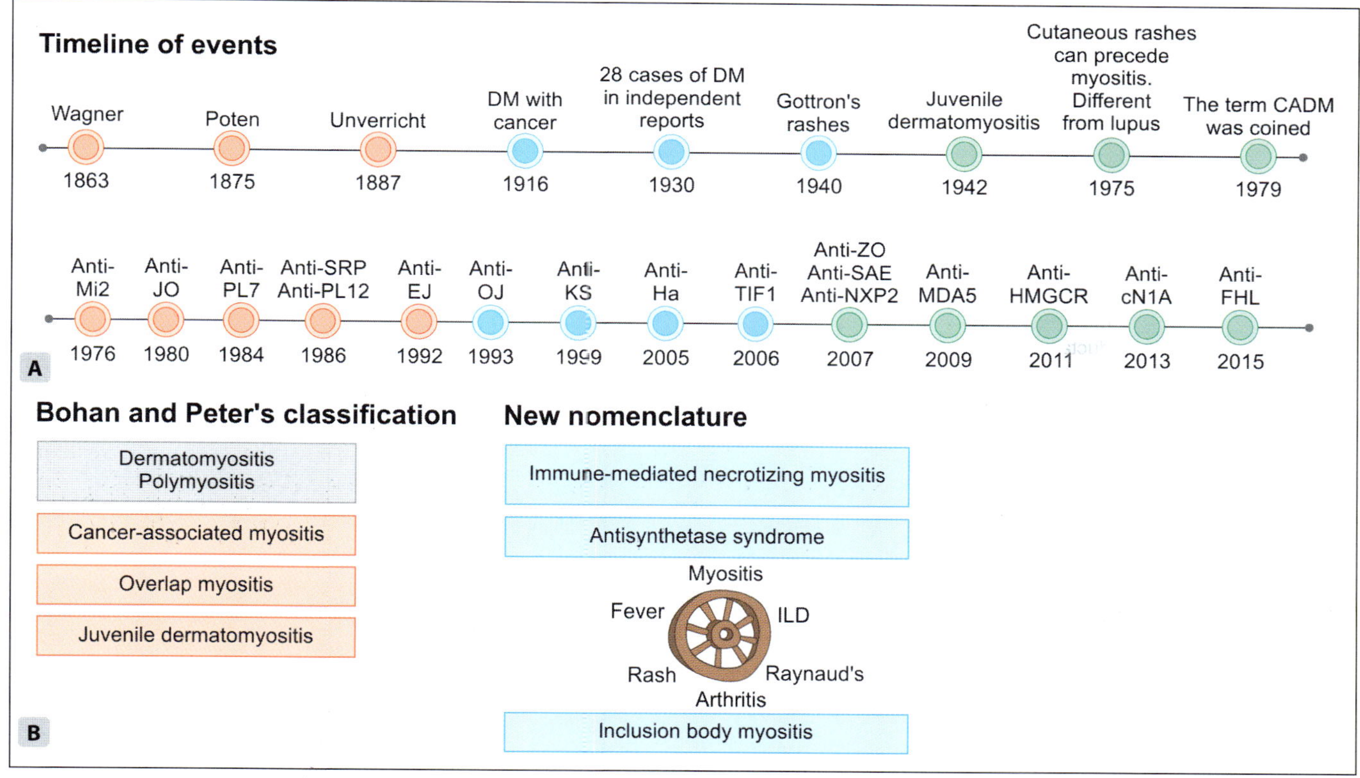

(ACR: American College of Rheumatology; CADM: clinically amyopathic dermatomyositis; EULAR: European League Against Rheumatism; ILD: interstitial lung disease; SRP: signal recognition particle)

FIGURES 1 A & B: History of discovery of the autoantibodies relevant to myositis along with the old (Bohan and Peter) and new (EULAR/ACR) classification of myositis. **(A)** The discovery and key milestones in the history of myositis along with the history of its nomenclature and the observance and hypothesis of correlation of various autoantibodies with myositis; and **(B)** The Peter and Bohan classification and the addition of other myositis manifestations as added in the new EULAR/ACR classification.

The heterogeneity of IIMs encompasses muscle weakness with rashes, namely dermatomyositis (DM), muscle inflammation alone, called as polymyositis (PM), cancer-associated myositis (CAM), overlap myositis (OM), when muscle weakness occurs in patients with other established connective tissue disorders (CTDs), and degenerative forms of myositis called the inclusion body myositis (IBM) and juvenile dermatomyositis (JDM). More recently, the identification of various autoantibodies has widely expanded the spectrum and led to a revised nomenclature of IIMs, with two new forms: (1) the antisynthetase syndrome (ASSD) and (2) immune-mediated necrotizing myopathies (IMNMs) being described.

EPIDEMIOLOGY

Nationwide, population-based studies suggest prevalence estimated 4–9 lacs cases per 10,000 of the population, though the estimates from India are still unknown. The IIMs exhibit a female predominance (female:male = 2.2:1), with the exception of IBM, which has a male predominance. The IIMs often manifest in the fourth to fifth decades of life, although OMs may be reported at an earlier age. Additionally, case series from India and the Middle East notes a younger average age of mid-30s.

CLASSIFICATION

In 1975, in a landmark paper, Dr Anthony Bohan and Dr James B Peter classified IIM into five categories (**Figs. 2 A** and **B**) consisted of DM, PM, OM, CAM, and JDM. This is the most commonly used classification of IIM by physicians for over four decades now (**Fig. 1**).

Bohan and Peter classification, however, had its drawbacks; DM and PM associated with vasculitis are not restricted to childhood ages and the overlap of myositis with other connective tissue disorders was not accurately defined. It did not include atypical myositis presentations such as IBM or those with amyopathic forms of IIM. On further studies, it was determined that the Bohan and Peter classification could be used only to distinguish between DM/PM and systemic lupus erythematosus (SLE) and systemic sclerosis (SSc).

The Bohan and Peter diagnostic criteria included five marked features: (1) symmetric proximal muscle weakness, (2) muscle biopsy changes, (3) a typical rash characteristic of DM, (4) elevated serum muscle enzymes, and (5) myopathic changes on electromyography (EMG).

However, the discovery of various autoantibodies and a greater understanding of previously described autoantibodies have led to better characterization of

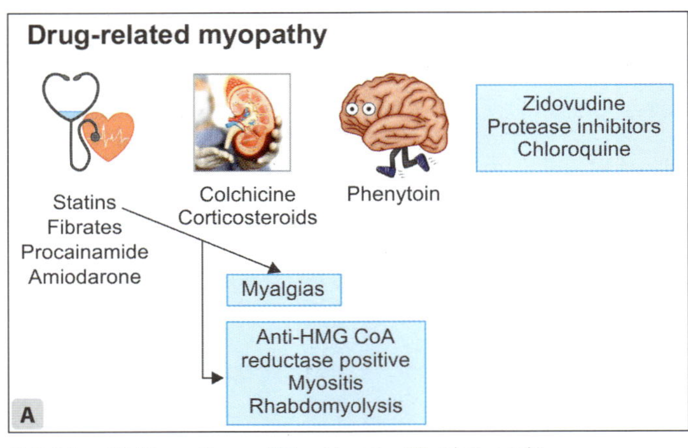

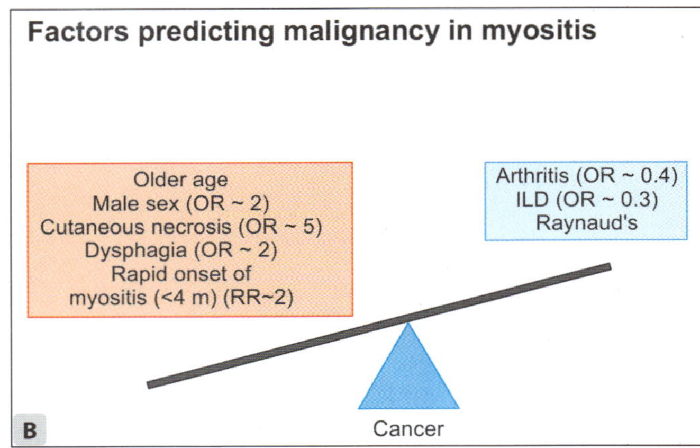

(ILD: interstitial lung disease; OR: odds ratio; RR: relative risk)

FIGURES 2 A & B: (A) The role of various drugs in the onset of myositis; and **(B)** The conditions that often pander to the incidence of malignancy with myositis.

many disease subsets (**Fig. 1**). In keeping with this, recent attempts have been made to revise the classification for better recruitment into clinical trials (**Fig. 1**).

The current European League Against Rheumatism/American College of Rheumatology (EULAR/ACR) IIM classification criteria include a weighted score, which determines the patient's probability of being classified as definite, probable, or possible IIM and includes anti-Jo1 antibodies as one of the criteria, with a heavy weightage to the various biopsy characteristics. Unfortunately, the study of the rarer disease subsets, which harbor the less prevalent autoantibodies, precludes better understanding of these and the criteria do not include these minor variants. Thus, the requirements may be revised at a later point when larger collaborative efforts may allow collection and formation of biorepositories and clinical registries of these rare subsets. Initiatives such as MyoIN–Pan-India collaborative network for myositis facilitate a collective growth and improvement in the understanding of myositis.

PATHOGENESIS

The exact pathogenesis of myositis is not known, although the onset of myositis after infections has been described. Like most other autoimmune disorders, there is a suggested predisposition due to genetic factors which may trigger the onset of IIM in the presence of an inciting stimulus from the environment. The list of proposed genetic and environmental predisposing factors is depicted in **Table 1**. The drug-related myopathies are shown in **Figures 2 A** and **B**. Recently, autoantibodies have become a reliable indicator and basis of classification of the various categories of myositis (**Table 2**).

TABLE 1 Predisposing genetic and environmental factors.

Genes		Environment
HLA	**Non-HLA**	
AH8.1 (ancestral haplotype) DRB103:01 DRB111:01 DRB107:01 DRB08:01 DRB113:01 DRB101:01 DRB108:03 DQA101:04 DQ2-DR3	PTPN22 Complement 4A STAT4 TRAF6 UBE2L3 PLCL1 BLK CCR5	• Infections ◦ Hepatitis B ◦ Hepatitis C ◦ HIV ◦ Myxoviruses (influenza) ◦ COVID-19 • Drugs, vaccines, and prosthesis/implants ◦ D-penicillamine ◦ Interferon-α ◦ anti-TNF agents ◦ Statins ◦ Vaccines containing aluminum hydroxide ◦ Collagen and silicone implants ◦ Silica • Smoking • Ultraviolet radiation

CLINICAL FEATURES

CUTANEOUS

The onset of DM is marked by the development of characteristic rashes in most cases, some of which are pathognomonic for the disease. The rashes impact in DM may be divided into those specific for a diagnosis of DM, suggestive of DM, and other forms. A picture gallery depicting some characteristic ones is presented in **Figure 3**, while the various types of rashes are detailed in **Table 3**.

The skin rashes may appear shortly before or at the same time as muscle weakness, though rarely, they may be the only marker of the underlying disease. They are erythematous, photosensitive, and may be spread across the neck, back, and shoulders (shawl sign). Heliotrope rash (violaceous erythema of the upper eyelids often with associated edema and telangiectasia) is common. Gottron's papules (erythematous to violaceous papules and plaques over the extensor surfaces of the

TABLE 2	Reliable antibodies indicating myositis.					
	Autoantibodies	**Target molecules**	**Functions**	**Disease association**	**Clinical association**	**Detection and significance in non-PM/-DM**
Myositis-specific autoantibodies	Anti-ARS antibodies, Jo-1, PL-7, PL-12, EJ, OJ, KS, Zo, and YRS	Various aminoacyl-tRNA synthetase	Biosynthesis of various proteins, including aminoacyl-tRNA. Glutamate, alanine, and aspartate metabolism	PM, DM, CADM, and ILD	Antisynthetase syndrome, myositis, ILD, arthritis, and Raynaud's phenomenon	Uncommon (anti-ARS can be in overlap syndrome and idiopathic ILD, hence, if found, indicates myopathy)
	Anti-signal recognition particle (SRP)	SRP	Regulates translocation of proteins across the endoplasmic reticulum	PM	Myositis (necrotizing)	
	Anti-Mi-2, anti-TIF1β, anti-NXP-2, and anti-SAE	Helicase protein	Transcriptional regulation and FNA metabolism	DM	DM with typical skin lesions and mild myositis, malignancy associated, and adult and JDM with severe skin disease	
	Anti-MDA5	MDA5	RNA-specific helicase that mediates the antiviral response	CADM/ADM	CADM, rapidly progressive ILD, and severe skin manifestations	
Myositis-associated autoantibodies	Anti-PM-Scl, anti-Ku, and anti-U1/U3RNP	Exosome protein complex (PM/Scl75/100), DNA-PK regulatory subunit, U1 small nuclear RNP, and fibrillarin, respectively		PM/DM, PM/DM-overlap syndrome, SSc, and SLE		Common and indicate myopathy
Other autoantibodies	Anti-Ro52, anti-Ro/SSA60, and anti-Su/argonaute-2 (Ago2)	Ro52/TRIM21, Ro60/SSA, and Ago2, respectively		Various SARD		Often but does not indicate myopathy

(ADM: amyopathic dermatomyositis; CADM: cancer-associated dermatomyositis; JDM: juvenile dermatomyositis; MDA5: melanoma differentiation-associated gene 5; PM: polymyositis; RNP: ribonucleoprotein; SARD: systemic autoimmune rheumatic disease; SSA: Sjögren's syndrome; SSc: systemic sclerosis)

metacarpophalangeal and interphalangeal joints) are usually accompanied with scales and may develop ulcerations. These resolve with dyspigmentation, atrophy, and scarring. Less often, patients may present with inverse Gottron's papules (rash on the volar aspect of hand) or rashes on the anterior chest wall (V-sign). Skin is not exposed to sun; like the scalp, lower back and inner thighs may also be involved and a specific examination may be revealing in the clinic.

Some patients may also exhibit cracked skin on dorsal and ventral surfaces of the hands (mechanic's hands). Those with mechanic's hands are likely to have ASSD [Raynaud's phenomenon, arthritis, myositis, and interstitial lung disease (ILD); presenting with "mechanic's hands", testing positive for antibodies to aminoacyl transfer of ribonucleic acid (RNA) synthetases]. Notably, incomplete forms of ASSD are way more common, making it imperative to have keen suspicion for diagnosis. Tender papules and plaques on the joint creases of the palms may depict mucin deposition on biopsy. Panniculitis, alopecia, and flagellate erythema are other rare pointers. Poikiloderma may be a sign of chronicity and damage. Calcinosis occurs largely in areas of trauma or inflammation, especially in JDM.

Over time, it was realized that some cutaneous signs of DM are the sine qua non for diagnosis and this heralded the recognition of amyopathic and hypomyopathic forms of DM, wherein the muscle involved was absent or subclinical (elevated enzymes or abnormal EMG or MRI of the muscle but no weakness on clinical examination). The recognition of JDM as a separate subset when it occurred in children <16 years of age was warranted by some cutaneous and systemic manifestations, which are way more frequent than

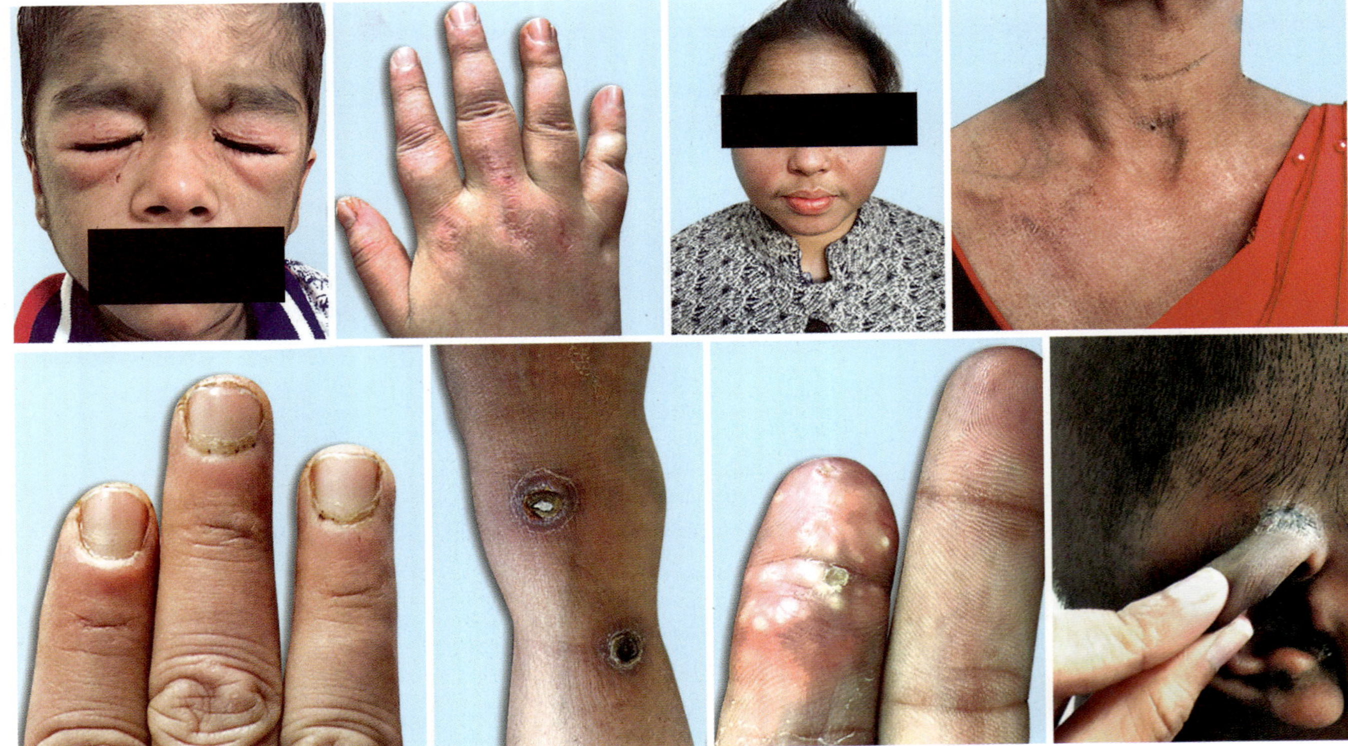

FIGURE 3: Characteristic cutaneous presentations of patients of myositis.

TABLE 3 Various types of rashes and cutaneous features seen in myositis.

Clinical features	Definition	Sites involved	Remarks
Diagnostic			
Heliotrope rash	Periorbital erythema, often accompanied by symmetrical edema	Upper eyelid	Also seen in SLE patients
Gottron's papules	Gottron's sign-like lesions, which are elevated and palpable	Often overlying the dorsolateral aspect of metacarpophalangeal joints, proximal interphalangeal joints, and/or distal interphalangeal joints (joint extensors)	Differentiating features—knuckle pad, verruca vulgaris, lichen planus, sarcoidosis, acanthosis nigricans, erythema elevatum diutinum, and multicentric reticulohistiocytosis
Gottron's sign	Erythematous to violaceous papules and plaques or macules (sign) over extensor surfaces of joints, which are sometimes scaly	At the joint extensors and bony prominences such as elbows, knees, and less commonly, the medial malleoli	
Suggestive			
Facial erythema	The entire face with nasolabial fold sparing		
Periungual changes	Erythema, dilated capillary loops, cuticular hemorrhages, and/or cuticular overgrowth	Periungual areas	Also seen in SSc and, rarely, SLE patients
Inverse Gottron's sign	Papules or erythema overlying the palmar surfaces of the hand joints		Associated with acute/subacute interstitial lung disease
V-neck sign	Violaceous erythema, probably caused by photosensitivity	V area of the neck and the upper chest	About 50% of DM patients suffer from severe photosensitivity (causes erythroderma). Long-standing inflammatory periods develop poikilodermatous changes

Continued...

Continued...

Clinical features	Definition	Sites involved	Remarks
Mechanic's hand	Hyperkeratosis, scaling, and fissuring of the fingers	The lesions are distributed along the ulnar aspect of the thumb and radial aspect of the fingers and are most prominent on the index and middle fingers, with infrequent extension to the palm	Characteristic cutaneous marker of the antisynthetase syndrome but seen in cases of polymyositis (PM), classic DM, and amyopathic DM not associated with antisynthetase antibody
Shawl's sign	Symmetrical violaceous erythema	Extends across the nape of the neck to the posterior aspects of the shoulders and upper back	
Flagellate erythema	Centripetal, patchy violaceous erythema, and/or poikilodermatous changes	On the back, lateral chest and/or upper buttocks	Rare in DM. Seen in adult-onset Still's disease, bleomycin-induced eruptions, and dermatitis from ingestion of shiitake mushrooms
Vesiculobullous eruptions	Multiloculated vesicles or bullous lesions	On the dorsal surfaces of the hands or forearms and other areas	May be caused by liquefaction degeneration of the epidermis, subepidermal edema with mucin deposition in the upper dermis, or complications from autoimmune bullous diseases
Alopecia	Mild-to-moderate nonscarring diffuse alopecia	Scalp	Even after the disease activity diminishes, the alopecia may persist
Panniculitis	Tender erythematous or violaceous nodules or depressions due to inflammation in the subcutaneous fat	Often occur on the buttocks and upper thighs	As a result of long-standing panniculitis and lipodystrophy may occur with JDM
Calcinosis cutis	Subcutaneous, deep, or visceral calcium deposits	Occurs in areas of panniculitis or poikilodermatous areas	Extrusion of calcium through the skin is associated with ulceration and infection. It is a major cause of morbidity in JDM patients
Skin ulcers	Associated with cutaneous vasculitis or with vascular damage due to panniculitis/calcification	Occur at the site of Gottron's sign, on the buttocks and thighs	Indicative of severe disease requiring aggressive immunosuppression
Holster sign	Violaceous erythema	Underlies the general area where a pistol holster is worn at a belt on the waist	
Poikiloderma	Circumscribed violaceous erythema containing telangiectasia, hypopigmentation, hyperpigmentation, and superficial atrophy	Posterior shoulder, upper arm, back, buttocks, and V neck area	May be seen in systemic sclerosis-associated fibrosing myopathy
Pruritus	In the early course of the skin lesions from DM	Anywhere at sites of inflammation	Often resistant to oral antihistaminics and corticosteroid ointments
Hyperpigmentation	Increased pigmentation on the body surface	At sites of previous erythema and inflammation	Tell-tale sequelae of previous inflammation and usually refractory to treatment
Sclerodactyly	Skin tightening with or without digital tapering and acro-osteolysis and pitting scars	It is limited to distal areas of the fingers and toes	Seen in overlap myositis, specifically MCTD and lcSsc
Sclerodactyly	Skin tightening with or without digital tapering and acro-osteolysis and pitting scars	It is limited to distal areas of the fingers and toes	Seen in overlap myositis, specifically MCTD and lcSsc
Skin thickening	Skin tightening	They are limited or diffuse in extent	In the distribution of scleroderma and related disorders

Continued...

Continued...

Clinical features	Definition	Sites involved	Remarks
Ocular sicca	Dryness of eye	Eye	Manifest as grittiness or gravel sensation in the eye or need to use eye drops for lubrication or previously diagnosed dry eye by an ophthalmologist
Oral sicca	Dryness of mouth	Mouth	Manifest as the inability to swallow solids without liquids, need to frequently take sips of water or using lubricative spray or lozenges
Photosensitivity	Abnormal cutaneous reaction to ultraviolet radiation and erythema	Involving the cheeks extending over the nasolabial bridge with concurrent involvement of the nasolabial folds	Involvement of the nasolabial fold is the key distinguishing feature from lupus, wherein the area is typically spared
Lipoatrophy	Loss of subcutaneous fat	Abdomen, lower limbs, or upper arm	May signify underlying vasculitis
Oral ulcers	Ulcers or discontinuity in the epithelium of oral mucosa	Hard and soft mucosa	Both major and minor aphthae can be seen
Gangrene	Death of body tissue due to lack of blood supply	Commonly affecting the digital tips	More marked in SSc and MCTD. Rarely reported in the anti-MDA5 positive disease

(DM: dermatomyositis; JDM: juvenile dermatomyositis; lcSsc: limited cutaneous systemic sclerosis; SSc: systemic sclerosis)

the others. It is now widely accepted that both calcinosis, a refractory and disabling complication of IIM, and vasculitis of the skin and the gut are more often seen in children than adults with DM.

MUSCLE

A diagnosis of IIM is frequently distinguished from other muscle disorders by a subacute onset, which runs into months rather than years. The dictum is that muscle weakness manifesting in days is typical of other causes, although more fulminant forms of IIM are increasingly recognized with the wider availability of autoantibody testing. The appearance of characteristic skin rashes is the most important clue to the timely diagnosis in those types of IIM where muscle weakness is either unremarkable or the presentation is more acute than typically expected.

The muscle weakness is of varying degrees, typically symmetrical and proximal muscle weakness followed by weakness in distal muscles. The weak muscles make it difficult for patients to carry out simple tasks such as rising from a chair, climbing up staircases, or combing one's hair. DM is usually painless, but along with the acute onset of the disease and subcutaneous calcifications, muscles may be painful on movement and touch.

LUNG

Patients with DM and ASSD may commonly present with ILD. They may present with dyspnea on exertion, cough, and decreased stamina for exercise. On the other hand, limited mobility due to related muscle disease or unrelated degenerative arthritis may impair the assessment of poor lung function and confound misdiagnosis.

The lung involvement in IIM may be varied, ranging from an acute and severe rapidly progressive ILD (RP-ILD) which may rarely exhibit classic features such as pneumomediastinum in anti-MDA5-positive disease, conferring a dismal prognosis with 60% 3-month mortality to more chronic slow forms with frequently missed diagnosis, albeit progressive as seen in ASSD. Pulmonary function tests reveal a restrictive disease pattern and decreased carbon monoxide diffusion capacity. Nodules, linear opacities, fibrosis with or without honeycombing, consolidation, traction bronchiectasis, and bronchiolectasis are characteristic high-resolution computed tomography (HRCT) finding of ILD.

CARDIAC

Cardiac manifestations, albeit described and relatively uncommon, though severe when present, mandating aggressive immunosuppression. Classic descriptions of myocarditis are well-described in anti-signal recognition particle (SRP)-positive severe and acute PM, though recent reports of cardiac involvement in antimitochondrial antibody-positive disease are emerging as well.

The subclinical cardiac manifestations are also described, ranging from congestive heart failure, arrhythmia to valvular diseases. Cardiac involvement is, however, a rare manifestation.

MALIGNANCY

It is noteworthy that sizeable proportions of individuals with certain specific clinical manifestations such as an extensive erythematous rash, severe muscle disease, early dysphagia, cutaneous vasculitis, and age-specific risk factors for cancer harbor a heightened risk for underlying malignancy (**Figs. 2 A** and **B**). In fact, the antitumor responses by the host immunity may be the key inciting event for autoimmunity on CAM, so much so that DM has now been classified as one of the paraneoplastic syndromes.

The occurrence of cancer clusters within 3 years of myositis, either preceding or after it. Since the diagnosis of CAM carries grievous prognostic implications, IIM patients with a negative autoantibody or anti-TIF1γ (anti-p155/140) positive should undergo age-specific cancer screening. Since the type of cancer varies by region and environmental as well as genetic risks, regional guidelines for cancer screening may be followed.

In line with this, Asians are advised pharyngeal examination for nasopharyngeal cancer and colonic cancer screen in the West. Notably, once the diagnosis is established, treatment of the underlying cancer is curative for myositis as the drivers of autoimmunity are managed. Autoimmunity may also confer a better tumor prognosis in terms of slower spread, possibly due to better antitumor immunity and counterintuitively mortality in CAM is due to progressive muscle disease rather than metastatic spread.

OTHER

Dysphagia due to esophageal or pharyngeal muscle involvement, hoarseness of voice, nasal speech, nasal regurgitation, and aspiration pneumonia are other features associated with pharyngeal muscle affliction. Manometry with low amplitude/absent pharyngeal contractions and decreased upper esophageal sphincter pressures confirm this diagnosis.

Gastrointestinal bleeding due to vasculopathy of the gut is reported in children with severe JDM and vasculitis. A careful gum examination may sometimes offer insight into the ongoing vascular disease. If more than two CTDs overlap, it is called an "overlap syndrome". It most commonly involves SSc, PM/DM, Sjögren's syndrome, and SLE. Other manifestations of IIM may be more marked in ASSD and overlap forms of IIM and seen in patients with other rheumatic diseases. These include Raynaud's phenomenon, fever, weight loss, fatigue, and inflammatory polyarthritis. The polyarthritis is usually nonerosive, except ASSD where erosions may be occasionally seen.

SPECIFIC FORMS OF IIM

INCLUSION BODY MYOSITIS (IBM)

Inclusion body myositis is a sporadic disease, which is more common in the elderly (>50 years) male (3:1) population. Inflammatory and degenerative changes characterize the onset of IBM. It has coexistent asymmetric involvement of both proximal and distal muscles.

The characteristic hallmark of IBM is slow and progressive quadriceps muscle weakness leading to falls and difficulty in getting out of a chair. Quadriceps weakening also causes loss of patellar weakness and atrophy. Due to the gradual onset, most patients present with asymmetric atrophy and weakness of wrist and finger flexors and quadriceps muscles, leading to dexterity and early falls. Less commonly, the involvement of flexors of fingers, ankle dorsiflexors (due to involvement of tibialis anterior muscle), and knee extensors are noted. Axial muscle involvement leads to a head drop and camptocormia. Rarely, instead of quadriceps, one may notice prominent forearm weakness.

Dysphagia is a common manifestation and occurs in more than half of all patients. Mild-to-moderate facial weakness may be frequently demonstrated. Uninterrupted progression of the disease may ultimately lead to wheelchair confinement due to weakness in the legs. IBM, even though a neurodegenerative disorder, may occasionally be associated with autoimmune disorders such as SLE, Sjögren's syndrome, thrombocytopenia, and sarcoidosis. Unlike PM and DM, it does not confer an increased risk of malignancy, cardiac disease, or ILD beyond those due to old age. It also presents with weaker wrist and finger flexors and knee extension weakness as compared to corresponding extensors and shoulder abductors in contrast with DM, PM, and neuromyositis (NM).

It has a similar presentation to amyotrophic lateral sclerosis; however, the sparing of thenar and hypothenar muscles (**Figs. 4 A** and **B**). Granulomatous myositis mimics IBM in weakness pattern and may be steroid responsive.

IMMUNE-MEDIATED NECROTIZING MYOPATHIES (IMNM)

The IMNMs are newly described and increasingly being recognized form of IIM, which manifest atypical presentation in contrast to the other subsets of IIM. These patients may present with acute onset muscle weakness, with remarkably elevated creatine kinase (CK) levels ranging over 10,000 IU/mL. IMNM is characterized by muscle necrosis and regeneration, causing proximal muscle weakness. Its onset may be idiopathic, following viral infections or the intake of statins (associated with autoantibodies directed against HMGCR) use. Unlike other forms of IIM, inflammatory infiltrates are not seen in IMNM patients. These are being diagnosed more frequently with the wider availability of anti-SRP and anti-HMGCR antibody. Rarely, IMNM may begin in those without a prior history of statin exposure; albeit with the specific anti-HMGCR antibodies, these cases being reported characteristically in young women who manifest a refractory form of autoimmune disease.

More recently, a chronic myopathy resampling limb-girdle muscle dystrophy is also described on occasion, particularly in children, which may be responsive to immunosuppressant therapy, particularly with intravenous immunoglobulin (IVIg) infusions. This raises the case for testing these antibodies in children where a diagnosis of nontreatable forms of muscle disease is being considered.

Management of patients suffering from IMNM is given in **Figures 4 A** and **B**.

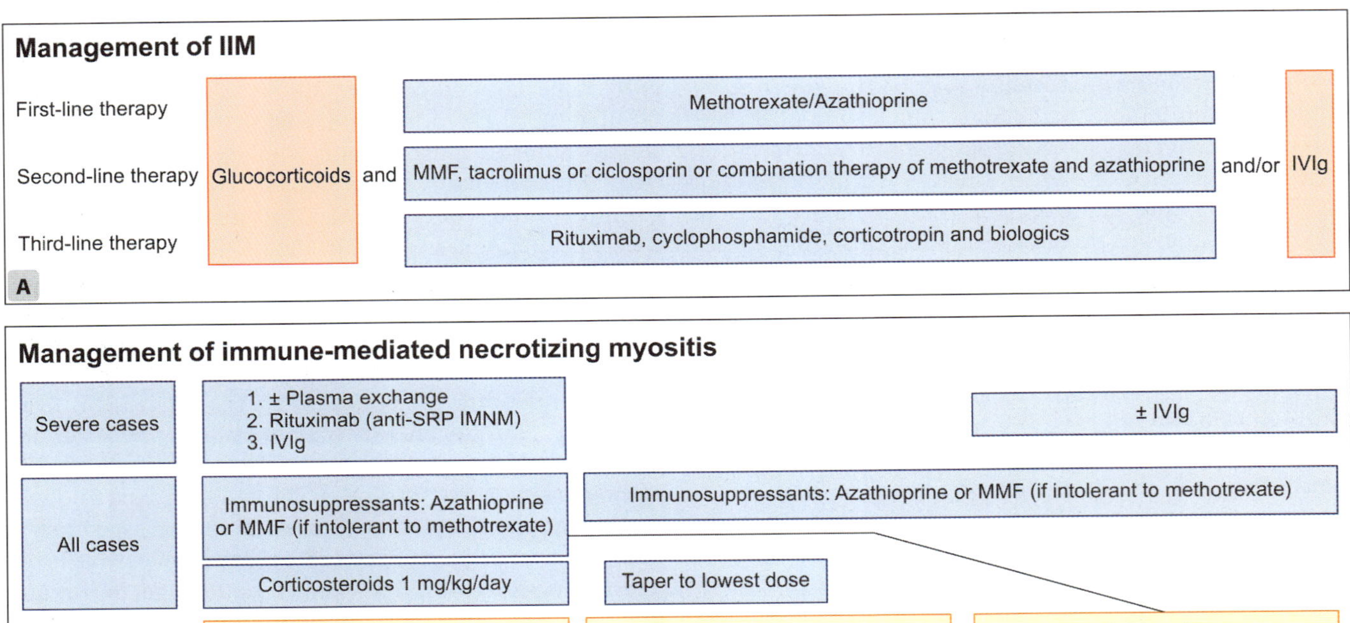

(IIM: idiopathic inflammatory myopathy; IVIg: intravenous immunoglobulin; MMF: mycophenolate mofetil; SRP: signal recognition particle)

FIGURES 4 A & B: Management of myositis. (A) General management of IIM; and **(B)** Management of immune-mediated necrotizing myositis.

ANTI-MDA5

This is a newer variant of myositis. Patients suffering from anti-MDA5 DM have been mainly reported from the Asian population and have different clinical features. They may encounter complications such as pneumomediastinum and macrophage activation syndrome. Patients presenting with rapidly progressive ILD are suspected of having MDA5 DM. IP can detect anti-MDA5 antibody, line immunoassay, or enzyme-linked immunosorbent assay (ELISA) and the ILD must be confirmed by an HRCT. Elevated ferritin, C-reactive protein and KL-6, and decreased T-helper subsets and serum CD206 are biomarkers for poor prognosis and high risk of mortality. This is the severe most form of DM and difficult to treat. It is managed by intensive immunosuppression comprising pulse corticosteroids (15–20 mg/kg/dose) for 3–5 days followed by oral corticosteroids (1 mg/kg) along with immunosuppressants.

DIAGNOSIS

The diagnosis is primarily clinical and history may be carefully visited for identifying intake of drugs, endocrine or metabolic disorders, and family history to suggest inherited disease. The key distinguishing clinical and biopsy characteristics are depicted in **Table 4**. Some noteworthy facts are listed below.

- Raised CK is sensitive for the diagnosis of IIM. Patients with a myositis spectrum disorder but no muscle disease may present with a normal CK value.
- Biopsies are an essential step to make a correct diagnosis and differentiate between various subtypes. MRI rules out muscular dystrophy and other forms of hereditary myopathy and end-stage tissue destruction. MRI helps to identify the best site for biopsy for diagnosis.
- Patients with antisynthetase autoantibodies and anti-CADM must undergo CT scans for detection of ILD.

MANAGEMENT

PHARMACOLOGICAL TREATMENT

Immunosuppressive agents:

Glucocorticoids: Glucocorticoids form the mainstay of therapy in IIM, with initial requirements of 1 mg/kg steroids for as long as 4–6 weeks before the first follow-up visit (**Figs. 4 A** and **B**). The muscle enzymes are neither sensitive nor entirely specific. Therefore, a clinical assessment of strength and mobility is preferred over chasing blood test for guiding management.

In adults having severe myositis or myositis with extramuscular manifestations (myocarditis or pharyngeal weakness), pulse therapy of 1,000 mg of methylprednisolone for 3 consecutive days is prescribed for rapid onset of action. These doses must be tapered by 20–25% of their current dose in a month with the final goal being 5–10 mg of prednisone within 6 months. They are used as first-line therapy in patients suffering from ILD (**Fig. 5**).

Methotrexate: Methotrexate (up to 25 mg/week subcutaneously or orally) is used in combination with GCs as first-line therapy for myositis patients and those that develop flares after glucocorticoid tapering (**Figs. 4** and **6**). The combination of methotrexate and prednisone is said to provide quicker remission in patients of JDM. These drugs,

TABLE 4 Diagnostic characteristics of the different myositis presentations.

	DM	PM	IBM	IMNM
Muscle biopsy findings				
Diagnostic	Perifascicular atrophy involving both type 1 and type 2 muscle fiber, affecting 2–10 layers	Presence of mononuclear inflammatory cells that surround, invade, and destroy healthy muscle fibers	Endomysial inflammation and muscle fiber degeneration	Randomly distributed necrotic muscle fibers along with fibers in various stages of regeneration, but in the absence of or sparse mononuclear cell infiltrates
Site of inflammatory infiltrates	Perivascular sites, within the interfascicular septae, rarely in the endomysium	Upregulation on the surface of fibers, perimysium, and rarely at perivascular sites	Nonnecrotic muscle fibers expressing MHC class I antigen on the sarcolemma	
Contents of inflammatory infiltrates	B cells accompanied by CD4+ T-helper cells, plasmacytoid dendritic cells and macrophages, CD8+ T cells are rare, and NK cells are sparse	Cytotoxic CD8+ T cells having granules containing cytotoxic molecules including perforin and granzymes with a lesser number of macrophages and few CD4+ T cells	Macrophages and CD8+ T cells	Mononuclear cell type,T and B cells are absent
Muscle fibers		Variation in fiber diameter, scattered necrotic and regenerating muscle fibers, and increase in perimysial and/or endomysial connective tissue	Irregular, eosinophilic cytoplasmic inclusions near or in rimmed vacuoles. Intracellular amyloid deposits in nonvacuolated areas (fluorescence-enhanced Congo red stain). Increased number of ragged red fibers and COX-negative fibers in mitochondria. Small, angulated muscle fibers, indicating the neurogenic process. PHFs, amyloid-like filaments, flocculomembranous and amorphous material, and protein deposition	Insufficient data
Blood vessels	Immunoglobulins and complement deposition. Reduced number of capillaries with endothelial hyperplasia and enlargement of the lumen. Presence of tubuloreticular inclusions within the endothelial cytoplasm of arterioles and capillaries			
Electromyography				
	Positive sharp waves, complex repetitive discharges, small polyphasic motor potentials, and increased spontaneous and insertional activity with fibrillation potentials	Spontaneous fibrillation at rest or after needle insertion, spontaneous high frequency discharges, and positive sharp waves	Mild sensory axonal peripheral polyneuropathy, mixed myopathic and neuropathic motor potential units, pseudoneurogenic changes due to reinnervation of denervated and split muscle fibers, and motor unit action potentials overshadowing myopathic changes falsely indicating motor neuron disease	Early confirmation of a myopathic pattern, ruling out other causes of muscle weakness (neuropathy or myasthenia gravis)

Continued...

Continued...

	DM	PM	IBM	IMNM
MRI findings				
	Muscle edema and atrophy (seen in later stages)	Slight muscle inflammation	Large lower limb muscle involvement. Hyperintensity with fatty atrophy in long finger flexors, anterior thigh muscles, and all the muscles of the lower leg	Muscle involvement is highest. Assesses fat replacement and active muscle edema (intramuscular hyperintensities) associated with inflammation and myofiber necrosis
Muscle enzyme				
	CK elevation to 700 IU/L; however, it is not a consistent finding	CK elevation; however, their levels may fluctuate in the late stages of the diseases or after treatment	CK elevated up to 10 times and can go up to 20 times. ANA positive and increased HLA-DR3*0301/0302 phenotype	Highest recorded CK elevations (4,700 IU/L)

(DM: dermatomyositis; IBM: inclusion body myositis; IMNM: immune-mediated necrotizing myopathy; NK: natural killer; PM: polymyositis)

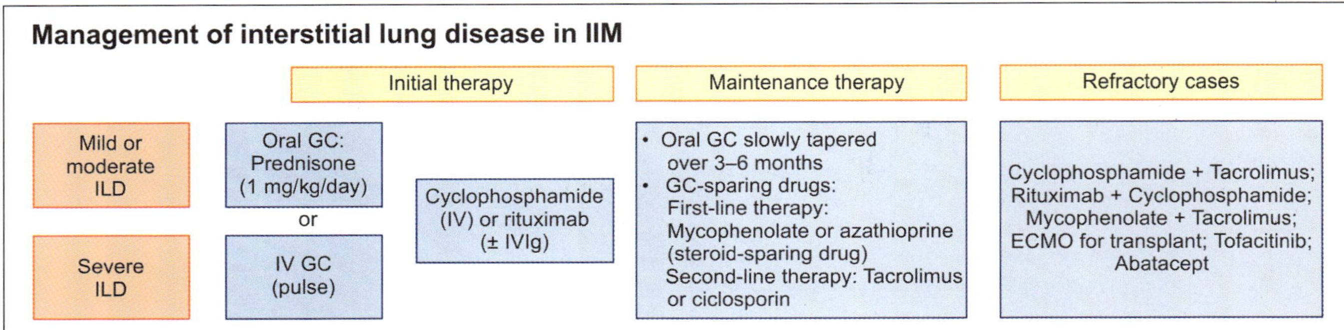

(GC: glucocorticoid; ECMO: extracorporeal membrane oxygenation; IIM: idiopathic inflammatory myopathy; IVIg: intravenous immunoglobulin)

FIGURE 5: Management of interstitial lung disease (ILD) in myositis.

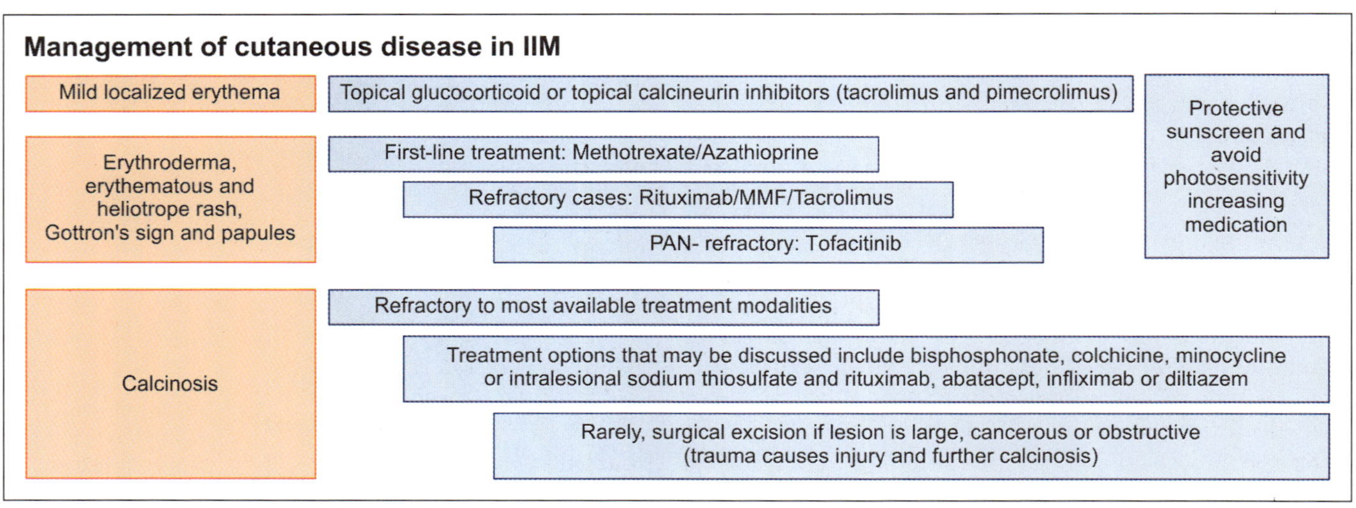

(IIM: idiopathic inflammatory myopathy; MMF: mycophenolate mofetil)

FIGURE 6: Management of cutaneous presentations of myositis.

along with cyclosporine, quicken remission and allow early prednisone discontinuation.

Azathioprine: Azathioprine is converted into 6-mercaptopurine, which is an effective immunosuppressant. Azathioprine and methotrexate have similar efficacies. However, azathioprine therapy is preferred in patients of liver disease or patients that are unwilling to abstain from alcohol or patients with severe ILD. Azathioprine, 2–3 mg/kg daily orally, in combination with prednisone 1 mg/kg/day, does not show any significant muscle strength or CK level improvement initially; however, in the long term, this combination is superior to monotherapy and improves functional status and reduces prednisone dosage in patients of PM.

Mycophenolate mofetil: Mycophenolate mofetil (MMF) (prodrug of mycophenolic acid) inhibits purine synthesis and impairing B-cell and T-cell proliferation. MMF (2,000–3,000 mg/daily, orally) along with IVIg has been seen to achieve complete remission in patients with refractory DM or PM.

Calcineurin inhibitors: Ciclosporin and tacrolimus are commonly used for management of refractory IIM. Ciclosporin blocks the production and release of interleukin-2 (IL-2) and IL-2-induced activation of T cells, whereas tacrolimus (second generation) binds to an intracellular protein, peptidyl-prolyl cis-trans isomerase FKBP12, leading to inhibition of T-cell activation. Tacrolimus has been proven to help patients of refractory myositis, PM, and DM that regain muscular strength and decrease serum creatine levels. However, due to the risk of toxicity, tacrolimus use is restricted for patients of refractory myositis.

Cyclophosphamide: This is an alkylating agent that interferes with cell growth and is used as oral or intravenous therapy of patients suffering from severe myositis, rapidly progressive ILD, overlapping systemic vasculitis, or patients refractory to second- or third-line therapies. However, it poses a risk of toxicity and malignancy (**Fig. 5**).

Biologic agents: Biologic agents are specific and target the immune cells or cytokines directly, in contrast with immunosuppressive agents that have a more generalized action.

Rituximab: Rituximab is proven to be effective in all patients of myositis, including those with severe or refractory IMNM associated with an anti-SRP autoantibody and those refractory to immunosuppressive agents having prominent muscle weakness during their first visit. It is also useful in patients suffering from the ASSD. Rituximab also has a considerable steroid-sparing effect and is well tolerated.

Tocilizumab: This is an IL-6 receptor antagonist and occasional reports suggest benefit in treating patients of refractory polymyositis, overlap syndrome (DM and SSc), and DM.

Abatacept: Abatacept inhibits T-cell costimulation and is undergoing phase III trials to the same effect.

Intravenous immunoglobulin: Intravenous immunoglobulin is administered at 2 g/kg monthly, but the dose depends on disease severity and subsequent therapeutic response of the patient. This therapy is used in adjunct with immunosuppressive agents in cases of infection or malignancy, but this therapy is expensive and is a long-term therapy thus, is unsuitable for most.

Treatment for inclusion body myositis: It is difficult to find an accurate therapy for IBM, as immunosuppressant treatment has proven to be ineffective and modestly exacerbate the disability progression. The lack of sample size, the slow and unpredictable progression rate, the need for expensive and long drawn out trials, and the absence of validated measures of strength limit the number of IBM clinical trials taking place. Furthermore, IBM is diagnosed years after the onset of symptoms, by which time, muscle damage is significant and treatment response is dismal.

Corticosteroids, methotrexate, and azathioprine: The use of these immunosuppressant therapies has been proven to show a fall in CK levels and reduce inflammation in muscle fibers; however, it was seen to be accompanied with a decrease in muscle strength and increase in the number of vacuolated and amyloid-positive fibers. However, the patients that received these therapies showed either stabilization or delayed progression as compared to the patients that did not receive any immunosuppressant medicines.

Calcineurin inhibitors: These pharmacological therapies have proven to show muscle strength improvement and maintained their clinical response even after removal of the medical therapy. However, this was seen in the early stages of the disease and, therefore, their efficacy in the chronic stages of the disease has not been proved.

Intravenous immunoglobulin: This has proven to improve dysphagia due to upper esophageal sphincter dysfunction. However, improvement in muscle strength is not observed. Patients refractory to IVIg are treated with cricopharyngeal myotomy with positive clinical improvement.

Interferon therapy: The treatment with interferon-β (IFN-β) therapy has shown considerable improvement in patients having IBM with hepatitis C.

Alemtuzumab: This has shown considerable slowing down in disease progression and maintenance of resolution after removal of therapy; however, blinded, placebo-controlled trials have not been done to confirm this finding.

Rituximab and antitumor necrosis factor: Drug therapies do not show any improvement in disease progression.

Exercise: Aerobic exercise programs with resistance training have proven to improve aerobic capacity and muscle strength in IBM patients.

Combined therapy of corticosteroids, methotrexate/azathioprine, and calcineurin inhibitors are said to be adequate for IBM patients.

Treatment for antisynthetase syndrome patients:

Corticosteroids: Their use is said to be based on its success with other IIM pathologies. It causes partial improvement and, therefore, must be used as a part of combination therapy. Prednisone (1 mg/kg/day) is used as first-line therapy.

Azathioprine (1 mg/day) and mycophenolate mofetil (500 mg twice a day): These are common second-line drugs and are used in combination with corticosteroids. Patients receiving azathioprine must undergo renal function tests periodically.

Tacrolimus (1 mg twice a day) and IVIg are used for add-on therapies.

Rituximab and cyclophosphamide (1–2 mg/kg/day orally or 500–1,000 mg IV every 4 weeks) are used as rescue therapy as required in the case of an acute respiratory distress syndrome (ARDS).

NONPHARMACOLOGICAL TREATMENT

Plasma exchange/leukapheresis: The use of plasmapheresis has been debated; however, hemoperfusion with polymyxin B in addition to the standard immunosuppressive treatment has shown positive results in patients having anti-MDA5 IIM with severe comorbid ILD.

Exercise: Exercise was contraindicated in IIM a few years back, due to scepticism regarding the possibility of worsened muscle inflammation, thereby increasing muscle weakness. However, now it is considered an important adjunct of therapy. It improves muscular metabolism, physical capacity, autonomy, and quality of life. The suggested exercise methods are treadmill walking, cycling, and resistance training. It is usually started with pharmacological treatment and can be monitored on a regular basis.

Funding: This study was not funded.

RECOMMENDED READINGS

1. Gupta L, Appani SK, Janardana R, Muhammed H, Lawrence A, Amin S, et al. Meeting report: MyoIN – Pan-India collaborative network for myositis research. Indian J Rheumatol. 2019;14:136-42.
2. Balakrishnan A, Aggarwal R, Agarwal V, Gupta L. Inclusion body myositis in the rheumatology clinic. Int J Rheum Dis. 2020;23:1126-35.
3. Naveen R, Anuja AK, Rai MK, Agarwal V, Gupta L. Development of the MyoCite biobank: Cost-efficient model of a public sector research biobank for idiopathic inflammatory myositis. Indian J Rheumatol. 2020;15:194-9.
4. Gupta L, Muhammed H, Naveen R, Kharbanda R, Gangadharan H, Misra DP, et al. Insights into the knowledge, attitude and practices for the treatment of idiopathic inflammatory myopathy from a cross-sectional cohort survey of physicians. Rheumatol Int. 2020;40:2047-55.
5. Naveen R, Sundaram TG, Agarwal V, Gupta L. Teleconsultation experience with the idiopathic inflammatory myopathies: a prospective observational cohort study during the COVID-19 pandemic. Rheumatol Int. 2021;41:67-76.
6. Muhammed H, Gupta L, Zanwar AA, Misra DP, Lawrence A, Agarwal V, et al. Infections Are Leading Cause of In-Hospital Mortality in Indian Patients With Inflammatory Myopathy. J Clin Rheumatol. 2021;27:114-9. [Online ahead of print].

CHAPTER 240

Vasculitis

Rohini Handa

ABSTRACT

Vasculitis is a broad group of immunoinflammatory conditions affecting primarily the blood vessels. The presentation is often multisystem with features ranging from mild purpuric skin lesions to life-threatening situations like pulmonary-renal syndrome. Physician awareness facilitates early diagnosis. While serology and radiology help to arrive at a diagnosis, definitive confirmation requires histopathologic demonstration of vasculitis. Treatment is based on disease activity and extent of organ involvement rather than the diagnostic label. Corticosteroids, methotrexate, azathioprine, and mycophenolate mofetil (MMF) are used to treat vasculitis. Not all vasculitides require steroids and those which require steroids do not need it all the time. Cyclophosphamide, despite being effective, is less frequently used because of the concern of adverse effects. Rituximab has emerged as an effective alternative to cyclophosphamide in several of the vasculitides.

"Medicine heals doubts as well as diseases"

—Karl Marx

INTRODUCTION

Vasculitis refers to inflammation of the blood vessels resulting in tissue ischemia, necrosis, or bleeding. The disease may arise as a primary process or may be secondary to another disease such as rheumatoid arthritis, lupus (**Fig. 1**) etc. Drugs and infections are also known to trigger vasculitis. The clinical presentation can be extremely varied and the disease may be confined to a single organ or multisystem. The symptoms generally reflect the organs involved. The classification and nomenclature are undergoing continual revisions.

NOMENCLATURE AND CLASSIFICATION

The Chapel Hill Consensus Conference (CHCC) nomenclature system is internationally accepted (**Table 1**). The nomenclature system is to be distinguished from classification criteria that subset patients into a specific category for research and study purposes. The classification is based on vessel size. Some overlap is not uncommon. Also, some forms of vasculitis involve more than one-sized vessel. These are grouped under the category of variable-vessel vasculitis. The American College of Rheumatology (ACR) criteria are available for classification of some of the vasculitides: giant-cell arteritis (GCA), Takayasu arteritis (TA), Wegener's granulomatosis (WG), Churg-Strauss syndrome (CSS), polyarteritis nodosa (PAN), Henoch-Schönlein purpura (HSP), and hypersensitivity vasculitis (HSV). These were proposed way back in 1990 and have not been updated. Both nomenclature and classification are different from diagnosis, the gold standard of which is physician's clinical judgment. The current nomenclature systems are adopting a shift away from eponyms as shown in **Table 2**.

WHEN TO SUSPECT

Systemic vasculitis is suspected when a patient presents with systemic or constitutional symptoms in combination with single or multiple organ dysfunctions (**Box 1**). Systemic manifestations include fever, anorexia, fatigue, weight loss, and arthralgias.

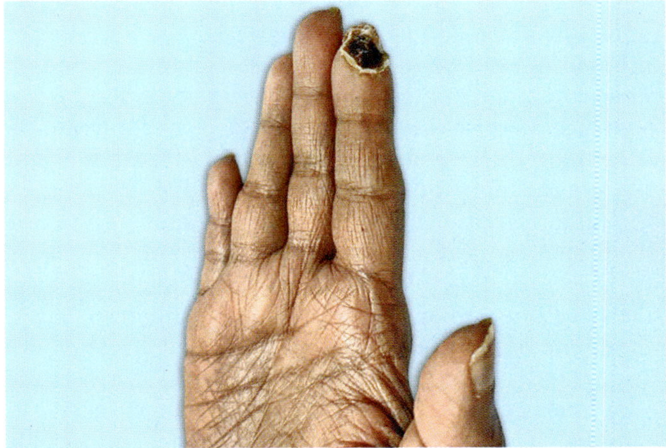

FIGURE 1: Digital gangrene in a patient with systemic lupus erythematosus (SLE).

WORK UP IN SUSPECTED VASCULITIS

This has to be tailored according to the clinical presentation. In general, the investigations can be divided into four categories:

TABLE 1 International Chapel Hill Consensus Conference on the Nomenclature of Vasculitides (CHCC 2012).

Type	Disease entities
Large-vessel vasculitis	• Takayasu's arteritis • Giant-cell arteritis (temporal arteritis)
Medium-vessel vasculitis	• Polyarteritis nodosa (PAN) • Kawasaki disease

Small-vessel vasculitis	• ANCA-associated vasculitis
	  ▪ Microscopic polyangiitis (MPA)
	  ▪ Wegener's granulomatosis (WG), or granulomatosis with polyangiitis (GPA)
	  ▪ Allergic granulomatosis, Churg–Strauss syndrome (CSS), or eosinophilic granulomatosis with polyangiitis (EGPA)
	• Immune complex vasculitis
	• Antiglomerular basement membrane (GBM) disease
	• Cryoglobulinemic vasculitis
	• IgA vasculitis (Henoch–Schönlein vasculitis)
	• Hypocomplementemic urticarial vasculitis (HUV) (anti-C1q vasculitis)

Variable vessel vasculitis	• Behçet syndrome • Cogan's syndrome
Vasculitis associated with systemic disease	*Examples:* rheumatoid vasculitis, lupus vasculitis etc.
Vasculitis associated with probable etiology	*Examples:* hepatitis B virus-associated vasculitis, hepatitis C virus-associated cryoglobulinemic vasculitis etc.
Single organ vasculitis	*Examples:* cutaneous vasculitis, central nervous system (CNS) vasculitis

(ANCA: antineutrophil cytoplasmic antibodies)

TABLE 2 Current nomenclature of eponymous vasculitides.

Eponym	Preferred nomenclature
Wegener's granulomatosis	Granulomatosis with polyangiitis (GPA)
Churg–Strauss syndrome	Eosinophilic granulomatosis with polyangiitis (EGPA)
Henoch–Schönlein purpura	Immunoglobulin A (IgA) vasculitis

BOX 1	Clinical clues that should arouse suspicion of systemic vasculitis.
• Eye inflammation, especially scleritis	
• ENT features such as epistaxis, persistent nasal stuffiness, nasal crusting, depressed bridge of nose, and hearing loss	
• Temporal headache	
• Skin manifestation in form of palpable purpura, skin necrosis, and skin ulcers	
• Lung involvement such as unexplained hemoptysis, pulmonary-renal syndrome	
• Kidney involvement, often paucisymptomatic, manifested by active urine sediment and rapidly progressive renal failure	
• Vascular involvement such as limb claudication, pulse or blood pressure inequality, absent pulses, bruits, and digital gangrene	
• Neurologic manifestations by way of acute foot drop or wrist drop, mononeuritis multiplex	
• Unexplained gastrointestinal bleed, severe pain abdomen	

1. Tests to assess inflammation
2. Tests to assess organ dysfunction
3. Tests to exclude mimics
4. Tests to confirm the diagnosis and extent of disease

Inflammation is assessed by erythrocyte sedimentation rate (ESR) and/or C-reactive protein (CRP), leukocytosis, thrombocytosis, and increase in serum globulins. Organ dysfunction is evaluated by complete blood count (CBC), kidney and liver function tests, urinalysis etc. The latter is invaluable in the detection of kidney disease. Mimics such as infections need appropriate investigations such as blood cultures, hepatitis serology etc.

Tests that aid in diagnosis include blood investigations such as antineutrophil cytoplasmic antibodies (ANCA), serum cryoglobulins, antinuclear antibodies etc. The testing for ANCA is done by indirect immunofluorescence (IIF) or enzyme immunoassay (EIA). IIF reveals two staining patterns: (1) cytoplasmic (c) and (2) perinuclear (p). The usual target antigen for cANCA is proteinase 3 (Pr-3) while it is myeloperoxidase (MPO) for pANCA. However, this is not invariable. Current guidelines advocate the use of EIAs for Pr-3 or MPO as the preferred testing method for ANCA. Titers of ANCA titers do not accurately predict disease activity and treatment decisions should not be based on ANCA levels alone.

Biopsy constitutes the gold standard for the diagnosis of vasculitis. Blind biopsies are discouraged. The site sampled depends on the organ involved. Possible sites include temporal artery biopsy in suspected GCA, skin biopsy in cutaneous vasculitis, renal biopsy in patients with glomerulonephritis, upper airway or lung biopsies in suspected granulomatosis with polyangiitis (GPA), sural nerve biopsy in vasculitic neuropathy etc. Adequate tissue should be obtained. Superficial biopsies of skin or needle biopsies from the lung may yield insufficient tissue and negative results. Direct immunofluorescence (DIF) should be performed in the case of renal and skin biopsies in addition to routine histopathology. DIF enables the identification of immunoglobulin and complement deposits within the tissue. DIF specimens cannot be sent in formalin. An appropriate transport medium has to be obtained from the laboratory. ANCA-associated vasculitides (AAV), in sharp contrast to lupus, are pauci-immune. A negative DIF in a patient with histopathologically confirmed vasculitis should draw attention to AAV. DIF is also essential to confirm perivascular immunoglobulin A (IgA) deposition in IgA vasculitis (HSP). Skin and renal tissue in HSP may reveal IgA deposition. Immunoglobulin M (IgM) deposition around vessel walls can be seen in vasculitis related to type 2 or type 3 cryoglobulinemia or rheumatoid vasculitis while hypocomplementemic urticarial vasculitis exhibits deposition of immunoglobulin G (IgG), complement, and fibrin on vessel walls and dermal–epidermal junction.

Imaging plays a major role in the diagnosis of large and medium vessel vasculitides. For Takayasu's arteritis, this may take the form of computed tomography (CT) angiography, magnetic resonance (MR) angiography, or even positron emission tomography (PET)-CT. Diseases like PAN need CT angiography to pick up aneurysms and/or stenosis. Imaging is unlikely to be helpful in small-vessel vasculitis because the affected vessels are beyond the resolution of the imaging modality. Ultrasound is being increasingly employed in GCA and Takayasu's arteritis. It is, however, operator dependent.

Investigations such as nerve conduction and electromyography, cerebrospinal fluid analysis, muscle biopsy etc., are employed on a case-to-case basis.

DIFFERENTIAL DIAGNOSIS

Infections (especially infective endocarditis), malignancies, and drugs can give rise to a clinical constellation mimicking vasculitis. Differential diagnosis requires clinical acumen and judicious use of investigations. Both vasculitis and infection may coexist adding to the challenge.

TREATMENT PRINCIPLES

The clinical course of vasculitis is punctuated by remissions and relapses. The treatment is, therefore, divided into two broad phases: (1) remission induction and (2) remission maintenance (relapse prevention). The disease activity and the nature of organs affected govern treatment rather than the primary diagnosis. Organ-threatening and life-threatening situations require aggressive treatment. The same disease, during a phase of quiescence, can be treated by minimal medication. Chronic rheumatic diseases, including vasculitis, need differentiation of active disease from damage. Disease activity refers to active immunoinflammation that may be reversed on treatment. In contradistinction, disease damage is irreversible. Immunosuppression is usually de-escalated in face of damage. Validated measures like the Birmingham vasculitis activity score (BVAS) and vasculitis damage index (VDI) are available. Comorbidities such as hypertension, accelerated atherosclerosis, osteoporosis etc., should be sought and addressed. Patients require constant vigil for disease recrudescence and drug toxicity.

Remission induction entails the use of medium to high doses of corticosteroids (0.5–1 mg/kg of prednisolone daily) along with additional immunosuppressive agents such as cyclophosphamide, rituximab, azathioprine, methotrexate, or MMF. While AAV may require aggressive treatment, vasculitis limited to skin may benefit from nonsteroidal anti-inflammatory drugs (NSAIDs), colchicine, or low dose steroids. Remission maintenance is initiated after remission has been achieved. The dose of steroids and other drugs is reduced gradually to limit adverse effects. The duration of treatment is usually 1–2 years after achieving remission.

SPECIFIC VASCULITIDES

LARGE-VESSEL VASCULITIS

TAKAYASU ARTERITIS

Takayasu arteritis is far more common in India as compared to GCA. The onset of the disease is usually before the age of 30 years. Patients may present in the prepulseless stage with nonspecific features such as fever, arthralgias, myalgias, high ESR etc. CT scans of the chest or abdomen done as a workup for fever may reveal inflammation of the aorta. Other presentations include renovascular hypertension, absent/unequal pulses, blood pressure inequality, vascular bruits, limb claudication, especially upper limb, carotidynia, aortic regurgitation, headaches, visual disturbances, transient ischemic attacks, strokes etc. While some patients have a monophasic and self-limited course, the majority have a relapsing and remitting course. The confirmation of the diagnosis is by vascular imaging. CT or MR angiography (which is less invasive than conventional angiography) is used. Imaging features include focal stenosis or occlusion with secondary collaterals. Regions of multisegmental dilation alternating with regions of the normal-appearing arterial wall and fusiform aneurysms can occur.

Corticosteroids along with methotrexate or azathioprine as steroid-sparing agents are employed in the treatment of TA. Other steroid-sparing agents are MMF and leflunomide. Tocilizumab and tumor necrosis factor (TNF) inhibitors are used for refractory disease. Low dose aspirin (75 mg/day) is frequently used in patients with critical stenosis of carotid or vertebral arteries. Endovascular intervention is used to tackle amenable stenotic lesions. Surgery may be needed for aneurysms, severe aortic regurgitation etc.

TEMPORAL ARTERITIS OR GIANT CELL ARTERITIS

Giant-cell arteritis is rare in Asians including Indians. The onset of the disease usually occurs in patients older than 50 years of age. Clinical features comprise headache, scalp tenderness, visual disturbances, and polymyalgia rheumatica (PMR). About 50% of patients with GCA have PMR, while ~15% of individuals with PMR develop GCA. The temporal artery may be visibly dilated and tender. Jaw claudication is an important clue. Vision loss due to anterior ischemic optic neuropathy is a dreaded complication of GCA. Elevated ESR, CRP, and platelets are characteristic of GCA. However, ESR may be normal in ~10% of patients. Superficial temporal artery biopsy is the gold standard for diagnosing GCA. Because of skip lesions, an adequate sample size of 2–3 cm is recommended. Temporal artery ultrasound with or without axillary artery ultrasound is recommended as the imaging modality of choice in patients with suspected GCA. A noncompressible "halo" suggests GCA.

Treatment is instituted with oral prednisolone 1 mg/kg/day. For patients with threatened or established visual loss, methylprednisolone pulses 500–1,000 mg intravenously daily for 3 days are recommended. The response to treatment is dramatic. Tapering of steroid dose begins after 2–4 weeks. The treatment is continued for at least a year. Patients with a relapsing disease that warrants prolonged or high-dose steroids are given tocilizumab or methotrexate. Subcutaneous tocilizumab has received the Food and Drug Administration (FDA) approval for GCA.

MEDIUM VESSEL VASCULITIS

POLYARTERITIS NODOSA

Classic polyarteritis nodosa (PAN or c-PAN) involves medium-sized and small muscular arteries. Hepatitis B virus (HBV) used to be an important cause of PAN earlier, accounting for one-third of cases. With the widespread adoption of hepatitis B vaccination, the incidence of HBV-PAN is declining. The clinical features include fever, weight loss, skin ulcers or nodules, arthralgias, myalgias, livedo reticularis, testicular pain, mononeuritis multiplex etc. The lungs are typically spared. ANCA is notably absent, and the urinalysis is unremarkable. Angiograms that include the celiac axis, superior mesenteric artery, and renal arteries show aneurysms, stenotic lesions, or occlusions. Tissue diagnosis is possible from the skin, sural nerve, and skeletal muscle, if affected.

Patients with mild disease are treated with steroids with or without azathioprine, methotrexate, or mycophenolate. This includes patients with cutaneous PAN, arthritis, and constitutional features. Cyclophosphamide is employed in moderate-to-severe disease. Rituximab may be used in refractory disease, although large trial data is not available to guide treatment decisions. The treatment of PAN associated with hepatitis B or C (HBV or HCV) entails the use of antivirals primarily.

KAWASAKI DISEASE

Kawasaki disease (KD), also called mucocutaneous lymph node syndrome, is common in children but rare in adults. It is usually a self-limited condition with fever and mucocutaneous involvement, viz., bilateral nonexudative conjunctivitis, erythema of the lips and oral mucosa, rash, and cervical lymphadenopathy. The average duration is

12 days. Infants are at greater risk for cardiovascular sequelae. A detailed discussion of KD is beyond the scope of this chapter.

SMALL VESSEL VASCULITIS

CUTANEOUS VASCULITIS

This includes diverse conditions with involvement of small- or medium-sized blood vessels of the skin or subcutaneous tissue. Thus, it is included both under small-vessel vasculitis or medium-vessel vasculitis depending on the specific condition. The morphology is quite variable. Small-vessel involvement manifests as petechiae, palpable purpura (**Fig. 2**), superficial ulcers, hemorrhagic bullae, or urticaria. Clinically, purpura due to hematologic causes like thrombocytopenia is nonpalpable while vasculitic purpura is palpable—a point that permits distinction at the bedside. Medium-vessel involvement may present with subcutaneous nodules, deep ulcers, livedo reticularis, livedo racemosa etc. Extracutaneous involvement should be diligently sought in every patient of cutaneous vasculitis because skin lesions may be the presenting feature of systemic disease.

Leukocytoclastic vasculitis (LCV) is a nonspecific pathologic term for neutrophilic small vessel vasculitis characterized by the breakdown of infiltrating neutrophils and the release of nuclear debris. It is also termed as hypersensitivity vasculitis—"HSV". LCV can be triggered by streptococcal sore throat, hepatitis B and C, HIV, drugs such as β-lactam antibiotics, erythromycin, sulfonamides, NSAIDs, oral pills etc. Other causes include malignancies or systemic diseases such as systemic lupus erythematosus, Sjögren syndrome etc.

Henoch–Schönlein purpura (IgA vasculitis) is the most frequent vasculitis in childhood. The typical presentation includes palpable purpura; gastrointestinal (GI) tract involvement in the form of abdominal pain, melena, or bloody diarrhea; arthralgias; and glomerulonephritis. Large joints such as the knees and ankles are affected.

Urticarial vasculitis, unlike the garden variety of urticaria, exhibits lesions that usually persist for >24 hours and are associated with a burning sensation or pain rather than pruritus, and hyperpigmentation after lesions heal.

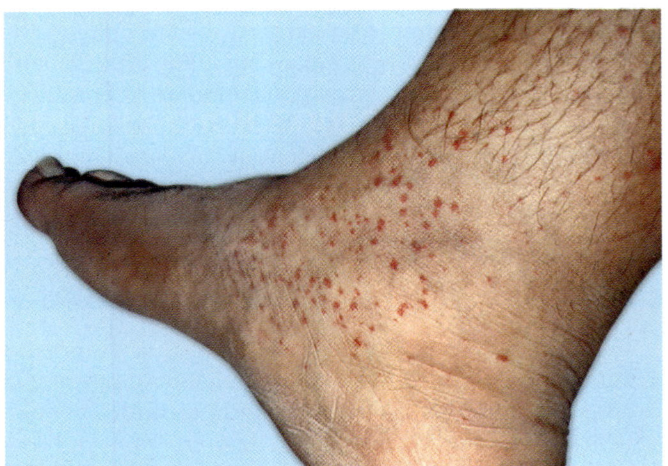

FIGURE 2: Cutaneous vasculitis.

A skin biopsy should be obtained in patients where cutaneous vasculitis is a diagnostic consideration. The type of biopsy determines how much tissue is available for interpretation. Shave biopsies should be avoided where vasculitis is suspected because it does not permit the evaluation of blood vessels in the mid-dermis and deep dermis. Punch biopsy allows for the evaluation of vessels throughout the dermis. It should be >4 mm in diameter. Subcutaneous nodules or ulcers require a wedge biopsy that includes the subcutaneous tissue or large punch biopsy (8–10 mm). For ulcers, the biopsy should be taken from the edge of the ulcer, rather than the ulcer itself. Tissue from the base of an ulcer may reveal incidental vascular injury that mimics vasculitis. Biopsy from the gangrenous area is unrewarding.

Skin biopsies are subjected to routine histopathology and DIF. Suitable lesions for biopsy are those between 24 and 48 hours old. Biopsies obtained before 24 hours may demonstrate some neutrophil infiltration but often do not reveal fibrinoid necrosis. Lesions older than 48 hours show neutrophils in the inflammatory infiltrate getting replaced by lymphocytes and macrophages. DIF is important in differentiating between immune complex-mediated vasculitides and pauci-immune vasculitis. DIF is best performed on fresh skin lesions <24 hours old. The inflammation evoked by immunoglobulin deposition may cause the destruction of the vessel wall and the immune complexes, resulting in negative immunofluorescence.

Treatment of cutaneous vasculitis involves the removal or treatment of an identifiable cause if present. Drug-induced cases respond to drug withdrawal. Since dependent areas are affected, leg elevation or compression stockings may be useful. Colchicine or dapsone is widely used to treat cutaneous vasculitis. Patients with extracutaneous severe visceral involvement may require high doses of corticosteroids (1 mg/kg/day) with or without an immunosuppressive agent (e.g., cyclophosphamide, azathioprine, methotrexate, MMF, and rituximab).

Henoch–Schönlein purpura is often a self-limiting condition and does not require treatment. Children do better than adults. Less than 1% of patients with HSP develop renal complications. Adults have a higher risk of developing significant renal disease. Some patients with severe bowel involvement and rapidly progressive renal failure need steroids and/or immunosuppressives.

ANTINEUTROPHIL CYTOPLASMIC ANTIBODIES-ASSOCIATED VASCULITIS

Antineutrophil cytoplasmic antibodies-associated vasculitis predominantly affects small vessels. The major variants of AAV include GPA-WG, microscopic polyangiitis (MPA), and eosinophilic granulomatosis with polyangiitis (EGPA). Some patients have a renal-limited disease.

Granulomatosis with polyangiitis (Wegener's Granulomatosis): Granulomatosis with polyangiitis characteristically produces granulomatous inflammation of the upper and lower respiratory tracts as well as necrotizing, pauci-immune glomerulonephritis. Cases without renal involvement are termed "Limited GPA" or "Limited WG". Clinical features include constitutional symptoms, purulent or bloody nasal discharge, nasal stuffiness, ear discharge, hearing loss, cough, shortness of breath, or hemoptysis. It is not uncommon for the patients to first present to the ear, nose, and throat (ENT) surgeon. The patients may develop saddle nose deformity (**Fig. 3**). Chest radiographs may show infiltrates, nodules, cavitary lesions, or any combination of these lesions (**Fig. 4**). Many patients receive an initial diagnosis of pulmonary tuberculosis. Careful examination of the urine is an inexpensive and rewarding investigation in this setting. Urinalysis reveals proteinuria, hematuria, and red blood cell (RBC) casts (active sediment). Eye involvement may take the form of proptosis, conjunctivitis, scleritis, episcleritis, uveitis, or optic nerve vasculitis. Nasolacrimal duct obstruction may be seen. Pr-3 ANCA is positive in 85–90% of patients with active GPA and 40% of patients in remission.

Tissue biopsy from the upper airways (sinuses or nasopharynx) usually reveals inflammation, necrosis, or granulomatous changes. Often, vasculitis is not present. Lung biopsies typically reveal both granuloma and vasculitis, while granulomas are rarely seen in a renal biopsy. The characteristic feature on a kidney biopsy is focal, segmental necrotizing pauci-immune glomerulonephritis. The treatment is discussed vide infra.

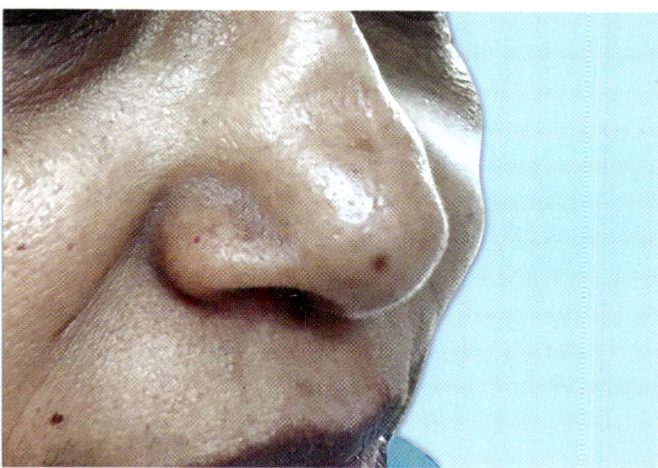

FIGURE 3: Depressed bridge of nose in granulomatosis with polyangiitis (Wegener's granulomatosis).

Microscopic polyangiitis: Microscopic polyangiitis is a necrotizing vasculitis that primarily affects capillaries, venules, or arterioles, with necrotizing glomerulonephritis and/or pulmonary capillaritis. Granulomatous inflammation is usually absent. Renal involvement is the central feature of MPA and takes the form of rapidly progressive glomerulonephritis (RPGN). Lung involvement takes the form of diffuse alveolar hemorrhage (**Fig. 5**). Pulmonary renal syndrome is a common presentation. Other clinical features include arthralgias, pain abdomen, GI bleeding, and peripheral neuropathy. Nearly 90% of patients are ANCA positive with >95% MPO positivity.

Eosinophilic granulomatosis with polyangiitis or Churg–Strauss syndrome: Eosinophilic granulomatosis with polyangiitis is a granulomatous necrotizing vasculitis characterized by chronic rhinosinusitis, asthma, and peripheral blood eosinophilia with ANCA in ~40% of patients, usually anti-MPO ANCA. Three phases are described:

1. *Prodromal phase*: Characterized by atopy, nasal polyposis, and asthma. This may last for several years.
2. *Peripheral blood and tissue eosinophilia*: In this phase, eosinophilia is a prominent feature.
3. *Systemic vasculitis*: It is heralded by fever, weight loss, and anorexia.

Asthma usually subsides when vasculitis emerges. All three phases may appear simultaneously. Skin lesions, peripheral neuropathy, and renal disease are also seen.

Treatment of ANCA-associated vasculitis (GPA, MPA, and EGPA): The treatment is divided into two phases: (1) induction of remission and (2) maintenance of remission. Induction of remission in severe AAV is achieved by corticosteroids (1 mg/kg of prednisolone

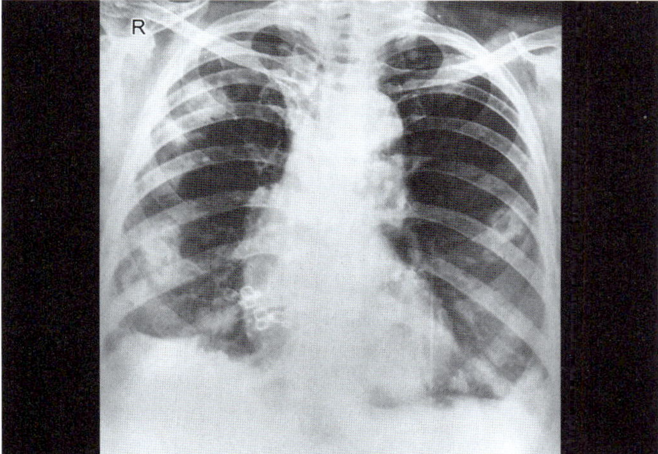

FIGURE 4: Chest radiograph in granulomatosis with polyangiitis (Wegener's granulomatosis) showing nodules and cavitatory lesions.

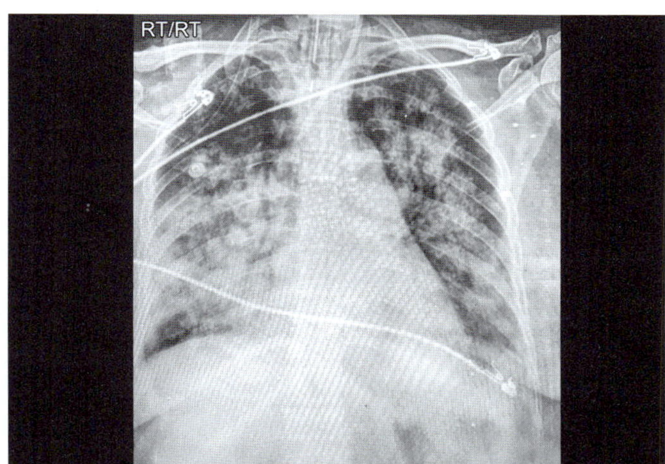

FIGURE 5: Diffuse alveolar hemorrhage in microscopic polyangiitis.

daily) and either cyclophosphamide or rituximab. Intravenous methylprednisolone pulses of 500–1,000 mg daily for 3–5 days are used in organ threatening or life-threatening situations. The dose employed for pulse intravenous cyclophosphamide is 15 mg/kg every month for 6 months. Oral cyclophosphamide is infrequently used nowadays because of the higher cumulative dose and fear of toxicity. Rituximab is employed as an alternative to cyclophosphamide in severe ANCA-associated vasculitis. The dose employed is 375 mg/m^2 of body surface area, once a week for four infusions or two doses of 1,000 mg each on day 1 and day 14. The choice between cyclophosphamide or rituximab is based on patient preference, cost considerations, and physician choice. Plasma exchange is used as a part of induction treatment in AAV in patients with RPGN and diffuse alveolar hemorrhage.

For remission-induction of nonorgan-threatening AAV, a combination of glucocorticoids and either methotrexate or MMF is used. The usual methotrexate dose employed is 15–25 mg/week, oral or parenteral. MMF is used in a dose of 2–3 g/day. Trimethoprim-sulfamethoxazole (80 mg/400 mg) tablet daily is administered as prophylaxis against infection, especially pneumocystis.

After successful induction, steroids are slowly and steadily reduced if the disease is quiescent. Maintenance doses of 5–10 mg prednisolone daily are continued for 12–18 months depending on the situation. Other agents used for maintenance therapy in AAV include rituximab, azathioprine (2 mg/KBW/day), methotrexate (15–25 mg/week), or MMF (2–3 g/day). Recent trial data shows that 500-mg rituximab infusion administered every 6 months is superior to azathioprine as maintenance therapy for ANCA-associated vasculitides, especially Pr-3 ANCA-positive patients. Remission-maintenance therapy for AAV is continued for 18–24 months following induction of sustained remission.

Relapses are common in AAV. Relapse may require reinduction with rituximab or cyclophosphamide. Patients with multiple relapses (>2 relapses) require indefinite treatment and lifelong monitoring.

CONCLUSION

The vasculitides represent multisystem diseases with a variable course. The diagnosis is clinico-serologic, clinico-histologic, or clinico-radiologic. A definite categorization into a particular type may not always be possible. While ANCA is a useful serologic marker for some vasculitides, ANCA positivity does not mean vasculitis. Transient ANCA positivity may be seen with infections. Treatment depends on the disease extent and activity. The relapsing and remitting nature of disease warrants long-term treatment and monitoring.

RECOMMENDED READINGS

1. Jennette JC, Falk RJ, Bacon PA, Basu N, Cid MC, Ferrario F, et al. 2012 revised International Chapel Hill Consensus Conference Nomenclature of Vasculitides. Arthritis Rheum. 2013;65:1.
2. Bossuyt X, Cohen Tervaert JW, Arimura Y, Blockmans D, Flores-Suárez LF, Guillevin L, et al. Position paper: Revised 2017 international consensus on testing of ANCAs in granulomatosis with polyangiitis and microscopic polyangiitis. Nat Rev Rheumatol. 2017;13:683-92.
3. Dejaco C, Ramiro S, Duftner C, Besson FL, Bley TA, Blockmans D, et al. EULAR recommendations for the use of imaging in large vessel vasculitis in clinical practice. Ann Rheum Dis. 2018;77:636-43.
4. Walsh M, Merkel PA, Peh CA, Szpirt WM, Puéchal X, Fujimoto S, et al. Plasma exchange and glucocorticoids in severe ANCA-associated vasculitis. N Engl J Med. 2020;382:622-31.
5. Guillevin L, Pagnoux C, Karras A, Khouatra C, Aumaître O, Cohen P, et al. Rituximab versus azathioprine for maintenance in ANCA-associated vasculitis. N Engl J Med. 2014;371:1771-80.

CHAPTER 241

Miscellaneous Rheumatic Diseases

Subramanian Shankar, Vivek Vasdev

ABSTRACT

Benign joint hypermobility syndrome is a noninflammatory and nonprogressive disorder with varied rheumatological and systemic manifestations. Musculoskeletal symptoms include polyarthralgia, recurrent ligament sprains and joint subluxations, or dislocations due to trivial trauma. It may also have associated fatigue, gastrointestinal, genitourinary, and dysautonomic cardiovascular symptoms. The condition is diagnosed using Brighton's criteria. Patient education is the most important aspect of the management and should stress on lifestyle modifications to prevent injuries and symptoms.

Adult onset Still's disease (AOSD) is characterized by fever, joint symptoms, and rash. It is frequently associated with lymph node enlargement and splenomegaly. The clinical course may be monophasic, intermittent, or chronic and the disease may mimic many infectious and noninfectious diseases. Many classification criteria have been developed of which Yamaguchi classification criteria is the most widely used. However, AOSD remains a diagnosis of exclusion. The treatment includes nonsteroidal anti-inflammatory drugs (NSAIDs) and immunosuppressive agents.

Behçet's disease is classified as primary variable vessel vasculitis and affects multiple organ systems. Mucocutaneous ulcerations in the form of recurrent orogenital ulcers are the most common symptoms. Human leukocyte antigen (HLA)-B51 is the strongest known genetic susceptibility factor. Treatment depends on symptom of severity and includes anti-inflammatory agents, anticoagulants, and immunosuppressants.

Chikungunya arthritis is a sequela of chikungunya, manifesting with prominent musculoskeletal features characterized by acute or chronic arthritis. Chikungunya is caused by arthropod-borne alphavirus (Vector-*Aedes* mosquito) and is a global public health problem. The management is mainly symptomatic and includes NSAIDs, conventional synthetic disease-modifying antirheumatic drugs (DMARDs), and occasionally, even biological DMARDs.

"In examining disease, we gain wisdom about anatomy and physiology and biology. In examining the person with disease, we gain wisdom about life"

—Oliver W Sacks

INTRODUCTION

This chapter entails a group of important rheumatology topics that have gained significant importance in current medical practice. On one hand, it deals with common conditions, such as benign joint hypermobility syndrome (BJHS) and chikungunya arthritis that are relatively benign and their knowledge is important to avoid misdiagnosis and initiating potentially harmful medicines. On the other hand, it also deals with relatively rare rheumatological conditions that need prompt diagnosis to avoid significant morbidity and mortality.

BENIGN JOINT HYPERMOBILITY SYNDROME

Benign joint hypermobility syndrome is one of the heritable connective tissue disorders characterized by chronic musculoskeletal symptoms attributable to joint hypermobility. Generalized joint hypermobility without systemic disease is commonly seen in healthy individuals with a recorded prevalence of 4–13%. The prevalence is higher in people of African, Asian, and Middle Eastern descent and in females as compared to males. Besides BJHS, hypermobility is also a feature of several heritable connective tissue disorders including Marfan's syndrome, Ehlers-Danlos syndrome (EDS), and osteogenesis imperfecta. It is also seen in chromosomal and genetic disorders such as Down syndrome and in metabolic disorders such as homocystinuria and hyperlysinemia. BJHS is often considered a milder variant of the most common variant of EDS hypermobility type.

CLINICAL FEATURES

The most common symptoms are muskuloskeletal in nature and attributable to generalized joint laxity such as acute pains from joint sprains, ligament, and tendon injuries. Joint subluxations or dislocations with minor trauma are also common. The commonly involved joints are knee, ankle, elbow, and small joints of hand. Unlike arthritic disorders, morning stiffness is not a feature of BJHS. At times, subjects may have symmetrical involvement of joints mimicking systemic arthritides. They may also experience muscle cramps, myalgias, joint stiffness, and nonarticular limb pain.

Extra-articular musculoskeletal manifestations may include scoliosis, pes planus lordosis, genu valgum, patellar dislocations, and Marfanoid habitus. Besides musculoskeletal symptoms, chronic fatigue and widespread pains due both to injuries and neuropathic pain are more commonly seen as compared to general population.

They may also have some systemic manifestations involving other organ systems. Skin manifestations are usually mild including hyperextensible fragile skin which is usually soft and silky with easy bruising and stretch marks. Some of the gastrointestinal and genitourinary symptoms may be attributable to connective tissue laxity including hiatus hernia with gastroesophageal reflux, irritable bowel syndrome, urinary urgency, frequency, urge, and stress incontinence. The cardiovascular manifestations may include palpitations, orthostatic symptoms, postural tachycardia, and syncope. The association of BJHS with mitral valve prolapse (MVP) is controversial. Eye abnormalities such as drooping eyelids and myopia may also be seen in a few cases.

DIAGNOSIS

Benign joint hypermobility syndrome should be suspected in young patients with polyarthralgias without overt features of inflammatory arthritides. The diagnosis is based upon the medical history and physical examination including use of the Beighton hypermobility score, by Brighton 1998 criteria. There are no diagnostic laboratory tests (e.g., blood tests, molecular genetic analyses, imaging, or pathology) for BJHS.

Beighton score depends on the presence of hypermobility in the hands, elbows, lumbar spine, and knees using specific examination techniques. One point is awarded for the ability to perform each of nine maneuvers. A score

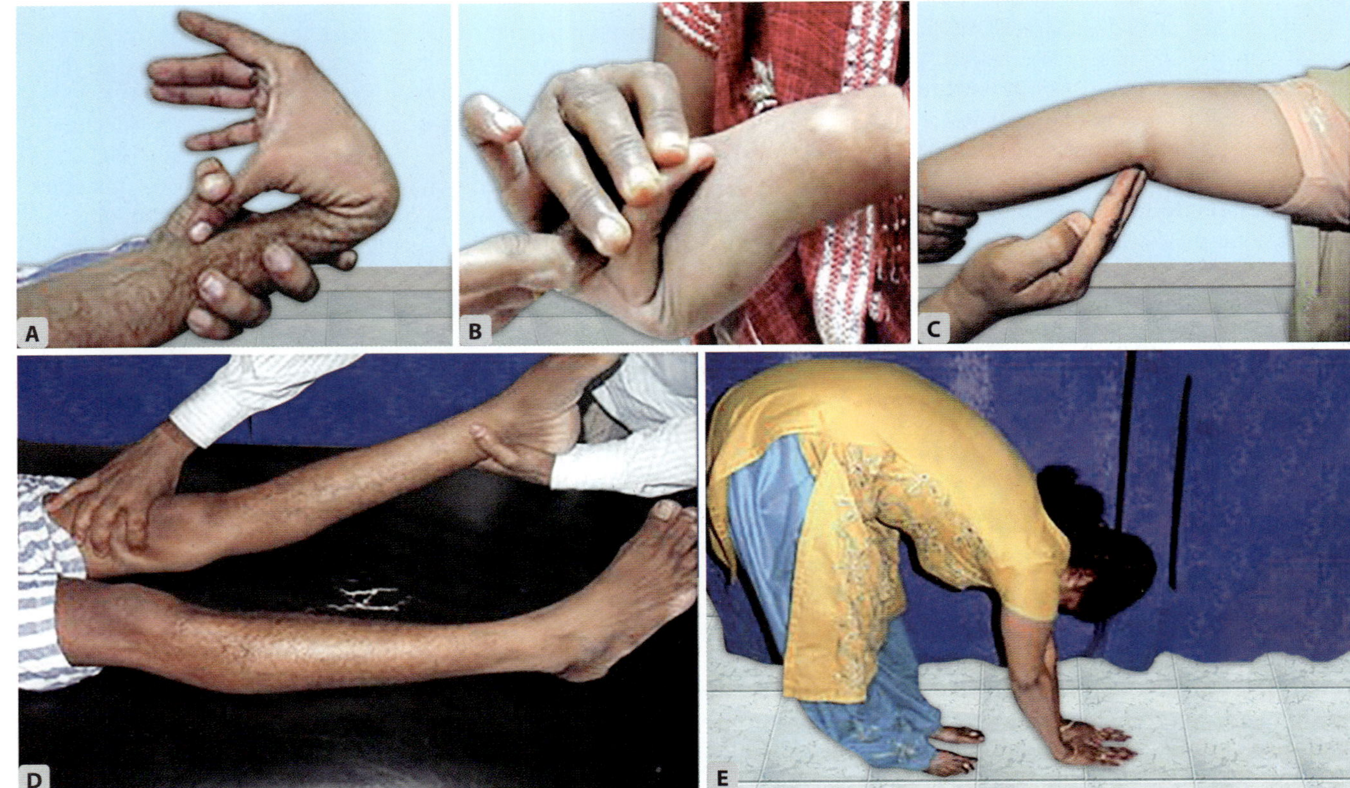

FIGURES 1 A to E: Maneuvers used to calculate the Beighton score. The Beighton score is calculated by adding the points obtained through each maneuvers, yielding a total maximum score of 9. A Beighton score of 4 or higher is a major criterion for the Brighton criteria.
Courtesy: Col Gautam Mullick.

of 4 or more points represents generalized hypermobility (**Figs. 1 A** to **E**). Brighton criteria comprise major and minor criteria. The major criteria include a Beighton score of 4/9 or greater and arthralgia for longer than 3 months in four or more joints. The minor criteria include a lower Beighton score, lesser number of painful joints, soft tissue rheumatism, Marfanoid habitus, thin hyperextensible skin, and certain eye signs such as drooping eyelids or myopia or antimongoloid slant. BJHS is diagnosed in the presence of the two major criteria, one major and two minor criteria, or four minor criteria. BJHS is excluded by the presence of Marfan or EDS, other than EDS hypermobility type (formerly EDS III).

MANAGEMENT

The management of BJHS is individualized based on the severity of symptoms, other medical conditions, and the presence of other extra-articular manifestations. Patient education is the first and most important aspect of management of BJHS. The patient needs to be aware of the benign nature of illness and lifestyle modifications to prevent overstretching of joints as well as injury. Muscle strengthening exercises would help in increasing the tone and strength of supporting muscles which, in turn, increases joint stability. Strengthening exercises and conditioning activities such as swimming, walking, and jogging help to improve joint strength. Braces, splints, or bandaging may be advised to prevent injury to the affected joints during activity. Acute symptoms following unaccustomed exercises may improve with physiotherapy massages, hot and cold therapy, and short wave diathermy as well as ultrasonic therapy.

Acute joint pain and swelling after unaccustomed activity can be reduced with short-term nonsteroidal anti-inflammatory drugs (NSAIDs). BJHS patients are more prone for joint dislocations, meniscal tears, tendon, and ligament damages. Appropriate orthopedic care may be required for specific conditions or complications.

ADULT ONSET STILL'S DISEASE

Adult onset Still's disease (AOSD) is an inflammatory disorder characterized by persistent high spiking fevers, joint involvement, and an evanescent rash. It is at the crossroads of autoinflammatory syndromes and autoimmune disorders. The gender distribution is nearly the same and majority of patients are 16–35 years of age. The etiology of AOSD is unknown and the precise pathogenesis is not established, but several factors including infectious agents, genetics, immune complexes, and environmental factors have been implicated. Whatever may be the triggering factor, the mechanism leads to an autoinflammatory systemic response with imbalance in production of proinflammatory cytokines such as interleukin (IL)-1, IL-6, IL-18, interferon-γ (IFN-γ), and tumor necrosis factor-α (TNF-α).

CLINICAL FEATURES AND DIAGNOSIS

High-spiking fever with one daily peak (rarely, two peaks) is usually the initial and most prominent symptom. Arthralgias or arthritis is less dramatic and commonly affects knees, wrists, ankles, and small joints of hands. The evanescent salmon-colored pink, macular, or maculopapular rash coincides with fever and mainly appears on the trunk and proximal limbs.

Up to 75% of cases develop lymph node enlargement with involvement of cervical lymph nodes being the most common. The enlargement of spleen and liver is also seen with the former being present in up to 60% of the cases.

Macrophage activation syndrome (MAS) is one of the life-threatening complications of AOSD that mimics the acute flare of the disease and needs to be differentiated (**Fig. 2**). Although, constitutional symptoms, raised acute phase reactants and serum ferritin levels are seen in both, MAS can be differentiated from acute flare of AOSD by presence of cytopenias (mainly leukopenia and thrombocytopenia) and raised serum triglycerides.

Laboratory findings are generally nonspecific with anemia and marked elevation of erythrocyte sedimentation rate (ESR), C-reactive protein (CRP), platelets, serum ferritin, and WBC count with neutrophilic leukocytosis. Serum transaminases are also frequently elevated. The other rheumatological markers, such as antinuclear antibodies, rheumatoid factor, and anticitrullinated peptide antibody are usually absent.

The clinical course of AOSD can be classified as monophasic, intermittent, or chronic with approximately one-third of patients falling in each category. Monophasic AOSD is characterized by a self-limited course lasting only weeks to months in most patients. Intermittent AOSD patients have one or more disease flares, with or without articular symptoms, and with complete remissions between episodes. Patients with chronic AOSD have persistently active disease in which articular symptoms usually predominate. The diagnosis of AOSD needs exclusion of infections, malignancies, and other rheumatic disease.

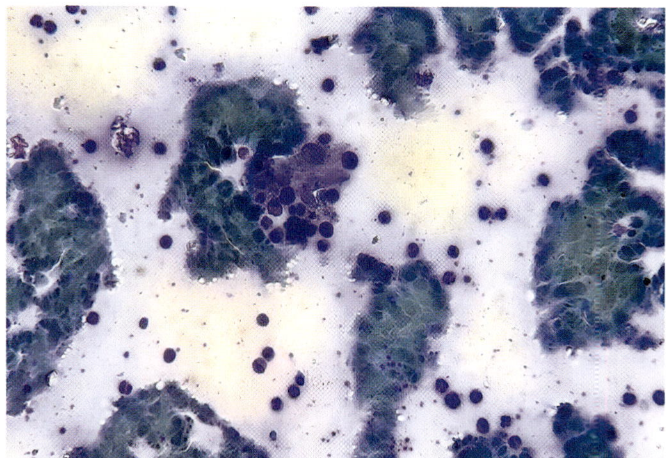

FIGURE 2: LG stain 400× macrophage ingesting lymphocytes and neutrophils in a case of Macrophage activation.

Although several sets of diagnostic criteria have been proposed, the Yamaguchi criteria are the most acceptable and widely practised. The major criteria include fever lasting 1 week, arthralgia or arthritis of >2 weeks, typical rash, and polymorphonuclear leukocytosis. The minor criteria include sore throat, lymphadenopathy, hepatosplenomegaly, and deranged liver function tests. To diagnose AOSD, five or more criteria are required, of whom two or more must be major.

Many conditions may have similar features seen in AOSD and in the absence of a definitive diagnostic criteria, intensive clinical and laboratory evaluation is required to make the diagnosis. The common differential diagnoses of AOSD include infections such as acute viral syndromes and bacterial sepsis and noninfectious conditions such as malignancies (lymphomas and leukemias), drug reactions, rheumatological diseases (lupus, idiopathic inflammatory myositis, and rheumatoid arthritis) vasculitis (polyarteritis nodosa) and autoinflammatory syndromes.

TREATMENT

Nonsteroidal anti-inflammatory drugs are the first-line treatment and responders usually have good prognosis. However, since liver function abnormalities are common during initial diagnosis of AOSD, a careful monitoring for NSAIDs related hepatotoxicity is mandatory. The usual second-line treatment is with corticosteroids (prednisolone 0.5–1 mg/kg) for 4–6 weeks. The patients who respond poorly to steroids or need prolonged therapy may require addition of a steroid sparing agent, such as methotrexate.

Biologic therapy may be considered in initial stages in severe form of disease or in patients where steroids with steroid sparing agents have failed to control the disease. Biologic therapy with IL-1 and IL-6 antagonists has been proved to be the most effective in AOSD. They should be supplemented with steroids and steroid sparing agents. While IL-1 blockers (anakinra) are more effective for the systemic manifestations, IL-6 antagonist (tocilizumab) has proved useful for both joint and systemic manifestations. Anti-TNF-α (infliximab) may be an attractive option in refractory AOSD with predominant articular pattern. An approach to the management of AOSD is shown in **Flowchart 1**. Long-term steroid use in AOSD demands careful supervision of bone health to prevent osteoporosis.

AOSD is a disease of young adults with tremendous impact on education, career, family life, and psychological well-being. Hence, a comprehensive treatment plan should include a caring physician, psychologist, and social support groups.

BEHÇET'S DISEASE

Behçet's disease (BD) is a primary variable vessel vasculitis with multisystem involvement, characterized by relapsing oral and genital aphthous ulcers and bilateral posterior or panuveitis as cardinal features. The syndrome has been named after Hulusi Behçet, a Turkish dermatologist, who described the symptom complex

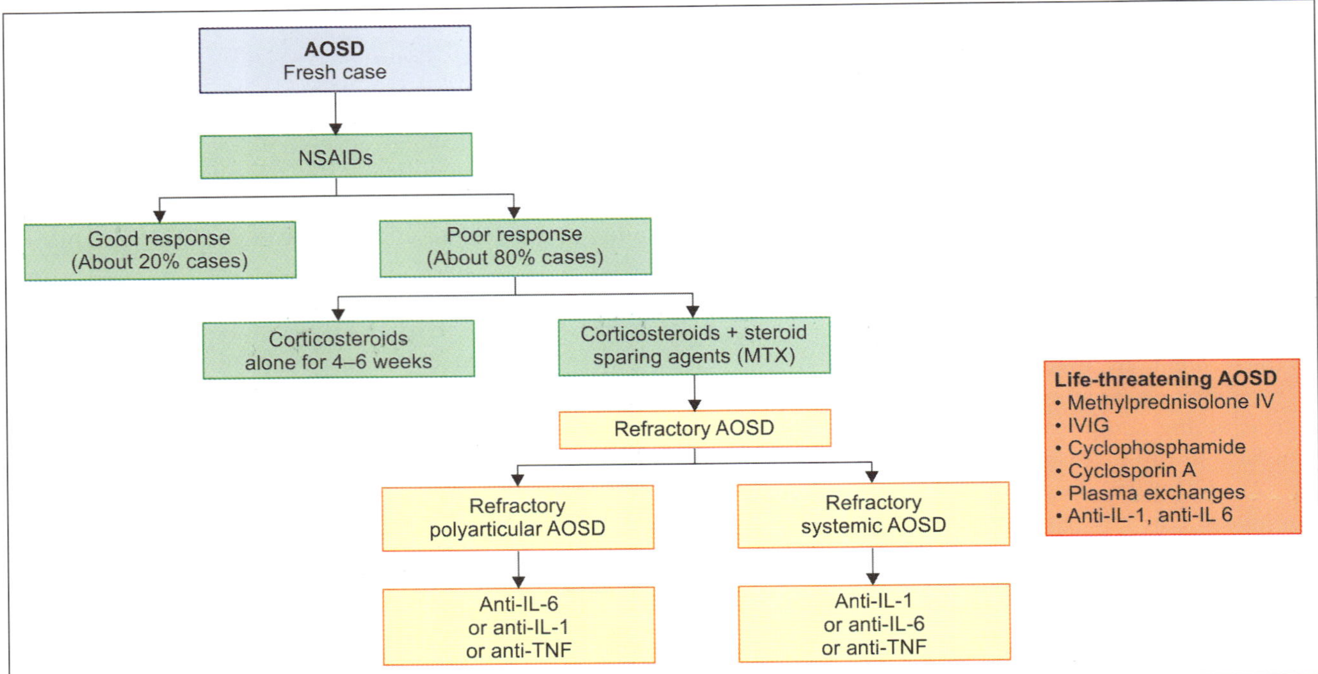

(IL: interleukin; IVIG: intravenous immunoglobulin; NSAIDs: nonsteroidal anti-inflammatory drugs; TNF: tumor necrosis factor)

FLOWCHART 1: Management of AOSD.

of recurrent aphthous ulcers, genital ulcers, and uveitis leading to blindness in 1937.

BD is relatively more common and severe along Eastern Asia to the Mediterranean (ancient silk route). The disease typically affects young adults with equal distribution among both genders. While most cases of BD are sporadic, familial clustering has also been reported, and there is increased risk for the disease in first-degree relatives of patients with BD.

BD is a multifactorial inflammatory disorder. HLA-B*51 is the strongest genetic susceptibility factor. Environmental factors have also been claimed as possible triggers of inflammatory flares, and *Streptococcus sanguis* and herpes simplex viruses have been extensively investigated in this regard.

CLINICAL MANIFESTATIONS

The presence of recurrent and usually painful mucocutaneous ulcers is the most common clinical feature in Behçet syndrome (**Fig. 3**). Other manifestations of this disorder vary among different populations. The highest morbidity and mortality occur with ocular, vascular, and central nervous system disease. Articular and cutaneous manifestations are common. Peripheral nervous system and renal involvement are rare compared to other vasculitides.

The most frequent and generally the initial manifestations of BD are recurrent aphthous oral ulcers that last for 1–2 weeks and rarely leave a scar. In contrast, genital ulcers are usually deep and heal with scarring. In ophthalmologic involvement, bilateral nongranulomatous posterior or panuveitis affects almost half of patients.

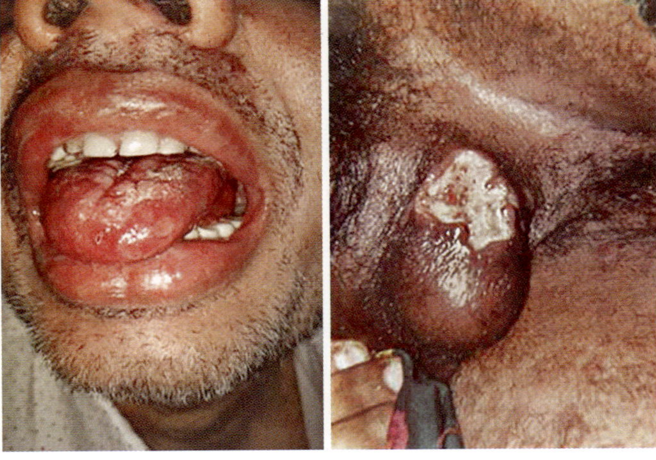

FIGURE 3: Patients of Behçets disease showing oral and scrotal aphthous ulcers.

The arthritis in BD is self-limiting, nonerosive, asymmetric acute mono or oligoarthritis, mainly affecting lower limb joints. BD affects all types and sizes of blood vessels and is classified as a variable vessel vasculitis. A small vessel involvement is the most common feature, but medium and large vessel disease may also be involved. Large vessel vascular involvement is seen in about one-third of patients with BD. Thrombotic occlusion of cerebral venous sinuses, hepatic veins, and caval veins can also be seen. Pulmonary artery aneurysm is the most common arterial lesion and is associated with a high mortality rate (25%). It usually presents with hilar opacities and massive hemoptysis. Neurologic involvement is seen in <10% of subjects in most clinical series. The parenchymal brain involvement is mainly due to focal parenchymal lesions and vascular thrombosis. Nonparenchymal involvement includes cerebral venous thrombosis, acute meningeal syndrome, intracranial hypertension syndrome, and uncommonly stroke due to arterial thrombosis, aneurysm or dissection. In gastrointestinal system, aphthous ulcers can occur throughout the gastrointestinal tract (GIT). They may manifest as abdominal pain, bleeding, and diarrhea. The patients of BD may suffer constitutional symptoms including low-grade fever and malaise. Some of the other less common manifestations include lung and cardiac involvement. The patients may develop parenchymal nodules, cavities, and organizing pneumonia. Cardiac involvement may include pericarditis, myocardial infarction, coronary artery aneurysms, conduction abnormalities, and valvular insufficiency including aortic regurgitation.

LABORATORY FEATURES

There is no confirmatory diagnostic test for BD. Skin pathergy reaction, although very helpful in diagnosis when positive, is less sensitive. HLA-B*51 is the strongest genetic susceptibility factor. It, however, has limited diagnostic value, particularly in endemic areas. Radiologic investigations are helpful in the evaluation of neurologic and vascular involvements and fundus fluorescein angiography is useful in managing uveitis.

Different sets of criteria have been developed for classification of BD, but all have certain limitations. The most recent and popular criteria is the "International Criteria for BD". All criteria for either diagnosis or classification of Behçet include clinical signs related to genital/oral aphthous ulcers, ocular lesions (anterior uveitis, posterior uveitis, or retinal vasculitis), skin lesions (pseudofolliculitis or erythema nodosum), vascular lesions (superficial phlebitis, deep vein thrombosis, large vein thrombosis, arterial thrombosis, or aneurysm), neurologic manifestations, and pathergy test (**Fig. 4**).

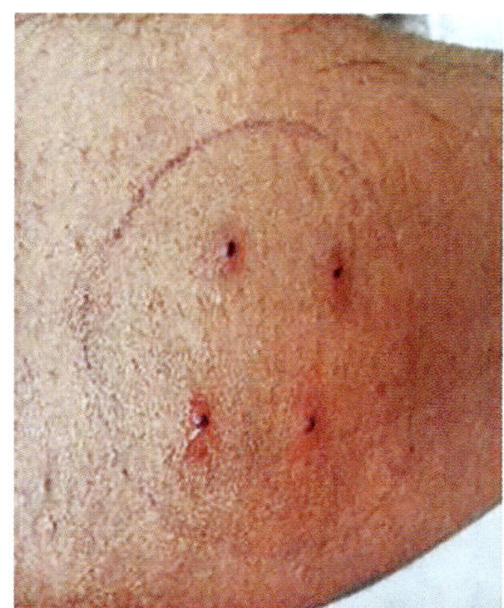

FIGURE 4: Positive pathergy test in a patient of Behçets disease.

TREATMENT

The therapeutic approach to BD is highly variable and is guided by the predominant disease manifestations. The management should be individualized based on age, sex, type, and severity of organ involvement as well as patient preferences. BD typically runs a remitting and relapsing course and the goal of treatment is to suppress inflammatory exacerbations/recurrences and prevent irreversible organ damage. Early management of flares is critical for averting permanent damages, especially in ocular, vascular, and neurologic involvements.

Mucocutaneous lesions are most frequent manifestations. Colchicine (1–2 mg/day) has been shown to be effective for genital ulcers and erythema nodosum like lesions. In refractory cases, low-dose corticosteroids and azathioprine are effective alternatives. Arthritis also responds to colchicine or low-dose corticosteroids and immunosuppressive drugs. Anti-TNF agents can also be considered in refractory cases.

Flares of a posterior or panuveitis require high-dose corticosteroids along with topical eye drops. INF-α and monoclonal anti-TNF agents (infliximab and adalimumab) can be considered for refractory or sight-threatening patients, as the first-line treatment. Deep vein thrombosis and arterial involvements are usually treated with anticoagulation, high-dose corticosteroids, and immunosuppressive agents, including cyclophosphamide for arterial aneurysms or high-risk venous disease.

CHIKUNGUNYA ARTHRITIS

Chikungunya is an arboviral disease caused by alpha virus and is spread by *Aedes* mosquito. In last two decades, chikungunya has spread rapidly affecting multiple regions and populations. India experienced the first outbreak of the chikungunya in 1963 in Kolkata followed by epidemics in Andhra Pradesh, Maharashtra, and Tamil Nadu.

Chikungunya is a systemic disorder with predominant involvement of musculoskeletal, gastrointestinal, and neurological systems. Musculoskeletal manifestations are the most prominent clinical feature, characterized by acute or chronic polyarthralgia/polyarthritis. Chronic arthritis related to chikungunya infection is described as an emerging rheumatological disorder which may require disease-modifying antirheumatic drugs (DMARDs).

CLINICAL FEATURES

The usual incubation period is 3–7 days and thereafter, acute infection manifests with fever and malaise. Joint symptoms often begin 2–5 days after fever onset and commonly involve multiple joints. Joints involvement is usually symmetric, involves distal joints more than proximal joints, and is associated with early morning stiffness. The duration of acute illness is usually 7–10 days. As many as 25–75% of patients develop chronic musculoskeletal manifestations following chikungunya infection. The chronic manifestations usually involve joints affected during the acute illness, including inflammatory polyarthritis, polyarthralgia, and tenosynovitis. Inflammatory arthritis can persist for weeks, months, or years.

CLASSIFICATION

Chikungunya arthritis can be divided according to different phases of the disease namely:

Acute arthritis (within first one month): In acute phase, the arthritis mainly involves the large and small joints of extremities (ankle, wrist, and phalanges).

Subacute arthritis (in second and third month of illness): In subacute phase, the arthritis of acute phase may persist and in addition there may be involvement of periarticular structures causing enthesitis, bursitis, tendinitis, capsulitis, and tenosynovitis.

Chronic arthritis (>3 months): In this stage, the arthritis can either resolve spontaneously or may persist to resemble chronic inflammatory rheumatism (CIR) or general musculoskeletal disorders (MSD). CIR is more debilitating with persistent monoarthritis, oligoarthritis, or polyarthritis and can even resemble peripheral spondyloarthropathy or rheumatoid arthritis. General MSD is more common than CIR but less debilitating and is characterized by recurrent joint pains without any evidence of synovitis.

There are multiple factors which may predispose individual to develop CIR. These include age >45 years, severe arthritis at presentation, female gender, past history of depression and raised chikungunya specific immunoglobulin G (IgG) titers in blood.

EVALUATION

Diagnosis of the illness is essentially clinical in the background of present or past chikugunya viral infection. In acute chikungunya arthritis, it is important to diagnose acute chikungunya viral infection by polymerase chain reaction (PCR)-based assay or antibody detections. In first 7 days, IgM antibodies may be elevated following which the IgG antibodies start rising.

In chronic chikungunya arthritis, IgG antibodies are usually raised. It is also important to evaluate HLA-B27, rheumatoid factor and anticyclic citrullinated peptide (CCP) in appropriate clinical settings to exclude rheumatoid arthritis and seronegative spondyloarthropathy.

MANAGEMENT

Management of chikungunya arthritis requires management of arthritis with medications along with non-pharmacological interventions like rest, hydration and physiotherapy. Acute chikungunya arthritis is usually managed with paracetamol, NSAIDs, weak opioids, and low-dose steroids. In case of acute synovitis or tenosynovitis, local infiltration with steroid injection can also be tried. Other pain modulation medicines such as tricyclic antidepressants and anticonvulsants such as pregabalin or gabapentin may be used. Management of chronic chikungunya arthritis is difficult and long-standing and may require DMARDs in addition to symptomatic management of the disease.

PROGNOSIS

It has been observed that almost all patients with musculoskeletal manifestations eventually recover, although the duration of chronic symptoms varies widely. The long-term chronic joint damage is still a controversial issue with no significant joint damage evidenced by radiography, but has been made appreciable by magnetic resonance imaging (MRI) in a subset of patients. *Aedes* mosquitoes are the vectors for chikungunya virus that primarily bite during the daytime. Measures to minimize mosquito bites and environmental control of the mosquito breeding are effective in prevention of chikungunya and its sequelae.

RECOMMENDED READINGS

1. Kumar B, Lenert P. Joint Hypermobility Syndrome: Recognizing a Commonly Overlooked Cause of Chronic Pain. Am J Med. 2017;130:640-7.
2. Gerfaud-Valentin M, Jamilloux Y, Iwaz J, Sève P. Adult-onset Still's disease. Autoimmun Rev. 2014;13:708-22
3. Yazici H, Seyahi E, Hatemi G, Yazici Y. Behçet syndrome: A contemporary view. Nat Rev Rheumatol. 2018;14:107-19.
4. Pathak H, Mohan MC, Ravindran V. Chikungunya arthritis. Clin Med (Lond). 2019;19:381-5.

MULTIPLE CHOICE QUESTIONS

To access the multiple choice questions of this Section online, kindly scan the QR code.